Neuroendocrine Tumours

Suayib Yalcin • Kjell Öberg
Editors

Neuroendocrine Tumours

Diagnosis and Management

2nd ed. 2024

Springer

Editors
Suayib Yalcin
Department of Medical Oncology
Hacettepe University Cancer Institute
Ankara, Türkiye

Kjell Öberg (Retired)
Department of Endocrine Oncology
Uppsala University Hospital
Uppsala, Sweden

ISBN 978-3-031-56967-8 ISBN 978-3-031-56968-5 (eBook)
https://doi.org/10.1007/978-3-031-56968-5

This Springer imprint is published by the registered company Springer Nature Switzerland AG
The registered company address is: Gewerbestrasse 11, 6330 Cham, Switzerland

Contents

Introduction to Neuroendocrine Tumors

1

Suayib Yalcin

1.1 Introduction

Including a wide range of clinicopathological entities, neuroendocrine tumors (NETs) are a group of diverse neoplasms arising from cells of a neuroendocrine origin dispersed throughout the body. Recently, significant progress has been observed not only in our understanding of the biology and genetics of NETs but also in their diagnosis and treatment [1, 2]. Besides, newer classification and staging systems have been adapted and guidelines published to help establish a more standardized approach [3, 4].

The incidence of NETs has been increasing in the last few years. The estimated incidence rate of 1.09/100,000 in 1973 increased to 5.25/100,000 in 2004 and reached 6.98/100,000 in 2012 [5, 6]. Although some series report a slightly higher incidence in men compared to women, there appears to be no significant difference in terms of gender [7]. The prevalence of the disease is, however, estimated to be much higher and ranks only second after colorectal cancers among gastrointestinal (GI) tumors in the United States [5, 8]. Although NETs may occur at any age, they are more common after the age of 50 and peak between the ages of 50 and 70. The incidence rate in patients 65 years or older is 25.3/100,000, and, in patients aged 50–64 years, it is 14.3/100,000; in patients younger than 50 years, the incidence was 1.75/100,000 in 2012 according to the Surveillance, Epidemiology, and End Results (SEER) database [6, 7]. NETs may be associated with familial genetic neuroendocrine tumor syndromes such as multiple endocrine neoplasia (MEN) syndromes (MEN-1 and MEN-2), neurofibromatosis type 1, Von Hippel–Lindau (VHL) disease, tuberous sclerosis, and Carney complex. In patients with these syndromes, the age of diagnosis is 15–20 years lower than those with sporadic NETs [5–8].

S. Yalcin (✉)
Department of Medical Oncology, Hacettepe University Cancer Institute, Ankara, Turkey

S. Yalcin, K. Öberg (eds.), *Neuroendocrine Tumours*,
https://doi.org/10.1007/978-3-031-56968-5_1

NETs are usually slow-growing tumors. They can arise from many organs but commonly from the GI tract, lungs, pancreas, thymus, and other endocrine organs. NETs may synthesize and secrete peptides and/or amines. These secreted peptides/amines can be used as tumor markers, and they may be responsible for the clinical signs and symptoms.

About 67% of NETs are located in the GI system, and these NETs are sometimes also called carcinoids or GI NETs. Carcinoids secrete numerous peptides, including serotonin (5-hydroxytryptamine (5-HT)) and tachykinins. About 10% of GI NETs metastasize to the liver and release 5-HT into the blood, resulting in carcinoid syndrome characterized by cutaneous flushing, diarrhea, and abdominal pain. After lung carcinoid tumors, pancreatic NETs comprise the next common group of NETs. These tumors may be either functional (~40%) or nonfunctional (~60%). Functional pancreatic NETs are usually defined by the predominant, clinically relevant hormone secretion of neuroendocrine biomarkers such as insulin, gastrin, glucagon, vasoactive intestinal peptide (VIP), etc.

NETs have some common histopathological characteristics. They show similar immune reactivity to pan-neuroendocrine markers, such as chromogranin A and synaptophysin [8]. Neuron-specific enolase (NSE), CD56, and CD57 are less specific markers; they can be used to identify poorly differentiated NETs. Immunohistochemical assessment of specific hormone expression is not routine in pathological evaluation, and a positive immune reaction for hormone expression in the tumor tissue does not indicate that the tumor is functional [9].

NETs are graded based on mitotic count and the Ki-67 index (Table 1.1). Grading should be combined with the organ-specific tumor, node, and metastasis (TNM) staging system. Primary localization, size and invasion depth of the tumor, and status of the surgical margin of the excision/resection material are also important [9, 10].

NETs usually express somatostatin receptors; therefore, somatostatin expression can be used both diagnostically and therapeutically [11]. Somatostatin receptor imaging with ^{111}In-DTPA-OCTREOTIDE or most preferably ^{68}Ga-DOTATATE can be used for initial staging, follow-up, and selecting patients for peptide receptor radionuclide therapy (PRRT) [12, 13]. According to the localization of the primary tumor, computerized tomography and/or magnetic resonance imaging (MRI) should also be used for diagnosis and staging. Ultrasound and endoscopic ultrasound can be used when necessary as complementary examinations.

Table 1.1 Grading system for neuroendocrine tumors

Mitosis index	Ki-67 index (%)	ENET/WHO definition	
<2	<3	NET	Grade I
2–20	3–20	NET	Grade II
>20	>20	NEC (small cell or large cell)	Grade III
		Mixed adenoneuroendocrine carcinoma (MANEC)	

NET neuroendocrine tumor, *NEC* neuroendocrine carcinoma, *ENET* European Neuroendocrine Tumor Society, *WHO* World Health Organization

5-Fluorodeoxyglucose-positron emission tomography (FDG-PET) can be used in the diagnosis, staging, and follow-up of aggressive, poorly differentiated NETs. FDG-PET may also show transformation to aggressive biological behavior [12, 13]. The role of newer PET tracers warrants further validation for routine clinical practice. Endoscopic evaluation of patients using esophagogastroduodenoscopy, colonoscopy, double-balloon enteroscopy, or capsule endoscopy is critical according to the localization of the primary tumor and also in patients with primary unknown metastatic neuroendocrine tumor or carcinoma.

Surgery is the only potentially curative treatment modality for low- and intermediate-grade NETs. Surgery should be considered for patients with early-stage disease, for those with locoregional and resectable metastatic disease, and for some selected symptomatic patients [14]. Resection of the primary tumor and metastasectomy should be considered for all suitable patients. However, surgery can be performed for only 20% of the patients because most patients are diagnosed at an advanced stage. Hence, medical treatment is necessary for both symptom and tumor control. Since somatostatin analogues provide critical symptom control, which was once the main reason for significant morbidity and mortality, now tumor bulk-related complications have become the leading cause of death [15]. The main clinical symptoms are pain, obstruction, diarrhea, hypoglycemia symptoms, hyperglycemia, weight loss, and carcinoid syndrome findings. Clinical symptoms may vary according to the functionality of the tumor and depend on the localization and size of the tumor. The majority of these findings can be eliminated by treatment of the tumor. If carcinoid symptoms are present, then somatostatin analogues, interferon, symptomatic treatment for diarrhea, mammalian target of rapamycin (mTOR) inhibition, and appropriate treatments can be used.

More patients are diagnosed at an earlier and asymptomatic stage, and more nonfunctional tumors are detected with the aid of widespread use of improved diagnostic and pathological tools, coupled with increased awareness of the public and medical community. However, this disease is still diagnosed more commonly at an advanced stage, making cure difficult to provide. The good side of the story is that the outcome of patients with NETs is becoming more favorable with increased survival rates, although cure is not possible [1].

In addition to an early diagnosis, improved surgical techniques can be used either aggressively or conservatively according to the presentation of the case [16, 17]. There are reported series of successful liver transplantation in selected cases, although the criteria for liver transplantation have not yet been fully established for NETs. Especially in cases with removed primary tumors, where surgery is not amenable, liver-directed therapies, ablation methods such as radiofrequency ablation (RFA), cryotherapy, radiosurgery or embolization, and bland or chemoembolization versus radioembolization can be offered. PRRT can be used in patients with well-differentiated low-grade NETs if positive for somatostatin receptor imaging. PRRT can be considered independently from the primary tumor site in both functional and nonfunctional tumors. ^{177}Lu-DOTA-Tyr3-octreotate is preferred as it has less renal toxicity and higher somatostatin receptor 2 affinity. Response rates are higher in PNETs in comparison to small intestine NETs [18].

Besides symptom control, somatostatin analogues improve the patient's quality of life and provide control of tumor progression in NETs [11]. Somatostatin analogues, namely, octreotide LAR and lanreotide, can be used in the treatment of functional and nonfunctional as well as well-differentiated gastrointestinal and pancreatic NETs due to their antiproliferative effects [19, 20]. For patients who have carcinoid syndrome refractory to somatostatin analogues, interferon and telotristat can be used.

Interferon (IFN) is used either alone or in combination with chemotherapy and somatostatin analogues for both symptom and tumor control. It can be used in selected cases as salvage therapy.

Systemic chemotherapy is more effective in patients with a rapidly progressive disease or a tumor with a high proliferation rate and aggressive pathological features, especially in pancreatic NETs. Combination chemotherapy is more effective than single-agent chemotherapy in NETs. Although the role of chemotherapy is relatively established for pancreatic NETs and for poorly differentiated tumors, there is a strong need for data to define the role of adjuvant treatment in low- or intermediate-degree tumors that are surgically resected [1].

Targeted agents have recently proven to show clinical activity [21, 22]. mTOR is a serine/threonine protein kinase that is a part of the phosphatidylinositol 3-kinase (PI3K)–AKT signaling pathway [21]. Everolimus is an mTOR inhibitor. Sunitinib is a multitargeted tyrosine kinase inhibitor, inhibiting vascular endothelial growth factor receptor (VEGFR)-1, -2, and -3 as well as platelet-derived growth factor (PDGF), KIT, and FMS-like tyrosine kinase 3 (FLT3) [21]. Both of these agents have shown clinical efficacy in phase three randomized studies in pancreatic NETs.

The follow-up of patients whose tumors are completely resected with surgery or endoscopy should be at 3- to 6-month intervals. Response evaluation in patients receiving systemic treatment should be performed at 3-month intervals. The imaging method to be used depends on the primary disease site, the course of the disease, and the best imaging method used at diagnosis.

References

1. Yalcin S (2011) Advances in the systemic treatment of pancreatic neuroendocrine tumors. Cancer Treat Rev 37:127–132
2. Burnik FS, Yalçin S (2009) NFKB1 -94 insertion/deletion ATTG polymorphism in gastroenteropancreatic neuroendocrine tumors. Chemotherapy 55:381–385
3. Rindi G, Arnold R, Bosman FT et al (2010) Nomenclature and classification of neuroendocrine neoplasms of the digestive system. In: Bosman FT, Carneiro F, Hruban RH, Theise ND (eds) WHO classification of tumours of the digestive system. IARC Press, Lyon, pp 13–14
4. Öberg K, Knigge U, Kwekkeboom D, Perren A (2012) Neuroendocrine gastro-entero pancreatic tumors: ESMO clinical practice guidelines for diagnosis, treatment and follow-up. Ann Oncol 23(7):124–130
5. Yao JC, Hassan M, Phan A et al (2008) One hundred years after "carcinoid": epidemiology of and prognostic factors for neuroendocrine tumors in 35,825 cases in the United States. J Clin Oncol 26:3063–3072
6. Dasari A, Shen C, Halperin D, Zhao B, Zhou S, Xu Y, Shih T, Yao JC (2017) Trends in the incidence, prevalence, and survival outcomes in patients with neuroendocrine tumors in the United States. JAMA Oncol 3:1335–1342

7. Yalcin S, Glasberg S, Abali H, Aykan F et al (2014) Gastroenteropancreatic neuroendocrine tumors (GEPNET) registry: update from an international collaboration. Ann Oncol 25(4):394–405. https://doi.org/10.1093/annonc/mdu345
8. National Cancer Institute. SEER cancer statistics review 1975-2004. Complete and limited-duration cancer prevalence estimates. http://seer.cancer.gov/csr/1975_2004/results_merged/topic_prevalence.pdf.
9. Klimstra DS, Modlin IR, Adsay NV et al (2010) Pathology reporting of neuroendocrine tumors: application of the Delphic consensus process to the development of a minimum pathology data set. Am J Surg Pathol 34:300–313
10. Klimstra DS, Modlin IR, Coppola D, Lloyd RV, Suster S (2010) The pathologic classification of neuroendocrine tumors: a review of nomenclature, grading, and staging systems. Pancreas 39:707–712
11. Keskin O, Yalcin S (2013) A review of the use of somatostatin analogs in oncology. Onco Targets Ther 6:471–483
12. Gabriel M, Decristofori C, Kendler D et al (2007) 68Ga-DOTA-Tyr 3-octreotide PET in neuroendocrine tumors: comparison with somatostatin receptor scintigraphy and CT. J Nucl Med 48:508–518
13. Buchmann I, Henze M, Engelbrecht S et al (2007) Comparison of ^{68}Ga-DOTATOC PET and ^{111}In-DTPAOC (Octreoscan) SPECT in patients with neuroendocrine tumours. Eur J Nucl Med Mol Imaging 34:1617–1626
14. Partelli S, Maurizi A, Tamburrino D, Baldoni A, Polenta V, Crippa S, Falconi M (2014) GEP-NETS update: a review on surgery of gastro-entero-pancreaticneuroendocrine tumors. Eur J Endocrinol 171:153–162
15. Oberg KE, Reubi JC, Kwekkeboom DJ, Krenning EP (2010) Role of somatostatins in gastroenteropancreatic neuroendocrine tumor development and therapy. Gastroenterology 139:742–753
16. Coppa J, Pulvirenti A, Schiavo M et al (2001) Resection versus transplantation for liver metastases from neuroendocrine tumors. Transplant Proc 33:1537–1539
17. Elvin A, Skogseid B, Hellman P (2005) Radiofrequency ablation of neuroendocrine liver metastases. Abdom Imaging 30:427–434
18. Bodei L, Kidd M, Paganelli G, Grana CM et al (2015) Long-term tolerability of PRRT in 807 patients with neuroendocrine tumours: the value and limitations of clinical factors. Eur J Nucl Med Mol Imaging 42:5–19
19. Rinke A, Müller HH, Schade-Brittinger C et al (2009) Placebo-controlled, double-blind, prospective, randomized study on the effect of octreotide LAR in the control of tumor growth in patients with metastatic neuroendocrine midgut tumors: a report from the PROMID Study Group. J Clin Oncol 27:4656–4663
20. Caplin ME, Pavel M, Ćwikła JB, Phan AT et al (2014) Lanreotide in metastatic enteropancreatic neuroendocrine tumors. N Engl J Med 371(3):224–233
21. Yao JC, Shah MH, Ito T et al (2011) Everolimus for advanced pancreatic neuroendocrine tumors. N Engl J Med 364:514–523
22. Raymond E, Dahan L, Raoul JL et al (2011) Sunitinib malate for the treatment of pancreatic neuroendocrine tumors. N Engl J Med 364:501–513

The Historical Evolution of Neuroendocrine Tumor Disease

2

Anna Malczewska, Alexander Mandel, Alexandra Kitz, Mark Kidd, and Irvin M. Modlin

2.1 Introduction

The recognition of neuroendocrine tumors (NETs) as a distinct oncological entity is relatively novel and represents a culmination of the early failure to recognize that the two physiological systems, neural and endocrine, had neoplastic implications as opposed to a purely regulatory role. Furthermore, since oncology was previously mostly focused upon organ-related tumors, the concept of a cancer arising from diffuse neural networks or isolated aggregations of endocrine cells was not initially appreciated. Limitations in the histology of neuroendocrine tumors of the early twentieth century have also contributed to the lack of understanding of their pathological basis. Moreover, the relative rarity of such lesions has resulted in a lack of focus on their unique differences to adenocarcinomas. The fact that NETs represent tumors within an organ that did not necessarily arise from the principal cell systems comprising an organ further obfuscated recognition of their unique differences from classical "organ cancers."

A. Malczewska
Department of Endocrinology and Neuroendocrine Tumors, Medical University of Silesia, Katowice, Poland

A. Mandel · A. Kitz · M. Kidd
Wren Laboratories, Branford, CT, USA
e-mail: am1061@exeter.ac.uk; akitz@wrenlaboratories.com; mkidd@wrenlaboratories.com

I. M. Modlin (✉)
School of Medicine, Yale University, New Haven, CT, USA
e-mail: imodlin@irvinmodlin.com

S. Yalcin, K. Öberg (eds.), *Neuroendocrine Tumours*,
https://doi.org/10.1007/978-3-031-56968-5_2

2.2 Concepts of Cell Regulation

2.2.1 Identification of Neural and Endocrine Regulatory Systems

In 1883, Pavlov (1849–1936) introduced the concept of nervism and proposed that the nervous system played a dominant role in the regulation of body function. This proposition was refuted to some extent by his failure to recognize the regulatory effect of the endocrine system. The latter system was identified in 1902 by Bayliss (1860–1924) and Starling (1866–1927), who challenged the concept of nervism in a series of animal experiments, which demonstrated that previously undescribed circulating agents ("chemical messengers" was their original term) are responsible for pancreatic secretion. They proposed the name "secretin" for the hypothetical chemical messenger involved and suggested a new class of chemical substances that they grouped together under the term "hormone" (derived from *hormonos* "I arouse to excitement"). This term was proposed by Hardy (1864–1934). Starling, in his Croonian Lectures of 1905, presciently noted the potential role of such agents in both secretion and as regulators of growth. The discovery of a "chemical messenger" initiated the development of endocrinology and the subsequent evolution of concepts that included the neurohumoral regulation of body function as well as the brain–gut axis. As a result, the consideration of nervism waned. Following the observations of Bayliss and Starling, numerous hormones and their cells of origin have been identified and their functions and complex interrelationships explored.

2.2.2 Recognition of Agents Secreted by Nerves (Neurotransmitters)

In 1905, Schiefferdecker (1849–1931) described the secretion of endocrine substances by neurons as a means of communication between a neuron and an effector cell in a muscle or a gland [1]. His observations were based on his own reflections and ideas initially propounded by Tigerstedt (1853–1923) ("automatic" irritation by metabolic products) [2]. Further support for this concept was provided in 1914 by Cannon (1871–1945), who used adrenaline to demonstrate that the adrenal medulla functioned not only as an endocrine gland but also as part of the autonomic nervous system in what is now termed "the flight or fight" survival response [3]. His experiments on chemical neurotransmission and search for "sympathins" bore some resemblance to those carried out by the Nobel laureate Loewi (1873–1961). The original idea of chemical transmission in the autonomic nervous system had been conceived by Elliott (1877–1961), who despairingly wrote, "I have tried in vain to discover an active principle in the muscle plates of striped muscles" [4]. In 1921, Loewi, a pharmacologist, established the chemical nature of nerve transmission by proving the theory of chemical intermediaries in nervous stimulation, and, by the 1930s, the secretory cells of the hypothalamus could be demonstrated to exert neurohormonal regulation of the anterior pituitary [5]. Thus, feedback mechanisms were identified and central nervous system regulation became a recognized part of hormonal regulation (Fig. 2.1).

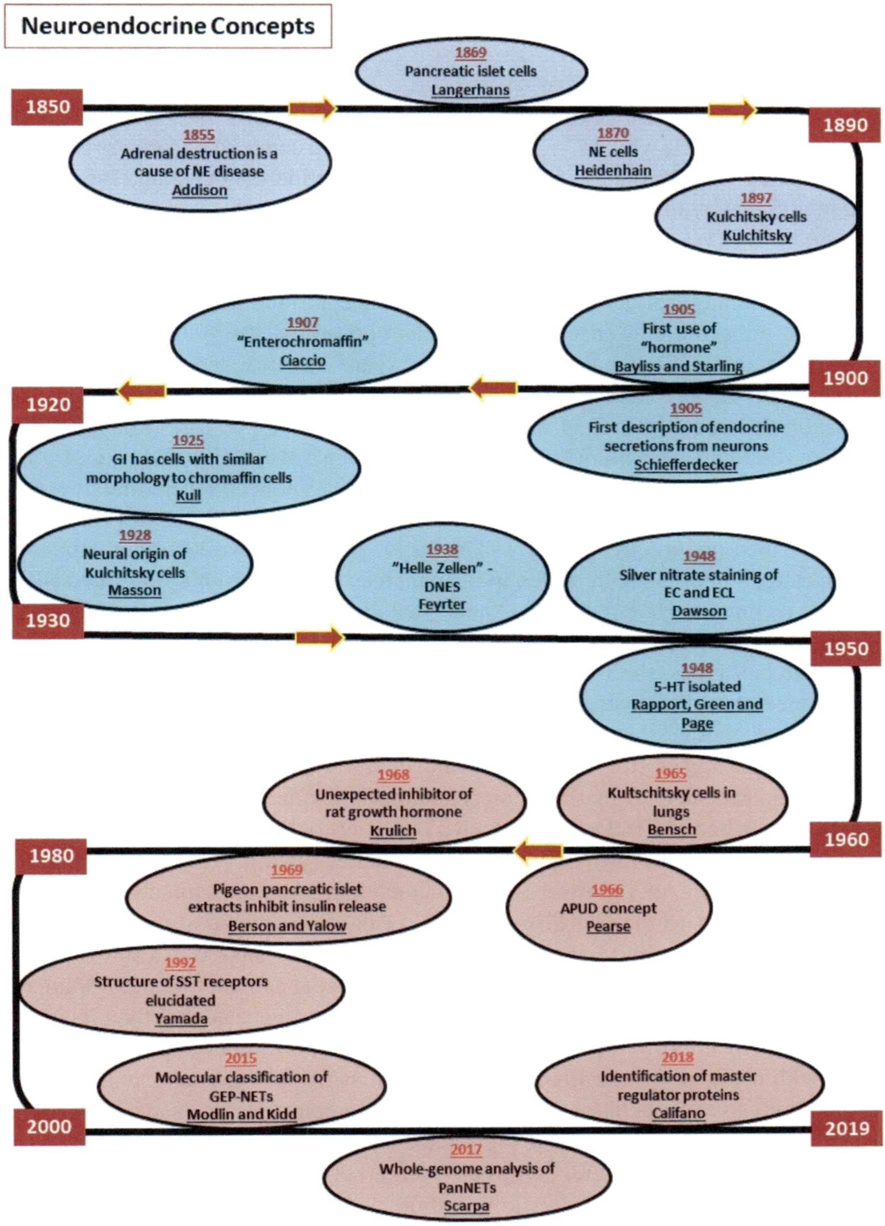

Fig. 2.1 A timeline of neuroendocrine concepts 1855–2018. *Dark blue*: 1850–1900; *light blue*: 1900–1950; and *red*: 1950–2019

2.2.3 Feyrter and the Concept of the Diffuse Neuroendocrine System (DNES)

The concept of a diffuse neuroendocrine system (DNES) was initially proposed by Feyrter (1895–1973) who, in 1938, put forward the existence of a regulatory system that included an interrelationship between nerves, endocrine cells, and the regulation of gut, motor, and secretory activities. Feyrter published *Über diffuse endocrine epitheliale Organe*, in which he summated the findings of the investigations of the endocrine system of the pancreas and gastrointestinal (GI) enterochromaffin cells [6]. In this manuscript, he established a new concept in the field of endocrinology, by proclaiming the existence of a DNES as opposed to the previously accepted dogma of ductless [7] glands and endocrine "organs." Feyrter described in detail the existence of "helle zellen," present in clusters throughout the duct epithelium and the "mucoid" ductal glands of the pancreas, which developed as a result of endophytism, budding, and branching. The "helle zellen" of the gastrointestinal tract, which comprised of the cornerstone of Feyrter's DNES concept, were first observed by Nicolas in lizards in 1891 [8] and rediscovered in 1905 by Schmidt [9] and further described in 1906 by Ciaccio (1877–1956) [10, 11]. Feyrter further expanded the investigation of the helle zellen in the pancreas using Masson's simplified silver staining technique. He envisaged a "new" cellular depiction of the pancreas, comprised of the exocrine duct epithelium, the exocrine mucoid duct gland, and two endocrine cell types, the islets of Langerhans and the clear cells, which classified the pancreas as a diffuse endocrine organ.

Feyrter suggested that the human endocrine system consisted of not only compact epithelial organs (that released hormones into the lymph and blood) but also scattered endocrine cells that were present either individually or in groups throughout the whole body [12]. Feyrter provided examples of the latter and correlated his findings in the pancreas with the intestinal epithelial "yellow cells" of Schmidt [9]. However, the latter cells showed similar characteristics to the clear cells of the pancreas with regard to their localization and formation within the mucosa. Feyrter noted that Schmidt's intestinal "yellow cells" only developed as a result of endophytism when induced by "inflammation" or "bourgeonnement" (budding), a term that had originally been used by Masson [13]. Feyrter suggested that the process of "bourgeonnement" provided the mechanism that led to the development of carcinoids within the gastrointestinal tract. The similarities of Feyrter's "helle zellen" and Schmidt's yellow cells, as well as the fact that carcinoids appeared to be derived from these cell types with variable prevalence throughout the intestine, suggested to Feyrter that there were different types of "yellow cells" with different functions and gastrointestinal epithelial localizations within.

More than half a century elapsed before cells from which carcinoids of the stomach (enterochromaffin-like (ECL) cells) and the intestine (enterochromaffin (EC) cells) were identified and related to tumorigenesis [14–17]. In addition, Feyrter suggested, in allusion to the structure of Meissner's and Auerbach's plexus, that the scattered endocrine cells were also connected within a neural network through the wall of the gastrointestinal tract. Supporting this theory were Masson's pathological findings describing the *appendicite neurogene*, drawing attention to the neural aggregations associated with appendicitis [18]. Feyrter compared the diffuse endocrine system to the neuroendothelial tissue found within the anatomic association of the inner zone of the adrenal cortex and the adrenal medulla and proposed that the DNES developed as a result of the "chemotactical migration" of the nervous tissue to specific sites of the body. As enunciated by Feyrter, the linked concept of a peripheral endocrine system, gastrointestinal carcinoids, and clear endocrine cells was by far the most comprehensive and integrated neuroendocrine-related hypothesis combining morphology, function, and pathology that arose during the first half of the twentieth century. The concept facilitated the development of neuroendocrinology, integrating two previously separate and distinct philosophies of neural and hormonal regulation. This concept proposed a paradigm shift, whereby regulation of organ function was based on a diffuse neuroendocrine regulatory system.

2.2.4 Cellular Basis of the Neuroendocrine System

In 1867, Langerhans (1847–1888) described previously unrecognized clusters of pancreatic cells embedded within sheets of pancreatic acinar cells (Fig. 2.2) but failed to identify their endocrine function. Laguesse (1861–1927) studied these

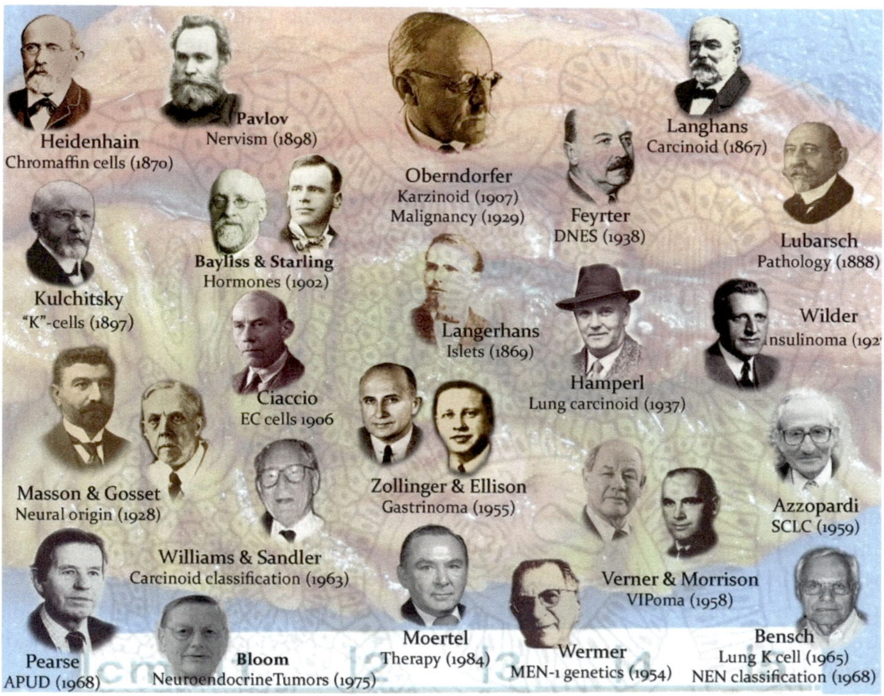

Fig. 2.2 The principal physiologists, anatomists, pathologists, and clinicians whose contributions led to advances in the identification and classification of gastrointestinal, pancreatic, and broncho-pulmonary neuroendocrine cells (left) and tumors (right). *APUD* amine precursor uptake and decarboxylation, *DNES* diffuse neuroendocrine system, *EC* enterochromaffin; *MEN* multiple endocrine neoplasia, *NEN* neuroendocrine neoplasia, *SCLC* small cell lung cancer

pancreatic cell clusters, postulated that they produce an internal secretion, and coined the term "islets of Langerhans" in memory of Langerhans who had contracted tuberculosis and died on the island of Madeira. In 1922, 30 years later, Banting (1891–1941) and Best (1899–1978) described the islets as the source of insulin. EC cells in the gastric mucosa of rabbits and dogs were first described in 1870 by Heidenhain (1834–1897) [19]. He noted that the cells contained acidophilic granules, and, 2 years later, he identified small, granular, yellow staining cells on the surface of gastric glands that are now understood to be histamine-secreting EC-like (ECL) cells. In 1891, Nikolas (1861–1939) reported the wide distribution of EC cells throughout the gastrointestinal (GI) tract [8]. In 1897, Kulchitsky (1856–1925) noted similar cells with granules with acidophilic properties in the crypts of Lieberkühn and the intestinal mucosa of cats and dogs and proposed that the cells were involved in the digestive process [20]. In 1906, Ciaccio identified the same cell type in the GI tract of humans and coined the term "EC cells." He also introduced the term "enterochromaffin" to depict the staining of the "helle zellen" with chromium salts. It, however, remained for Masson (1880–1959) in 1914 to suggest that the endocrine cells of the gut formed a diffuse endocrine organ and corresponded to the enterochromaffin cells described by Ciaccio [11]. In his manuscript, *La glande endocrine de l'intestin chez l'homme* [13] (The endocrine glands of the gut in man), and in his collaboration with Gosset (1872–1944) in *Les tumeurs endocrines de l'appendice* (Endocrine tumors of the appendix), Masson proposed that these cells could be aggregated into a single functional unit [21]. In addition, based on their affinity for silver stain, he classified them as the cell of origin of carcinoid tumors, thereby implicating the latter as an endocrine neoplasm. Later in 1928, he proposed that EC cells were of a neural origin and that their secretion of "substances" is responsible for carcinoid syndrome [22]. Similarly, Erös [23–25] and Kahlau [26], using animal experimental studies, also opined that clear endocrine cells possessed endocrine function and produced hormone-like substances.

Building on the theory of the integrated DNES proposed by Feyrter, Pearse (1915–2003) developed the amine precursor uptake and decarboxylation (APUD) concept, linking together endocrine cells with common cytochemical characteristics. The APUD concept suggested that all neuroendocrine cells are APUD cells and derive from the neural crest. However, the neural crest origin of the DNES proved to be incorrect and has been replaced by the concept of the endodermal origin of the neuroendocrine cells of the GI tract. Thus, as the result of overlapping chemical, histological, and physiological studies, the endocrinology of the gastrointestinal tract became a focus of considerable attention and advanced relatively rapidly. Indeed, the initial observation of Bernard (1813–1878) followed by those of Brown-Séquard (1817–1894), Bayliss, and Starling in concert with the evolution of staining techniques resulted in a complete reassessment of the concept of organ regulation.

2.3 Initial Steps in the Recognition of the Neuroendocrine Tumor System

In 1907, Oberndorfer (1876–1944) was the first to coin the term "carcinoid" and describe the idiosyncratic nature of these tumors (Fig. 2.3). However, such lesions had in fact been observed during the nineteenth century by a number of physicians (Fig. 2.4), including Langhans (1839–1915) (in 1867), Lubarsch (1860–1933) (in 1888), and Ransom (1860–1890) (in 1890). Theodor Langhans, a former pupil of Recklinghausen (1833–1910), was the first to describe a carcinoid tumor. The lesion had been identified at autopsy in a 50-year-old woman who had perished of tuberculosis. Langhans described a firm, mushroom-shaped submucosal tumor that projected into the lumen of the small intestine and commented on the extremely sharp borders without any evidence of peritumoral invasion. In addition, he commented on the histological nature of the tumor cells, which he described as resembling a poorly differentiated glandular tissue arranged in "nests" with a rich, thick, fibrous stroma. His manuscript, published in 1867, chiefly focused on the histological features of the tumor and did not address the clinical and growth behavior of this previously undocumented neoplasm. Two decades would pass before this obscure and unexplained entity was revisited by Otto Lubarsch. In 1888, the 28-year-old Lubarsch described two cases of ileal tumors discovered at autopsy [27]. In one case (a 49-year-old male), the ileum contained numerous tubercular ulcers and tubercular nodules on the mucous membrane; the second case (a 52-year-old male), which was also tubercular, was marked by six scattered small, carcinomatous growths in the ileum and a cirrhotic liver. Interestingly, diarrhea had been a prominent symptom in the latter patient, quite possibly as a manifestation of carcinoid syndrome, although Lubarsch made no mention of metastatic disease in either case. Microscopically, he noted a low-grade penetration of the tumor into the muscularis circularis and hyperplasia of the adjacent muscularis mucosae.

Lubarsch evaluated the records of 35 cases of intestinal carcinomas occurring near the ileocecal valve and opined that in his estimation, several of these were not "true" carcinomas. William Bramwell Ransom was the third to describe a lesion resembling carcinoid tumors [27]. In the 1890 issue of *The Lancet*, Ransom described a case involving a 50-year-old woman who initially presented with two egg-sized lumps in the lower part of her abdomen, menorrhagia, and severe diarrhea. Her symptomatology was mainly attributed to uterine fibroids, and her symptoms had improved only somewhat by the time she left the hospital several weeks later. The diarrhea persisted for the next 2 years, at which time the patient presented with a large, palpable abdominal mass and distinct cachexia. Of particular interest was the observation of severe attacks of wheezing and diarrhea on eating, arguably the first reported sign of carcinoid syndrome. After the patient's death soon thereafter, autopsy revealed several small nodules in the ileum located 6 inches above the ileocecal valve as well as extensive hepatic tumors (presumably metastases). Ransom noted that the tumor cells were arranged in small nests that formed small tubes or solid bars and that scarcely any remains of villi or crypts of Lieberkühn were visible near the free surfaces of the tumor. Ransom also noted hyperplasia of

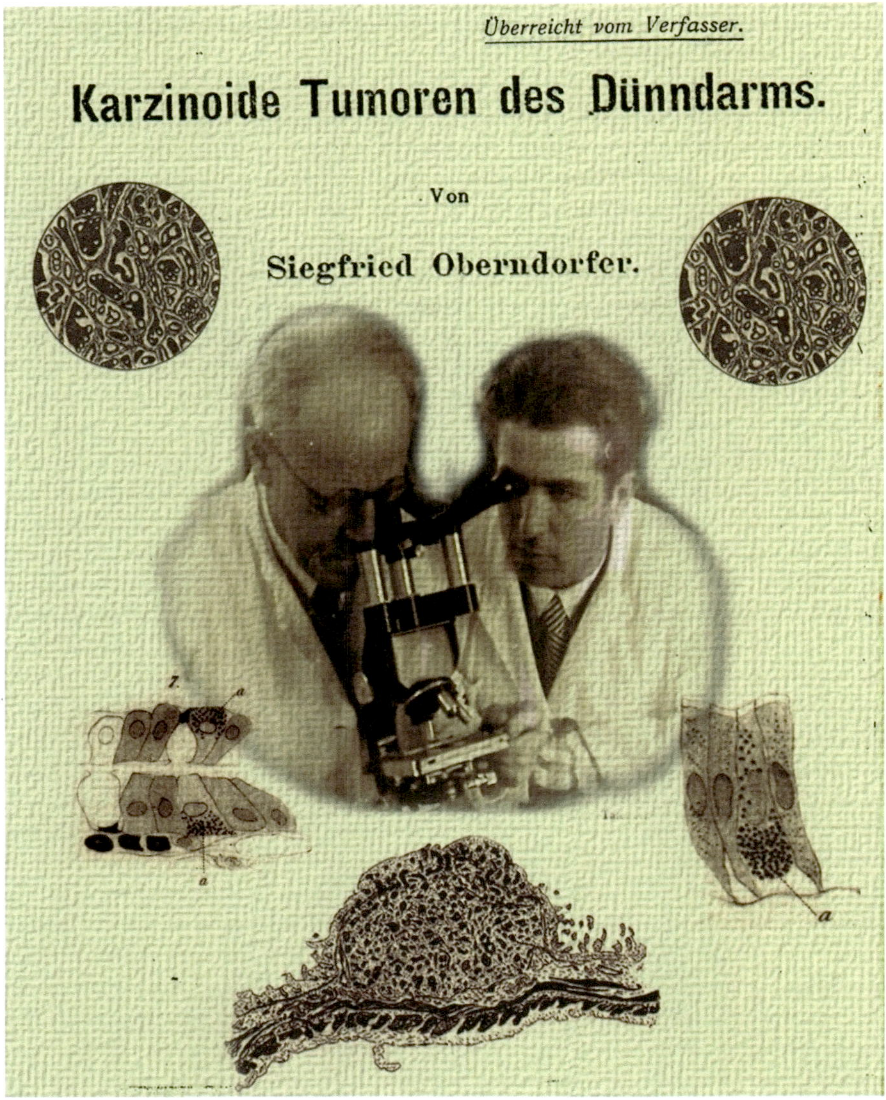

Fig. 2.3 Siegfried Oberndorfer, a pathologist originally from Munich *(center left)*, in 1907 described tumors that resembled "less aggressive carcinomas" and introduced the term "*karzinoide*" into the lexicon of medicine. This image is with his Turkish pathology fellow at the University of Istanbul where he was forced to flee, having been evicted by the Nazi regime in 1939

the adjacent muscularis mucosae and astutely commented that these tumors resembled carcinomas only histologically and "may remain undetected for a long time." These tumors demonstrate a very slight local malignancy or the tendency to infiltrate or destroy their surrounding tissues. In concluding his remarks, Ransom proposed that the tumors' malignant potential largely depends on local conditions

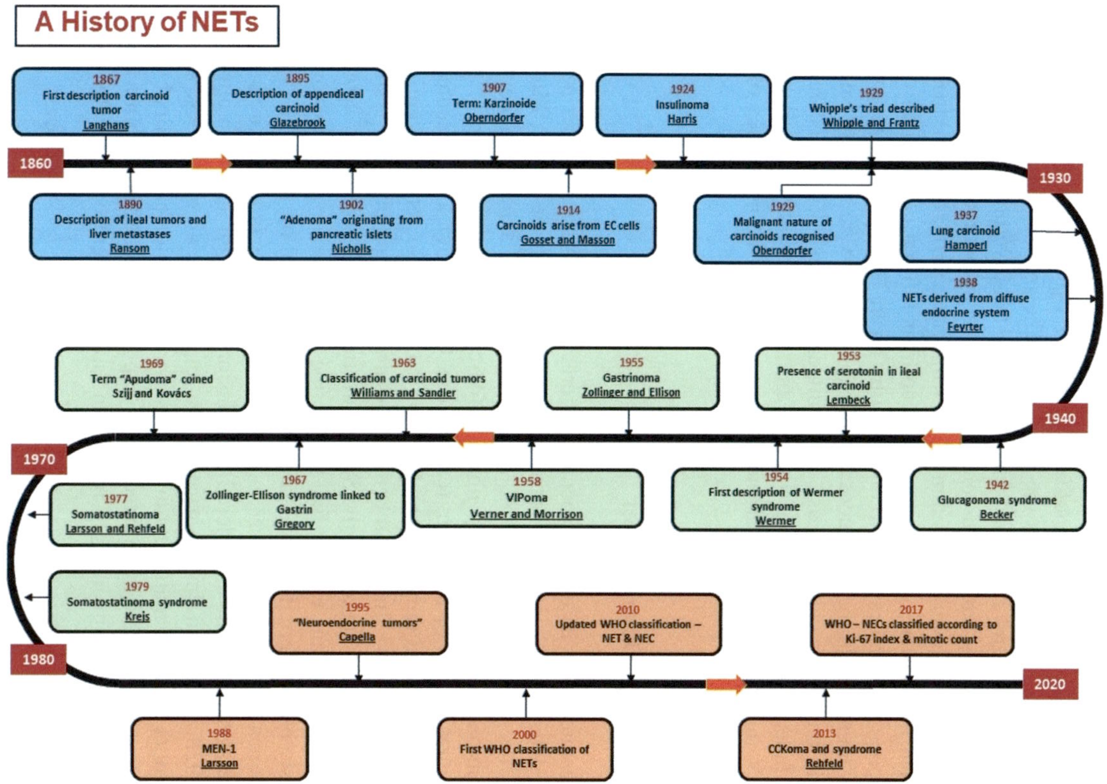

Fig. 2.4 The historical evolution of neuroendocrine tumor description: 1867–2013. *Blue*: 1860–1940; *green*: 1940–1980; and *orange*: 1980–2020. The timeline begins in 1867 with Langhans' initial description of a carcinoid tumor and details the identification over time of the recognition of cells and tumors that currently comprise the landscape of neuroendocrine tumor disease. The novel neoplastic proposal of the disease "*karzinoide*" was introduced by Oberndorfer in 1907 and was thereafter followed by the recognition of different tumors and their syndromes. A variety of classifications have been introduced culminating with the WHO NETs classification of 2017

(i.e., vascular supply and resistance) of the peritumoral tissues and referred to the lesions as “glandular carcinomas,” although their peculiar appearance, caused by penetrating blood vessels into the tumor, led him to propose a resemblance to cylindromas (uncommon benign adnexal tumors). In fact, he believed that this angiogenesis was more consistent with the behavior of sarcomas than that of carcinomas.

In 1895, Notthafft described three tumors of the upper jejunum found at autopsy in a patient who had died of pneumonia [27]. The first pinhead-sized tumor was found approximately 10 cm beyond the duodenum. The second and third tumors, both pea-sized, were found 10 cm and 15 cm distal to the first tumor, respectively. They had a whitish color and a hard consistency with a smooth surface. Notthafft noted rampant tumor growth in the submucosa, which rose strongly above the level of the adjacent mucous membrane, and small cellular infiltration in much of the adjacent mucous membranes and into the muscular layer. The tumors were uncharacteristically identified in the submucosa and histologically were not true carcinomas; Notthafft thus referred to them as “beginning carcinomas” [27]. The carcinoid tumor then faded into obscurity once more, and 12 more years passed before Oberndorfer’s initial attempt to characterize and delineate the properties of this enigmatic neoplasm was presented.

2.3.1 The Role of Oberndorfer

At much the same time as the gastroenteropancreatic (GEP) neuroendocrine cell system was described, Siegfried Oberndorfer, a German pathologist in Munich, reported a series of unusual tumors (Fig. 2.3). He recognized the difference between cancerous tumors of the ileocolonic junction (carcinomas) and a group of more benign-behaving lesions of the ileum (carcinoids). Oberndorfer first presented his observation on carcinoid tumors at the German Pathologic Society Convention in Dresden, Germany, 1907. In December of the same year, he published a similar article titled “Carcinoid Tumors of the Small Intestine” in the *Frankfurt Journal of Pathology* [28]. This article was the first to describe and characterize the tumor that had previously been referred to as a carcinoma; it was based on six similar cases with multiple pea-sized tumors. Oberndorfer used the term “*karzinoide*” (carcinoma-like) because at that time he considered these lesions as benign and not malignant tumors. In 1928, he revised this observation in a review, indicating that these small intestinal tumors could be malignant and metastasize. Oberndorfer’s seminal work in this field was prematurely terminated by his expulsion by the Nazi regime from Germany. He spent the remainder of his life in Istanbul where he ironically died from a thymic carcinoid.

2.3.2 The Chemical Basis for Tumor Symptomatology

That the EC cell is the cell of origin of carcinoid tumors was strongly argued by Feyrter in 1938. EC cells were chemically active, and Dawson (1892–1968) developed a technique (silver nitrate) for the staining of EC and ECL cells in 1948 [29].

The same year, serotonin was isolated and described by Rapport (1919–2011) [30]. In 1953, Lembeck (1922–2014) biochemically confirmed the presence of serotonin in an ileal carcinoid tumor, confirming the assumption that human EC cells contain this bioactive amine [31]. In 1952, Biörck et al. [32] established the relationship between carcinoid heart disease and carcinoid tumors and the secretion of serotonin. In 1954, Pernow and Waldenström added that paroxysmal flushing was part of the syndrome [33]. Oates et al. demonstrated the release of kallikrein from some carcinoid tumors [34]. In 1986, Norheim et al. [35] published the concept that tachykinins in carcinoid tumors were possibly involved in carcinoid flushing. In 1956, Haverback and Sjoerdsma [36] reported on the presence of the serotonin metabolite 5-hydroxyindoleacetic acid (5-HIAA) in urine.

2.3.3 Recognition of Carcinoid Syndrome

In 1927, Postma (1892–1960) described the first case of flushing in a 45-year-old male, who was later shown to suffer from a metastatic ileal carcinoid. Postma designated the disease as "hemangioma planum extensum" [37, 38]. In 1931, Scholte performed a postmortem examination on the patient and identified an ileal tumor as well as extensive hepatic metastases and stenosis of the pulmonary ostium and thickening of the leaflets of the tricuspid valve [39]. In the same year, Cassidy (1880–1949) described a case of a 31-year-old male patient who presented with diarrhea and flushing, a systolic heart murmur, and right-sided heart failure, and, at autopsy, liver metastases of an "adenocarcinoma" and tricuspid valve stenosis were identified. In addition, extensive pelvic fibrosis was noted but no tumor was identified [40, 41]. At that time, the relationship between gastrointestinal NETs, carcinoid syndrome, and fibrosis was not evident. In 1952, prior to the identification of the relationship between serotonin and carcinoid syndrome, Biörck et al. suggested a relationship between carcinoid tumors and carcinoid heart disease [32, 42–44]. In 1954, serotonin and its urinary metabolite 5-hydroxyindoleacetic acid (5-HIAA) were identified by Page as plasma and urine markers of carcinoid syndrome (1901–1991) [45, 46]. This was confirmed by Sjoerdsma (1924–2014) and colleagues in 1956 [34, 47–52].

2.4 Evolution of NETs as an Oncological Discipline

2.4.1 Cellular and Secretory Basis

Although the concept of neuroendocrine tumors (NETs) was initiated by Oberndorfer in 1907, observations remained anecdotal and ill-understood until the unifying theories of Sandler (1926–2014) and Pearse were introduced in the late 1960s. The former described different tumors in the fore, hind, and midgut, and the latter introduced the concept of a common APUD-derived cell system. Between 1960 and 1970, the true NET concept was established with the development of radioimmunoassays for peptides and hormones and the introduction of computerized tomography

(CT) [53]. The former contributions mostly reflected the work of Bloom and Polak, who at a peptide and histological level further refined the syndromic and immunohistopathological nature of the tumors and developed diagnostic radioimmunoassays (RIAs) for their identification. Histopathology now included immunohistochemistry with specific antibodies, and chromogranin A (CgA) was established as a general marker of NETs, both in cytochemistry and as a circulating biomarker.

2.4.1.1 The Recognition and Role of Somatostatin Receptors (SSTRs)

In 1968, Krulich (1925–2005) and McCann (1925–2007) discovered a hypothalamic factor that inhibited the secretion of the growth hormone [54]. Five years later, in 1973, Guillemin isolated a peptide from sheep hypothalami, which could inhibit the release of the growth hormone, and named it somatostatin (somatotropin release–inhibiting factor (SRIF)) [55]. Guillemin received the Nobel Prize for this discovery in conjunction with Schally and Yalow (1921–2011). Further studies indicated that somatostatin had a wide range of inhibitory actions, and, in 1978, Vale (1941–2012) described a short octapeptide somatostatin analogue with full somatostatin biological activity [56]. An analogue, SMS 201-995 octreotide acetate, was developed by Bauer and became widely used to control carcinoid syndrome and the diarrhea of VIPoma syndrome [57]. Kvols described its efficacy, and, subsequently, Rubin reported the utility of a long-acting octreotide acetate preparation [58, 59]. Reubi described the different somatostatin receptor subtypes and developed methods to detect or visualize them [60, 61]. On March 25, 1988, the first female multiple endocrine neoplasia (MEN)-1 patient underwent a scan using ^{125}I-tyr-3-octreotide at University Hospital Rotterdam, The Netherlands. The scan not only demonstrated a neuroendocrine pancreatic tumor and its lymph node metastases but also several previously undetected meningiomas [62]. In 1991, ^{111}In-pentetreotide scintigraphy was first performed in the same hospital by Krenning et al. [63]. This product became commercially available in 1994 and was named OctreoScan®. More recently, ^{68}Gallium (Ga)-DOTATOC and ^{68}Ga-DOTATATE have been developed as positron emission tomography (PET) tracers for somatostatin receptor imaging [64, 65]. The first peptide receptor radiotherapy (PRRT) using the Auger electron emitter ^{111}In-pentetreotide was performed in 1994 [66]. ^{90}Yt- and ^{177}Lu-labeled somatostatin analogues were subsequently introduced, and a phase 3 trial using ^{177}Lu-octreotide has recently finished its patient enrollment [67].

2.4.2 Biomarkers

The evolution of biomarker development for NETs ranges from purely functional assays that measured the activity of a hormone to highly sensitive antibody-based assays that detected and quantified the level of a specific hormone. The latter is best typified by the development of radioimmunoassays in the 1960s and 70s by Yalow and Berson (1918–1972) and is now exemplified by the time-resolved amplified cryptate emission immune approach that significantly amplifies an immune ligand complex (Fig. 2.5).

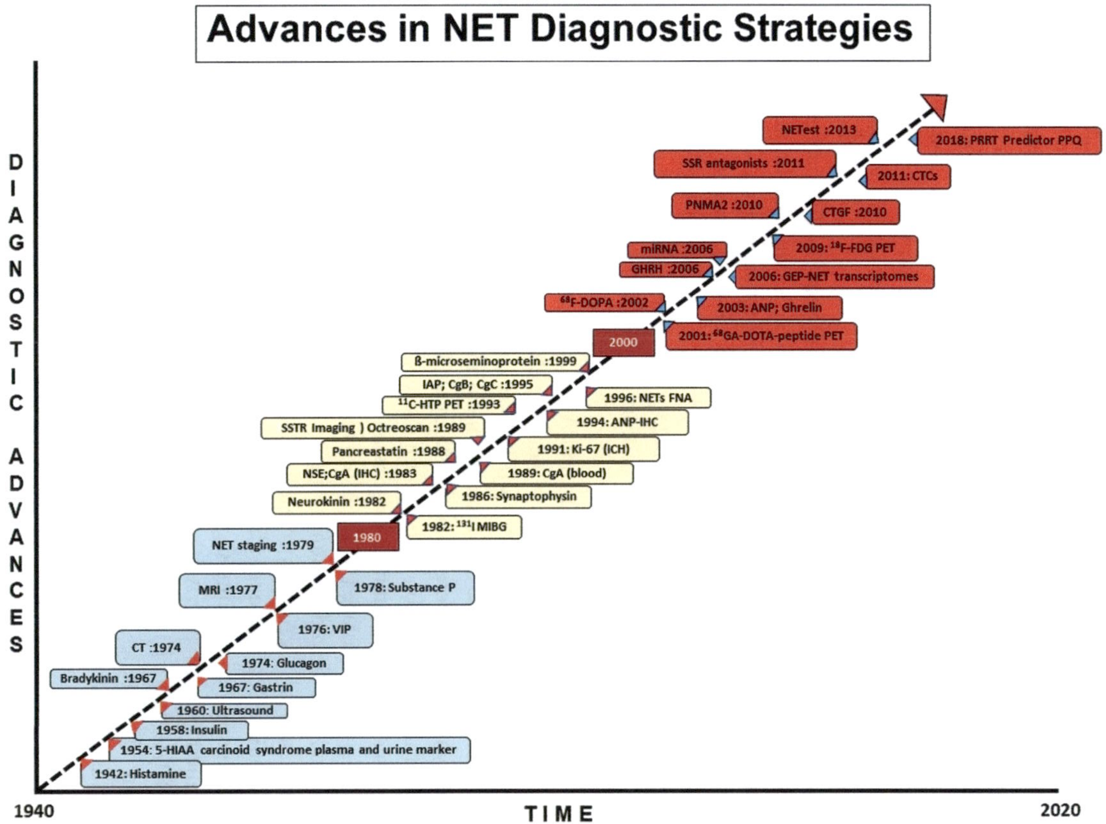

Fig. 2.5 NET diagnostic strategy timeline: 1942–2018. The linear scale delineates advances in imaging and biomarkers and is color coded by time periods: *blue*: 1940–1980; *yellow*: 1980–2000, and *red*: 2000–2018. The earliest biomarker was histamine in 1942 with the most recent being circulating gene transcripts (NETest). Diagnostic imaging became effective with the introduction of CT in 1974 and currently is best exemplified by ^{68}Gallium-DOTA peptide scanning

In 1942, histamine was detected via functional assays using isolated guinea pig gut. Radioenzymatic assays became available in 1966, which had the advantage of not requiring prior isolation of histamine from a sample. These provided a sensitive evaluation of histamine conversion to histidine, providing an indirect measure of the hormone. RIAs (1980s) and enzyme-linked immunosorbent assays (ELISAs) (1990) were subsequently developed for histamine. In 1954, serotonin and 5-HIAA were identified in plasma and urine using colorimetric and spectrophotometric methods. This methodology has evolved with time and currently utilizes quantitative high-performance liquid chromatography-tandem mass spectrometry or standard ELISAs for quantification. Urine remains the principal compartment for 5-HIAA measurements, which can be undertaken typically using a 24-h collection or, more recently, a 1-h collection test. Platelet-free serum provides another option, but both approaches require dietary restrictions or fasting and extensive pre-analytical sample preparation.

The first insulin RIA was developed in 1958. Subsequent approaches include radioreceptor and enzyme immune electrode assays as well as immunometric assays, though these have mostly been supplanted by quantitative chemiluminescent immunoassays and rapid, point-of-care finger prick-based assays. Both gastrin and bradykinin measurements were introduced in 1967 using RIAs. Accurate bradykinin measurement required a pre-chromatography Sephadex cleanup. In order to effectively identify different gastrin isoforms, biotinylated derivatives were developed.

With the increased interest in NETs and APUDomas during the 1970s, a series of RIAs for tumor hormonal products were developed. These included glucagon (1974), vasoactive intestinal peptide (VIP) (1976), and substance P and somatostatin (1978). These peptides are still typically measured using quantitative RIAs. The subsequent synthesis of different somatostatin analogues allowed for the development of quantitative extraction with immunoassays. Further developments included the measurement of neurokinin A (or substance K) in 1982 (RIA) and thereafter in 1983 neuron-specific enolase (NSE). More recently, NSE has been measured using quantitative enzyme-linked immunosorbent assays (ELISAs).

Chromogranin A (CgA) was initially identified in 1967 as a protein released from the stimulated calf adrenal gland [68]. Thereafter, a family of uniquely acidic proteins, the granins, including CgB, secretogranin II (SGII), 7B2, and NESP 55, were identified. The first CgA RIA was introduced in 1984, and, subsequently, a variety of RIAs and ELISAs have been developed for diagnostic and prognostic purposes. In addition, assays for CgA fragments such as pancreastatin (1988) and the other granin family members (e.g., CgB) have been developed.

Given the recognition of the limitations of monoanalyte measurements of secretory peptides and amines, more sophisticated strategies have been addressed since 2013. These include circulating transcripts (messenger RNA (mRNA)), microRNA (miRNA), and circulating tumor cells (CTCs). The measurement of miRNA has proven problematic given the analytical difficulties of quantifying small miRNAs. The methodology for CTC capture has technological limitations and is limited to an epithelial cell adhesion molecule (EpCAM) approach, which is nonspecific for

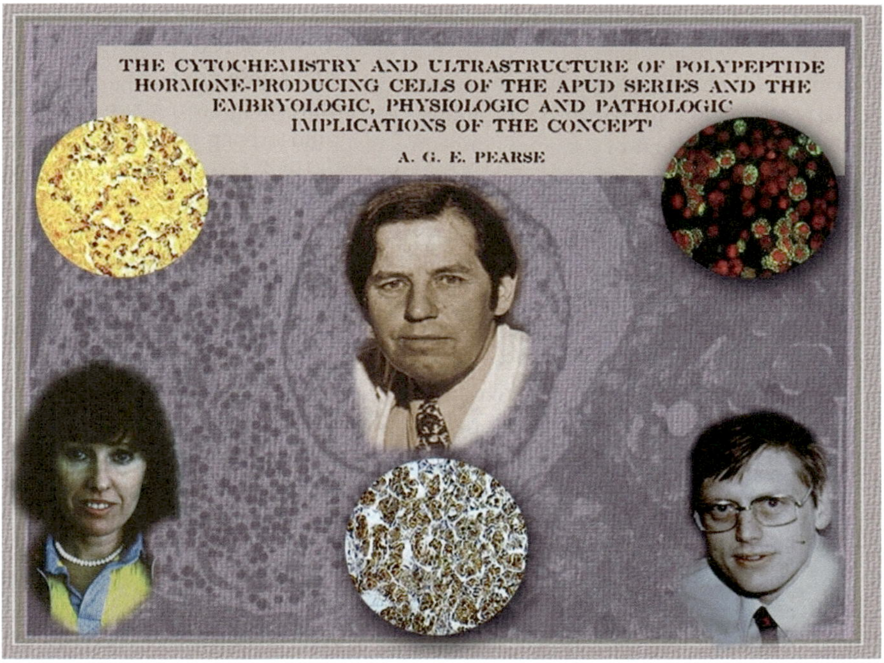

Fig. 2.6 The concept of APUDomas and the immunohistochemical identification (*circles*) of neuroendocrine tumors. Steven Bloom (*bottom right*), Julia Polak (*bottom left*), and Everson Pearse (*center*) of Hammersmith Hospital, London, were pivotal in the development of these advances. Pearse elucidated the APUD concept, which laid the foundation for the understanding of the cell systems that comprised neuroendocrine neoplasia

neuroendocrine cells. As an alternative, blood-based polymerase chain reaction (PCR) assays (mRNA) have been developed both for NET diagnosis (NETest) and for prediction of therapeutic response [69]. These are robust and currently provide the state-of-the-art diagnostic approach. The accuracy of transcript-based measurement is significantly more sensitive and accurate than either an RIA or an ELISA/ enzyme immunoassay (EIA) (Fig. 2.6). Since the assay provides a multi-genomic assessment of the disease, it provides a spectrum of tumor biological information, including tumor proliferation and progression as opposed to a measurement of tumor secretion [70]. The latter event is usually of limited value in determining disease outcome.

2.4.3 Classification of Tumor Types

Carcinoid tumors were initially classified in 1963 according to the foregut, midgut, or hindgut derivation by Williams and Sandler. This stratification was developed prior to the elucidation of the different NE cell types and the appreciation that an embryological classification had little mechanistic or physiological validity [71]. This concept was supplanted in 1966 by Pearse who identified and described common chemical characteristics in the endocrine cells of the gastrointestinal tract, particularly the uptake of 5-hydroxytryptophan and its conversion to 5-HT [72], and established the concept of a shared amine precursor uptake cell type [73]. In 1969, Szijj of Kovács's group introduced the term "APUDoma" when describing a patient with an adrenocorticotrophin (ACTH)-producing medullary carcinoma of the thyroid [74]. In 1995, the Italian pathologist Capella and other European NET expert pathologists published a revised classification of NETs and suggested avoiding the term "carcinoid tumors" and instead using the term "neuroendocrine tumors" to include all NETs [75]. Thereafter, a more formalized approach was adopted by the World Health Organization (WHO), which resulted in a series of classifications embodying histopathological information. The first (2000) WHO classification for NETs suggested the following categories: (a) well-differentiated endocrine tumors characterized by a low grade of malignancy and (b) well-differentiated endocrine carcinomas. It was generally agreed that the term "carcinoid" should no longer be used for gastroenteropancreatic NETs. In 2010, the WHO classification for gastroenteropancreatic NETs was updated and the general terms "neuroendocrine tumor (NET)" and "neuroendocrine carcinoma (NEC)" were introduced [76]. The current classification for pancreatic NETs recognizes a subset of well-differentiated grade 3 (Ki-67 >20%) tumors and defines it as a basis for treatment strategy. The most up-to-date 2015 WHO classification of lung tumors grouped four histological neuroendocrine subtypes (typical carcinoids, atypical carcinoids (ACs), large cell neuroendocrine carcinoma, and small cell lung carcinoma) together to improve taxonomy or diagnostic recognition [77] and indicated a role of Ki-67 in separation of the high-grade tumors from well-differentiated carcinoids, especially in small biopsies [78].

2.4.4 Imaging

Tumor imaging, which had been previously limited to standard radiography and ultrasound, was further refined during the 1970s and 1980s. Initially, this related to the introduction of CT scanning and thereafter molecular imaging, first with somatostatin receptor (SSTR) scintigraphy and later with PET using gallium-labeled radiochemicals. CT was developed by Hounsfield (1919–2004) and Cormack (1924–1998) [79], who received the 1979 Nobel Prize. Spiral (helical CT) with multidetector (MD)-CT scanners became widely available, and the introduction of MD-CT techniques with intravenous contrast media facilitated the acquisition of contrast enhancement phases [80]. Subsequently, magnetic resonance imaging (MRI) was introduced by the chemist Lauterbur (1929–2007) and the physician Mansfield (1933–2017) who received the 2003 Nobel Prize for its development. MRI became of particular utility in the identification of metastatic disease; it has significantly improved in the last few decades, becoming especially valuable in the identification of hepatic metastatic disease. The introduction of nuclear medicine techniques using radiolabeled peptides represented a great advance in NET identification. The overexpression of SSTRs on NETs provided a significant opportunity to identify such lesions. The first radiolabeled somatostatin analogue approved for scintigraphy of NETs was indium (In)-111, DTPA-octreotide (OctreoScan), which was introduced by Krenning et al. in 1989 [81]. The next-generation somatostatin analogues, DOTATOC, DOTATATE, and DOTANOC, were developed and labeled with different radionuclides (Ga-68, yttrium [Y]-90, lutetium [Lu]-177) for imaging as well as for therapy [82, 83]. DOTATATE showed the highest affinity for SSTR2 and became the standard [84, 85]. The next developments were the third-generation somatostatin analogues, such as DOTANOC, which improved affinity for SSTR2 as well as for SSTR3 and SSTR4 [82]. To further improve molecular imaging, single-photon emission CT-PET was developed during the 1980s and 1990s. The original octreotide scans with ^{111}In were subsequently supplanted by ^{68}Gallium due to greater accuracy. The development of ^{18}F-fluorodeoxyglucose (FDG) allowed for identification of high-grade lesions based upon their glycolytic metabolic activity.

2.4.5 Therapy

Somatostatin analogues were introduced in the early 1980s for treatment of patient's NETs with clinical symptoms. In 1983, Öberg described the beneficial effects of alpha interferon in the treatment of carcinoid syndrome [86], and, 2 years later in 1986, Kvols and Moertel (1928–1994) reported on the successful control of carcinoid syndrome using octreotide [87]. Their usage as effective antiproliferative therapies has, however, proved disappointing and has resulted in the development of a variety of therapies of modest benefit (Fig. 2.7).

Initially, interferon seemed promising but has modest efficacy with often substantial adverse effects. Some of the agents utilized are nonspecific cytotoxic drugs and others have been proposed as "targeted" drugs. The efficacy of the pharmacological strategies has been modest (~30%) and is associated with substantial adverse events. Cytotoxic agents (capecitabine, temozolomide, streptozotocin, etc.) are nonspecific, and the target (mammalian target of rapamycin (mTOR)) of the "targeted" agents (everolimus) is putative and is not identified prior to therapy. More recently, the adoption of PRRT has evoked considerable enthusiasm since the target of the isotopic radiation can be identified prior to the administration of therapy and the efficacy predicted using blood-based molecular strategies.

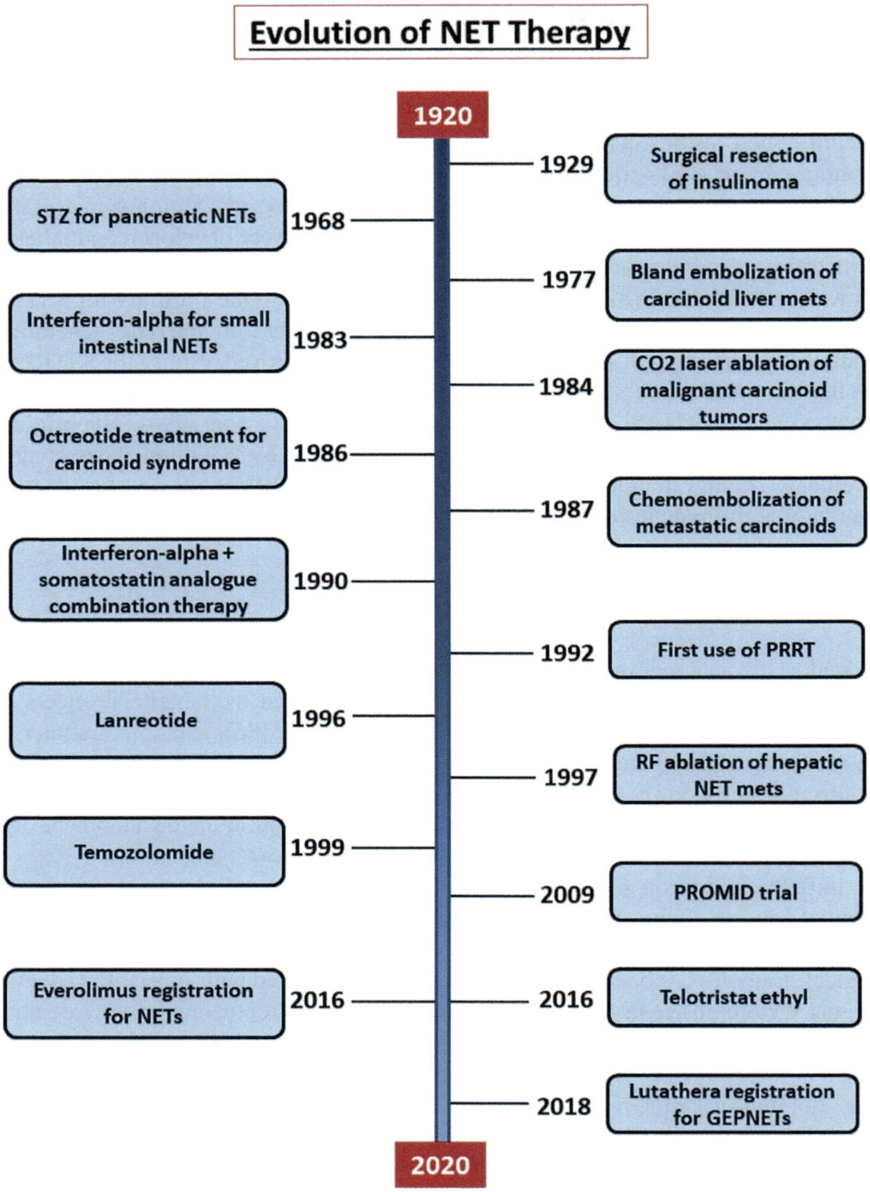

Fig. 2.7 The Introduction of NET therapy: 1929–2018. The first effective therapy was resection of a neuroendocrine tumor (insulinoma) in 1929, and the most current therapeutic advance is the registration and use of peptide radioreceptor therapy in 2018

2.5 Tumor Types, Hormonal Release, and Symptomatology

2.5.1 Bronchopulmonary Tumors

The initial descriptions of bronchopulmonary NETs date from the nineteenth century. A report by Laennec (1781–1826) in 1831 of an intrabronchial mass probably represents the first written description of a bronchial carcinoid tumor. Mueller, in 1882, had described a bronchial adenoma at autopsy, followed by Heine (in 1927) and Reisner (1928). In 1930, Kramer presciently noted that such "growths" may have malignant potential, and, shortly thereafter, Geipel (1931) described the histological basis of bronchial *Basalzellkrebs* ("bronchial adenomata") [88]. In 1937, Hamperl (1899–1976) determined that bronchial adenoma comprised of two pathological variants, a cylindroid group and "carcinoids," comprising neuroendocrine or "Kulchitsky" cells (Fig. 2.2). Thereafter, pathologists began to consider pulmonary tumors to reflect neuroendocrine cell-derived (now known as "typical" carcinoids) neoplasia as well as lesions where neuroendocrine cells were a component of the tumor, e.g., oat cell carcinomas (current terminology, "small cell lung cancer").

In 1968, Bensch et al. recognized that oat cell carcinoma and carcinoid tumors were histogenetically related [89]. Four years later, in 1972, Arrigoni et al. from the Mayo Clinic noted that although "carcinoids" generally have a good prognosis, some metastasized and progressed to systemic spread with eventual death [90]. This led to the description of the so-called "atypical" carcinoids. Ten years later, Mills described a group of atypical carcinoids (ACs), which more closely resembled small cell lung cancer [91]. DeLellis in 1984 [92] noted that bronchopulmonary carcinoids closely resembled the "benign" carcinoid lesions of the small intestine initially described by Oberndorfer in 1907 [28]. These observations have formed the basis for the concept of a spectrum of bronchopulmonary lesions. There is now common acceptance that typical (well-differentiated) carcinoids represent one end of the neoplastic spectrum and the typical small cell (oat cell) carcinoma (small cell lung cancer) the other end [78].

2.5.2 Gastrinoma (Zollinger–Ellison Syndrome)

On April 29, 1955, the US surgeons Zollinger (1903–1992) and Ellison (1918–1970) presented the case histories of two females with extremely severe peptic ulcer disease and associated pancreatic (neuroendocrine) tumors to the American Surgical Association in Philadelphia (Fig. 2.2) [46]. They postulated that these tumors produced an ulcerogenic humoral factor but erroneously speculated that this was glucagon [46]. Despite the fact that from 1946 to 1952, at least six different reports described patients with peptic ulcer disease, acid hypersecretion, and NETs of the pancreas [93–99], the eponym remained. Zollinger was of the opinion that the secretagogue responsible for the peptic ulceration and diarrhea was secretin. However, in 1967, the British physiologist Gregory (1913–1990) and coworkers extracted gastrin from a pancreatic NET [51], and, thereafter, the tumor was recognized as a gastrinoma.

2.5.3 Insulinoma

Pancreatic islet cells were first described by Langerhans (1847–1888) in 1869 while undertaking his doctorate studies as a medical student [100]. At that time, Langerhans could only speculate on their function. In 1902, Nicholls (1870–) first described a tumor—which he named "adenoma"—as originating from the pancreatic islets [101]. In 1922, Macleod (1876–1935), Banting (1891–1941), and the medical student Best (1899–1978) isolated insulin from an extract of a dog's pancreas [102, 103]. In reality, however, Paulescu (1869–1931) had identified insulin earlier but was never credited for this [104]. In 1924, Harris (1870–1957), after visiting Banting and having observed the clinical effects of insulin overdosing, was the first to identify a case of endogenous hyperinsulinism [105, 106]. In 1926, Mayo (1861–1939) performed an exploratory laparotomy on a 39-year-old orthopedic surgeon suffering from recurrent severe hypoglycemia and found an unresectable pancreatic tumor with multiple liver, lymph node, and mesenteric metastases [107].

In 1927, Wilder (1885–1959) et al. reported on the necropsy of this patient (Fig. 2.2). Extracts of a liver metastasis produced marked lowering of blood glucose levels when injected into rabbits. It seems likely that Mayo's and Wilder's patient had multiple endocrine neoplasia type 1 (MEN-1) since he also had renal stones and his cousin had had similar symptoms and died 6 years earlier [108]. In 1954, Wermer (1898–1975) reported disorders of one or more endocrine glands in five members of one family in 1954. This familial syndrome was once called Wermer syndrome but is nowadays better known as MEN-1 [109]. In 1929, the first cure of hyperinsulinism by removal of an insulinoma was undertaken by the surgeon Graham (1890–1948) and reported by his colleague, the occupational therapist Howland (1875–1950) and coworkers [110, 111]. In 1939, it was reported that this patient was still disease-free [112]. The US surgeon Whipple (1881–1963) and the pathologist Frantz (1896–1967) identified the diagnostic hallmark of insulinoma called Whipple's triad: (1) symptoms known or likely to be caused by hypoglycemia, (2) a low plasma glucose measured at the time of the symptoms, and (3) relief of symptoms when the glucose is raised to normal [113].

2.5.4 Glucagonoma

In 1923, a hyperglycemic factor named glucagon was isolated by the physiologists Kimball and Murlin (1874–1960) [114–116]. Almost two decades later, in 1942, the dermatologist Becker (1894–1964) described the typical glucagonoma skin eruption in a patient with a pancreatic tumor [117]. The relationship between glucagon and the tumor was confirmed in 1963 by Unger (1924–) who recovered glucagon from extracts of pancreatic NETs found at autopsy [118]. In 1966, McGavran (1923–1999), a pathologist, published the first report on a patient with a glucagonoma. This 42-year-old woman presented with diabetes mellitus, anemia, an unusual skin eruption, and a metastatic pancreatic tumor. Subsequently elevated plasma glucagon levels were noted, and the tumor was resected by Polk Jr. [119].

The characteristic cutaneous lesion, which occurs in association with glucagonoma syndrome, was first described by the dermatologist Church in 1967 (1922–2007) [120]. The dermatologist Wilkinson (1919–2009) named this lesion "necrolytic migratory erythema" in 1971 [121].

2.5.5 VIPoma

In 1958, the pathologist Morrison (1922–2008) and the physician Verner Jr. first described the watery diarrhea syndrome in association with islet cell tumors identified on laparotomy or autopsy [48] that had also been known as pancreatic cholera (Fig. 2.2). Apart from the chronic, profuse, watery diarrhea, this syndrome is also accompanied by achlorhydria, hyperglycemia, and episodic flushing and became known as the watery diarrhea, hypokalemia, and achlorhydria (WDHA) syndrome [48]. More than a decade later, in 1970, vasoactive intestinal peptide (VIP) was isolated from pig upper small intestine by the physician Said (1928–2013) and the biochemist Mutt (1923–1998) [122]. Evidence that VIP is the mediator of the watery diarrhea syndrome was produced by the British physicians Bloom (1942–), Julia Polak, and Anthony Pearse in 1973 [123]. Medical management of the tumor was reported by Oberg in 1985 using alpha interferon, and, in the same year, Maton described the beneficial effects of octreotide [124, 125].

2.5.6 CCK-oma

In 1928, Ivy (1893–1978) and Oldberg (1901–1986) found evidence of a gallbladder-emptying hormone in extracts of the small intestine and referred to it as cholecystokinin (CCK) [126]. In 1943, Raper (1882–1951) discovered a stimulator of pancreatic enzyme secretion in small intestinal extracts and named it pancreozymin [127]. In the 1960s, Jorpes (1894–1973) and Mutt (1923–1998) recognized that CCK and pancreozymin are the same substance [128, 129]. In 2013, Rehfeld described a syndrome characterized by non-watery diarrhea, severe weight loss, and gallbladder and peptic ulcer disease, which they named the CCK-oma syndrome [130].

2.5.7 Somatostatinoma

In 1977, Larsson and Jens Rehfeld and Ganda reported the first two cases of pancreatic somatostatinoma [131–133]. In 1979, a full description of the somatostatinoma syndrome caused by a periampullary tumor was reported by the Austrian gastroenterologist Krejs et al. (1945–) [134]. Somatostatinomas generally arise from the pancreas or the periampullary region in the duodenum. They are associated with diabetes mellitus, cholelithiasis, weight loss, steatorrhea and diarrhea, hypochlorhydria, or achlorhydria.

2.5.8 Genetic Tumor Syndromes

Although most NETs are sporadic, multiple inherited syndromes associated with NETs exist, including multiple endocrine neoplasia (MEN) types 1 and 2, von Hippel–Lindau (VHL) disease, neurofibromatosis 1 (NF1), and tuberous sclerosis.

2.5.8.1 Wermer (MEN-1) Syndrome

MEN-1 In 1903, Erdheim (1874–1937) was the first to describe a patient with tumors in two different endocrine organs (pituitary and parathyroid tumors). In 1953, Underdahl published eight cases featuring tumors in the pituitary, parathyroids, and pancreatic islets. In 1954, Wermer was the first to report that the cases reported by Underdahl and colleagues must be genetic disorders with autosomal dominant inheritance (MEN-1) (Wermer syndrome). It was not until 1988 that Larsson and fellow researchers at Uppsala University Hospital and the Karolinska Institute in Stockholm mapped the *MEN1* gene to the long arm of chromosome 11 (11q13). Finally, in 1997, a group at the National Institutes of Health isolated the *menin* gene, a tumor suppressor. Functionally, *menin* is linked to more than a hundred different signaling pathways, including epigenetic remodeling. Phenocopy reduction results in abrogation in vital cell activities, including transcriptional regulation, cell division, cell proliferation, and genome stability.

2.5.8.2 Sipple (MEN-2A) Syndrome

In 1959, Sipple (1930–) reported on an association between carcinoma of the thyroid and pheochromocytoma. MEN-2A is an autosomal dominant disease resulting in pheochromocytoma, medullary carcinoma of the thyroid, and parathyroid adenomas. In 1987, the causative gene was mapped to chromosome 10, the receptor tyrosine kinase gene protooncogene, which is involved in the transforming growth factor beta (TGF-beta) signaling system. Typically, a rearranged during transfection (RET) mutation results in a gain-of-function genotype affecting the neural tissue. A variant of MEN-2A was described in 1989. This variant also has patches of cutaneous amyloidosis in the mid/upper back. RET mutations are uncommon in NETs.

2.5.8.3 Other Genetic Syndromes

VHL

In 1904, von Hippel (1867–1939) first described retinal angiomas, and, in 1927, Lindau (1892–1958) described hemangiomas of the central nervous system. VHL disease includes hemangioblastomas, clear cell renal carcinoma, pancreatic NETs, pheochromocytomas, and endolymphatic sac tumors of the middle ears. The *VHL* gene is a tumor suppressor gene located on chromosome 3p (mapped in 1988, sequenced in 1993). The protein encoded by the gene is a component of the protein complex that is involved in the ubiquitination and degradation of the hypoxia-inducible factor (HIF), which is a transcription factor that plays a central role in the regulation of gene expression by oxygen. Loss of function results in abnormalities in angiogenesis and the development of lesions that require less oxygen to grow.

NF1

In 1882, von Recklinghausen (1833–1910) first described a syndrome characterized by neurofibromas, pheochromocytomas, and periampullary somatostatinomas. The *NF1* gene, which encodes for neurofibrin, is located on chromosome 17q11.2. It was mapped to chromosome 17 in 1987 and subsequently sequenced in 1990. It functions as a GTPase-activating protein that negatively regulates the RAS/mitogen-activated protein kinase (MAPK) pathway activity. There are currently five isoforms. *M*utations in *NF1* can alter cellular growth control and neural development, resulting in the development of cutaneous neurofibromas, café au lait pigment spots, plexiform neurofibromas, skeletal defects, and optic nerve gliomas.

TSC (Tuberous Sclerosis Complex)

Tuberous sclerosis complex (TSC) is a multisystem autosomal dominant disease initially described by Bourneville (1840–1909) (in 1880) that includes pancreatic NETs. TSC is a rare inherited autosomal dominant syndrome caused by mutations in two tumor suppressor genes, *TSC1* mapped to chromosome 9q34 and *TSC2* mapped to chromosome 16p13.3, encoding for the proteins hamartin and tuberin, respectively. The complex regulates both cell growth and proliferation.

2.6 CODA

It has been almost 150 years since Heidenhain and Kulchitsky identified chromaffin cells and initiated the cellular basis for understanding the endocrine system. Feyrter provided a unifying concept of a diffuse neuroendocrine network, while Pavlov, Starling, and Bayliss enunciated its functional and regulatory basis. Gosset and Masson identified the neoplastic potential of the cells, and Oberndorfer recognized the prototypical tumors in his seminal pathological description of carcinoid disease. Thereafter, the peptides and amines based on the syndromic aspects of neuroendocrine disease were identified for individual tumors of the pancreas, small bowel, and lungs. Berson developed a radioimmunoassay, and this technique allowed diagnostic measurements of CgA, serotonin, and other implicated bioactive agents. Identification of the somatostatin receptor system led to the development of symptom-controlling agents and thereafter isotope linkage initially enabled tumor visualization (OctreoScan) and then therapeutic applications of yttrium and lutetium (PRRT) by Krenning. Surgical resection was pioneered by Wilder (insulinoma) and reached its apogee (sic) with the application of the Whipple technique. Specific therapeutic agents exemplified by everolimus have remained disappointing and toxic, and no effective agents have been identified to date. Recent advances in molecular identification of tumors by Scarpa, identification of the molecular circulosome of neuroendocrine neoplasia by Modlin and Kidd, and identification of key oncogenic dependencies by Califano have provided novel advances that may initiate the next chapter in the history of neuroendocrine tumor disease. In a century, the field has progressed from proliferating cells with unclear functions and ill-understood secretory products to tumors whose molecular biology and genomic regulation is becoming apparent.

References

1. Schiefferdecker P (1905) İber die Neuronen und die innere Sekretion. Sitzgsber Niedderrhein Ges Naturheilkd, pp 46–54
2. Tigerstedt R, Bergman P (1898) Niere und Kreislauf, skandinav. Arch Phys Ther 8:223–271
3. Cannon WB (1914) The emergency function of the adrenal medulla in pain and the major emotions. Am J Physiol 33(2):356–372
4. Elliott TR (1907) The innervation of the bladder and urethra. J Physiol 35(5-6):367–445
5. Loewi O (1921) Über humorale übertragbarkeit der Herznervenwirkung. Arch Eur J Physiol 189(1):239–242
6. Feyrter F (1938) Über diffuse endokrine epitheliale Organe. Zbl Inn Med 545:561
7. Frilling A, Modlin I, Kidd M, Russell C, Breitenstein S, Salem R et al (2014) Recommendations for management of patients with neuroendocrine liver metastases. Lancet Oncol 15(1):8–21
8. Nicolas A (1891) Recherches sur l'épithélium de l'intestin grêle. Intern Monatssch Anat Physiol 8:1
9. Schmidt JE (1905) Beiträge zur normalen und pathologischen Histologie einiger Zellarten der Schleimhaut des tnenschlichen Darmkanales. Arch Mikrosk Anat 66(1):12–40
10. Ciaccio C (1906) Ricerche istologiche e citologiche sul timo degli Uccelli. Anat Anz 29(597-600):32
11. Ciaccio C (1906) Sur une nouvelle espèce cellulaire dans les glandes de Lieberkühn. C R Soc Biol 1:76
12. Feyrter F (1934) Karzinoid und Karzinom. Ergebn Allg Pathol Anat 29:305–489
13. Masson P (1914) La glande endocrine de l'intestin chez l'homme. C R Acad Sci 158:59–61
14. Modlin IM, Kidd M, Latich I, Zikusoka MN, Shapiro MD (2005) Current status of gastrointestinal carcinoids. Gastroenterology 128(6):1717–1751
15. Modlin IM, Kidd M, Pfragner R, Eick GN, Champaneria MC (2006) The functional characterization of normal and neoplastic human enterochromaffin cells. J Clin Endocrinol Metabol 91(6):2340–2348
16. Capella C, Polak JM, Timson CM, Frigerio B, Solcia E (1980) Gastric carcinoids of argyrophil ECL cells. Ultrastruct Pathol 1(3):411–418
17. Håkanson R, Sundler F (1979) APUD cells in rat oxyntic mucosa. Gastroenterology 77(4):800–803
18. Masson P (1924) Appendicite neurogène et carcinoides. Ann d'Anat Pathol 1:1–59
19. Heidenhain R (1870) Untersuchungen über den Bau der Labdrüsen. Arch Mikrosk Anat 6(1):368–406
20. Kulchitsky N, Anat AM (1897) Zur Frage über den bau des Darmkanals. Arch Mikroskop Anat 49:7–35
21. Gosset A (1914) Tumeurs endocrines de l'appendice. Presse Med 22:37–40
22. Masson P (1928) Carcinoids (argentaffin-cell tumors) and nerve hyperplasia of the appendicular mucosa. Am J Pathol 4(3):181
23. Erös G (1932) Eine neue Darstellungsmethode der sogenannten "gelben" argentaffinen Zellen des Magendarmtraktes. Zbl Allg Path Anat 54:385–391
24. Erös G (1931) Über die Bedeutung der argentaffinen Zellen. Frankf Z Pathol 40:155
25. Erös G (1928) Über die argentaffinen Zellen der Schleimhaut des Magen-und Darmtraktes. Frankf Z Pathol 36:2
26. Kahlau G (1932) Versuche zur Beeinflussung der "gelben Zellen" des Darmes durch Hormone. Res Exp Med 80(1):190–205
27. O'Connor DT, Bernstein KN (1984) Radioimmunoassay of chromogranin a in plasma as a measure of exocytotic sympathoadrenal activity in normal subjects and patients with pheochromocytoma. N Engl J Med 311(12):764–770
28. Oberndorfer S (1907) Karzinoide Tumoren des Dünndarms. Frankf Z Pathol 1:426–432

29. Dawson AB (1948) Argentophile and argentaffin cells in the gastric mucosa of the rat. Anat Rec 100(3):319–329
30. Rapport MM, Green AA, Page IH (1948) Partial purification of the vasoconstrictor in beef serum. J Biol Chem 174(2):735–741
31. Lembeck F (1953) 5-Hydroxytryptamine in a carcinoid tumour. Nature 172(4385): 910–911
32. Biörck G, Axén O, Thorson Å (1952) Unusual cyanosis in a boy with congenital pulmonary stenosis and tricuspid insufficiency. Fatal outcome after angiocardiography. Am Heart J 44(1):143–148
33. Pernow B, Waldenström J (1954) Paroxysmal flushing and other symptoms caused by 5-hydroxytryptamine and histamine in patients with malignant tumours. Lancet 264(6845):951
34. Oates J, Melmon Albert Sjoerdsma K, Gillespie L, Mason D (1964) Release of a kinin peptide in the carcinoid syndrome. Lancet 283(7332):514–517
35. Norheim I, Theodorsson-Norheim E, Brodin E, Oberg K (1986) Tachykinins in carcinoid tumors: their use as a tumor marker and possible role in the carcinoid flush. J Clin Endocrinol Metabol 63(3):605–612
36. Haverback BJ, Sjoerdsma A, Terry LL (1956) Urinary excretion of the serotonin metabolite, 5-hydroxyindoleacetic acid, in various clinical conditions. N Engl J Med 255(6):270–272
37. Postma C (1927) Een geval van haemangioma planum extensum. Ned Tijdschr Geneeskd 71:1842–1846
38. Snapper I (1961) Connection between postma's "Haemangioma Planum Extensum" and carcinoid syndrome. JAMA 175(9):811–812
39. Scholte AJ (1931) Ein fall von angioma teleangiectaticum cutis mit chronischer endocarditis und malignem dünndarmcarcinoid. Beitr Pathol Anat 86:440–443
40. Cassidy MA (1931) Post-mortem findings in case shown on October 10, 1930, as one of abdominal carcinomatosis with probable adrenal involvement. Proc R Soc Med 24(7):920–921
41. Cassidy MA (1930) Abdominal carcinomatosis, with probable adrenal involvement. Proc R Soc Med 24(2):139–141
42. Thorson Å, Biörck G, Björkman G, Waldenström J (1954) Malignant carcinoid of the small intestine with metastases to the liver, valvular disease of the right side of the heart (pulmonary stenosis and tricuspid regurgitation without septal defects), peripheral vasomotor symptoms, broncho-constriction, and an unusual type of cyanosis: a clinical and pathologic syndrome. Am Heart J 47(6):795–817
43. Hutcheson JD, Setola V, Roth BL, Merryman WD (2011) Serotonin receptors and heart valve disease—it was meant 2B. Pharmacol Ther 132(2):146–157
44. Goble AJ, Hay DR, Sandler M (1955) 5-hydroxytryptamine metabolism in acquired heart-disease associated with argentaffin carcinoma. Lancet 266(6898):1016–1017
45. Eiseman B, Maynard RM (1956) A non-insulin producing islet cell adenoma associated with progressive peptic ulceration (the Zollinger-Ellison syndrome). Gastroenterology 31(3):296–304
46. Zollinger RM, Ellison EH (1955) Primary peptic ulcerations of the jejunum associated with islet cell tumors of the pancreas. Ann Surg 142(4):709–728
47. Becker ER (1942) The Iowa academy of science. Science 95(2478):651–652
48. Verner JV, Morrison AB (1958) Islet cell tumor and a syndrome of refractory watery diarrhea and hypokalemia. Am J Med 25(3):374–380
49. McGuigan JE, Trudeau WL (1968) Immunochemical measurement of elevated levels of gastrin in the serum of patients with pancreatic tumors of the Zollinger-Ellison variety. N Engl J Med 278(24):1308–1313
50. Komarov SA (1942) Studies on gastrin. I. Method of isolation of a specific gastric secretagogue from the pyloric mucous membrane and its properties. Rev Can Biol 1:191–205
51. Gregory RA, Grossman MI, Tracy H, Bentley PH (1967) Nature of the gastric secretagogue in Zollinger-Ellison tumours. Lancet 290(7515):543–544

52. Sakula A (1988) Paul Langerhans (1847-1888): a centenary tribute. J R Soc Med 81(7):414–415
53. Ambros V (2004) The functions of animal microRNAs. Nature 431(7006):350–355
54. Krulich L, Dhariwal APS, McCann SM (1968) Stimulatory and inhibitory effects of purified hypothalamic extracts on growth hormone release from rat pituitary in vitro. Endocrinology 83(4):783–790
55. Brazeau P, Vale W, Burgus R, Ling N, Butcher M, Rivier J et al (1973) Hypothalamic polypeptide that inhibits the secretion of immunoreactive pituitary growth hormone. Science 179(4068):77–79
56. Vale W, Rivier J, Ling N, Brown M (1978) Biologic and immunologic activities and applications of somatostatin analogs. Metabolism 27(9):1391–1401
57. Bauer W, Briner U, Doepfner W, Haller R, Huguenin R, Marbach P et al (1982) SMS 201–995: a very potent and selective octapeptide analogue of somatostatin with prolonged action. Life Sci 31(11):1133–1140
58. Rubin J, Ajani J, Schirmer W, Venook AP, Bukowski R, Pommier R et al (1999) Octreotide acetate long-acting formulation versus open-label subcutaneous octreotide acetate in malignant carcinoid syndrome. J Clin Oncol 17(2):600–606
59. O'Dorisio TM, Anthony LB (2015) A 25-year experience of gastroenteropancreatic neuroendocrine tumors and somatostatin (congeners) analogs: from symptom control to antineoplastic therapy. Front Horm Res 44:177–192
60. Reubi JC, Krenning E, Lamberts SWJ, Kvols L (1992) In vitro detection of somatostatin receptors in human tumors. Metabolism 41(9):104–110
61. Reubi JC, Waser B, Kvols LK, Moertel C, Nagorney DM, Charboneau JW et al (1990) Detection of somatostatin receptors in surgical and percutaneous needle biopsy samples of carcinoids and islet cell carcinomas. Cancer Res 50(18):5969–5977
62. Krenning EP, Breeman WAP, Kooij PPM, Lameris JS, Bakker WH, Koper JW et al (1989) Localisation of endocrine-related tumours with radioiodinated analogue of somatostatin. Lancet 333(8632):242–244
63. Krenning EP, Kwekkeboom DJ, Reubi JC, Van Hagen PM, van Eijck CHJ, Oei HY et al (1992) 111In-octreotide scintigraphy in oncology. Metabolism 41(9):83–86
64. Bodei L, Sundin A, Kidd M, Prasad V, Modlin IM (2015) The status of neuroendocrine tumor imaging: from darkness to light? Neuroendocrinology 101(1):1–17
65. Sundin A (2012) Radiological and nuclear medicine imaging of gastroenteropancreatic neuroendocrine tumours. Best Pract Res Clin Gastroenterol 26(6):803–818
66. Krenning EP, Kooij PPM, Bakker WH, Breeman WAP, Postema PTE, Kwekkeboom DJ et al (1994) Radiotherapy with a radiolabeled somatostatin analogue, [111In-DTPA-d-Phe1]-octreotide. Ann N Y Acad Sci 733(1):496–506
67. Van Der Zwan WA, Bodei L, Mueller-Brand J, De Herder WW, Kvols LK, Kwekkeboom DJ (2015) Radionuclide therapy in neuroendocrine tumors. Eur J Endocrinol 172(1):R1–R8
68. Blaschko H, Comline RS, Schneider FH, Silver M, Smith AD (1967) Secretion of a chromaffin granule protein, chromogranin, from the adrenal gland after splanchnic stimulation. Nature 215(5096):58–59. https://doi.org/10.1038/215058a0
69. Modlin IM, Kidd M, Malczewska A, Drozdov I, Bodei L, Matar S et al (2018) The NETest: the clinical utility of multigene blood analysis in the diagnosis and management of neuroendocrine tumors. Endocrinol Metab Clin N Am 47(3):485–504. https://doi.org/10.1016/j.ecl.2018.05.002
70. Kidd M, Drozdov I, Modlin I (2015) Blood and tissue neuroendocrine tumor gene cluster analysis correlate, define hallmarks and predict disease status. Endocr Relat Cancer 22(4):561–575. https://doi.org/10.1530/ERC-15-0092. Epub 2015 Jun 2
71. Williams ED, Sandler M (1963) The classification of carcinoid tumours. Lancet 281(7275):238–239
72. Pearse A (1966) 5-Hydroxytryptophan uptake by dog thyroid 'C' cells, and its possible significance in polypeptide hormone production. Nature 211(5049):598–600

73. Pearse AG (1974) The APUD cell concept and its implications in pathology. Pathol Annu 9:27–41
74. Szijj I, Csapó Z, László FA, Kovács K (1969) Medullary cancer of the thyroid gland associated with hypercorticism. Cancer 24(1):167–173
75. Capella C, Heitz PU, Höfler H, Solcia E, Klöppel G (1995) Revised classification of neuroendocrine tumours of the lung, pancreas and gut. Virchows Arch 425(6):547–560
76. Bosman FT, Carneiro F, Hruban RH, Theise ND (2010) WHO classification of tumours of the digestive system. World Health Organization, Geneva
77. Pelosi G, Sonzogni A, Harari S, Albini A, Bresaola E, Marchiò C et al (2017) Classification of pulmonary neuroendocrine tumors: new insights. Transl Lung Cancer Res 6(5):513–529
78. Travis WD, Brambilla E, Nicholson AG, Yatabe Y, Austin JH, Beasley MB et al (2015) The 2015 World Health Organization classification of lung tumors: impact of genetic, clinical and radiologic advances since the 2004 classification. J Thorac Oncol 10(9):1243–1260. https://doi.org/10.1097/JTO.0000000000000630
79. Hounsfield GN (1973) Computerized transverse axial scanning (tomography): Part 1. Description of system. Br J Radiol 46(552):1016–1022
80. Mamdani H, Induru R, Jalal SI (2015) Novel therapies in small cell lung cancer. Transl Lung Cancer Res 4(5):533–544
81. Krenning EP, Kwekkeboom DJ, Bakker WH, Breeman WAP, Kooij PPM, Oei HY et al (1993) Somatostatin receptor scintigraphy with [111In-DTPA-d-Phe1]- and [123I-Tyr3]-octreotide: the Rotterdam experience with more than 1000 patients. Eur J Nucl Med 20(8):716–731
82. Krausz Y, Freedman N, Rubinstein R, Lavie E, Orevi M, Tshori S et al (2011) 68Ga-DOTA-NOC PET/CT imaging of neuroendocrine tumors: comparison with ^{111}In-DTPA-octreotide (OctreoScan®). Mol Imaging Biol 13(3):583–593
83. Maecke HR, Hofmann M, Haberkorn U (2005) 68Ga-labeled peptides in tumor imaging. J Nucl Med 46:172S
84. Yang J, Kan Y, Ge BH, Yuan L, Li C, Zhao W (2014) Diagnostic role of Gallium-68 DOTATOC and Gallium-68 DOTATATE PET in patients with neuroendocrine tumors: a meta-analysis. Acta Radiol 55(4):389–398
85. Velikyan I, Sundin A, Sörensen J, Lubberink M, Sandström M, Garske-Román U et al (2014) Quantitative and qualitative intrapatient comparison of 68Ga-DOTATOC and 68Ga-DOTATATE: net uptake rate for accurate quantification. J Nucl Med 55(2):204–210
86. Öberg K, Funa K, Alm G (1983) Effects of leukocyte interferon on clinical symptoms and hormone levels in patients with mid-gut carcinoid tumors and carcinoid syndrome. N Engl J Med 309(3):129–133
87. Kvols LK, Moertel CG, O'Connell MJ, Schutt AJ, Rubin J, Hahn RG (1986) Treatment of the malignant carcinoid syndrome. N Engl J Med 315(11):663–666
88. Geipel P (1931) Concerning our knowledge of benign bronchial tumors. Frankf Z Pathol 42:516
89. Bensch KG, Corrin B, Pariente R, Spencer H (1968) Oat-cell carcinoma of the lung. Its origin and relationship to bronchial carcinoid. Cancer 22(6):1163–1172
90. Arrigoni MG, Woolner LB, Bernatz PE (1972) Atypical carcinoid tumors of the lung. J Thorac Cardiovasc Surg 64(3):413–421
91. Mills SE, Cooper PH, Walker AN, Kron IL (1982) Atypical carcinoid tumor of the lung. A clinicopathologic study of 17 cases. Am J Surg Pathol 6(7):643–654
92. DeLellis RA, Dayal Y, Wolfe HJ (1984) Carcinoid tumors. Changing concepts and new perspectives. Am J Surg Pathol 8(4):295–300
93. Cunningham L, Hawe P, Evans RW (1952) Islet-celled tumour of the pancreas with unusual clinico-pathological features. BJS 39(156):319–324
94. Forty F, Barrett GM (1952) Peptic ulceration of the third part of the duodenum associated with islet-cell tumours of the pancreas. BJS 40(159):60–63
95. Janowitz HD, Crohn BB (1951) Hyperinsulinism and duodenal ulcer: a rare clinical combination. Gastroenterology 17(4):578–580
96. Howard RW (1950) Folic acid and pernicious anaemia. Br Med J 2(4675):417

97. Brown CH, Neville WE, Hazard JB (1950) Islet-cell adenoma, without hypoglycemia, causing duodenal obstruction. Surgery 27(4):616–620
98. Sailer S, Zinninger MM (1946) Massive islet cell tumor of the pancreas without hypoglycemia. Surg Gynecol Obstet 82:301–305
99. Stabile BE (1997) Gastrinoma before zollinger and ellison. Am J Surg 174(3):232–236
100. Langerhans P; Fakultät KF-W-UzBM (1869) Beiträge zur mikroskopischen Anatomie der Bauchspeicheldrüse: Buchdruckerei von Gustav Lange
101. Nicholls AG (1902) Simple adenoma of the pancreas arising from an island of Langerhans. J Med Res 8(2):385–395
102. Bliss M (2013) The discovery of insulin. University of Chicago Press, Chicago
103. Banting FG, Best CH (1922) The internal secretion of the pancreas By FG banting, MB, and CH Best, BA. J Lab Clin Med 7:465–480
104. Paulesco N (1921) Recherches sur le rôle du pancréas dans l'assimilation nutritice. Arch Int Physiol 17:85–109
105. Harris S (1933) Hyperinsulinism, a definite disease entity: etiology, pathology, symptoms, diagnosis, prognosis and treatment of spontaneous insulogenic hypoglycemia (hyperinsulinism). JAMA 101(25):1958–1965
106. Harris S (1924) Hyperinsulinism and dysinsulinism. JAMA 83(10):729–733
107. Van Heerden JA, Churchward MM (1999) Dr Dickinson Ober Wheelock—a case of sporadic insulinoma or multiple endocrine neoplasia type 1? Mayo Clin Proc 74(7):735–738
108. Wilder RM, Allan FN, Power MH, Robertson HE (1927) Carcinoma of the islands of the pancreas: hyperinsulinism and hypoglycemia. JAMA 89(5):348–355
109. Wermer P (1954) Genetic aspects of adenomatosis of endocrine glands. Am J Med 16(3):363–371
110. Howland G, Campbell WR, Maltby EJ (1929) Dysinsulinism: convulsions and coma due to islet-cell tumor of pancreas: operation and cure. Trans Am Neurol Assoc 55:551–556
111. Howland G, Campbell WR, Maltby EJ, Robinson WL (1929) Dysinsulinism: convulsions and coma due to islet cell tumor of the pancreas, with operation and cure. JAMA 93(9):674–679
112. Campbell W, Graham R, Robinson W (1939) Islet cell tumors of the pancreas. Am J Med Sci 198(4):445–454
113. Whipple AO, Frantz VK (1935) Adenoma of islet cells with hyperinsulinism: a review. Ann Surg 101(6):1299–1335
114. Foa PP, Galansino G, Pozza G (1957) Glucagon, a second pancreatic hormone. Recent Prog Horm Res 13:473–503; discussion 10
115. Unger RH (1971) Glucagon. Physiology and pathophysiology. N Engl J Med 285:443
116. Kimball CP, Murlin JR (1923) Aqueous extracts of pancreas. III. Some precipitation reactions of insulin. J Biol Chem 58:337–346
117. Becker SW, Kahn D, Rothman S (1942) Cutaneous manifestations of internal malignant tumors. JAMA Dermatol 45(6):1069–1080
118. Unger R, Eisentraut A, Lochner J (1963) Glucagon-producing tumors of the islets of Langerhans. J Clin Invest 42:987–988
119. McGavran MH, Unger RH, Recant L, Polk HC, Kilo C, Levin ME (1966) A glucagon-secreting alpha-cell carcinoma of the pancreas. N Engl J Med 274(25):1408–1413
120. And RC, Crane W (1967) A cutaneous syndrome associated with islet-cell carcinoma of the pancreas. Br J Dermatol 79(5):284–286
121. Wilkinson DS (1971) Necrolytic migratory erythema with pancreatic carcinoma. Proc R Soc Med 64(12):1197–1198
122. Said SI, Mutt V (1970) Potent peripheral and splanchnic vasodilator peptide from normal gut. Nature 225(5235):863–864
123. Bloom SR, Polak J, Pearse AGE (1973) Vasoactive intestinal peptide and watery-diarrhoea syndrome. Lancet 302(7819):14–16
124. Maton PN, O'Dorisio TM, Howe BA, McArthur KE, Howard JM, Cherner JA et al (1985) Effect of a long-acting somatostatin analogue (SMS 201–995) in a patient with pancreatic cholera. N Engl J Med 312(1):17–21

125. Öberg K, Lindström H, Alm G, Lundqvist G (1985) Successful treatment of therapy-resistant pancreatic cholera with human leucocyte interferon. Lancet 325(8431):725–727
126. Ivy AC, Oldberg E (1928) A hormone mechanism for gall-bladder contraction and evacuation. Am J Physiol 86(3):599–613
127. Harper AA, Raper HS (1943) Pancreozymin, a stimulant of the secretion of pancreatic enzymes in extracts of the small intestine. J Physiol 102(1):115–125
128. Mutt V, Jorpes JE (1968) Structure of porcine cholecystokinin-pancreozymin. Eur J Biochem 6(1):156–162
129. Jorpes E, Mutt V (1966) Cholecystokinin and pancreozymin, one single Hormone? Acta Physiol Scand 66(1-2):196–202
130. Rehfeld JF, Federspiel B, Bardram L (2013) A neuroendocrine tumor syndrome from cholecystokinin secretion. N Engl J Med 368(12):1165–1166
131. Ganda OP, Soeldner JS (1977) Somatostatinoma: follow-up studies. N Engl J Med 297(24):1352–1353
132. Ganda OP, Weir GC, Soeldner JS, Legg MA, Chick WL, Patel YC et al (1977) Somatostatinoma: a somatostatin-containing tumor of the endocrine pancreas. N Engl J Med 296(17):963–967
133. Larsson LI, Holst JJ, Kühl C, Lundqvist G, Hirsch MA, Ingemansson S et al (1977) Pancreatic somatostatinoma: clinical features and physiological implications. Lancet 309(8013):666–668
134. Krejs GJ, Orci L, Conlon JM, Ravazzola M, Davis GR, Raskin P et al (1979) Somatostatinoma syndrome. N Engl J Med 301(6):285–292

Neuroendocrine Tumors: Epidemiology 3

Eric H. Liu

3.1 Introduction

An accurate assessment of the epidemiology of neuroendocrine tumors (NETs) around the world is elusive and dynamic. Based on a history of a poor understanding of the disease and confusing nomenclature, the impact of neuroendocrine tumors on human health has only recently been better-defined, and, globally, the general conclusion is that more people are being affected by the disease. For those with experience caring for patients with neuroendocrine tumors, it is no surprise that there is an increasing trend in both their incidence and prevalence. Moreover, as more data are collected and our understanding of the disease grows, neuroendocrine cancer is emerging as a broad collection of diseases with a wide spectrum of biological behaviors that require subtle clinical appreciation to provide the best care. Epidemiological studies and accurate data will bring attention to the field so that adequate resources can be allocated to treating this once "rare" disease.

3.2 Challenges to Neuroendocrine Epidemiology

"Neuroendocrine tumor" is a relatively recent term that describes a family of malignancies that went by several names over the past century. First described by Sigfried Oberndorfer as "*karzinoide tumoren,*" for decades the dominant term was "carcinoid tumors" [1, 2]. Unfortunately, since they were relatively rare, there was a poor general understanding and many health-care professionals considered them a "benign" disease. As a result, early International Classification of Diseases (ICD)

E. H. Liu (✉)
Rocky Mountain Cancer Centers, Denver, CO, USA

U.S. Oncology, Denver, CO, USA

S. Yalcin, K. Öberg (eds.), *Neuroendocrine Tumours*,
https://doi.org/10.1007/978-3-031-56968-5_3

coding systems from the World Health Organization (WHO) used the term "carcinoids" to describe these diffuse endocrine malignancies [3, 4]. In the 1960s, as the biochemical nature of these tumors was discovered, the molecular feature "amine precursor uptake and decarboxylation" emerged as a new moniker to describe gastrointestinal (GI)/lung/pancreatic endocrine tumors as well as medullary thyroid carcinomas, melanomas, and pheochromocytomas [5, 6]. It was not until the year 2000 that WHO organized these tumors under the term "neuroendocrine" to provide an improved structure and nomenclature for pathologists [7–9]. The term "neuroendocrine" derives from the theory that these tumors originated from the embryonic neural crest. This theory was disproved, but, because they still have pathological features of neural and epithelial cells, the term "neuroendocrine" was adopted [10]. In 2004, 2010, and 2017, the terminology was updated for pancreatic neuroendocrine tumors and the term "neuroendocrine neoplasm" was added and the grading system adjusted [11–14]. These terms are now widely accepted, except for those neuroendocrine tumors that derive from the bronchopulmonary (BP) system, which still use the term "carcinoid" [15].

Given these changes in terminology and classification, comparing studies over time can be complicated, especially in different countries. Cancer registries may use different coding systems, and they may not meet the current WHO classification. The International Classification of Diseases for Oncology (ICD-O) system still contains the terms "carcinoid tumor," "APUDoma," and "oat cell carcinoma," which are essentially never used in modern clinical pathology reports but may be necessary for historical data capture [16]. Using these codes, most of the modern, robust national databases capture neuroendocrine cases. The types of studies available for review include a mixture of national registries, provincial registries, consortium databases, and single institution reports. The general epidemiology of neuroendocrine tumors has been extensively reviewed [17–21].

Large national cancer registries provide the broadest examination of neuroendocrine tumors. In the United States, the Surveillance, Epidemiology, and End Results (SEER) database is the largest and the most carefully studied in the world. Because it includes all types of cancer, it has extremely well-structured protocols and procedures for reporting. However, the most recent iteration, SEER 18, still only covers 34.6% of the US population from 1975 to 2017 [22]. In addition, up to 1986, carcinoid tumors that were considered "benign" were not reported in this database. Other national registries from Europe, Asia, and Australia have not been reported on in several years. The differences in reporting complicate the analysis over time and between countries but provide the best sense of the general trends of the disease. Regional studies may provide a more focused analysis in certain subpopulations.

Most of the data come from single-center analyses of their "experience" with neuroendocrine tumors. These reports obviously come with significant biases given the country of origin, referral patterns, data culling protocols, and analyses. However, these data still illuminate practice patterns and general distributions of diseases and their outcomes. It is also extremely important to consider that all of these reports were generally taken from registries before the age of modern neuroendocrine imaging. The rapid conversion of imaging technology from traditional cross-sectional imaging, to somatostatin receptor scintigraphy, to the most modern, widely available somatostatin positron emission tomography (PET) imaging makes some of the previous information less certain in reporting the true nature of the disease, thus likely underreporting the true stage of the disease. In addition, modern multimodal therapies will continue to change and affect survival. Thankfully, the interest in neuroendocrine tumors is increasing as evidenced by the fact that NET publications have increased by 60%, but continual study and reporting are absolutely necessary to continuing documenting trends [20].

3.3 General Trends

There are some general trends that can be seen across all neuroendocrine populations. In all reports, the incidence rate of neuroendocrine tumors has increased over the decades. Survival rates have increased with new treatments, especially somatostatin analogues. The distribution of primary neuroendocrine tumors varies greatly depending on geography and presumably genetic predisposition. Survival, as expected, was associated with the grade of the tumors and the extent of the metastases, but it also varied greatly depending on the primary type.

3.4 Trends by Geography

3.4.1 The United States

Documentation of the epidemiology of neuroendocrine tumors exists because of the availability of the Surveillance, Epidemiology, and End Results (SEER) database in the United States, which captures meaningful information about many types of cancers. It is a population-based cancer registry that collects data from major geographic areas across the country starting from 1973 [22]. Hundreds of studies have extracted data on neuroendocrine cancer from the SEER database to examine various aspects of the disease [23–27]. The most recent analyses have covered the years 1973–2014 [23, 24].

Gender differences show that women have a slightly higher risk of NETs (52.7%), and the majority are low-grade (G1 = 51%, G2 = 16%, G3/4 = 32%). A high proportion of them are metastatic (localized = 52%, regional = 20%, distant metastatic = 27%) [23]. The annual incidence of the disease has increased over sixfold from 1973 to 2012 (1.09 per 100,000 in 1973 to 6.98 per 10,000 in 2012), with the most dramatic increase in patients 65 years and older, and has been consistent across all sites, stages, and grades. Certain primary tumors saw a greater increase, especially the stomach, which saw a 15-fold increase. When analyzed by primary, the lung and small intestine had the highest incidences (lung = 1.49, small intestine = 1.05, rectum = 1.04, pancreas = 0.48, unknown primary = 0.84, all per 100,000). The estimated prevalence also increased to 171,321. The racial distribution was predominantly White (White = 79.9%, Black = 14.0%, others = 6.1%) [24]. In Whites, the primary prevalence was lung > small intestine > colon > rectum > pancreas > stomach. For Blacks, the primary prevalence was rectum > small intestine> lung > colon > pancreas > stomach. For other races: rectum> lung > pancreas > colon > small intestine > stomach.

Survival was generally long for NETs, with a median overall survival of 9.3 years [23]. It was clearly associated with grade (G1 = 16.2 years, G2 = 8.3 years, G3/4 = 10 months). By primary, the rectum and appendix had the best survivals, whereas the pancreas and lung had the worst (rectum = 24.6 years, appendix = 30 years, pancreas =3.6 years, lung = 5.5 years). In cases with metastatic disease, the small intestine had the best survival, whereas the lung and colon were the worst (small intestine = 5.83 years, lung = 6 months, colon = 4 months). Survival has increased over time, with a 21.3% reduction in the risk of death from the periods 2000–2004 to 2009–2012. Metastatic pancreatic NETs saw the biggest improvements.

In terms of treatments, surgery was common (57.2%), but external beam radiation (7.5%) and chemotherapy (15%) were not. Patients who underwent surgery had the best median survival (52 months) [24].

An interesting study examined neuroendocrine epidemiology based on US commercial insurance claims [28]. It confirmed that even in patients not included in the SEER database, the incidence was increasing and that women had a slightly higher number. One interesting observation was that in the commercial database, the incidence rate was between 65 and 124% greater than what was reported in the SEER database.

3.4.2 Europe

The types of epidemiological reporting that describe neuroendocrine tumors in Europe vary greatly. Ranging from national registries to single institutional reviews, it is difficult to make general observations. Overall, there is also an increasing incidence rate and improved survival [29–31]. The distribution of primaries varies depending on the country. In Norway, Sweden, United Kingdom, and France, the most common NETs were appendiceal and small intestinal (SI) [32–34]. In Italy and Spain, it was lung NETs [30, 35]. In Switzerland, it was colorectal NETs, and in The Netherlands, it was appendiceal and lung NETs [36, 37]. For small intestinal NETs, the incidence, while highest in Norway (1.01 per 100,000) and Sweden (0.7 per 100,000), was still somewhat lower than in the United States at 1.05 per 100,000. The 5-year survival of SI NETs ranges from 55 to 64%, with better survival in northern and western Europe [38]. However, those data were extracted from 1985 to 1994, prior to the creation of professional societies and centers of excellence in Europe. A population study from the UK found that 21.2% of their cases were "small cell tumors" but that survival had not improved from 1986 to 2001 [39].

In a study of multiple cancer registries across Europe, covering the period 1985–1994, the overall 5-year survival was 47.5%, with 58.1% for well-differentiated and only 8.1% for poorly differentiated disease [38]. There was also a geographical difference, with survival rates of 60.3% in northern Europe, 53.6% in western Europe, 42.5% in UK, and only 37.6% in eastern Europe. However, this was during a period before the creation of neuroendocrine centers of excellence.

An analysis of the RARECARE database, which includes 76 population-based cancer registries from 1978 to 2002, found that the overall incidence in Europe for NETs was 2.5 per 100,000 [40]. The overall 5-year survival was 50%. The primary distribution sites were the small intestine (18%), thyroid (8.6%), pancreas (8.0%), colon (7.0%), stomach (6.9%), appendix (5.5%), and rectum (5.3%). In 2008, an estimated 100,000 people were living with neuroendocrine tumors. The relative overall 5-year survival for pancreatic and nonfunctioning digestive neuroendocrine tumors was 64%. Still, the best survival rates were observed for appendiceal and thyroid cancers.

For metastatic neuroendocrine disease in Sweden, 23% of cases had distant metastatic disease, with the liver as the most common site of metastases. Bone was commonly a metastatic site for rectal NETs (27%). In 41% of small intestinal cases, the disease was already metastatic. These data were collected prior to the wide use of somatostatin receptor PET imaging, so it may be a general underestimation of the true nature of the disease.

Certain NET types are clearly increasing, supporting the overall rise in the disease. A study of the Netherlands cancer registry reports that there are more cases of pancreatic neuroendocrine tumors, especially nonfunctional ones, in older people. The metastatic rate was 44–53%, and the 5-year survival rate was 53%. Surgery was the best treatment even in the setting of metastatic disease, followed by peptide receptor radionuclide therapy (PRRT) [41, 42].

The most complete analysis comes from Norway, where all cases from 1993 to 2015 were analyzed. In their database, the 5-year survival rate was 64.8%, with females having a higher survival rate than males. The incidence rate had increased from 2.35 per 100,000 from 1993 to 1997 to 4.06 per 10,000 from 2000 to 2004. Survival had also improved significantly over time, regardless of gender, age, and tumor stage [31].

A French study from the Digestive Cancer Registry of Burgundy identified 229 cases from 1976 to 1999 with increasing incidences over time (0.76 for men, 0.50 for women), although still rare (0.8% in men and 1.1% in women of all digestive cancers). The primary sites were the small intestine (38.9%), colon (27.1%), pancreas (20.5%), and stomach (6.1%). Surgery was performed in 74.1% of cases. Metastases were common, with 20.1% having regional lymph node disease and 53.3% having distant metastases. The overall 5-year survival rate was 42.7%.

A German neuroendocrine registry found the most common gastroenteropancreatic (GEP) NETs were those of the pancreas (34.2%), midgut (5.8%), stomach (6.5%), bowel (6.9%), and duodenum (4.8%). Metastatic disease was found in 46% and functional tumors in 46.7%. The most common treatment was surgery (78%), somatostatin analogues (28%), and PRRT (19%). The 5-year survival rate was approximately 85% but was highly correlated with grade [43].

In Spain, several careful analyses have been performed, providing a more detailed description of the disease at different levels. For the national registry, there was a general twofold increase in the diagnosis rate [30]. Here, only 42% were female with a mean age of 62 years at diagnosis [30]. Well-differentiated disease was 47%, whereas poorly differentiated was 43%. Metastatic disease occurred in 43%. The most common primary site was the lung. Interestingly, the average cost per year for treatment was Euros (€), with most expenses being a major surgery: pancreatic resection, intestinal surgery, cholecystectomy, hepatic resection, and splenectomy. Chemotherapy cost was much lower.

In a subgroup of just digestive neuroendocrine tumors, small intestinal tumors were the most common (55%), followed by pancreatic nonfunctional tumors (20%) [29]. Metastatic disease was also present in 44% of the cases. The metastatic sites included the liver (42%), distant lymph nodes (10%), peritoneum (7%), bone (5%), and lung (3%). Surgery was performed in 79% of patients, and 44% had systemic treatment, with somatostatin analogues used most frequently (29%). The overall survival was 12 years.

In a local registry study from Girona, Spain, from the eastern region near France, bronchopulmonary neuroendocrine tumors were the most common with small cell lung carcinoma being the most frequent. Low-grade neuroendocrine tumors of the lung were only 0.32 per 100,000, and GEP NETs were 1.07 per 100,000.

3.4.3 Asia/Australia

The same trends can be seen in Asia and Australia but with different distributions of primary tumors. In Australia, there was an increase in the annual incidence of neuroendocrine tumors from 1.7 in 1980–1989 to 3.3 in 2000–2006 [44]. The common sites were the lung (25.9%), large bowel (23.3%) (40.9% were the appendix), small intestine (20.6%), unknown primary (15.0%), pancreas (6.5%), and stomach (3.7%). The 5-year rate survival was 68.5%.

For East Asian nations, the disease distribution was quite different. A detailed analysis from the Taiwan nationwide cancer registry showed that 62% of the cases were males and that the incidence rate had increased from 0.3 per 100,000 in 1996 to 1.51 per 10,000 in 2008. The most common site was the rectum (25.4%), lung (20%), and stomach (7.4%). In this population, the small intestine only accounted for 5.3% and the pancreas only 6%. The 5-year overall survival was 50.4%, which was higher in women. This study highlights and compares the differences in primary distribution among northern Europeans and White Americans (small intestine and lung), Black Americans (rectum and small intestine), and US Asian-Pacific Islanders (rectum and lung) [33, 45].

A Japanese study gathered data by sending out surveys to major medical centers about GEP NETs only. With two studies, one in 2005 and another in 2010, they were able to assess the change at two time points [46–48]. There was a 20% increase in the patients treated with pancreatic NETs, with a prevalence of 2.69 per 100,000 and an incidence of 1.27 per 100,000, with two-thirds nonfunctional. Insulinoma was the most common at 20.9%. In all, 20% presented with metastatic disease. For GI NETs, there was an 80% increase over 5 years. The prevalence was 6.42 per 100,000. As in other Asian studies, the highest prevalence rates were for hindgut tumors (4.52 per 100,000), then foregut (1.67 per 100,000), and lastly midgut (0.23 per 100,000). The incidence of GI NETs was 3.51 per 100,000.

A Korean study pooled the pathology reports from the major university and general hospitals in Korea from 2000 to 2009 [49]. They specifically looked at GET NETs and found them to be a rare cancer, with more cases in men. However, the incidence increased linearly from 2000 to 2009. The majority of cases were rectal (48%), followed by stomach (14.6%), pancreatic (8.7%), small intestinal (7.7%), and appendiceal (2.5%). These findings are similar to those of a single institutional study in which the rectum was the most common primary site (79.8%) with the duodenum (5.6%), pancreas (4.8%), stomach (3.2%), and appendix (0.8%) much farther behind. There were no cases of small intestinal neuroendocrine tumors. At another Korean institution, hindgut NETs were the most common (38.3%), followed by pancreatic (16.2%) and foregut NETs (13.5%) [50]. In this study, the 5-year disease-free survival (DFS) rate was 72.4%, 75.9%, and 93.9% for pancreatic, GI, and pulmonary NETs. The recurrence rate was 20.9% in pancreatic NETs, 11.9% in Gl NETs, and 2.9% in pulmonary NETs.

Another single institutional study out of South China found that GEP NETs were quite uncommon, with only 178 cases in 17 years, mostly in men (60.7%) [51]. The pancreas was the most common site of involvement (34.8%), followed by the rectum (20.2%), stomach (14%), and duodenum (7.3%). There were only four cases from the small intestine and six from the appendix. The mean overall survival for pancreatic NETs was 11.1 years and that of GI NETs was 6.7 years. Another single institutional study from Zhengzhou, central China, found a different distribution of primary tumors: the stomach (24.3%), rectum (24.1), pancreas (20.5%), esophagus (12.3%), duodenum (6.1%), appendix (1.8%), and small intestine (1.8%) [52].

A single institutional study from Mumbai, India, of 74 patients over 7 years focusing on GEP NETs showed a male preponderance with the primary distribution sites in the stomach (30.2%), pancreas (23.3%), and duodenum (18.9%). Metastatic disease was seen in 18.9% of the cases.

3.4.4 Other Regions

Several other single institutional studies report their experience with neuroendocrine cancer. In Brazil, a registry of 1000 patients found that the bronchopulmonary system was the most common primary site (71.6%) [53]. In Egypt, the rate of NETs was extremely low compared to those of other malignancies (0.86%) with the lung being the most common (38.5%). The incidence rate of small cell carcinoma was extremely high (68.6%) [54].

3.5 Trends by the Primary Subtype and Others

An analysis of particular organ subtypes is limited by the data reported. Most studies do not provide specific data based on primary tumors. Moreover, the parameters vary greatly based on geography and study type. We provide general observations of each subtype.

3.5.1 The Bronchopulmonary Tract

Neuroendocrine tumors of the BP tract still utilize an older pathological scheme that divides them into typical carcinoid tumors, atypical carcinoids, large cell neuroendocrine carcinoma, and small cell lung cancer. They do tend to be the most prominent in certain parts of the world, with their incidence rate ranging from 25 to 31% of all neuroendocrine tumors, especially in those countries where they show a common increase in incidence, for example, rising from 0.32 per 100,000 from 1973 to 1991 to 1.3 from 2000 to 2004 in the United States [45]. The United States, Switzerland, Australia, Norway, and Brazil saw high rates in lung neuroendocrine tumors [23, 33, 34, 44]. Some of those studies included small cell carcinoma. In the United States, Sweden, and Australia, lower-grade neuroendocrine tumors were more common in women. Survival was always associated with grade, but the 5-year survival for typical carcinoids and atypical carcinoids varied from 70 to 90%.

3.5.2 The Small Intestine

The incidence rate of small intestinal neuroendocrine tumors varies widely with geography, with the highest rates in the United States and northern Europe and the lowest in East Asia. They were the most common NETs in the UK, Sweden, and Norway, with a high incidence in the Netherlands, Switzerland, and Germany. In all the countries with prominent cases of SI NETs, there has been a consistent increase in incidence over time. The mean age of diagnosis is between 59 and 65 years of age, and the majority have some metastatic disease (58–71%). Moreover, survival has been increasing over time. In the United States, the median overall survival for local disease was 14 years, whereas distant metastatic disease was 5.83 years. For G3 and G4 NETs, the survival was only 30 months.

In Sweden, the small intestine was the most common source of NET metastases. The metastases tended to be multifocal and mostly to the liver. In all, 41% of SI NET patients had metastatic disease. In Norway, SI NET patients had the highest relative survival rate in distant disease but had among the poorest relative survival rates in localized disease.

3.5.3 The Pancreas

The incidence of pancreatic lesions is significantly increasing. Improved detection may be contributing to this fact, with the increased use of high-resolution computed tomography (CT) scans and endoscopic ultrasound. In the United States, an analysis of the SEER database from 1988 to 2009 demonstrated a 710.4% increase in pancreatic NETs <2 cm. Even small tumors had extrapancreatic extension (17.9%), nodal metastases (27.3%), and distant metastases (9.1%). Survival was associated with race (worse for Blacks and Asians) and increasing grade.

The general incidence of pancreatic neuroendocrine tumors in the United States was 0.48 per 100,000 [23]. Depending on the study, the rates of pancreatic NETs can be between 8 and 34%. Their incidence peaks between the sixth and eighth decades, and they frequently have distant spread (77–86%). Multiple endocrine neoplasia type 1 (MEN1) syndrome is associated with pancreatic NETs and contributes to the number of cases.

Survival varies greatly and is often treated by surgical resection. Survival ranged from 8.5% to 78% and depended heavily on the geographic source.

3.5.4 The Rectum

Rectal neuroendocrine tumors are the most common in certain populations, especially in East Asians and Black Americans. The incidence of rectal NETs is also increasing, presumably due to increased use of lower endoscopy. Most patients present with local disease, with extremely high survival because of the high rate of the local disease.

3.5.5 The Appendix

Like small intestinal NETs, given the fact that they both derive from the midgut embryologically, the incidence of appendiceal neuroendocrine tumors varies dramatically depending on the population. They are quite high in Europe but low in Asia. The incidence of appendiceal neuroendocrine tumors has increased over time, but some of that may be the inclusion of benign lesions in many registries. Unlike most other NETs, appendiceal NETs present at a younger age and mostly at incidental appendectomy. The rates are higher in females, presumably because of incidental appendectomy secondary to gynecological intervention.

In a study of three referral centers in England and Poland, out of 14,850 appendectomies, 1.45% had histologically confirmed appendiceal NETs. Lymph node metastases were found in 24.5% of patients at the time of right hemicolectomy, and <1% had liver metastases. The 10-year survival rate was 99%.

3.5.6 Gastric

The relative frequency of gastric neuroendocrine tumors varied greatly, again with geography. Moreover, the subtypes of gastric neuroendocrine tumors can introduce variability. They tend to be less common, though their incidence is increasing throughout the world, which may be associated with the increased use of upper endoscopy as well as the inclusion of benign lesions in cancer registries. Most patients present with local disease. As with other NETs, there is an improvement in survival.

3.5.7 Pediatrics

There is generally very little information about neuroendocrine tumors in children. An analysis of the SEER database showed 481 cases from 1973 to 2005, with most in the soft tissue, then the lung, thyroid, appendix, and colon [55]. The 5-year survival rate was the best in colorectal, appendiceal, thyroid, and lung tumors. Children <5 years of age and belonging to the Black race had the worst survival. Tumors of the appendix, lung, and thyroid had >95% 5-year survival, whereas those of the soft tissue and ovary had poor survival.

3.5.8 Brain Metastases

Brain metastases are relatively uncommon findings in neuroendocrine tumors. When they occur, they often arise from primary lung tumors (45.1%) and have true neuroendocrine carcinoma (60.8%) with Ki-67 >55% [56]. Nearly all had metastatic disease at the time of diagnosis (96.1%). Most have multiple lesions (41.2%). The median overall survival after diagnosis of brain metastases was 11 months [56].

3.6 Conclusions

It is nearly impossible to accurately describe the evolving epidemiological landscape of neuroendocrine tumors around the world. However, there are clear epidemiological trends in neuroendocrine tumors that can be seen across all geographical regions. The total numbers of cases in terms of both incidence and prevalence rates are increasing over time. The primary tumor-type distribution seems relatively consistent within but varies between geographic areas. Survival continues to be associated with the grade of the disease and total tumor burden. However, with improvements in high-sensitivity functional imaging, especially the increased use of somatostatin receptor PET imaging, there may be a shift to even more metastatic disease at the time of diagnosis and fewer unknown primaries as they may identify the source. Moreover, as the detection rates of incidental neuroendocrine adenomas increase, it will be critical to develop new methods of determining which patients

Table 3.1 Summary of important data from SEER 18 (up to 2012) [23]

Total	64,971	
Female	34,233	52.7%
Male	30,738	47.3%
G1	51.03%	
G2	16.36%	
G3	32.58%	
Local	52.43%	
Regional	20.16%	
Distant	27.41%	
Incidence		
Overall	6.98/100,000	
Age 0–15	1.75/100,000	
51–64	14.3/100,000	
>65	25.3/100,000	
Lung	1.49/100,000	
Small intestine	1.05/100,000	
Rectum	1.04/100,000	
Pancreas	0.48/100,000	
Unknown	0.84/100,000	
Overall survival		
G1	Rectum and appendix	>30 years
G3	Small intestine	30 months
G3	Appendix	33 months
Metastatic distant	Colon	14 months
Metastatic distant	Lung	24 months
Metastatic distant	Stomach	29 months
Metastatic distant	Rectum	33 months
Metastatic distant	Pancreas	60 months
Metastatic distant	Cecum	98 months
Metastatic distant	Small intestine	103 months

Survival over time (hazard ratio)			
	Overall	Small intestine	Pancreas
2000–2004	1	1	1
2005–2008	0.83	0.76	0.76
2009–2012	0.79	0.71	0.56

are at the greatest risk of disease-specific mortality. It will be most interesting to review new studies that "revisit" the epidemiology of NETs to see how major advances in diagnosis and treatments affect overall survival (Table 3.1).

References

1. Oberndorfer S (1907) Karzinoid Tumoren des Dunndarms. Frankf Z Pathol 1:426–432
2. Oberndorfer S (1928) Karzinoide Handbuch der Speziellen. In: Handbuch der Speziellen Pathologischen Anatomie und Histologie. Springer, Berlin, pp 814–847

3. Liu EH, Oberg K (2010) The history and development of the gastroenteropancreatic endocrine axis. Endocrinol Metab Clin N Am 39(4):697–711
4. Williams ED, Sandler M (1963) The classification of carcinoid tum ours. Lancet 1(7275):238–239
5. Pearse AG (1968) Common cytochemical and ultrastructural characteristics of cells producing polypeptide hormones (the APUD series) and their relevance to thyroid and ultimobranchial C cells and calcitonin. Proc R Soc Lond B Biol Sci 170(1018):71–80
6. Temple WJ, Sugarbaker EV, Ketcham AS (1981) The APUD system and its apudomas. Int Adv Surg Oncol 4:255–276
7. Capella C, Sorbin LH et al (2000) Endocrine tumours of the colon and rectum. In: Hamilton AL (ed) Pathology and genetics of tumours of the digestive system. IARC Press, Lyon, pp 137–139
8. Capella C, Sorbin LH et al (2000) Endocrine tumours of the small intestine. In: Hamilton AL (ed) Pathology and genetics of tumours of the digestive system. IARC Press, Lyon, pp 77–82
9. Capella C, Sorbin LH et al (2000) Endocrine tumours of the stomach. In: Hamilton AL (ed) Pathology and genetics of tumours of the digestive system. IARC Press, Lyon, pp 53–57
10. Klimstra DS et al (2010) The pathologic classification of neuroendocrine tumors: a review of nomenclature, grading, and staging systems. Pancreas 39(6):707–712
11. Rindi G, Bosman F et al (2010) Nomenclature and classification of digestive neuroendocrine tumours. In: Bosman FT, Hruban R et al (eds) WHO classification of tumours, pathology and genetics of tumours of the digestive system. IARC Press, Lyon, pp 10–12
12. Heitz PU, Perren A et al (2004) Pancreatic endocrine tumours: introduction. In: DeLellis LR, Heitz PU, Eng C (eds) Pathology and genetics of tumours of endocrine organs. IARC Press, Lyon, pp 177–182
13. Klimstra D, Oberg K et al (2004) Pancreatic endocrine tumours: non-functioning tumours and microadenomas. In: DeLellis LR, Heitz PU, Eng C (eds) Pathology and genetics of tumours of endocrine organs. IARC Press, Lyon, pp 201–204
14. Kloppel G, Hruban R et al (2017) Neuroendocrine neoplasms of the pancreas. In: Lloyd RV, Kloppel G et al (eds) WHO classification of tumours of endocrine organs. IARC Press, Lyon, pp 210–239
15. Brambilla E, Austin JH et al (2015) Neuroendocrine tumours. In: Travis WD, Burke AP et al (eds) WHO classification of tumours of the lung, pleura, thymus and heart. IARC Press, Lyon
16. Fritz AG (2000) International classification of diseases for oncology: ICD-O, 3rd edn. World Health Organization, Geneva, p 240
17. Fraenkel M, Faggiano A, Valk GD (2015) Epidemiology of neuroendocrine tumors. Front Horm Res 44:1–23
18. Fraenkel M et al (2014) Incidence of gastroenteropancreatic neuroendocrine tumours: a systematic review of the literature. Endocr Relat Cancer 21(3):R153–R163
19. Fraenkel M et al (2012) Epidemiology of gastroenteropancreatic neuroendocrine tumours. Best Pract Res Clin Gastroenterol 26(6):691–703
20. Huguet I, Grossman AB, O'Toole D (2017) Changes in the epidemiology of neuroendocrine tumours. Neuroendocrinology 104(2):105–111
21. Modlin IM et al (2008) Gastroenteropancreatic neuroendocrine tumours. Lancet Oncol 9(1):61–72
22. SEER Incidence Data. 1975-2017. 2020. Available from https://seer.cancer.gov/data/.
23. Dasari A et al (2017) Trends in the incidence, prevalence, and survival outcomes in patients with neuroendocrine tumors in the United States. JAMA Oncol 3(10):1335–1342
24. Man D et al (2018) Prognosis of patients with neuroendocrine tumor: a SEER database analysis. Cancer Manag Res 10:5629–5638
25. Modlin IM, Lye KD, Kidd M (2003) A 5-decade analysis of 13,715 carcinoid tumors. Cancer 97(4):934–959
26. Tsikitis VL, Wertheim BC, Guerrero MA (2012) Trends of incidence and survival of gastrointestinal neuroendocrine tumors in the United States: a seer analysis. J Cancer 3:292–302

27. Maggard MA, O'Connell JB, Ko CY (2004) Updated population-based review of carcinoid tumors. Ann Surg 240(1):117–122
28. Broder MS et al (2018) Incidence and prevalence of neuroendocrine tumors of the lung: analysis of a US commercial insurance claims database. BMC Pulm Med 18(1):135
29. Garcia-Carbonero R et al (2010) Incidence, patterns of care and prognostic factors for outcome of gastroenteropancreatic neuroendocrine tumors (GEP-NETs): results from the National Cancer Registry of Spain (RGETNE). Ann Oncol 21(9):1794–1803
30. Darba J, Marsa A (2019) Exploring the current status of neuroendocrine tumours: a population-based analysis of epidemiology, management and use of resources. BMC Cancer 19(1):1226
31. Boyar Cetinkaya R et al (2018) Survival in neuroendocrine neoplasms: a report from a large Norwegian population-based study. Int J Cancer 142(6):1139–1147
32. Ellis L, Shale MJ, Coleman MP (2010) Carcinoid tumors of the gastrointestinal tract: trends in incidence in England since 1971. Am J Gastroenterol 105(12):2563–2569
33. Hauso O et al (2008) Neuroendocrine tumor epidemiology: contrasting Norway and North America. Cancer 113(10):2655–2664
34. Hemminki K, Li X (2001) Incidence trends and risk factors of carcinoid tumors: a nationwide epidemiologic study from Sweden. Cancer 92(8):2204–2210
35. Caldarella A, Crocetti E, Paci E (2011) Distribution, incidence, and prognosis in neuroendocrine tumors: a population based study from a cancer registry. Pathol Oncol Res 17(3):759–763
36. Levi F et al (2000) Epidemiology of carcinoid neoplasms in Vaud, Switzerland, 1974-97. Br J Cancer 83(7):952–955
37. Quaedvlieg PF et al (2001) Epidemiology and survival in patients with carcinoid disease in The Netherlands. An epidemiological study with 2391 patients. Ann Oncol 12(9):1295–1300
38. Lepage C et al (2010) European disparities in malignant digestive endocrine tumours survival. Int J Cancer 126(12):2928–2934
39. Lepage C, Rachet B, Coleman MP (2007) Survival from malignant digestive endocrine tumors in England and Wales: a population-based study. Gastroenterology 132(3):899–904
40. van der Zwan JM et al (2013) Rare neuroendocrine tumours: results of the surveillance of rare cancers in Europe project. Eur J Cancer 49(11):2565–2578
41. Kuiper P et al (2010) Pathological incidence of duodenopancreatic neuroendocrine tumors in the Netherlands: a Pathologisch Anatomisch Landelijk Geautomatiseerd Archief study. Pancreas 39(8):1134–1139
42. Genc CG et al (2018) A nationwide population-based study on the survival of patients with pancreatic neuroendocrine tumors in The Netherlands. World J Surg 42(2):490–497
43. Begum N et al (2014) Neuroendocrine tumours of the GI tract–data from the German NET Registry. Zentralbl Chir 139(3):276–283
44. Luke C et al (2010) Epidemiology of neuroendocrine cancers in an Australian population. Cancer Causes Control 21(6):931–938
45. Yao JC et al (2008) One hundred years after "carcinoid": epidemiology of and prognostic factors for neuroendocrine tumors in 35,825 cases in the United States. J Clin Oncol 26(18):3063–3072
46. Ito T et al (2015) Epidemiological trends of pancreatic and gastrointestinal neuroendocrine tumors in Japan: a nationwide survey analysis. J Gastroenterol 50(1):58–64
47. Ito T et al (2010) Epidemiological study of gastroenteropancreatic neuroendocrine tumors in Japan. J Gastroenterol 45(2):234–243
48. Ito T et al (2007) Preliminary results of a Japanese nationwide survey of neuroendocrine gastrointestinal tumors. J Gastroenterol 42(6):497–500
49. Gastrointestinal Pathology Study Group of Korean Society of Pathologists (2012) Current trends of the incidence and pathological diagnosis of gastroenteropancreatic neuroendocrine tumors (GEP-NETs) in Korea 2000-2009: multicenter study. Cancer Res Treat 44(3):157–165
50. Kim SJ et al (2012) Clinical course of neuroendocrine tumors with different origins (the pancreas, gastrointestinal tract, and lung). Am J Clin Oncol 35(6):549–556

51. Wang YH et al (2012) Relationship between clinical characteristics and survival of gastroenteropancreatic neuroendocrine neoplasms: a single-institution analysis (1995-2012) in South China. BMC Endocr Disord 12:30
52. Zhang M et al (2017) Clinicopathological features and prognosis of gastroenteropancreatic neuroendocrine neoplasms in a Chinese population: a large, retrospective single-centre study. BMC Endocr Disord 17(1):39
53. Younes RN, GETNE (2008) Neuroendocrine tumors: a registry of 1000 patients. Rev Assoc Med Bras 54(4):305–307
54. Saber M et al (2018) Neuroendocrine tumors of the lung: a five-year retrospective experience of Egyptian NCI (2010-2014). J Egypt Natl Canc Inst 30(4):151–158
55. Allan B et al (2013) Malignant neuroendocrine tumors: incidence and outcomes in pediatric patients. Eur J Pediatr Surg 23(5):394–399
56. Krug S et al (2019) Brain metastases in patients with neuroendocrine neoplasms: risk factors and outcome. BMC Cancer 19(1):362

Neuroendocrine Neoplasms (NENs) in Complex Genetic Disorders

4

Wouter W. de Herder

4.1 Introduction

Neuroendocrine neoplasms (NENs) can occur either sporadically or in association with multisystem inherited genetic disorders (Table 4.1) [1, 2]. The four most common endocrine tumour syndromes are multiple endocrine neoplasia type 1 (MEN1), multiple endocrine neoplasia type 2 (MEN2a and MEN2b), von Hippel–Lindau (VHL) disease and Carney complex (CNC). Less commonly, endocrine tumours of the pancreas and adrenal glands have been observed in neurofibromatosis type 1 (NF-1) and tuberous sclerosis complex (TSC) (Table 4.1) [3–10]. This review will only focus on tumour syndromes associated with NENs of the digestive tract, pancreas, lungs and thymus.

W. W. de Herder (✉)
ENETS Center of Excellence for Neuroendocrine Tumours, Erasmus MC, Rotterdam, The Netherlands

Department of Internal Medicine, Sector of Endocrinology, Erasmus MC, Rotterdam, The Netherlands

Erasmus MC Cancer Institute, Rotterdam, The Netherlands
e-mail: w.w.deherder@erasmusmc.nl

S. Yalcin, K. Öberg (eds.), *Neuroendocrine Tumours*,
https://doi.org/10.1007/978-3-031-56968-5_4

Table 4.1 Hereditary tumour syndromes associated with neuroendocrine tumours

Name neuroendocrine tumour (NET) (frequency)
MEN1 syndrome (MEN1) (MIM 131100) pituitary adenoma (5–65%)
(Wermer syndrome) pancreatic NENs (80–100%)
Thymic carcinoid (mostly ♂) (<10%)
Lung carcinoid (20–25%)
Gastric, type 2, NENs (Zollinger Ellison syndrome (ZES)-related) (5–35%)
MEN2a syndrome (MEN2a) (MIM 171400) medullary thyroid carcinoma
(Sipple syndrome) pheochromocytoma
MEN2b syndrome (MEN2b) (MIM 162300) medullary thyroid carcinoma
Pheochromocytoma
Familiarly medullary thyroid carcinoma medullary thyroid carcinoma
(FMTC) (MIM 155240)
von Hippel–Lindau (VHL) syndrome pancreatic NENs (5–10%)
(MIM 193300) pheochromocytoma (10–20%)
Neurofibromatosis I (NF-1, MIM 162200) periampullary NENs (somatostatinoma)
Pheochromocytoma
Tuberous sclerosis (TSC, MIM 191100) pituitary adenoma??
(Bourneville's disease) pancreatic NENs?
Carney complex I (CNC1, MIM 160980) pituitary adenoma
Aryl hydrocarbon receptor-interacting protein Pituitary adenoma
(AIP) mutations (MIM 605555)
Chromosome Xq26.3 duplication syndrome acrogigantism (pituitary)
(X-LAG)
Carney–Stratakis syndrome (MIM 606864) paraganglioma
MEN4 (MEN-X) syndrome (MIM 610755) pituitary adenoma
Familial paraganglioma syndromes paraganglioma pheochromocytoma
(MIM 115310, MIM 168000, MIM 601650, MIM 605373, MIM 614165)
MAX deletions (MIM 154950) pituitary adenoma
Pheochromocytoma
Thyroid tumour
Mahvash disease/pancreatic NENs/mutant P86S glucagon receptor (GCGR) pancreatic α-cell hyperplasia
MAFA mutation (MIM 147630) insulinomatosis

4.2 MEN1

MEN1 (MIM 131100) is an autosomal dominant inherited genetic disorder characterized by hyperplasia and/or multiple adenomas of the parathyroid glands, single or multiple functional/non-functional NENs of the pancreas and/or duodenum and stomach, adenomas of the anterior pituitary, NENs of the thymus and lungs and functioning and non-functioning hyperplasia or adenomas of the adrenal cortex. Less common lesions associated with MEN1 include cutaneous lesions like angiofibroma, collagenoma, lipoma and melanoma and peripheral or central nervous system (CNS) tumours such as ependymoma and meningioma and breast cancer (in female patients) [4, 11–15].

The prevalence of MEN1 syndrome is approximately 0.002–0.02%. MEN1 should be suspected in patients with characteristic endocrine pathology in two out of the three characteristically affected organs or with a characteristic endocrine disorder in one of these organs plus a first-degree relative affected by MEN1 syndrome [13–18].

MEN1 syndrome is the result of an inactivating mutation of the MEN1 tumour suppressor localized on chromosome 11q13. The *MEN1* gene encodes for the 67-kd tumour suppressor protein menin, consisting of 610 amino acids [19, 20]. More than 300 MEN1 germline mutations have been identified thus far [21, 22]. There is yet no clearly recognizable genotype/phenotype relation between germline MEN1 mutations. Somatic MEN1 mutations have also been reported in sporadic forms of endocrine tumours with variable incidence of 20–40% in pancreatic and lung NENs [15, 23]. MEN1 patients carrying the p27 rs2066827 variant of the *p27* tumour suppressor gene are more likely to have tumours in more endocrine glands (in –two to three glands) than are those who are not gene carriers (in –one to two glands) [24]. Missense mutations involving loss of interaction with checkpoint suppressor 1 (FOXN3/CHES1) (associated with DNA repair) correlate with a more aggressive disease course of pancreatic NENs and, therefore, increased NEN-related mortality in MEN1 patients [25]. Similarly, it has been shown that MEN1 patients with mutations in the JunD interacting domain have a higher risk of MEN1-related death [26].

Clinical screening of patients remains a prerequisite of genetic analysis [13–17]. Patients with MEN1 have a shorter life expectancy than does the general population. Nowadays, this is mainly caused by MEN1-related NENs [27]. The estimated 20-year survival of MEN1 patients is 64% [13–16, 27, 28].

Gastroenteropancreatic (GEP) NENs occur in about 30–80% of MEN1 patients and are the second most frequent clinical manifestation of MEN1 [13–16, 29, 30]. Unlike sporadic GEP NENs, functional GEP NENs are frequently characterized by multiple tumours that are usually diagnosed a decade earlier than sporadic GEP NENs. About two-thirds of these tumours are clinically active (=functional) = producing one or more peptides/hormones, which can result in distinct clinical syndromes. The most common functional pancreatic NENs are insulinomas (15%) [13–16]. (Multiple) insulinomas in MEN1 patients are usually diagnosed before the age of 40—many times in association with gastrinomas—which is generally earlier than the diagnosis of sporadic insulinomas [31]. Gastrinomas represent more than half of all functional GEP NENs in MEN1. The great majority of (multiple) gastrinomas (>90%) in MEN1 patients is located in the duodenum. In MEN1 patients, these tumours can manifest with the typical symptoms of Zollinger–Ellison syndrome usually also before the age of 40 and are generally diagnosed when metastases have occurred [29, 30, 32]. Gastrinomas represent one of the major causes of morbidity and mortality in MEN1 patients and are associated with a poor prognosis [32–34]. Variants of MEN1 syndrome have been described. One of these, MEN1 Burin is characterized by a low incidence of gastrinomas (10%) [35]. Glucagonomas have also been reported in only a few MEN1 cases. Thymic NENs almost exclusively occur in male patients with MEN1. Their prevalence is between 3 and 4%, and the 10-year survival of patients with these tumours is approximately 25%.

Lung NENs = carcinoids occur in 20–25% of MEN1 patients. MEN1 patients with lung carcinoids, as compared to those with thymic carcinoids, have a much better 10-year survival (>70%) [28, 33, 36, 37].

The therapies for NENs in MEN1 patients are essentially not different from those for their sporadic counterparts. However, there are discussions as to whether gastrinoma surgery should be generally attempted in MEN1 patients [32, 38–40]. Gastric NENs in MEN1 patients almost exclusively develop in the presence of Zollinger–Ellison syndrome [41]. They are generally characterized as type 2 enterochromaffin-like (ECL)-omas or gastric carcinoids/NENs. These generally well-differentiated lesions usually show a benign clinical course [41]. Surgery for non-functioning pancreatic NENs in MEN1 patients is associated with relatively high rates (up to 33%) of major short- and long-term complications [42]. It is generally recommended that MEN1 patients with non-functioning pancreatic NENs of diameter <2 cm can be managed by watchful waiting, hereby avoiding major surgery without loss of oncological safety. The beneficial effect of a surgery in non-functioning pancreatic NENs with a diameter between 2 and 3 cm in MEN1 requires further research. In MEN1 patients with non-functioning pancreatic NENs with a diameter >3 cm, or those increasing in size, surgery is generally recommended [43–45].

Periodic screening for tumour manifestations and subsequent treatment of asymptomatic MEN1 mutation carriers can prevent complications and may lead to a more favourable course of the disease. Therefore, according to the recently published Clinical Practice Guidelines for MEN1, periodic (biochemical) radiological screening for pancreatic NENs and thymic and lung carcinoids has been recommended every 1–2 years using thoracic and abdominal computed tomography (CT) or magnetic resonance imaging (MRI) [16]. There might also be a role for ^{68}Ga-DOTATOC or ^{68}Ga-DOTATATE positron emission tomography (PET)/CT in the follow-up of MEN1 patients [46–48]. In experienced hands, endoscopic ultrasonography (EUS) appears to be the most sensitive localization technique for pancreatic NENs in MEN1 [49]. According to the current guidelines, MEN1 germline mutation testing should be offered to index patients with MEN1 and to their—many times asymptomatic—first-degree relatives from the age of 5 years [14, 50].

4.3 von Hippel–Lindau Disease

von Hippel–Lindau (VHL, MIM 193300) disease is a multisystem autosomal dominant inherited genetic disorder that may manifest with retinal angiomas, central nervous system haemangioblastomas (involving the cerebellum, spinal cord or brainstem), clear cell renal carcinoma, uni- or bilateral pheochromocytoma(s), pancreatic lesions (see later), endolymphatic sac tumours of the middle ear and papillary cystadenomas of the epididymis and broad ligament [8, 51–54]. The prevalence of VHL syndrome is approximately 0.003% [8].

The *VHL* gene is a tumour suppressor gene located on chromosome 3p25–26. The VHL protein binds to elongin C and elongin B, thereby inhibiting transcription elongation, Cul2 and Rbx1 and degrading the α-subunits of hypoxia-inducible factors (HIFs). This mechanism is influenced by oxygen. In absence of the VHL protein, lack of degradation of HIFs results in uncontrolled production of factors, like vascular endothelial growth factor (VEGF), which promote formation of new blood vessels and tumour development [8, 9]. Germline mutations in the *VHL* gene are now identifiable in virtually all VHL families [8]. *VHL* gene sequencing has been useful in VHL disease for presymptomatic diagnosis [8]. The exact molecular mechanism of development of NENs in VHL is yet unknown.

Patients with VHL may be divided into two groups, namely, type 1 and type 2, both leading to a specific phenotype. Patients with type 1 VHL do not develop pheochromocytoma(s), whereas those with type 2 disease are at a high risk of developing pheochromocytoma(s). Type 2 VHL is further divided into types 2A, 2B and 2C. Patients with type 2A VHL have a low risk of renal clear cell carcinoma in contrast with those with type 2B VHL, and patients with type 2C VHL develop pheochromocytomas only [8, 9].

Approximately 60% of VHL patients can develop pancreatic disease, including true cysts, serous cystadenomas, metastases (from renal carcinoma) and NENs (in 15%), which can also be cystic [29, 30, 55, 56]. Studies also suggest that VHL-related pancreatic NENs are mostly non-functional [57, 58]. VHL-related pancreatic NENs might be distinguished from MEN1-related NENs based on (1) the absence of duodenal tumours, (2) frequent clinically non-functional tumours and (3) frequent occurrence of cystic adenomas around the pancreatic NENs. In VHL patients, for pancreatic NENs with a diameter ≤1 cm, an annual follow-up with CT or MRI is recommended. For pancreatic NENs between 1 and 3 cm in VHL patients, a personalized approach is recommended. NENs >3 cm that are symptomatic or functional or lesions that are increasing in size should be considered for resection [59–61]. For the imaging of pancreatic NENs in VHL patients, not only CT or MRI can be used but both ^{68}Ga-DOTATOC/^{68}Ga-DOTATATE PET-CT and EUS also show high detection rates [62, 63].

4.4 Neurofibromatosis Type 1

Neurofibromatosis type 1 (NF-1), (von Recklinghausen disease, MIM 162200) is a multisystem autosomal dominant inherited genetic disorder characterized by neurofibromas, multiple cafe-au-lait spots, axillary and inguinal freckling, iris haematomas (Lisch nodules), skeletal abnormalities, CNS gliomas, pheochromocytomas and paragangliomas and occasionally with periampullary somatostatinomas [64]. The prevalence of NF-1 is about 0.03%.

The *NF-1* gene is located on chromosome 17q11.2. It encodes for the protein neurofibromin, which inhibits the intracellular phosphoinositide 3-kinase–protein kinase B–mammalian target of rapamycin (PI3K–AKT–mTOR) pathway, which is important in apoptosis. Loss of function of the *NF-1* gene results in mTOR upregulation and tumour development [10, 65].

Approximately 40% of the periampullary somatostatinomas are associated with NF-1 [64].

4.5 Tuberous Sclerosis Complex

Tuberous sclerosis complex (TSC) (OMIM 191100) is a multisystem autosomal dominant inherited genetic disorder, which is characterized by hamartomas in several organs, including the brain, heart, skin, eyes, kidneys, lungs and liver. The prevalence of TSC is approximately 0.015%.

TSC is caused by inactivating mutations in either of the two genes: *TSC1* (located on chromosome 9q34 and encoding for the protein hamartin) or *TSC2* (located on chromosome 16p13.3 and encoding for the gene product tuberin). Mutations of the *TSC1* and *TSC2* genes result in an impaired function of the hamartin–tuberin complex, which results in the upregulation of the PI3K–AKT–mTOR pathway [7, 65].

Pancreatic NENs, mostly insulinomas or non-functioning tumours, appear to be more frequent in TSC patients than in the general population. However, it is still unclear whether pancreatic NENs should be considered as a feature of TSC. Current clinical recommendations for TSC do not include routine investigation for pancreatic NENs [29, 30, 66, 67].

4.6 Summary

NENs represent a group of neoplasms arising from the neuroendocrine cells of the diffuse endocrine system. The majority of gastrointestinal, pancreatic, lung and thymic NENs are sporadic. However, some of the NENs may occur as part of multisystem autosomal dominant inherited genetic disorders, such as MEN1 syndrome, VHL, NF-1 and TSC. Over the last three decades, the genetic basis of tumourigenesis in the context of these familial syndromes has been unravelled, thus providing clinicians with useful screening tools for affected families.

References

1. de Herder WW, Lamberts SW (2004) Clinical endocrinology and metabolism. Gut endocrine tumours. Best Pract Res Clin Endocrinol Metab 18(4):477–495
2. Modlin IM, Oberg K, Chung DC, Jensen RT, de Herder WW, Thakker RV et al (2008) Gastroenteropancreatic neuroendocrine tumours. Lancet Oncol 9(1):61–72
3. Brandi ML, Gagel RF, Angeli A, Bilezikian JP, Beck-Peccoz P, Bordi C et al (2001) Consensus: guidelines for diagnosis and therapy of MEN type 1 and type 2. J Clin Endocrinol Metab 86(12):5658–5671
4. Thakker RV (2001) Multiple endocrine neoplasia. Horm Res 56(1):67–72
5. Carney JA (1995) Carney complex: the complex of myxomas, spotty pigmentation, endocrine overactivity, and schwannomas. Semin Dermatol 14(2):90–98
6. Stratakis CA (2001) Clinical genetics of multiple endocrine neoplasias, Carney complex and related syndromes. J Endocrinol Investig 24(5):370–383
7. Orlova KA, Crino PB (2010) The tuberous sclerosis complex. Ann N Y Acad Sci 1184:87–105. https://doi.org/10.1111/j.1749-6632.2009.05117.x
8. Hes FJ, Hoppener JW, Luijt RB, Lips CJ (2005) Von hippel-lindau disease. Hered Cancer Clin Pract 3(4):171–178

9. Chou A, Toon C, Pickett J, Gill AJ (2013) von Hippel-Lindau syndrome. Front Horm Res 41:30–49. https://doi.org/10.1159/000345668
10. Larizza L, Gervasini C, Natacci F, Riva P (2009) Developmental abnormalities and cancer predisposition in neurofibromatosis type 1. Curr Mol Med 9(5):634–653
11. Dreijerink KM, Goudet P, Burgess JR, Valk GD (2014) Breast-cancer predisposition in multiple endocrine neoplasia type 1. N Engl J Med 371(6):583–584
12. van Leeuwaarde RS, Dreijerink KM, Ausems MG, Beijers HJ, Dekkers OM, de Herder WW et al (2017) MEN1-dependent breast cancer: indication for early screening? Results from the Dutch MEN1 Study Group. J Clin Endocrinol Metab 102(6):2083–2090
13. Marini F, Falchetti A, Del Monte F, Carbonell SS, Gozzini A, Luzi E et al (2006) Multiple endocrine neoplasia type 1. Orphanet J Rare Dis 1:38. https://doi.org/10.1186/1750-1172-1-38
14. Thakker RV (2014) Multiple endocrine neoplasia type 1 (MEN1) and type 4 (MEN4). Mol Cell Endocrinol 386(1-2):2–15
15. Leotlela PD, Jauch A, Holtgreve-Grez H, Thakker RV (2003) Genetics of neuroendocrine and carcinoid tumours. Endocr Relat Cancer 10(4):437–450
16. Thakker RV, Newey PJ, Walls GV, Bilezikian J, Dralle H, Ebeling PR et al (2012) Clinical practice guidelines for multiple endocrine neoplasia type 1 (MEN1). J Clin Endocrinol Metab 97(9):2990–3011
17. de Laat JM, van der Luijt RB, Pieterman CR, Oostveen MP, Hermus AR, Dekkers OM et al (2016) MEN1 redefined, a clinical comparison of mutation-positive and mutation-negative patients. BMC Med 14(1):182–0708
18. van Leeuwaarde RS, van Nesselrooij BP, Hermus AR, Dekkers OM, de Herder WW, van der Horst-Schrivers AN et al (2016) Impact of delay in diagnosis in outcomes in MEN1: results from the Dutch MEN1 Study Group. J Clin Endocrinol Metab 101(3):1159–1165
19. Larsson C, Skogseid B, Oberg K, Nakamura Y, Nordenskjold M (1988) Multiple endocrine neoplasia type 1 gene maps to chromosome 11 and is lost in insulinoma. Nature 332(6159):85–87
20. Chandrasekharappa SC, Guru SC, Manickam P, Olufemi SE, Collins FS, Emmert-Buck MR et al (1997) Positional cloning of the gene for multiple endocrine neoplasia-type 1. Science 276(5311):404–407
21. Lemos MC, Thakker RV (2008) Multiple endocrine neoplasia type 1 (MEN1): analysis of 1336 mutations reported in the first decade following identification of the gene. Hum Mutat 29(1):22–32
22. Concolino P, Costella A, Capoluongo E (2016) Multiple endocrine neoplasia type 1 (MEN1): An update of 208 new germline variants reported in the last nine years. Cancer Genet 209(1-2):36–41
23. Jiao Y, Shi C, Edil BH, de Wilde RF, Klimstra DS, Maitra A et al (2011) DAXX/ATRX, MEN1, and mTOR pathway genes are frequently altered in pancreatic neuroendocrine tumors. Science 331(6021):1199–1203
24. Longuini VC, Lourenco DM Jr, Sekiya T, Meirelles O, Goncalves TD, Coutinho FL et al (2014) Association between the p27 rs2066827 variant and tumor multiplicity in patients harboring MEN1 germline mutations. Eur J Endocrinol 171(3):335–342
25. Bartsch DK, Slater EP, Albers M, Knoop R, Chaloupka B, Lopez CL et al (2014) Higher risk of aggressive pancreatic neuroendocrine tumors in MEN1 patients with MEN1 mutations affecting the CHES1 interacting MENIN domain. J Clin Endocrinol Metab 99(11):E2387–E2391
26. Thevenon J, Bourredjem A, Faivre L, Cardot-Bauters C, Calender A, Murat A et al (2013) Higher risk of death among MEN1 patients with mutations in the JunD interacting domain: a Groupe d'etude des Tumeurs Endocrines (GTE) cohort study. Hum Mol Genet 22(10):1940–1948
27. Conemans EB, Nell S, Pieterman CRC, de Herder WW, Dekkers OM, Hermus AR et al (2017) Prognostic factors for survival of MEN1 patients with duodenopancreatic tumors metastatic to the liver: results from the DMSG. Endocr Pract 23(6):641–648
28. de Laat JM, Pieterman CR, van den Broek MF, Twisk JW, Hermus AR, Dekkers OM et al (2014) Natural course and survival of neuroendocrine tumors of thymus and lung in MEN1 patients. J Clin Endocrinol Metab 99(9):3325–3333

29. Philips S, Shah SN, Vikram R, Verma S, Shanbhogue AK, Prasad SR (2012) Pancreatic endocrine neoplasms: a current update on genetics and imaging. Br J Radiol 85(1014):682–696
30. Alexakis N, Connor S, Ghaneh P, Lombard M, Smart HL, Evans J et al (2004) Hereditary pancreatic endocrine tumours. Pancreatology 4(5):417–433
31. de Herder WW, Niederle B, Scoazec JY, Pauwels S, Kloppel G, Falconi M et al (2006) Well-differentiated pancreatic tumor/carcinoma: insulinoma. Neuroendocrinology 84(3):183–188
32. Jensen RT (1998) Management of the Zollinger-Ellison syndrome in patients with multiple endocrine neoplasia type 1. J Intern Med 243(6):477–488
33. Ito T, Igarashi H, Uehara H, Berna MJ, Jensen RT (2013) Causes of death and prognostic factors in multiple endocrine neoplasia type 1: a prospective study: comparison of 106 MEN1/Zollinger-Ellison syndrome patients with 1613 literature MEN1 patients with or without pancreatic endocrine tumors. Medicine 92(3):135–181
34. Doherty GM, Thompson NW (2003) Multiple endocrine neoplasia type 1: duodenopancreatic tumours. J Intern Med 253(6):590–598
35. Hao W, Skarulis MC, Simonds WF, Weinstein LS, Agarwal SK, Mateo C et al (2004) Multiple endocrine neoplasia type 1 variant with frequent prolactinoma and rare gastrinoma. J Clin Endocrinol Metab 89(8):3776–3784
36. Pieterman CR, Conemans EB, Dreijerink KM, de Laat JM, Timmers HT, Vriens MR et al (2014) Thoracic and duodenopancreatic neuroendocrine tumors in multiple endocrine neoplasia type 1: natural history and function of menin in tumorigenesis. Endocr Relat Cancer 21(3):R121–R142
37. de Laat JM, Tham E, Pieterman CR, Vriens MR, Dorresteijn JA, Bots ML et al (2012) Predicting the risk of multiple endocrine neoplasia type 1 for patients with commonly occurring endocrine tumors. Eur J Endocrinol 167(2):181–187
38. MacFarlane MP, Fraker DL, Alexander HR, Norton JA, Lubensky I, Jensen RT (1995) Prospective study of surgical resection of duodenal and pancreatic gastrinomas in multiple endocrine neoplasia type 1. Surgery 118(6):973–979
39. Norton JA, Alexander HR, Fraker DL, Venzon DJ, Gibril F, Jensen RT (2001) Comparison of surgical results in patients with advanced and limited disease with multiple endocrine neoplasia type 1 and Zollinger-Ellison syndrome. Ann Surg 234(4):495–505
40. Thompson JC, Lewis BG, Wiener I, Townsend CM Jr (1983) The role of surgery in the Zollinger-Ellison syndrome. Ann Surg 197(5):594–607
41. O'Toole D, Delle FG, Jensen RT (2012) Gastric and duodenal neuroendocrine tumours. Best Pract Res Clin Gastroenterol 26(6):719–735
42. Nell S, Borel R, Verkooijen HM, Bonsing BA, van Eijck CH, van Goor H et al (2018) Early and late complications after surgery for MEN1-related nonfunctioning pancreatic neuroendocrine tumors. Ann Surg 267(2):352–356
43. Triponez F, Simon S, Robert J, Andereggen E, Ussel M, Bouchardy C et al (2001) Thyroid cancers: the Geneva experience. Ann Chir 126(10):969–976
44. Triponez F, Wong M, Sturgeon C, Caron N, Ginzinger DG, Segal MR et al (2006) Does familial non-medullary thyroid cancer adversely affect survival? World J Surg 30(5):787–793
45. Nell S, Verkooijen HM, Pieterman CR, de Herder WW, Hermus AR, Dekkers OM et al (2017) Management of MEN1 related nonfunctioning pancreatic NETs: a shifting paradigm: results from the DutchMEN1 Study Group. Ann Surg 10:1155–1160
46. Albers MB, Librizzi D, Lopez CL, Manoharan J, Apitzsch JC, Slater EP et al (2017) Limited value of Ga-68-DOTATOC-PET-CT in routine screening of patients with multiple endocrine neoplasia type 1. World J Surg 41(6):1521–1527
47. Morgat C, Velayoudom-Cephise FL, Schwartz P, Guyot M, Gaye D, Vimont D et al (2016) Evaluation of (68)Ga-DOTA-TOC PET/CT for the detection of duodenopancreatic neuroendocrine tumors in patients with MEN1. Eur J Nucl Med Mol Imaging 43(7):1258–1266
48. Froeling V, Elgeti F, Maurer MH, Scheurig-Muenkler C, Beck A, Kroencke TJ et al (2012) Impact of Ga-68 DOTATOC PET/CT on the diagnosis and treatment of patients with multiple endocrine neoplasia. Ann Nucl Med 26(9):738–743

49. van Asselt SJ, Brouwers AH, van Dullemen HM, van der Jagt EJ, Bongaerts AH, Kema IP et al (2015) EUS is superior for detection of pancreatic lesions compared with standard imaging in patients with multiple endocrine neoplasia type 1. Gastrointest Endosc 81(1):159–167
50. van Leeuwaarde RS, Pieterman CRC, Bleiker EMA, Dekkers OM, van der Horst-Schrivers AN, Hermus AR et al (2018) High fear of disease occurrence is associated with low quality of life in patients with multiple endocrine neoplasia type 1 (MEN1): results from the Dutch MEN1 Study Group. J Clin Endocrinol Metab 103(6):2354–2361
51. Lonser RR, Glenn GM, Walther M, Chew EY, Libutti SK, Linehan WM et al (2003) von Hippel-Lindau disease. Lancet 361(9374):2059–2067
52. Gossage L, Eisen T, Maher ER (2015) VHL, the story of a tumour suppressor gene. Nat Rev Cancer 15(1):55–64
53. Nielsen SM, Rhodes L, Blanco I, Chung WK, Eng C, Maher ER et al (2016) Von Hippel-Lindau disease: genetics and role of genetic counseling in a multiple neoplasia syndrome. J Clin Oncol 34(18):2172–2181
54. Maher ER, Neumann HP, Richard S (2011) von Hippel-Lindau disease: a clinical and scientific review. Eur J Hum Genet 19(6):617–623
55. Charlesworth M, Verbeke CS, Falk GA, Walsh M, Smith AM, Morris-Stiff G (2012) Pancreatic lesions in von Hippel-Lindau disease? A systematic review and meta-synthesis of the literature. J Gastrointest Surg 16(7):1422–1428
56. van Asselt SJ, de Vries EG, van Dullemen HM, Brouwers AH, Walenkamp AM, Giles RH et al (2013) Pancreatic cyst development: insights from von Hippel-Lindau disease. Cilia 2(1):3–2
57. de Mestier L, Hammel P (2015) Pancreatic neuroendocrine tumors in von Hippel-Lindau disease. Scand J Gastroenterol 50(8):1054–1055
58. Hammel PR, Vilgrain V, Terris B, Penfornis A, Sauvanet A, Correas JM et al (2000) Pancreatic involvement in von Hippel-Lindau disease. The Groupe Francophone d'Etude de la Maladie de von Hippel-Lindau. Gastroenterology 119(4):1087–1095
59. Libutti SK, Choyke PL, Bartlett DL, Vargas H, Walther M, Lubensky I et al (1998) Pancreatic neuroendocrine tumors associated with von Hippel Lindau disease: diagnostic and management recommendations. Surgery 124(6):1153–1159
60. Blansfield JA, Choyke L, Morita SY, Choyke PL, Pingpank JF, Alexander HR et al (2007) Clinical, genetic and radiographic analysis of 108 patients with von Hippel-Lindau disease (VHL) manifested by pancreatic neuroendocrine neoplasms (PNETs). Surgery 142(6):814–818
61. Keutgen XM, Hammel P, Choyke PL, Libutti SK, Jonasch E, Kebebew E (2016) Evaluation and management of pancreatic lesions in patients with von Hippel-Lindau disease. Nat Rev Clin Oncol 13(9):537–549
62. Prasad V, Tiling N, Denecke T, Brenner W, Plockinger U (2016) Potential role of (68) Ga-DOTATOC PET/CT in screening for pancreatic neuroendocrine tumour in patients with von Hippel-Lindau disease. Eur J Nucl Med Mol Imaging 43(11):2014–2020
63. van Asselt SJ, Brouwers AH, van Dullemen HM, van der Jagt EJ, Bongaerts AH, Koopmans KP et al (2016) Potential value of EUS in pancreatic surveillance of VHL patients. Eur J Endocrinol 174(5):611–620
64. Relles D, Baek J, Witkiewicz A, Yeo CJ (2010) Periampullary and duodenal neoplasms in neurofibromatosis type 1: two cases and an updated 20-year review of the literature yielding 76 cases. J Gastrointest Surg 14(6):1052–1061
65. Franz DN, Weiss BD (2012) Molecular therapies for tuberous sclerosis and neurofibromatosis. Curr Neurol Neurosci Rep 12(3):294–301
66. Yates JR, Maclean C, Higgins JN, Humphrey A, le Marechal K, Clifford M et al (2011) The tuberous sclerosis 2000 study: presentation, initial assessments and implications for diagnosis and management. Arch Dis Child 96(11):1020–1025
67. Yates JR (2006) Tuberous sclerosis. Eur J Hum Genet 14(10):1065–1073

Pathological Evaluation and Classification of Digestive Neuroendocrine Neoplasms

5

Anne Couvelard

5.1 The Pathological Diagnosis of Digestive NENs

Neuroendocrine neoplasms (NENs) arise from neuroendocrine cells, which are distributed in the mucosa of the gastrointestinal (GI) tract and in the pancreas. There are several diagnostic tools to perform the diagnosis of NENs, including imaging, serological tests, and endoscopy, but the diagnosis should be formally confirmed by a pathological investigation. The histological feature of NENs, which is generally characteristic in most cases, at least for well-differentiated NENs, must be confirmed by immunohistochemistry and allows categorizing these tumors as either NETs (neuroendocrine tumors) or NECs (neuroendocrine carcinomas) according to the international World Health Organization (WHO) classifications [1–4]. This is extremely important to assess the tumor prognosis and to guide patient therapy.

5.1.1 Morphology

The characteristic histopathological features of digestive NENs are held in common. By morphology, there is a clear distinction to be made, at all digestive locations, between well-differentiated and poorly differentiated tumors. This distinction is important, since their morphology, prognosis, and response to treatments are all extremely different. However, a relatively small percentage of tumors is not easy to classify into well-differentiated or poorly differentiated groups because they share some morphological characteristics. Well-differentiated tumors (called "neuroendocrine tumors" (NETs), according to the 2010, 2017, and 2019 WHO classifications, as discussed below) are composed of tumor cells possessing round nuclei with "salt-and-pepper"

A. Couvelard (✉)
Department of Pathology, Bichat Hospital AP-HP, Université Paris Cité and INSERM U1149, Paris, France
e-mail: anne.couvelard@aphp.fr

S. Yalcin, K. Öberg (eds.), *Neuroendocrine Tumours*,
https://doi.org/10.1007/978-3-031-56968-5_5

chromatin. Their cytoplasm is eosinophilic and granular. They show regular insular, trabecular, or sheet-like patterns, depending on the site of the primary, with the insular pattern being more frequent in the ileum and palisading of the peripheral cell layers. Poorly differentiated tumors (called "neuroendocrine carcinomas" (NECs), according to the 2010, 2017, and 2019 WHO classifications, as discussed below) are classified as small or large cell carcinomas, according to the histological morphology of their cells. The small cells are, as their name implies, small, round ovoid, or spindle-shaped, with extremely scant cytoplasm; their chromatin is fine and granular without nucleoli. In contrast, large cell carcinomas are composed of medium- or large-sized cells; their nuclei are atypical with evident nucleoli. These morphological characteristics are similar to those used to classify lung neuroendocrine tumors according to the lung 2004, 2015, and 2021 WHO classifications [3, 5, 6].

5.1.2 Immunohistochemistry

The morphological diagnosis of digestive NENs must be confirmed by immunohistochemistry, as first proposed by the European Neuroendocrine Tumor Society (ENETS), and by the last digestive 2019 WHO classification [2, 3, 7–9]. Among the several neuroendocrine markers, chromogranin A and synaptophysin are the most common and those that are required to confirm the diagnosis of NENs according to ENETS recommendations and WHO classifications of digestive tumors [1–3, 8, 9]. The neural cell adhesion molecule (NCAM) CD56 is also useful, especially in poorly differentiated tumors, because they may either weakly or not at all express chromogranin A, but its specificity is low. Hindgut rectal NENs may be negative for chromogranin A and only express chromogranin B. The diagnosis of rectal NETs should not be ruled out in the case of negativity of chromogranin A. INSM1 (insulinoma-associated protein 1), a transcription factor, is a more recent neuroendocrine marker, increasingly used in lung NENs and expressed in the nucleus of most NENs, which can be of help, especially in NECs that express low levels of chromogranin A [10–12]. In addition to these diagnostic biomarkers, the only currently used prognostic biomarker in digestive NETs is proliferative activity, best assessed by Ki-67. In pancreatic NETs (PanNETs), DAXX/ATRX, which can help identify the site of origin and have prognostic relevance, could be implemented in routine in the next future, by immunohistochemistry (loss of expression corresponding to genetic alteration). Other biomarkers can be of help, to distinguish G3 NETs from NECs, such as RB and p53 (global loss of RB and/or aberrant p53 indicate molecular alterations in favor of NECs) [13, 14].

5.2 The Pathological Classification of Digestive NETs

5.2.1 Introduction

In 2000, WHO published a classification for the histological typing of digestive neuroendocrine tumors (NETs) [15]. This classification remained unchanged following WHO's 2004 revision and was used until 2010 [16]. A new classification of digestive neuroendocrine neoplasms, based on grading (G) and differentiation, has been formulated in the 2010 revision of the WHO classification of tumors of the digestive system [1]. The terminology and principles were greatly modified in this classification as compared to those used before: three main grading categories were recognized, irrespective of the site in the digestive system (neuroendocrine tumors of grade 1 (G1), neuroendocrine tumors of grade 2 (G2), and neuroendocrine carcinomas of small or large cell types of grade 3 (G3)). For pancreatic NENs in 2017 and then for all digestive NENs in 2019, the WHO classification was modified, introducing a fourth subgroup: neuroendocrine tumors of grade G3 [2, 3]: neuroendocrine tumors grade 1 or NET G1 (Fig. 5.1a, b); neuroendocrine tumors grade 2 or NET G2; neuroendocrine tumors grade 3 or NET G3 (Fig. 5.1c, d); neuroendocrine carcinomas or NECs of large or small cell types; NECs of grade G3 (Fig. 5.1e, f); and mixed neuroendocrine non-neuroendocrine neoplasms (MiNENs) (Table 5.1).

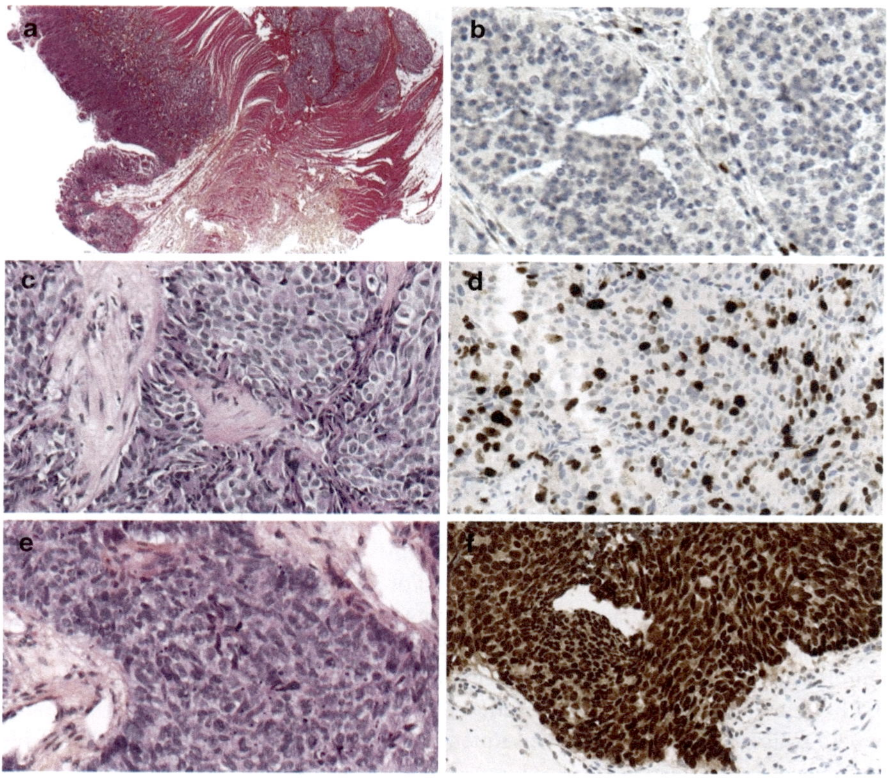

Fig. 5.1 A well-differentiated (**a**) neuroendocrine tumor (NET) of grade 1 (Ki-67 <1%) (**b**) of the ileum; a well-differentiated (**c**) neuroendocrine tumor (NET) of grade 3 (Ki-67 = 27%) (**d**) of the pancreas; and a small cell poorly differentiated (**e**) neuroendocrine carcinoma (NEC) of the colon metastatic to the liver, strongly expressing thyroid transcription factor 1 (TTF1) (**f**)

Table 5.1 General neuroendocrine neoplasm categories in the WHO 2019 classification

1	Neuroendocrine tumor, NET G1
2	Neuroendocrine tumor, NET G2
3	Neuroendocrine tumor, NET G3
3	Neuroendocrine carcinoma, NEC (small or large cell type)
4	Mixed neuroendocrine non-neuroendocrine neoplasm, MiNEN

Adapted from Lokuhetty [3]

Table 5.2 Grading for digestive neuroendocrine tumors, according to WHO Classification of Tumours Editorial Board [4]

Grade	Mitotic count (/2 mm^2)[a]	Ki-67 index (%)[b]
G1	<2	<3
G2	2–20	3–20
G3	>20	>20

Adapted from WHO Classification of Tumours Editorial Board [4]

[a] A total of 10 high power field (HPF), 40× magnification = 2 mm^2. It is recommended to count mitoses in at least 50 fields at ×40 magnification in areas of highest mitotic density and to divide the total number of mitoses by 5

[b] MIB-1 antibody; percentage of at least 500–2000 tumor cells in areas of highest labeling

5.2.2 Basis of the Grading

The histological grading into G1, G2, and G3 is performed on the basis of the assessment of the proliferation fraction according to the ENETS scheme that was first published in 2006 [8]. In the current WHO 2019 classification (Table 5.2), it is required to count mitosis in 50 HPF (high power field) (1 HPF = 0.2 mm^2) in a total area of 10 mm^2, and mitotic rates are expressed as the number of mitoses/2 mm^2. It is recommended to count the Ki-67 index using the MIB-1 antibody as a percentage of at least 500–2000 cells in areas of higher staining (hot spots). Grade 1 tumors have a mitotic count <2/2 mm^2 (10 HPF) and <3% Ki-67. Grade 2 tumors have a mitotic count between 2 and 20/2 mm^2 and/or 3 and 20% Ki-67. Grade 3 tumors have a mitotic count >20/2 mm^2 and/or Ki-67 >20%. If the grade differs for mitosis and Ki-67 evaluation, then it is suggested to consider the higher grade [2, 3]. It is of importance to note that in order to perform a proper evaluation of the mitotic count, the pathological specimen must have a minimal size: indeed, 50 HPFs represent 10 mm^2. The mitotic count is not feasible in a biopsy specimen where evaluation of Ki-67 is consequently required. The prognostic value of this grading was demonstrated for foregut, midgut, and hindgut NETs [17–25]. It has been suggested that Ki-67 is a better prognosis marker and predictor of metastases than mitoses [26], and the European Neuroendocrine Tumor Society (ENETS) recommendations suggest at least analyzing Ki-67 if possible; adding mitotic count could be optional [27].

5.2.3 Definitions of the Five Categories of the 2019 WHO Classification

(1) Neuroendocrine tumors grade 1: These tumors are well-differentiated and possess a low proliferation rate of grade 1 (see above). (2) Neuroendocrine tumors grade 2: These tumors are well-differentiated and possess an intermediate proliferation rate of grade 2 (see above). (3) Neuroendocrine tumors grade 3: These tumors are well-differentiated on morphology and possess a high proliferation rate of grade 3 (see above). (4) Neuroendocrine carcinomas of large or small cells: These tumors are poorly differentiated and malignant and are composed of small or large cells expressing the neuroendocrine markers chromogranin A and synaptophysin (staining might be faint or focal, especially for chromogranin). They are not formally graded but are considered high-grade by definition. It is important to note that the high-grade G3 group is heterogeneous, containing both well-differentiated NETs and poorly differentiated NECs, with the former being less aggressive with a lower Ki-67 index (frequently but not always <50%) and a lower response rate to cisplatin-based chemotherapy [28–34]. Morphological differentiation is a major criterion, which must be clearly specified in pathology reports. 5. MiNENs (mixed neuroendocrine non-neuroendocrine neoplasms) replace the previous adenoneuroendocrine carcinomas (MANECs), with the same description (30% of each component must be at least identified for this definition). MiNENs are classified as high-, intermediate-, or low-grade malignancies depending on the metastatic potential of the tumor components [35]. The frequency of MiNENs and the type of exocrine or neuroendocrine component depends on the location in the digestive system. For example, in the colon, MiNENs are more frequent and often contain a poorly differentiated neuroendocrine component [35, 36].

5.2.4 The 2017 American Joint Cancer Committee/International Union Against Cancer (AJCC/UICC) Tumor, Node, Metastasis (TNM)

5.2.4.1 Introduction

In 2009, the seventh edition of the American Joint Cancer Committee (AJCC) TNM classification was published [37], including digestive neuroendocrine tumors for the first time. It followed the first TNM classification, which was proposed in 2006 (for NETs of the stomach, duodenum, and pancreas) and in 2007 (for NETs of the ileum, colon/rectum, and appendix) by a working group of ENETS [8, 9]. In December 2017, a new edition of the AJCC classification (eighth edition) was published, with

Table 5.3 T categories in the UICC (eighth edition) of digestive neuroendocrine tumors, in the pancreas, stomach, duodenum/ampulla of Vater, jejunum/ileum, appendix, and colon/rectum

Pancreas	
TX	Tumor cannot be assessed
T1	Tumor limited to the pancreas, <2 cm
T2	Tumor limited to the pancreas, 2–4 cm
T3	Tumor limited to the pancreas, >4 cm or the invading duodenum or bile duct
T4	Tumor invading the adjacent organs (stomach, spleen, colon, adrenal glands) or the wall of large vessels (coeliac axis or superior mesenteric artery)
Stomach	
TX	Tumor cannot be assessed
T0	No evidence of primary tumor
T1	Tumor invading the mucosa or submucosa and ≤1 cm
T2	Tumor invading the muscularis propria or >1 cm
T3	Tumor invading the subserosa
T4	Tumor invading the visceral peritoneum (serosal) or adjacent structures
Duodenum and ampulla of Vater	
TX	Tumor cannot be assessed
T1	Tumor invading only the mucosa or submucosa and ≤1 cm (duodenal tumor) Tumor ≤1 cm and confined within the sphincter of Oddi (ampullary tumor)
T2	Tumor invading the muscularis propria or >1 cm (duodenal tumor) Tumor invading through the sphincter into the duodenal submucosa or muscularis propria or >1 cm (ampullary tumor)
T3	Tumor invading the pancreas or the peripancreatic adipose tissue
T4	Tumor invading the visceral peritoneum (serosa) or other organs
Jejunum and ileum	
TX	Tumor cannot be assessed
T0	No evidence of primary tumor
T1	Tumor invading the mucosa or submucosa, ≤1 cm
T2	Tumor invading the muscularis propria or >1 cm
T3	Tumor invading the subserosa
T4	Tumor invading the visceral peritoneum (serosal) or other organs or adjacent structures
Appendix	
TX	Tumor cannot be assessed
T0	No evidence of primary tumor
T1	Tumor ≤2 cm
T2	Tumor 2–4 cm
T3	Tumor >4 cm or invading the subserosa or mesoappendix
T4	Tumor perforating the serosa or invading other adjacent organs or structures (excluding direct mural extension to the adjacent subserosa of the adjacent bowel), e.g., the abdominal wall and skeletal muscle
Colon/rectum	
TX	Tumor cannot be assessed
T0	No evidence of primary tumor

(continued)

Table 5.3 (continued)

T1	Tumor invading the mucosa or submucosa and is ≤2 cm
T1	T1a: Tumor <1 cm
	T1b: Tumor 1–2 cm
T2	Tumor invading the muscularis propria or >2 cm
T3	Tumor invading the subserosa
T4	Tumor invading the visceral peritoneum (serosal) or other organs or adjacent structures

Extension into the peripancreatic adipose tissue is not a basis for staging
If the number of tumors is known, use T(#); if it is unavailable or too numerous, use the m suffix, T(m)
Note: According to the UICC, poorly differentiated NECs are classified as exocrine tumors
Adapted from Brierley [38]
Note: If the number of tumors is known, use T(#); if it is unavailable or too numerous, use the m suffix, T(m). For multiple tumors with different T, use the highest

Table 5.4 N and M categories of AJCC TNM

Definition of regional lymph node (N)	
NX	Regional lymph nodes cannot be assessed
N0	No regional lymph node metastasis
N1	Regional lymph node metastasis
Definition of regional lymph node (N) for the small bowel	
N1	Regional lymph node metastasis <12 nodes
N2	Large mesenteric masses (>2 cm) and/or extensive nodal deposits (12 or greater), especially those that encase the superior mesenteric vessels
Definition of distant metastasis	
M0	No distant metastasis
M1	Distant metastasis
M1a	Metastasis confined to the liver
M1b	Metastasis in at least one extrahepatic site (e.g., lung, ovary, non-regional lymph node, peritoneum, bone)
M1c	Both hepatic and extrahepatic metastases

Adapted from Brierley [38]

substantial modifications as compared to the previous one (Tables 5.3 and 5.4) [38]. The duodenum/ampulla of Vater and jejunum/ileum locations are now separated. The M1 category (distant metastasis) is now separated into three groups: M1a metastasis confined to the liver, M1b extrahepatic (lung, ovary, non-regional lymph node, peritoneum, or bone) metastasis, and M1c both hepatic and extrahepatic metastases. The N1 category also changed for small bowel location (classified as N1 or N2). Importantly, as in the seventh edition, high-grade (poorly differentiated) NECs are classified separately, using the exocrine classification established in respective sites. It is important to document the pathological features, such as invasion and tumor size, to allow the translation of the staging between the successive classifications [39].

5.2.4.2 TNM Staging at Different Digestive Locations (Table 5.3)

The Pancreas
In this location, the International Union Against Cancer (UICC) is comparable to the TNM proposed by ENETS [8] and highly different from the previous seventh edition UICC TNM [37, 38]. The classification is mainly based on tumor size (cutoff of 2 cm and 4 cm). This size cutoff of 4 cm was reported to be an important prognostic factor [24].

The Stomach
T is (T in situ) stage was suppressed in the current classification. T1 tumors are ≤1 cm in size and do not invade the muscularis propria. Tumors invading the subserosa are T3.

The Duodenum and Ampulla of Vater
This location was not previously individualized in the seventh edition (it was included in "small intestine"). The invasion of the sphincter of Oddi and duodenal submucosa or muscularis propria is described for ampullary tumors.

The Jejunum and Ileum
In this location, the N1 category changed and was classified as either N1 (regional lymph node metastasis <12 nodes) or N2 (large mesenteric masses (>2 cm) and/or extensive nodal deposits (≥12), especially those that encase the superior mesenteric vessels). The T2 and T3 stages apply to tumors invading the muscularis propria or >1 cm (T2) and the subserosal tissue, respectively, whereas T4 tumors penetrate the visceral peritoneum or other organs or adjacent structures.

The Appendix
Tumor size below 2 cm is not a criterion included in the current classification, despite the importance of describing size below 1 cm or between 1 and 2 cm for patient management. A tumor invading the subserosa or mesoappendix is classified as T3. The ENETS classification can be added to analyze the importance of the invasion of the mesoappendix.

The Colon and Rectum
In the colon and rectum, T1 is separated into T1a and T1b, according to size (<1 cm or 1–2 cm). This parameter is important for endoscopic resection of rectal tumors.

5.3 Specificities of Pathological Diagnosis According to the Different Digestive Locations

5.3.1 The Pancreas

Pancreatic NETs represent an extremely heterogeneous group of tumors, depending on the functional status, the presence of inherited syndromes, or tumor differentiation [2, 40, 41]. Functional tumors are associated with clinical syndromes caused by inappropriate secretion of insulin, glucagon, somatostatin, gastrin, or vasoactive intestinal peptide (VIP). Nonfunctioning tumors are often discovered incidentally or when they become clinically apparent due to their large size, invasion of adjacent organs, or occurrence of metastases. Most PanNETs are solitary and well-differentiated; when tumors are multiple, multiple endocrine neoplasia type 1 (MEN1) or von Hippel–Lindau (VHL) syndromes should be suspected. Well-differentiated NETs are usually well-circumscribed; they may present different histological patterns (such as solid, trabecular, gland-like, oncocytic). The first metastasis is usually found in the regional lymph nodes and the liver. Poorly differentiated NECs are infrequent in the pancreas, mostly represented by large cell NECs [42]. The molecular landscape of pancreatic NETs has been studied, describing germline mutations, including the DNA repair genes *MUTYH*, *CHEK2* and *BRCA2*, and *MEN1* and *VHL*, and somatic mutations involved in chromatin remodeling, DNA damage repair, activation of mammalian target of rapamycin (mTOR) signaling, and telomere maintenance [43]. When morphological diagnosis of high-grade pancreatic neuroendocrine neoplasms, which include NETs and NECs, is challenging, the protein expression of DAXX, ATRX, p53, and Rb, detected by immunohistochemistry, may help pathologists. Loss of DAXX or ATRX protein expression favor a well-differentiated NET, whereas abnormal p53 and/or Rb expression favor a poorly differentiated NEC [2, 3, 44].

Among functional pancreatic NETs, insulinomas are the most frequent. In 4–6% of cases, they are associated with MEN1 [45]. They are frequently discovered while still small and most are <2 cm, due in part to their earlier detection [46]. A relatively characteristic histological feature is the stroma with deposition of amyloid. Pancreatic gastrinomas are associated with the sporadic form of Zollinger–Ellison syndrome, as compared to duodenal ones, which are more frequent, smaller, and more often associated with MEN1 syndrome [45]. The histological aspect of gastrinomas has no distinctive features with other functioning or nonfunctioning pancreatic NETs. Glucagonomas are usually large and solitary tumors more frequent in the tail. They cause functional syndromes, including skin rash (necrolytic migratory erythema). They represent 8–13% of functioning tumors [2, 3].

Inherited diseases, mostly MEN1 and VHL disease, are responsible for multiple PanNETs, associated with microtumors (<0.5 mm in size), which are more frequent and numerous in MEN1. In VHL disease, pancreatic NETs occur in about 10–17% of patients, whereas VHL is prevalent in about 0.5% of pancreatic NETs [47–49]. The presence of microtumors is not constant in pancreatic specimens resected for NETs; tumor cells are frequently large with a clear foamy cytoplasm (Fig. 5.2a, b) [50]. Compared to sporadic NETs, VHL NETs present a lower malignancy rate [49, 51]. A new associated genetic syndrome was first described in the WHO classification for pancreatic NENs [2]: Mahvash disease, or glucagon cell adenomatosis, caused by inactivating glucagon receptor mutation. Microadenomas and tumors, usually <2 cm, are numerous, without glucagonoma syndrome [52].

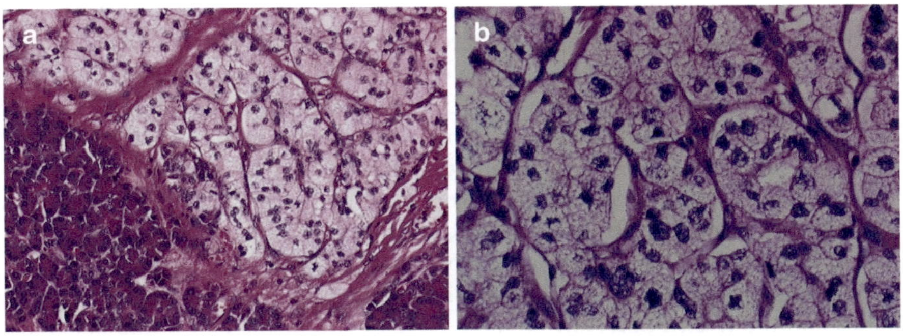

Fig. 5.2 A well-differentiated clear cell NET of grade 1 in a patient with von Hippel–Lindau disease (**a**). At high magnification, the tumor cells are frequently atypical with irregular large and hyperchromatic nuclei (**b**)

5.3.2 The Stomach

Well-differentiated gastric NETs are classified into types 1, 2, and 3. Type 4 NETs correspond to neuroendocrine carcinomas [13, 45, 53]. Type 1 NETs are the most common NETs (70–80%). They are related to fundic atrophic gastritis and hypergastrinemia secondary to the deficient production of gastric acid. They occur in the fundus, are multifocal, small (mostly <1 cm), and polypoid, usually G1 or, less frequently, G2 tumors [13]. They are composed of enterochromaffin (EC)-like (ECL) cells and associated with ECL cell hyperplasia in the adjacent mucosa. The prognosis of type 1 gastric NETs is excellent; their small size allows an endoscopic resection in most cases (Fig. 5.3a–d). Type 2 tumors are rare. They are associated with Zollinger–Ellison syndrome. Hypergastrinemia causes fundic ECL cell hyperplasia and, in the setting of MEN1, small fundic neuroendocrine tumors, which are numerous and multifocal. Type 2 tumors are highly similar to type 1 tumors, associated with gastrinomas and MEN1 but not with fundic atrophic gastritis (Fig. 5.3e, f). Moreover, lymph node metastases are more frequent than in type 1 NETs [45, 53]. Type 3 NETs, often called "sporadic NETs," occur in any part of the stomach and are not associated with atrophic gastritis, hypergastrinemia, ECL cell hyperplasia, or MEN1. They are well-differentiated, solitary, and larger than type 1 or 2 tumors, with a more aggressive course and more frequent local or distant metastases [54]. Type 4 gastric NENs are poorly differentiated, large, ulcerated tumors of poor prognosis, occurring in any part of the stomach [45] (Fig. 5.4a–c). Poorly differentiated NECs are rare in the stomach. There is a fifth infrequent subtype of NETs, recently described, secondary to long-term use of proton pump inhibitors (PPI), fundic, and possibly multifocal, and possibly associated with parietal cell and ECL cell hyperplasia [55, 56]. Analysis of the gastric antral and fundic mucosa is of utmost importance to better classify gastric NETs.

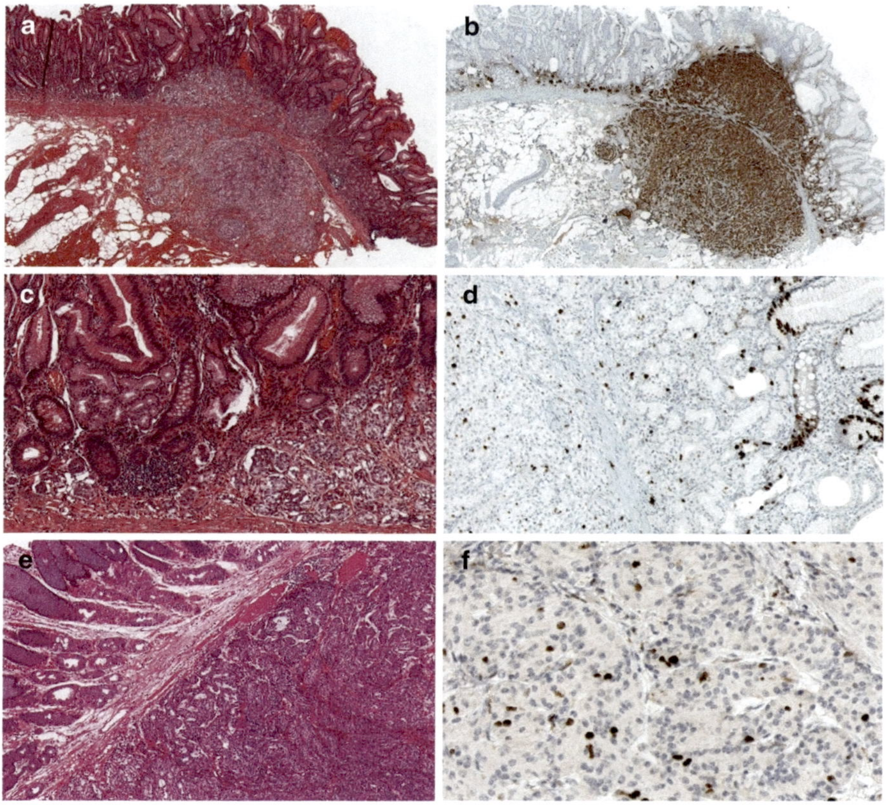

Fig. 5.3 A well-differentiated NET of grade 2 of the stomach, of type 1 (**a**–**d**) infiltrating the submucosa (**a**, **b**, chromogranin A-positive) in fundic atrophic autoimmune gastritis (**c**). The tumor is of grade 2 (**d**) (Ki-67 = 4%). A well-differentiated NET of type 2 (**e**, **f**) associated with a gastrinoma in a patient with multiple endocrine neoplasia of type 1; see the non-atrophic overlying mucosa (**e**). The tumor is of grade 2 (**f**) (Ki-67 = 6%)

5.3.3 The Small Intestine

5.3.3.1 The Duodenum

In the duodenum, well-differentiated NETs are of five main types: (1) gastrinomas or gastrin-producing NETs with or without MEN1 syndrome, (2) somatostatinomas or somatostatin-producing NETs with or without neurofibromatosis type 1, (3) non-functioning NETs, (4) gangliocytic paragangliomas (now classified as composite gangliocytoma/neuroma and neuroendocrine tumors (CoGNETs), and (5) poorly differentiated NECs [4, 13].

Gastrin-producing NETs mainly occur in the proximal duodenum, whereas somatostatin-producing NETs mainly occur in the ampulla of Vater [57].

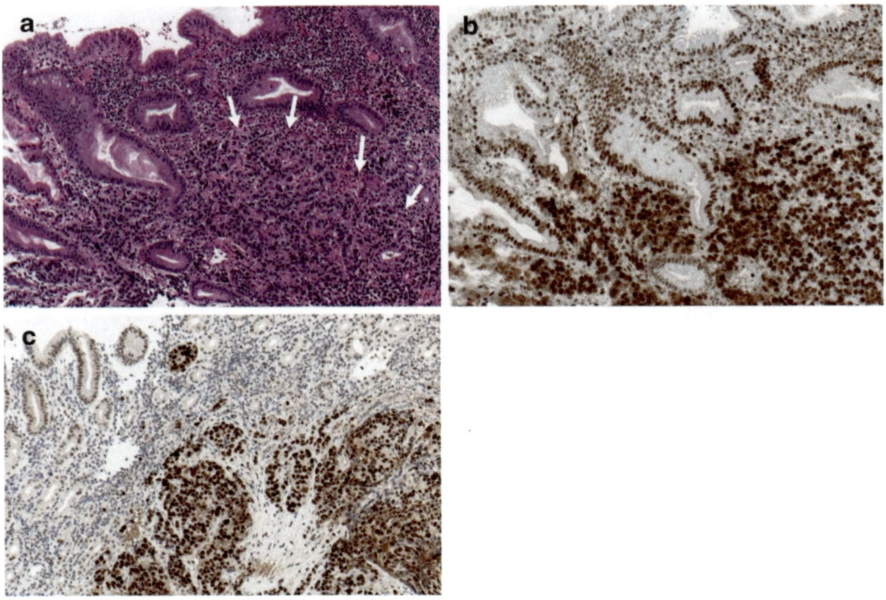

Fig. 5.4 A poorly differentiated gastric NEC (**a**, arrows) of type 4, of a large cell type and of grade 3 (**b**) (Ki-67 >95%), strongly expressing p53 (**c**)

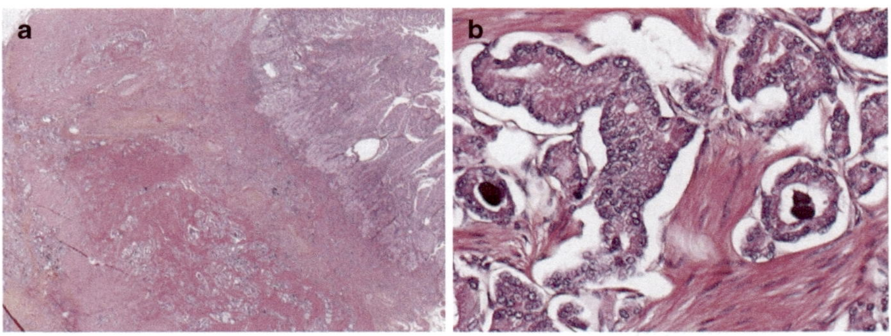

Fig. 5.5 A well-differentiated NET of the ampulla expressing somatostatin, infiltrating the sphincter of Oddi (**a**) in a patient with neurofibromatosis type 1. At high magnification, the tumor cells form small tubes with psammomas (**b**)

Somatostatinoma syndrome does not usually develop. Histologically, the pseudoglandular pattern with psammoma bodies is characteristic and may be mistaken for adenocarcinoma; neurofibromatosis type 1 syndrome should be suspected (Fig. 5.5a, b). Both gastrin- and somatostatin-producing NETs can be associated with MEN1. In this case, there is hyperplasia of gastrin or somatostatin cells, in the adjacent non-neoplastic mucosa. Most duodenal gastrinomas are confined to the mucosa and submucosa, but lymph node metastases are frequent, and often much larger than the duodenal primary, whereas liver metastases are rare [45, 58]. Composite gangliocytoma/neuroma and neuroendocrine tumors (CoGNETs) possess triphasic cellular differentiation with neuroendocrine cells, ganglion cells, and Schwann-like cells. They mainly occur in the papilla of Vater. Duodenal gastrinomas can be sporadic or associated with MEN1 (in 20–30% of the cases). They frequently metastasize to the regional lymph nodes, but liver metastases are less frequent than in patients with pancreatic gastrinomas. Duodenal NECs, which are infrequent, most commonly occur in the ampulla of Vater [45].

5.3.3.2 The Jejunum

Jejunal NETs are heterogeneous, and "upper" and "lower" jejunal tumors could be grouped, for prognostic purposes, with, respectively, duodenal and ileal NETs [59]. In the eighth edition AJCC TNM, duodenal and ileal NETs are classified separately.

5.3.3.3 The Ileum

Most of the ileal NETs are serotonin-producing EC tumors. Carcinoid syndrome, due to the effect of serotonin, is present when tumors are of significant size, usually with liver metastases. These NETs are not associated with any of the known inherited syndromes (i.e., MEN1, von Hippel–Lindau disease, neurofibromatosis, etc.). However, familial cases have been described [35, 60–62]. Ileal NETs occur in the distal part of the ileum and can present as multiple tumors in some cases [63]. Histologically, they present an insular growth pattern with frequent palisading at their periphery and a fibrosclerotic stroma. They often deeply invade the intestinal wall and cause lymph node and liver metastasis, whereas their proliferative index is usually low [20] (Fig. 5.1a, b). The presence of mesenteric tumor deposits is frequent and could be indicators of poor prognosis and survival [64].

5.3.4 The Appendix

Appendiceal NETs are frequent, often diagnosed after an appendiceal surgical rejection because of symptoms of acute appendicitis. Most are EC NETs, comparable to ileal EC NETs and arise at the tip (>70% of cases) of the appendix [65] (Fig. 5.6). A Tubular carcinoid is an histological variant that is difficult to diagnose, which should not been misdiagnosed as adenocarcinoma. The goblet cell carcinoid is now classified as an exocrine tumor, called "goblet cell adenocarcinoma" [3]. Most NETs of the appendix are <2 cm (>80%) and infiltrate the appendix wall [66], so most of them are classified as T3, according to the eighth edition of UICC TNM. Poorly differentiated tumors are exceptional. The risk of metastases increases with size and deep invasion of the appendix. Moertel et al. reported metastatic disease in 31% of patients with tumors >2 cm. Patients with tumors >2 cm should be treated by right hemicolectomy [66, 67]. The invasion of the mesoappendix was included in the ENETS TNM proposal, but not in the eighth edition of UICC TNM

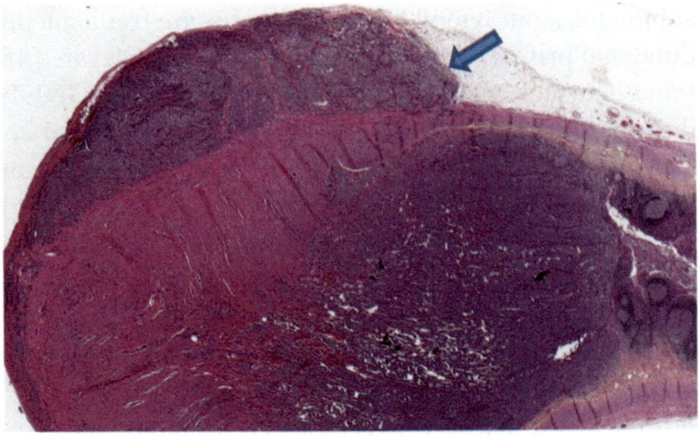

Fig. 5.6 A well-differentiated NET of the tip of the appendix, infiltrating the mesoappendix through the muscularis propria (arrow)

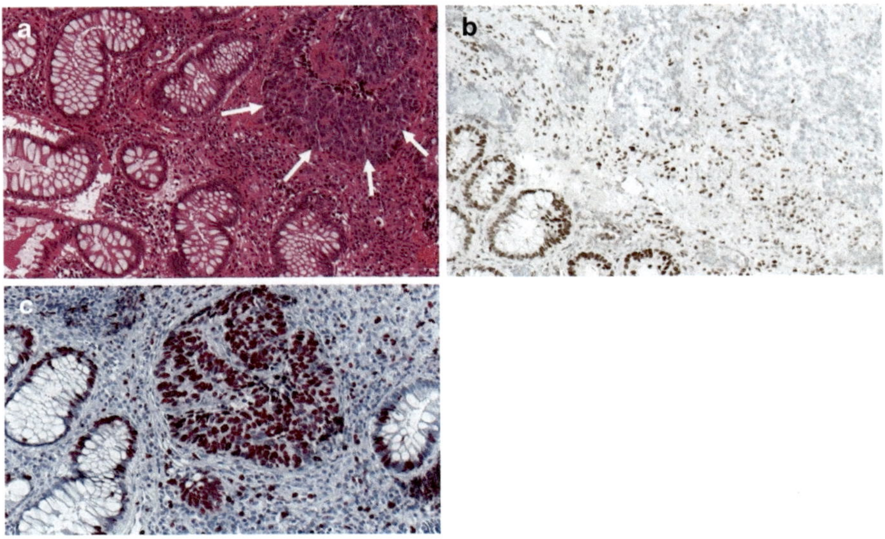

Fig. 5.7 A poorly differentiated large cell NEC of the rectum (**a**, arrows); tumor cells undergo loss of Rb expression, in contrast to the positive surrounding non-tumor cells (**b**), and strongly express p53 (**c**)

[38]. Its prognostic impact is still controversial, but McGillivray et al. reviewed 414 appendiceal NETs and found that the mesoappendiceal invasion was related to metastatic disease [68].

5.3.5 The Colon and Rectum

In the colon, neuroendocrine carcinomas are more frequent than in the rectum and in other digestive locations, except the esophagus. Large cell NECs are the most common type [69]. (Fig. 5.7a–c). Mixed tumors are not infrequent. The component of poorly differentiated neuroendocrine carcinomas may be deep and infiltrant [36]. Some NECs can present a lymphoid component and microsatellite instability (MSI), with better survival [70]. There are important diagnostic issues with adenocarcinomas in this location. Colon adenocarcinoma may express neuroendocrine markers, especially synaptophysin, and this has been reported to be more frequent in V600E BRAF-mutated colorectal cancers and to be associated with adenocarcinomas of worse prognosis [71, 72].

Rectal NETs are more frequent than are colonic NETs and are often solitary, sessile, and incidentally discovered on colonoscopy. They are increasing in incidence, probably due to an increase in the reporting of small polyps at endoscopy. The average tumor size is <1 cm, and G1 tumors account for >80% of cases [25]. Rectal NETs are frequently negative for chromogranin A but are frequently stained by SATB2, which can be helpful in the metastatic setting [73]. They can be treated by endoscopic resection, depending on their size and on tumor invasion, as determined by endoscopic ultrasound (in general if <2 cm and no invasion of the muscularis propria) [74, 75]. Evaluation of the margin and grading is important in such specimens as well as vascular invasion and tumor budding that could be a factor associated with lymph node metastasis in grades 1–2 rectal NETs [25, 76].

5.4 Conclusions

Despite a certain degree of morphological and immunohistochemical homogeneity of well-differentiated digestive NETs, these tumors are heterogeneous regarding their presentation (functional status, presence of inherited syndromes), prognosis, and staging according to their location in the digestive system. Because of frequent modifications in the nomenclature, grading, and staging, it is important to identify the minimal data that should be reported in all pathology reports [77] in order to ensure optimal reproducible and uniform data to aid in both clinical management and stratification in therapeutic trials. The use of the eighth edition of the international UICC TNM is recommended in all digestive locations. The histological differentiation should clearly appear in pathology reports in order to avoid problems with the previous "carcinoma" category, used before the 2010 WHO classification. It is important to provide the exact value of the proliferation rate to make comparison possible and to better stratify patient groups. It is now clear that the Ki-67 index is not optional, and is extremely important especially in biopsy specimens, which do not allow to properly assess the mitotic counts [2, 27, 78]. It is important to standardize the pathological diagnosis and the grading and staging of neuroendocrine tumors in the clinical management of patients and also to provide a uniform basis for research trials.

References

1. Bosman FT, Carneiro F, Hruban RH, Theise ND (eds) (2010) WHO classification of tumors of the digestive system, 4th edn. Lyon, IARC
2. Lloyd RV, Osamura RY, Klöppel G, Rosai J (2017) WHO classification of tumours of endocrine organs, 4th edn. IARC Press, Lyon

3. Lokuhetty D, White V, Watanabe R, Cree I (2019) WHO classification of tumours – digestive system tumours, 5th edn. IARC Press, Lyon
4. WHO Classification of Tumours Editorial Board (2022) Endocrine and neuroendocrine tumours. International Agency for Research on Cancer, Lyon
5. Travis WD, Brambilla E, Müller-Hermelink HK, Harris CC (eds) (2004) WHO classification of tumours. Pathology and genetics. Tumours of the lung, pleura, thymus and heart. IARC, Lyon
6. Travis WD, Brambilla E, Burke AP, Marx A, Nicholson AG (2015) WHO classification of tumours of the lung, pleura, thymus and heart. IARC Press, Lyon
7. Rindi G, Klimstra DS, Arnold R, Klöppel G, Bosman FT, Komminoth K, Capella C, Solcia E (2010) Nomenclature and classification of neuroendocrine neoplasms of the digestive system. In: Bosman FT, Carneiro F, Hruban RH, Theise ND (eds) WHO classification of tumors of the digestive system, 4th edn. IARC, Lyon, pp 13–14
8. Rindi G, Klöppel G, Alhman H, Caplin M, Couvelard A, de Herder WW, Erikssson B, Falchetti A, Falconi M, Komminoth P, Körner M, Lopes JM, McNicol AM, Nilsson O, Perren A, Scarpa A, Scoazec JY, Wiedenmann B, Frascati Consensus Conference Participants; European Neuroendocrine Tumor Society (ENETS) (2006) TNM staging of foregut (neuro)endocrine tumors: a consensus proposal including a grading system. Virchows Arch 449:395–401
9. Rindi G, Klöppel G, Couvelard A, Komminoth P, Körner M, Lopes JM, McNicol AM, Nilsson O, Perren A, Scarpa A, Scoazec JY, Wiedenmann B (2007) TNM staging of midgut and hindgut (neuro)endocrine tumors: a consensus proposal including a grading system. Virchows Arch 451:757–762
10. González I, Lu HC, Sninsky J, Yang C, Bishnupuri K, Dieckgraefe B, Cao D, Chatterjee D (2019) INSM1 expression in primary and metastatic neuroendocrine neoplasms of the gastrointestinal and pancreatobiliary tracts. Histopathology. https://doi.org/10.1111/his.13899
11. Kim D, Viswanathan K, Goyal A, Rao R (2020) Insulinoma-associated protein 1 (INSM1) is a robust marker for identifying and grading pancreatic neuroendocrine tumors. Cancer Cytopathol 128:269–277
12. Zhang Q, Huang J, He Y, Cao R, Shu J (2021) Insulinoma-associated protein 1(INSM1) is a superior marker for the diagnosis of gastroenteropancreatic neuroendoerine neoplasms: a meta-analysis. Endocrine 74(1):61–71
13. Rindi G, Mete O, Uccella S, Basturk O, La Rosa S, Brosens LAA, Ezzat S, de Herder WW, Klimstra DS, Papotti M, Asa SL (2022) Overview of the 2022 WHO classification of neuroendocrine neoplasms. Endocr Pathol 33(1):115–154
14. Singhi AD, Liu TC, Roncaioli JL, Cao D, Zeh HJ, Zureikat AH, Tsung A, Marsh JW, Lee KK, Hogg ME, Bahary N, Brand RE, McGrath KM, Slivka A, Cressman KL, Fuhrer K, O'Sullivan RJ (2017) Alternative lengthening of telomeres and loss of DAXX/ATRX expression predicts metastatic disease and poor survival in patients with pancreatic neuroendocrine tumors. Clin Cancer Res 23(2):600–609
15. Solcia E, Klöppel G, Sobin LH (eds) (2000) Histological typing of endocrine tumours. WHO international histological classification of tumours, 2nd edn. Springer, Berlin
16. DeLellis RA, Lloyd RV, Heitz PU et al (eds) (2004) Pathology and genetics of tumours of endocrine organs. IARC Press, Lyon
17. Ekeblad S, Skogseid B, Dunder K, Oberg K, Eriksson B (2008) Prognostic factors and survival in 324 patients with pancreatic endocrine tumor treated at a single institution. Clin Cancer Res 14:7798–7803
18. Fischer L, Kleeff J, Esposito I, Fischer L, Kleeff J, Esposito I, Hinz U, Zimmermann A, Friess H, Büchler MW (2008) Clinical outcome and long-term survival in 118 consecutive patients with neuroendocrine tumours of the pancreas. Br J Surg 95:627–635
19. Hochwald SN, Zee S, Conlon KC, Colleoni R, Louie O, Brennan MF, Klimstra DS (2002) Prognostic factors in pancreatic endocrine neoplasms: an analysis of 136 cases with a proposal for low-grade and intermediate-grade groups. J Clin Oncol 20:2633–2642
20. Jann H, Roll S, Couvelard A, Hentic O, Pavel M, Müller-Nordhorn J, Koch M, Röcken C, Rindi G, Ruszniewski P, Wiedenmann B, Pape UF (2011) Neuroendocrine tumors of midgut

and hindgut origin: tumor-node-metastasis classification determines clinical outcome. Cancer 117:3332–3341
21. La Rosa S, Klersy C, Uccella S, Dainese L, Albarello L, Sonzogni A, Doglioni C, Capella C, Solcia E (2009) Improved histologic and clinicopathologic criteria for prognostic evaluation of pancreatic endocrine tumors. Hum Pathol 40:30–40
22. Pape UF, Berndt U, Müller-Nordhorn J, Böhmig M, Roll S, Koch M, Willich SN, Wiedenmann B (2008) Prognostic factors of long-term outcome in gastroenteropancreatic neuroendocrine tumours. Endocr Relat Cancer 15:1083–1097
23. Pape UF, Jann H, Müller-Nordhorn J, Bockelbrink A, Berndt U, Willich SN, Koch M, Röcken C, Rindi G, Wiedenmann B (2008) Prognostic relevance of a novel TNM classification system for upper gastroenteropancreatic neuroendocrine tumors. Cancer 113:256–265
24. Scarpa A, Mantovani W, Capelli P, Beghelli S, Boninsegna L, Bettini R, Panzuto F, Pederzoli P, delle Fave G, Falconi M (2010) Pancreatic endocrine tumors: improved TNM staging and histopathological grading permit a clinically efficient prognostic stratification of patients. Mod Pathol 23:824–833
25. Weinstock B, Ward SC, Harpaz N, Warner RR, Itzkowitz S, Kim MK (2013) Clinical and prognostic features of rectal neuroendocrine tumors. Neuroendocrinology 98:180–187
26. Lowe K, Khithani A, Liu E, Winston T, Christian D, Saad J, Jeyarajah DR (2012) Ki-67 labeling: a more sensitive indicator of malignant phenotype than mitotic count or tumor size? J Surg Oncol 106:724–727
27. Perren A, Couvelard A, Scoazec JY, Costa F, Borbath I, Delle Fave G, Gorbounova V, Gross D, Grossma A, Jense RT, Kulke M, Oeberg K, Rindi G, Sorbye H, Welin S, Antibes Consensus Conference Participants (2017) ENETS consensus guidelines for the standards of care in neuroendocrine tumors: pathology: diagnosis and prognostic stratification. Neuroendocrinology 105(3):196–200
28. Basturk O, Yang Z, Tang LH, Hruban RH, Adsay V, McCall CM et al (2015) The high-grade (WHO G3) pancreatic neuroendocrine tumor category is morphologically and biologically heterogenous and includes both well differentiated and poorly differentiated neoplasms. Am J Surg Pathol 39:683–690
29. Coriat R, Walter T, Terris B, Couvelard A, Ruszniewski P (2016) Gastroenteropancreatic well-differentiated grade 3 neuroendocrine tumors: review and position statement. Oncologist 21:1191–1199
30. de Mestier L, Lamarca A, Hernando J, Zandee W, Alonso-Gordoa T, Perrier M, Walenkamp AM, Chakrabarty B, Landolfi S, Van Velthuysen MF, Kats-Ugurlu G, Caminoa A, Ronot M, Manoharan P, Garcia-Alvarez A, Brabander T, García Gómez-Muriel MI, Cadiot G, Couvelard A, Capdevila J, Pavel ME, Cros J (2021) Treatment outcomes of advanced digestive well-differentiated grade 3 NETs. Endocr Relat Cancer 28(8):549–561
31. Heetfeld M, Chougnet CN, Olsen IH, Rinke A, Borbath I, Crespo G et al (2015) Characteristics and treatment of patients with G3 gastroenteropancreatic neuroendocrine neoplasms. Endocr Relat Cancer 22:657–664
32. Lacombe C, De Rycke O, Couvelard A, Turpin A, Cazes A, Hentic O, Gounant V, Zalcman G, Ruszniewski P, Cros J, de Mestier L (2021) Biomarkers of response to etoposide-platinum chemotherapy in patients with grade 3 neuroendocrine neoplasms. Cancer 13(4):643
33. Tang LH, Untch BR, Reidy DL, Eileen O'Reilly E, Dhall D, Jih L et al (2015) Well differentiated neuroendocrine tumors with a morphologically apparent high grade component: a pathway distinct from poorly differentiated neuroendocrine carcinomas. Clin Cancer Res 22(4):1011–1017
34. Vélayoudom-Céphise FL, Duvillard P, Foucan L, Hadoux J, Chougnet CN, Leboulleux S, Malka D, Guigay J, Goere D, Debaere T, Caramella C, Schlumberger M, Planchard D, Elias D, Ducreux M, Scoazec JY, Baudin E (2013) Are G3 ENETS neuroendocrine neoplasms heterogeneous? Endocr Relat Cancer 20:649–657
35. de Mestier L, Cros J, Neuzillet C, Hentic O, Egal A, Muller N, Bouché O, Cadiot G, Ruszniewski P, Couvelard A, Hammel P (2017) Digestive system mixed neuroendocrine-non-neuroendocrine neoplasms. Neuroendocrinology 105(4):412–425

36. Li Y, Yau A, Schaeffer D, Magliocco A, Gui X, Urbanski S, Waghray R, Owen D, Gao ZH (2011) Colorectal glandular-neuroendocrine mixed tumor: pathologic spectrum and clinical implications. Am J Surg Pathol 35:413–425
37. Sobin LH, Gospodarowicz MA, Wittekind C (eds) (2009) TNM classification of malignant tumors, 7th edn. Springer, Heidelberg
38. Brierley JD, Gospodarowicz MA, Wittekind C (eds) (2016) TNM classification of malignant tumors, 8th edn. Wiley, Hoboken
39. Klöppel G, Rindi G, Perren A, Komminoth P, Klimstra DS (2010) The ENETS and AJCC/UICC TNM classifications of the neuroendocrine tumors of the gastrointestinal tract and the pancreas: a statement. Virchows Arch 456:595–597
40. Klimstra DS, Modlin IR, Adsay NV, Chetty R, Deshpande V, Gönen M, Jensen RT, Kidd M, Kulke MH, Lloyd RV, Moran C, Moss SF, Oberg K, O'Toole D, Rindi G, Robert ME, Suster S, Tang LH, Tzen CY, Washington MK, Wiedenmann B, Yao J (2010) Pathology reporting of neuroendocrine tumors: application of the Delphic consensus process to the development of a minimum pathology data set. Am J Surg Pathol 34:300–313
41. Klimstra DS, Arnold R, Capella C, Hruban RH, Klöppel G, Komminoth P, Solcia E, Rindi G (2010) Neuroendocrine neoplasm of the pancreas. In: Bosman FT, Carneiro F, Hruban RH, Theise ND (eds) WHO classification of tumors of the digestive system, 4th edn. IARC, Lyon
42. Basturk O, Tang L, Hruban RH, Adsay V, Yang Z, Krasinskas AM, Vakiani E, La Rosa S, Jang KT, Frankel WL, Liu X, Zhang L, Giordano TJ, Bellizzi AM, Chen JH, Shi C, Allen P, Reidy DL, Wolfgang CL, Saka B, Rezaee N, Deshpande V, Klimstra DS (2014) Poorly differentiated neuroendocrine carcinomas of the pancreas: a clinicopathologic analysis of 44 cases. Am J Surg Pathol. 38(4):437–447
43. Scarpa A, Chang DK, Nones K, Corbo V, Patch AM, Bailey P, Lawlor RT, Johns AL, Miller DK, Mafficini A, Rusev B, Scardoni M, Antonello D, Barbi S, Sikora KO, Cingarlini S, Vicentini C, McKay S, Quinn MC, Bruxner TJ, Christ AN, Harliwong I, Idrisoglu S, McLean S, Nourse C, Nourbakhsh E, Wilson PJ, Anderson MJ, Fink JL, Newell F, Waddell N, Holmes O, Kazakoff SH, Leonard C, Wood S, Xu Q, Nagaraj SH, Amato E, Dalai I, Bersani S, Cataldo I, Dei Tos AP, Capelli P, Davì MV, Landoni L, Malpaga A, Miotto M, Whitehall VL, Leggett BA, Harris JL, Harris J, Jones MD, Humphris J, Chantrill LA, Chin V, Nagrial AM, Pajic M, Scarlett CJ, Pinho A, Rooman I, Toon C, Wu J, Pinese M, Cowley M, Barbour A, Mawson A, Humphrey ES, Colvin EK, Chou A, Lovell JA, Jamieson NB, Duthie F, Gingras MC, Fisher WE, Dagg RA, Lau LM, Lee M, Pickett HA, Reddel RR, Samra JS, Kench JG, Merrett ND, Epari K, Nguyen NQ, Zeps N, Falconi M, Simbolo M, Butturini G, Van Buren G, Partelli S, Fassan M, Khanna KK, Gill AJ, Wheeler DA, Gibbs RA, Musgrove EA, Bassi C, Tortora G, Pederzoli P, Pearson JV, Waddell N, Biankin AV, Grimmond SM (2017) Whole-genome landscape of pancreatic neuroendocrine tumours. Nature 543(7643):65–71
44. Tang LH, Basturk O, Sue JJ, Klimstra DS (2016) A practical approach to the classification of WHO grade 3 (G3) well-differentiated neuroendocrine tumor (WD-NET) and poorly differentiated neuroendocrine carcinoma (PD-NEC) of the pancreas. Am J Surg Pathol 40(9):1192–1202
45. Klöppel G (2011) Classification and pathology of gastroenteropancreatic neuroendocrine neoplasms. Endocr Relat Cancer 18(1):1–16
46. Komminoth A, Perren A, Öberg K, Rindi G, Heitz PU, Klöppel G (2004) Insulinoma. In: DeLellis RA, Lloyd RV, Heitz PU et al (eds) Pathology and genetics. Tumours of endocrine organs. IARC Press, Lyon
47. Blansfield JA, Choyke L, Morita SY, Choyke PL, Pingpank JF, Alexander HR, Seidel G, Shutack Y, Yuldasheva N, Eugeni M, Bartlett DL, Glenn GM, Middelton L, Linehan WM, Libutti SK (2007) Clinical, genetic and radiographic analysis of 108 patients with von Hippel-Lindau disease (VHL) manifested by pancreatic neuroendocrine neoplasms (PNETs). Surgery 142:814–818
48. Charlesworth M, Verbeke CS, Falk GA, Walsh M, Smith AM, Morris-Stiff G (2012) Pancreatic lesions in von Hippel-Lindau disease? A systematic review and meta-synthesis of the literature. J Gastrointest Surg 16:1422–1428

49. Erlic Z, Ploeckinger U, Cascon A, Hoffmann MM, von Duecker L, Winter A, Kammel G, Bacher J, Sullivan M, Isermann B, Fischer L, Raffel A, Knoefel WT, Schott M, Baumann T, Schaefer O, Keck T, Baum RP, Milos I, Muresan M, Peczkowska M, Januszewicz A, Cupisti K, Tönjes A, Fasshauer M, Langrehr J, von Wussow P, Agaimy A, Schlimok G, Lamberts R, Wiech T, Schmid KW, Weber A, Nunez M, Robledo M, Eng C, Neumann HP, VHL-ICT Consortium; German NET Registry (2010) Systematic comparison of sporadic and syndromic pancreatic islet cell tumors. Endocr Relat Cancer 17:875–883
50. Périgny M, Hammel P, Corcos O, Larochelle O, Giraud S, Richard S, Sauvanet A, Belghiti J, Ruszniewski P, Bedossa P, Couvelard A (2009) Pancreatic endocrine microadenomatosis in patients with von Hippel-Lindau disease: characterization by VHL/HIF pathway proteins expression. Am J Surg Pathol 33:739–748
51. de Mestier L, Gaujoux S, Cros J, Hentic O, Vullierme MP, Couvelard A, Cadiot G, Sauvanet A, Ruszniewski P, Richard S, Hammel P (2015) Long-term prognosis of resected pancreatic neuroendocrine tumors in von Hippel-Lindau disease is favorable and not influenced by small tumors left in place. Ann Surg 262(2):384–388
52. Sipos B, Sperveslage J, Anlauf M, Hoffmeister M, Henopp T, Buch S, Hampe J, Weber A, Hammel P, Couvelard A, Höbling W, Lieb W, Boehm BO, Klöppel G (2015) Glucagon cell hyperplasia and neoplasia with and without glucagon receptor mutations. J Clin Endocrinol Metab 100(5):E783–E788
53. Rindi G, Luinetti O, Cornaggia M, Capella C, Solcia E (1993) Three subtypes of gastric argyrophil carcinoid and the gastric neuroendocrine carcinoma: a clinicopathologic study. Gastroenterology 104:994–1006
54. Rindi G, Azzoni C, La Rosa S, Klersy C, Paolotti D, Rappel S, Stolte M, Capella C, Bordi C, Solcia E (1999) ECLcell tumor and poorly differentiated endocrine carcinoma of the stomach: prognostic evaluation by pathological analysis. Gastroenterology 116:532–542
55. Rais R, Trikalinos NA, Liu J, Chatterjee D (2022) Enterochromaffin-like cell hyperplasia-associated gastric neuroendocrine tumors may arise in the setting of proton pump inhibitor use: the need for a new clinicopathologic category. Arch Pathol Lab Med 146(3):366–371
56. Trinh VQ-H, Shi C, Ma C (2020) Gastric neuroendocrine tumours from long-term proton pump inhibitor users are indolent tumours with good prognosis. Histopathology 77:865–876
57. Garbrecht N, Anlauf M, Schmitt A, Henopp T, Sipos B, Raffel A, Eisenberger CF, Knoefel WT, Pavel M, Fottner C, Musholt TJ, Rinke A, Arnold R, Berndt U, Plöckinger U, Wiedenmann B, Moch H, Heitz PU, Komminoth P, Perren A, Klöppel G (2008) Somatostatin-producing neuroendocrine tumors of the duodenum and pancreas: incidence, types, biological behavior, association with inherited syndromes, and functional activity. Endocr Relat Cancer 15:229–241
58. Anlauf M, Enosawa T, Henopp T, Schmitt A, Gimm O, Brauckhoff M, Dralle H, Musil A, Hauptmann S, Perren A, Klöppel G (2008) Primary lymph node gastrinoma and occult duodenal microgastrinoma. Am J Surg Pathol. 32:1101–1105
59. Chopin-Laly X, Walter T, Hervieu V, Poncet G, Adham M, Guibal A, Chayvialle JA, Lombard-Bohas C, Scoazec JY (2013) Neuroendocrine neoplasms of the jejunum: a heterogeneous group with distinctive proximal and distal subsets. Virchows Arch 462:489–499
60. de Mestier L, Pasmant E, Fleury C, Brixi H, Sohier P, Féron T, Diebold MD, Clauser E, Cadiot G, Groupe d'Étude des Tumeurs Endocrines (2017) Familial small-intestine carcinoids: chromosomal alterations and germline inositol polyphosphate multikinase sequencing. Dig Liver Dis 49(1):98–102
61. Hiripi E, Bermejo JL, Sundquist J, Hemminki K (2009) Familial gastrointestinal carcinoid tumours and associated cancers. Ann Oncol 20:950–954
62. Kharazmi E, Pukkala E, Sundquist K, Hemminki K (2013) Familial risk of small intestinal carcinoid and adenocarcinoma. Clin Gastroenterol Hepatol 11:944–949
63. Yantiss R, Odze RD, Farraye FA, Rosenberg AE (2003) Solitary versus multiple carcinoid tumors of the ileum: a clinical and pathologic review of 68 cases. Am J Surg Pathol 27:811–817
64. Gonzalez RS, Liu EH, Alvarez JR, Ayers GD, Washington MK, Shi C (2014) Should mesenteric tumor deposits be included in staging of well-differentiated small intestine neuroendocrine tumors? Mod Pathol 27(9):1288–1295

65. Carr N, Sobin LH (2004) Neuroendocrine tumors of the appendix. Semin Diagn Pathol 21:108–119
66. Plöckinger U, Couvelard A, Falconi M, Sundin A, Salazar R, Christ E, de Herder WW, Gross D, Knapp WH, Knigge UP, Kulke MH, Pape UF, Frascati Consensus Conference Participants (2008) Consensus guidelines for the management of patients with digestive neuroendocrine tumours: well-differentiated tumour/carcinoma of the appendix and goblet cell carcinoma. Neuroendocrinology 87:20–30
67. Pape UF, Perren A, Niederle B, Gross D, Gress T, Costa F, Arnold R, Denecke T, Plöckinger U, Salazar R, Grossman A, Barcelona Consensus Conference Participants (2012) ENETS Consensus Guidelines for the management of patients with neuroendocrine neoplasms from the jejuno-ileum and the appendix including goblet cell carcinomas. Neuroendocrinology 95:135–156
68. MacGillivray DC, Heaton RB, Rushin JM, Cruess DF (1992) Distant metastasis from a carcinoid tumor of the appendix less than one centimeter in size. Surgery 111(4):466–471
69. Shia J, Tang LH, Weiser MR, Brenner B, Adsay NV, Stelow EB, Saltz LB, Qin J, Landmann R, Leonard GD, Dhall D, Temple L, Guillem JG, Paty PB, Kelsen D, Wong WD, Klimstra DS (2008) Is nonsmall cell type high-grade neuroendocrine carcinoma of the tubular gastrointestinal tract a distinct disease entity? Am J Surg Pathol 32:719–731
70. Chetty R, Capo-Chichi JM, Serra S (2019) Colorectal large cell neuroendocrine carcinoma with lymphoid stroma: further evidence confirming a unique sub-type associated with MLH-1/PMS2 protein loss, BRAF mutation, EBV-negativity and possible better prognosis. Histopathology 75(2):247–253. https://doi.org/10.1111/his.13875
71. Digiacomo N, Bolzacchini E, Veronesi G, Cerutti R, Sahnane N, Pinotti G, Bregni M, Artale S, Verusio C, Crivelli F, Capella C, Sessa F, Furlan D (2019) Neuroendocrine differentiation, microsatellite instability, and tumor-infiltrating lymphocytes in advanced colorectal cancer with BRAF mutation. Clin Colorectal Cancer 18(2):e251–e260
72. Fassan M, Milione M, Maddalena G, Cremolini C, Schirripa M, Pietrantonio F, Pella N, Dell'Aquila E, Sperti E, Zichi C, Bergamo F, Volante M, Boccaccino A, Morano F, Cortiula F, De Maglio G, Rimassa L, Smiroldo V, Calvetti L, Aprile G, Salvatore L, Santini D, Salmaso R, Centonze G, Biason P, Borga C, Lonardi S, Zagonel V, Dei Tos AP, Di Maio M, Loupakis F (2021) Synaptophysin expression in V600EBRAF-mutated advanced colorectal cancers identifies a new subgroup of tumours with worse prognosis. Eur J Cancer 146:145–154
73. Zhao L-H, Chen C, Mao C-Y, Xiao H, Fu P, Xiao HL, Wang G (2019) Value of SATB2, ISL1, and TTF1 to differentiate rectal from other gastrointestinal and lung well-differentiated neuroendocrine tumors. Pathol Res Pract 215:152448
74. de Mestier L, Brixi H, Gincul R, Ponchon T, Cadiot G (2013) Updating the management of patients with rectal neuroendocrine tumors. Endoscopy 45:1039–1046
75. Ramage JK, Goretzki PE, Manfredi R, Komminoth P, Ferone D, Hyrdel R, Kaltsas G, Kelestimur F, Kvols L, Scoazec JY, Garcia MI, Caplin ME, Frascati Consensus Conference Participants (2008) Consensus guidelines for the management of patients with digestive neuroendocrine tumours: well-differentiated colon and rectum tumour/carcinoma. Neuroendocrinology 87:31–39
76. Chida K, Watanabe J, Hirasawa K, Inayama Y, Misumi T, Kunisaki C, Endo I (2020) A novel risk-scoring system for predicting lymph node metastasis of rectal neuroendocrine tumors. Ann Gastroenterol Surg 4(5):562–570
77. van Velthuysen MF, Couvelard A, Rindi G, Fazio N, Hörsch D, Nieveen van Dijkum EJ, Klöppel G, Perren A (2022) ENETS standardized (synoptic) reporting for neuroendocrine tumour pathology. J Neuroendocrinol 34(3):e13100
78. Klöppel G, Couvelard A, Perren A et al (2009) ENETS consensus guidelines for the standards of care in neuroendocrine tumors: towards a standardized approach to the diagnosis of gastroenteropancreatic neuroendocrine tumors and their prognostic stratification. Neuroendocrinology 90:162–166

6 The NETest: A Multigene Liquid Biopsy for Diagnosis and Management of Neuroendocrine Tumors

Anna Malczewska, Mark Kidd, Kjell Öberg, Lisa Bodei, Alexander Mandel, Alexandra Kitz, and Irvin M. Modlin

6.1 The Current Status of Neuroendocrine Tumor (NET) Blood-Borne Biomarkers

The management of neuroendocrine neoplasms (NENs) remains a perplexing problem due to the lack of knowledge of the biology of the disease, its late presentation, the relative insensitivity of imaging modalities, and a critical limitation posed by the lack of accurate biomarkers to guide management and monitor the efficacy of therapy [1]. Current clinical practice involves the mutual consideration of both imaging and biomarkers. Simple monoanalyte measurements, however, often do not correlate with radiological evaluation [2, 3].

From testing urine through invention of a microscope to molecular testing, diagnostic techniques have come a long way (from empirical to experimental) [4] and continue to advance to meet the needs of the emerging era of precision medicine and the modern concept of cancer biomarkers (Fig. 6.1).

A. Malczewska
Department of Endocrinology and Neuroendocrine Tumors, Medical University of Silesia, Katowice, Poland

M. Kidd · A. Mandel · A. Kitz
Wren Laboratories, Branford, CT, USA
e-mail: mkidd@wrenlaboratories.com; am1061@exeter.ac.uk; akitz@wrenlaboratories.com

K. Öberg
Department of Endocrine Oncology, Uppsala University Hospital, Uppsala, Sweden
e-mail: kjell.oberg@medsci.uu.se

L. Bodei
Molecular Imaging and Therapy Service, Department of Radiology, Memorial Sloan Kettering Cancer Center, New York, NY, USA
e-mail: bodeil@mskcc.org

I. M. Modlin (✉)
School of Medicine, Yale University, New Haven, CT, USA

S. Yalcin, K. Öberg (eds.), *Neuroendocrine Tumours*,
https://doi.org/10.1007/978-3-031-56968-5_6

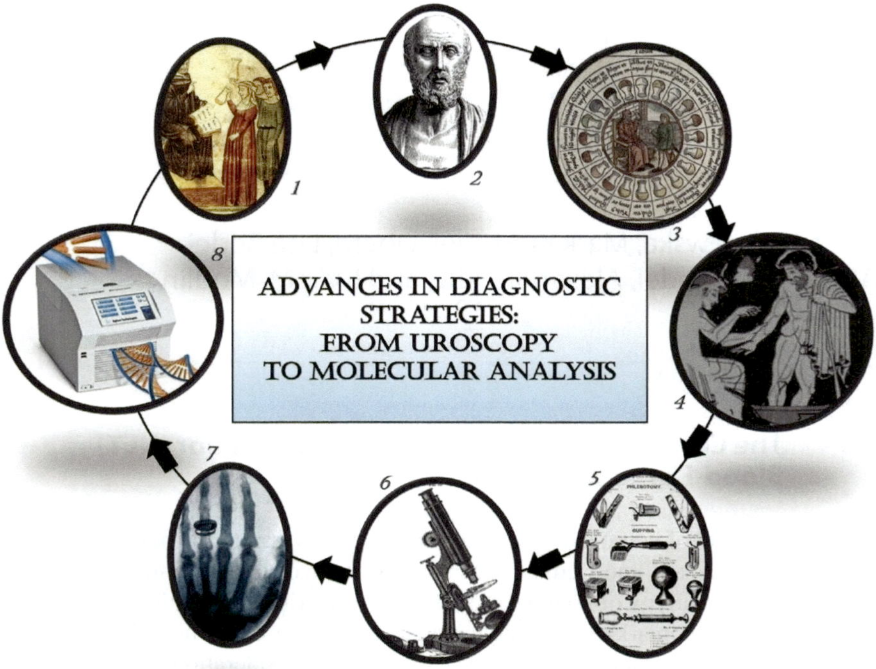

Fig. 6.1 Historical advances in diagnostic strategies from empirical to experimental. (**a**) Ancient visual examination of urine, the first bodily fluid to be utilized for diagnostics. (**b**) Hippocrates, the father of medicine, promoted the theory of humoral pathology and attributed all disease to disorders of bodily fluids. (**c**) A medieval uroscopy chart listing various urine colors to guide disease diagnosis. (**d**) Bloodletting; modern phlebotomy has its ancient roots in bloodletting. (**e**) Early bloodletting devices. (**f**) Microscope invention in ~1590; its concept is attributed to the Dutch spectacle makers Zaccharias Janssen and Hans Lipperhey, although Leeuwenhoek and Spinoza played key roles in lens grinding. (**g**) X-ray technology introduced by Wilhelm Conrad Röntgen in 1895; image of the first X-ray of Röntgen's wife's hand. (**h**) The PCR machine invented in 1983 by Kary Mullis, following the discovery of nucleic acids in 1868 by the Swiss physician Friedrich Miescher

Biomarkers play an important role in disease diagnosis, monitoring, and/or treatment outcome prediction. They are cellular, biochemical, or molecular alterations measurable in biological media, such as tissues, cells, or fluids [5]. To function effectively, they are required to exhibit metrics of sensitivity ≥80%, specificity ≥90%, and positive and negative predictive values of each ≥80% [6].

Some general biomarkers are used in NENs, though their clinical utility has not proved sustainable. These include chromogranin A (CgA) and urinary 5-hydroxyindoleacetic acid (5-HIAA) [7]. More effective secretory (monoanalyte) biomarkers for functional tumors such as insulin, gastrin, and vasoactive intestinal polypeptide (VIP) are accurate measurements of tumor secretory activity. However, their utility is significantly restricted since they are mostly effective in pancreatic tumors that comprise an extremely small group of NETs (<5%).

CgA is a component of neuroendocrine cell secretory granules and is measurable in the blood and tissue. Some reports consider it to correlate with tumor biology and size and to provide information with respect to outcome [8]. More recently, the enthusiasm for the clinical use of CgA has much diminished, as rigorous studies have demonstrated its low utility [9–13]. Of particular concern is the inability of the different assays to produce comparable data [14–19]. A major limitation is that CgA sensitivity ranges from 43 to 100%, whereas the metrics for specificity are <50% [6]. These low metrics reflect abnormal CgA elevations related to acid-suppressive medications (e.g., proton pump inhibitors (PPIs)), kidney failure, heart disease, and other cancers [19–21]. Given the complexity and multidimensionality of the neoplastic process itself, the heterogeneity of neuroendocrine tumors (NETs), and the interaction of the tumor microenvironment, it is not unexpected that no single (monoanalyte) biomarker has proven to be effective. Secretory products of a tumor cell into the blood alone cannot adequately define the state or progression of the neoplastic process nor the efficacy of therapy [1]. Such products are unable to adequately define the cellular activity of a tumor since they do not encompass the numerous biological processes that define neoplasia and its progression (growth factor signaling, metabolic status, and cell cycling) [6].

Thus, logic dictates that no single measured parameter can capture the pathobiological diversity of neoplasia and that monoanalytes cannot define the multiple variables (proliferation, metabolic activity, invasive potential, and metastatic propensity) that constitute tumor growth. Thus far, most biomarkers, whether in a tissue or the blood/urine, have been single analytes with varying degrees of sensitivity and specificity and, in general, have failed to exhibit robust metrics or lacked methodological rigor [1].

The conclusion of a number of consensus meetings and authorities in the field is that a multifactorial measurement that is effective in real time is required to evaluate the molecular topography of a tumor. Thus, the "hallmarks of cancer," proposed by Hanahan et al., can probably be best assessed by a liquid biopsy, which describes and measures the molecular genomic mechanisms of a tumor cell in the circulating blood. Such tools would provide more detailed information reflecting the biology of the tumor as it evolves, thus facilitating its management [6].

The development of a technique whereby blood-based molecular information could be integrated with functional imaging would be a substantial clinical advance. The ideal goal would be to deliver noninvasive, real-time, multidimensional information that defines the clinical and molecular functionality of a tumor. Thus, a liquid biopsy, which is a precise diagnostic, correlates with imaging, and reduces exposure to radiation (and/or cost), would be of clinical value [22].

6.2 The Concept of a Multianalyte Liquid Biopsy for Neuroendocrine Tumors

During cancer progression and treatment, multiple subclonal populations of tumor cells compete with one another, with selective pressures leading to the emergence of predominant tumor clones that replicate and spread most proficiently and are less susceptible to treatment. At present, the molecular landscapes of solid tumors are established using surgical or biopsy tissue samples. Tissue-based tumor profiles are, however, subject to sampling bias, provide only a snapshot of tumor heterogeneity, and cannot be obtained repeatedly [23]. They are invasive in nature and are associated with many limitations, including patient risk, sample preparation, sensitivity and accuracy, procedural costs, and invasive testing. This makes the procedure incompatible for clinical longitudinal monitoring. Furthermore, a significant limitation of tissue biopsies is that they fail to capture intra-tumoral and inter-metastatic genetic heterogeneity, thus impacting the accuracy of the assessment [24].

While previously focus was on the histology of a tumor, there is now substantial interest in the identification and quantification of tumor products in the blood compartment broadly described as the "tumor circulome." This group colliquation represents a variety of tumor-derived components, including circulating tumor DNA (ctDNA), circulating tumor cells (CTCs), messenger RNA (mRNA), extracellular vesicles, or "tumor-educated" platelets [24]. Indeed, the rapid turnover of cancer cells is postulated to result in the release of a constant tumor cell product (DNA, mRNA) into circulation, and viable tumor cells can also separate from the tumor to enter the bloodstream [23]. The possibility of probing the molecular landscape of solid tumors via a blood sample, with major implications for research and patient care, has attracted substantial interest among the oncology community [23]. Analyses of circulating nucleic acids, commonly referred to as "liquid biopsies," can be used to monitor response to treatment, assess the emergence of drug resistance, and quantify minimal residual disease [23]. These data can then be integrated using systems biology for better delineation of the molecular biology of a specific tumor and to define mutations, master regulators, and oncogenic check points [25]. Overall, the future will certainly include the introduction of molecular technologies to more accurately demarcate the biological status of a cancer cell. The likely way forward will include identification of mutations in ctDNA or transcriptional profiles, including mRNA and signal pathway analyses [22, 26, 27] to limit invasive biopsies, define therapeutic targets, and provide a real-time monitoring tool to evaluate disease status [28].

Each of the tumor circulome components can provide various levels of information [24]. Identification of actionable mutation events, e.g., BRAF mutations in ctDNA, allows for patient stratification (e.g., as a companion diagnostic), screening, or monitoring treatment responses. Examples include identification of mutation *T790M* in ctDNA, which allows for monitoring of treatment responses to epidermal growth factor receptor (EGFR) inhibitors in lung cancer [29, 30]. Measurements of ctDNA levels have been successfully used for the detection of minimal residual disease after surgery/recurrence, e.g., in colon cancer [31].

Unlike the majority of cancers, NENs exhibit infrequent activating mutations [25] and most tumors exhibit somatic mutations (when identified) in tumor suppressor genes, e.g., *MEN-1* that is a predominant pancreatic mutation [32]. The clinical usefulness of other alterations, e.g., in *ATRX*, *DAXX* [33], or *YY1* [34] (all identified as sporadic mutations in pancreatic NENs (PNENs)) remains unproven. In addition, the clinical usefulness of copy number and chromosomal imbalances as well as chemical-based DNA modifications, e.g., methylation, require further elucidation before they can be shown to have clinical utility [25]. To date, the clinical utility of the measurement of molecular signals such as ctDNA or methylated gene targets has therefore been of limited value in NENs [32]. Similarly, the measurement of microRNA (miRNA) remains complex and is not adequately standardized for clinical usage [35]. CTCs, though intuitively attractive as a direct measurement of tumor cell-related events, have to date failed to provide evidence of clinical utility in NENs [36]. The focus in NENs has thus switched to mRNA-based liquid biopsy approaches, which have been demonstrated to have utility in other diseases. For example, FibroSure (FibroTest) is a blood-based, biochemical, algorithmic test for liver damage used to detect hepatitis C [37]. It is a repeatable, noninvasive gene expression test, with high accuracy and without complications related to a liver biopsy.

Dynamic characterization of tumor behavior based upon blood-derived genomic information can be derived from assessment of circulating real-time multianalyte genetic information (NETest). As a clinically available mRNA liquid biopsy, the NETest has been specifically developed for management of NENs disease. Blood-based transcriptomic analysis and interrogation of the specific genomic drivers of a tumor provide a liquid biopsy, which is an optimal platform to assess tumor status on a real-time basis [38]. In the era of precision medicine, it is probable that therapeutic individualization (stratification into responders and nonresponders by a predictive biomarker) will become the standard of care. The efficacy of treatment will be identified by genomic characterization to target specific molecular features of an individual tumor prior to use of the therapeutic agent (Fig. 6.2) [22].

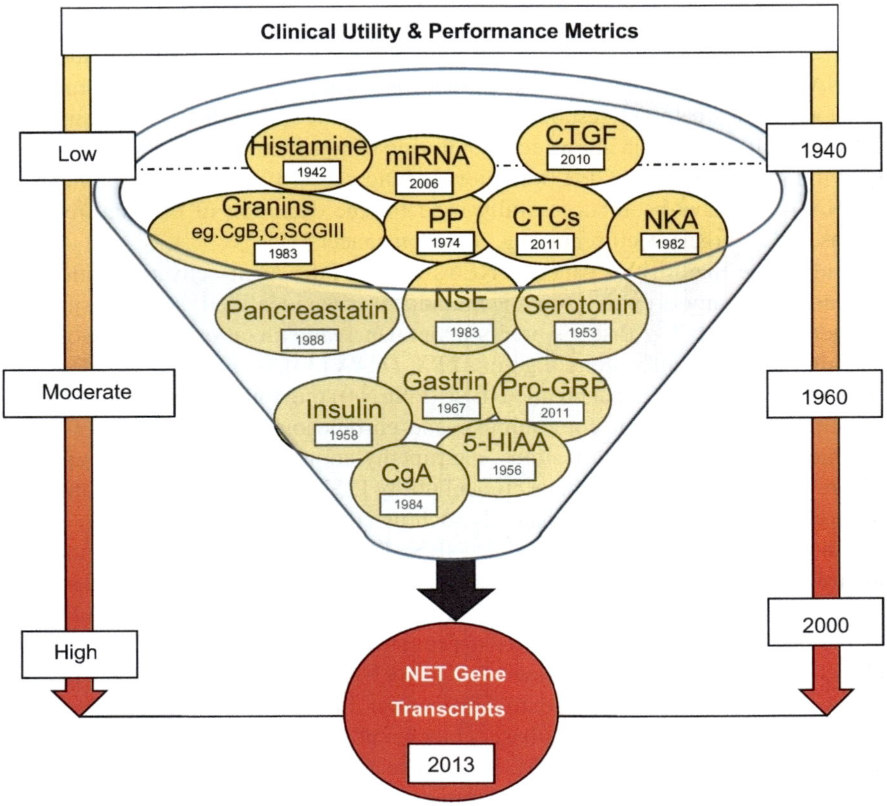

Fig. 6.2 Assessment of advances in NET biomarker development. The left arrow indicates increasing clinical utility and performance metrics. The right arrow indicates NET biomarker advancements between the 1940s and 2019. In 1942, histamine was described and, in the 1950s, other monoanalytes, e.g., 5-HIAA and insulin. More recently, techniques include microRNAs (2006) or CTCs (2011) and NET transcripts (NETest) (2013). Insulin and gastrin have clinical utility in a subset of functional tumors. NSE, pancreatic polypeptide, NKA, pancreastatin, and CTGF all display nonoptimal performance metrics. Serotonin, urinary 5-HIAA, and CgA have moderate utility but variable metrics. *CgA* chromogranin A, *CTGF* connective tissue growth factor, *NSE* neuron-specific enolase, *PP* pancreatic polypeptide, *Pro-GRP* progastrin-releasing peptide, *u5-HIAA* urinary 5-hydroxyindoleacetic acid

6.3 The Scientific Basis of Blood-Based Multi-Genomic Assay (NETest)

In 1996, the detection of circulating tumor-associated mRNA was first described in the blood of patients with melanoma [39]. The presence of tumor-derived mRNA in the blood is of clinical relevance since it enables the identification of tumor-specific gene expression profiles. Somatic mutations in DNA only represent a subset of the molecular alterations associated with cancers and do not fully recapitulate changes in

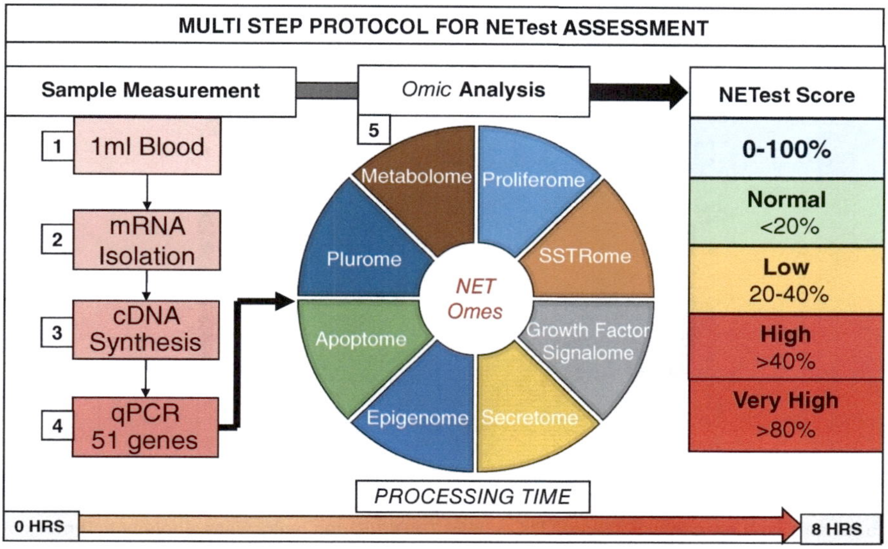

Fig. 6.3 The multistep NETest protocol to provide a multigene expression score. A two-step protocol (mRNA isolation and cDNA synthesis) is undertaken prior to quantitative PCR gene expression. NET omes are analyzed and normalized, and the 51-marker signature is interrogated using mathematical algorithms to provide a scaled score of 0–100 (the NETest score). The NETest delineates in a specific patient, irrespective of whether the tumor falls into a category of low ($\leq$40), intermediate (41–79), or high ($\geq$80) risk of disease activity

gene expression profiles that might result from epigenetic alterations, the effects of miRNAs, or other mechanisms. Thus, blood-based RNA profiling of a specific tumor can provide unique biological information directly relevant to the individual [23].

The NETest signature is based on transcriptomic evaluation of NETs per gene discovery, followed by evaluation and validation of the assay in training and independent sets [40]. The basis of the assay is provided by mRNA isolation from stabilized whole blood with subsequent complementary DNA (cDNA) production measured by polymerase chain reaction (PCR) (Fig. 6.3) [40]. The final results are expressed as an activity index (a NETest score) ranging from 0 (low activity) to 100 (high activity) [38, 41, 42]. This score provides a prediction of the clinical status of an individual tumor based on NET gene expression levels. The normal score cutoff is $\leq$20. Scores between 20 and 40 represent a low biological activity associated with "stable" disease. Values 41–100 identify progressive disease [5, 38, 43–48]. Clinical studies have confirmed the utility of the NETest for the assessment of disease status (stable/progressive); a concordance of 85–95% was identified [5, 48].

The metrics of this signature as a diagnostic exhibit a sensitivity/specificity of 90–97% [5, 48]. Comparative studies have confirmed the utility of the NETest as a diagnostic. Significantly better metrics were determined for the multigene approach (area under the curve (AUC): 0.95–0.98) versus commonly used biomarkers like CgA (AUC: 0.64), pancreastatin (0.58), or neurokinin A (0.63) [5, 49].

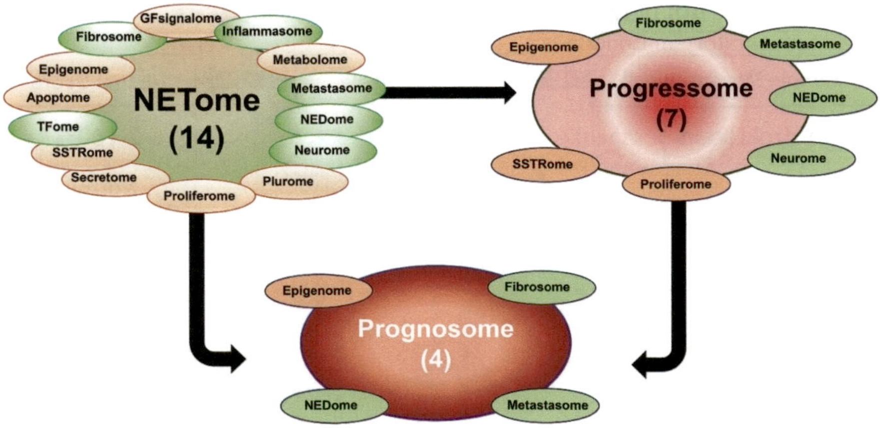

Fig. 6.4 Omics gene expression in the NETest. The NETest amplifies 51 genes, which comprises "14 omes" (left: NETome). Seven omes are consistently elevated above the upper limit of normal in patients with progressive disease. These omes constitute the molecular pathology hallmarks of progressive disease (right: progressome) and define progressive disease (PD). Prognostic information (bottom) can be derived from four omes that constitute the prognosome (epigenome, fibrosome, metastasome, and NEDome). This omics group can be used in conjunction with the NETest as a proctor of progressive disease

To expand the utility of the test from a pure diagnostic to a tool that could capture the biology of neuroendocrine neoplasia, regulatory network analysis was undertaken (Fig. 6.4). Briefly, this approach involves mapping NET-specific genes to a database of human protein–protein interactions, thus visualizing marker genes in the context of their respective biological function. This strategy identified 14 biologically relevant gene "omics" clusters, which define the NENs "fingerprint" and constitute the "oncobiome" of the NET cell [50]. The oncobiome is overall constituted by gene expression in the apoptome, epigenome, fibrosome, growth factor (GF)-signalome, inflammasome, metabolome, metastasome, NEDome, neuroma, plurome, proliferome, secretome, SSTRome, and TFome.

Differential analysis of gene expression in seven of the clusters (epigenome, fibrosome, metastasome, NEDome, neurome, proliferome, and SSTRome) can then be mathematically analyzed to deduce the "progressome," which differentiates stable from progressive disease [50]. These constitute a molecular representation of the "biological signature" of an individual tumor, and this strategy captures the biology of a specific NENs and defines the molecular status of an individual tumor [38]. Progressive tumors exhibit elevated expression of genes in the progressome, which correlates with the NETest scores >40. The higher the score, the greater the number of omes that are upregulated in the progressome. Further analysis of the progressome demonstrated a set of four omics clusters that can be used as a prognostic. Expression levels of the epigenome, fibrosome, metastasome, and NEDome can be used to predict those patients with a low score (NETest ≤40) that will develop progressive disease (Fig. 6.4) [50].

The multianalyte algorithmic analysis procedure has been validated [51] and is undertaken in Clinical Laboratory Improvement Amendments (CLIA)-certified clinical laboratories in London and Connecticut (state of CT: 07D2081388, Sarah Cannon laboratory in London UK). The inter-assay variability is 2.14 ± 1.14%, and the intra-assay variability is 1.02 ± 0.74% [51]. In clinical studies, the intra-assay reproducibility ranges from 0.4% to 1% for individual gene expression. Assessment of PCR cycle times, normalized gene expression, and scoring demonstrate high correlation levels (Spearman >0.90). Consecutive daily analysis of NENs samples had a Spearman's correlation for scored expression of 0.96 ($p < 0.001$, coefficient of variation (CV) <5%). The summated NETest data assessed in ~100,000 samples from ~100 different institutions (USA and Europe) and ~250 physicians indicate that the day-to-day variability for the test is extremely low (<2%) and that the test is highly reproducible (sample concordance >95%).

Measurement of the NETest signature in the blood is robust and not affected by food intake [51]. Assessment of the gene expression measurements using unsupervised hierarchical clustering failed to identify intrinsic relationships between feeding and gene expression, and the NETest was not altered over a 4-h period following a test meal [51]. No relationship between age, sex and ethnicity, and PPI usage was identifiable [51]. The latter is a particular issue in the measurement of CgA since PPIs significantly increase CgA levels [52]. NETest scores are not affected by long-term PPI treatment (>1 year). Overall, the test was demonstrated to exhibit a reliably high level of sensitivity and specificity (both >95%) [40], to be standardized and reproducible (inter- and intra-assay CV <2%) [51], and to be unaffected by age, gender, ethnicity, fasting, or PPI medication [51, 53]. The pre-spotted PCR plate protocol for the NETest has been established and prospectively tested in clinical samples. It is highly reproducible, has similar metrics (CV, categorization by control or NETs) to the standard PCR assay, and generates clinically concordant (>96%) NETest results. Moreover, it functions significantly more accurately than CgA (Fig. 6.5) [54].

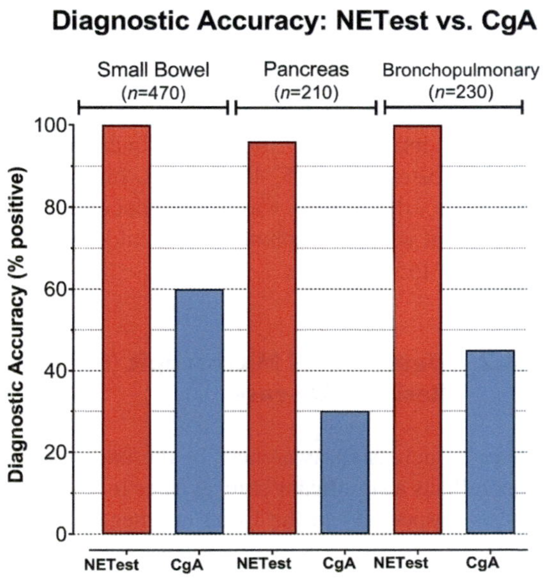

Fig. 6.5 Comparison of the accuracy of circulating NET transcript measurement (NETest) to chromogranin A. The NETest is positive in 96–100% of bronchopulmonary, pancreatic, and small bowel NETs. CgA, in contrast, is significantly less accurate. It is positive (elevated) in only ~30–60%. In PNETs, CgA is elevated in only 30% of tumors. Overall, CgA levels are normal in 40–70% of patients with NENs, thus significantly limiting its clinical utility as a biomarker

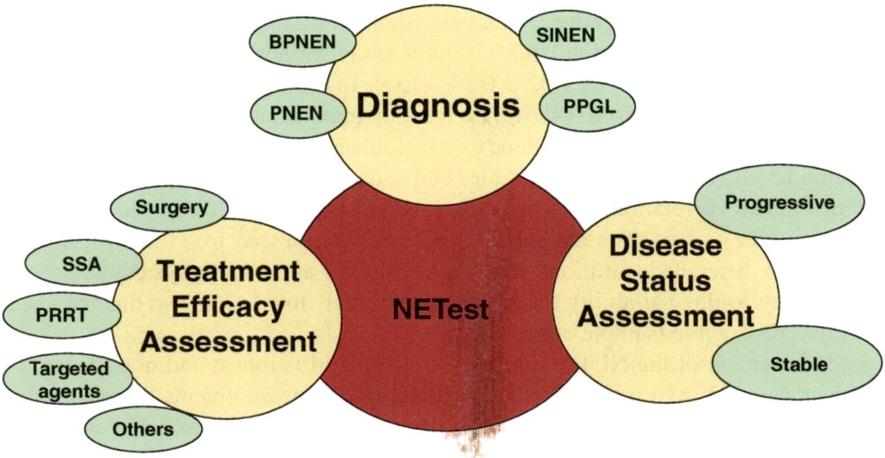

Fig. 6.6 Clinical applications of the NETest. The NETest, a novel multigene liquid biopsy, is as an accurate NET diagnostic (all NET sites, gastroenteropancreatic and bronchopulmonary NETs, paragangliomas, and pheochromocytomas). The assay identifies progressive versus stable disease and facilitates real-time assessment of the treatment efficacy (surgery, SSA, PRRT, etc.). *GEP NETs* gastroenteropancreatic NETs, *BPNETs* bronchopulmonary NETs

6.4 Diagnostic Applications of the NETest

6.4.1 Correlation with Imaging and Disease Status

Although imaging exhibits limitations in NET management, it remains the critical arbiter of NET disease diagnostic workup and monitoring (Fig. 6.6). A liquid biopsy, which would correlate, or *ideally* outperform it, would have substantial clinical utility given the opportunity to decrease radiation exposure and costs. A recent independent validation study [55] has assessed the concordance of the NETest liquid biopsy with anatomical and functional imaging [55]. The NETest accurately correlated with imaging, and the concordances was: computed tomography/magnetic resonance imaging (CT/MRI) 92%, functional imaging 94%, and when all modalities were used 96% [45, 46, 55, 56]. In image-positive disease (macroscopically detectable), the NETest was 100% concordant with anatomical imaging and 98% concordant with ^{68}Ga-somatostatin analogue (SSA) positron emission tomography (PET)/CT [55].

6.4.2 Detection of Microscopic (Occult Metastatic) or Residual Disease

There is increasing awareness of the underestimation of disease burden [57–59]. This reflects a significant clinical issue in terms of treatment delay. Since metastatic disease (especially in the liver) is a negative prognostic factor, failure to identify would be predicted to negatively impact outcome. Thus, the failure to initiate timely therapy can be expected to adversely impact outcome. Based upon the limitations in spatial resolution <2–4 mm (CT/MRI) or ~5 mm (^{68}Ga-SSA PET/CT or ^{18}F-fludeoxyglucose PET/CT), it can be inferred that low-volume disease will not be detected. In contrast, circulating *NET* genes can identify as little as one tumor cell/milliliter [5]. Thus, it is predictable that the presence of micrometastatic disease is more likely to be identified by sophisticated molecular amplification (gene expression PCR) techniques. In support of this assertion, it has been demonstrated that the NETest could detect occult liver metastatic disease that was undetectable by imaging or monoanalyte biomarkers but confirmed by histology [60]. The assay also enabled monitoring disease progression and response to given therapies (peptide receptor radionuclide therapy (PRRT), SSA) [60]. Furthermore, the NETest has been shown to precede the alterations on imaging by 6–24 months, which enables early implementation of effective treatment [5, 41, 44–46, 60, 61]. This paradigm shift in the levels of disease detection opens a novel clinical discussion as to how one may treat disease that is undetectable by imaging but identified by more sensitive molecular technology. What will be the criteria for the treatment of invisible disease and would it be monitored by molecular tools as opposed to the previous norm, represented by imaging? More specifically, will NET experts be able to advance from palliation to cure, if the disease can be captured earlier?

6.4.3 Identification of Gastroenteropancreatic (GEP) NENs

6.4.3.1 Small Intestinal NENs (SINENs)

The NETest has a high accuracy level (~95%) in the diagnosis of NETs of the small intestine. Furthermore, it can accurately (>95%) distinguish a neuroendocrine bowel tumor from adenocarcinoma of the small and large intestines. A prospective analysis demonstrated an accuracy of 100% in the identification of small intestinal NENs, with three false positives being colorectal cancers [62]. CgA levels were elevated in 80%, but 29% ($n = 7$) of colorectal tumors had increased CgA levels. Metastatic small intestinal NENs exhibited increased NETest levels compared to localized disease. Overall, NETest levels in SINENs were more accurate (76–80%) than were CgA levels (20–32%) for detecting disease [62]. In a recent, independent validation study, in a GEP NET cohort (pancreatic NENs, $n = 67$, SINENs, $n = 44$), the diagnostic accuracy, sensitivity, and specificity of the NETest were 97, 99, and 95%, respectively. The overall accuracy of the NETest (a cutoff of 40) for differentiating progressive from stable disease based on Response Evaluation Criteria in Solid Tumors (RECIST) 1.1 criteria was 95% [55].

6.4.3.2 Pancreatic NENs (PNENs)

Pancreatic disease is sometimes difficult to accurately diagnose since fibrosis and cystic disease confound clinical and imaging interpretations. The NETest can accurately differentiate (94%) these conditions by identification of PNENs [62]. Elevations of blood CgA were identifiable in 29% of PNENs, providing an overall diagnostic accuracy of 56% [62]. The NETest identified 6% (2/31) of intra-pancreatic mucinous neoplasia as positive. This is consistent with the coexistence of PNENs and mucinous pancreatic disease (Fig. 6.6) [63].

6.4.4 Bronchopulmonary Neuroendocrine Neoplasms (BPNENs)

The NETest can identify neuroendocrine lung lesions in ~90% and differentiate neuroendocrine lung tumors from controls with ~95% accuracy and a receiver operating characteristic (ROC) analysis AUC of 0.96–0.99 [56, 64]. In contradistinction, the monoanalyte biomarker CgA was increased in only 19–33%. NETest sensitivity and specificity range from 93 to 95% and 82 to 93%, respectively [65]. A clinical analysis indicated that stable disease levels (33 ± 17) were significantly lower than progressive disease levels (72 ± 23) irrespective of the histology. Surgical resection considered decreased curative levels of 10 ± 5, whereas localized disease had levels of 45 ± 21 compared to disseminated tumors with levels of 63 ± 26. Quantification of the clinical value of NETest vs. CgA using decision curve analysis indicated a >75% standardized clinical net benefit up to a risk threshold of 90% for gene expression analysis as compared to CgA. Overall, CgA as a lung NET marker displayed a net clinical benefit in <30% of patients.

In a recent, multicenter, and multinational independent validation study, elevated NETest levels were diagnostic of bronchopulmonary NETs and tumor tissue gene expression was correlated with blood levels [56]. The levels were consistent with imaging data and accurately defined disease progression [55]. The NETest was significantly increased in lung carcinoids ($n = 99$, 45 ± 25) compared to control subjects (9 ± 8, $p < 0.0001$); the ROC AUC was 0.96 ± 0.01. The metrics of the test were overall accuracy (92%), sensitivity (84%), and specificity (100%). Levels in stable disease were 36 ± 18 as compared to 61 ± 26 in progressive disease ($p < 0.0001$). Disseminated tumor exhibited NETest elevation regardless of histological subtype (atypical carcinoid (AC): $p < 0.02$; typical carcinoid (TC): $p = 0.0006$). The NETest was also elevated in small cell lung cancer (SCLC) (42 ± 32) and large cell neuroendocrine carcinoma (28 ± 7). In non-endocrine lung cancers, adenocarcinoma (18 ± 21) and squamous cell carcinoma (SCC) (12 ± 11) levels were significantly lower than in lung NETs (carcinoids, $p < 0.001$). Benign lung disease, such as idiopathic pulmonary fibrosis, exhibited increased levels (18 ± 25). The paired comparability of the tumor with the blood levels of gene expression indicates significant correlation for lung NETs (carcinoids; R: 0.83, $p < 0.0001$) and SCLC (R: 0.68) but not for SCC and adenocarcinoma (ACC) (R: 0.25–0.31). This is consistent with the interpretation that the gene signature originates in the tumor.

6.4.5 Paragangliomas and Pheochromocytomas (PPGLs)

The NETest accuracy for tumor identification was identified as 100% in one series [66]. Analysis of the ROC area under the curve demonstrated a value of 0.98 in distinguishing these neural crest-derived lesions from controls. Local disease had lower NETest levels (43 ± 7) than did multicentric (64 ± 9) or metastatic disease (80 ± 9) ($p < 0.04$). Gene expression levels distinguished stable (41 ± 2) from progressive disease (86 ± 2) $p < 0.0001$) [66]. Moreover, there was a significant relationship between gene expression and PPGL molecular subtyping; cluster II tumors (*SDHx* mutations) exhibited higher NETest scores than did cluster I tumors (*MEN2/VHL* and *NF-2* mutations) consistent with their more aggressive phenotype [66]. The overall diagnostic accuracy of the NETest for PPGLs was ~95%.

6.4.6 Validation Studies

Independent validation studies are important in biomarker implementation. The NETest has been independently validated in clinical GEP [55, 67, 68] and lung [56] cohorts, providing further evidence for >90% sensitivity, specificity, and accuracy [5]. In 2018, the biological basis of the signature was validated in an independent genomic-based multicenter National Institutes of Health (NIH)-funded study (10,224 tumor specimens from 32 different tumor types) that demonstrated that the NETest gene panel was significantly and specifically related to neuroendocrine tumors [69]. A recent meta-analysis has confirmed that the test was an effective diagnostic (94.9–96% accurate), a marker of natural history (90.2–93.6%), and exhibited excellent metrics as an interventional/response biomarker (93.7–97.4%) [48].

6.5 The NETest for Assessment of Therapy Efficacy

6.5.1 Surgical Resection/Detection of Residual Disease

6.5.1.1 GEPNENs

Alteration in NETest levels pre- and post-tumor resection provides objective evidence of complete tumor resection or identifies residual disease. A prospective analysis of 30 pancreatic NENs reported that all exhibited elevated NETest levels pre-surgery, whereas only 9 had increased CgA levels [70]. Successful removal of the tumor reduced transcript levels from 45 ± 27 to 25 ± 24 ($p < 0.0001$). Alterations in CgA did not correlate with tumor resection. Of the 26 patients that had R0 resections, 4 still had increased NETest levels at 1 month. At 6 months post-surgery, all four had image-positive evidence of tumor recurrence.

6.5.1.2 BPNENs

Alteration in NETest levels pre- and post-lung tumor resection provides objective evidence of complete tumor resection or identifies residual disease.

In a prospective study of 37 NENs lung resections, all had elevated levels pre-surgery (68 ± 15). The NETest levels at 6 months had returned to normal in 28 patients [65]. Nine patients, however, had elevated levels post-surgery (66 ± 8%) and image evidence of disease recurrence. The 28 patients assessed as "disease-free" exhibited a significant decrease in the NETest levels to 23 ± 5 ($p = 0.0002$). CgA, in contrast, was not effective as a measure of effective surgical resection.

Separately, an evaluation in other lung cancers undergoing surgery identified that the NETest levels, as expected, were low in these cancers and not affected by surgical procedures. Measurements of NETest levels in BPNENs provide objective evidence of tumor removal and identify residual disease or recurrence accurately.

6.5.2 Somatostatin Analogue (SSA) Efficacy

The NETest is effective in assessing the efficacy of SSA therapy irrespective of whether sandostatin or lanreotide is used. In a prospective, blinded investigation ($n = 28$), it was compared to CgA to assess treatment failure [44]. Therapy response could be predicted using univariate analysis of tumor grade and the NETest. Using multiple regression analysis, only the NETest predicted disease progression during SSA usage ($p = 0.0002$). Of note was the observation that blood levels of transcripts preceded imaging changes [46]. Analysis of CgA data indicated that it had no predictive value. In a separate study, progression could be identified in 100% of patients using the NETest [46].

There has been concern that investigative studies do not accurately capture "real-world" conditions in which most medical doctors (MDs) function [71, 72]. However, a US Registry study (NCT02270567) designed to assess the utility of the NETest under such conditions demonstrated considerable efficacy [46]. A US prospective observational investigation of SSA-treated patients ($n = 51$) demonstrated with a low score (≤40%) that all ($n = 37$) patients could be managed without any treatment modification (type or dose). Conversely, those ($n = 24$) with an elevated score (≥80%) experienced a treatment modification (86%). This second high NETest-level group ($n = 24$) was all identified to have disease progression indicative of failed SSA therapy. In this group 21/24) underwent treatment change (dose escalation of SSA, different brand of SSA or addition of other therapy such as liver embolization or PRRT). All ($n = 21$) were then reported to have image-based stable disease after 6 months. In the low-score group, the median progression free survival (PFS) was not demonstrable, whereas in the high-score group, an median progrssion free survival (mPFS) of 5 months was identified (chi-squared = 27.7, hazard ratio (HR) 60, $p < 0.0001$) (Fig. 6.7).

6.5.3 Peptide Receptor Radionuclide Therapy (PRRT)

This modality of therapy has now obtained the Food and Drug Administration (FDA)'s approval and is effective in certain groups of patients [73]. The standard technique for stratifying such patients for PRRT is based upon image-based subjective assessment of somatostatin receptor uptake [74, 75]. Nevertheless, only ~60% of individuals with the most promising characteristics for PRRT at somatostatin receptor imaging respond to the therapy [73]. NETest levels in PRRT patients demonstrate that the NETest correlated accurately (94%) with PRRT responders (97%) vs. nonresponders (91%) [41]. Of note was that alterations in NETest scores during PRRT exhibited (89%, $p < 10^{-6}$) concordance with the clinical assessment of response (RECIST). Alterations in CgA levels were concordant in 24% [41].

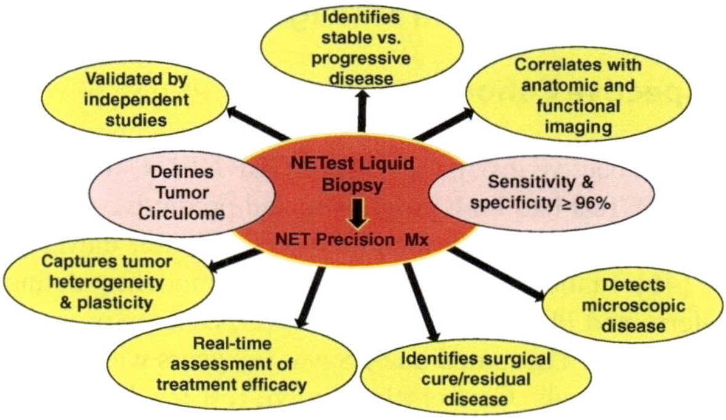

Fig. 6.7 The NETest liquid biopsy as a NET precision management tool. The NETest is a multigene liquid biopsy, which measures the neuroendocrine tumor circulome and captures in real time tumor heterogeneity and plasticity (tumor biology). Its clinical utility encompasses diagnosis of NETs at different sites, including gastroenteropancreatic NETs, bronchopulmonary NETs, paragangliomas, and pheochromocytomas, as well as identification of disease progression and microscopic disease. The assay correlates with anatomical and functional imaging and facilitates real-time assessment of residual disease and treatment efficacy (surgery, SSA, PRRT, etc.)

Since somatostatin receptor expression is a subjective assessment and not highly accurate in predicting PRRT efficacy, a gene-based positive predictive quotient in the blood was developed to accurately stratify patients. This is based upon a blood-based analysis and integration genes from the NET metabolome and growth factor signalome with Ki-67 levels [41].

The growth factor and the metabolomic genes used in the signature are related to oxidative stress, metabolism, and hypoxic signaling [76–78]. The elevated expression of these genes in the blood probably identifies tumors that are more radiosensitive given the role of hypoxia, oxidative stress, and loss of DNA repair associated with radiation responsivity [79]. The specificity of PRRT efficacy prediction therefore reflects the identification of molecular mechanisms related to radiation response-associated genes, which modulate tumor response to PRRT [80].

The PRRT predictive quotient (PPQ) was prospectively evaluated in three independent PRRT studies ($n = 158$) [42]. It is a binary predictive tool, which identifies a patient as either positive (PRRT-responsive) or negative (PRRT-nonresponsive). Analysis of the data from 158 PRRT-treated patients using decision curve analysis identified a >90% predictive benefit up to a risk threshold of 80% for the PPQ test. A comparison of CgA or grade as predictors demonstrated that neither was of any benefit (<10% across comparable risk thresholds). PPQ was in aggregate of the 3 studies 94–97% accurate in the prediction of PRRT efficacy. Clinical correlation of the accuracy of prediction demonstrated that predicted nonresponders had an mPFS of 8–14 months, whereas the mPFS in responders did not reach 31 months after treatment. Hazard ratio calculation demonstrated a value of 47 for the PPQ. NETest levels and PPQ assessment of PRRT therapy demonstrated a >90% efficacy for prediction and treatment monitoring [41].

6.6 Monitoring Long-Term Management

6.6.1 Retrospective Cohort Analysis

Assessment of a prospective group ($n = 34$) of GEP NENs studied for 5 years demonstrated that the NETest had both prognostic and predictive utility in GEP NENs. Image-based progression was only identified ~1 year after elevated NETest levels were detectable [45]. In the assessment of PFS, Cox modeling defined that the only variable that determined PFS was the NETest level. Disease progression was definable by the NETest level. Thus, median PFS was 0.7 years with levels >80 compared to 2.8 years with ≤40 levels. Conversely, if a NETest level was >40 in individuals clinically classified as stable, the value was 100% prognostic for progression. If the baseline NETest level was ≤40, then it accurately predicted stability (100%) over 5 years. CgA values in comparison had no value. Thus, a chi-squared analysis evaluating the NETest levels to CgA assessed the NETest to be 96% more instructive than CgA ($p < 0.001$) in predicting alteration in disease status [45].

6.6.2 Prospective Observational Registry Study

This was undertaken to assess whether a NETest level could be used as an adjunct to management decisions in a prospective observational study. Analysis of 100 patients (Registry study: NCT02270567) [46] provided prospective information with regard to management strategy. In a watch-and-wait program ($n = 28$), a low NETest score defined conservative management. All 28 patients remained stable at 12 months follow-up. In the high-score group (NETest ≥80; $n = 12$), all were considered to be clinically progressive and underwent treatment intervention. At 12 months, all had disease stabilization (imaging interpretation or symptom diminution). The high-score group had an mPFS of 3 months, which was significantly less than that of the low-score group (chi-squared = 28, HR 30, $p < 0.0001$). CgA in comparison was of no clinical value by McNemar's test (comparison of two biomarkers in paired sample sets) in decision-making. Of interest in the final assessment was the observation that a low NETest score decreased the utilization of imaging by ~40%.

6.7 Conclusions

The NETest multigene measurement has been analytically and clinically validated in >10,000 patients, in multicenter studies worldwide, both prospectively and independently. The platform (quantitative PCR (qPCR)) is highly sensitive, detection of tumor-related genes is rapid, reproducible, and cost-effective, and protocols are standardized, even in pre-spotted PCR plate technology. Conventional biomarkers are typically elevated at advanced/extensive disease stage, whereas circulating *NET* genes can be identified in as few as one tumor cell/milliliter. One of the challenges of utilization of circulating mRNA had been the need for cautious handling (time, immediate cooling/freezing protocols). This has now been supplanted by the development of a stabilization protocol that enables mRNA to be usable for 1 week at room temperature. The published data identify the value of transcriptomic analysis in the diagnostic and monitoring setting of a variety of therapeutic modalities, particularly in conjunction with other clinical and imaging parameters to monitor disease progression. We predict that future strategies for refining and improving the evaluation of therapy will be provided by incorporating imaging modalities and the blood-based molecular information provided by tumor transcriptomic analysis.

6.8 CODA

There is a clear need for accurate and sophisticated novel biomarkers. The strategy that is most likely to fulfill such criteria is represented by liquid biopsy as opposed to tissue biopsy. The former technique is noninvasive, can be repeated as information is desired, and provides real-time information without the potential adverse events associated with tissue biopsy. Such a strategy would provide information adjunctive to imaging and probably decrease the need for an intensive use of the latter. Of particular interest would be the opportunity to incorporate into liquid biopsies, information that can identify an appropriate therapy for a particular tumor. This would obviate the use of drugs that fail, which could lead to adverse events and place an unnecessary burden on the health economic system. A good example is provided by circulating RNA-based PRRT-predictive signature. A predictor strategy is of importance not only for forecasting drug efficacy but also for identifying potential drug toxicity. Although PRRT is in general well-tolerated, kidney toxicity is a small but significant issue, whereas rare bone marrow toxicity can be lethal. Both adverse events are not predictable, their pathogenesis is undefined, and there is a need to understand who may be at risk. The identification of transcriptional profiles for the blood or kidney that can monitor such emerging risks or predict them is an important developmental goal.

Omics analysis is predicted to facilitate further stratification of the tumors based on their aggressiveness, propensity to progress, and predicted response to various treatments. These novel biomarkers should have three abilities, which should embrace the diagnosis, prediction, and assessment of disease prognosis. In clinical terms, this would facilitate early identification of disease, forecast with certitude the likelihood of therapeutic efficacy, and be able to accurately monitor disease status. Furthermore, minimization of a blood sample required for analysis (<1 ml) would be of great practicality, and current strategies enable the use of ~100 uL to accurately identify tumors with equal facility to 1 ml of venous blood.

References

1. Modlin IM, Bodei L, Kidd M (2016) Neuroendocrine tumor biomarkers: from monoanalytes to transcripts and algorithms. Best Pract Res Clin Endocrinol Metab 30(1):59–77
2. Kulke MH, Siu LL, Tepper JE, Fisher G, Jaffe D, Haller DG et al (2011) Future directions in the treatment of neuroendocrine tumors: consensus report of the National Cancer Institute Neuroendocrine Tumor clinical trials planning meeting. J Clin Oncol 29(7):934–943
3. Kidd M, Bodei L, Modlin IM (2015) Chromogranin A: any relevance in neuroendocrine tumors? Curr Opin Endocrinol Diabetes Obes 30:30
4. Berger D (1999) A brief history of medical diagnosis and the birth of the clinical laboratory. Part 1–ancient times through the 19th century. MLO 31(7):28–30
5. Modlin IM, Kidd M, Malczewska A, Drozdov I, Bodei L, Matar S et al (2018) The NETest: the clinical utility of multigene blood analysis in the diagnosis and management of neuroendocrine tumors. Endocrinol Metab Clin N Am 47(3):485–504
6. Oberg K, Modlin IM, De Herder W, Pavel M, Klimstra D, Frilling A et al (2015) Consensus on biomarkers for neuroendocrine tumour disease. Lancet Oncol 16(9):e435–ee46
7. Modlin IM, Oberg K, Taylor A, Drozdov I, Bodei L, Kidd M (2014) Neuroendocrine tumor biomarkers: current status and perspectives. Neuroendocrinology 100(4):265–277
8. Yao JC, Pavel M, Phan AT, Kulke MH, Hoosen S, St Peter J et al (2011) Chromogranin A and neuron-specific enolase as prognostic markers in patients with advanced pNET treated with everolimus. J Clin Endocrinol Metab 96(12):3741–3749. Epub 2011 Oct 12
9. Marotta V, Zatelli MC, Sciammarella C, Ambrosio MR, Bondanelli M, Colao A et al (2018) Chromogranin A as circulating marker for diagnosis and management of neuroendocrine neoplasms: more flaws than fame. Endocr Relat Cancer 25(1):R11–R29
10. Pulvirenti A, Rao D, McIntyre CA, Gonen M, Tang LH, Klimstra DS et al (2018) Limited role of chromogranin A as clinical biomarker for pancreatic neuroendocrine tumors. HPB 21(5):612–618
11. Rossi RE, Ciafardini C, Sciola V, Conte D, Massironi S (2018) Chromogranin A in the follow-up of gastroenteropancreatic neuroendocrine neoplasms: is it really game over? A systematic review and meta-analysis. Pancreas 47(10):1249–1255
12. Malczewska A, Kidd M, Matar S, Kos-Kudla B, Bodei L, Oberg K et al (2019) An assessment of circulating Chromogranin A as a biomarker of bronchopulmonary neuroendocrine neoplasia: a systematic review and meta-analysis. Neuroendocrinology 110(3-4):198–216
13. Matar S, Malczewska A, Oberg K, Bodei L, Aslanian H, Lewczuk-Myslicka A et al (2019) Blood chromogranin A is not effective as a biomarker for diagnosis or management of bronchopulmonary NET/NET. Neuroendocrinology 110(3-4):185–197
14. Stridsberg M, Eriksson B, Oberg K, Janson ET (2003) A comparison between three commercial kits for chromogranin A measurements. J Endocrinol 177(2):337–341
15. Italian Network for Quality Assessment of Tumor Biomarkers Group (2005) An Italian program of external quality control for chromogranin A (CgA) assay: state of the art of CgA measurement. Int J Biol Markers 20(4):264–268
16. Leon A, Torta M, Dittadi R, Degli Uberti E, Ambrosio MR, Delle Fave G et al (2005) Comparison between two methods in the determination of circulating chromogranin A in neuroendocrine tumors (NETs): results of a prospective multicenter observational study. Int J Biol Markers 20(3):156–168
17. Verderio P, Dittadi R, Marubini E, Pizzamiglio S, Gion M, De Apollonia L et al (2007) An Italian program of external quality control for chromogranin A (CgA) assay: performance evaluation of CgA determination. Clin Chem Lab Med 45(9):1244–1250
18. Zatelli MC, Torta M, Leon A, Ambrosio MR, Gion M, Tomassetti P et al (2007) Chromogranin A as a marker of neuroendocrine neoplasia: an Italian Multicenter Study. Endocr Relat Cancer 14(2):473–482
19. Oberg K, Couvelard A, Delle Fave G, Gross D, Grossman A, Jensen RT et al (2017) ENETS consensus guidelines for standard of care in neuroendocrine tumours: biochemical

markers. Neuroendocrinology 105(3):201–211. https://doi.org/10.1159/000472254. Epub 2017 Apr 8
20. Modlin IM, Gustafsson BI, Moss SF, Pavel M, Tsolakis AV, Kidd M (2010) Chromogranin A–biological function and clinical utility in neuro endocrine tumor disease. Ann Surg Oncol 17(9):2427–2443
21. Gut P, Czarnywojtek A, Fischbach J, Baczyk M, Ziemnicka K, Wrotkowska E et al (2016) Chromogranin A - unspecific neuroendocrine marker. Clinical utility and potential diagnostic pitfalls. Arch Med Sci 12(1):1–9
22. Malczewska AK-KB, Kidd M, Drozdov I, Bodei L, Matar S, Oberg K, Modlin IM (2019) The clinical applications of a multigene liquid biopsy (NETest) in neuroendocrine tumors. Adv Med Sci 65(1):18–29
23. Siravegna G, Marsoni S, Siena S, Bardelli A (2017) Integrating liquid biopsies into the management of cancer. Nat Rev Clin Oncol 14(9):531–548
24. De Rubis G, Rajeev Krishnan S, Bebawy M (2019) Liquid biopsies in cancer diagnosis, monitoring, and prognosis. Trends Pharmacol Sci 40(3):172–186
25. Kidd M, Modlin I, Bodei L, Drozdov I (2015) Decoding the molecular and mutational ambiguities of gastroenteropancreatic neuroendocrine neoplasm pathobiology. Cell Mol Gastroenterol Hepatol 1:131–153
26. Walenkamp A, Crespo G, Fierro Maya F, Fossmark R, Igaz P, Rinke A et al (2014) Hallmarks of gastrointestinal neuroendocrine tumours: implications for treatment. Endocr Relat Cancer 21(6):R445–R460. https://doi.org/10.1530/ERC-14-0106
27. Wang E, Zaman N, McGee S, Milanese JS, Masoudi-Nejad A, O'Connor-McCourt M (2014) Predictive genomics: a cancer hallmark network framework for predicting tumor clinical phenotypes using genome sequencing data. Semin Cancer Biol 18(14):50–59
28. Siravegna G, Marsoni S, Siena S, Bardelli A (2017) Integrating liquid biopsies into the management of cancer. Nat Rev Clin Oncol 2(10):14
29. Oxnard GR, Paweletz CP, Kuang Y, Mach SL, O'Connell A, Messineo MM et al (2014) Noninvasive detection of response and resistance in EGFR-mutant lung cancer using quantitative next-generation genotyping of cell-free plasma DNA. Clin Cancer Res 20(6):1698–1705. https://doi.org/10.1158/1078-0432.CCR-13-2482. Epub 014 Jan 15
30. Remon J, Caramella C, Jovelet C, Lacroix L, Lawson A, Smalley S et al (2017) Osimertinib benefit in EGFR-mutant NSCLC patients with T790M-mutation detected by circulating tumour DNA. Ann Oncol 28(4):784–790. https://doi.org/10.1093/annonc/mdx017
31. Reinert T, Scholer LV, Thomsen R, Tobiasen H, Vang S, Nordentoft I et al (2015) Analysis of circulating tumour DNA to monitor disease burden following colorectal cancer surgery. Gut 4:308859
32. Kidd M, Modlin I, Oberg K (2016) Towards a new classification of gastroenteropancreatic neuroendocrine neoplasms. Nat Rev Clin Oncol 13(11):691–705. https://doi.org/10.1038/nrclinonc.2016.85. Epub 16 Jun 7
33. Jiao Y, Shi C, Edil BH, de Wilde RF, Klimstra DS, Maitra A et al (2011) DAXX/ATRX, MEN1, and mTOR pathway genes are frequently altered in pancreatic neuroendocrine tumors. Science 331(6021):1199–1203
34. Shay JW, Reddel RR, Wright WE (2012) Cancer and telomeres–an ALTernative to telomerase. Science 336(6087):1388–1390
35. Malczewska A, Kidd M, Matar S, Kos-Kudla B (2018) A comprehensive assessment of the role of miRNAs as biomarkers in gastroenteropancreatic neuroendocrine tumors. Neuroendocrinology 107(1):73–90
36. Oberg K, Modlin I, DeHerder W, Pavel M, Klimstra D, Frilling A et al (2015) Biomarkers for neuroendocrine tumor disease: a delphic consensus assessment of multianalytes, genomics, circulating cells and monoanalytes. Lancet Oncol 16:e435046
37. Patel K, Friedrich-Rust M, Lurie Y, Grigorescu M, Stanciu C, Lee CM et al (2011) FibroSURE and FibroScan in relation to treatment response in chronic hepatitis C virus. World J Gastroenterol 17(41):4581–4589. https://doi.org/10.3748/wjg.v17.i41.4581

38. Kidd M, Drozdov I, Modlin I (2015) Blood and tissue neuroendocrine tumor gene cluster analysis correlate, define hallmarks and predict disease status. Endocr Relat Cancer 22(4):561–575. https://doi.org/10.1530/ERC-15-0092. Epub 2015 Jun 2
39. Stevens GL, Scheer WD, Levine EA (1996) Detection of tyrosinase mRNA from the blood of melanoma patients. Cancer Epidemiol Biomarkers Prev 5(4):293–296
40. Modlin IM, Drozdov I, Kidd M (2013) The identification of gut neuroendocrine tumor disease by multiple synchronous transcript analysis in blood. PLoS One 8(5):e63364
41. Bodei L, Kidd M, Modlin IM, Severi S, Drozdov I, Nicolini S et al (2016) Measurement of circulating transcripts and gene cluster analysis predicts and defines therapeutic efficacy of peptide receptor radionuclide therapy (PRRT) in neuroendocrine tumors. Eur J Nucl Med Mol Imaging 43(5):839–851. https://doi.org/10.1007/s00259-015-3250-z. Epub 2015 Nov 23
42. Bodei L, Kidd MS, Singh A, van der Zwan WA, Severi S, Drozdov IA et al (2018) PRRT genomic signature in blood for prediction of 177Lu-octreotate efficacy. EJNMMI 45(7):1155–1169
43. Modlin I, Drozdov I, Kidd M (2013) A multitranscript blood neuroendocrine tumor molecular signature to identify treatment efficacy and disease progress. J Clin Oncol 31:A4137
44. Cwikla JB, Bodei L, Kolasinska-Cwikla A, Sankowski A, Modlin IM, Kidd M (2015) Circulating transcript analysis (NETest) in GEP-NETs treated with somatostatin analogs defines therapy. J Clin Endocrinol Metab 100(11):E1437–E1445
45. Pavel M, Jann H, Prasad V, Drozdov I, Modlin IM, Kidd M (2017) NET blood transcript analysis defines the crossing of the clinical rubicon: when stable disease becomes progressive. Neuroendocrinology 104(2):170–182
46. Liu E, Paulson S, Gulati A, Freudman J, Grosh W, Kafer S et al (2018) Assessment of NETest clinical utility in a U.S. Registry-Based Study. Oncologist 24(6):783–790
47. Liu E, Paulson S, Gulati A, Freudman J, Kafer S, Wickremesinghe P et al (2019) Assessment of NETest clinical utility in a US Registry-based study. Oncologist 24(6):783–790
48. Oberg K, Califano A, Strosberg J, Ma S, Pape U, Bodei L et al (2019) A meta-analysis of the accuracy of a neuroendocrine tumor mRNA genomic biomarker (NETest) in blood. Blood Ann Oncol 31(2):202–212
49. Modlin IM, Drozdov I, Alaimo D, Callahan S, Teixiera N, Bodei L et al (2014) A multianalyte PCR blood test outperforms single analyte ELISAs (chromogranin A, pancreastatin, neurokinin A) for neuroendocrine tumor detection. Endocr Relat Cancer 21(4):615–628
50. Kidd M, Kitz A, Drozdov I, Modlin I (2020) Neuroendocrine tumor omic gene cluster analysis amplifies the prognostic accuracy of the NETest. Neuroendocrinology 111(5):490–504
51. Modlin I, Drozdov I, Kidd M (2014) Gut neuroendocrine tumor blood qPCR fingerprint assay: characteristics and reproducibility. Clin Chem 52(3):419–429
52. Giusti M, Sidoti M, Augeri C, Rabitti C, Minuto F (2004) Effect of short-term treatment with low dosages of the proton-pump inhibitor omeprazole on serum chromogranin A levels in man. Eur J Endocrinol 150(3):299–303
53. Modlin IM, Aslanian H, Bodei L, Drozdov I, Kidd M (2014) A PCR blood test outperforms chromogranin A in carcinoid detection and is unaffected by PPIs. Endocr Connect 14:14
54. Kidd M, Drozdov IA, Matar S, Gurunlian N, Ferranti NJ, Malczewska A et al (2019) Utility of a ready-to-use PCR system for neuroendocrine tumor diagnosis. PLoS One 14(6):e0218592
55. Malczewska A, Witkowska M, Makulik K, Bocian A, Walter A, Pilch-Kowalczyk J et al (2019) NETest liquid biopsy is diagnostic of small intestine and pancreatic neuroendocrine tumors and correlates with imaging. Endocr Connect 8(4):442–453
56. Malczewska A, Oberg K, Bodei L, Aslanian H, Lewczuk A, Filosso PL et al (2019) NETest liquid biopsy is diagnostic of lung neuroendocrine tumors and identifies progressive disease. Neuroendocrinology 17:000497037
57. Elias D, Lefevre JH, Duvillard P, Goere D, Dromain C, Dumont F et al (2010) Hepatic metastases from neuroendocrine tumors with a "thin slice" pathological examination: they are many more than you think. Ann Surg 251(2):307–310
58. Clift AK, Faiz O, Al-Nahhas A, Bockisch A, Liedke MO, Schloericke E et al (2016) Role of staging in patients with small intestinal neuroendocrine tumours. J Gastrointest Surg 20(1):180–188. discussion 88.

59. Gibson WE, Gonzalez RS, Cates JMM, Liu E, Shi C (2018) Hepatic micrometastases are associated with poor prognosis in patients with liver metastases from neuroendocrine tumors of the digestive tract. Hum Pathol 79:109–115
60. Malczewska A, Bodei L, Kidd M, Modlin IM (2019) Blood mRNA Measurement (NETest) for neuroendocrine tumor diagnosis of image-negative liver metastatic disease. J Clin Endocrinol Metab 104(3):867–872
61. Modlin IM, Frilling A, Salem RR, Alaimo D, Drymousis P, Wasan HS et al (2016) Blood measurement of neuroendocrine gene transcripts defines the effectiveness of operative resection and ablation strategies. Surgery 159(1):336–347. https://doi.org/10.1016/j.surg.2015.06.056. Epub 15 Oct 9
62. Modlin IM, Kidd M, Bodei L, Drozdov I, Aslanian H (2015) The clinical utility of a novel blood-based multi-transcriptome assay for the diagnosis of neuroendocrine tumors of the gastrointestinal tract. Am J Gastroenterol 110(8):1223–1232. https://doi.org/10.1038/ajg.2015.160. Epub 15 Jun 2
63. Ishida M, Shiomi H, Naka S, Tani T, Okabe H (2013) Concomitant intraductal papillary mucinous neoplasm and neuroendocrine tumor of the pancreas. Oncol Lett 5(1):63–67. Epub 2012 Oct 3
64. Kidd M, Modlin IM, Drozdov I, Aslanian H, Bodei L, Matar S et al (2018) A liquid biopsy for bronchopulmonary/lung carcinoid diagnosis. Oncotarget 9(6):7182–7196
65. Filosso PL, Kidd M, Roffinella M, Lewczuk A, Chung KM, Kolasinska-Cwikla A et al (2018) The utility of blood neuroendocrine gene transcript measurement in the diagnosis of bronchopulmonary neuroendocrine tumours and as a tool to evaluate surgical resection and disease progression. Eur J Cardiothorac Surg 53(3):631–639
66. Peczkowska M, Cwikla J, Kidd M, Lewczuk A, Kolasinska-Cwikla A, Niec D et al (2017) The clinical utility of circulating neuroendocrine gene transcript analysis in well-differentiated paragangliomas and pheochromocytomas. Eur J Endocrinol 176(2):143–157. Epub 2016 Nov 9
67. van Treijen MJC, Korse CM, van Leeuwaarde RS, Saveur LJ, Vriens MR, Verbeek WHM et al (2018) Blood transcript profiling for the detection of neuroendocrine tumors: results of a large independent validation study. Front Endocrinol 9:740
68. Al-Toubah TE, Cives M, Valone T, Blue K, Strosberg JR (2019) Sensitivity and specificity of the NETest: a validation study. J Clin Oncol 37(4):222
69. Chen F, Zhang Y, Gibbons DL, Deneen B, Kwiatkowski DJ, Ittmann M et al (2018) Pan-cancer molecular classes transcending tumor lineage across 32 cancer types, multiple data platforms, and over 10,000 cases. Clin Cancer Res 24(9):2182–2193. https://doi.org/10.1158/078-0432.CCR-17-3378. Epub 2018 Feb 9
70. Partelli S, Andreasi V, Muffatti F, Schiavo Lena M, Falconi M (2020) Circulating neuroendocrine gene transcripts (NETest): a postoperative strategy for early identification of the efficacy of radical surgery for pancreatic neuroendocrine tumors. Ann Surg Oncol 27(10):3928–3936
71. Ginsburg GS, Kuderer NM (2012) Comparative effectiveness research, genomics-enabled personalized medicine, and rapid learning health care: a common bond. J Clin Oncol 30(34):4233–4242. https://doi.org/10.1200/JCO.2012.42.6114. Epub 2012 Oct 15
72. Malik SM, Pazdur R, Abrams JS, Socinski MA, Sause WT, Harpole DH Jr et al (2014) Consensus report of a joint NCI thoracic malignancies steering committee: FDA workshop on strategies for integrating biomarkers into clinical development of new therapies for lung cancer leading to the inception of "master protocols" in lung cancer. J Thorac Oncol 9(10):1443–1448. https://doi.org/10.1097/JTO.0000000000000314
73. Strosberg J, El-Haddad G, Wolin E, Hendifar A, Yao J, Chasen B et al (2017) Phase 3 trial of ^{177}Lu-dotatate for midgut neuroendocrine tumors. N Engl J Med 376(2):125–135. https://doi.org/10.1056/NEJMoa1607427
74. Bodei L, Kidd M, Paganelli G, Grana C, Drozdov I, Cremonesi M et al (2014) Clinical features are not reliable in predicting long-term toxicity after PRRT - evidence from >800 patients to support genetic screen development. Endocrinol Metab Clin N Am 47(3):485–504
75. Brabander T, van der Zwan WA, Teunissen JJM, Kam BLR, de Herder WW, Feelders RA et al (2017) Pitfalls in the response evaluation after peptide receptor radionuclide therapy

with [(177)Lu-DOTA(0),Tyr(3)]octreotate. Endocr Relat Cancer 24(5):243–251. https://doi.org/10.1530/ERC-16-0524. Epub 2017 Mar 20
76. Olsson AH, Yang BT, Hall E, Taneera J, Salehi A, Nitert MD et al (2011) Decreased expression of genes involved in oxidative phosphorylation in human pancreatic islets from patients with type 2 diabetes. Eur J Endocrinol 165(4):589–595. https://doi.org/10.1530/EJE-11-0282. Epub 2011 Jul 20
77. Valli A, Rodriguez M, Moutsianas L, Fischer R, Fedele V, Huang HL et al (2015) Hypoxia induces a lipogenic cancer cell phenotype via HIF1alpha-dependent and -independent pathways. Oncotarget 6(4):1920–1941
78. Day TF, Mewani RR, Starr J, Li X, Chakravarty D, Ressom H et al (2017) Transcriptome and proteome analyses of TNFAIP8 knockdown cancer cells reveal new insights into molecular determinants of cell survival and tumor progression. Methods Mol Biol 1513:83–100
79. Hill RP (2017) The changing paradigm of tumour response to irradiation. Br J Radiol 90(1069):20160474. https://doi.org/10.1259/bjr.74. Epub 2016 Aug 2
80. Kidd M, Modlin IM (2017) Therapy: the role of liquid biopsies to manage and predict PRRT for NETs. Nat Rev Gastroenterol Hepatol 14(6):331–332

Radiological Imaging

7

Andrea Rockall, Shema Hameed, and Mark Wills

7.1 Introduction

Neuroendocrine tumours (NETs) may arise from the gastrointestinal tract, pancreas—now collectively known as gastroenteropancreatic neuroendocrine tumours (GEP-NETs) and from neuroendocrine cells scattered in other tissues. Non-functioning tumours, in which there is no recognizable clinical syndrome, often present late with a large lesion that may cause mass effect, although small non-functioning lesions may be detected when screening family groups with genetic disorders associated with NETs. Functioning tumours usually present relatively early due to the clinical symptoms and signs and may be a challenge for the radiologist to localize as they are often small. The malignant potential of NETs varies, with malignancy being more common in some types.

As surgery may be the only form of curative treatment, imaging is essential in order to select patients for surgery and plan the procedure. Imaging is primarily directed at accurate localization and staging of the tumour. However, research into the predictive or prognostic features on imaging, such as radiomic or texture features, is active research areas. Preoperative localization increases the chances of successful surgical resection and reduces the likelihood of surgical complications. Nuclear imaging techniques are also a key part of the imaging workup and are

A. Rockall (✉)
Imperial College London, London, UK

Imperial College Healthcare NHS Trust and at The Royal Marsden Hospital, London, UK
e-mail: a.rockall@imperial.ac.uk

S. Hameed
Evelina London Children's Hospital, Guy's and St Thomas' NHS Foundation Trust, London, UK
e-mail: shema.hameed@gstt.nhs.uk

M. Wills
Consultant Gastrointestinal & Abdominal Radiologist, Salisbury District Hospital, Wiltshire, UK
e-mail: mark.wills@nhs.net

S. Yalcin, K. Öberg (eds.), *Neuroendocrine Tumours*,
https://doi.org/10.1007/978-3-031-56968-5_7

discussed in chapter X. Cross-sectional imaging is also valuable in the context of patient follow-up, for evaluating treatment response, and in the detection of recurrent or metastatic disease. The imaging workup for NETs does vary depending on the local availability of particular techniques and expertise, although guidelines are available that make recommendations [1]. This chapter will describe the cross-sectional imaging techniques and appearances of NETs.

7.2 Medullary Thyroid Carcinoma

These tumours arise from the parafollicular C-cells of the thyroid gland and secrete calcitonin. They account for 1–2% of all thyroid cancers, with 25% occurring in association with a genetic syndrome due to a germline mutation in the RET proto-oncogene, including familial autosomal dominant medullary thyroid cancer (MTC), MEN IIA and B syndromes [2, 3]. Clinical course is highly variable ranging from an indolent course to aggressive disease with high mortality. Clinical presentation includes a solitary thyroid nodule or presumed multi-nodular goitre, unless metastatic disease is present by which time the patient may experience flushing and diarrhoea. Tumours are often firm, encapsulated masses, thereby appearing as well-circumscribed masses on both US and CT.

Ultrasound is the modality of choice for initial assessment, and a skilled US is recommended, allowing for identification of non-palpable nodules in familial cases [4, 5]. Pre-operative neck US is considered the gold standard for surgical planning. Lesions may appear ill-defined on US, with a spiculated border. They are typically round or ovoid, internally solid and markedly hypoechoic in comparison to surrounding thyroid tissue and strap muscles. The presence of multifocal lesions, regional lymph nodes and extra-thyroid tumour extension is more frequent at presentation in aggressive malignant cases (m-MTC) than in indolent cases (b-MTC) [5]. Micro- or macrocalcifications are found in approximately half of cases (Fig. 7.1) [6]. Fine-needle aspiration cytology (FNAC) of suspicious nodules should be performed promptly, ideally at the time of examination to ensure rapid diagnosis. Although some studies have shown calcitonin

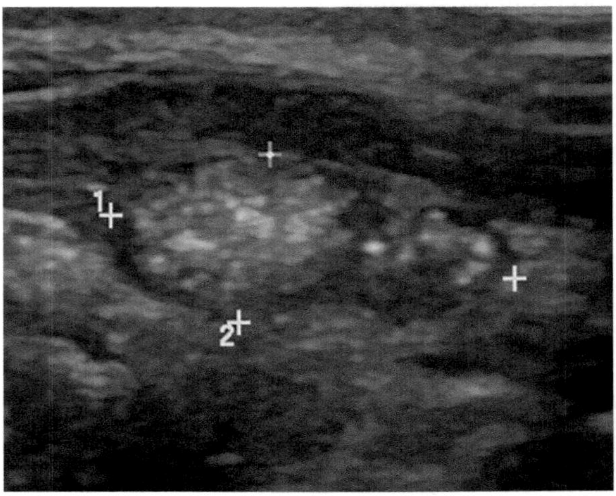

Fig. 7.1 Ultrasound demonstrating a medullary carcinoma of thyroid in a patient with MEN2B. Bright speckles of calcification are demonstrated within the hypoechoic lesion

levels to be more sensitive at diagnosing medullary thyroid carcinoma than FNAC [7], hypercalcitoninemia is also associated with C-cell hyperplasia and thyroiditis; therefore, biochemistry and imaging should be complimentary [8].

CT may be performed for staging purposes, particularly in cases if postoperative calcitonin level remains elevated [3]. MTC appears as a well-circumscribed, heterogeneously enhancing mass. Inherited forms are likely to have multi-focal disease, with numerous nodules within the thyroid gland and lymph node metastases with similar enhancement characteristics [9]. Metastatic lesions beyond the regional nodes are typically present in the mediastinal nodes, lungs, bones and liver. Lung lesions may be micronodular and may calcify.

MRI can be used to localize MTC and is particularly useful in determining local invasion and detecting lymph node metastases, although nuclear medicine techniques may be preferrable where available. On MRI, MTC lesions are isointense to hyperintense on T1-weighted (TIW) imaging and hyperintense on T2-weighted (T2W) imaging and show marked enhancement post contrast administration. Although T2 hyperintensity is highly suggestive of MTC, this is not specific to MTC; diagnosis is therefore only possible with a confirmed hypercalcitoninemia [3, 4]. MRI using diffusion weighted imaging (DWI) and dynamic contrast enhancement is sensitive for the detection of liver, and bone metastases are sensitively demonstrated on DWI and T1-weighted sequences. These techniques are particularly useful in evaluating response to treatment [3].

7.3 Adrenal Tumours

7.3.1 Adrenocortical Carcinoma

Adrenocortical carcinoma is an aggressive tumour arising from the adrenal cortex. It is rare, with an annual incidence of 1 case per million in the United States, and a median age of 55 years at diagnosis [10]. Although most are sporadic, they may arise in association with various familial cancer syndromes [11]. Approximately 60% of adrenocortical carcinomas (ACCs) are functional, secreting a variety of hormones including cortisol, androgens, oestrogens and aldosterone, and often in combination. Co-secretion of cortisol with androgens is highly suggestive of malignancy [12]. Functional tumours typically present with Cushing's syndrome, virilization or a combination of the two, with Conn's syndrome also being a feature in children. Non-functioning tumours usually present late with pain and compressive symptoms together with an adrenal mass. Incidental detection of ACC is becoming more frequent but is still relatively unusual [13]. Most tumours are unilateral. Up to 30% have metastatic disease to regional and para-aortic lymph node metastases, lung, liver and bone lesions at presentation [10, 14].

7.3.2 CT

Imaging features suggestive of an ACC include a suprarenal mass measuring >4 cm, with approximately 70% of tumours larger than 6 cm at the time of diagnosis (Fig. 7.2) [15]. Typical features include irregular margins, central intratumoral

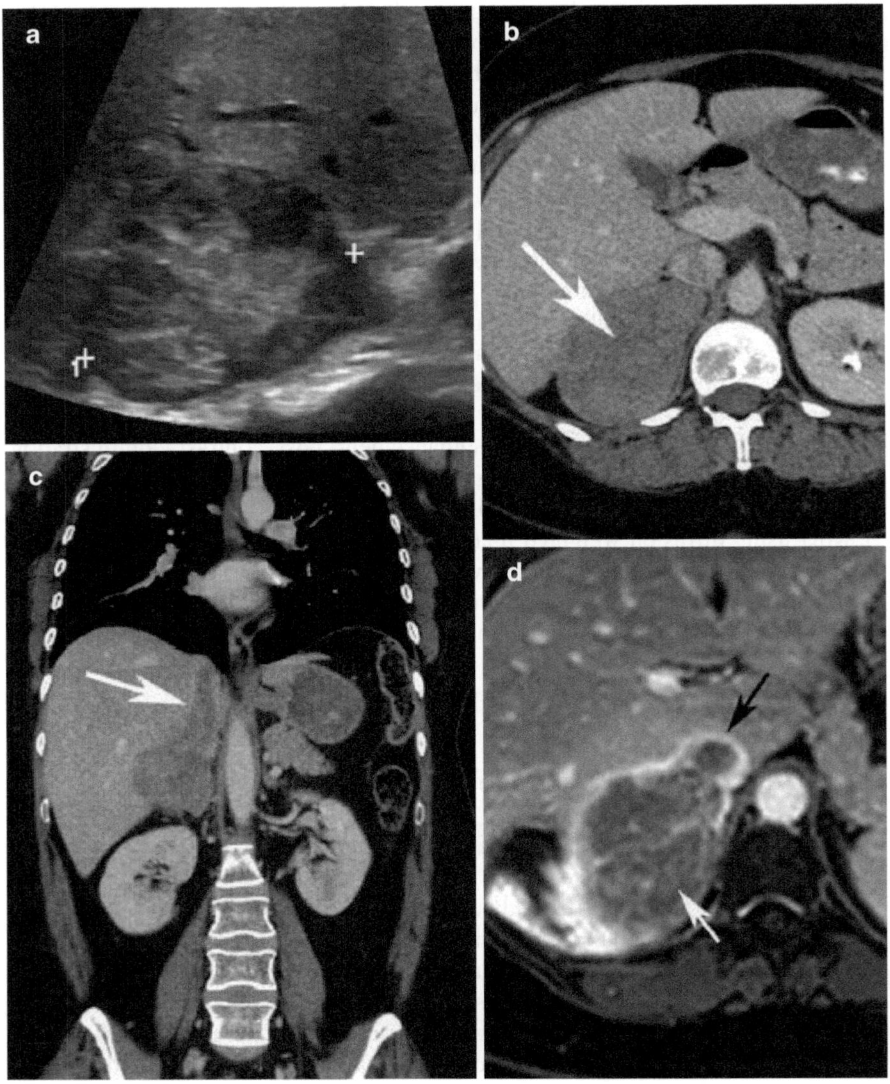

Fig. 7.2 Adrenocortical carcinoma. A 39-year-old lady presented with Cushing's syndrome and right-sided flank pain. (**a**) Ultrasound showed a large solid right suprarenal mass (between calipers) abutting the liver, with heterogeneous internal echoes. (**b**) Contrast-enhanced CT demonstrates a 7-cm-diameter heterogeneous hypodense right suprarenal lesion (*arrow*) abutting the right lobe of the liver. (**c**) Enhancing tumour extending into the IVC (*white arrow*). (**d**) Dynamic contrast-enhanced MRI showed slightly atypical gradual patchy and heterogeneous enhancement, with poor enhancement internally (*white arrow*) and avid rim enhancement (*black arrow*) after 5 min. Restricted diffusion is demonstrated by high signal on the b500 DWI (**e**) and low signal on the ADC map, (**f**) typical of malignancy (*arrow*). The lesion was excised via thoracotomy

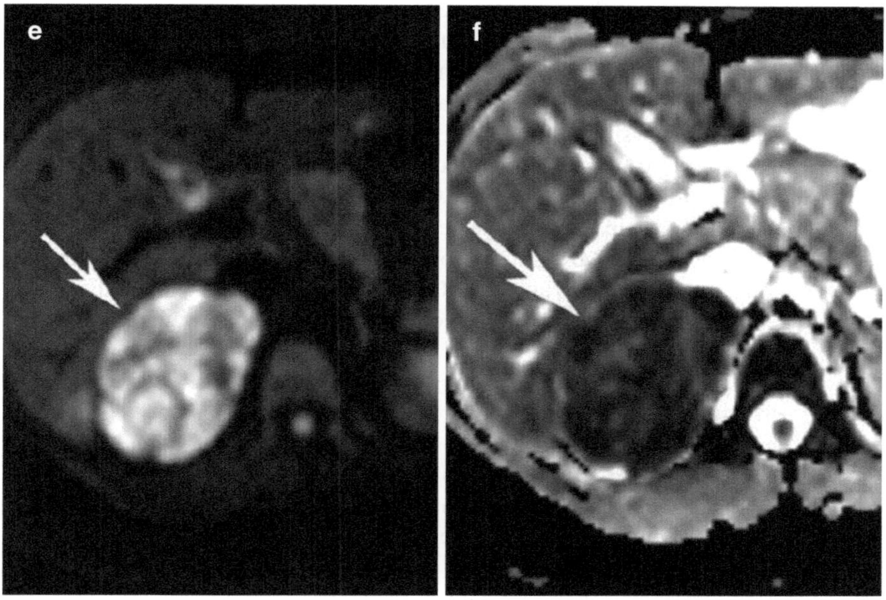

Fig. 7.2 (continued)

necrosis or haemorrhage, heterogeneous enhancement and fatty regions due to intracytoplasmic lipid, calcification (present in 30%), invasion into adjacent structures and venous extension into the IVC and renal vein, more commonly found with right-sided lesions. Metastases to lymph nodes, lungs, liver and bone are frequently present on initial imaging, with staging of disease according to the European Network for the Study of Adrenal Tumors (ENSAT) system [16].

In smaller lesions, measuring the density of adrenal lesions on both unenhanced and enhanced CT is a well-established tool that aids in differentiating benign from potentially malignant adrenal lesions. Adrenal lesions that have a Hounsfield unit (HU) of $\leq$10 are adenomas [17], in contrast to ACCs that will almost always have a HU of >10 on the unenhanced study. Following intravenous contrast administration, ACCs retain contrast for longer than a benign adenoma would, with an absolute percentage washout of <60% and relative washout of <40% at 10 min, although washout should only be considered in homogeneous lesions.

7.3.3 MRI

Lesions are typically heterogeneous in signal intensity and iso- or very slightly hypointense to normal liver parenchyma on T1W images. High T1 signal areas may be seen within the lesion due to haemorrhage. On T2W images, lesions are usually hyperintense to liver parenchyma with a heterogeneous appearance due to intratumoral cysts and haemorrhage. Lesions usually demonstrate avid enhancement throughout with slow washout on delayed imaging; however, other enhancement patterns have been described in small numbers, including peripheral mural-based enhancing nodules (Fig. 7.2d–f) [18]. Chemical shift imaging, which is now routinely performed to differentiate benign adrenal adenomas from malignancy, typically shows no loss of signal in ACCs. However in <30% of functioning lesions, small irregular regions of signal drop-out are demonstrated due to the scattered intracytoplasmic lipid found in these ACCs [18, 19]. Diffusion-weighted imaging has not been found to help differentiate benign from malignant lesions, due to overlapping appearances [11]. MR spectroscopy may be a potentially useful method of differentiating between lesions such as ACC, pheochromocytoma, adrenal metastases and adrenal adenomas although the technique is not widely available [20].

7.3.4 Pheochromocytoma

These rare catecholamine-secreting tumours arise from the chromaffin cells of the adrenal medulla. Extra-adrenal pheochromocytomas can also be found in the paraspinal paraganglia, where they are termed paragangliomas, discussed separately below.

Phaeochromocytomas are usually unilateral and benign; however, 10% are bilateral and 10% are malignant [21]. Bilateral phaeochromocytomas are usually found in MEN II (50–80%), von Hippel–Lindau disease (40–80%), and rarely in sporadic cases. Hypertension is the commonest presenting symptom; however, less than 1% of hypertensive patients are found to have a phaeochromocytoma.

Pheochromocytomas often have relatively non-specific imaging features that overlap with other benign and malignant adrenal tumours [22, 23]. Functional imaging is therefore often required for characterization. Although generally large at presentation, there is marked variability in reported sizes, from 1.2 to 15 cm, although phaeochromocytoma are typically larger than adrenal adenomas [24, 25]. Lesion size may also affect the imaging characteristics of the tumour, with smaller lesions typically appearing more homogeneous and larger lesions heterogeneous, usually due to intratumoral haemorrhage [24].

Ultrasound may locate moderately sized adrenal tumours, but it can be technically challenging and is operator dependent. The majority of lesions are completely solid, round and well-defined with either a homogeneous echotexture which may be iso or hyperechoic to liver, and therefore similar to that of adjacent renal parenchyma [26]. However, approximately half of the solid tumours will appear complex, demonstrating a heterogeneous appearance with interspersed hyper and hypoechoic regions. This correlates with macroscopic findings of intratumoral haemorrhage and necrosis, respectively [26]. Cystic tumours appear as primarily anechoic lesions with posterior acoustic enhancement confirming their liquid property, correlating with old, evolved haemorrhage and necrotic debris at pathology.

CT An adrenal protocol scan (unenhanced, 60 s portal-venous phase and 15-min post contrast phase) is usually performed in order to quantify the intracellular lipid content of the lesion and to measure contrast enhancement and wash-out characteristics. Pheochromocytomas vary widely in appearance on non-contrast CT, with a range of densities from low to soft-tissue. Although the majority will have an attenuation value of around 40–50 Hounsfield units (HU), very rare cases have been reported of pheochromocytomas which demonstrate much lower densities of less than 10 HU, due to intracellular lipid, similar to benign adenomas [27]. Conversely higher density lesions are found in cases of intratumoral haemorrhage. Approximately 10% of lesions are reported to contain calcification, with nearly a quarter of symptomatic lesions being calcified. Following contrast administration, these tumours typically show avid enhancement of their solid components and may show homogeneous or variable heterogeneous enhancement depending on how complex their composition and relative amounts of internal haemorrhage and necrosis. Lesions show an absolute washout of less than 60% and a relative percentage washout of less than 40% at 15 min, or an absolute washout of less than 50% and a relative percentage washout of less than 40% at 10 min [28] (Fig. 7.3). However, variations can occur, and studies have shown pheochromocytomas to have similar washout patterns to adenomas [25, 29].

MRI Pheochromocytomas have been described as having a classical 'light-bulb' bright appearance on T2, being brighter than fat and comparable with CSF [30], and isointense to muscle, hypointense to liver on T1WI. However, variations in

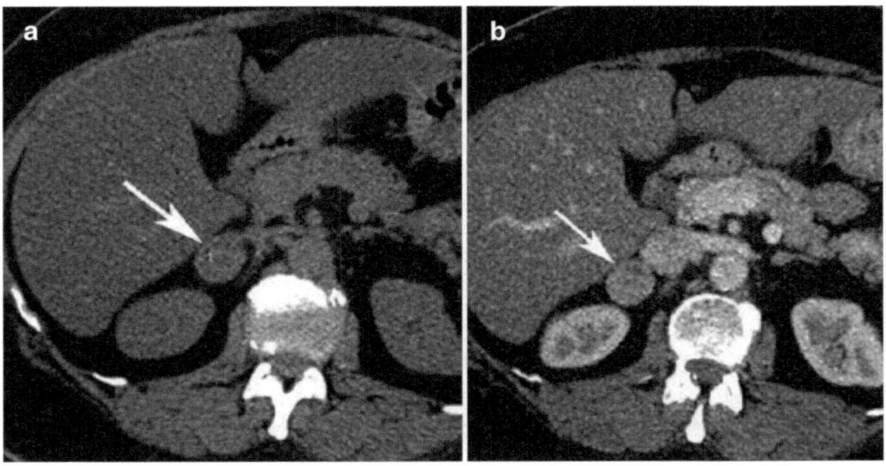

Fig. 7.3 Pheochromocytoma (adrenal protocol CT). A 58-year-old female presented with refractory high blood pressure and palpitations. (**a**) Non-contrast CT demonstrates a 2.7 cm spherical solid lesion arising from the lateral limb of the right adrenal gland with a HU of 25 and no sign of fat or calcification (*arrow*). (**b**) It enhances heterogeneously with a HU of 92 on the first phase and 60 on the delayed phase. This gives the lesion a relative washout of 35 % and absolute washout of 48 %, in keeping with a non-adenomatous lesion. Histology proved this to be a phaeochromocytoma following surgical resection

appearance occur (Fig. 7.4). This may be due to the often complex haemorrhagic and necrotic components of these lesions. Haemorrhage of varying ages can have different signal characteristic on T1-weighted images, with methaemoglobin in sub-acute haemorrhage resulting in high T1W and low T2W signal. The rare cases that contain intracellular lipid will show loss of signal intensity on chemical-shift images (dual-echo in and out of phase T1-weighted MRI). Pheochromocytomas demonstrate avid contrast enhancement post gadolinium administration, with a heterogeneous appearance when there are haemorrhagic, necrotic or cystic components, which will not enhance [24].

7.4 Paraganglioma

These tumours (also known as extra-adrenal phaeochromocytoma) arise from neuroectodermally derived paraganglionic cells anywhere within the body. Paragangliomas arising from the sympathetic chain typically secrete catecholamines, with common sites including the carotid body, jugular foramen, posterior mediastinum and abdominal paraaortic region including Zuckerkandl's body [1]. Clinical presentation is typically with headache, palpitations and sweating, with potentially fatal cardiovascular effects including sudden myocardial infarction, malignant hypertension and cerebral haemorrhage [31]. Parasympathetic paragangliomas tend to be non-secretory tumours and therefore present insidiously with an enlarging palpable mass or pain related to the site of tumour. These lesions include aortic body tumours found in the aortico-pulmonary window, as well as those found within the head and neck regions, including carotid body, jugular foramen and middle ear [31]. The majority of cases of paragangliomas are solitary and sporadic; however, familial paraganglioma are recognized in 10% of cases, including patients with succinate dehydrogenase B (SDHB) mutation where tumours can be multiple and have a higher rate of malignancy [32].

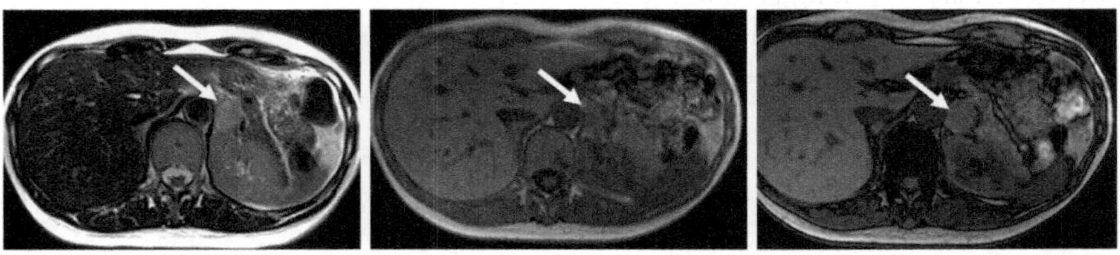

Fig. 7.4 MRI of left phaeochromocytoma. (**a**) T2-weighted image demonstrates a round lesion with high T2 signal intensity. (**b**) T1-weighted image in-phase demonstrates intermediate signal intensity. (**c**) T1-weighted image out-of-phase demonstrates no loss of signal intensity, ruling out intra-cellular lipid

7.4.1 Head and Neck Paragangliomas

The carotid body is the commonest site, followed by jugular foramen, middle ear and along the distribution of the vagus nerve. Less common sites include the orbit, nasal cavity, nasopharynx, thyroid gland, pineal gland and cheek [31, 32]. The carotid body is within the medial aspect of each carotid bifurcation and is the largest compact collection of paraganglia in the head and neck. Carotid body tumours appear as a well-defined soft-tissue mass within the carotid space of the infrahyoid neck, splaying the internal and external carotid arteries. On CT, these lesions demonstrate avid homogeneous enhancement post contrast administration due to their marked hypervascularity (Fig. 7.5a, b) [31]. Occasionally, particularly in larger tumours, haemorrhage and necrosis will result in heterogeneous non-enhancing regions. CT can be used to aid surgical planning [33]. On MRI, they are typically of intermediate signal intensity on T1W and high signal on T2W imaging (Fig. 7.5c, d). A classical feature is the so-called 'salt-and-pepper' appearance, characterized by multiple punctate and serpiginous areas of signal void due to the high-velocity flow of internal vessels, interspersed with high-signal regions due to slow flow or haemorrhage, and MR angiographic techniques can be helpful in delineating the vascular anatomy [34].

7.4.2 Thoracic Paragangliomas

These constitute 1–2% of all paragangliomas and occur predominantly in mediastinal compartments, with less common sites being trachea, lung, heart and oesophagus. Aorticopulmonary paragangliomas, which are located within the anterior mediastinum, tend to present late as incidental lesions on chest radiographs, whereas the posterior mediastinal lesions present earlier with symptoms related to catecholamine secretion [31]. On CT, lesions appear as well-enhancing typically homogeneous masses; however, in cases where there has been haemorrhage or cystic degeneration, patchy areas of low-attenuation within the lesion may be seen [31]. Angiography demonstrates marked hypervascularity with multiple feeding vessels; pre-operative embolization may be considered in cases of bulky or surgically challenging tumours [35]. On MRI, lesions are homogeneous or heterogeneous intermediate signal intensity similar to liver parenchyma on T1W imaging and are of hyperintense signal intensity compared to liver parenchyma on T2W images (Fig. 7.5e) [36].

7.4.3 Abdominal Paragangliomas

Retroperitoneal paragangliomas are most commonly seen in the tissues surrounding the aorta and inferior mesenteric artery. CT demonstrates a soft-tissue mass with either homogeneous enhancement or central areas of low attenuation. Focal areas of

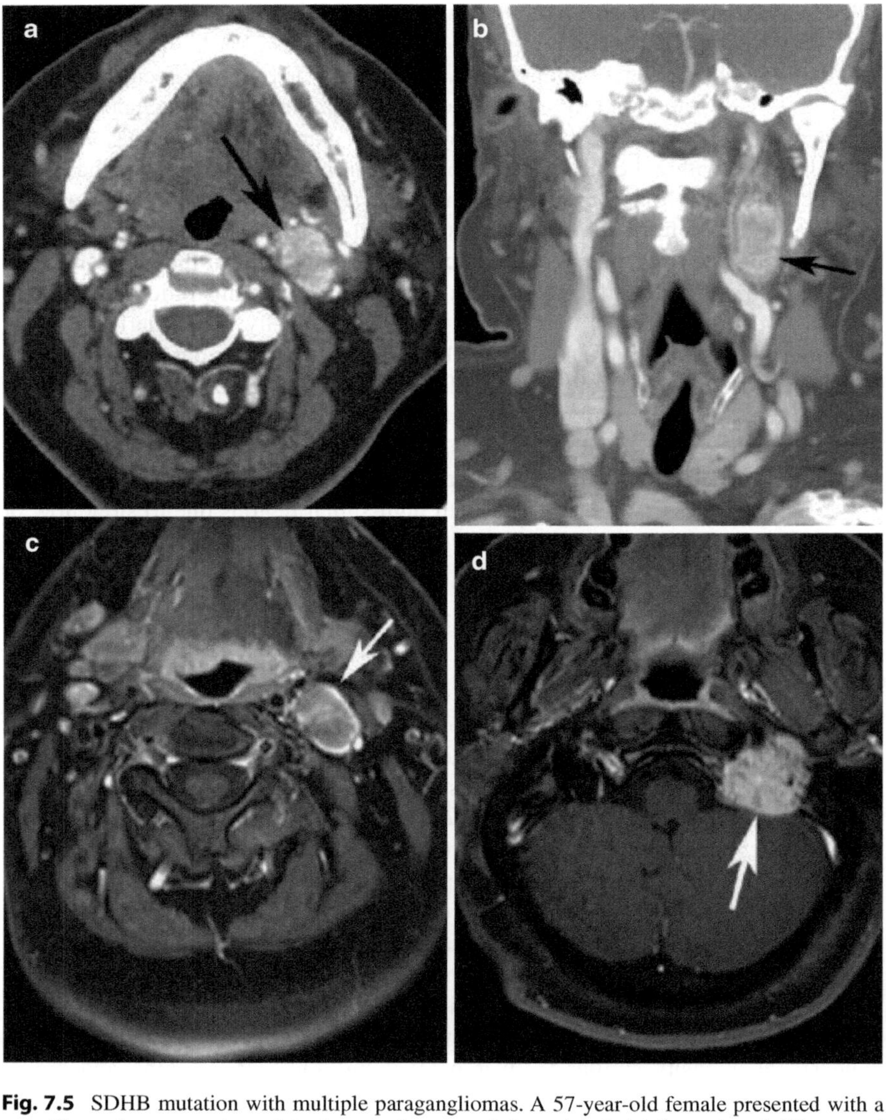

Fig. 7.5 SDHB mutation with multiple paragangliomas. A 57-year-old female presented with a pulsatile neck mass and persistently raised metanephrines. (**a**) Axial (*arrow*) and (**b**) coronal (*arrow*) reformatted arterial-phase CT demonstrates an avid arterially enhancing lesion at the left carotid bifurcation in keeping with a carotid body paraganglioma. (**c**) Post-contrast T1 fat-suppressed image showing the avidly enhancing paraganglioma at the carotid bifurcation, which slightly splays the bifurcation and extends posterior to the common and external carotid arteries. (**d**) Post-contrast fat-suppressed T1-weighted image shows a large avidly enhancing lesion within the left jugular foramen which has eroded and destroyed adjacent bone. Histology following surgical removal confirmed a glomus jugulotympanicum. (**e**) T2-weighted imaging through the thorax revealed a 3 cm hyperintense left paraspinal lesion (*arrow*). The lesion was not PET avid and was proven to be a paraganglioma on histology

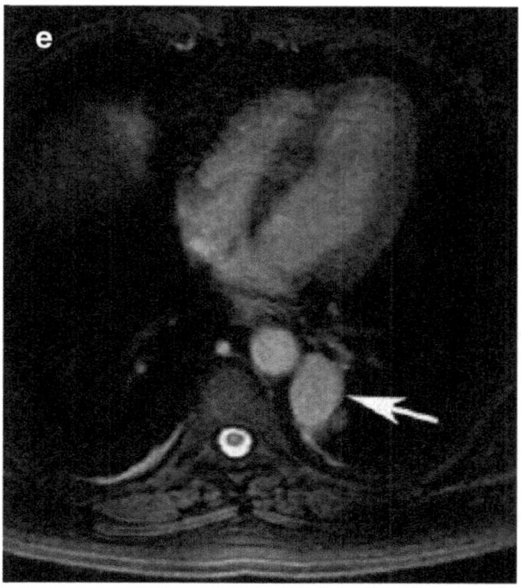

Fig. 7.5 (continued)

high density or punctate calcification due to haemorrhage may also be seen [37]. On MRI, lesions appear isointense or hypointense compared to liver on T1W imaging and are markedly hyperintense on T2W imaging [38].

7.5 Pancreatic Neuroendocrine Tumours (pNETs)

Pancreatic endocrine tumours (pNETs) arise from the islet cells of Langerhans and include functioning tumours (insulinoma, gastrinoma, VIPoma, glucagonoma and somatostatinoma) and non-functioning tumours (including pancreatic polypeptidoma (PPoma) and tumours with no associated clinical syndrome).

Insulinomas are the commonest pNET. Diagnosis is based on clinical presentation and biochemical findings (Whipple's triad). Lesions are typically benign (90%), solitary and almost always intrapancreatic (>90%), being equally distributed between the head, body and tail of pancreas Due to their early presentation, they are often small at diagnosis, with 90% measuring <2 cm and 40% <1 cm in diameter [39].

Gastrinomas are the second commonest pNET. Clinical presentation is usually with the Zollinger–Ellison syndrome (ZES), due to gastrin-driven gastric acid secretion; the diagnosis is usually confirmed biochemically. The majority of gastrinomas are malignant with approximately 60% of patients having hepatic metastases at presentation and an even higher incidence of malignancy when associated with MEN1 [39]. Hepatic and peripancreatic lymph node metastases are typical, and bone metastases have also been reported in approximately 30% of cases [40]. The 'gastrinoma triangle,' which is where more than 90% of lesions are found, is formed by the junction between the neck and body of the pancreas medially, the second and third parts of the duodenum inferiorly, and the junction of the cystic and common bile ducts superiorly [40]. Gastrinomas may be very small in size, measuring as little as 3 mm at presentation, and are more often extrapancreatic and less vascular [40].

Other functioning pNETs are very rare, frequently associated with MEN1 and frequently malignant (between 50 and 80%) [39, 41].

VIPomas comprise 3% of all pNETs and are usually in the pancreatic tail. However, 20% of lesions are extrapancreatic, predominantly in the retroperitoneal sympathetic chain and adrenal medulla.

Glucagonomas usually arise within the body or tail of pancreas and are often large (2–10 cm) at the time of diagnosis. Glucagonomas tend to present late and have a poor prognosis, usually with hepatic and mesenteric lymph node metastases.

Somatostatinomas are intra-pancreatic (usually in head of pancreas), in over half of cases, the remainder being located in the duodenum and jejunum, usually in association with neurofibromatosis. Somatostatinomas are slow-growing and present with relatively mild non-specific symptoms and therefore tend to be very large at presentation, with metastases in liver, lymph nodes and bones in up to 90% of malignant somatostatinomas.

Nonfunctioning pNETS including PPoma and tumours with no clinical syndrome tend to be sporadic and slow-growing, presenting late as large tumours causing mass effect [42]. They usually lie in the pancreatic head, and thus presentation may be with biliary obstruction; 60–90% are malignant. In MEN1, nonfunctional pancreatic tumours are the most frequently diagnosed and surveillance may be undertaken using a combination of endoscopic ultrasound and MRI [43]. These tumours may also be seen in von Hippel–Lindau syndrome.

7.6 Localization of Pancreatic NETs on Imaging

A wide variety of imaging methods are available for the localization of the primary tumour, reflecting the difficulties encountered in detection. Local expertise also dictates the type of imaging used.

7.7 Ultrasound

7.7.1 Transabdominal Ultrasound

Transabdominal ultrasound (US) is widely available, non-invasive and has a high specificity but low sensitivity for localizing small pNETs in the range of 20–86%. Optimization of the technique is achieved by filling the stomach with water, providing an acoustic window. Scanning the patient in both the standing and posterior oblique lying positions allows a more complete assessment. As with most of the imaging techniques available, sensitivity increases with the size of the lesion [39].

Sonographic appearances are usually of a well-defined round mass, which is homogeneously hypoechoic in comparison to the relatively hyperechoic normal pancreatic tissue, and may also exhibit a hyperechoic halo. Hypervascularity is typical on Doppler imaging. Tumours that lie along the surface of the pancreas or in the duodenum are less conspicuous on ultrasound.

Contrast-enhanced ultrasound (CEUS) has shown a high specificity of 90–100% in differentiating pancreatic ductal adenocarcinoma from other solid neoplastic masses, including pNETs [44]. Ductal adenocarcinomas are characteristically hypovascular in relation to the surrounding avidly enhancing pancreatic parenchyma post-contrast medium administration. Conversely, iso- or hypervascularity is characteristic of pNETs [45]. CEUS has shown promising results in detecting small pNETs, with a sensitivity of 94% and specificity of 96% [46].

7.7.2 Endoscopic Ultrasound

Endoscopic ultrasound (EUS) has been shown to have the highest mean sensitivity (90%, range 77–100%) for detection of small functioning pNETs [40].

EUS with a high frequency probe (7.5–10 mHz) results in superior image resolution due to the close proximity of the transducer to the pancreas. Contrast enhancement may also be used. The probe is positioned within the stomach for visualization of the pancreatic body and tail, and in the duodenum for the head and duodenum. The advantages include localization of: small tumours, particularly in the pancreatic head which may be difficult to palpate at surgery; multiple tumours, in cases of MEN1; tumours arising in the duodenal wall; and accurate depiction of the relations between tumour and vascular and biliary structures. FNAC can also be undertaken which has a close correlation with the final histology [47]. EUS can identify regional nodal enlargement, but it cannot fully assess the liver. It is technically challenging and highly specialized, therefore not widely available. Detection of lesions in the tail or extra-pancreatic can be challenging. It may also not be suitable for all patients, for example, where there is duodenal scarring in ZES.

7.7.3 Intraoperative Ultrasound

Intraoperative ultrasound (IOUS) has similar advantages to EUS and may improve the intraoperative sensitivity to 92–97% for identifying small lesions in the head and multiple lesions in the gland and is a useful adjunct to palpation [48]. It has been shown to change operative management by identifying multiple gastrinomas or by demonstrating the malignant nature of a lesion in up to 10% of ZES cases. IOUS has the advantage over EUS of being able to assess the liver, although it is not as sensitive as surgical palpation in detecting extra-pancreatic lesions. Disadvantages of the technique include increasing the time and complexity of operation, as complete mobilization of the pancreas is required, specialist experience for performing and interpreting the scan and poor sensitivity in detecting extrapancreatic/duodenal lesions.

7.7.4 CT

Multidetector CT is the most widely used diagnostic tool for the localization and staging of pNETs. It is widely available and is not subject to the difficulties encountered with US and is not operator-dependent.

7.7.5 CT Technique

The patient should be fasted to ensure that the stomach and duodenum are emptied of their contents. The stomach is then distended with water just prior to scanning, and an IV anti-peristaltic agent is administered. An initial pre-contrast scan is performed at the level of the pancreas followed by biphasic scanning. Depending on the contrast medium used, around 150 ml should be administered at a rate of 3–5 ml/s. Arterial-phase scanning should be performed either by bolus tracking or after a delay of 25–30 s, followed by portal venous scanning after 60–70 s with a section thickness ≤5 mm, and the entire liver should be included in both phases. The images are then reconstructed to 1–2 mm in slice thickness, and coronal or sagittal reformats should be reviewed. Images should also be viewed on narrow window settings in order to augment the difference between the enhancing tumour and pancreatic tissue [49, 50].

7.7.6 CT Appearance

Functioning pNETs are usually small and subtle at presentation, appearing isodense to normal pancreatic tissue on precontrast images with no distortion of the contour of the pancreas. The majority of pNETs are hypervascular and will only be seen after IV contrast medium. Some tumours are seen more easily on arterial phase and others on portal phase images (Fig. 7.6). Biphasic imaging is therefore recommended. Rarely, insulinomas may be hypovascular or cystic and will therefore appear hypodense to the surrounding pancreas (Fig. 7.7) [50, 51]. Cystic pNETs are usually benign and non-functioning; they cannot be reliably differentiated from other cystic pancreatic neoplasms on imaging alone [47]. In patients with a suspected gastrinoma, particular attention should be given to the 'gastrinoma triangle' and duodenal wall, where lesions are commonly found (Fig. 7.8).

Large tumours are more likely to be nonfunctioning and malignant, with signs of necrosis, (central non-enhancing low density), calcifications and overt infiltration of the surrounding retroperitoneal structures such as vessels [39].

7.7.7 Diagnostic Performance of CT

Biphasic multidetector CT with multiplanar thin reformats has improved the sensitivity for detection of the primary tumour, particularly insulinomas, with

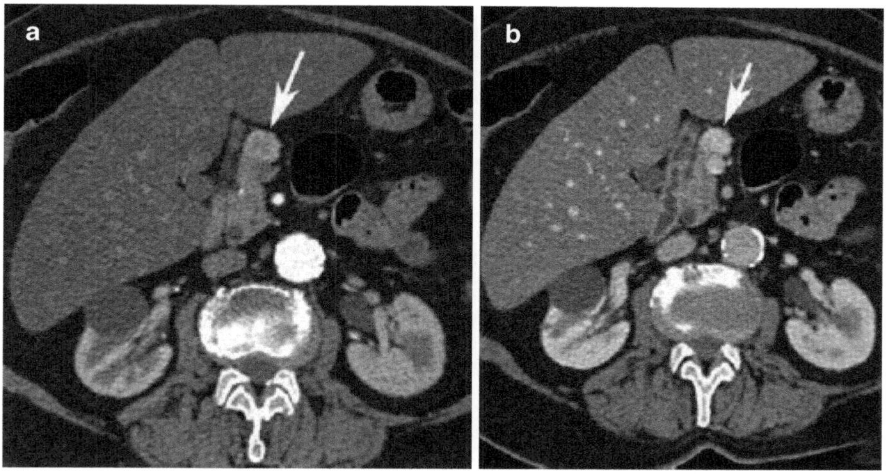

Fig. 7.6 Insulinoma in neck of the pancreas. An 81-year-old female presented with hyperinsulinaemia. (**a**) Arterial-phase CT shows an 18 mm arterially enhancing lesion in the neck of the pancreas (*arrow*) and (**b**) portal-venous-phase CT shows that the lesion remained avidly enhancing (*arrow*)

sensitivities of over 90% on MDCT alone [52]. Detection is directly related to tumour size, with significant difficulty in detecting tumours <1 cm, detection of 30% of tumours between 1 cm and 3 cm, and 95% of tumours >3 cm. Tumours within the head and body have a higher detection rate than those in the tail. Small duodenal tumours <1 cm are often missed on CT, and CT sensitivity for the detection of extrahepatic and extrapancreatic gastrinomas, which are often small at presentation, is only 30–50% [40]. The use of radiomic quantitative analysis may help to characterize pancreatic lesions, and this is an area of current research interest [51].

7.7.8 Magnetic Resonance Imaging

Marked advances in MR technology have improved the diagnostic performance in lesion detection, with several studies having shown this to equal and even exceed that of CT [53, 54]. A sensitivity of 94% for pancreatic lesions, but less for extra-pancreatic lesions, has been reported [54]. Tumour detection increases with tumour size, and small multiple tumours in patients with MEN1 remain difficult to detect.

Optimal technique is needed for high sensitivity as degradation of images due to artifact from movement or body size leads to difficulty in detection. The imaging sequences should include axial images on T1, T2, T1 fat-suppressed spin echo and gradient echo, dynamic contrast-enhancement and diffusion weighted imaging (DWI).

Lesions are usually of low signal intensity on T1W and high on T2W sequences in relation to normal pancreatic tissue, appearing most conspicuous on the

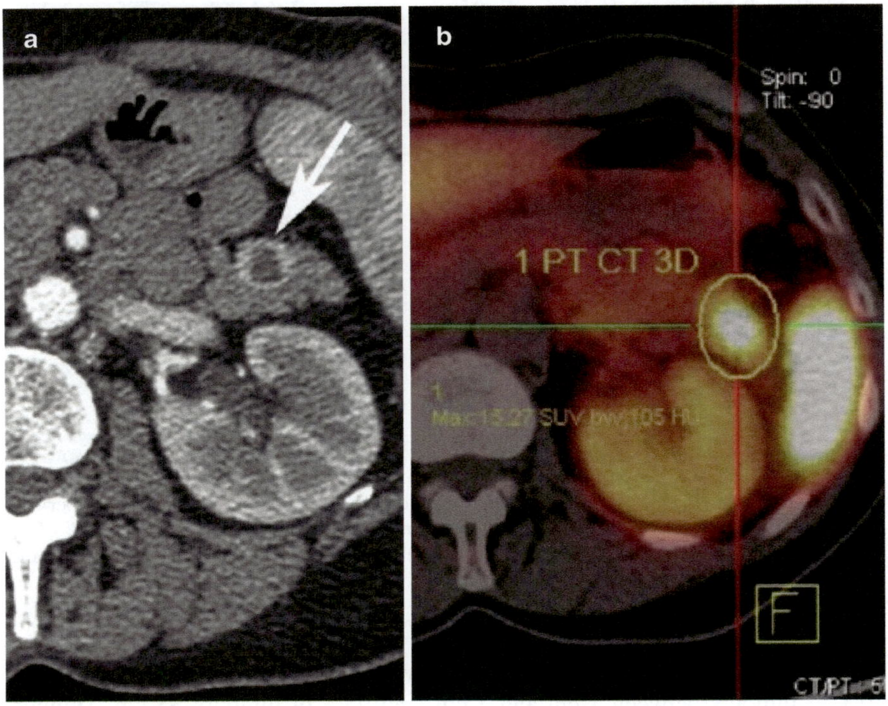

Fig. 7.7 Cystic pancreatic NET. A 61-year-old female. (**a**) Incidental 16 mm lesion in the tail of the pancreas which demonstrated increased vascularity peripherally, suggestive of a cystic NET (*arrow*). (**b**) Gallium PET demonstrated avidity in keeping with a NET

fat-suppressed T1W images (spin-echo or gradient-recalled) (Fig. 7.9) [53, 54]. Rarely, tumours contain a high collagen or fibrous tissue content and therefore return low T2 signal intensity [55]. Following IV gadolinium, characteristic marked homogeneous enhancement is demonstrated. Cystic lesions may demonstrate rim enhancement [54].

DWI is an MRI technique that measures water diffusivity in biological tissues, generating the quantifiable apparent diffusion coefficient (ADC). Small benign tumours show high ADC values, whereas malignant pNETs may show low ADC values (which is seen as corresponding high signal intensity of high b value DWI), consistent with dense tumour cellularity. Although there is overlap, DWI is deemed potentially useful in distinguishing benign from malignant lesions [51, 56].

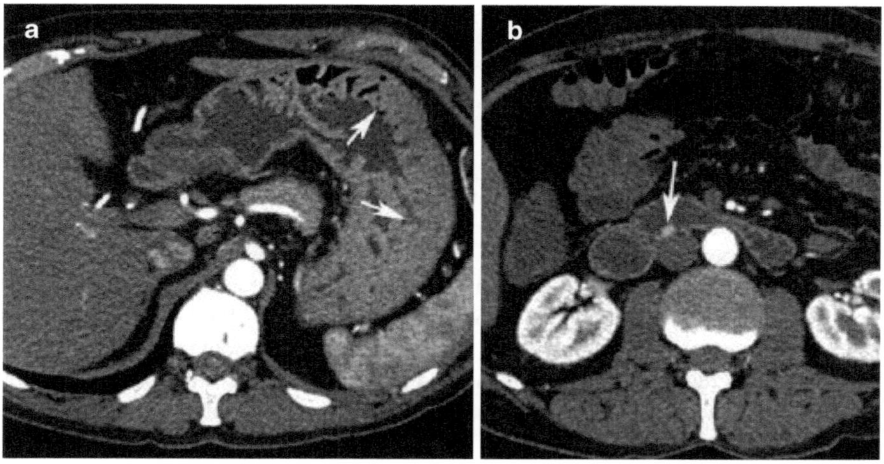

Fig. 7.8 Duodenal gastrinoma. A 49-year-old gentleman presented with Zollinger-Ellison syndrome. (**a**) Arterial-phase CT shows generalized gastric rugal hypertrophy consistent with hypergastrinaemia. (**b**) A small hypervascular lesion on the posterior wall of the third part of the duodenum was identified consistent with a gastrinoma, shown here on axial CT (*white arrow*)

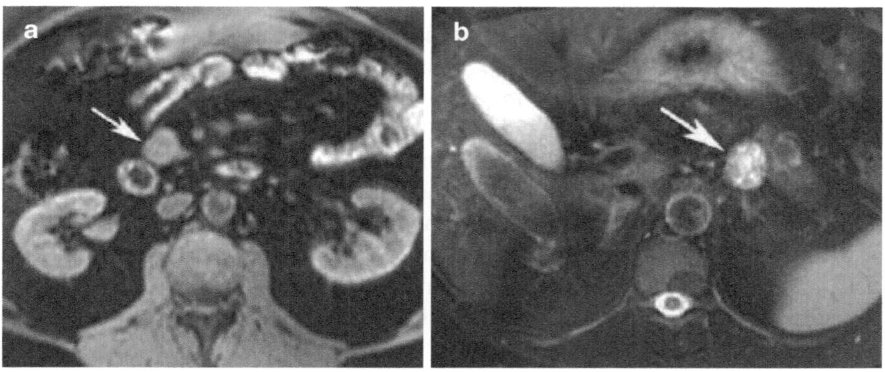

Fig. 7.9 Multiple pancreatic NETs in patient with MEN1. MRI evaluation. (**a**) T1W fat saturated demonstrates a lesion in the uncinate process; (**b**) T2W fat-saturated images shows a high-signal-intensity lesion arising from the tail of the pancreas

7.8 Angiography

Diagnostic angiography is used in selected cases in specialist centres and is combined with venous sampling (see below). Detailed assessment of the vasculature includes selective catheterization of all the branches of the coeliac and superior mesenteric arteries. Primary tumours and liver metastases are seen (with high sensitivity) as a well-defined blush in the capillary and early venous phase. Diagnostic difficulties can arise if a tumour is very small, multiple, hypovascular, or when a lesion lies adjacent to a loop of bowel or spleen and the blush is not separately visible. False positives arise from the blush of a splenunculus or normal pancreas or bowel.

7.8.1 Transhepatic Portal Venous Sampling

Transhepatic portal venous sampling (TSPVS) involves percutaneous catheterization of a portal venous branch. Blood is sampled from the splenic vein, superior and inferior mesenteric veins, pancreatic veins and portal trunk, with the principle that one of these veins will be draining the tumour and therefore contain high concentrations of the secreted hormone. This method is only useful for functioning tumours, although false-negative results occur if hormone secretion is intermittent.

7.8.2 Arterial Stimulation and Venous Sampling

Arterial stimulation venous sampling (ASVS) combines simultaneous hepatic venous sampling with selective arterial injection of a pancreatic secretagogue, a technique that is less invasive than THPVS. Although several different specific secretagogues have been used in the past, calcium gluconate is usually used regardless of the specific secretory product. Following injection of the secretagogue, hepatic venous sampling is performed every 30 s for 2 min. A two to threefold increase in the level of hormone indicates the presence of tumour. Tumour region is well depicted as with THPVS. This technique is most useful in cases where the tumour remains occult on other imaging modalities, predominantly with very small functional tumours. It can be performed as part of pancreatic angiography and is liable to some of the risks associated with THPVS, such as hepatic arteriovenous fistulae, haematoma and superior mesenteric arterial occlusion. Reported sensitivities are as high as over 90%, and the stimulation technique improves the sensitivity of angiography alone [57].

7.9 Gastro-Intestinal Neuroendocrine Tumours

Gastro-intestinal NETs (previously known as carcinoids) are traditionally classified according to their site of origin. The secretory products and therefore the clinical manifestations and immunohistochemical staining patterns are similar for tumours arising from different anatomical sites. 'Foregut carcinoids' include NETs arising from the thymus, bronchus, gastric or duodenal mucosa, and pancreas; 'midgut carcinoids' arise in the jejunum, ileum and proximal colon; while 'hindgut' NETs arise in the distal colon and rectum. The most commonly reported sites are bronchus (32.5%), jejuno-ileum (20%), appendix (8%) and rectum (10%). They are usually highly vascular tumours, resulting in their characteristic brightly enhancing appearances on imaging.

7.9.1 Bronchial Neuroendocrine Tumours

Bronchopulmonary NETs arise from Kulschitsky cells, neuroepithelial bodies or pluripotential bronchial epithelial stem cells in the bronchial epithelium. There are four groups (World Health Organization), according to malignant potential: Low-grade typical carcinoid tumour (classical or benign bronchial carcinoid), intermediate-grade atypical carcinoid tumour, high-grade malignancy including large cell neuroendocrine carcinoma (LCNEC) and small-cell carcinoma (SCLC) [58, 59].

The imaging features vary depending on whether the tumour is located in the airways of the central/middle third of the lung (80% of cases) or in the peripheral airways [60]. Plain radiography may demonstrate a well-demarcated round or ovoid mass, which is often notched. Centrally located tumours will appear as a central mediastinal or hilar mass, usually measuring 2–5 cm in diameter. These lesions may result in airways obstruction, with recurrent infection and/or lobar collapse. However, as they are frequently small, CT scanning is the most sensitive cross-sectional technique [61]. Lesions are seen within the bronchial lumen, usually with both an intra- and extraluminal component being visible. Collapse or air trapping beyond the lesion may be seen due to ball-valve obstruction of the bronchial lumen. Peripheral bronchial NETs are seen in 20% of cases, appearing as solitary pulmonary nodules, typically round or ovoid with a smooth or lobulated border, commonly with punctate or diffuse calcification (Fig. 7.10). Cavitation and hilar adenopathy are rare in well differentiated bronchial NETs, although aggressive lesions (large or small cell carcinomas) may demonstrate direct mediastinal invasion. Typically lesions demonstrate intense homogeneous enhancement, although this may not be seen in all cases. The marked enhancement may mimic a pulmonary varix or pulmonary artery aneurysm, making diagnosis challenging [60]. In patients with occult ectopic ACTH secretion, bronchial NETs are the most common source; however, these can be elusive and difficult to identify.

7.9.2 Thymic Neuroendocrine Tumours

NETs of the thymus are extremely rare, typically presenting with an anterior mediastinal mass. Thought to arise from thymic cells of neural crest origin (Kulchitsky cells), these tumours are not too dissimilar to those arising from the bronchi, with a range of differentiations including typical carcinoid, atypical carcinoid, large cell neuroendocrine and small cell carcinoma [62]. Approximately 50% of tumours are functioning, frequently secreting ACTH resulting in Cushing's syndrome [58]. These patients tend to have much smaller lesions at the time of diagnosis. Patients with nonfunctioning tumours usually present with large lesions in the anterior

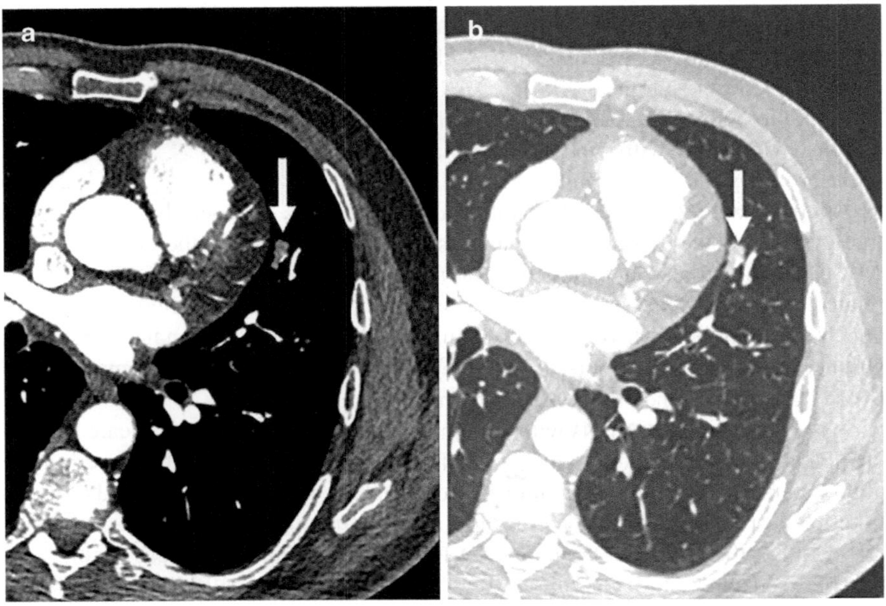

Fig. 7.10 Atypical carcinoid in lingula, Ki67 6–8%. (**a**) Arterial phase CT on soft tissue window settings demonstrates ovoid sub-cm lesion (arrow) with small fleck of calcification. (**b**) Appearance on the lung window settings. Review of CT from 10 years previously demonstrated a tiny 2 mm nodule at this site, confirming the slow rate of growth

mediastinum, with signs and symptoms related either to mass effect and/or local invasion (Fig. 7.11) [63]. Lesions are heterogeneous on CT and may show calcification and necrosis (Fig. 7.12). Assessment of the SVC for obstruction is vital. Invasive disease as evidenced by extension into the pleura, pericardium, great vessels or regional lymph nodes, is also frequently seen in this group of patients. Bilateral adrenal hyperplasia may be present in those with functioning ACTH-secreting tumours. Metastatic disease in lungs, liver and bone, which may be sclerotic, may also be present at the time of diagnosis [58, 64].

7.9.3 Gastric Neuroendocrine Tumours

Gastric carcinoid is rare, representing about 7% of all carcinoid tumours but less than 1% of stomach neoplasms [65]. As gastric neuroendocrine tumours are luminal, they are usually diagnosed by endoscopy, with endoscopic US to aid in detection of depth of tumour invasion, regional nodal evaluation and for fine-needle aspiration [65, 66]. The role of CT is predominantly to detect regional and distant metastatic disease. Administration of an anti-peristaltic agent and a negative oral contrast agent (water) may also improve detection of the gastric NETs. CT should

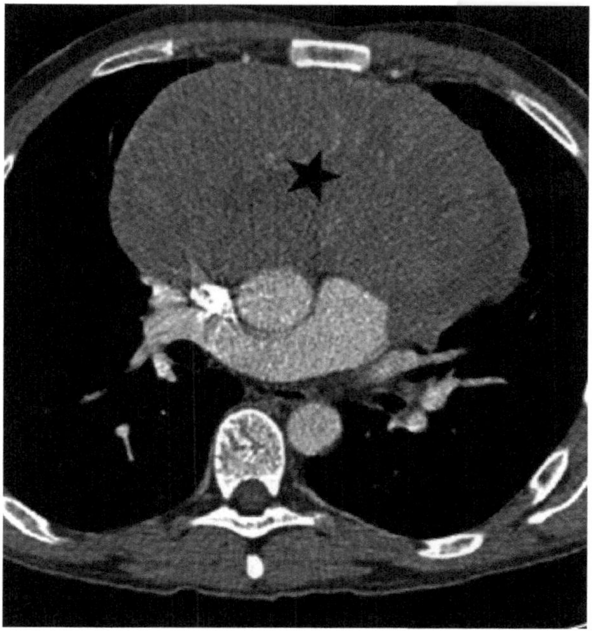

Fig. 7.11 Neuroendocrine tumour of the thymus. A 37-year-old man presented with recurrent chest pain for several years and a previous episode of pericarditis. Chest radiograph showed a large lobulated mediastinal mass. The patient proceeded to a CT scan, which demonstrates a 16 cm heterogeneously enhancing anterior mediastinal mass (*star*), displacing the aorta and pulmonary trunk posteriorly. Functional imaging in the form of gallium-68 DOTATAE showed the lesion to be somatostatin receptor positive. The lesion was unsuitable for resection, and the patient underwent lutetium-177 therapy

include an arterial phase acquisition at 25–30 s following the injection of contrast agent at a rate of 4–5 ml/s, followed by a delayed portal venous phase at 60 s [67].

Type I gastric NETs, associated with atrophic gastritis, are poorly seen on CT and MR, being multicentric and typically <1 cm in size. The disease is almost always benign, with metastases present in only 2% of cases. Type II gastric NETs, the least common, are associated with MEN1. There are typically multiple lesions within the gastric wall, which is thickened due to the association with the ZES. There is an increased tendency to metastasise to regional lymph nodes, although the prognosis is generally good. Type I and type II tumours may appear similar to other gastric tumours and polyps as numerous enhancing submucosal lesions [68]. Type III sporadic gastric NETs are usually solitary, large lesions with an irregular contour and diffuse margins that may ulcerate. Local invasion with extension into the surrounding gastric fat, as well as metastases, is common at presentation [69].

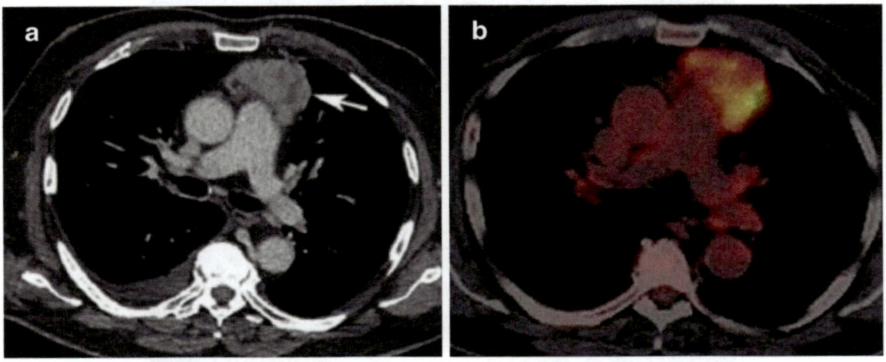

Fig. 7.12 Thymic NET. (**a**) A 77-year-old male presented with chest sepsis. CT chest revealed an incidental 5 cm lobulated, heterogeneously enhancing anterior mediastinal mass with hypodense regions suggestive of necrosis and tiny calcific foci. (**b**) F-18 FDG PET shows metabolic activity within the lesion. Histology showed neuroendocrine carcinoma, with an atypical marker profile

7.10 'Midgut' Neuroendocrine Tumours

Midgut NETs arise beyond the ligament of Treitz to the level of the mid-transverse colon. They are the commonest primary malignant tumour of the small bowel, as well as being the commonest location of all gastrointestinal NETs [41]. Patients present with abdominal pain and gastrointestinal bleeding, usually with associated colic and diarrhoea, or with symptoms of obstruction that may be due to the primary tumour or due to intussusception (Fig. 7.13) [70]. Tumour-associated desmoplastic mesenteric fibrosis due to the local production of fibrogenic agents results in tethering and kinking of the small bowel mesentery that can also result in obstruction. Metastases are often present at diagnosis, in approximately a quarter of cases, most frequently to nodes, liver, bone and lung [71]. The incidence of metastases increases with tumour size. Staging includes CT, MR and nuclear medicine techniques (described elsewhere) [49].

7.10.1 CT

7.10.1.1 Primary Tumour

Detection of the primary tumour on conventional CT is extremely challenging, as these are usually small lesions not easily detected against the bowel from which they arise and may only be detected due to a complication such as intussusception into the caecum (as in Fig. 7.13). CT enterography (CTE) is a superior and more reliable imaging technique for diagnosing small bowel lesions, with good potential

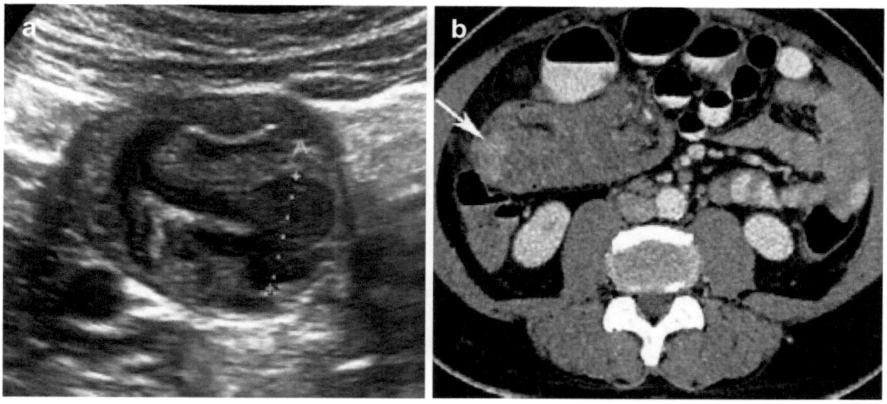

Fig. 7.13 Intussusception due to small bowel NET. (**a**) Ultrasound demonstrates an intussusception, and the lead point is a small bowel NET, shown here between the calipers. (**b**) CT demonstrates the enhancement of the primary lesion

for diagnosing small bowel NET (95% on CTE compared to 45% on CT) and may be complimentary to PET/CT techniques [70, 72]. The small bowel is distended with 2.5 l of water (negative contrast) through a nasojejunal tube. An antispasmodic drug is given to reduce peristalsis, and an arterial and portal-venous phase CT is performed, allowing visualization of the entire small bowel, including intra and extraluminal lesions [49].

NETs are seen as a solitary focal nodular mass, a smooth submucosal mass within the bowel wall or an intraluminal polyp (Fig. 7.14). If detected early, tumours may only manifest as subtle wall-thickening with most lesions demonstrating avid contrast-enhancement. Larger lesions may cause distortion and fixation of the bowel loop and surrounding mesentery, with a pathognomonic appearance on CT of mesenteric strands radiating from the nodule due to a desmoplastic reaction (Fig. 7.14) [73]. CT enteroclysis has high reported sensitivities and specificities greater than 90% [70]. NETs as small as 5 mm in diameter may be detected due to the excellent distension of bowel lumen. Multiplanar reformats optimize visualization of the bowel wall allowing high diagnostic accuracy for transmural and extramural lesions. The disadvantage of CT enteroclysis include patient discomfort and the radiation dose, as the NJ tube requires insertion under fluoroscopic guidance and there are a minimum of two phases of CT image acquisition. Wireless capsule enteroscopy has been shown to detect more bowel lesions; however, it is limited to intraluminal evaluation [74]. A recent large single centre retrospective cohort study has found that there has been a marked increase in detection of small bowel neuroendocrine neoplasms by CTE over the past 20 years; and cases detected by CTE, as well as small tumours detected at endoscopy, had longer disease-free survival after surgical resection [70].

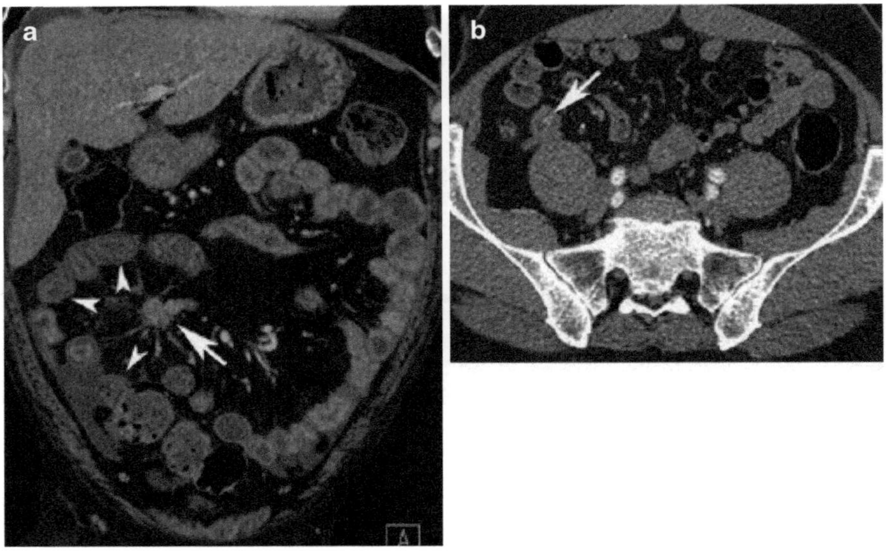

Fig. 7.14 Mesenteric mass secondary to small bowel NET. (**a**) A 56-year-old man presented with a 2-month history of weight loss and rectal bleeding. Contrast-enhanced CT, coronal reformat, shows a 3-cm-diameter soft tissue mass within the small bowel mesentery which contains tiny foci of calcification. The lesion (*arrow*) is causing a desmoplastic reaction, with in-drawing of surrounding bowel loops (*arrowheads*) which demonstrates mural thickening and hyperenhancement. There are a few small adjacent lymph nodes. (**b**) A focal nodular enhancement was thought to represent the primary tumour

7.11 Mesenteric Masses

Mesenteric masses occur in 50–75% of small bowel NET and appear as soft-tissue density lesions, usually identified on CT imaging. These masses typically demonstrate a 'spoke-wheel' appearance, i.e. radiating strands of soft-tissue density, reflecting the fibrosis that occurs secondary to the production of hormonally active substances such as serotonin (Fig. 7.14) [73].

Calcification often occurs within the mesenteric mass (40–70%), appearing either as small stippled calcifications or as more bulky, conglomerate foci of calcification [73]. The superior mesenteric artery and vein may also be encased by the contracted mesentery, resulting in vascular compromise and possible bowel ischaemia [75].

Diffuse peritoneal metastatic disease occurs with a smaller percentage (10–30%) of patients with GI NET and is associated with poor prognosis [76]. On CT, this appears as foci of irregular nodularity throughout the mesentery and on the peritoneal surfaces, often with ascites and abdominal distension. In advanced cases, peritoneal disease may result in bowel obstruction.

7.11.1 MR

MRI of the small bowel is now established in inflammatory small bowel disease, but there is less published evidence in non-inflammatory conditions. The examination is costly and time-consuming, requires bowel preparation and may be poorly tolerated by some patients and so the use of MRI is determined by local expertise [77]. Patients must be able to breath-hold, as fast sequences are crucial for good image quality, in addition to adequate bowel distension. Sequences include breath-hold T2W (single-shot fast spin echo, single shot turbo spin echo and a balanced gradient echo sequence such as true fast imaging with steady-state precession) and T1W pre- and post-gadolinium fat-suppressed sequences. Axial and coronal images are obtained.

MR enterography and MR enteroclysis are two techniques that allow distension of the small bowel lumen, which is essential for accurate detection of NETs. Enterography involves the patient drinking a large volume (approximately 2 l) of fluid; an easy, quick and well-tolerated method. Enteroclysis is the distension of small bowel via a nasojejunal tube as described above [77, 78]. Most studies have concluded that enteroclysis results in more adequate and uniform luminal distension of the entire small bowel [79]. However, there is limited data directly comparing the diagnostic performance of these two techniques in the detection of small bowel neoplasms. Both have the advantage of the ability to evaluate indirectly the state of the bowel wall, detecting submucosal and extramural primary lesions or extension of small bowel disease, as well as resolving the limitations caused by overlapping bowel loops [80].

Dynamic sequences in MR enterography also allow evaluation of small bowel peristalsis and distensibility, and imaging may be performed following further oral contrast administration to reassess possible regions of narrowing or suspected intraluminal masses.

As with CT, small bowel NETs typically appear as a focal nodular region of bowel wall thickening, or a smooth submucosal mass [81]. Focal wall thickening of more than 3 mm in a well-distended small-bowel loop should be considered abnormal. On the unenhanced T1W images, lesions are isointense to muscle and appear iso or mildly hyperintense to muscle on T2W images, occasionally exhibiting radiating spiculated strands. Multifocal enhancing polypoid lesions segmentally distributed and numerous tiny enhancing nodules have also been described. Mesenteric masses are low signal on both T1- and T2-weighted imaging and show no or negligible enhancement (Fig. 7.15).

The diagnostic accuracy of small bowel MR enteroclysis at detecting all small bowel neoplasms has been reported to be very high, with sensitivities and specificities greater than 90% [78].

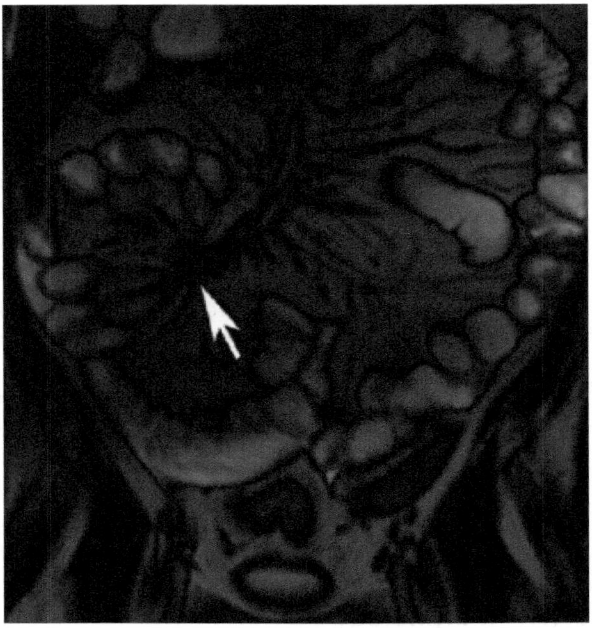

Fig. 7.15 Mesenteric mass secondary to small bowel NET. T2W coronal MRI shows a soft tissue mesenteric mass which is of low T2 signal intensity (*arrow*). The locally tethered adjacent small bowel loops may represent the site of primary disease, but the primary lesion could not be seen

7.12 Hindgut NETs

Hindgut NETs include tumours arising from the mid-transverse colon extending distally to the rectum, the commonest hindgut NET. Hindgut NETs have increased in incidence over the last decade, accounting for 12% of all carcinoids [82, 83]. The tumours are usually slow-growing and are frequently diagnosed at endoscopy, including screening colonoscopy. Small low-grade neoplasms may be treated with minimally invasive surgical techniques, with an excellent 5-year survival rate [82, 83]. Metastases are uncommon but are more common in patients with atypical histology and as would be expected, the incidence increases with the size of the tumour [82, 83].

Imaging may be used to identify cases suitable for local resection, including stage T1 (tumour is confined to the mucosa and submucosa) and T2 (invasion of muscularis propria) disease, with no evidence of extension to the serosa. Endoscopic US may be useful in demonstrating invasion of the full rectal wall (T3) and invasion into adjacent structures (T4) with the primary lesion appearing as a homogeneously hypoechoic submucosal mass. MR may have a role in local staging, appearing as a discrete mass or asymmetric wall thickening localized to the submucosa, isointense to muscle on T1 and iso- to hyperintense on T2 with homogeneous contrast enhancement [84]. Both CT and MR can be used to stage local lymph node disease and distant metastatic disease in preoperative planning.

7.13 Appearances of NET Metastatic Disease

Nodal metastases are the most frequent metastatic site at histology, but liver metastases are the most frequently identified metastases on imaging. Mesenteric disease is described in the section on small bowel NETs. The lungs and bones are other common sites of metastatic disease.

7.14 Liver Metastases from GEP-NET

7.14.1 Ultrasound

The ultrasound technique used to assess for liver metastases is the transabdominal (TA) approach, which allows visualization of all or most of the liver, for most patients. Endoscopic ultrasound (EUS) does not allow full visualization of the liver, although the principles of lesion characterization would be identical for any liver lesion identified at EUS.

Whereas metastases from adenocarcinomas (e.g. colorectal, lung) tend to appear hypoechoic on ultrasound, NETs are typically seen on ultrasound as hyperechoic foci within the liver parenchyma, which have irregular and poorly defined margins. In some cases, these appearances may mimic a liver haemangioma and additional imaging will be required to further characterize the lesion. In the context of hepatic steatosis (where the liver has a generalized increase in its echotexture), the presence of a hyperechoic liver metastasis may be masked. Less commonly, liver metastases from GEP-NETs may appear as hypoechoic foci, with or without a hyperechoic halo [49].

CEUS is a technique used to characterize focal liver lesions on ultrasound following intravenous injection of a microbubble contrast agent. NET liver metastases classically demonstrate avid enhancement in the arterial phase followed by washout to appear as a non-enhancing defect in the late phase. This contrasts to adenocarcinoma metastases, which do not typically demonstrate avid arterial enhancement. Although traditionally used as a tool for lesion characterization, CEUS is comparable to contrast enhanced CT for response assessment of NET liver metastases following radiopeptide therapy [49].

Sensitivity for detection of liver metastases is reported to be 88% for US and 82% for CEUS. US may be complimentary to CT or other imaging techniques and is useful for directing biopsy [49].

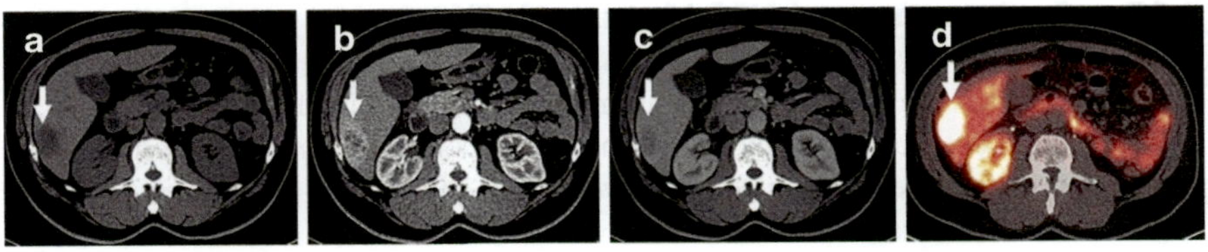

Fig. 7.16 Hepatic metastasis from a pancreatic NET. (**a**) Non contrast CT, (**b**) arterial phase CT, (**c**) portal venous phase CT and (**d**) Gallium scan demonstrate a lesion in segment VI of the liver (arrow). This is low attenuation prior to contrast administration, then demonstrates bright enhancement in the arterial phase, becoming less conspicuous on portal venous phase. The lesion is avid on the Gallium scan

7.14.2 CT

NET hepatic metastases are often masked by appearing isointense to normal enhancing liver parenchyma on portal venous phase (PVP) CT imaging and are therefore best imaged using 'triple-phase' CT scanning, i.e. pre-contrast, hepatic arterial phase (HAP) and PVP (Fig. 7.16) [49].

On the precontrast imaging, liver metastases are not well delineated and may not be identifiable. They may appear of lower attenuation than normal liver parenchyma or occasionally contain foci of calcification. Larger lesions may become necrotic and appear of fluid density.

NET hepatic metastases typically demonstrate avid enhancement during the HAP imaging, hyperintense with respect to liver parenchyma, though not all lesions have bright arterial enhancement. During the PVP, the metastases may become isointense to liver parenchyma (reducing their conspicuity) or may washout to appear as a hypointense lesion.

7.14.3 MRI

MRI of the liver is advocated by ENETs and NANETs for detection of metastases from GEP-NET and for surveillance [49, 85]. On MR imaging, the majority of NET liver metastases are of low signal intensity on T1W and of intermediate/high signal intensity on T2W imaging (Fig. 7.17). Following contrast administration, these hypervascular lesions typically demonstrate avid enhancement in the HAP and a proportion of these lesions will be solely identifiable in this phase [49]. The use of hepatobiliary contrast media with 20-minute hepatobiliary phase imaging has been reported to ensure the best interreader variability for the size of NET liver lesions [86]. DWI has been demonstrated to be more sensitive than T2W imaging for the detection of NET metastases, although it does not reliably differentiate between metastases of different tumour types.

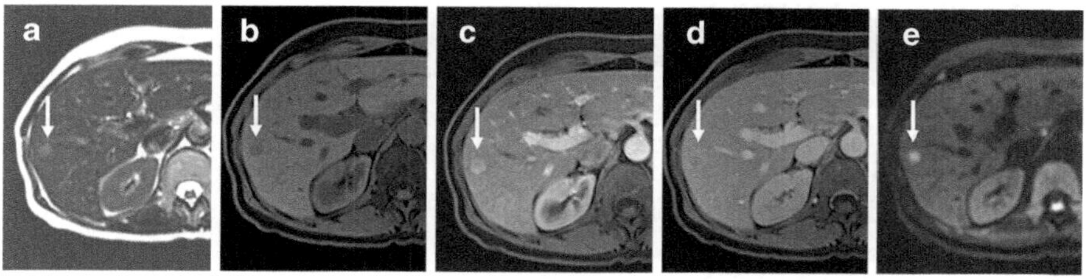

Fig. 7.17 Liver metastasis from small bowel NET. MRI sequences (**a**) T2 weighted the lesion is moderately high signal intensity, (**b**) T1 with fat saturation, low signal, (**c**) arterial phase bright enhancement, (**d**) portal venous phase wash-out and (**e**) b800 bright signal intensity. This was low on the ADC map confirming restricted diffusion

7.15 Lymph Node Metastases

Features suggestive of malignant involvement include a rounded rather than oval appearance, loss of the normal fatty hilum and an increase in the short-axis diameter above that considered to be the upper limit of normal. For most lymph nodes, this upper limit is taken as 10 mm, although this should be used with caution as smaller lymph nodes may still be malignant, and larger lymph nodes may be 'reactive' and thus not contain any malignant cells. Involved lymph nodes in NET may also contain foci of calcification, although this finding is not specific for malignancy. Morphologic criteria are not accurate enough to allow confident diagnosis of involvement in most cases [68]. Retroperitoneal and mesenteric lymph node enlargement is commonly seen in patients with midgut NET (20–30%) and may result in retroperitoneal fibrosis [49].

7.16 Lung Metastases

The diagnosis of lung metastases arising from NETs is made on CT, manifest by rounded pulmonary nodules of non-uniform sizes in a bronchovascular distribution which enlarge with progression of disease.

Following local metastatectomy for pulmonary metastases, follow-up CT studies of the thorax evaluate for local disease recurrence, identified as a new soft tissue mass at the resection margin, or new/enlarging pulmonary metastases.

7.17 Bone Metastases

The presence of metastatic bone disease is associated with a poor prognosis, particularly in the presence of metastatic disease elsewhere. NET bone metastases typically involve the axial skeleton, are usually multiple, are frequently sclerotic, often appearing as small punctate deposits (Fig. 7.18a, b) [87]. Less commonly, bone

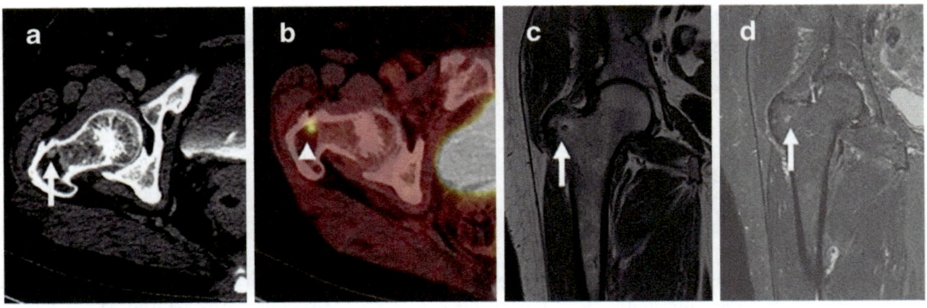

Fig. 7.18 Bone metastasis from a NET of the terminal ileum. (**a**) axial CT demonstrates a sclerotic area (arrow), (**b**) Gallium Dotatate scan demonstrates the lesion to be avid, (**c**) coronal T1 weighted MR the lesion is low in signal intensity, (**d**) coronalT2 weighted MR with fat saturation the lesion is high in signal intensity

metastases appear as mixed osteolytic/osteosclerotic lesions, and a minority appear as purely osteolytic. Treated bony metastases may become more sclerotic and thus be misdiagnosed as disease progression.

Whole-body MR imaging has been found to have a sensitivity of 86% in the detection of bone metastases in patients with GEP-NET cancer, similar to that of somatostatin receptor scintigraphy (81%) [87, 88]. Nuclear medicine studies for the detection of bony metastatic disease are discussed in other chapters.

On MRI, bone metastases typically appear as lesions of reduced signal on T1W imaging, with variable signal intensity on T2W imaging dependent upon the extent of associated oedema (Fig. 7.18c, d). Bone metastases from NETs may enhance following gadolinium administration and demonstrate restricted diffusion [87].

7.18 Response to Treatment

Response of metastatic NETs to medical treatment is traditionally assessed according to Response Evaluation Criteria In Solid Tumors (RECIST) criteria and is defined by changes in size of target metastatic lesions, usually on CT or MRI. This method remains the most widely used system for evaluating response in NET. However, more research is needed into novel ways to evaluate response, particularly in light of the increasing use of targeted chemotherapy agents, which may offer improved patient outcome in the absence of a RECIST response [49].

Surgical resection is the only curative technique in GEP NETs. However, palliation of symptoms may be achieved by radiofrequency ablation or embolization/chemoembolization of liver metastases.

Radio-frequency ablation (RFA) is a technique employed to induce thermal coagulation necrosis within hepatic metastases. Following ablation, the lesion will typically appear as a focus of necrosis on CT (i.e. an area of lower attenuation than the surrounding liver) with smooth margins. Immediately following treatment, the area of necrosis is expected to be slightly larger than the pre-treatment tumour.

There may be peripheral enhancement following contrast administration, but the central necrotic part of the tumour would not be expected to enhance. On subsequent imaging, the defect should remain stable or reduce in size, indicating stable disease or a response to treatment. An increase in size or enhancement within the lesion itself suggests disease recurrence or incomplete therapy [89].

Transcatheter chemoembolization (TACE) is an Interventional Radiology technique that selectively embolises and delivers chemotherapy to the branches of the hepatic artery supplying the hypervascular liver lesions. A CT performed following treatment will demonstrate very high-density material within the liver metastasis due to the lipiodol administered during chemoembolization. Response to treatment may be assessed by a change in the size of the lesion on subsequent CT imaging, with an increase in tumour size indicating disease progression. Additionally, response to TACE may be assessed on contrast enhanced MRI and DWI, demonstrated by a reduction in the percentage enhancement of the lesions and a reduction in the extent of restricted diffusion [90].

References

1. Vinik AI, Woltering EA, Warner RR, Caplin M, O'Dorisio TM, Wiseman GA et al (2010) NANETS consensus guidelines for the diagnosis of neuroendocrine tumor. Pancreas 39(6):713–734
2. Chen H, Sippel RS, O'Dorisio MS, Vinik AI, Lloyd RV, Pacak K et al (2010) The North American Neuroendocrine Tumor Society consensus guideline for the diagnosis and management of neuroendocrine tumors: pheochromocytoma, paraganglioma, and medullary thyroid cancer. Pancreas 39(6):775–783
3. Kushchayev SV, Kushchayeva YS, Tella SH, Glushko T, Pacak K, Teytelboym OM (2019) Medullary thyroid carcinoma: an update on imaging. J Thyroid Res 2019:1893047
4. Kloos RT, Eng C, Evans DB, Francis GL, Gagel RF et al (2009) Medullary thyroid cancer: management guidelines of the American Thyroid Association. Thyroid 19(6):565–612
5. Trimboli P, Giovanella L, Valabrega S, Andrioli M, Baldelli R, Cremonini N et al (2014) Ultrasound features of medullary thyroid carcinoma correlate with cancer aggressiveness: a retrospective multicenter study. J Exp Clin Cancer Res 33:87
6. Kim SH, Kim BS, Jung SL, Lee JW, Yang PS, Kang BJ et al (2009) Ultrasonographic findings of medullary thyroid carcinoma: a comparison with papillary thyroid carcinoma. Korean J Radiol 10(2):101–105
7. Elisei R (2008) Routine serum calcitonin measurement in the evaluation of thyroid nodules. Best Pract Res Clin Endocrinol Metab 22(6):941–953
8. Papi G, Corsello SM, Cioni K, Pizzini AM, Corrado S, Carapezzi C et al (2006) Value of routine measurement of serum calcitonin concentrations in patients with nodular thyroid disease: a multicenter study. J Endocrinol Investig 29(5):427–437
9. Aiken AH (2012) Imaging of thyroid cancer. Semin Ultrasound CT MR 33(2):138–149
10. Sharma E, Dahal S, Sharma P, Bhandari A, Gupta V, Amgai B et al (2018) The characteristics and trends in adrenocortical carcinoma: a United States Population Based Study. J Clin Med Res 10(8):636–640
11. Ahmed AA, Thomas AJ, Ganeshan DM, Blair KJ, Lall C, Lee JT et al (2020) Adrenal cortical carcinoma: pathology, genomics, prognosis, imaging features, and mimics with impact on management. Abdom Radiol 45(4):945–963
12. Allolio B, Fassnacht M (2006) Clinical review: adrenocortical carcinoma: clinical update. J Clin Endocrinol Metab 91(6):2027–2037

13. Fassnacht M, Arlt W, Bancos I, Dralle H, Newell-Price J, Sahdev A et al (2016) Management of adrenal incidentalomas: European Society of Endocrinology Clinical Practice Guideline in collaboration with the European Network for the Study of Adrenal Tumors. Eur J Endocrinol 175(2):G1–G34
14. Luton JP, Cerdas S, Billaud L, Thomas G, Guilhaume B, Bertagna X et al (1990) Clinical features of adrenocortical carcinoma, prognostic factors, and the effect of mitotane therapy. N Engl J Med 322(17):1195–1201
15. Bharwani N, Rockall AG, Sahdev A, Gueorguiev M, Drake W, Grossman AB et al (2011) Adrenocortical carcinoma: the range of appearances on CT and MRI. AJR Am J Roentgenol 196(6):706–714
16. Fassnacht M, Johanssen S, Quinkler M, Bucsky P, Willenberg HS, Beuschlein F et al (2009) Limited prognostic value of the 2004 International Union Against Cancer staging classification for adrenocortical carcinoma: proposal for a Revised TNM Classification. Cancer 115(2):243–250
17. Pennanen M, Raade M, Louhimo J, Sane T, Heiskanen I, Arola J et al (2013) Adrenocortical tumours: high CT attenuation value correlates with eosinophilia but does not discriminate lipid-poor adenomas from malignancy. J Clin Pathol 66(12):1076–1080
18. Schlund JF, Kenney PJ, Brown ED, Ascher SM, Brown JJ, Semelka RC (1995) Adrenocortical carcinoma: MR imaging appearance with current techniques. J Magn Reson Imaging 5(2):171–174
19. Ilias I, Sahdev A, Reznek RH, Grossman AB, Pacak K (2007) The optimal imaging of adrenal tumours: a comparison of different methods. Endocr Relat Cancer 14(3):587–599
20. Melo HJ, Goldman SM, Szejnfeld J, Faria JF, Huayllas MK, Andreoni C et al (2014) Application of a protocol for magnetic resonance spectroscopy of adrenal glands: an experiment with over 100 cases. Radiol Bras 47(6):333–341
21. Mayo-Smith WW, Boland GW, Noto RB, Lee MJ (2001) State-of-the-art adrenal imaging. Radiographics 21(4):995–1012
22. Woo S, Suh CH, Kim SY, Cho JY, Kim SH (2018) Pheochromocytoma as a frequent false-positive in adrenal washout CT: a systematic review and meta-analysis. Eur Radiol 28(3):1027–1036
23. Mohammed MF, ElBanna KY, Ferguson D, Harris A, Khosa F (2018) Pheochromocytomas versus adenoma: role of venous phase CT enhancement. AJR Am J Roentgenol 210(5):1073–1078
24. Jacques AE, Sahdev A, Sandrasagara M, Goldstein R, Berney D, Rockall AG et al (2008) Adrenal phaeochromocytoma: correlation of MRI appearances with histology and function. Eur Radiol 18(12):2885–2892
25. Schieda N, Alrashed A, Flood TA, Samji K, Shabana W, McInnes MD (2016) Comparison of quantitative MRI and CT washout analysis for differentiation of adrenal pheochromocytoma from adrenal adenoma. AJR Am J Roentgenol 206(6):1141–1148
26. Bowerman RA, Silver TM, Jaffe MH, Stuck KJ, Hinerman DL (1981) Sonography of adrenal pheochromocytomas. AJR Am J Roentgenol 137(6):1227–1231
27. Blake MA, Krishnamoorthy SK, Boland GW, Sweeney AT, Pitman MB, Harisinghani M et al (2003) Low-density pheochromocytoma on CT: a mimicker of adrenal adenoma. AJR Am J Roentgenol 181(6):1663–1668
28. Szolar DH, Korobkin M, Reittner P, Berghold A, Bauernhofer T, Trummer H et al (2005) Adrenocortical carcinomas and adrenal pheochromocytomas: mass and enhancement loss evaluation at delayed contrast-enhanced CT. Radiology 234(2):479–485
29. Park BK, Kim CK, Kwon GY, Kim JH (2007) Re-evaluation of pheochromocytomas on delayed contrast-enhanced CT: washout enhancement and other imaging features. Eur Radiol 17(11):2804–2809
30. Elsayes KM, Mukundan G, Narra VR, Lewis JS Jr, Shirkhoda A, Farooki A et al (2004) Adrenal masses: MR imaging features with pathologic correlation. Radiographics 24(1):73–86
31. Lee KY, Oh YW, Noh HJ, Lee YJ, Yong HS, Kang EY et al (2006) Extraadrenal paragangliomas of the body: imaging features. AJR Am J Roentgenol 187(2):492–504

32. Magliulo G, Zardo F, Varacalli S, D'Amico R (2003) Multiple paragangliomas of the head and neck. An Otorrinolaringol Ibero Am 30(1):31–38
33. Deng Y, Wang XM, Wu LB, Sun C, Duan YH, Cheng ZP et al (2010) Significance of the preoperative guidance of dual-source CT in carotid body tumor. Chin Med J 123(20):2816–2819
34. van den Berg R, Schepers A, de Bruine FT, Liauw L, Mertens BJ, van der Mey AG et al (2004) The value of MR angiography techniques in the detection of head and neck paragangliomas. Eur J Radiol 52(3):240–245
35. Rakovich G, Ferraro P, Therasse E, Duranceau A (2001) Preoperative embolization in the management of a mediastinal paraganglioma. Ann Thorac Surg 72(2):601–603
36. Sahin-Akyar G, Erden I, Yagci C, Akyar S, Erekul S (1997) Magnetic resonance imaging findings of a nonfunctional mediastinal paraganglioma with an unusual presentation. Eur Radiol 7(7):1114–1116
37. Hayes WS, Davidson AJ, Grimley PM, Hartman DS (1990) Extraadrenal retroperitoneal paraganglioma: clinical, pathologic, and CT findings. AJR Am J Roentgenol 155(6):1247–1250
38. Tabakin AL, Weintraub MA, Radadia KD, Salazar CG, Sadimin E, Singer EA (2019) Metastatic retroperitoneal paraganglioma: case report and review of the literature. Clin Oncol 4:1589
39. Singh A, Hines JJ, Friedman B (2019) Multimodality imaging of the pancreatic neuroendocrine tumors. Semin Ultrasound CT MR 40(6):469–482
40. Malla S, Kumar P, Madhusudhan KS (2020) Radiology of the neuroendocrine neoplasms of the gastrointestinal tract: a comprehensive review. Abdom Radiol 46(3):919–935
41. Patel N, Barbieri A, Gibson J (2019) Neuroendocrine tumors of the gastrointestinal tract and pancreas. Surg Pathol Clin 12(4):1021–1044
42. Rockall AG, Reznek RH (2007) Imaging of neuroendocrine tumours (CT/MR/US). Best Pract Res Clin Endocrinol Metab 21(1):43–68
43. van Treijen MJC, van Beek DJ, van Leeuwaarde RS, Vriens MR, Valk GD (2018) Diagnosing nonfunctional pancreatic NETs in MEN1: the evidence base. J Endocr Soc 2(9):1067–1088
44. Dietrich CF, Ignee A, Braden B, Barreiros AP, Ott M, Hocke M (2008) Improved differentiation of pancreatic tumors using contrast-enhanced endoscopic ultrasound. Clin Gastroenterol Hepatol 6(5):590–597
45. Oshikawa O, Tanaka S, Ioka T, Nakaizumi A, Hamada Y, Mitani T (2002) Dynamic sonography of pancreatic tumors: comparison with dynamic CT. AJR Am J Roentgenol 178(5):1133–1137
46. Rickes S, Monkemuller K, Malfertheiner P (2006) Contrast-enhanced ultrasound in the diagnosis of pancreatic tumors. JOP 7(6):584–592
47. Baker MS, Knuth JL, DeWitt J, LeBlanc J, Cramer H, Howard TJ et al (2008) Pancreatic cystic neuroendocrine tumors: preoperative diagnosis with endoscopic ultrasound and fine-needle immunocytology. J Gastrointest Surg 12(3):450–456
48. Nikfarjam M, Warshaw AL, Axelrod L, Deshpande V, Thayer SP, Ferrone CR et al (2008) Improved contemporary surgical management of insulinomas: a 25-year experience at the Massachusetts General Hospital. Ann Surg 247(1):165–172
49. Sundin A, Arnold R, Baudin E, Cwikla JB, Eriksson B, Fanti S et al (2017) ENETS Consensus Guidelines for the Standards of Care in neuroendocrine tumors: radiological, nuclear medicine & hybrid imaging. Neuroendocrinology 105(3):212–244
50. Fidler JL, Fletcher JG, Reading CC, Andrews JC, Thompson GB, Grant CS et al (2003) Preoperative detection of pancreatic insulinomas on multiphasic helical CT. AJR Am J Roentgenol 181(3):775–780
51. Saleh M, Bhosale PR, Yano M, Itani M, Elsayes AK, Halperin D et al (2020) New frontiers in imaging including radiomics updates for pancreatic neuroendocrine neoplasms. Abdom Radiol 47(9):3078–3100
52. Zhu L, Xue H, Sun H, Wang X, Wu W, Jin Z et al (2017) Insulinoma detection with MDCT: is there a role for whole-pancreas perfusion? AJR Am J Roentgenol 208(2):306–314
53. Thoeni RF, Mueller-Lisse UG, Chan R, Do NK, Shyn PB (2000) Detection of small, functional islet cell tumors in the pancreas: selection of MR imaging sequences for optimal sensitivity. Radiology 214(2):483–490

54. Owen NJ, Sohaib SA, Peppercorn PD, Monson JP, Grossman AB, Besser GM et al (2001) MRI of pancreatic neuroendocrine tumours. Br J Radiol 74(886):968–973
55. Ichikawa T, Peterson MS, Federle MP, Baron RL, Haradome H, Kawamori Y et al (2000) Islet cell tumor of the pancreas: biphasic CT versus MR imaging in tumor detection. Radiology 216(1):163–171
56. Wang Y, Chen ZE, Yaghmai V, Nikolaidis P, McCarthy RJ, Merrick L et al (2011) Diffusion-weighted MR imaging in pancreatic endocrine tumors correlated with histopathologic characteristics. J Magn Reson Imaging 33(5):1071–1079
57. Zhao K, Patel N, Kulkarni K, Gross JS, Taslakian B (2020) Essentials of insulinoma localization with selective arterial calcium stimulation and hepatic venous sampling. J Clin Med 9(10):3091
58. Oberg K, Hellman P, Kwekkeboom D, Jelic S (2010) Neuroendocrine bronchial and thymic tumours: ESMO Clinical Practice Guidelines for diagnosis, treatment and follow-up. Ann Oncol 21(Suppl 5):220–222
59. Caplin ME, Baudin E, Ferolla P, Filosso P, Garcia-Yuste M, Lim E et al (2015) Pulmonary neuroendocrine (carcinoid) tumors: European Neuroendocrine Tumor Society expert consensus and recommendations for best practice for typical and atypical pulmonary carcinoids. Ann Oncol 26(8):1604–1620
60. Jeung MY, Gasser B, Gangi A, Charneau D, Ducroq X, Kessler R et al (2002) Bronchial carcinoid tumors of the thorax: spectrum of radiologic findings. Radiographics 22(2):351–365
61. Caplin M, Sundin A, Nillson O, Baum RP, Klose KJ, Kelestimur F et al (2012) ENETS consensus guidelines for the management of patients with digestive neuroendocrine neoplasms: colorectal neuroendocrine neoplasms. Neuroendocrinology 95(2):88–97
62. Marx A, Chan JK, Coindre JM, Detterbeck F, Girard N, Harris NL et al (2015) The 2015 World Health Organization Classification of tumors of the thymus: continuity and changes. J Thorac Oncol 10(10):1383–1395
63. Wagner-Bartak NA, Baiomy A, Habra MA, Mukhi SV, Morani AC, Korivi BR et al (2017) Cushing syndrome: diagnostic workup and imaging features, with clinical and pathologic correlation. AJR Am J Roentgenol 209(1):19–32
64. Phan AT, Oberg K, Choi J, Harrison LH Jr, Hassan MM, Strosberg JR et al (2010) NANETS consensus guideline for the diagnosis and management of neuroendocrine tumors: well-differentiated neuroendocrine tumors of the thorax (includes lung and thymus). Pancreas 39(6):784–798
65. Gluckman CR, Metz DC (2019) Gastric neuroendocrine tumors (carcinoids). Curr Gastroenterol Rep 21(4):13
66. Roberto GA, Rodrigues CMB, Peixoto RD, Younes RN (2020) Gastric neuroendocrine tumor: a practical literature review. World J Gastrointest Oncol 12(8):850–856
67. Baumann T, Rottenburger C, Nicolas G, Wild D (2016) Gastroenteropancreatic neuroendocrine tumours (GEP-NET) - imaging and staging. Best Pract Res Clin Endocrinol Metab 30(1):45–57
68. Sahani DV, Bonaffini PA, Fernandez-Del Castillo C, Blake MA (2013) Gastroenteropancreatic neuroendocrine tumors: role of imaging in diagnosis and management. Radiology 266(1):38–61
69. Ba-Ssalamah A, Prokop M, Uffmann M, Pokieser P, Teleky B, Lechner G (2003) Dedicated multidetector CT of the stomach: spectrum of diseases. Radiographics 23(3):625–644
70. Kim S, Marcus R, Wells ML, Sheedy SP, Hansel SL, Bruining DH et al (2020) The evolving role of imaging for small bowel neuroendocrine neoplasms: estimated impact of imaging and disease-free survival in a retrospective observational study. Abdom Radiol 45(3):623–631
71. Scarpa M, Prando D, Pozza A, Esposti ED, Castoro C, Angriman I (2010) A systematic review of diagnostic procedures to detect midgut neuroendocrine tumors. J Surg Oncol 102(7):877–888
72. Sharma A, Das CJ, Makharia GK, Arora G, Kumar R (2020) Comparison of contrast-enhanced CT + CT enterography and ^{68}Ga-DOTANOC PET/CT in gastroenteropancreatic neuroendocrine tumors. Clin Nucl Med 45(11):848–853

73. Druce MR, Bharwani N, Akker SA, Drake WM, Rockall A, Grossman AB (2010) Intra-abdominal fibrosis in a recent cohort of patients with neuroendocrine ('carcinoid') tumours of the small bowel. QJM 103(3):177–185
74. Noujaim MG, Green J, Min M, Schlieve CR, Patel K, Cahan M et al (2017) Carcinoids and capsules: a case series highlighting the utility of capsule endoscopy in patients with small bowel carcinoids. Gastroenterology Res 10(6):347–351
75. Sundin A, Vullierme MP, Kaltsas G, Plockinger U, European Neuroendocrine Tumor S (2009) ENETS consensus guidelines for the standards of care in neuroendocrine tumors: radiological examinations. Neuroendocrinology 90(2):167–183
76. Benhaim L, Faron M, Hadoux J, Gelli M, Sourrouille I, Burtin P et al (2020) Long term results after surgical resection of peritoneal metastasis from neuroendocrine tumors. Neuroendocrinology 111(6):599–608
77. Amzallag-Bellenger E, Oudjit A, Ruiz A, Cadiot G, Soyer PA, Hoeffel CC (2012) Effectiveness of MR enterography for the assessment of small-bowel diseases beyond Crohn disease. Radiographics 32(5):1423–1444
78. Masselli G, Casciani E, Polettini E, Laghi F, Gualdi G (2013) Magnetic resonance imaging of small bowel neoplasms. Cancer Imaging 13:92–99
79. Masselli G, Polettini E, Casciani E, Bertini L, Vecchioli A, Gualdi G (2009) Small-bowel neoplasms: prospective evaluation of MR enteroclysis. Radiology 251(3):743–750
80. Masselli G, Gualdi G (2013) CT and MR enterography in evaluating small bowel diseases: when to use which modality? Abdom Imaging 38(2):249–259
81. Masselli G, Polettini E, Laghi F, Monti R, Gualdi G (2014) Noninflammatory conditions of the small bowel. Magn Reson Imaging Clin N Am 22(1):51–65
82. Storino A, Wong D, Ore AS, Gaytan-Fuentes IA, Fabrizio A, Cataldo T et al (2020) Recurrence and survival of neuroendocrine neoplasms of the rectum: single-center experience. J Gastrointest Surg 25(9):2398–2400
83. Zhao B, Hollandsworth HM, Lopez NE, Parry LA, Abbadessa B, Cosman BC et al (2020) Outcomes for a large cohort of patients with rectal neuroendocrine tumors: an analysis of the national cancer database. J Gastrointest Surg 25(2):484–491
84. Rouse HC, Godoy MC, Lee WK, Phang PT, Brown CJ, Brown JA (2008) Imaging findings of unusual anorectal and perirectal pathology: a multi-modality approach. Clin Radiol 63(12):1350–1360
85. Howe JR, Merchant NB, Conrad C, Keutgen XM, Hallet J, Drebin JA et al (2020) The North American Neuroendocrine Tumor Society consensus paper on the surgical management of pancreatic neuroendocrine tumors. Pancreas 49(1):1–33
86. Luersen GF, Wei W, Tamm EP, Bhosale PR, Szklaruk J (2016) Evaluation of magnetic resonance (MR) biomarkers for assessment of response with response evaluation criteria in solid tumors: comparison of the measurements of neuroendocrine tumor liver metastases (NETLM) with various MR sequences and at multiple phases of contrast administration. J Comput Assist Tomogr 40(5):717–722
87. Altieri B, Di Dato C, Martini C, Sciammarella C, Di Sarno A, Colao A et al (2019) Bone metastases in neuroendocrine neoplasms: from pathogenesis to clinical management. Cancer 11(9):1332
88. Leboulleux S, Dromain C, Vataire AL, Malka D, Auperin A, Lumbroso J et al (2008) Prediction and diagnosis of bone metastases in well-differentiated gastro-entero-pancreatic endocrine cancer: a prospective comparison of whole body magnetic resonance imaging and somatostatin receptor scintigraphy. J Clin Endocrinol Metab 93(8):3021–3028
89. Choi H, Loyer EM, DuBrow RA, Kaur H, David CL, Huang S et al (2001) Radio-frequency ablation of liver tumors: assessment of therapeutic response and complications. Radiographics 21:41–54
90. Liapi E, Geschwind JF, Vossen JA, Buijs M, Georgiades CS, Bluemke DA et al (2008) Functional MRI evaluation of tumor response in patients with neuroendocrine hepatic metastasis treated with transcatheter arterial chemoembolization. AJR Am J Roentgenol 190(1):67–73

8 Nuclear Medicine Imaging in Neuroendocrine Tumors

Andreas Kjaer

8.1 Introduction

With the paradigm of personalized medicine in cancer, it has increasingly become necessary to diagnose and characterize tumors at the molecular level. Whereas this is possible through invasive methods, for example, analyses of biopsies, it can also be achieved in a noninvasive manner using nuclear medicine imaging methods [1]. These image-based methods for phenotyping tumors have several advantages over invasive methods. First, they are not prone to sampling error as they are analyses based on tissue samples that often turn out not to be representative of the entire disease. Accordingly, WHO grading is based on the measurement of proliferation, for example, Ki67, in biopsies [2]. However, there is no guarantee that such biopsies are taken from the areas with highest proliferation, which is likely to determine the destiny of the patient. Based on experience with nuclear medicine imaging, indeed large regional variation in uptake of functional tracers is seen. Moreover, exact phenotyping of therapeutic targets is important before initiating treatment. Accordingly, somatostatin receptor scintigraphy prior to PRRT reveals if the whole or only part of the tumor burden in a neuroendocrine tumor (NET) patient will be targeted and thereby predicts the likelihood of success. In many ways, PRRT and somatostatin receptor imaging using the same ligands have been the proof-of-concept of theranostics within cancer.

For reasons mentioned above, somatostatin receptor scintigraphy based on gamma camera technique has been used extensively and on a routine basis for decades in NET. However, recent developments within nuclear medicine are increasingly moving the field toward the use of PET due to the higher sensitivity, better spatial resolution, and quantitative nature. Accordingly, most guidelines now recommend the use

A. Kjaer (✉)
Department of Clinical Physiology and Nuclear Medicine, Cluster for Molecular Imaging, Rigshospitalet, University of Copenhagen, Copenhagen, Denmark
e-mail: akjaer@sund.ku.dk

S. Yalcin, K. Öberg (eds.), *Neuroendocrine Tumours*,
https://doi.org/10.1007/978-3-031-56968-5_8

of PET and not SPECT for somatostatin receptor imaging. In addition, the use of non-somatostatin receptor PET imaging in particular FDG-PET may become increasingly important in the future, especially for therapy selection and monitoring with early detection of non-responders that may then be changed in therapy.

8.2 Somatostatin Receptors as Target for Imaging in NET

Most gastro-entero-pancreatic (GEP) and broncho-pulmonary NETs, which are the focus of this chapter, overexpress somatostatin receptors and especially the subtype 2 receptor [3, 4]. Therefore, somatostatin receptor imaging is effective in diagnosing, staging, and re-staging of NET. However, in vitro measurements have shown that the proportion of NETs that express somatostatin receptors varies with high proportion of approximately 90% of carcinoids and but only approximately 70% of insulinomas [5]. However, since high expressing NETs, for example, carcinoids, are much more abundant than low expressing NET types, for example, insulinomas, the overall expression rate for NETs is close to 90%. Overexpression of somatostatin receptors is also used as a target for therapy using long-acting somatostatin analogs as well as PRRT with beta-emitting somatostatin receptor ligands, for example, ^{177}Lu-DOTATATE and ^{90}Y-DOTATOC [6]. Due to this, somatostatin receptor imaging is also used for selecting patients suited for therapy and to monitor therapy response.

8.3 From SPECT to PET Imaging

The field of nuclear medicine is increasingly moving into use of PET, and many tracers that served well for many years in gamma camera-based imaging and SPECT are substituted with new PET tracers visualizing the same characteristics. There are major advantages using PET-based imaging compared to SPECT-based imaging.

Firstly, the sensitivity of PET is at least 100-fold higher than that of SPECT allowing for better count statistics with less noise in images obtained at lower tracer doses. This in general translates into less radiation burden.

Secondly, the spatial resolution is typically twofold better and around 4–5 mm for state-of-the-art PET scanners vs. 8–10 mm for SPECT scanners. However, it should be noted that spatial resolution does not refer to the minimal detectable lesion but whether foci can be discriminated from each other. Accordingly, a small, for example, 2 mm foci, with high tracer accumulation can be detected but will be represented as a larger focus (blurred). However, due to the averaging of activity in the image, increasing amounts of activity are necessary for detection when spatial resolution drops.

Thirdly, due to the physics in PET, an accurate attenuation correction can be performed which leads to the ability to quantify tracer uptake in absolute terms. In contrast, uptake in SPECT has to be expressed in relative terms, for example, relative to liver as used for somatostatin receptor imaging using the Krenning scale. With PET, it is possible to follow absolute uptake over time and typically the reproducibility allows for detection of changes of 10% or more between two scans. This can be and is used for therapy response monitoring.

Another challenge in PET imaging is the necessity of a cyclotron and radiochemistry laboratories. However, recently, generator-based PET isotopes have become available most notably ^{68}Ga thereby making production of PET isotopes possible without an expensive on-site cyclotron. Also, the use of PET isotopes with long half-lives, for example, ^{64}Cu with 13h half-life, has made it possible to centralize the production of tracers for distribution to PET centers. In part, this is also possible, if logistics is in place, with ^{18}F-labeled compounds, since ^{18}F has a half-life of 110 min. Therefore, at present, Nuclear Medicine departments may implement PET technology by installing PET scanners without the need of creating a whole PET center with cyclotrons and advanced radiochemistry facilities. This has lowered the entry barrier to perform PET scans considerably.

8.4 PET-Based Imaging of Somatostatin Receptors

8.4.1 ^{68}Ga-DOTATATE, ^{68}Ga-DOTATOC, and Other ^{68}Ga-labeled PET Tracers

Considering the obvious advantages of using PET for somatostatin receptor imaging and the convenience of ^{68}Ga labeling using a generator, several new PET tracers targeted toward the somatostatin receptor have recently been introduced. The majority is based on the same peptides as used for SPECT imaging, that is, octreotide and octreotate using DOTA as the chelator. The affinity for the different subtypes of somatostatin receptors is dependent both on radionuclide, chelator and peptide. Discussion on which PET tracer is best includes the affinity for the somatostatin receptor subtype 2 as well as affinity for other somatostatin receptors, especially subtype 5. However, we have shown on a gene-expression level that somatostatin 2 receptors are expressed to a much higher level on NETs than any other of the receptors [3], so we suggest that affinities toward the other 4 receptor subtypes are of limited interest. The three most commonly used ^{68}Ga-labeled somatostatin receptor PET tracers are ^{68}Ga-DOTATATE, ^{68}Ga-DOTATOC, and ^{68}Ga-DOTANOC of which the first two have gained marketing authorizations. These tracers are all somatostatin receptor agonists. Table 8.1 summarizes in vitro affinities of the different PET

Table 8.1 In vitro binding affinities (IC50 in nM ± SEM) of ^{68}Ga-labeled, chelated somatostatin analogs

Name	SST_1	SST_2	SST_3	SST_4	SST_5
Ga-DOTATATE	>10,000	0.2 ± 0.04	>10,000	300 ± 140	377 ± 18
Ga-DOTATOC	>10,000	2.5 ± 0.5	613 ± 140	>1000	73 ± 21
Ga-DOTANOC	>10,000	1.9 ± 0.4	40 ± 5.8	260 ± 74	7.2 ± 1.6
Ga-NODAGA-JR11	>1000	1.2 ± 0.2	>1000	>1000	>1000

Data from [7–9]. *SST* somatostatin receptor, *Ga-DOTATATE* Ga-DOTA-tyr^{3}Octreotate, *Ga-DOTATOC* Ga-DOTA-tyr^3-Octreotide, *Ga-DOTANOC* Ga-DOTA-l-Nal^3-Octreotide tracers toward the five somatostatin receptor subtypes as reported in the literature [7, 8]. ^{68}Ga-DOTATATE has a tenfold higher affinity for the somatostatin 2 receptor and a very low affinity toward the somatostatin 5 receptor compared to the other two tracers. ^{68}Ga-DOTANOC has the highest affinity toward the somatostatin 5 receptor, which we believe is of minor importance in NETs. A difference between the three tracers in normal tissue distribution could lead to differences in tumor-to-background ratios and thereby easiness to detect lesions. However, for most organs, the tumor-to-background ratios are comparable [4].

Performance of the three ^{68}Ga-based PET tracers has recently been reviewed [10]. For ^{68}Ga-DOTATATE, sensitivity on a patient basis was reported to be 72–96% in 6 smaller studies including between 18 and 38 patients (total of 144 patients) [11–15]. The study with the median sensitivity reported 93% (CI: 70–99%; 20 patients) [14]. For ^{68}Ga-DOTATOC, sensitivity on a patient basis was found to be 92–100% in 6 small or medium sized studies including between 8 and 84 patients (total of 211 patients) [16–21]. The largest study with 84 patients reported a sensitivity of 97% (CI: 90–100%) [19]. Finally, for ^{68}Ga-DOTANOC, patient-based sensitivity was reported to be 68–100% from 9 studies including 11–1239 patients (total of 1677 patients) [14, 15, 22–27]. The study with 1239 patients reported a sensitivity of 92% (CI: 90–94%) [27].

Taking into consideration that the number of patients as well as the composition of the groups evaluated with the different ^{68}Ga-based tracers varied, it seems fair to conclude that no major differences have been documented. Especially, the populations studied varied between the investigations. So far, only three studies have compared these tracers pair-wise on a head-to-head basis [14, 15, 28]. In all these studies, comparisons were undertaken lesion-based rather than patient-based since only minor differences were expected and since the superiority of one tracer could be the ability to detect more lesions. Two studies compared ^{68}Ga-DOTATATE with ^{68}Ga-DOTANOC [14, 15] and one compared ^{68}Ga-DOTATATE with ^{68}Ga-DOTATOC [28]. Although minor differences were reported, many were nonsignificant on a patient basis and considering clinical relevance in our view, there were no major differences favoring use of one of these three tracers. Local availability, experience, and wish to theranostic pairing, for example, use of ^{68}Ga-DOTATATE before ^{177}Lu-DOTATATE is to be used for PRRT, may decide which tracer to use. Absolute uptake of tracer between the tracers did vary although not systematically. However, if comparing absolute values as SUV longitudinally, for example, in therapy response monitoring, the same tracer has to be used.

Another ^{68}Ga-labeled PET somatostatin receptor PET tracer, ^{68}Ga-DOTA-lantreotide (^{68}Ga-DOTALAN), was introduced mainly as a companion diagnostic for ^{90}Y-labeled lantreotide. Two studies compared ^{68}Ga-DOTALAN on a head-to-head basis with ^{68}Ga-DOTATOC [29] and ^{68}Ga-DOTATATE [30], separately. Both studies found substantially less lesions visualized with ^{68}Ga-DOTALAN questioning the usefulness of this tracer as a stand-alone imaging agent.

More recently, a somatostatin receptor antagonist, ^{68}Ga-NODAGA-JR11 (OPS202), has been tested clinically in patients [31]. The theoretical advantages of using an antagonist rather than an agonist are binding to somatostatin receptors independently of their activation state [32]. In a small study comparing with ^{68}Ga-DOTATOC, ^{68}Ga-NODAGA-JR11 demonstrated a higher lesion detection rate and tumor-to-background ratio for liver lesions [33].

8.4.2 ^{64}Cu-DOTATATE and Other ^{64}Cu-labeled PET Tracers

As an alternative to ^{68}Ga-labeled PET tracers, we introduced the somatostatin receptor PET tracer ^{64}Cu-DOTATATE for human use [34, 35]. Theoretical advantages compared to ^{68}Ga-labeled tracers include the longer half-life of ^{64}Cu (13h) compared to ^{68}Ga (68 min) allowing for delayed imaging. Indeed, we recently showed that imaging is possible from 1 to 3 h post injection with ^{64}Cu-DOTATATE with the same lesion detection ability [36] (Fig. 8.1). Also, the positron range which is the distance a positron travels from emission until it is annihilated and sends out two photons differ between the radionuclides. Since the PET scanner detects the coincident photons and not where the emission took place, which is really what should be visualized, the image is off-focus (blurred). For ^{64}Cu, the average positron range is only 1 mm, whereas it is 4 mm for ^{68}Ga. This translates into better resolution and potentially better detection of small foci using ^{64}Cu as radionuclide. In accordance with this, we demonstrated in a head-to-head comparison with ^{68}Ga-DOTATOC a better lesion-detection rate using ^{64}Cu-DOTATATE [37] (Fig. 8.2). Finally, the long half-life and a shelf life of >24 h of ^{64}Cu-DOTATATE allow for central production and distribution, which has logistical advantages.

Taken together, ^{64}Cu-DOTATATE seems promising for clinical use and following a pivotal phase III study performed in the US [38], the tracer was approved by FDA on September 2020.

Another ^{64}Cu-labeled somatostatin receptor PET tracer is ^{64}Cu-SARTATE, where promising first-in-humans data from 10 NET patients were published recently [39]. Apart from imaging, the tracer is to be used for prospective dosimetry for its therapeutic counterpart ^{67}Cu-SARTATE.

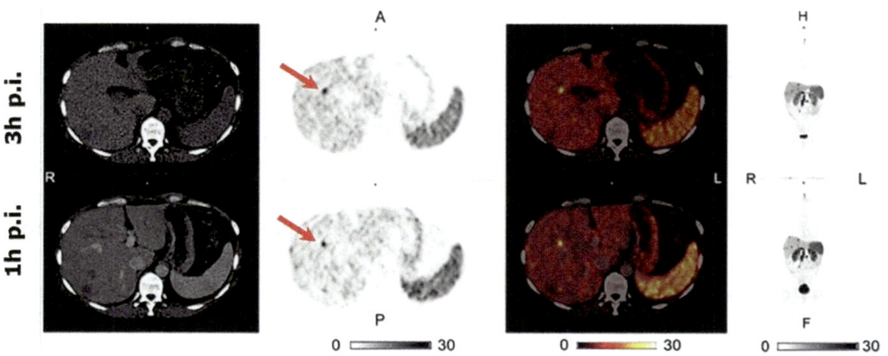

Fig. 8.1 Example of ^{64}Cu-DOTATATE PET/CT performed in the same NET patient 1 h p.i. and 3 h p.i. Note the similar images obtained throughout the period. From study of Loft et al. [36]

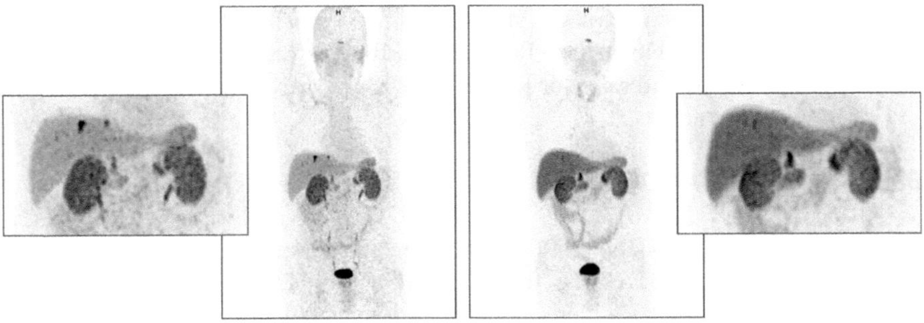

Fig. 8.2 Head-to-head comparison of ^{64}Cu-DOTATATE and ^{68}Ga-DOTATOC in a NET patient with liver lesions. Please note the better image resolution obtained with ^{64}Cu-DOTATATE probably due to lower image resolution. Image from prospective study of Johnbeck et al. [37]

8.4.3 Other Somatostatin Receptor-Targeting PET Tracers

In addition to ^{68}Ga and ^{64}Cu-labeled tracers, development of ^{18}F-labeled somatostatin receptor PET tracers is ongoing. Advantages include short positron range on par with ^{64}Cu. Most recently, a first-in-humans study testing ^{18}F-SiFA*lin*-TATE in 13 patients with NET has been published with promising results [40].

8.5 Catecholaminergic and Serotonergic Pathways for Imaging of NETs

Neuroendocrine tumors have the ability for uptake of amine precursors the *L*-type large neutral amino acid transport system (LAT) transporter and through further metabolism including decarboxylation to form catecholamines and serotonin.

8.5.1 ^{18}F-DOPA

The PET tracer and dopamine precursor ^{18}F-L-dihydroxyphenylalanine (^{18}F-DOPA) are taken up by neuroendocrine tumor cells by LAT, transported into the cytoplasm and metabolized (decarboxylated) to dopamine, which is then transported into secretory vesicles by VMAT. In the secretory vesicles, dopamine is further metabolized to noradrenaline and adrenaline.

Whereas early studies showed promising results for ^{18}F-DOPA in GEP and bronchopulmonary NETs with sensitivities on a patient basis ranging from 65 to 96% based on 4 studies with total of 116 patients (meta-analysis sensitivity: 87%; CI: 80–93%) [41], even higher sensitivities were found for pheochromocytomas and paragaglioma that are, however, not the focus of this chapter. Performance in abdominal NETs was in general superior when compared to gamma camera-based somatostatin receptor scintigraphy. However, since PET-based somatostatin receptor imaging is superior as well, the question arises whether ^{18}F-DOPA is better and valuable compared to the ^{68}Ga-labeled somatostatin receptor PET tracers. Two studies with a total of 28 patients compared on a head-to-head basis ^{18}F-DOPA with ^{68}Ga-DOTANOC or ^{68}Ga-DOTATOC, respectively. In both studies, ^{68}Ga-DOTANOC or ^{68}Ga-DOTATOC visualized considerably more lesions than ^{18}F-DOPA even in pheochromocytomas [22, 42]. One study with 25 patients compared ^{18}F-DOPA with ^{68}Ga-DOTATATE, and also here it was found that ^{68}Ga-DOTATATE had a much higher sensitivity [13].

Taken together, although ^{18}F-DOPA performs pretty well in GEP and bronchopulmonary NETs when compared with modern PET tracers targeting somatostatin receptors, they are inferior. In general, it therefore seems that this tracer is not necessary for routine use if somatostatin receptor PET is available.

8.6 $^{123/131}$I-MIBG and ^{18}F-MFBG

A reuptake mechanism exists at the catecholaminergic terminals for noradrenaline. This reuptake mechanism can be visualized using the false neurotransmitter metaiodobenzylguanidine (MIBG) of metafluorobenzylguanidine (MFBG) which is also a substrate for the reuptake mechanism. MIBG can be labeled with radioiodine and is most commonly used for SPECT as ^{123}I-MIBG or ^{131}I-MIBG, where the latter may also be used for therapy due to concomitant beta-emission. For PET imaging, ^{18}F-MFBG may be used [43].

For imaging of GEP and bronchopulmonary NETs, the sensitivity of $^{123/131}$I-MIBG gamma camera imaging is somewhat disappointing based on two studies with a total of 125 patients: 63% (CI: 54–72%) [41]. For pheochromocytomas, neuroblastomas, and paragangliomas, the same meta-analysis found sensitivities of 79% (9 studies; $n = 161$; CI: 68–82%), 84% (5 studies; $n = 204$; CI: 79–89%), and 69% (4 studies; $n = 87$; CI: 58–78%), respectively. Again, the question arises whether $^{123/131}$I-MIBG imaging has any role when somatostatin receptor imaging and FDG-PET are available. In a recent prospective study, we therefore performed ^{111}In-DTPA-octreotide SPECT, ^{123}I-MIBG and FDG-PET for head-to-head comparison in a total of 96 consecutive patients [44]. We found an overall sensitivity on a patient-basis of 52% and ^{111}In-DTPA-octreotide detected more than twice the number of lesions compared to ^{123}I-MIBG. Of the 96 patients, three were ^{123}I-MIBG positive and ^{111}In-DTPA-octreotide negative. However, all of them were also FDG-PET positive. Accordingly, when somatostatin receptor scintigraphy and FDG-PET are available, we found no additional value of ^{123}I-MIBG. Therefore, we doubt that there is any future role of ^{123}I-MIBG imaging in NETs apart from companion diagnostics if ^{131}I-MIBG treatment is planned. For this reason, we do no longer offer ^{123}I-MIBG as a routine method at our department. ^{18}F-MFBG has only been tested in 10 patients with neuroblastoma and 5 patients with paraganglioma/pheochromocytoma [43].

8.7 ^{11}C-5-HTP

The PET tracer and serotonin precursor ^{11}C-5-hyroxytryptophan (^{11}C-5-HTP) are transported into the neuroendocrine tumor cells via LAT, decarboxylized to serotonin and transported into secretory vesicles by VMAT.

The PET tracer is labeled with ^{11}C, which has a half-life of 20 min. This demands an on-site cyclotron and that synthesis is made in close relation to the scan. Accordingly, the capacity of ^{11}C-5-HTP PET scans is limited and only available in few centers. Maybe for this reason, data on performance is also somewhat limited. A total of 54 patients were studied in 3 different investigations [45–47] and when data were pooled, a sensitivity of 87% (CI: 75–95%) was found [41]. One of these studies compared the performance with ^{18}F-DOPA and ^{111}In-DTPA-octreotide and found ^{18}F-DOPA best for staging in carcinoids (n = 24), whereas ^{11}C-5-HTP was best in pancreatic islet cell tumors (n = 23) [47]. In another study with 42 consecutive NET patients in comparison with ^{111}In-DTPA-octreotide, ^{11}C-5-HTP found more lesions in 58% of patients and it was concluded that ^{11}C-5-HTP could be used as an universal imaging method for detection of NETs [46]. However, no other PET-based imaging was included in this study, and the superiority found was probably largely due to difference between SPECT and PET performance. Moreover, no studies until now have compared ^{11}C-5-HTP with PET-based somatostatin receptor scintigraphy and FDG-PET. Accordingly, at present, it is unsettled whether ^{11}C-5-HTP would be the method of choice in unclear NET cases. One could speculate if combined somatostatin receptor PET and FDG-PET would not solve most such cases in an easier way?

8.8 ^{18}F-FDG

^{18}F-2-deoxy-glucose (FDG) is a glucose analogue transported into the cells by means of GLUT transporters, in cancer mainly GLUT-1. In the cell, FDG is phosphorylated by hexokinases and once phosphorylated it is not further metabolized and therefore metabolically trapped in the cell. In this way, FDG accumulated to a degree reflecting the glycolytic activity of cancer cells. It should be noted that it visualizes aerobic glycolysis seen in cancer cells, also known as the Warburg effect, indirectly due to the increased glucose uptake. A high uptake of glucose for oxidative phosphorylation, for example, in muscles will also accumulate high amounts of FDG. For comprehensive visualization of the Warburg effect we recently developed the new imaging concept of hyperPET using a hybrid PET/MR scanner [48–51].

The sensitivity for detection of NETs is rather low for FDG. We found in a prospective study of 98 consecutive NET patients a sensitivity of 58% [44]. However, the sensitivity depended largely on proliferation index, and accordingly we found the sensitivity to be 41% for NETs with Ki67 <2% but 92% for Ki67 at or above 15%. Since most somatostatin receptor negative tumors have high proliferation index, FDG-PET may be of value in these tumors. In support of this, we found that of the 11 out of 96 ^{111}In-DTPA-octreotide negative patients, 7 were FDG-PET positive. Therefore, we suggest that FDG-PET could be used in these somatostatin receptor imaging negative cases. However, the main application may not lie in diagnosing and stating of NETs but in the strong prognostic value of FDG-PET. In line with this, we found that FDG-PET positivity was a stronger prognostic marker than Ki67, presence of liver metastases and chromogranin A [52, 53]. Since aggressiveness of NETs is a major determinant for selection of therapy [6], one could speculate whether FDG uptake could serve as a relevant grouping parameter alone or in addition to proliferation index. Also FDG-PET, as with other cancer forms, may be used as an early indicator for detection of response or failure to therapy in NET patients.

8.9 ^{18}F-FLT

As the Ki-67 proliferation index is currently used as a key marker for grading, prognostication, and selection of therapy, a noninvasive PET measure of proliferation would serve the same purpose. Accordingly, we investigated the prognostic value of ^{18}F-fluorothymidine prospectively in 100 NET patients [54]. In univariate models, ^{18}F-FLT had prognostic value both with regard to overall survival (OS) and progression free survival (PFS). However, when adding ^{18}F-FDG and Ki-67 to multivariate models, ^{18}F-FLT only remained of prognostic value in PFS. Accordingly, it seems that ^{18}F-FLT has no major role in NET prognostication if ^{18}F-FDG is available.

8.10 Conclusion

Somatostatin receptor imaging targeting the subtype 2 receptor is a key in the diagnostic workup and staging in NET patients. Three PET tracers, ^{68}Ga-DOTATATE, ^{68}Ga-DOTATOC, and ^{64}Cu-DOTATATE, have so far been approved by the authorities in the US and/or EU. In addition to somatostatin receptor PET imaging, imaging of metabolism using FDG-PET seems to have a major role in the diagnostic workup, phenotyping, prognostication, and planning as well as monitoring of therapy.

References

1. Kjaer A (2006) Molecular imaging of cancer using PET and SPECT. Adv Exp Med Biol 587:277–284
2. Hamilton S, Aaltonen L (2000) Pathology and genetics of tumors of the digestive system. IARC, Lyon
3. Binderup T, Knigge U, Mellon Mogensen A, Palnaes Hansen C, Kjaer A (2008) Quantitative gene expression of somatostatin receptors and noradrenaline transporter underlying scintigraphic results in patients with neuroendocrine tumors. Neuroendocrinology 87(4):223–232

4. Reubi JC, Waser B, Schaer JC, Laissue JA (2001) Somatostatin receptor sst1-sst5 expression in normal and neoplastic human tissues using receptor autoradiography with subtype-selective ligands. Eur J Nucl Med 28(7):836–846
5. Krenning EP, Kwekkeboom DJ, Bakker WH, Breeman WA, Kooij PP, Oei HY (1993) Somatostatin receptor scintigraphy with [^{111}In-DTPA-D-Phe1]- and [^{123}I-Tyr3]-octreotide: the Rotterdam experience with more than 1000 patients. Eur J Nucl Med 20(8):716–731
6. Öberg K, Knigge U, Kwekkeboom D, Perren A, ESMO Guidelines Working Group (2012) Neuroendocrine gastro-entero-pancreatic tumors: ESMO clinical practice guidelines for diagnosis, treatment and follow-up. Ann Oncol 23(Suppl 7):124–130
7. Reubi JC, Schär JC, Waser B, Wenger S, Heppeler A, Schmitt JS (2000) Affinity profiles for human somatostatin receptor subtypes SST1-SST5 of somatostatin radiotracers selected for scintigraphic and radiotherapeutic use. Eur J Nucl Med 27(3):273–282
8. Antunes P, Ginj M, Zhang H, Waser B, Baum RP, Reubi JC (2007) Are radiogallium-labelled DOTA-conjugated somatostatin analogues superior to those labelled with other radiometals? Eur J Nucl Med Mol Imaging 34(7):982–993
9. Fani M, Braun F, Waser B, Beetschen K, Cescato R, Erchegyi J (2012) Unexpected sensitivity of sst2 antagonists to N-terminal radiometal modifications. J Nucl Med 53(9):1481–1489
10. Johnbeck CB, Knigge U, Kjær A (2014) PET tracers for somatostatin receptor imaging of neuroendocrine tumors: current status and review of the literature. Future Oncol 10(14):2259–2277
11. Kayani I, Bomanji JB, Groves A, Conway G, Gacinovic S, Win T (2008) Functional imaging of neuroendocrine tumors with combined PET/CT using ^{68}Ga-DOTATATE (DOTA-DPhe1,Tyr3-octreotate) and ^{18}F-FDG. Cancer 112(11):2447–2455
12. Kayani I, Conry BG, Groves AM, Win T, Dickson J, Caplin M (2009) A comparison of ^{68}Ga-DOTATATE and ^{18}F-FDG PET/CT in pulmonary neuroendocrine tumors. J Nucl Med 50(12):1927–1932
13. Haug A, Auernhammer CJ, Wängler B, Tiling R, Schmidt G, Göke B (2009) Intraindividual comparison of ^{68}Ga-DOTA-TATE and ^{18}F-DOPA PET in patients with well-differentiated metastatic neuroendocrine tumours. Eur J Nucl Med Mol Imaging 36(5):765–770
14. Kabasakal L, Demirci E, Ocak M, Decristoforo C, Araman A, Ozsoy Y (2012) Comparison of ^{68}Ga-DOTATATE and ^{68}Ga-DOTANOC PET/CT imaging in the same patient group with neuroendocrine tumours. Eur J Nucl Med Mol Imaging 39(8):1271–1277
15. Wild D, Bomanji JB, Benkert P, Maecke H, Ell PJ, Reubi JC, Caplin ME (2013) Comparison of ^{68}Ga-DOTANOC and ^{68}Ga-DOTATATE PET/CT within patients with gastroenteropancreatic neuroendocrine tumors. J Nucl Med 54(3):364–372
16. Hofmann M, Maecke H, Börner R, Weckesser E, Schöffski P, Oei L (2001) Biokinetics and imaging with the somatostatin receptor PET radioligand (^{68})Ga-DOTATOC: preliminary data. Eur J Nucl Med 28(12):1751–1757
17. Koukouraki S, Strauss LG, Georgoulias V, Schuhmacher J, Haberkorn U, Karkavitsas N (2006) Evaluation of the pharmacokinetics of ^{68}Ga-DOTATOC in patients with metastatic neuroendocrine tumours scheduled for ^{90}Y-DOTATOC therapy. Eur J Nucl Med Mol Imaging 33(4):460–466
18. Buchmann I, Henze M, Engelbrecht S, Eisenhut M, Runz A, Schäfer M (2007) Comparison of ^{68}Ga-DOTATOC PET and ^{111}In-DTPAOC (Octreoscan) SPECT in patients with neuroendocrine tumours. Eur J Nucl Med Mol Imaging 34(10):1617–1626
19. Gabriel M, Decristoforo C, Kendler D, Dobrozemsky G, Heute D, Uprimny C (2007) 68Ga-DOTA-Tyr3-octreotide PET in neuroendocrine tumors: comparison with somatostatin receptor scintigraphy and CT. J Nucl Med 48(4):508–518
20. Putzer D, Gabriel M, Henninger B, Kendler D, Uprimny C, Dobrozemsky G (2009) Bone metastases in patients with neuroendocrine tumor: ^{68}Ga-DOTA-Tyr3-octreotide PET in comparison to CT and bone scintigraphy. J Nucl Med 50(8):1214–1221
21. Versari A, Camellini L, Carlinfante G, Frasoldati A, Nicoli F, Grassi E (2010) Ga-68 DOTATOC PET, endoscopic ultrasonography, and multidetector CT in the diagnosis of duodenopancreatic neuroendocrine tumors: a single-centre retrospective study. Clin Nucl Med 35(5):321–328

22. Ambrosini V, Tomassetti P, Castellucci P, Campana D, Montini G, Rubello D (2008) Comparison between ^{68}Ga-DOTA-NOC and ^{18}F-DOPA PET for the detection of gastro-entero-pancreatic and lung neuro-endocrine tumours. Eur J Nucl Med Mol Imaging 35(8):1431–1438
23. Ambrosini V, Castellucci P, Rubello D, Nanni C, Musto A, Allegri V (2009) 68Ga-DOTA-NOC: a new PET tracer for evaluating patients with bronchial carcinoid. Nucl Med Commun 30(4):281–286
24. Naswa N, Sharma P, Kumar A, Nazar AH, Kumar R, Chumber S (2011) Gallium-68-DOTA-NOC PET/CT of patients with gastroenteropancreatic neuroendocrine tumors: a prospective single-center study. AJR Am J Roentgenol 197(5):1221–1228
25. Krausz Y, Freedman N, Rubinstein R, Lavie E, Orevi M, Tshori S (2011) 68Ga-DOTA-NOC PET/CT imaging of neuroendocrine tumors: comparison with ^{111}In-DTPA-octreotide (OctreoScan®). Mol Imaging Biol 13(3):583–593
26. Naswa N, Sharma P, Soundararajan R, Karunanithi S, Nazar AH, Kumar R (2013) Diagnostic performance of somatostatin receptor PET/CT using ^{68}Ga-DOTANOC in gastrinoma patients with negative or equivocal CT findings. Abdom Imaging 38(3):552–560
27. Ambrosini V, Campana D, Tomassetti P, Fanti S (2012) 68Ga-labelled peptides for diagnosis of gastroenteropancreatic NET. Eur J Nucl Med Mol Imaging 39(1):52–60
28. Poeppel TD, Binse I, Petersenn S, Lahner H, Schott M, Antoch G (2011) 68Ga-DOTATOC versus ^{68}Ga-DOTATATE PET/CT in functional imaging of neuroendocrine tumors. J Nucl Med 52(12):1864–1870
29. Putzer D, Kroiss A, Waitz D, Gabriel M, Traub-Weidinger T, Uprimny C (2013) Somatostatin receptor PET in neuroendocrine tumours: ^{68}Ga-DOTA0,Tyr3-octreotide versus ^{68}Ga-DOTA0-lanreotide. Eur J Nucl Med Mol Imaging 40(3):364–372
30. Demirci E, Ocak M, Kabasakal L, Araman A, Ozsoy Y, Kanmaz B (2013) Comparison of Ga-68 DOTA-TATE and Ga-68 DOTA-LAN PET/CT imaging in the same patient group with neuroendocrine tumours: preliminary results. Nucl Med Commun 34(8):727–732
31. Nicolas GP, Beykan S, Bouterfa H, Kaufmann J, Bauman A, Lassmann M (2018) Safety, biodistribution, and radiation dosimetry of ^{68}Ga-OPS202 in patients with gastroenteropancreatic neuroendocrine tumors: a prospective phase I imaging study. J Nucl Med 59(6):909–914
32. Ginj M, Zhang H, Waser B, Cescato R, Wild D, Wang X (2006) Radiolabeled somatostatin receptor antagonists are preferable to agonists for in vivo peptide receptor targeting of tumors. Proc Natl Acad Sci USA 103(44):16436–16441
33. Nicolas GP, Schreiter N, Kaul F, Uiters J, Bouterfa H, Kaufmann J (2018) Sensitivity comparison of ^{68}Ga-OPS202 and ^{68}Ga-DOTATOC PET/CT in patients with gastroenteropancreatic neuroendocrine tumors: a prospective phase II imaging study. J Nucl Med 59(6):915–921
34. Pfeifer A, Knigge U, Mortensen J, Oturai P, Berthelsen AK, Loft A (2012) Clinical PET of neuroendocrine tumors using ^{64}Cu-DOTATATE: first-in-humans study. J Nucl Med 53(8):1207–1215
35. Pfeifer A, Knigge U, Binderup T, Mortensen J, Oturai P, Loft A (2015) 64Cu-DOTATATE PET for neuroendocrine tumors: a prospective head-to-head comparison with ^{111}In-DTPA-octreotide in 112 patients. J Nucl Med 56(6):847–854
36. Loft M, Carlsen EA, Johnbeck CB, Johannesen HH, Binderup T, Pfeifer A (2020) 64Cu-DOTATATE PET in patients with neuroendocrine neoplasms: prospective, head-to-head comparison of imaging at 1 hour and 3 hours post-injection. J Nucl Med 62(1):73–80
37. Johnbeck CB, Knigge U, Loft A, Berthelsen AK, Mortensen J, Oturai P (2017) Head-to-head comparison of (64)Cu-DOTATATE and (68)Ga-DOTATOC PET/CT: a prospective study of 59 patients with neuroendocrine tumors. J Nucl Med 58(3):451–457
38. Delpassand ES, Ranganathan D, Wagh N, Shafie A, Gaber A, Abbasi A (2020) 64Cu-DOTATATE PET/CT for imaging patients with known or suspected somatostatin receptor-positive neuroendocrine tumors: results of the first U.S. Prospective, Reader-Masked Clinical Trial. J Nucl Med 61(6):890–896
39. Hicks RJ, Jackson P, Kong G, Ware RE, Hofman MS, Pattison DA (2019) 64Cu-SARTATE PET imaging of patients with neuroendocrine tumors demonstrates high tumor uptake and

retention, potentially allowing prospective dosimetry for peptide receptor radionuclide therapy. J Nucl Med 60(6):777–785
40. Ilhan H, Lindner S, Todica A, Cyran CC, Tiling R, Auernhammer CJ (2020) Biodistribution and first clinical results of ^{18}F-SiFAlin-TATE PET: a novel ^{18}F-labeled somatostatin analog for imaging of neuroendocrine tumors. Eur J Nucl Med Mol Imaging 47(4):870–880
41. Koopmans KP, Neels ON, Kema IP, Elsinga PH, Links TP, de Vries EGE (2009) Molecular imaging in neuroendocrine tumors: molecular uptake mechanisms and clinical results. Crit Rev Oncol Hematol 71(3):199–213
42. Putzer D, Gabriel M, Kendler D, Henninger B, Knoflach M, Kroiss A (2010) Comparison of (68)Ga-DOTA-Tyr(3)-octreotide and (18)F-fluoro-L-dihydroxyphenylalanine positron emission tomography in neuroendocrine tumor patients. Q J Nucl Med Mol Imaging 54(1):68–75
43. Pandit-Taskar N, Zanzonico P, Staton KD, Carrasquillo JA, Reidy-Lagunes D, Lyashchenko S (2018) Biodistribution and dosimetry of ^{18}F-meta-fluorobenzylguanidine: a first-in-human PET/CT imaging study of patients with neuroendocrine malignancies. J Nucl Med 59(1):147–153
44. Binderup T, Knigge U, Loft A, Mortensen J, Pfeifer A, Federspiel B (2010) Functional imaging of neuroendocrine tumors: a head-to-head comparison of somatostatin receptor scintigraphy, ^{123}I-MIBG scintigraphy, and ^{18}F-FDG PET. J Nucl Med 51(5):704–712
45. Orlefors H, Sundin A, Ahlström H, Bjurling P, Bergström M, Lilja A (1998) Positron emission tomography with 5-hydroxytryprophan in neuroendocrine tumors. J Clin Oncol 16(7):2534–2541
46. Orlefors H, Sundin A, Garske U, Juhlin C, Oberg K, Skogseid B (2005) Whole-body (11) C-5-hydroxytryptophan positron emission tomography as a universal imaging technique for neuroendocrine tumors: comparison with somatostatin receptor scintigraphy and computed tomography. J Clin Endocrinol Metab 90(6):3392–3400
47. Koopmans KP, Neels OC, Kema IP, Elsinga PH, Sluiter WJ, Vanghillewe K (2008) Improved staging of patients with carcinoid and islet cell tumors with ^{18}F-dihydroxy-phenyl-alanine and ^{11}C-5-hydroxy-tryptophan positron emission tomography. J Clin Oncol 26(9):1489–1495
48. Hansen AE, Gutte H, Holst P, Johannesen HH, Rahbek S, Clemmensen AE (2018) Combined hyperpolarized ^{13}C-pyruvate MRS and ^{18}F-FDG PET (hyperPET) estimates of glycolysis in canine cancer patients. Eur J Radiol 103:6–12
49. Gutte H, Hansen AE, Johannesen HH, Clemmensen AE, Ardenkjær-Larsen JH, Nielsen CH (2015) The use of dynamic nuclear polarization (13)C-pyruvate MRS in cancer. Am J Nucl Med Mol Imaging 5(5):548–560
50. Gutte H, Hansen AE, Larsen MME, Rahbek S, Henriksen ST, Johannesen HH (2015) Simultaneous hyperpolarized ^{13}C-Pyruvate MRI and ^{18}F-FDG PET (HyperPET) in 10 dogs with cancer. J Nucl Med 56(11):1786–1792
51. Gutte H, Hansen AE, Larsen MME, Rahbek S, Johannesen HH, Ardenkjaer-Larsen J (2015) In vivo phenotyping of tumor metabolism in a canine cancer patient with simultaneous (18) F-FDG-PET and hyperpolarized (13)C-pyruvate magnetic resonance spectroscopic imaging (hyperPET): mismatch demonstrates that FDG may not always reflect the Warburg effect. Diagnostics 5(3):287–289
52. Binderup T, Knigge U, Loft A, Federspiel B, Kjaer A (2010) 18F-fluorodeoxyglucose positron emission tomography predicts survival of patients with neuroendocrine tumors. Clin Cancer Res 16(3):978–985
53. Johnbeck CB, Knigge U, Langer SW, Loft A, Berthelsen AK, Federspiel B (2016) Prognostic value of ^{18}F-FLT PET in patients with neuroendocrine neoplasms: a prospective head-to-head comparison with ^{18}F-FDG PET and Ki-67 in 100 patients. J Nucl Med 57(12):1851–1857
54. Binderup T, Knigge U, Johnbeck CB, Loft A, Berthelsen AK, Oturai P, Mortensen J, Federspiel B, Langer SW, Kjaer A (2021) ^{18}F-FDG PET is Superior to WHO Grading as a Prognostic Tool in Neuroendocrine Neoplasms and Useful in Guiding PRRT: A Prospective 10-Year Follow-up Study. J Nucl Med 62(6);808–815. https://doi.org/10.2967/jnumed.120.244798

Neuroendocrine Tumors of the Lung

9

Dan Granberg

9.1 Introduction

Lung neuroendocrine tumors, which belong to the foregut group of neuroendocrine tumors, have traditionally been divided into typical and atypical carcinoids [1], large cell neuroendocrine carcinomas (LCNECs), and small cell lung carcinomas (SCLCs), but several other classifications have subsequently been proposed [2–5]. A new WHO classification was introduced in 1999 [6] based on the work by Travis et al. [7]. This classification was revised in 2004 and apart from the grading also includes a staging system. Typical carcinoids contain fewer than 2 mitoses per 2 mm^2 and lack necroses, while atypical carcinoids have 2–10 mitoses per 2 mm^2 and/or necroses. Large cell neuroendocrine carcinomas and small cell lung carcinomas have more than 10 mitoses per 2 mm^2. Areas of necroses are common [8]. Typical carcinoids are usually considered as fairly benign tumors, while atypical carcinoids have a considerable malignant potential, while LCNEC and SCLC are highly malignant. Recently, a new grading system has been proposed for lung neuroendocrine tumors, based on the frequency of mitoses, proliferative rate (Ki67), and presence/absence of necroses [9]. In addition, two other conditions, lung carcinoid tumorlets and diffuse idiopathic neuroendocrine cell hyperplasia (DIPNECH), have been recognized. The most common neuroendocrine tumor in the lung is SCLC (20%) followed by LCNEC (3%), typical carcinoid (2%), and atypical carcinoid (0.2%). This chapter provides an overview of clinical features, diagnosis, and a framework of the currently available therapeutic measures for neuroendocrine tumors of the lung.

D. Granberg (✉)
Department of Medical Sciences, Division of Endocrine Oncology, Uppsala University, University Hospital, Uppsala, Sweden
e-mail: dan.granberg@medsci.uu.se

S. Yalcin, K. Öberg (eds.), *Neuroendocrine Tumours*,
https://doi.org/10.1007/978-3-031-56968-5_9

9.2 Carcinoid Tumorlets and Neuroendocrine Cell Hyperplasia

Neuroendocrine cell hyperplasia refers to the hyperplasia of neuroendocrine cells in the airways. The cells may be arranged as scattered single cells, clusters, or linear arrays but are confined to the basement membrane. In contrast, the cells in tumorlets extend beyond the respiratory epithelial basement membrane [8]. Tumorlets are morphologically identical to typical carcinoids but have a maximum size of 5 mm. Neuroendocrine cell hyperplasia may be reactive, found in patients living at high altitudes, heavy smokers, or in chronic lung diseases such as bronchiectasis or fibrosis. When there is hyperplasia of neuroendocrine cells without predisposing conditions, it is called DIPNECH. Symptoms of DIPNECH include cough, dyspnea, and wheezing. The condition is usually found in middle-aged women. Both tumorlets and DIPNECH may be found in patients with lung carcinoids. The preferable treatment of patients with DIPNECH is not well known, but possible alternatives include bronchodilators, inhaled corticosteroids, surgical excision of the dominant lesion, and somatostatin analogs. In about half of the patients, DIPNECH is stable, and in another half it progresses. Somatostatin analogs have been effective in stabilizing the condition. Metastatic disease has been described [10, 11].

9.3 Lung Carcinoids

9.3.1 Epidemiology, Etiology

Lung carcinoids are rare tumors, although the incidence has increased during the last decades. The reason for this is not known. The incidence is about 0.7/100,000 in Caucasians and 0.5/100,000 in black people. The disease is slightly more common in women than in men [12]. The disease is most frequent in middle ages but occurs in all ages, even in children. An increased incidence of neuroendocrine tumors has been reported [12, 13], which in part may be due to an increased awareness and better diagnostic tools. Carcinoid is the most common respiratory tumor in children and adolescents. The etiology is unknown, except that patients with multiple endocrine neoplasia type 1 have a higher risk. Smoking is not a proven risk factor.

9.3.2 Pathology

9.3.2.1 Macroscopic Findings

Lung carcinoids may be located centrally (60–84%) in the main or lobar bronchi, or peripherally. Central carcinoids may be seen at bronchoscopy as a polypoid, highly vascular, cherry-red, white-yellow, or brownish-yellow endobronchial tumor (Fig. 9.1). The tumor often infiltrates the surrounding lung parenchyma. Peripheral carcinoids, which are located in segmental bronchi or more distally, are not accessible by bronchoscopy. They may be multiple and surrounded by small satellite

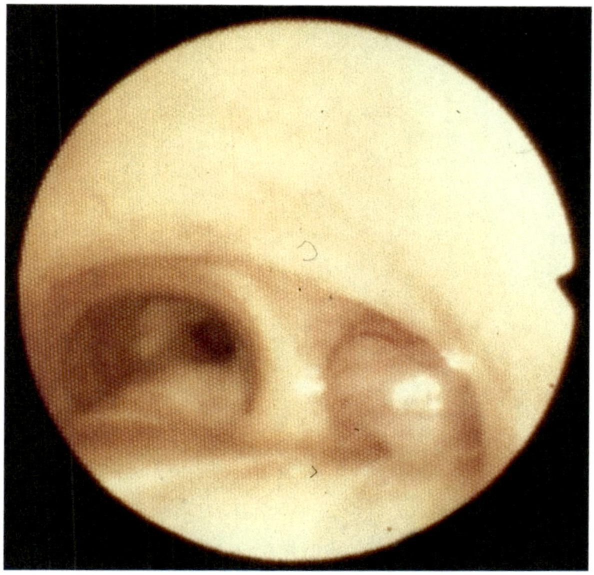

Fig. 9.1 Bronchoscopic visualization of intrabronchial typical carcinoid

lesions, tumorlets. Typical carcinoids may be located anywhere in the lungs, while atypical carcinoids are more often peripheral.

9.3.2.2 Histopathology and Immunohistochemistry

Typical carcinoids are characterized by organoid, trabecular, insular, palisading, ribbon, or rosette-like growth patterns separated by a fibrovascular stroma. The tumor cells are small and polyhedral with small, round, or oval nuclei and eosinophilic, finely granular cytoplasm. Mitoses are rare or absent, and the proliferative rate is usually low. Atypical carcinoids are characterized by nuclear pleomorphism, hyperchromatism, abnormal nuclear to cytoplasmic ratio, prominent nucleoli, and areas of increased cellularity with disorganized architecture. Mitoses are more frequent, and necroses may be found (Figs. 9.2a–c). At electron microscopy, typical carcinoids have abundant membrane-bound secretory granules, while atypical carcinoids have fewer granules, distributed in the cytoplasm [14].

Lung carcinoids are epithelial in origin and stain positive for cytokeratin. Most of the tumors are also stain positive for the neuroendocrine markers chromogranin A (Fig. 9.2d), synaptophysin, and neuron-specific enolase. In addition, positive immunohistochemistry for various hormones, including serotonin, gastrin-releasing peptide (mammalian bombesin), pancreatic polypeptide, gastrin, human chorionic gonadotropin alpha subunit, leucine enkephalin, VIP, somatostatin, calcitonin, ACTH, and growth-hormone-releasing hormone is found in a majority of tumors. Positive staining for multiple hormones is not uncommon [14, 15]. Expression of S-100 protein may occur, usually in peripheral tumors [16, 17]. The standard (hematopoietic) form of the adhesion molecule CD44 (CD44s) is usually expressed in lung carcinoids and may be used for prognostic evaluation in typical carcinoids

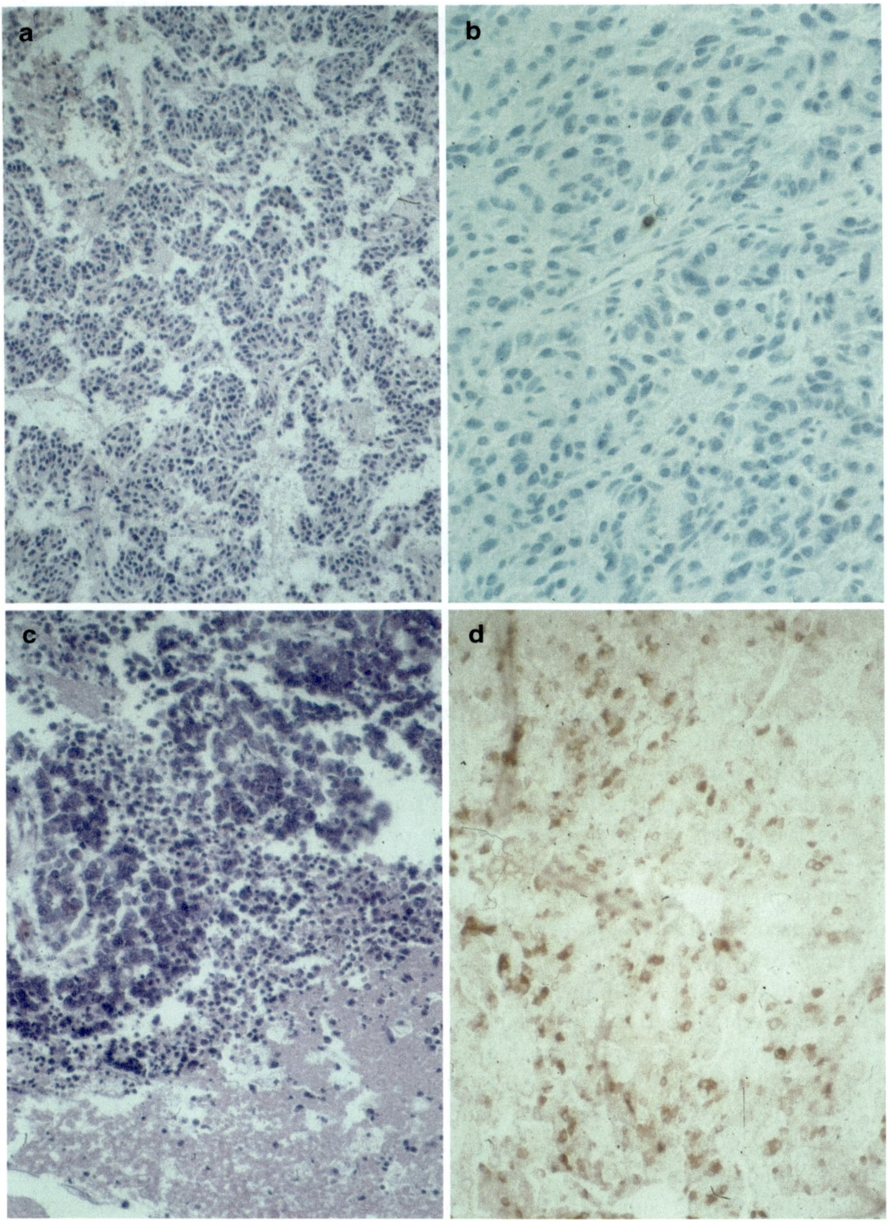

Fig. 9.2 (**a**) Typical lung carcinoid. Hematoxylin–eosin stain. Magnification, ×200. (**b**) Typical lung carcinoid. Ki67 stain, low proliferation. Magnification, ×400. (**c**). Atypical lung carcinoid. Hematoxylin–eosin stain. Magnification, ×200. (**d**) Typical lung carcinoid. Chromogranin A stain, strong positive. Magnification, ×200

[18]. Positive staining for the retinoblastoma gene protein is also common in typical carcinoids [19, 20]. The oncoproteins *p53* and *bcl-2*, however, are usually negative in typical carcinoids but more frequently positive in atypical carcinoids [21, 22]. Thyroid transcription factor-1 (TTF-1) is positive in 28–69% of lung carcinoids [23, 24] and may help to differentiate a primary lung carcinoid from a metastasis from a neuroendocrine tumor originating elsewhere.

9.3.3 Genetic Alterations

Deletions in the *MEN1* locus at 11q are common both in typical and atypical carcinoids [25]. Homozygous somatic inactivation of the *MEN1* gene is detected in 36% of sporadic lung carcinoids [26]. Atypical carcinoids frequently have deletions in 10q or 13q [25]. Aneuploidy has been reported in 5–32% of typical carcinoids and 17–79% of atypical carcinoids [4, 27–29].

9.3.4 Clinical Presentation

A substantial number of patients (13–51%) are asymptomatic, and the tumor is diagnosed incidentally on routine chest X-ray or CT scan. Common symptoms on presentation include cough, hemoptysis, wheezing, recurrent pneumonias with or without persisting lung infiltrate on chest X-ray, dyspnea, and chest pain [15, 30–32]. Some patients may have several year's delay in the correct diagnosis due to misdiagnosis as asthma. Like other neuroendocrine tumors, lung carcinoids may secrete hormones. Endocrine symptoms are however rare. Despite serotonin immunoreactivity is present in up to 84% of the tumors, the classical carcinoid syndrome with flush, diarrhea, bronchoconstriction, right-sided valvular heart disease, and elevated urinary 5-hydroxyindolacetic acid is seen in only about 2–12% of the patients, usually when liver metastases are present [33–35]. This low frequency may in part be due to the high pulmonary content of monoamine oxidase, which metabolizes serotonin, but also to the fact that most lung carcinoids do not give rise to distant metastases. An atypical carcinoid syndrome with generalized flushing, edema, lacrimation, asthma, and diarrhea may occasionally be seen. This syndrome, which must not be confused with atypical carcinoids, is caused by secretion of histamine. An ectopic Cushing's syndrome, caused by the production of adrenocorticotropic hormone (ACTH) or corticotropin-releasing factor, may be seen in 2–6% of patients with lung carcinoids. These tumors are often small and difficult to detect with conventional radiologic imaging. Acromegaly, caused by secretion of growth hormone-releasing hormone, is infrequent [36, 37].

Typical carcinoids metastasize in 5–20% of patients, while up to 70% of patients with atypical carcinoids develop metastases. Metastases most frequently occur in regional lymph nodes but also distantly to the liver, bones, brain, subcutaneous tissue, mammary glands, eyes, and adrenals [1, 33, 38, 39]. Metastases may occur late, up to 30 years after surgery for the primary tumor.

9.3.5 Diagnosis

In more than 60% of the patients, the tumor is visible on chest X-ray. Peripheral tumors are seen as round or oval nodules. Patients with central tumors may have signs of bronchial obstruction, with peripheral atelectasis or pneumonic infiltrates which may be persistent. CT scan (Fig. 9.3a) is more sensitive than chest X-ray and should always be performed in order to identify enlarged lymph nodes, delineate tumor growth, and detect satellite lesions (tumorlets). MRI may be an alternative to CT scan but is less sensitive in detecting small intrapulmonary lesions.

About 70–80% of lung carcinoids express somatostatin receptors and are demonstrable on Octreoscan (scintigraphy with ^{111}In-octreotide) [40]. Positron emission tomography (PET) with ^{68}Ga-DOTATOC or ^{68}Ga-DOTATATE (Fig. 9.3b) is a newer, more sensitive method to detect somatostatin-receptor positive neuroendocrine tumors. ^{68}Ga-PET should always be performed preoperatively for staging of the disease and clarify whether this method may be used for post-operative follow-up to detect recurrence or metastases. Patients with Cushing's syndrome often have small tumors, which is difficult to detect on CT scan. Up to 12 years delay have been described in localizing the tumor [41]. In these patients, PET with ^{68}Ga is especially

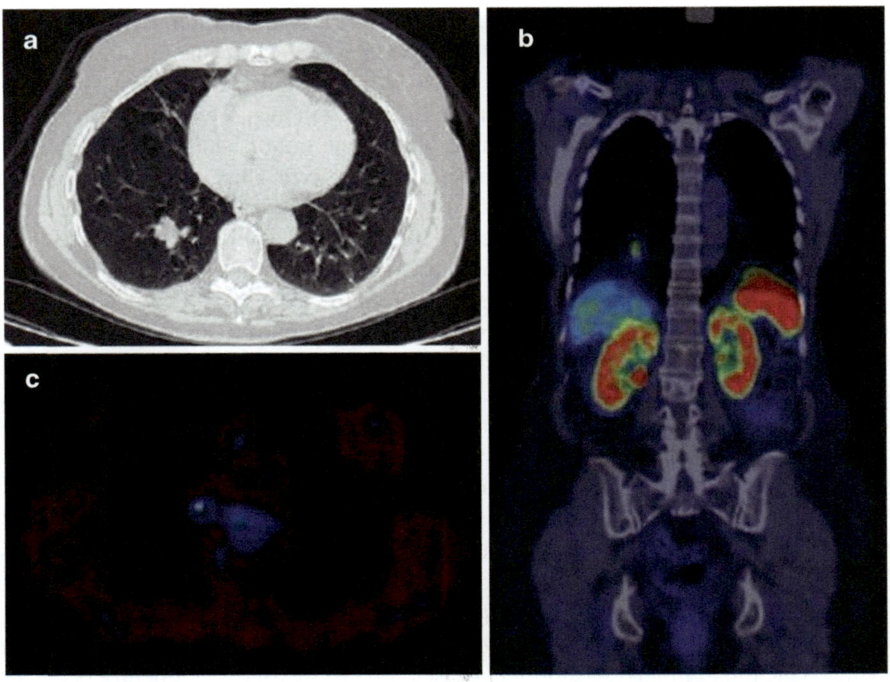

Fig. 9.3 (**a**) CT scan showing a carcinoid in the right lung. (**b**) PET with ^{68}Ga-DOTATATE showing a carcinoid in the right lung. (**c**) PET with ^{11}C-5-HTP showing a right hilar lymph node metastasis from a typical carcinoid in the right lung, 9 years after primary surgery

useful to obtain the correct diagnosis. An alternative is PET with ^{11}C-5-HTP (Fig. 9.3c), which is a sensitive tool for detection of neuroendocrine tumors [42]. The value of PET with ^{18}F-fluorodeoxyglucose (FDG) is controversial. Some authors claim that it is of limited value in detecting lung carcinoids, since these tumors often display lower uptake than expected for malignant tumors [43, 44], while others have found this method useful in patients with both typical and atypical carcinoids [45].

Central tumors are accessible via bronchoscopy (Fig. 9.1), which is performed in most patients. Since the tumor is often covered by a layer of normal mucosa, brushing or sputum cytology is frequently negative. To obtain a preoperative diagnosis, it is thus important to take biopsies, despite the risk of bleeding. It is generally safe to take biopsies, both through a flexible and a rigid bronchoscope [46]. Peripheral tumors may be reached by transthoracic CT-guided core-needle biopsy, although misdiagnosis is not uncommon, since the differential diagnosis to small cell lung carcinoma may be difficult. Staining the tissue sample for the proliferation marker Ki67 may aid in the differential diagnosis between these entities [47, 48].

Plasma chromogranin A should always be measured preoperatively but is usually normal if the tumor is confined to the lung. If chromogranin A is elevated, intense search for distant metastases is warranted. Measurement of urinary 5-hydroxyindolacetic acid, urinary cortisol, and plasma ACTH is not recommended routinely but is only indicated if the patient has endocrine symptoms.

9.3.6 Differential Diagnosis

Alternative diagnoses when a tumor is found on chest X-ray or CT scan include other benign or malignant lung neoplasms, hamartoma, and metastasis from another primary tumor. The histopathological differentiation, both via bronchoscopy and transthoracically, between atypical carcinoid and SCLC may sometimes be difficult but is important since patients with carcinoids are often cured by surgery, which is generally not performed in patients with SCLC. High proliferative rate, Ki67 > 25%, favors the diagnosis of SCLC, while a low Ki67 index indicates lung carcinoid [47, 48].

9.3.7 Treatment

The main treatment for patients with lung carcinoids is surgery, which offers the only chance for cure. External radiotherapy is mainly used for palliation of bone or brain metastases. Patients with metastatic disease or inoperable tumors can be treated with various chemotherapy combinations, peptide receptor radionuclide therapy (PRRT) with ^{177}Lu-DOTA-octreotate or ^{90}Y-DOTA-octreotide, and biotherapy (somatostatin analogs, alpha-interferon) or newer targeted therapies such as everolimus or sunitinib. Patients with liver metastases may undergo hepatic arterial embolization with particles, chemotherapeutic agents, or ^{90}Y-labeled microspheres

(SIR-Spheres® or TheraSpheres®). Symptomatic treatment for patients with carcinoid syndrome includes somatostatin analogs and alpha-interferon. Patients with metastatic tumors and Cushing's syndrome are generally subjected to bilateral adrenalectomy; symptom relief may be obtained with ketoconazole, metyrapone, somatostatin analogs, or mitotane.

9.3.7.1 Surgery

Radical surgery should be considered in all patients with lung carcinoids confined to the thorax and is curative in most patients. The principles of surgery include complete removal of the primary tumor, preservation of as much healthy lung parenchyma as possible and a thorough lymph node dissection, aided by frozen sections, with removal of all affected nodes. Possible surgical procedures include bronchotomy with resection of the tumor and bronchoplasty, sleeve resection, wedge or segmental resection, lobectomy, bilobectomy, and pneumonectomy. Wide resection margins are not necessary, but in patients with atypical carcinoids, it is recommended to perform at least a lobectomy. Endoscopic removal of the tumor by YAG-laser has previously not been recommended, since lung carcinoids often grow deeply into the surrounding tissue (the "iceberg" phenomenon), and radical removal thus is difficult to obtain by laser resection. Two studies however questioned this opinion and found initial bronchoscopic laser treatment to be a safe and effective therapy for patients with intrabronchial typical carcinoids. In 36–46% of the patients, open surgery was nevertheless later required [49, 50]. One indication for endoscopic tumor removal by YAG laser is palliation of obstructive symptoms in patients with high cardiopulmonary operative risk and short life expectancy. In a limited number of patients, surgery may be considered after previous laser treatment to reduce the tumor and allow post-obstructive infiltrates to resolve. Adjuvant chemotherapy has not shown any beneficial effect after radical surgery [51].

9.3.7.2 Radiotherapy

Patients with bone or brain metastases may have palliation from external radiotherapy. This may also be considered in cases with inoperable tumors or incomplete resection. PRRT is an interesting option in patients with metastatic or inoperable tumors and high expression of somatostatin receptors. Four uncontrolled studies have shown promising results. In a small study, 5/9 patients treated with ^{177}Lu-DOTA-octreotate had a radiological response lasting median 31 months [52], and in another report, 24/84 patients (29%) receiving ^{90}Y-DOTA-octreotide responded radiologically [53]. Since there was a high frequency (9.5% of all patients) of severe permanent decrease in renal function in patients treated with ^{90}Y-DOTA-octreotide, it may be preferable to choose ^{177}Lu-DOTA-octreotate for PRRT. Ianniello et al. evaluated 34 patients with progressing lung carcinoids (15 typical, 19 atypical) treated with 4–5 cycles of ^{177}Lu-DOTA-octreotate up to a cumulated activity of 18.5 or 27.8 GBq. In the patients with typical carcinoids, disease control rate was 80% (6% complete response, 27% partial response, and 47% stable disease) and median PFS was

20.1 months, while in the patients with atypical carcinoids, disease control rate was 47.5% (all stable disease) and median PFS was 15.7 months [54]. In another, more comprehensive retrospective study including 114 patients, three different protocols were compared: ^{90}Y-DOTATOC, ^{177}Lu-DOTATATE, and ^{90}Y-DOTATOC +^{177}Lu-DOTATATE. Median overall survival (evaluated in 94 patients) was 58.8 months, and median progression-free survival (PFS) was 28.0 months. The highest response rate (38.1%) was seen in the patients receiving the combination of ^{90}Y-DOTATOC and ^{177}Lu-DOTATATE [55].

9.3.7.3 Chemotherapy

The treatment of patients with metastatic lung carcinoids depends on the histopathology (typical versus atypical carcinoid), proliferative rate (Ki67 index), somatostatin receptor expression, extent of disease, performance status of the patient, and renal and bone marrow function. Various chemotherapy combinations have been tried with limited success, including cisplatin or carboplatin + etoposide, docetaxel or paclitaxel ± doxorubicin, streptozotocin + 5-fluorouracil or doxorubicin, oxaliplatin + capecitabine, 5-fluorouracil + dacarbazine + epirubicin, and 5-fluorouracil + cisplatin + streptozotozin [56–60]. A non-randomized study however confirmed earlier observations that temozolomide as monotherapy may be active in these patients. A significant tumor reduction was seen in 14% and stabilization of progressive disease in 52%. All patients with partial response had atypical carcinoids, but stabilization was observed in typical as well as atypical carcinoids [61, 62]. Combining temozolomide with capecitabine and/or bevacizumab may have better effect, but this has not been studied. These combinations are mainly used in patients with higher proliferation or if progression occurs on monotherapy with temozolomide. Patients with high Ki67 often receive platinum-based chemotherapy as first-line treatment.

9.3.7.4 Biotherapy

Somatostatin analogs (octreotide, lanreotide) have shown anti-tumoral activity in gastrointestinal and pancreatic neuroendocrine tumors [63, 64] but are less well studied in lung carcinoids. In a recent retrospective evaluation including 61 patients, 47 (77%) had stable disease as best response. Median duration of response was 13.7 months, median PFS was 17.4 months, and median OS was 58.4 months. Significantly longer PFS was seen in patients with slow progressive disease prior to start of the somatostatin analog and in patients with functioning tumors [65]. The ongoing double-blind SPINET trial, randomizing patients with somatostatin-receptor positive typical and atypical carcinoids 2:1 to Lanreotide autogel 120 mg s.c. or placebo every 4 weeks, will hopefully clarify the antiproliferative effect of somatostatin analogs in patients with lung carcinoids. Another indication for somatostatin analogs is symptomatic relief of a classical carcinoid syndrome or an atypical carcinoid syndrome. Sometimes, the addition of alpha-interferon is necessary to control the carcinoid syndrome.

9.3.7.5 Targeted Therapies

During recent years, new drugs targeting signal pathways or membrane receptors have proven to be active in patients with neuroendocrine tumors. Both everolimus, an mTOR inhibitor and sunitinib, inhibiting vascular endothelial growth factor receptor (VEGFR), platelet-derived growth factor receptor (PDGFR), and c-kit have shown to prolong PFS in patients with pancreatic endocrine tumors. In a subanalysis from the randomized, placebo-controlled RADIANT-2 study, everolimus + octreotide LAR was found to prolong PFS in patients with lung carcinoids from 5.6 to 13.6 months compared with placebo + octreotide LAR. The difference was however not significant. Minor response was seen in 67% in the everolimus group and 27% in the placebo group [66]. A recent subanalysis encompassing 90 patients from the randomized phase 3 RADIANT-4 study comparing everolimus 10 mg daily ($n = 63$) with placebo ($n = 27$) found median PFS to be 9.2 months in the everolimus group vs 3.6 months in the placebo group. Tumor shrinkage was seen in 58% of the patients treated with everolimus vs 13% among those receiving placebo [67]. The results from the LUNA study comparing everolimus ($n = 42$), long-acting pasireotide (another somatostatin analog; $n = 41$), and everolimus + pasireotide ($n = 41$) in patients with well-differentiated lung and thymic carcinoids have recently been published. At the evaluation after 9 months, tumor control rate (complete response + partial response + stable disease) was 33.3% in the everolimus group, 39.0% in the long-acting pasireotide group, and 58.5% in the combination group [68]. Hence, everolimus seems to have antitumor activity in patients with lung carcinoids, yet further studies are necessary to confirm the efficacy of combining everolimus with a somatostatin analog. Sunitinib has not been studied in lung carcinoids, but many lung carcinoids express the tyrosine kinase receptors PDGFRα, PDGFRβ, c-kit, and EGFR [69]. This makes it possible that sunitinib and other tyrosine kinase inhibitors may have activity in lung carcinoids.

9.3.7.6 Immune Therapy

Immune checkpoint inhibitor antibodies such as pembrolizumab and nivolumab, targeting the interaction between programmed death receptor 1 (PD-1) and its ligand PD-L1, have shown activity in several tumor types. A recent report found no expression of PD-L1 in typical and atypical carcinoids, but expression was present in 10.4% of LCNEC and 5.8% of SCLC [70]. Atezolizumab, a monoclonal antibody targeting PD-L1, has shown antitumor activity in patients with non-small-cell lung cancer regardless of PD-L1 expression [71]. Spartalizumab, a humanized anti-PD-1 antibody blocking PD-L1 and PD-L2, was investigated in a phase 2 study encompassing 116 patients with advanced non-functioning well- and poorly differentiated neuroendocrine tumors (33 pancreatic NET, 32 gastrointestinal NET, 30 thoracic NET, and 21 NEC) who had progressed on prior therapy. Partial response was seen in 20% and stable disease in 53.3% of the patients with thoracic NET; all responses were seen in patients with atypical tumors. In the other patient groups, the clinical effect was marginal [72]. Further testing spartalizumab, atezolizumab, and other immune checkpoint inhibitors in patients with lung carcinoids in more comprehensive clinical trials would be highly interesting.

9.3.8 Prognosis

Most patients with typical lung carcinoids are cured by surgery, even in the presence of lymph node metastases, and have an excellent prognosis. Five- and 10-year survival is 87–100% and 82–95%, respectively [7, 15, 73–75]. Poor prognostic factors include lymph node metastases at diagnosis, presence of tumorlets, and high Ki67 index. On the other hand, positive immunohistochemistry for the standard form of the adhesion molecule CD44 (Fig. 9.4a), as well as positive nuclear staining for the metastasis suppressor gene *nm23* (Fig. 9.4b) correlate with decreased risk for distant metastases and death [18, 76]. The prognosis for patients with atypical carcinoids is worse, although many of these patients are also cured by surgery. Five- and 10-year survival is 40–69% and 31–59%, respectively [15, 31, 74, 77]. Since metastases may develop late, up to 30 years after primary surgery, patients with lung carcinoids must be followed for a long time, at least 10–15 years. The follow-up should include measurement of plasma chromogranin A, CT scan of the thorax and abdomen, and PET with ^{68}Ga-DOTATOC/DOTATATE (in patients with somatostatin-receptor positive tumors) or MRI of the vertebral column. In selected patients, repeated bronchoscopies are indicated. Special attention should be paid to patients with atypical carcinoids or high proliferative rate.

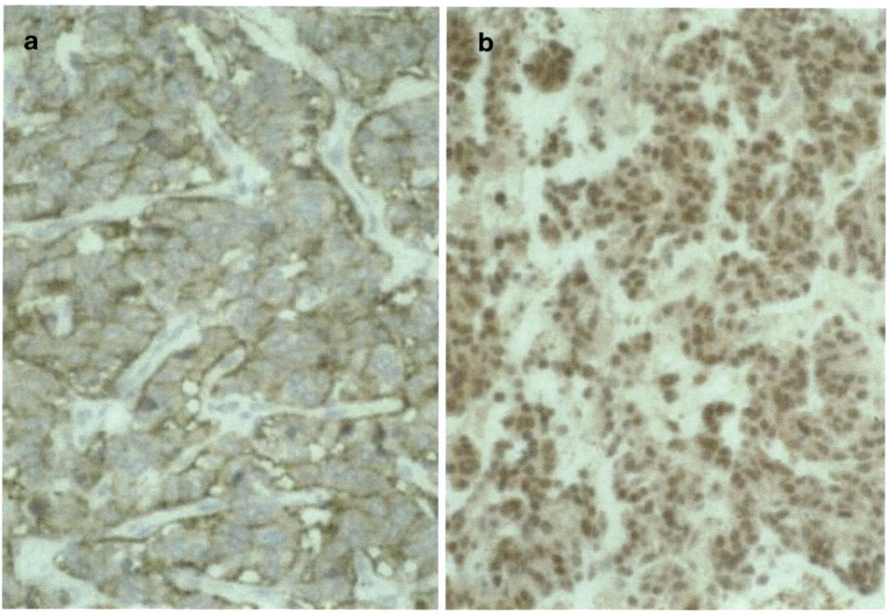

Fig. 9.4 (**a**) Typical lung carcinoid. CD44s stain, strong positive. Magnification, ×400. (**b**) Typical lung carcinoid. *nm23* stain, strong positive. Magnification, ×400

9.4 Large Cell Neuroendocrine Carcinoma

Large cell neuroendocrine carcinomas constitute about 3% of all lung cancers. Almost all patients are smokers. The disease is most frequent in older patients; mean age is between 59 and 66 years. Men are affected more often than women and constitute 55–86% of the cases [4, 78, 79].

9.4.1 Pathology

LCNEC are usually peripheral, seen as large masses on X-ray. The tumor consists of large cells with moderate to abundant finely granular, eosinophilic cytoplasm and frequent nucleoli. The cells are arranged in organoid, palisading, trabecular, or rosette-like patterns (Fig. 9.5a). The mitotic rate is high, ≥11 (average 75) per 2 mm^2. Large areas of necroses are frequent. The proliferative rate is high. Aneuploidy is found in 75% of the tumors. Positive immunohistochemistry for neuroendocrine markers such as chromogranin A (Fig. 9.5b), synaptophysin, and neuron-specific enolase is less frequent than in lung carcinoids. One positive marker is enough for the diagnosis. TTF-1 is positive in about 50% of the tumors [8]. Positive staining for *p53* and *bcl-2* is common [80], but retinoblastoma protein is usually not present by immunohistochemistry [20]. *K-ras* mutations occur in the

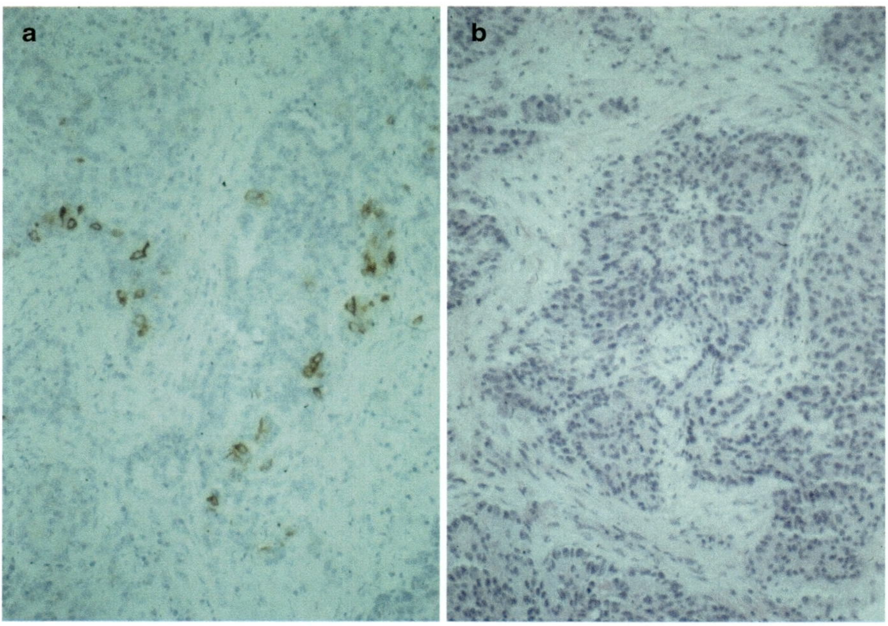

Fig. 9.5 (**a**) Large cell neuroendocrine carcinoma. Hematoxylin–eosin stain. Magnification, ×200. (**b**) Large cell neuroendocrine carcinoma. Chromogranin A stain, weak positive. Magnification, ×200

same frequency as in other non-small cell lung cancers [8]. At electron microscopy, the ultrastructural appearance is variable. The majority of tumors have only few cytoplasmic neurosecretory granules.

9.4.2 Clinical Presentation

Common presenting symptoms in patients with LCNEC include cough, dyspnea, hemoptysis, obstructive pneumonias, or constitutional symptoms such as weight loss and malaise. Some patients are asymptomatic and diagnosed incidentally by an abnormal chest X-ray. Endocrine symptoms due to ectopic hormone production have not been described. Metastases occur in 71–100% of the patients with LCNEC, most often to hilar or mediastinal lymph nodes. Distant metastases occur to pleura, liver, brain, bones, adrenal glands, pericardium, and abdominal lymph nodes.

9.4.3 Diagnosis

Many tumors are detectable on chest X-ray. CT scan of the chest and abdomen, as well as PET with FDG, is of value for staging. Histopathological diagnosis may be obtained by surgery or trans-thoracic core-needle biopsy.

9.4.4 Treatment

There is no consensus regarding the treatment of patients with LCNEC. Surgery is indicated in patients with stage 1. Since the risk for recurrence and distant metastases is high, surgery must be combined with adjuvant chemotherapy. Active combinations include cisplatin + etoposide, cisplatin + irinotecan, and nadaplatin + irinotecan. Several studies have reported the response to cisplatin-based chemotherapy to be comparable in patients with advanced LCNEC and SCLC [81–85]. Amrubicin as monotherapy has also some activity in LCNEC [86]. Patients with widespread disease may receive the same chemotherapy regimens. The role of radiotherapy is more controversial. Patients with EGFR mutations may obtain partial responses with gefitinib [87, 88]. Octreotide, which prolongs progression-free survival in patients with slow-growing neuroendocrine tumors, may be used as adjuvant treatment after surgery for LCNEC [89]. Sunitinib and other agents targeting VEGFR and c-kit are possible new drugs for treatment of LCNEC [90].

9.4.5 Prognosis

The prognosis for patients with LCNEC is dismal. The reported 5-year survival varies between 15% and 57% [79, 91–97]. Patients with stage 1 tumors have slightly better 5-year survival, 27–67% [92, 94, 95, 97–99].

9.5 Small Cell Lung Carcinoma

9.5.1 Epidemiology and Etiology

Small cell lung carcinoma, which is the most aggressive form of lung malignancy, accounts for 14–20% of all cases of lung cancer. It is most common in the seventh and eighth decades. There is a clear male preponderance, but this discrepancy may decrease due to the increasing smoking habits among women. Almost all patients with SCLC are smokers, which represents the main risk factor. Other known etiologic factors include ionizing radiation, asbestos, aromatic hydrocarbons (in particular chloromethyl ethers), and various metals [100].

9.5.2 Pathology

A majority of SCLC are centrally located, appearing as hilar or perihilar masses, spreading early to hilar and mediastinal lymph nodes [8]. Only about 5% are seen as a peripheral solitary mass [101]. Distant metastases occur to the brain, liver, bone marrow, bones, adrenal glands, and pancreas. Brain metastases are seen in 10–20% on presentation but occur later as the disease progresses in 25% of patients not receiving prophylactic cranial irradiation [102]. In total, 50–80% of the patients will develop brain metastases [103].

9.5.2.1 Light Microscopy

Small cell lung carcinoma consists of small cells, usually less than the diameter of 3 small resting lymphocytes. The cells are round to fusiform and have a high nuclear to cytoplasmic ratio and finely granular, hyperchromatic nuclei with inconspicuous or absent nucleoli. Histologic patterns include trabeculae, spindling, nesting, palisading, rosettes, or solid sheet-like growth, with indistinct cell borders. The mitotic rate is high, ≥ 11 per 2 mm^2, median 80 per 2 mm^2. Necroses and crush artifacts are frequent. The proliferative rate is high (Fig. 9.6). Combined small cell lung carcinoma is defined as small cell carcinoma combined with an additional component, usually adenocarcinoma, squamous cell carcinoma, or large cell carcinoma [8].

9.5.2.2 Immunohistochemistry

The neuroendocrine markers chromogranin A, synaptophysin, and NSE stain positive in most SCLC and TTF-1 are positive in up to 90% of the tumors [104, 105]. Hormonal immunoreactivity, most often for ACTH, bombesin, and serotonin, may also be found, but staining for multiple hormones is less common than in lung carcinoids [4, 5]. Gastrin-releasing peptide has been shown to function as a growth factor for SCLC [106]. Positive immunostaining for *p53* is common [19, 21, 80] as is *bcl-2* immunoreactivity [80, 107, 108]. Retinoblastoma gene protein is usually negative at immunohistochemistry [19, 20, 109].

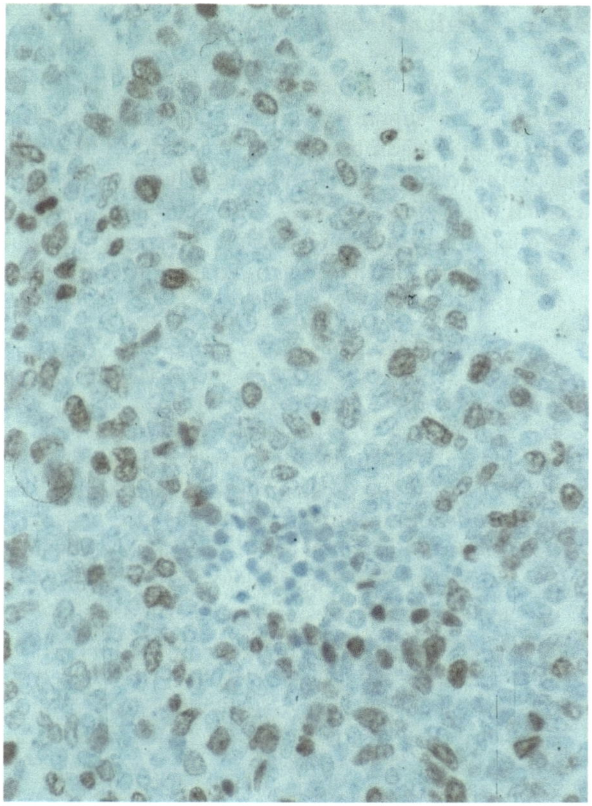

Fig. 9.6 Small cell lung carcinoma. Ki67 stain, high proliferation. Magnification, ×400

9.5.2.3 Electron Microscopy

Neurosecretory granules, about 100 nm in size, are found in at least 60–70% of cases [8]. Basal lamina are scarce or absent [5].

9.5.3 Genetic Alterations

All SCLCs are aneuploid. The multistep process for development of invasive SCLC encompass activations of several proto-oncogenes such as *kit*, *SCF*, and *myc* (*c*-, *N*-, and *L*-) and inactivation of several suppressor genes [110]. Some of the most common allelic deletions are various loci on 3p (present in nearly 100%), 4, 5q, 10q, 13q, and 17p. DNA gains are seen on 3q, 5p, 6p, 8q, 17q, 19, and 20q [111]. The *p53* gene is homozygously mutated in 90% of SCLC [112]. The retinoblastoma protein is absent or abnormal in an equally high percentage of tumors. Other characteristic features of SCLC are amplification of *MYC* [113] and methylation of caspase-8 DNA [114]. DNA gain on 17q24–q25 is a potential marker for development of brain metastases [115].

9.5.4 Clinical Presentation

Presenting symptoms include cough, weight loss, dyspnea, chest pain, hoarseness, dysphagia, and superior vena cava syndrome. Endocrine syndromes or paraneoplastic neurologic syndromes are not uncommon on presentation. SIADH (syndrome of inappropriate secretion of antidiuretic hormone) is seen in 11–46%, ectopic ACTH-production leading to Cushing's syndrome, typically causing peripheral edema, proximal myopathy, hypertension, glucose intolerance, and metabolic alkalosis occurs in 2–5% and the Eaton–Lambert myasthenic syndrome in 3% of patients [116, 117].

9.5.5 Staging

Although a TNM classification has been proposed for SCLC [118, 119], since this tumor is not considered as a surgical disease, the TNM classification may not be applicable. Another system is recommended by the Veterans Administration Lung Cancer Study Group based on the feasibility of including all known tumor locations in one radiation field. Thus, limited-stage (LS) disease is defined as tumor confined to one hemithorax, with or without hilar, ipsilateral/contralateral mediastinal and/or supraclavicular lymph node metastases, with/without ipsilateral pleural effusion, while extensive-stage (ES) disease is tumor outside the thorax or in the contralateral lung [120]. About 60–70% of the patients have extensive disease when diagnosed.

9.5.6 Diagnosis

Apart from chest X-ray, CT scan of the thorax, abdomen, and brain as well as PET with FDG is of value for staging. Octreoscan is of limited value, since metastases are depicted only in about 50% of the patients, yet nearly all primary tumors are found [121–123]. Although sputum cytology is positive in 75–80% of patients with SCLC [100], the diagnosis should be based on acquiring enough tissue material for histologic diagnosis. Bronchoscopy, transthoracic core-needle biopsy, mediastinoscopy or surgical excision of a supraclavicular lymph node can make the diagnosis. It may sometimes be difficult to differentiate between SCLC and atypical carcinoid tumors. Staining of the tissue sample for Ki67 may aid in this differential diagnosis [47, 48].

9.5.7 Treatment

Surgery has little role in the treatment of patients with SCLC, unless in rare patients in whom the diagnosis is made early. The main treatment is chemotherapy and radiotherapy. Earlier schemes included combinations of cyclophosphamide, doxorubicin, and vincristine. Today, platinum-based chemotherapy is used as first-line treatment, with 60–70% response rates [124]. Patients with limited-stage disease are usually treated with cisplatin or carboplatin + etoposide combined with thoracic radiotherapy. Patients who respond receive prophylactic cranial irradiation. Up to 20% of patients will have long-term disease control, but a majority will recur. Patients with extended-stage disease are treated with chemotherapy alone, usually cisplatin/carboplatin + etoposide, or platinum + irinotecan. Prophylactic cranial irradiation is given to patients who respond. Second-line treatment in relapsing or not responding patients include topotecan, paclitaxel, docetaxel, irinotecan, vinorelbine, gemcitabine, and temozolomide, but response rates are limited or poor [124]. Immune checkpoint inhibitors are potential new treatment alternatives for these patients. In one study, nivolumab alone and nivolumab + iplimumab (a monoclonal antibody activating the immune system by targeting CTLA-4) showed antitumoral activity with durable responses and acceptable safety in patients with pretreated SCLC. Objective responses were seen in 10% of patients receiving nivolumab as monotherapy and in 19–33% of patients receiving the combination [125]. In a more recent report, pembrolizumab showed antitumor activity in 24 patients with previously treated, PD-L1-expressing SCLC. One patient had a complete response and seven had partial responses, yielding an overall response rate of 33% [126]. Atezolizumab, a monoclonal anti-PD-L1 antibody blocking the PD-1 and B7.1 receptors and thereby restoring PD-L1/PD1-mediated tumor-specific T-cell immunity, has been investigated in treatment naïve SCLC patients with extensive disease. Patients were randomized 1:1 to four cycles of carboplatin and etoposide plus either atezolizumab ($n = 201$) or placebo ($n = 202$), followed by maintenance with either atezolizumab or placebo according to the previous assignment. Median overall survival was 12.3 months in the atezolizumab group and 10.3 months in the placebo group ($p = 0.007$), and PFS was 5.2 months in the atezolizumab group vs 4.3 months in the placebo group ($p = 0.02$) [127]. These results are highly promising, yet further, more comprehensive trials, are urgently warranted.

9.5.8 Prognosis

The prognosis for patients with SCLC is dismal. Overall 5-year-survival is <7% [124]. Patients with limited-stage disease have significantly better prognosis (median survival 16–22 months, 5-year survival around 25% and about 20% cured) than patients with extensive-stage disease (median survival 10 months, 2-year survival <5%) [124, 128]. The main poor prognostic factors are more widespread disease (even within the stages), poor performance status, male gender, and old age [129].

9.6 Concluding Remarks

Lung carcinoids are generally slow growing tumors, yet harboring malignant potential. The main treatment is surgery with resection of the primary tumor and affected lymph nodes. Maximal preservation of normal lung parenchyma is warranted. There

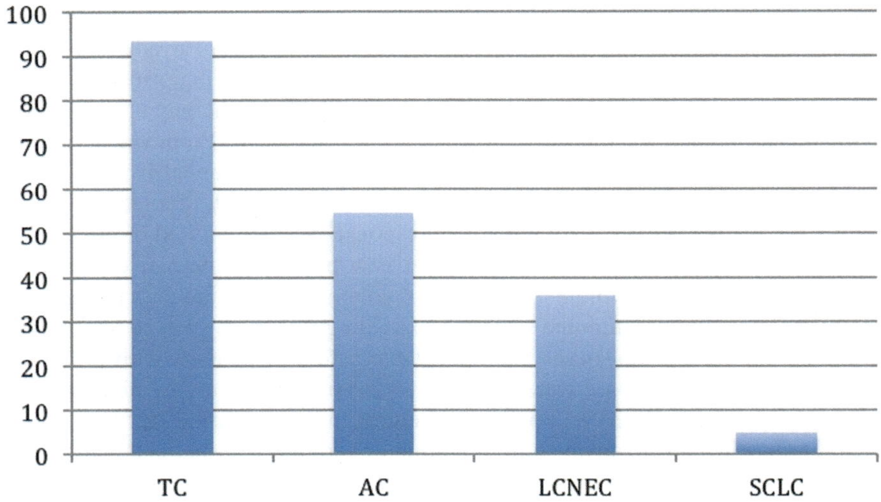

Fig. 9.7 Median 5-year survival in patients with typical carcinoids (TCs), atypical carcinoids (ACs), large cell neuroendocrine carcinomas (LCNECs), and small cell lung carcinomas (SCLCs)

is no scientific evidence for post-operative adjuvant treatment. Long-term follow-up is necessary, since recurrences may occur late, after several decades. Atypical carcinoids have a more malignant behavior than typical. Large cell neuroendocrine carcinomas are highly malignant tumors with poor prognosis. If possible, radical surgery should be performed, followed by adjuvant chemotherapy. Small cell lung carcinomas are highly aggressive tumors, rapidly spreading to distant organs. Intensive platinum-based chemotherapy, in patients with limited-stage disease combined with concurrent thoracic radiotherapy, should be started as soon as possible. Patients who respond to initial treatment should be offered prophylactic cranial irradiation. The prognosis is nevertheless dismal, with short expected survival (Fig. 9.7).

References

1. Arrigoni MG, Woolner LB, Bernatz PE (1972) Atypical carcinoid tumors of the lung. J Thorac Cardiovasc Surg 64:413–421
2. Capella C, Heitz PU, Höfler H et al (1994) Revised classification of neuroendocrine tumors of the lung, pancreas and gut. Digestion 55(suppl 3):11–23
3. Paladugu RR, Benfield JR, Pak HY et al (1985) Bronchopulmonary Kulchitzky cell carcinomas. Cancer 55:1303–1311
4. Travis WD, Linnoila RI, Tsokos MG et al (1991) Neuroendocrine tumors of the lung with proposed criteria for large-cell neuroendocrine carcinoma. An ultrastructural, immunohistochemical, and flow cytometric study of 35 cases. Am J Surg Pathol 15:529–553
5. Warren WH, Gould VE, Faber LP et al (1985) Neuroendocrine neoplasms of the bronchopulmonary tract. A classification of the spectrum of carcinoid to small cell carcinoma and intervening variants. J Thorac Cardiovasc Surg 89:819–825

6. Travis WD, Colby TV, Corrin B et al (1999) World Health Organization. Histological typing of lung and pleural tumours, 3rd edn. Springer, Berlin
7. Travis WD, Rush W, Flieder DB et al (1998) Survival analysis of 200 pulmonary neuroendocrine tumors with clarification of criteria for atypical carcinoid and its separation from typical carcinoid. Am J Surg Pathol 22:934–944
8. Travis WD, Brambilla E, Müller-Hermelink HK, Harris CC (eds) (2004) World Health Organization classification of tumours, pathology & genetics. Tumours of the lung, pleura, thymus and heart. IARCPress, Lyon
9. Rindi G, Klersy C, Inzani F et al (2014) Grading the neuroendocrine tumors of the lung: an evidence-based proposal. Endocr Relat Cancer 21:1–16
10. Gorshtein A, Gross DJ, Barak D et al (2012) Diffuse idiopathic pulmonary neuroendocrine cell hyperplasia and the associated lung neuroendocrine tumors: clinical experience with a rare entity. Cancer 118:612–619
11. Nassar AA, Jaroszewski DE, Helmers RA et al (2011) Diffuse idiopathic pulmonary neuroendocrine cell hyperplasia: a systematic overview. Am J Respir Crit Care Med 184:8–16
12. Modlin IM, Lye KD, Kidd M (2003) A 5-decade analysis of 13,715 carcinoid tumors. Cancer 97:934–959
13. Dasari A, Shen C, Halperin DM et al (2017) Trends in the incidence, prevalence, and survival outcomes in patients with neuroendocrine tumors in the United States. JAMA Oncol 3:1335–1342
14. Warren WH, Memoli VA, Gould VE (1984) Immunohistochemical and ultrastructural analysis of bronchopulmonary neuroendocrine neoplasms. I. carcinoids. Ultrastruct Pathol 6:15–27
15. McCaughan BC, Martini N, Bains MS (1985) Bronchial carcinoids—review of 124 cases. J Thorac Cardiovasc Surg 89:8–17
16. Barbareschi M, Frigo B, Mosca L et al (1990) Bronchial carcinoids with S-100 positive Sustentacular cells. A comparative study with gastrointestinal carcinoids, pheochromocytomas and paragangliomas. Pathol Res Pract 186:212–222
17. El-Salhy M, Lundqvist M, Wilander E (1986) Bronchial carcinoids and pheochromocytomas—a comparative study with special emphasis on S-100 protein, serotonin and neuron-specific enolase (NSE) immunoreactivity. Acta Pathol Microbiol Immunol Scand A 94:229–235
18. Granberg D, Wilander E, Öberg K, Skogseid B (1999) Decreased survival in patients with CD44-negative typical bronchial carcinoid tumors. Int J Cancer (Pred Oncol) 84:484–488
19. Barbareschi M, Girlando S, Mauri FA et al (1992) Tumour suppressor gene products, proliferation, and differentiation markers in lung neuroendocrine neoplasms. J Pathol 166:343–350
20. Gouyer V, Gazzeri S, Bolon I et al (1998) Mechanism of retinoblastoma gene inactivation in the Spectrum of neuroendocrine lung tumors. Am J Respir Cell Mol Biol 18:188–196
21. Coppola D, Clarke M, Landreneau R et al (1996) Bcl-2, p53, CD44, and CD44v6 isoform expression in neuroendocrine tumors of the lung. Mod Pathol 9:484–490
22. Lohmann D, Pütz B, Reich U et al (1993) Mutational Spectrum of the p53 gene in human small-cell lung cancer and relationship to clinicopathological data. Am J Pathol 142:907–915
23. Cai Y-C, Banner B, Glickman J, Odze RD (2001) Cytokeratin 7 and 20 and thyroid transcription factor 1 can help distinguish pulmonary from gastrointestinal carcinoid and pancreatic endocrine tumors. Hum Pathol 32:1087–1093
24. Du EZ, Goldstraw P, Zacharias J et al (2004) TTF-1 expression is specific for lung primary in typical and atypical carcinoids: TTF-1-positive carcinoids are predominantly in peripheral location. Hum Pathol 35:825–831
25. Walch AK, Zitzelsberger HF, Aubele MM et al (1998) Typical and atypical carcinoid tumors of the lung are characterized by 11q deletions as detected by comparative genomic hybridization. Am J Pathol 153:1089–1098
26. Debelenko LV, Brambilla E, Agarwal SK et al (1997) Identification of MEN1 gene mutations in sporadic carcinoid tumors of the lung. Hum Mol Genet 6:2285–2290

27. El-Naggar AK, Ballance W, Abdul Karim FW et al (1991) Typical and atypical bronchopulmonary carcinoids—a Clinicopathologic and flow cytometric study. Am J Clin Pathol 95:828–834
28. Jones DJ, Hasleton PS, Moore N (1988) DNA ploidy in bronchopulmonary carcinoid tumours. Thorax 43:195–199
29. Thunnissen FBJM, van Eijk J, Baak JPA et al (1988) Bronchopulmonary carcinoids and regional lymph node metastases—a quantitative pathologic investigation. Am J Pathol 132:119–122
30. Bertelsen S, Aasted A, Lund C et al (1985) Bronchial carcinoid tumors—a clinicopathologic study of 82 cases. Scand J Thorac Cardiovasc Surg 19:105–111
31. Harpole DH Jr, Feldman JM, Buchanan S et al (1992) Bronchial carcinoid tumors: a retrospective analysis of 126 patients. Ann Thorac Surg 54:50–55
32. Mårtensson H, Böttcher G, Hambraeus G et al (1987) Bronchial carcinoids: an analysis of 91 cases. World J Surg 11:356–364
33. Davila DG, Dunn WF, Tazelaar HD, Pairolero PC (1993) Bronchial carcinoid tumors. Mayo Clin Proc 68:795–803
34. Dusmet ME, McKneally MF (1996) Pulmonary and thymic carcinoid tumors. World J Surg 20:189–195
35. Ricci C, Patrassi N, Massa R et al (1973) Carcinoid syndrome in bronchial adenoma. Am J Surg 126:671–677
36. Ezzat S, Asa SL, Stefaneanu L et al (1994) Somatotroph hyperplasia without pituitary adenoma associated with a long standing growth hormone-releasing hormone-producing bronchial carcinoid. Endokrina Tumörer—MEN 1 78:555–560
37. Huber RM, Schopohl J, Losa M et al (1991) Growth-hormone releasing hormone in a bronchial carcinoid. Cancer 67:2538–2542
38. Colby TV (1994) Carcinoid and other neuroendocrine tumors. In: Tumors of the lower respiratory tract. Armed Forces Instute of Pathology, Bethesda, pp 287–317
39. Okike N, Bernatz PE, Woolner LB (1976) Carcinoid tumors of the lung. Ann Thorac Surg 22:270–277
40. Granberg D, Sundin A, Janson ET et al (2003) Octreoscan in patients with bronchial carcinoid tumours. Clin Endocrinol 59:793–799
41. Vaidya B, Richardson D, Hilton CJ, Kendall-Taylor P (1997) Adrenocorticotropin-secreting carcinoid tumour identified and treated 12 years after presentation with Cushing's syndrome. Postgrad Med J 73:737–739
42. Örlefors H, Sundin A, Garske U et al (2005) Whole-body 11C-5-hydroxytryptophan positron emission tomography as a universal imaging technique for neuroendocrine tumors—comparison with somatostatin receptor scintigraphy and computed tomography. J Clin Endocrinol Metab 90:3392–3400
43. Chong S, Lee KS, Kim BT et al (2007) Integrated PET/CT of pulmonary neuroendocrine tumors: diagnostic and prognostic implications. AJR Am J Roentgenol 188:1223–1231
44. Erasmus JJ, McAdams HP, Patz EF Jr et al (1998) Evaluation of primary pulmonary carcinoid tumors using FDG PET. AJR Am J Roentgenol 170:1369–1373
45. Daniels CE, Lowe VJ, Aubry MC et al (2007) The utility of fluorodeoxyglucose positron emission tomography in the evaluation of carcinoid tumors presenting as pulmonary nodules. Chest 131:255–260
46. Hurt R, Bates M (1984) Carcinoid tumours of the bronchus: a 33 year experience. Thorax 39:617–623
47. Aslan DL, Gulbahce HE, Pambuccian SE et al (2005) Ki-67 immunoreactivity in the differential diagnosis of pulmonary neuroendocrine neoplasms in specimens with extensive crush artifact. Am J Clin Pathol 123:874–878
48. Pelosi G, Rodriguez J, Viale G, Rosai J (2005) Typical and atypical pulmonary carcinoid tumor overdiagnosed as small-cell carcinoma on biopsy specimens: a major pitfall in the management of lung cancer patients. Am J Surg Pathol 29:179–187

49. Brokx HA, Risse EK, Paul MA et al (2007) Initial bronchoscopic treatment for patients with intraluminal bronchial carcinoids. J Thorac Cardiovasc Surg 133:973–978
50. Neyman K, Sundset A, Naalsund A et al (2012) Endoscopic treatment of bronchial carcinoids in comparison to surgical resection: a retrospective study. J Bronchology Interv Pulmonol 19:29–34
51. Anderson KL Jr, Mulvihill MS, Speicher PJ et al (2017) Adjuvant chemotherapy does not confer superior survival in patients with atypical carcinoid tumors. Ann Thorac Surg 104:1221–1230
52. van Essen M, Krenning EP, Bakker WH et al (2007) Peptide receptor radionuclide therapy with (177)Lu-octreotate in patients with foregut carcinoid tumours of bronchial, gastric and thymic origin. Eur J Nucl Med Mol Imaging 34:1219–1227
53. Imhof A, Brunner P, Marincek N et al (2011) Response, survival, and long-term toxicity after therapy with the radiolabeled somatostatin analogue [90Y-DOTA]-TOC in metastasized neuroendocrine cancers. J Clin Oncol 29:2416–2423
54. Ianniello A, Sansovini M, Severi S et al (2016) Peptide receptor radionuclide therapy with (177)Lu-DOTATATE in advanced bronchial carcinoids: prognostic role of thyroid transcription factor 1 and (18)F-FDG PET. Eur J Nucl Med Mol Imaging 43:1040–1046
55. Mariniello A, Bodei L, Tinelli C et al (2016) Long-term results of PRRT in advanced bronchopulmonary carcinoid. Eur J Nucl Med Mol Imaging 43:441–452
56. De Dosso S, Bajetta E, Procopio G et al (2007) Pulmonary carcinoid tumours: indolent but not benign. Oncology 73:162–168
57. Granberg D, Eriksson B, Wilander E et al (2001) Experience in treatment of metastatic pulmonary carcinoid tumors. Ann Oncol 12:1383–1391
58. Turner NC, Strauss SJ, Sarker D et al (2010) Chemotherapy with 5-fluorouracil, cisplatin and streptozocin for neuroendocrine tumours. Br J Cancer 102:1106–1112
59. Wirth LJ, Carter MR, Jänne PA, Johnson BE (2004) Outcome of patients with pulmonary carcinoid tumors receiving chemotherapy or chemoradiotherapy. Lung Cancer 44:213–220
60. Chong CR, Wirth LJ, Nishino M et al (2014) Chemotherapy for locally advanced and metastatic pulmonary carcinoid tumors. Lung Cancer 86:241–246
61. Crona J, Fanola I, Lindholm DP et al (2013) Effect of Temozolomide in patients with metastatic bronchial carcinoids. Neuroendocrinology 98:151–155
62. Ekeblad S, Sundin A, Tiensuu Janson E et al (2007) Temozolomide as monotherapy is effective in treatment of advanced malignant neuroendocrine tumors. Clin Cancer Res 13:2986–2991
63. Caplin ME, Pavel M, Cwikla JB et al (2014) Lanreotide in metastatic enteropancreatic neuroendocrine tumors. N Engl J Med 371:224–233
64. Rinke A, Müller HH, Schade-Brittinger C et al (2009) Placebo-controlled, double-blind, prospective, randomized study on the effect of octreotide LAR in the control of tumor growth in patients with metastatic neuroendocrine midgut tumors: a report from the PROMID Study Group. J Clin Oncol 27:4656–4663
65. Sullivan I, Le Teuff G, Guigay J et al (2017) Antitumour activity of somatostatin analogues in sporadic, progressive, metastatic pulmonary carcinoids. Eur J Cancer 75:259–267
66. Fazio N, Granberg D, Grossman A et al (2012) Everolimus plus octreotide LAR in patients with advanced lung neuroendocrine tumors: analysis of the phase III, randomized, placebo-controlled RADIANT-2 study. Chest
67. Fazio N, Buzzoni R, Delle Fave G et al (2017) Everolimus in advanced, progressive, well-differentiated, non-functional neuroendocrine tumors: RADIANT-4 lung subgroup analysis. Cancer Sci
68. Ferolla P, Brizzi MP, Meyer T et al (2017) Efficacy and safety of long-acting pasireotide or everolimus alone or in combination in patients with advanced carcinoids of the lung and thymus (LUNA): an open-label, multicentre, randomised, phase 2 trial. Lancet Oncol 18:1652
69. Granberg D, Wilander E, Öberg K (2006) Expression of tyrosine kinase receptors in lung carcinoids. Tumour Biol 27:153–157
70. Tsuruoka K, Horinouchi H, Goto Y et al (2017) PD-L1 expression in neuroendocrine tumors of the lung. Lung Cancer 108:115–120

71. Rittmeyer A, Barlesi F, Waterkamp D et al (2017) Atezolizumab versus docetaxel in patients with previously treated non-small-cell lung cancer (OAK): a phase 3, open-label, multicentre randomised controlled trial. Lancet 389:255–265
72. Yao JC, Strosberg J, Fazio N et al (2018) Activity & safety of spartalizumab (PDR001) in patients (pts) with advanced neuroendocrine tumors (NET) of pancreatic (Pan), gastrointestinal (GI), or thoracic (T) origin, & gastroenteropancreatic neuroendocrine carcinoma (GEP NEC) who have progressed on prior treatment (Tx). *Ann Oncol* **29**:vIII467–vIvIII8
73. Chughtai TS, Morin JE, Sheiner NM et al (1997) Bronchial carcinoid—twenty years' experience defines a selective surgical approach. Surgery 122:801–808
74. Soga J, Yakuwa Y (1999) Bronchopulmonary carcinoids: an analysis of 1,875 reported cases with special reference to a comparison between typical carcinoids and atypical varieties. Ann Thorac Cardiovasc Surg 5:211–219
75. Thomas CF Jr, Tazelaar HD, Jett JR (2001) Typical and atypical pulmonary carcinoids : outcome in patients presenting with regional lymph node involvement. Chest 119:1143–1150
76. Granberg D, Wilander E, Öberg K, Skogseid B (2000) Prognostic markers in patients with typical bronchial carcinoid tumors. Endokrina Tumörer—MEN 1 85:3425–3430
77. Beasley MB, Thunnissen FBJM, Brambilla E et al (2000) Pulmonary atypical carcinoid: predictors of survival in 106 cases. Hum Pathol 31:1255–1265
78. Dresler CM, Ritter JH, Patterson GA et al (1997) Clinical-pathologic analysis of 40 patients with large cell neuroendocrine carcinoma of the lung. Ann Thorac Surg 63:180–185
79. Jiang S-X, Kameya T, Shoji M et al (1998) Large cell neuroendocrine carcinoma of the lung: a histologic and immunohistochemical study of 22 cases. Am J Surg Pathol 22:526–537
80. Brambilla E, Negoescu A, Gazzeri S et al (1996) Apoptosis-related factors p53, Bcl_2, and Bax in neuroendocrine lung tumors. Am J Pathol 149:1941–1952
81. Yamazaki S, Sekine I, Matsuno Y et al (2005) Clinical responses of large cell neuroendocrine carcinoma of the lung to cisplatin-based chemotherapy. Lung Cancer 49:217–223
82. Tokito T, Kenmotsu H, Watanabe R et al (2014) Comparison of chemotherapeutic efficacy between LCNEC diagnosed using large specimens and possible LCNEC diagnosed using small biopsy specimens. Int J Clin Oncol 19:63–67
83. Sun JM, Ahn MJ, Ahn JS et al (2012) Chemotherapy for pulmonary large cell neuroendocrine carcinoma: similar to that for small cell lung cancer or non-small cell lung cancer? Lung Cancer 77:365–370
84. Shimada Y, Niho S, Ishii G et al (2012) Clinical features of unresectable high-grade lung neuroendocrine carcinoma diagnosed using biopsy specimens. Lung Cancer 75:368–373
85. Igawa S, Watanabe R, Ito I et al (2010) Comparison of chemotherapy for unresectable pulmonary high-grade non-small cell neuroendocrine carcinoma and small-cell lung cancer. Lung Cancer 68:438–445
86. Yoshida H, Sekine I, Tsuta K et al (2011) Amrubicin monotherapy for patients with previously treated advanced large-cell neuroendocrine carcinoma of the lung. Jpn J Clin Oncol 41:897–901
87. De Pas TM, Giovannini M, Manzotti M et al (2011) Large-cell neuroendocrine carcinoma of the lung harboring EGFR mutation and responding to gefitinib. J Clin Oncol 29:e819–ee22
88. Kozuki T, Fujimoto N, Ueoka H et al (2005) Complexity in the treatment of pulmonary large cell neuroendocrine carcinoma. J Cancer Res Clin Oncol 131:147–151
89. Filosso PL, Ruffini E, Oliaro A et al (2005) Large-cell neuroendocrine carcinoma of the lung: a clinicopathologic study of eighteen cases and the efficacy of adjuvant treatment with octreotide. J Thorac Cardiovasc Surg 129:819–824
90. Iyoda A, Travis WD, Sarkaria IS et al (2011) Expression profiling and identification of potential molecular targets for therapy in pulmonary large-cell neuroendocrine carcinoma. Exp Ther Med 2:1041–1045
91. Asamura H, Kameya T, Matsuno Y et al (2006) Neuroendocrine neoplasms of the lung: a prognostic spectrum. PDF-artiklar, Somatuline 24:70–76
92. Battafarano RJ, Fernandez FG, Ritter J et al (2005) Large cell neuroendocrine carcinoma: an aggressive form of non-small cell lung cancer. J Thorac Cardiovasc Surg 130:166–172

93. Iyoda A, Hiroshima K, Toyozaki T et al (2001) Clinical characterization of pulmonary large cell neuroendocrine carcinoma and large cell carcinoma with neuroendocrine morphology. Cancer 91:1992–2000
94. Paci M, Cavazza A, Annessi V et al (2004) Large cell neuroendocrine carcinoma of the lung: a 10-year clinicopathologic retrospective study. Ann Thorac Surg 77:1163–1167
95. Rossi G, Cavazza A, Marchioni A et al (2005) Role of chemotherapy and the receptor tyrosine kinases KIT, PDGFRalpha, PDGFRbeta, and met in large-cell neuroendocrine carcinoma of the lung. J Clin Oncol 23:8774–8785
96. Skuladottir H, Hirsch FR, Hansen HH, Olsen JH (2002) Pulmonary neuroendocrine tumors: incidence and prognosis of histological subtypes. A population-based study in Denmark. Lung Cancer 37:127–135
97. Veronesi G, Morandi U, Alloisio M et al (2006) Large cell neuroendocrine carcinoma of the lung: a retrospective analysis of 144 surgical cases. Lung Cancer 53:111–115
98. Iyoda A, Hiroshima K, Moriya Y et al (2006) Prognostic impact of large cell neuroendocrine histology in patients with pathologic stage Ia pulmonary non-small cell carcinoma. J Thorac Cardiovasc Surg 132:312–315
99. Takei H, Asamura H, Maeshima A et al (2002) Large cell neuroendocrine carcinoma of the lung: a clinicopathologic study of eighty-seven cases. J Thorac Cardiovasc Surg 124:285–292
100. Cook RM, Miller YE, Bunn PA Jr (1993) Small cell lung cancer: etiology, biology, clinical features, staging, and treatment. Curr Probl Cancer 17:69–141
101. Curran WJ Jr (2001) Combined-modality therapy for limited-stage small cell lung cancer. Semin Oncol 28:14–22
102. Komaki R, Byhardt RW, Anderson T et al (1985) What is the lowest effective biologic dose for prophylactic cranial irradiation? Am J Clin Oncol 8:523–527
103. Samson DJ, Seidenfeld J, Simon GR et al (2007) Evidence for management of small cell lung cancer: ACCP evidence-based clinical practice guidelines (2nd edition). Chest 132:314S–323S
104. Folpe AL, Gown AM, Lamps LW et al (1999) Thyroid transcription factor-1: immunohistochemical evaluation in pulmonary neuroendocrine tumors. Mod Pathol 12:5–8
105. Kaufmann O, Dietel M (2000) Expression of thyroid transcription factor-1 in pulmonary and extrapulmonary small cell carcinomas and other neuroendocrine carcinomas of various primary sites. Histopathology 36:415–420
106. Cuttitta F, Carney DN, Mulshine J et al (1985) Bombesin-like peptides can function as autocrine growth factors in human small-cell lung cancer. Nature 316:823–826
107. Ben-Ezra JM, Kornstein MJ, Grimes MM, Krystal G (1994) Small cell carcinomas of the lung express the Bcl-2 protein. Am J Pathol 145:1036–1040
108. Jiang S-X, Kameya T, Sato Y et al (1996) Bcl-2 protein expression in lung cancer and close correlation with neuroendocrine differentiation. Am J Pathol 148:837–846
109. Cagle PT, el-Naggar AK, Xu H-J et al (1997) Differential retinoblastoma protein expression in neuroendocrine tumors of the lung. Potential diagnostic implications. Am J Pathol 150:393–400
110. Vuitch F, Sekido Y, Fong K et al (1997) Neuroendocrine tumors of the lung. pathology and molecular biology. Chest Surg Clin N Am 7:21–47
111. Balsara BR, Testa JR (2002) Chromosomal imbalances in human lung cancer. Oncogene 21:6877–6883
112. Onuki N, Wistuba II, Travis WD et al (1999) Genetic changes in the spectrum of neuroendocrine lung tumors. Cancer 85:600–607
113. Johnson BE, Russell E, Simmons AM et al (1996) MYC family DNA amplification in 126 tumor cell lines from patients with small cell lung cancer. J Cell Biochem Suppl 24:210–217
114. Shivapurkar N, Toyooka S, Eby MT et al (2002) Differential inactivation of caspase-8 in lung cancers. Cancer Biol Ther 1:65–69
115. Petersen I, Hidalgo A, Petersen S et al (2000) Chromosomal imbalances in brain metastases of solid tumors. Brain Pathol 10:395–401

116. Planchard D, Le Pechoux C (2011) Small cell lung cancer: new clinical recommendations and current status of biomarker assessment. Eur J Cancer 47(Suppl 3):S272–S283
117. van Meerbeeck JP, Fennell DA, De Ruysscher DK (2011) Small-cell lung cancer. Lancet 378:1741–1755
118. Detterbeck FC, Boffa DJ, Tanoue LT (2009) The new lung cancer staging system. Chest 136:260–271
119. Mirsadraee S, Oswal D, Alizadeh Y et al (2012) The 7th lung cancer TNM classification and staging system: review of the changes and implications. World J Radiol 4:128–134
120. Micke P, Faldum A, Metz T et al (2002) Staging small cell lung cancer: Veterans Administration Lung Study Group versus International Association for the Study of Lung Cancer—what limits limited disease? Lung Cancer 37:271–276
121. O'Byrne KJ, Ennis JT, Freyne PJ et al (1994) Scintigraphic imaging of small-cell lung cancer with [^{111}In]pentetreotide, a radiolabelled somatostatin analogue. Br J Cancer 69:762–766
122. Reisinger I, Bohuslavitzki KH, Brenner W et al (1998) Somatostatin receptor scintigraphy in small-cell lung cancer: results of a multicenter study. J Nucl Med 39:224–227
123. Valkema R, Steens J, Cleton F, Pauwels E (1996) The diagnostic utility of somatostatin receptor scintigraphy in oncology. J Cancer Res Clin Oncol 122:513–532
124. Byers LA, Rudin CM (2015) Small cell lung cancer: where do we go from here? Cancer 121:664–672
125. Antonia SJ, Lopez-Martin JA, Bendell J et al (2016) Nivolumab alone and nivolumab plus ipilimumab in recurrent small-cell lung cancer (CheckMate 032): a multicentre, open-label, phase 1/2 trial. Lancet Oncol 17:883–895
126. Ott PA, Elez E, Hiret S et al (2017) Pembrolizumab in patients with extensive-stage small-cell lung cancer: results from the phase Ib KEYNOTE-028 study. J Clin Oncol 35:3823–3830
127. Horn L, Mansfield A, Szczęsna A et al (2018) First-line Atezolizumab plus chemotherapy in extensive-stage small-cell lung cancer. N Engl J Med 379:2220–2229
128. Simon GR, Turrisi A, American College of Chest P (2007) Management of small cell lung cancer: ACCP evidence-based clinical practice guidelines (2nd edition). Chest 132:324S–339S
129. Foster NR, Mandrekar SJ, Schild SE et al (2009) Prognostic factors differ by tumor stage for small cell lung cancer: a pooled analysis of North Central Cancer Treatment Group trials. Cancer 115:2721–2731

Update of Neuroendocrine Tumors, Diagnosis, and Management

10

Suayib Yalcin and Kjell Öberg

10.1 Overview of Gastrointestinal Neuroendocrine Tumors

10.1.1 Introduction

Intestinal neuroendocrine tumors (NETs/NENs) constitute a heterogenous group of malignant disorders including duodenal, small intestinal, colonic, rectal, and gastric tumors. In the most recent SEER register (C17), gastroenteropancreatic NETs constitute more than 60% of all NETs with the highest frequency being in the rectum (17.7%), small intestinal (17.3%), and colon (10.1%) [1]. The tumor biology varies with the location of the primary tumors as well as with the grade and staging of the tumors. The malignant potential ranges from the most benign types of tumors, such as small intestinal tumors (carcinoids) to colonic neuroendocrine carcinoma (NEC) with very malignant behavior [2]. Tumors are graded according to the classification system of the World Health Organization (WHO), where a new classification system just has been introduced in 2019 (to be published). The tumors are divided into grade 1 NET-G1 with a proliferation of <3%, NET-G2 with a proliferation between 3 and 20%, NET-G3 which is a new group with Ki-67 > 20%, and finally NEC-G3 exhibiting a Ki-67 of >20% as well, however usually >50%. The difference between NET-G3 and NEC-G3 is mainly the degree of differentiation; NET-G3 is well-differentiated tumors, often with the expression of somatostatin receptors. NEC-G3 is poorly differentiated tumors that usually lack expression of somatostatin receptors [3]. Furthermore, the tumors are classified according to the staging system from

S. Yalcin (✉)
Department of Medical Oncology, Hacettepe University Cancer Institute, Ankara, Turkey
e-mail: syalcin@hacettepe.edu.tr

K. Öberg
Department of Endocrine Oncology, Uppsala University Hospital, Uppsala, Sweden
e-mail: adm-oberg@medsci.uu.se; kjell.oberg@medsci.uu.se

S. Yalcin, K. Öberg (eds.), *Neuroendocrine Tumours*,
https://doi.org/10.1007/978-3-031-56968-5_10

ENETS and UICC (Union of International Cancer Control)/AJCC (American Joint Committee of Cancer) depending on the spread of the disease [4].

Genetic background information of intestinal NET is still limited. It is well known that small intestinal NET displays chromosomal losses on chromosome 18 and cyclin-dependent kinase inhibitor mutations [5]. However, genetic changes such as mutations are very rare in this group of tumors. When they become more malignant, such as NEC-G3, more genetic changes are found, for example, RB and TP53 mutations [6]. Epigenetic changes (DNA methylation) are noticed in methylguanine methyl transferase (MGMT), RAS association domain family 1A (RASSF1A), and cyclin-dependent kinase inhibitor (CDKN2A) [7–9]. Intestinal NET expresses a number of G-protein couple receptors where the somatostatin receptors are the most frequent and target for the correct staging of disease, evaluation, therapeutic responses, and treatment [10, 11].

10.2 Esophageal Neuroendocrine Tumors

NETs of the esophagus are rare, around 1%. The mean age at diagnosis is close to 60 years with a male predominance. Dysphagia is the most predominant clinical manifestation followed by weight loss and pain. Nearly half of the tumors occur in the lower third of the esophagus, and the tumors are usually larger than 5 cm in diameter [12, 13]. Histologically, there are two types, typical and atypical; immunohistochemical staining shows the expression of CEA, NSE, and chromogranin-A. Metastases are frequent at presentation of atypical esophageal NETs, primarily in the lymph nodes, liver, bone, and lung [14]. The five-year survival rate for patients with atypical esophageal NETs is 0%, whereas for those with typical, it is around 30% [14]. Most tumors are removed surgically.

10.3 Gastric Neuroendocrine Tumors

Gastric NETs represent the most frequent digestive NET and are increasingly detected due to expanding indications of upper gastrointestinal endoscopy [15, 16]. Gastric NETs are classified into three types [17, 18]. Correct classification into these types is based on biopsies that are taken both from antrum and body/fundus. It is also recommended that the proliferation Ki-67 index, mitotic index, and ENETS differentiation grade should also be assessed [18].

Type 1 gastric neuroendocrine tumor is the most common type, is in general small and multiple, and occurs in patients with chronic atrophic gastritis with or without pernicious anemia [17]. Type 1 gastric carcinoids are not infrequent asymptomatic and are detected when a patient is evaluated for iron deficiency anemia or pernicious anemia [17]. Type 1 gastric NET usually appears as polypoid lesions, associated with mucosal atrophy. Histological type 1 gastric carcinoids are well differentiated and always associated with a varying degree of gastric ECL cell hyperplasia [17, 19]. The ECL hyperplasia is driven by hypergastrinemia caused by loss of the feedback inhibition by gastric acid on gastrin cells. Type 1 gastric NETs are nearly minimally invasive and limited to the mucosa and the submucosa; only 9% invade the muscularis propria. Metastases to lymph nodes or liver are rare and uncommon [19, 20].

Type 2 gastric carcinoids are the least frequent type and occur almost exclusively in patients with MEN1/Zollinger–Ellison syndrome [17]. They occur in 20–30% of patients with MEN1/ZES, invariable with hyperparathyroidism. Type 2 gastric NETs are like type 1, in general multiple but they tend to be larger, sometimes more than 2 cm in size. They appear as polypoid lesions, well differentiated or more invasive than type 1 tumors, and the 5-year survival is lower than that in type 1 tumors (60–90% vs 100%) [17–19]. Metastases are also more common in type 2 than in type 1 gastric NETs [17].

Type 3 gastric NETs differ from the other two types, in that they are not associated with hypergastrinemia or alterations in acid secretion [17]. They are solitary sporadic NETs, not associated with other diseases of the stomach. Endoscopically, type 3 gastric carcinoids are usually single, large, infiltrating lesions that in some cases are ulcerating [17, 19]. Histologically, they are generally well differentiated; however, their Ki-67 index may exceed 3%. At the time of diagnosis, most type 3 gastric carcinoids are already invasive and the 5-year overall survival rate is close to 50% [17–19].

The carcinoid syndrome occurs in a small percentage of patients with type 1 and type 3 gastric carcinoids. Atypical flush may occur in these patients, which is a prolonged red/purple flush involving the trunk and extremities. This flushing might be related to the release of unprocessed serotonin (5-HTP) or in rare cases also histamine which might result in bronchospasm, itching, contagious flushing, and lacrimation [17]. Poorly differentiated gastric NETs in the stomach are included in some classifications as type 4 gastric NETs. They comprise 3–8% of all gastric carcinoids [19]. They are generally solitary larger tumors, poorly differentiated G-3 tumors with normal fasting gastrin levels and gastric pH. They are associated with metastases in 80-100% of the cases [19]. These tumors are treated like other poorly differentiated GI-NETs in other locations. Type 1 and type 2 gastric NETs are usually treated endoscopically if there are 5 or fewer lesions without adverse risk factors such as muscular wall infiltration, increased proliferative Ki-67 index, or angioinvasion [21, 22]. For type 1 or 2 gastric carcinoids that infiltrate the submucosa, it is recommended that endoscopic mucosal resection (EMR) can be considered [23]. Surgical resection is recommended in patients with larger tumors and with infiltration of the muscularis wall and angioinvasion. Long-term treatment with somatostatin analog may result in disappearance of small gastric carcinoids. However, the tumors will reoccur when the treatment is stopped [24]. Type 3 gastric carcinoids, if they are small, <1 cm can be treated conservatively with endoscopic mucosectomy. Larger tumors need to be removed surgically [19].

10.4 Duodenal NETs

Duodenal NETs have an annual incidence of 0.19/100.000 in the United States and constitute 5% of all gastrointestinal neuroendocrine tumors [25]. The incidence is somewhat higher in Japan compared to the western countries. Most duodenal NETs arise from the first or second part of the duodenum with about 20% occurring in the periampullary region [26]. Duodenal somatostatinomas and gangliocytic paragangliomas show a preference for the periampullary region, and the former may be particularly associated with NF1 [26]. Duodenal NETs are generally small with a diameter of 1–1.5 cm and mostly limited to the mucosa or submucosa, but they can still metastases to lymph nodes; liver metastases occur in less than 10%. Most duodenal NETs are solitary, but they are multiple in patients with MEN1 which comprise 6% of all patients with duodenal NETs, for example, in MEN1/ZES patients, 80% of gastrinomas are in the duodenum, they invariable are multiple [27]. Duodenal NETs can be divided into five subtypes: Duodenal gastrinomas (40–60%), somatostatinomas (15–40%), nonfunctioning NET (20%), gangliocytic paraganglioma (<2%), and poly-differentiated neuroendocrine carcinoma (<3%) [26]. Although various GI-hormones are frequently found in the duodenal NETs, no clinical syndrome is seen in 60–90% of the patients. Most duodenal NETs are well differentiated neuroendocrine tumors, and only about 3% or less are poorly differentiated [26, 28]. They stain positive for the typical NET features, such as CGA, NSE, and synaptophysin. Paragangliomas also stain for S-100 protein, positive in Schwann cells. Most frequent functional syndromes are Zollinger–Ellison syndrome 10% and carcinoid syndrome 4% [26, 29]. Even though duodenal somatostatinomas are the second most frequent type of duodenal NET, they are only very rarely associated with somatostatinomas syndrome [26]. Periampullary NETs present in 5% with jaundice and may also cause pain, nausea/vomiting, and diarrhea [26]. The 5-year survival in patients with well differentiated duodenal NETs is 80-95% [25, 26, 29].

10.5 Small Intestinal NETs (Jejunal/Ileal)

NETs originating in the small intestine are reported with an incidence of 0.32/100.000 up to 1.22/100.000 in Sweden [16, 30]. Mean age at initial diagnosis is in the late 50-ies in several cohorts; it is equally distributed between males and females. The incidence of small intestinal NETs may be lower in persons of Asian descent [31] and somewhat higher in African American's according to the SEER database. The true incidence of small intestinal NETs in post-mortem studies is much higher, 1.22/100.000 and suggests that these NETs may be much more abundant at early or very early stages but do not manifest themselves clinically and are not diagnosed during life [30]. Familial clustering of jejunal and ileal NETs is described but rare [32]. Abdominal pain is the most frequent initial symptoms in patients presenting with NETs from the small bowel. The presence of the carcinoid syndrome is about

20-30% in patients with metastases higher than previously stated. Small bowel ischemia can be another cause of diarrhea and pain, not only hormone hypersecretion-related diarrhea. In the literature, flushing is reported to be a more frequent symptom than diarrhea (90% vs 80%) [32–34]. It is emphasized that carcinoid syndrome is usually seen in patients with liver metastases. Excess tachykinin or serotonin production from retroperitoneal metastases or ovarian tumor/metastases can bypass the liver and enter the systemic circulation and cause the typical carcinoid syndrome (see later). The survival rate strongly depends on histopathological WHO classification and TNM stage [35, 36]. Five-year survival for all stages reaches between 50% and 60%. However, in NETs with only locally and limited disease, the five-year survival is 80-100%. For only regional lymph node involvement, it is 70–80%. In patients with liver metastases, the five-year survival is around 35–60% [32, 33, 35, 37, 38]. Ki-67 rating is an important prognostic stratifier and is therefore mandatory in pathological reporting.

10.6 Appendiceal NETs

Appendiceal NETs are reported in the literature with an incidence of 0.15/100.000 per year. They are diagnosed slightly more often in females than in male patients at an average age of 40-50 years [16, 39]. Appendiceal NETs are however much more frequently diagnosed incidentally during appendectomies with a rate of approximately 3–5/1000 appendectomies. Survival is extremely good (local disease) with five-year survival, 95–100%. Regional disease, 85-100% [39]. It is noticed that an appendiceal NEN with a size of less than 1 cm with invasion up to the sub-serosa or meso-appendiceal invasion of up to 3 mm and clear surgical margins, there is no further risk of recurrence after appendectomy. Most tumors (70%) are located at the tip of the appendix. However, tumors at the base of the appendix and tumors above 2 cm in size, deep meso-appendiceal invasion or margin invasion there is a high risk of recurrence. Further surgical procedure is warranted although no data have proven survival benefit by more aggressive surgery [39–43]. NETs of the appendix are rarely symptomatic; however, tumors with extensive local disease or distant metastases may appear symptomatic with abdominal pain and signs of bowel obstruction. An association with the carcinoid syndrome is extremely rare and indicates metastatic disease [39].

Goblet cell carcinoids are rare appendiceal tumors which must be differentiated from appendiceal NETs and are considered as a MANEC or MINEN and approximately 2/3 of cases there are incidental findings on appendectomy or ileocecal resection [44, 45]. Biologically, they are a subtype of adenocarcinoma. Most goblet cells carcinoids, when located in the mid third of the appendix may cause appendicitis. At diagnosis, approximately 10% of the tumors are already wide-spread with distant metastases to the liver, ovaries, and the peritoneum [46, 47]. The limited stage in survival is better in local regional disease, 50–80%, but in cases with distant metastases, the five-year survival is less than 20% [48].

10.7 Colonic Carcinoids

Colonic carcinoids (excluding the rectum and the appendix) occur with an annual incidence of 0.1–1.19/100.000 [16]. Colonic NETs comprise 4–8% of all carcinoids. The majority of the colonic carcinoid occur in the cecum with the reminder arising in the ascending, transverse, descending, and sigmoid colon [49]. Colonic NETs tend to be large with more than 50% being larger than 5 cm. These tumors are often malignant with metastases to lymph nodes, liver, mesentery, and omentum [50, 51]. Histologically, the colonic NETs have positive staining for chromogranin A and NSE as well as synaptophysin. The tumors are composed of EC-cells and L-cells. The serotonin producing EC-cell type is mainly found in the right colon and is generally a grade 1 tumor. L-cell NETs are found in the distal colon and rectum and produce GLP, PP, and PYY [50] Some colonic NETs are classified as neuroendocrine carcinomas and are poorly differentiated, high-grade G3, large or small cell malignant tumors [52, 53]. The overall survival rate for patients with colonic carcinoid is 30-70%, and the survival varies considered by stage [52, 53]. Colonic NETs are often asymptomatic and found on cancer screening. Carcinoid syndrome occurs in 5–12% of patients with colonic carcinoids [49].

10.8 Rectal NETs

Rectal NETs comprise 25% of all gastrointestinal NETs and 16% of all NETs in the United States [16, 49]. They are increasing in incidence. It is unclear whether there is a true increased incidence or if these tumors simply have increased detection due to wide-spread use of lower GI endoscopy for cancer screening and other indications [54]. Early detection of rectal carcinoid tumors may explain the decrease in size of the typical rectal carcinoid over the past decades [55]. Studies from Japan and other Asian countries, rectal carcinoids account for 60-90% of all GI-NETs [56]. Rectal NETs are often diagnosed in the sixth decade of life and are usually asymptomatic. The carcinoid syndrome is very uncommon (0.7%) in patients with rectal NETs. Rectal NETs are characteristically small polypoid lesions (mean dm <1 cm). Most rectal NETs are well differentiated, grade 1 (72%) tumors. Nearly 80% of the tumors invade no deeper than the submucosa with some invading into the muscularis layer [55, 57]. Metastases from rectal carcinoid are related to size. For tumors that exceed 2 cm in size, the metastatic rate jumps up to 60–80% [57]. Overall five-year survival with the rectal NETs is 80% with a survival very much dependent of the stage of the disease [58]. Patients with colorectal NETs have a higher risk of second cancer than the control population. This second cancer may originate in the colon or rectum, small bowel, esophagus, stomach, lung and urinary tract as well as prostate. Most secondary GI cancer was synchronous, whereas secondary outside the GI tract was most commonly metachronous tumors [49].

References

1. Lawrence B, Gustafsson BI, Chan A, Svejda B, Kidd M, Modlin IM (2011) The epidemiology of gastroenteropancreatic neuroendocrine tumors. Endocrinol Metab Clin N Am 40:1–18. vii
2. Tang LH, Untch BR, Reidy DL et al (2016) Well-differentiated neuroendocrine tumors with a morphologically apparent high-grade component: a pathway distinct from poorly differentiated neuroendocrine carcinomas. Clin Cancer Res 22:1011–1017
3. Kloppel G (2011) Classification and pathology of gastroenteropancreatic neuroendocrine neoplasms. Endocr Relat Cancer 18(Suppl 1):S1–S16
4. Kloppel G, Rindi G, Perren A, Komminoth P, Klimstra DS (2010) The ENETS and AJCC/UICC TNM classifications of the neuroendocrine tumors of the gastrointestinal tract and the pancreas: a statement. Virchows Arch 456:595–597
5. Francis JM, Kiezun A, Ramos AH et al (2013) Somatic mutation of CDKN1B in small intestine neuroendocrine tumors. Nat Genet 45:1483–1486
6. Tang LH, Contractor T, Clausen R et al (2012) Attenuation of the retinoblastoma pathway in pancreatic neuroendocrine tumors due to increased cdk4/cdk6. Clin Cancer Res 18:4612–4620
7. La Rosa S, Marando A, Furlan D, Sahnane N, Capella C (2012) Colorectal poorly differentiated neuroendocrine carcinomas and mixed adenoneuroendocrine carcinomas: insights into the diagnostic immunophenotype, assessment of methylation profile, and search for prognostic markers. Am J Surg Pathol 36:601–611
8. Stricker I, Tzivras D, Nambiar S et al (2012) Site- and grade-specific diversity of LINE1 methylation pattern in gastroenteropancreatic neuroendocrine tumours. Anticancer Res 32:3699–3706
9. Dammann R, Schagdarsurengin U, Strunnikova M et al (2003) Epigenetic inactivation of the Ras-association domain family 1 (RASSF1A) gene and its function in human carcinogenesis. Histol Histopathol 18:665–677
10. Reubi JC (2003) Peptide receptors as molecular targets for cancer diagnosis and therapy. Endocr Rev 24:389–427
11. Reubi JC, Waser B (2003) Concomitant expression of several peptide receptors in neuroendocrine tumours: molecular basis for in vivo multireceptor tumour targeting. Eur J Nucl Med Mol Imaging 30:781–793
12. Brenner S, Heimlich H, Widman M (1969) Carcinoid of esophagus. N Y State J Med 69:1337–1339
13. Ready AR, Soul JO, Newman J, Matthews HR (1989) Malignant carcinoid tumour of the oesophagus. Thorax 44:594–596
14. Lindberg GM, Molberg KH, Vuitch MF, Albores-Saavedra J (1997) Atypical carcinoid of the esophagus: a case report and review of the literature. Cancer 79:1476–1481
15. O'Connor JM, Marmissolle F, Bestani C et al (2014) Observational study of patients with gastroenteropancreatic and bronchial neuroendocrine tumors in Argentina: results from the large database of a multidisciplinary group clinical multicenter study. Mol Clin Oncol 2:673–684
16. Yao JC, Hassan M, Phan A et al (2008) One hundred years after "carcinoid": epidemiology of and prognostic factors for neuroendocrine tumors in 35,825 cases in the United States. J Clin Oncol 26:3063–3072
17. Rindi G, Bordi C, Rappel S, La Rosa S, Stolte M, Solcia E (1996) Gastric carcinoids and neuroendocrine carcinomas: pathogenesis, pathology, and behavior. World J Surg 20:168–172
18. La Rosa S, Inzani F, Vanoli A et al (2011) Histologic characterization and improved prognostic evaluation of 209 gastric neuroendocrine neoplasms. Hum Pathol 42:1373–1384
19. Rindi G, Azzoni C, La Rosa S et al (1999) ECL cell tumor and poorly differentiated endocrine carcinoma of the stomach: prognostic evaluation by pathological analysis. Gastroenterology 116:532–542
20. Grozinsky-Glasberg S, Thomas D, Strosberg JR et al (2013) Metastatic type 1 gastric carcinoid: a real threat or just a myth? World J Gastroenterol 19:8687–8695

21. Merola E, Sbrozzi-Vanni A, Panzuto F et al (2012) Type I gastric carcinoids: a prospective study on endoscopic management and recurrence rate. Neuroendocrinology 95:207–213
22. Uygun A, Kadayifci A, Polat Z et al (2014) Long-term results of endoscopic resection for type I gastric neuroendocrine tumors. J Surg Oncol 109:71–74
23. Kim HH, Kim GH, Kim JH, Choi MG, Song GA, Kim SE (2014) The efficacy of endoscopic submucosal dissection of type I gastric carcinoid tumors compared with conventional endoscopic mucosal resection. Gastroenterol Res Pract 2014:253860
24. Jianu CS, Fossmark R, Syversen U, Hauso O, Fykse V, Waldum HL (2011) Five-year follow-up of patients treated for 1 year with octreotide long-acting release for enterochromaffin-like cell carcinoids. Scand J Gastroenterol 46:456–463
25. Mullen JT, Wang H, Yao JC et al (2005) Carcinoid tumors of the duodenum. Surgery 138:971–977. discussion 7-8
26. Soga J (2003) Endocrinocarcinomas (carcinoids and their variants) of the duodenum. An evaluation of 927 cases. J Exp Clinical Cancer Research: CR 22:349–363
27. Pipeleers-Marichal M, Donow C, Heitz PU, Kloppel G (1993) Pathologic aspects of gastrinomas in patients with Zollinger-Ellison syndrome with and without multiple endocrine neoplasia type I. World J Surg 17:481–488
28. Capella C, Riva C, Rindi G, Usellini L, Chiaravalli A, Solcia E (1990) Endocrine tumors of the duodenum and upper jejunum. A study of 33 cases with clinico-pathological characteristics and hormone content. Hepato-Gastroenterology 37:247–252
29. Kolby L, Nilsson O, Ahlman H (2004) Gastroduodenal endocrine tumours. Scand J Surg 93:317–323
30. Berge T, Linell F, Carcinoid tumours. (1976) Frequency in a defined population during a 12-year period. Acta Pathol Microbiol Scand A Pathol 84:322–330
31. Ito T, Sasano H, Tanaka M et al (2010) Epidemiological study of gastroenteropancreatic neuroendocrine tumors in Japan. J Gastroenterol 45:234–243
32. Modlin IM, Oberg K, Chung DC et al (2008) Gastroenteropancreatic neuroendocrine tumours. Lancet Oncol 9:61–72
33. Garcia-Carbonero R, Capdevila J, Crespo-Herrero G et al (2010) Incidence, patterns of care and prognostic factors for outcome of gastroenteropancreatic neuroendocrine tumors (GEP-NETs): results from the National Cancer Registry of Spain (RGETNE). Ann Oncol 21:1794–1803
34. Jann H, Roll S, Couvelard A et al (2011) Neuroendocrine tumors of midgut and hindgut origin: tumor-node-metastasis classification determines clinical outcome. Cancer 117:3332–3341
35. Klimstra DSAR, Capella C et al (2010) WHO classification of tumours of the digestive system. IACR, Lyon
36. Niederle MB, Niederle B (2011) Diagnosis and treatment of gastroenteropancreatic neuroendocrine tumors: current data on a prospectively collected, retrospectively analyzed clinical multicenter investigation. Oncologist 16:602–613
37. Norlen O, Stalberg P, Oberg K et al (2012) Long-term results of surgery for small intestinal neuroendocrine tumors at a tertiary referral center. World J Surg 36:1419–1431
38. Niederle B, Pape UF, Costa F et al (2016) ENETS consensus guidelines update for neuroendocrine neoplasms of the jejunum and ileum. Neuroendocrinology 103:125–138
39. Pape UF, Niederle B, Costa F et al (2016) ENETS consensus guidelines for neuroendocrine neoplasms of the appendix (excluding goblet cell carcinomas). Neuroendocrinology 103:144–152
40. In't Hof KH, van der Wal HC, Kazemier G, Lange JF (2008) Carcinoid tumour of the appendix: an analysis of 1,485 consecutive emergency appendectomies. J Gastrointest Surg 12:1436–1438
41. Hsu C, Rashid A, Xing Y et al (2013) Varying malignant potential of appendiceal neuroendocrine tumors: importance of histologic subtype. J Surg Oncol 107:136–143
42. Shapiro R, Eldar S, Sadot E, Papa MZ, Zippel DB (2011) Appendiceal carcinoid at a large tertiary center: pathologic findings and long-term follow-up evaluation. Am J Surg 201:805–808

43. Bamboat ZM, Berger DL (2006) Is right hemicolectomy for 2.0-cm appendiceal carcinoids justified? Arch Surg (Chicago, Ill : 1960) 141:349–352. discussion 52
44. Holt N, Gronbaek H (2013) Goblet cell carcinoids of the appendix. TheScientificWorldJOURNAL 2013:543696
45. Pape UF, Perren A, Niederle B et al (2012) ENETS Consensus Guidelines for the management of patients with neuroendocrine neoplasms from the jejuno-ileum and the appendix including goblet cell carcinomas. Neuroendocrinology 95:135–156
46. Tang LH, Shia J, Soslow RA et al (2008) Pathologic classification and clinical behavior of the spectrum of goblet cell carcinoid tumors of the appendix. Am J Surg Pathol 32:1429–1443
47. Tang LH (2010) Epithelial neoplasms of the appendix. Arch Pathol Lab Med 134:1612–1620
48. Lamarca A, Nonaka D, Lopez Escola C et al (2016) Appendiceal goblet cell carcinoids: management considerations from a reference peritoneal tumour service centre and ENETS Centre of Excellence. Neuroendocrinology 103:500–517
49. Ramage JK, De Herder WW, Delle Fave G et al (2016) ENETS consensus guidelines update for colorectal neuroendocrine neoplasms. Neuroendocrinology 103:139–143
50. Smith JD, Reidy DL, Goodman KA, Shia J, Nash GM (2014) A retrospective review of 126 high-grade neuroendocrine carcinomas of the colon and rectum. Ann Surg Oncol 21:2956–2962
51. Li Y, Yau A, Schaeffer D et al (2011) Colorectal glandular-neuroendocrine mixed tumor: pathologic spectrum and clinical implications. Am J Surg Pathol 35:413–425
52. Sorbye H, Strosberg J, Baudin E, Klimstra DS, Yao JC (2014) Gastroenteropancreatic high-grade neuroendocrine carcinoma. Cancer 120:2814–2823
53. Sorbye H, Welin S, Langer SW et al (2013) Predictive and prognostic factors for treatment and survival in 305 patients with advanced gastrointestinal neuroendocrine carcinoma (WHO G3): the NORDIC NEC study. Ann Oncol 24:152–160
54. Taghavi S, Jayarajan SN, Powers BD, Davey A, Willis AI (2013) Examining rectal carcinoids in the era of screening colonoscopy: a surveillance, epidemiology, and end results analysis. Dis Colon Rectum 56:952–959
55. Gleeson FC, Levy MJ, Dozois EJ, Larson DW, Wong Kee Song LM, Boardman LA (2014) Endoscopically identified well-differentiated rectal carcinoid tumors: impact of tumor size on the natural history and outcomes. Gastrointest Endosc 80:144–151
56. Yangong H, Shi C, Shahbaz M et al (2014) Diagnosis and treatment experience of rectal carcinoid (a report of 312 cases). Int J Surg (London, England) 12:408–411
57. Al Natour RH, Saund MS, Sanchez VM et al (2012) Tumor size and depth predict rate of lymph node metastasis in colon carcinoids and can be used to select patients for endoscopic resection. J Gastrointest Surg 16:595–602
58. McDermott FD, Heeney A, Courtney D, Mohan H, Winter D (2014) Rectal carcinoids: a systematic review. Surg Endosc 28:2020–2026

Overview of Functioning Pancreatic Neuroendocrine Tumors (F-panNETs) 11

Nicola Fazio and Anna Koumarianou

11.1 Introduction

Functioning pancreatic neuroendocrine tumors (F-panNETs) are rare malignancies developing from the hormone-producing cells (islet cells) of the pancreas. They are distinguished from the nonfunctioning panNETs because of the presence of a clinical syndrome depending on one or more hormones or substances secreted by the tumor cells.

A panNET can be *nonfunctioning* and at the same time *secreting*, but not *functioning* if *not secreting*. Therefore, the diagnosis of a F-panNET is clinical, rather than biochemical.

11.2 Epidemiology

Incidence of panNETs has been reported as <1 new cases per year/100,000 although it varies among the several registries across the world [1–5]. As reported for other NETs, incidence of panNETs has been dramatically increasing over the last decades, particularly for localized stage and low grade [5, 6].

Functioning panNETs have been reported to be much rarer than nonfunctioning (NF) panNETs [7, 8] although it is very difficult to find specific data in the main epidemiological reports and databases. For instance, in the RARECARE website, F-panNETs are included in the functioning GEP NETs item and they overall account

N. Fazio (✉)
Division of Gastrointestinal Medical Oncology and Neuroendocrine Tumors, European Institute of Oncology, IEO, IRCCS, Milan, Italy
e-mail: nicola.fazio@ieo.it

A. Koumarianou
Hematology Oncology Unit, Fourth Department of Internal Medicine, 'Attikon' University Hospital, National and Kapodistrian University of Athens, Athens, Greece

S. Yalcin, K. Öberg (eds.), *Neuroendocrine Tumours*,
https://doi.org/10.1007/978-3-031-56968-5_11

for 0.026 new cases per year/100,000 (RARECARENet website). Insulinomas and gastrinomas are the most common subtypes of F-panNET with an incidence of 1 to 3/million population/year and 0.5 to 2/million population/year, respectively [9]. Carcinoid syndrome is less commonly related to panNETs compared to small intestinal NETs. From a large carcinoid series, the carcinoid syndrome was calculated as 23.3% (34/146) deriving from F-panNETs, compared with 35.8% (406/1134; $P < 0.01$) in the small intestine and 24.1% (20/83: without significant statistical difference) in the ileocecal region [10].

11.3 Genetic Features

Genomic literature data are not specific for F-panNETs, so we refer to panNETs in general. Whole-exome (WE) and whole-genome sequencing (WGS), mainly performed on surgical samples from the primary site, much improved our knowledge about pathogenesis of panNETs over the last decade. Alterations of *DAXX/ATRX*, *MEN-1*, and *mTOR* pathway represent the most common genetic features of advanced panNETs [11]. From an outstanding paper recently published in the Nature, we learned that four main genetic settings resulted alteration in a series of 102 primary panNETs studied with WGS, such as *MEN-1, DAXX/ATRX, mTOR*, and DNA damage repair [12]. Particularly, the authors described a new mutational mechanism involving *MUTYH* inactivation, new *mTOR* pathway mechanisms *DEPDC5* inactivation, and *EWSR1* fusion events. Interestingly, germline mutations in *MUTYH* and *BRCA2* were detected in this series of sporadic panNETs [12].

11.4 Classification

There are several recognized functional syndromes related to panNETs (Table 11.1).

Table 11.1 Clinical syndromes and secreted substances associated with panNETs

panNET	Name of the syndrome	Hormone/substance
Insulinoma	Hypoglycemia	Insulin
Gastrinoma	Zollinger–Ellison	Gastrin
VIPoma	Verner–Morrison	Vasoactive intestinal peptide (VIP)
Glucagonoma	Hyperglycemia	Glucagon
Somatostatinoma		Somatostatin (SS)
PPoma		Pancreatic polypeptide (PP)
GRFoma		Growth hormone-releasing factor (GHRH)
ACTHoma	Ectopic Cushing	Adrenocorticotropic hormone (ACTH)
PanNET with hypercalcemia	PTHrPoma	Parathormone-related protein (PTHrP)
Pancreatic carcinoids	Carcinoid syndrome	Serotonin

Functioning panNETs are sporadic in the vast majority of cases as it is for NF-panNETs. Multiple endocrine neoplasia (MEN)-1, Von Hippel Lindau (VHL), tuberous sclerosis complex (TSC), and neurofibromatosis (NF)-1 represent the main known familial syndrome associated with panNETs [13].

The histological classification of F-panNETs is similar to that of the NF-panNETs, that is the WHO 2019 [14]. Four categories were recognized, including panNET G1, panNET G2, panNET G3, and panNEC based on Ki-67/mitotic index and tumor morphology. The F-panNETs are usually G1-G2, which is low/intermediate rather than high-grade neoplasms.

11.5 Prognosis

Survival related to panNETs as a whole has been reported to be improved more than other NETs over the last decades, particularly for distant metastasis stage [6].

Specific prognostic information for F-panNETs is lacking. However, in the past, functioning NETs, including F-panNETs, were associated with high morbidity and mortality due to the lack of specific treatments. The positive turning point was represented by the introduction of somatostatin analogs (SSAs) in clinical practice [15, 16]. Of course, this is just related to the prognostic role of the syndrome; however, whether or not F-panNETs have a different prognosis compared with NF-panNETs also due to a different tumor growth or tumor response to the same therapies is not clear.

11.6 Treatment

The treatment goals of a F-panNET are the syndrome control ± tumor growth control.

In accordance with the European Neuroendocrine Tumor Society (ENETS) [7] and European Society of Medical Oncology (ESMO) [17], surgical resection is recommended for all patients with a localized or locally advanced radically resectable sporadic F-panNET. For all localized F-PanNETs, gastrinoma surgery should be considered [9].

Primary tumor resection in the presence of unresectable liver metastases from a panNET may be beneficial in selected cases, including patients with F-panNET for syndrome control [18]. On the other hand, liver metastases resection ± ablation has been reported to be successful for syndrome control and potential better survival in patients with F-panNET [19]. Liver-directed treatment, such as trans-arterial embolization (TAE) or chemoembolization (TACE), radioembolization (TARE), can be considered to the same goal [8].

For gastrinoma patients, the critical therapy is represented by proton pump inhibitors (PPIs), which showed to be highly effective to control the secretory syndrome related to excessive gastrin secretion [20].

Diazoxide is a drug used for hypoglycemia from insulinoma, as it suppresses insulin secretion from insulinoma cells via ATP-sensitive potassium channels. Its schedule has to be often adapted due to its several side effects [21]. Treatment of hypoglycemia with an SSA can be challenging in patients with insulinoma as the SSA can worsen hypoglycemia. This can happen especially in patients without SSTR-2 expression, which is quite common in insulinoma. However, patients with malignant metastatic insulinoma often have a positive ^{68}GaPET/CT-DOTA-peptide or somatostatin receptor scintigraphy (SRS), and they can also benefit from peptide receptor radionuclide therapy (PRRT) [22]. Everolimus can be a good option to treat patients with insulinoma as it can control both the tumor growth and hypoglycemia [17]. Somatostatin analogs are also recommended in other F-panNETs, such as VIPoma and glucagonoma [17].

Over the last years, the treatment field carcinoid syndrome has evolved dramatically and ENETs have recently issued guidelines for the management of this clinical syndrome that may also compromise significantly patient's quality of life [23, 24].

11.7 Conclusion

Although much rarer that NF, the F-panNETs represent a challenging entity in clinical practice and research. First of all, it should be taken in mind that the clinical syndrome represents the real clinical priority for prognosis. Thus, the best treatment for syndrome control should be promptly applied. To some extent, F-panNETs are managed similarly to NF-panNETs. For instance, the approved anticancer systemic therapies are the same. With regard to the locoregional treatments, surgical and nonsurgical, the presence of the syndrome represents a specific indication to proceed compared with NF-panNETs.

References

1. Boyar Cetinkaya R, Aagnes B, Thiis-Evensen E, Tretli S, Bergestuen DS, Hansen S (2017) Trends in incidence of neuroendocrine neoplasms in Norway: a report of 16,075 cases from 1993 through 2010. Neuroendocrinology 104:1–10
2. Gastrointestinal Pathology Study Group of Korean Society of, P, Cho MY, Kim JM, Sohn JH, Kim MJ, Kim KM, Kim WH, Kim H, Kook MC, Park DY, Lee JH, Chang H, Jung ES, Kim HK, Jin SY, Choi JH, Gu MJ, Kim S, Kang MS, Cho CH, Park MI, Kang YK, Kim YW, Yoon SO, Bae HI, Joo M, Moon WS, Kang DY, Chang SJ (2012) Current trends of the incidence and pathological diagnosis of gastroenteropancreatic neuroendocrine tumors (GEP-NETs) in Korea 2000-2009: multicenter study. Cancer Res Treat 44:157–165
3. Ito T, Igarashi H, Nakamura K, Sasano H, Okusaka T, Takano K, Komoto I, Tanaka M, Imamura M, Jensen RT, Takayanagi R, Shimatsu A (2015) Epidemiological trends of pancreatic and gastrointestinal neuroendocrine tumors in Japan: a nationwide survey analysis. J Gastroenterol 50:58–64
4. Tsai HJ, Wu CC, Tsai CR, Lin SF, Chen LT, Chang JS (2013) The epidemiology of neuroendocrine tumors in Taiwan: a nation-wide cancer registry-based study. PLoS One 8:e62487

5. Yao JC, Hassan M, Phan A, Dagohoy C, Leary C, Mares JE, Abdalla EK, Fleming JB, Vauthey JN, Rashid A, Evans DB (2008) One hundred years after "carcinoid": epidemiology of and prognostic factors for neuroendocrine tumors in 35,825 cases in the United States. J Clin Oncol 26:3063–3072
6. Dasari A, Shen C, Halperin D, Zhao B, Zhou S, Xu Y, Shih T, Yao JC (2017) Trends in the incidence, prevalence, and survival outcomes in patients with neuroendocrine tumors in the United States. JAMA Oncol 3:1335–1342
7. Falconi M, Eriksson B, Kaltsas G, Bartsch DK, Capdevila J, Caplin M, Kos-Kudla B, Kwekkeboom D, Rindi G, Kloppel G, Reed N, Kianmanesh R, Jensen RT, p. Vienna Consensus Conference (2016) ENETS consensus guidelines update for the management of patients with functional pancreatic neuroendocrine tumors and non-functional pancreatic neuroendocrine tumors. Neuroendocrinology 103:153–171
8. Oberg K (2018) Management of functional neuroendocrine tumors of the pancreas. Gland Surg 7:20–27
9. Jensen RT, Bodei L, Capdevila J et al (2019) Unmet needs in functional and non functional pancreatic neoplasms. Neuroendocrinology 108:26–36
10. Soga J (2005) Carcinoids of the pancreas: an analysis of 156 cases Cancer 104(6):1180–7. https://doi.org/10.1002/cncr.21291
11. Raj N, Shah R, Stadler Z, Mukherjee S, Chou J, Untch B, Li J, Kelly V, Saltz LB, Mandelker D, Ladanyi M, Berger MF, Klimstra DS, Reidy-Lagunes D, Osoba M (2018) Real-time genomic characterization of metastatic pancreatic neuroendocrine tumors has prognostic implications and identifies potential germline actionability. JCO Precis Oncol 2018:PO.17.00267. https://doi.org/10.1200/PO.17.00267. Epub 2018 Apr 19
12. Scarpa A, Chang DK, Nones K, Corbo V, Patch AM, Bailey P, Lawlor RT, Johns AL, Miller DK, Mafficini A, Rusev B, Scardoni M, Antonello D, Barbi S, Sikora KO, Cingarlini S, Vicentini C, McKay S, Quinn MC, Bruxner TJ, Christ AN, Harliwong I, Idrisoglu S, McLean S, Nourse C, Nourbakhsh E, Wilson PJ, Anderson MJ, Fink JL, Newell F, Waddell N, Holmes O, Kazakoff SH, Leonard C, Wood S, Xu Q, Nagaraj SH, Amato E, Dalai I, Bersani S, Cataldo I, Dei Tos AP, Capelli P, Davi MV, Landoni L, Malpaga A, Miotto M, Whitehall VL, Leggett BA, Harris JL, Harris J, Jones MD, Humphris J, Chantrill LA, Chin V, Nagrial AM, Pajic M, Scarlett CJ, Pinho A, Rooman I, Toon C, Wu J, Pinese M, Cowley M, Barbour A, Mawson A, Humphrey ES, Colvin EK, Chou A, Lovell JA, Jamieson NB, Duthie F, Gingras MC, Fisher WE, Dagg RA, Lau LM, Lee M, Pickett HA, Reddel RR, Samra JS, Kench JG, Merrett ND, Epari K, Nguyen NQ, Zeps N, Falconi M, Simbolo M, Butturini G, Van Buren G, Partelli S, Fassan M, I. Australian Pancreatic Cancer Genome, Khanna KK, Gill AJ, Wheeler DA, Gibbs RA, Musgrove EA, Bassi C, Tortora G, Pederzoli P et al (2017) Whole-genome landscape of pancreatic neuroendocrine tumours. Nature 543:65–71
13. Metz DC, Jensen RT (2008) Gastrointestinal neuroendocrine tumors: pancreatic endocrine tumors. Gastroenterology 135:1469–1492
14. Nagtegaal ID, Odze RD, Klimstra D, Paradis V, Rugge M, Schirmacher P, Washington KM, Carneiro F, Cree IA, W. H. O. C. o. T. E. Board (2020) The 2019 WHO classification of tumours of the digestive system. Histopathology 76:182–188
15. Kvols LK, Martin JK, Marsh HM, Moertel CG (1985) Rapid reversal of carcinoid crisis with a somatostatin analogue. N Engl J Med 313:1229–1230
16. Modlin IM, Pavel M, Kidd M, Gustafsson BI (2010) Review article: somatostatin analogues in the treatment of gastroenteropancreatic neuroendocrine (carcinoid) tumours. Aliment Pharmacol Ther 31:169–188
17. Pavel M, Oberg K, Falconi M, Krenning E, Sundin A, Perren A, Berruti A, E. G. Committee (2020) Gastroenteropancreatic neuroendocrine neoplasms: ESMO clinical practice guidelines for diagnosis, treatment and follow-up. Ann Oncol 31(7):844–860. https://doi.org/10.1016/j.annonc.2020.03.304. Epub 2020 Apr 6
18. Andreasi V, Muffatti F, Guarneri G, Falconi M, Partelli S (2020) Surgical principles in the management of pancreatic neuroendocrine neoplasms. Curr Treat Options in Oncol 21:48

19. Mayo SC, Herman JM, Cosgrove D, Bhagat N, Kamel I, Geschwind JF, Pawlik TM (2013) Emerging approaches in the management of patients with neuroendocrine liver metastasis: role of liver-directed and systemic therapies. J Am Coll Surg 216:123–134
20. Ito T, Igarashi H, Uehara H, Jensen RT (2013) Pharmacotherapy of Zollinger-Ellison syndrome. Expert Opin Pharmacother 14:307–321
21. Dimitriadis GK, Weickert MO, Randeva HS, Kaltsas G, Grossman A (2016) Medical management of secretory syndromes related to gastroenteropancreatic neuroendocrine tumours. Endocr Relat Cancer 23:R423–RR36
22. Veltroni A, Cosaro E, Spada F, Fazio N, Faggiano A, Colao A, Pusceddu S, Zatelli MC, Campana D, Piovesan A, Pia A, Grossrubatscher EM, Filice A, Bianchi A, Razzore P, Toaiari M, Cingarlini S, Landoni L, Micciolo R, Davi MV (2020) Clinico-pathological features, treatments and survival of malignant insulinomas: a multicenter study. Eur J Endocrinol 182:439–446
23. Grozinsky-Glasberg S, Davar J, Hofland J, Dobson R, Prasad V, Pascher A, Denecke T, Tesselaar MET, Panzuto F, Albage A, Connolly HM, Obadia JF, Riechelmann R, Toumpanakis C (2022) European Neuroendocrine Tumor Society (ENETS) 2022 guidance paper for carcinoid syndrome and carcinoid heart disease. J Neuroendocrinol 34:e13146
24. Koumarianou A, Daskalakis K, Tsoli M, Kaltsas G, Pavel M (2022) Efficacy, safety and unmet needs of evolving medical treatments for carcinoid syndrome. J Neuroendocrinol 34:e13174

Insulinoma

12

Kira Oleinikov, David J. Gross, Harold Jacob, Haggi Mazeh, and Simona Grozinsky-Glasberg

12.1 Introduction

Insulinoma, the most common functioning pancreatic neuroendocrine tumor (pNET), represents a rare neoplasm that originates from pancreatic beta cells, with an incidence of about 1–3 per million per year [1–3]. The median age of the patient at the time of diagnosis is 50 years (range: 17–86 years), with a slightly higher female preponderance [3].

Insulinomas are usually smaller than 2 cm in diameter (84%) and mostly (90%) are solitary lesions that are located in the pancreas in an equal distribution between the pancreatic head, body, and tail [4]. The majority (>90%) of insulinomas are sporadic and non-metastatic at presentation and therefore can be surgically cured [5]. In about 5–10% of patients, the insulinoma is part of the Multiple Endocrine Neoplasia type 1 (MEN-1) syndrome: these patients often present with one or more insulinomas as well as with other functioning or nonfunctioning neuroendocrine tumors [6]. Finally, a rare condition is malignant insulinoma, which is also found in less than 10% of insulinoma patients [2].

K. Oleinikov · D. J. Gross · S. Grozinsky-Glasberg (✉)
Neuroendocrine Tumor Unit, ENETS Center of Excellence, Hadassah-Hebrew University Medical Center, Jerusalem, Israel

Division of Medicine, Hadassah-Hebrew University Medical Center, Jerusalem, Israel
e-mail: simonag@hadassah.org.il

H. Jacob
Division of Medicine, Hadassah-Hebrew University Medical Center, Jerusalem, Israel

Department of Gastroenterology, Hadassah-Hebrew University Medical Center, Jerusalem, Israel

H. Mazeh
Division of Medicine, Hadassah-Hebrew University Medical Center, Jerusalem, Israel

Department of Surgery, Hadassah-Hebrew University Medical Center, Jerusalem, Israel

S. Yalcin, K. Öberg (eds.), *Neuroendocrine Tumours*,
https://doi.org/10.1007/978-3-031-56968-5_12

The aim of this review is to summarize the existing literature on insulinoma with regard to diagnosis (clinical, biochemical, and localization methods), therapy (surgery, ablative techniques, and medical therapies), and long-term medical strategies in patients with disseminated or inoperable disease.

12.2 Clinical and Laboratory Manifestations of Insulinomas (Endogenous Hyperinsulinism-Related Hypoglycemia)

12.2.1 Clinical Manifestations

The clinical symptoms of insulinomas are heterogeneous and related to hyperinsulinemic–hypoglycemia. Hypoglycemia results in autonomic and neuroglycopenic symptoms [7, 8].

Autonomic symptoms comprise *adrenergic symptoms*, such as palpitations and tremor, and *cholinergic symptoms*, with sweating, hunger, and/or paresthesias [9]. These clinical features are the consequence of sympathetic, parasympathetic, and sympatho-adrenal systems activation—a counter-regulatory response to the falling blood sugar. Hypoglycemia provokes secretion of glucagon, epinephrine, norepinephrine, pancreatic polypeptide, cortisol, and growth hormone. Critical role in detection of incipient hypoglycemia plays glucose-sensing neurons located in ventromedial hypothalamus [10]. However, with recurrent and prolonged hypoglycemic episodes, an adaptation of adrenergic system can appear, which results in lower glycemic threshold for activation of autonomic response. This phenomenon known as "hypoglycemia-associated autonomic failure," has been described in patients with insulinomas and may cause misattribution of symptoms to neurological or psychiatric disorders when patients present with vague neuroglycopenic symptoms only [11–13].

Neuroglycopenic symptoms comprise severe weakness as well as a wide variety of psychiatric and neurological manifestations, most commonly behavioral changes, confusion, agitation or slow reaction patterns, blurred vision, seizures, transient loss of consciousness, or hypoglycemic coma [14]. Hypoglycemic coma is usually sudden, preceded by agitation, hypothermia, and sometimes pyramidal signs; it may be profound and prolonged, leading occasionally to brain death. The combination of autonomic and neuroglycopenic symptoms strongly suggests the diagnosis of hypoglycemia [8]. As autonomic symptoms may often be lacking, it is important to remember that neuroglycopenic symptoms are more specific of insulinoma-related hypoglycemia. Therefore, measurement of plasma glucose concentrations should be recommended in all patients with such symptoms. Hypoglycemic spells typically occur after a period of fasting, several hours after the last meal, or after physical exercise. However, sometimes hypoglycemia may occur within hours following a meal, or even without any relationship with meal time. As a result of the variable relationship between meals and hypoglycemia, it is important to remember that symptoms occurring in non-fasting patients do not exclude the diagnosis of insulinoma. In a series of 214 insulinoma patients, symptoms of hypoglycemia were reported exclusively in the fasting state in 73%, postprandial state alone in 6%, and both fasting and postprandial state in 21% [3]. Weight gain is also reported in 25% of patients.

In rare pregnant patients with insulinoma, symptoms may mimic those of emesis in early pregnancy, may disappear in late pregnancy as a consequence of insulin resistance, and then return after delivery [15, 16].

Because insulinoma symptoms are not specific and can mimic other pathological conditions, a broad differential diagnosis should be considered. Excluding the diagnosis of noninsulinoma pancreatogenous hypoglycemia (NIPHS), use of oral hypoglycemic agents and presence of circulating insulin antibodies, are of major importance [17–19].

12.2.2 Laboratory/Biochemical Diagnosis of Insulinomas

12.2.2.1 Whipple's Triad

The combination of symptoms of hypoglycemia, documented low plasma glucose level, and symptomatic relief with administration of glucose (known as **Whipple's triad**) is fundamental for the diagnosis of insulinoma.

12.2.2.2 Plasma Glucose and Insulin Concentrations

Glucose

The lack of diagnostic specificity of the clinical symptoms in patients with insulinomas requires evidence of low plasma glucose concentration, ideally during clinical symptoms, and must be performed in venous blood samples with a reliable laboratory method.

The threshold to define hypoglycemia is controversial: according to expert recommendations, a 0.55 g/L threshold is a must. However, the glycemic threshold that can cause clinical symptoms is highly variable among individuals, and a plasma concentration of glucose <0.7 g/L at the time of clinical symptoms is considered sufficient to warrant further investigation [19]. Since even values below 0.55 g/L can be found in some healthy individuals, it is also recommended by the expert consensus that such levels justify further evaluation only in patients who had presented with Whipple's triad. On the other hand, an extremely rare insulinoma patient may be asymptomatic and not fulfill Whipple's triad [20]. Furthermore, in many insulinoma patients, the clinical symptoms may appear only at very low glucose levels, so that these patients may be asymptomatic at the time of plasma glucose concentrations below 0.45 g/L.

Insulin

The evidence for inappropriate insulin secretion at the time of hypoglycemia is mandatory for the diagnosis of insulinoma. The criteria include requirement for non-suppressed levels of endogenous hormone; serum insulin concentration is ≥3 mIU/L, serum C-peptide concentration is ≥0.6 ng/mL, and serum proinsulin concentration is ≥5 pmol/L, at the time of venous plasma glucose concentrations <0.55 g/L [21].

An important prerequisite for a valid diagnosis of insulinoma is a careful processing of the blood samples for insulin in order to obtain reliable biochemical data for evaluation. Identical serum and plasma samples measured in different laboratories may produce widely disparate insulin values, unacceptable for comparison [22]. Assay characteristics such as linearity, recovery, accuracy, and cross-reactivity to proinsulin vary among the laboratories; therefore, a rigorous quality control and ongoing quality improvement are mandatory to maintain reliability of the insulin measurement [23].

Though the 3 mIU/L threshold was established for insulin-specific assays, it is known now that the finding of low insulin levels with such assays cannot rule out the diagnosis of insulinoma [24].

12.2.2.3 Other Markers

C-Peptide, Proinsulin and Beta-Hydroxybutyrate

C-peptide and proinsulin levels at the time of hypoglycemia have better diagnostic accuracy than insulin levels. A serum C-peptide level of ≥0.6 ng/mL with a concomitant plasma glucose of ≤0.55 g/L is required criteria for defining endogenous hyperinsulinism hypoglycemia [19, 23].

Another valuable tool for the diagnosis of insulinoma is measurement of fasting plasma beta-hydroxybutyrate levels. As insulin suppresses ketogenesis, a progressive rise in beta-hydroxybutyrate of >2.7 mmol/L may augment in excluding the diagnosis of insulinoma when blood glucose levels were 0.50–0.60 g/L during a 72-h fast [19].

Most of the insulin metabolism takes place in the liver and in the kidney. The kidney also removes 70% of C-peptide by renal filtration. So, measuring insulin and C-peptide levels in patients with severe renal insufficiency is not helpful. In these patients, it has been recommended to use beta-hydroxybutyrate levels and glucose response to glucagon at the end of a fast test to provide evidence for insulin-related hypoglycemia [25].

12.2.2.4 The Prolonged (72 h) Fast

One of the most robust standard tests used for establishing a biochemical diagnosis of insulinoma is the prolonged (72 h) fast, which is recommended if a venous sample cannot be collected when hypoglycemia occurs spontaneously. There is a detailed protocol for the fast test [17, 19]. Currently, it is recommended that a prolonged, supervised fast be performed in the hospital setting, for at least 48 h if not for 72 h. The absence of hypoglycemia after a 72-h fast should exclude the diagnosis. However, although the sensitivity of the 72-h fast is high and the test plays an important role in the diagnosis of an insulinoma, a "normal" test result should be interpreted in light of clinical symptoms [20]. The patient is allowed to drink calorie-free beverages, blood samples are collected every 6 h until the plasma glucose concentration is less than 0.6 g/L if the patient remains asymptomatic, then the frequency of sampling is increased to every 1–2 h. Serum insulin, C-peptide, proinsulin, and beta-hydroxybutyrate are measured in all the samples taken at the same time when plasma glucose concentration drops below 0.6 g/L. It is recommended that at the end of the fast test, a sample should be collected to measure oral hypoglycemic agents. Insulin antibodies should also be measured. The fast test can be stopped: (1) when Whipple's triad is observed; (2) when plasma glucose concentrations drop below 0.55 g/L in a patient who had previously experienced Whipple's triad; and (3) if plasma beta-hydroxybutyrate levels rise above 2.7 mmol/L. In most insulinoma patients, plasma glucose concentrations below 0.45 g/L are usually reached within the first 48 h of the test, though the 72 h-fast test was reported to be necessary to provide a clear diagnostic conclusion in a few patients [17, 19].

12.2.2.5 Glucagon Test

The glucagon test may be used to better clarify the etiology and distinguish between insulin-mediated and IGF-2-mediated hypoglycemia. In insulin-related hypoglycemia, hepatic glucose production is increased with sufficient reserve of hepatic glycogen stores, even after the prolonged fasting [26, 27].

An increase in plasma glucose of at least 0.25 g/L after intravenous glucagon suggests insulin-induced hypoglycemia. The test should be performed at the end of a prolonged fast test: at the time of symptomatic hypoglycemia with concomitant fall of plasma glucose to $\leq$0.45 g/L, or after 72 h of fast and measuring plasma glucose at 10 min-intervals for 30 min showing higher glucose in insulinomas [8, 19].

In summary, clinical and laboratory diagnosis of insulinoma patients, as recommended also by European Neuroendocrine Tumor Society (ENETS) guidelines, can be established using the following six strict criteria: a documented blood glucose levels $\leq$40 mg/dL; a concomitant insulin levels $\geq$6 U/L ($\geq$ 36 pmol/L; $\geq$ 3 U/L by ICMA); C-peptide levels $\geq$200 pmol/L; proinsulin levels $\geq$5 pmol/L; hydroxybutyrate levels $\leq$2.7 mmol/L; and absence of sulfonylurea (metabolites) in the plasma and/or urine [28].

12.3 Differential Diagnosis of Insulinoma (Table 12.1)

12.3.1 Reactive "Functional Hypoglycemia"

Reactive "functional hypoglycemia" is a controversial entity, and it is now known that many organic disorders may result both in fasting and reactive hypoglycemia. Many patients present with dizziness or other minor autonomic symptoms within the hours following a meal, but most do not meet the criteria for hypoglycemia or for Whipple's triad. Rarely, insulinoma can present as reactive hypoglycemia [26, 29, 30].

Table 12.1 Differential diagnosis of endogeneous hyperinsulinemic hypoglycemia

Congenital
Transient neonatal hyperinsulinism
Focal hyperinsulinism (K_{ATP} channel disorders)
• Paternal SUR1 mutation with clonal loss of heterozygosity of 11p15
• Paternal Kir6.2 mutation with clonal loss of heterozygosity of 11p15
Diffuse hyperinsulinism
• K_{ATP} channel disorders (SUR1 and Kir6.2 mutations)
• Glucokinase gain-of –function mutations
• Hyperammonemic hyperinsulinism
• Short chain acyl coenzyme A dehydrogenase deficiency
• Carbohydrate-deficient glycoprotein syndrome (Jaeken disease)
• Beckwith-Wiedemann syndrome
Acquired
Postprandial hyperinsulinemic hypoglycemia
• Dumping syndrome
• Post-gastric bypass surgery
• Insulin autoimmune syndrome
Insulinoma
• Sporadic
• Multiple endocrine neoplasia type 1
Adult nesidioblastosis
Drugs (quinine etc.*)*
Factitious use of oral anti-hyperglycemic drugs (sulfonylurea etc.*)*
Adrenal insufficiency

12.3.2 Hyperinsulinemic Hypoglycemia

12.3.2.1 Drug-Induced Hypoglycemia

The first step in the evaluation of hypoglycemia is to check if the patient is treated with medications that can cause hypoglycemia. There are a large variety of drugs implicated in hypoglycemia (e.g., aspirin, pentamidine, quinine, disopyramide, etc.) [31, 32].

12.3.2.2 Hypoglycemia Related to Insulin and Insulin Analogues (High Insulin Levels with Low C-Peptide and Proinsulin Levels, Exogenous Hyperinsulinism)

The finding of high insulin levels with concomitant low C-peptide and proinsulin levels is almost specific of the diagnosis of surreptitious insulin injections [19]. Importantly, insulin assays that can identify the presence of insulin analogues are to be preferred [33, 34].

12.3.2.3 Factitious Hypoglycemia Related to Sulfonylureas or Glinides (High Insulin, C-Peptide, and Proinsulin Levels)

At the time of symptomatic hypoglycemia, in order to distinguish factitious (or accidental) hypoglycemia from the endogenous abnormal insulin secretion (observed in patients with insulinomas and nesidioblastosis), it is mandatory to collect a plasma sample to measure oral hypoglycemic agents (sulfonylureas and glinides). This diagnosis is difficult and usually suspected in patients whose relatives are diabetic or health or professionals [35].

12.3.2.4 Idiopathic Noninsulinoma Pancreatogenous Hypoglycemia Syndrome (Endogenous Hyperinsulinism)

The noninsulinoma pancreatogenous hypoglycemia syndrome (NIPHS) identifies a group of hyperinsulinemic hypoglycemic patients with unique clinical, diagnostic, surgical, and pathologic features. These patients experience predominantly postprandial hypoglycemia and have nesidioblastosis with islet cell hypertrophy, findings different from those in patients with insulinomas [36, 37].

12.4 The Histopathological Diagnosis of Insulinomas

According to the latest 2017 WHO criteria, pancreatic neuroendocrine neoplasms classified as well-differentiated tumors, called pancreatic neuroendocrine tumors (pNETs), and poorly differentiated neoplasms, called small or large cell pancreatic neuroendocrine carcinomas (pNECs). The well-differentiated pancreatic NETs are graded into low-grade (G1, Ki-67 index <3%), intermediate-grade (G2, Ki-67 index 3–20%), and high grade (G3, Ki-67 > 20%) categories according to proliferative rate. While the term pancreatic neuroendocrine carcinoma (NEC) is reserved for highly proliferative tumors with poorly differentiated morphology [38]. This morphology-based division of Grade 3 neoplasms reflects heterogeneity of this group in terms of prognosis and probably treatment [39]. Most insulinomas are well-differentiated endocrine tumors, WHO Grade 1; however, occasionally they belong to higher grade groups.

For the appropriate histological diagnosis of insulinoma, a detailed macroscopic and microscopic description, an immunohistochemical staining for neuroendocrine tumor markers (chromogranin A and synaptophysin), as well as for insulin, proinsulin and amyloid, are all recommended. However, the immunohistochemical determination of insulin expression by tumor cells does not appear to be an absolute need for diagnosis, as some insulinomas do not stain positively for insulin due to a rapid release of insulin from the insulin-producing cells. Evaluation of the mitotic index and Ki67 index is required to define the grade of the tumor and the related patient prognosis and treatment approach [38].

In 5–10%, insulinomas may be malignant [1–3]. Whereas the clinical and biological diagnostic criteria of insulinoma do not differ from those of benign insulinomas, the histological diagnosis of malignancy is difficult and actually the only definite criteria for malignancy are the presence of invasive and/or metastatic disease. However, in clinical practice, a malignant insulinoma is generally described as a single large tumor, and in most cases, there are synchronous metastases, generally located in lymph nodes or in the liver. Suspicion of aggressive tumor behavior, apart from metastases, includes invasion of adjacent organs, a tumor size >2 cm, angioinvasion, and high proliferative activity [3, 40–42].

Rarely, metastatic nonfunctioning pancreatic NETs may change their biological behavior in parallel with tumor progression, with insulinoma transformation, together with a clinical picture of endogenous hyperinsulinemic hypoglycemia [43].

12.5 The Role of Imaging and Nuclear Medicine in the Diagnosis of Insulinomas (Table 12.2)

As a rule, imaging should be performed only after the biochemical diagnosis of insulinoma has been established. The role of imaging is to detect the anatomical localization and to stage the tumor prior to surgery or other intervention [28]. Multimodality approach may be necessary to identify characteristically small (most being ≤2 cm at presentation) and therefore extremely difficult to localize radiologically [44].

Two different modes of the localizing techniques are performed: preoperative and/or intraoperative. Further, the preoperative localization can be divided into noninvasive and invasive. The noninvasive studies include 3-phase computed tomography (CT), gadolinium-enhanced dynamic magnetic resonance imaging (MRI), and functional imaging including radiolabeled analogues such as somatostatin receptor (SSTR), glucagon-like peptide1 receptor (GLP-1R), etc.

If noninvasive methods fail to localize the tumor, invasive studies are applied such as endoscopic ultrasound (EUS) and selective intra-arterial injection of calcium with hepatic venous insulin gradients (IACIG). The IACIG may serve as a complementary technique in specific situations, such as tumor localization in

Table 12.2 Summary of the literature regarding detection rates of insulinomas by diagnostic modality

Localization modality	Mean detection rate %, (range)	Patients (*n*)	Studies (*n*)	References
Non-Invasive				
CT	83 (63–96)	317	5	[47–50]
MRI	87 (72–100)	144	4	[50–53]
SSTR PET/CT	52 (22–90)	64	4	[74, 75, 77, 78]
GLP-1R PET/CT[1]	96 (94–98)	95	2	[80, 81]
Invasive				
EUS	86 (57–100)	250	12	[54–65]
IOUS	92 (84–100)	264	9	[61, 66–73]
IACIG	87 (84–93)	107	4	[74, 83–85]

[1]Data exclude series with malignant insulinomas

patients with MEN1 who frequently have multiple pancreatic tumors, not all being insulinomas [45].

Intraoperative or endoscopic ultrasound examination of the pancreas is thought to be the best methods to detect insulinomas [44]. The glucagon-like peptide-1 receptor (GLP-1R) PET/CT, though not widely available, shows promising data and may emerge as the most sensitive noninvasive diagnostic modality in the near future [46].

Intraoperatively ultrasound tumor localization remains mandatory, but to date careful pre-operative radiological examination must be performed in an attempt to localize the tumor before surgery and to avoid reoperations [44]. Unfortunately, there is a wide discrepancy in the use of localization techniques between different centers, as a result of the specialist expertise and the availability of imaging equipment (Table 12.2).

12.5.1 Computed Tomography (CT)

High definition multidetector helical 3-phase CT-scan is the first examination recommended to be performed to localize insulinomas. A multiphasic CT exam is mandatory, as sensitivities of lesion detection may vary by phase: most small insulinomas are isodense with the pancreas on pre-contrast images and tend to be best visualized as sharply delineated, evenly contrast—enhanced on arterial phase, but occasionally are more easily detected on portal venous phase images. In rare cases, the tumors are hypodense to the pancreas after injection of contrast medium and may have nodular calcification or cystic compartments. Detection rate is optimized by evaluation of all phases. Exceptionally rare, ectopic insulinomas are located in the proximity of the pancreas or of the liver. CT also stages the disease in case of regional lymph node involvement and presence of distant metastases. Liver metastases tend to be hypervascular; therefore, the arterial phase better identifies the number and size of liver metastases. A meticulous CT exam technique is mandatory, and mean detection rate shown in studies is 83% (range 63–96) [47–51].

12.5.2 Magnetic Resonance Imaging (MRI)

MRI is superior to CT for the detection of small insulinoma, by including multiple sequences; it offers more opportunities to detect tumor within normal pancreatic tissue. The enhancement pattern of insulinomas on MRI is related to the degree of their vascularity which correlates with malignant potential; usually, indolent insulinomas are hypervascular. On fat-suppressed T1-weighted images, they depicted as low in signal intensity and moderately high in signal intensity on fat-suppressed T2-weighted images [47–50]. Magnetic resonance cholangiopancreatography (MRCP) is advantageous to optimally evaluate the relation of the tumor to the pancreatic and the main bile ducts.

With reported mean detection rate of 87% (range 72–100), the benefit is the absence of ionizing radiation, that of particular importance in younger patients who may require surveillance [50–53].

12.5.3 Ultrasound

The ultrasound modalities are highly operator-dependent technique leading to wide variation in terms of sensitivity, specificity, and detection rate.

Trans-abdominal ultrasound examination is considered to be of low sensitivity with a mean detection of 39% for pancreatic neuroendocrine tumors like insulinomas.

Endoscopic ultrasound (EUS) is currently considered the best preoperative procedure to localize insulinomas with a reported mean detection rate of 86% (range 57–100), mainly for lesions located in the head and body of the pancreas, and less for the lesion in the tail [54–65]. These tumors usually appear as hypoechoic and hypervascular lesions.

Even if recent CT-scan techniques lead to localization of most insulinomas, EUS permits a better evaluation of the lesions (especially if they are multiple), their proximity to vital structures (pancreatic duct, splenic vessels) enables the operator to take biopsies and combined with CT imaging increases detection sensitivity up to 100% [49]. Furthermore, the contrast-enhanced harmonic technology combined with EUS allows real-time perfusion imaging without Doppler-related artifacts and has improved the diagnostic yield of EUS-guided fine needle aspiration (EUS-FNA) for a very small lesions.

Intraoperative Ultrasound (IOUS) is mandatory during surgery. IOUS is also highly useful in defining the relationship of the tumor to the adjacent pancreatic and bile ducts, and blood vessels. Moreover, it is exquisite in patients in whom multiple lesions are suspected, e.g., in Multiple Endocrine Neoplasia type 1 (MEN1) syndrome patients. In experienced hands, IOUS was reported to identify insulinomas with a mean rate of 92% (range 84–100) [61, 66–73].

Despite the high sensitivity of IOUS, detailed preoperative imaging studies are necessary in order to carefully plan the procedure of choice. Such planning may increase the success rate of laparoscopic surgery as well as minimize the risk of re-operation.

12.5.4 Functional Imaging

Oftentimes challenging insulinoma localization with conventional anatomic imaging was substantially augmented with the introduction of somatostatin receptor imaging (SRI) that had implications not only for diagnosis but also for understanding tumor biology and for treatment planning.

Particularly with small tumors, such as most insulinomas, the value of SRI increased with better spatial resolution, evolving from basic planar scintigraphy with adequate accuracy only for tumors of several centimeters toward PET/CT technology that enables to identify sub-centimeter lesions. Currently, three traces are widely used with varying somatostatin receptor (SSTR) subtype specificity: ^{68}Ga-DOTATATE, ^{68}Ga-DOTATOC, and ^{68}Ga-DOTANOC, with highest affinity for $SSTR_2$, $SSTR_5$, and $SSTR_{3/5}$, respectively. Several small retrospective series demonstrated successful insulinoma localization with SSTR PET/CT imaging with mean detection rate 52% (range 22–90), including syndromic forms and metastatic disease [74–78].

Arguably, the most substantial progress in molecular imaging of insulinomas has emerged from in vitro autoradiography study assessing the expression of various peptide receptors in 27 insulinoma tissue samples [79]. Among the tested peptide receptors in insulinoma tumors, glucagon-like peptide-1 receptor (GLP-1R) had the highest density in 93% of tissue samples, compared to less densely expressed $SSTR_2$ with incidence of 69%. Exenedin-4 is a long acting GLP-1 analog which has been successfully radiolabeled and is implemented in clinical practice with reported mean detection rate 96% (range 94–98) for benign insulinomas [80, 81].

A prospective cohort study demonstrated ^{68}Ga-NOTA-exendin-4 to be efficient in detecting insulinoma in 42 of 43 patients. In this study, GLP-1R PET/CT sensitivity of 97.7% was compared with CT, MRI, EUS, and SRS modalities, with reported sensitivities 73.3%, 56%, 84.6%, and 16.3%, respectively [80]. Interestingly, only a false negative result was found in a patient with Grade 2 insulinoma that was photopenic on GLP-1R PET/CT and positive on SRS modality, suggestive of notion that insulinomas may have either GLP-1R or $SSTR_2$ expression status [46]. Prospectively evaluated tracer ^{68}Ga-DOTA-exendin-4 PET/CT was compared with ^{111}In-DOTA-exendin-4 SPECT/CT, and MRI was found to be superior in terms of sensitivity and accuracy in 38 patients with histologically confirmed insulinoma [81]. Transient exacerbation of hypoglycemia is often seen after radiolabeled-exendin-4 imaging and routine glucose infusion should be considered in all patients to reduce this risk.

PET imaging of benign insulinomas with ^{18}F-fluorodeoxyglucose (^{18}F-FDG) is of less diagnostic value, presumably because of their low proliferative potential, but more relevant in setting of malignant insulinomas. Notably, in malignant insulinomas, the relative distribution of SSTR subtypes is different from benign tumors with a higher rate of scan-positivity. It has been conceptualized that the above-mentioned tracers sensitivity GLP-1R $<$ SSTR $<$ FDG may represent a spectrum of differentiation of insulinomas, from benign to higher grade disease [46].

12.5.5 Selective Angiography

The selective intra-arterial injection of calcium with hepatic venous insulin gradients (IACIGs) is based on the phenomenon that calcium stimulates the release of insulin selectively from hyperfunctional (as in case with insulinoma) but not from normal beta cells.

In this technique, stimulation is performed with selective angiography and injection of calcium gluconate into the major pancreatic arteries including gastroduodenal, proper hepatic, splenic, and superior mesenteric arteries with subsequent insulin blood sampling of the hepatic veins. A greater than two to three-fold rise in the venous insulin concentration following calcium stimulation suggests insulinoma presence in that territory. This method is used in patients with non-localized tumors by other modalities, successfully mapping the region of the tumor location with mean rate of 87% (range 84–93) [74, 82–85].

12.6 Therapy of Insulinomas

12.6.1 Surgical Therapy

As most sporadic insulinomas are small and solitary, their surgical excision is considered a treatment of choice [86]. Owing to tumor benign nature in the majority of cases, surgical resection carries a high cure rates and long-term remission can be achieved in 95% of patients [87]. Granted that pre- and intraoperative decision-making may be challenging, patients with insulinomas should be referred to high-volume endocrine surgeons.

Over the past 25 years, surgical approach for insulinomas has greatly evolved. Targeted, tissue-preserving resection became a common practice due to more effective tumor localization modalities. This focused, imaging-guided approach replaced blind distal pancreatectomy that was associated with a high failure rate (>20%) [5, 61, 88].

Most insulinomas are smaller than 20 mm (84%) and distributed almost equally in the pancreas. Therefore, often times, the most demanding and critical step for successful surgery is an accurate tumor localization.

Previously practiced open surgical approach allowed surgeons to bypass pre-operative localization and rely on intra-operative bi-digital palpation and intra-operative ultrasound (IOUS) [89, 90]. Currently recommended laparoscopic approach enables limited tactile feedback thus increasing the role of pre-operative localization [91, 92]. The mandatory practice of IOUS use in combination with pre-operative imaging increases localization accuracy to almost 100% [93]. A number of studies demonstrated that the laparoscopic approach can be safely applied with shorter recovery, hospital stay, and non-inferior cure rates when compared to open approach [94–97].

Several considerations dictate the extent of surgery. The surgeon must carefully evaluate the preoperative anatomic imaging studies and identify the tumor location, size, relation to the pancreatic duct and splenic vessels, as well as evaluate the risk for multiple lesions. In general, enucleation is the preferred approach for lesions located in the pancreatic head or neck in order to avoid the need for a Whipple's procedure. Lesions that involve or in close proximity to the pancreatic duct may not be suitable for enucleation due to the high rate of postoperative pancreatic fistula. Lesions located at the body/tail of pancreas are usually located closer to the pancreatic duct; therefore, the procedure of choice is spleen-preserving distal pancreatectomy [98].

In patients with MEN1-related insulinomas, surgical exploration should be performed. The laparoscopic approach is possible in appropriate cases after careful evaluation for the presence of multiple lesions, and tissue preserving resection is recommended in such cases [28, 99]. The utility of IOUS by an experienced endocrine surgeon cannot be underscored in these patients. Blind pancreatectomy is no longer advocated in cases where an insulinoma is not detected. In such cases, the advised approach is to stop the operation and to perform additional investigations for tumor localization [100].

Importantly, an open approach with extended resection is always the rule for insulinomas that are suspected to be malignant. Where the disease at presentation is unresectable and uncontrolled with medical therapy, debulking surgery may provide symptomatic relief [101].

12.6.1.1 Perioperative Management

Insulinoma patients with clinically significant hypoglycemia should be referred to surgery as soon as possible [102]. Generally, diazoxide pre-treatment is not recommended for benign insulinoma. Episodes of hypoglycemia can be treated with dextrose, glucagon, and potassium administration. Intravenous glucose infusion may be required shortly before the surgery. During the surgery, glucose infusion should be discontinued to allow monitoring and observation of expectant glucose level rise within minutes to an hour after insulinoma resection [5]. In the case of bulky/metastatic disease with anticipated severe hypoglycemia during the surgery, octreotide infusion may be considered. However, it should be established before the surgery whether it has a suppressive effect on insulin. Furthermore, in some patients, octreotide was shown to induce more severe hypoglycemia, caused by suppression of the counter-regulatory hormones [103].

12.6.2 Ablative Techniques (Fig. 12.1)

In recent years, there is a growing interest in new therapeutic approaches, mainly for the patients with a small localized lesion and for those who are not fit for surgery. Minimally invasive cytoreductive modalities using direct tumor ablation such as Endoscopic Ultrasound-Guided Ethanol Ablation or Endoscopic Ultrasound-Guided Radiofrequency Ablation (EUS-RFA) have been applied in patients with insulinomas [104].

Radiofrequency use causing controlled thermo-coagulative necrosis of the target lesions has been successfully implemented as a locally ablative technique for solid tumors in various organs, including the treatment of liver neuroendocrine metastases [105–107]. The application of RFA for treatment of pancreatic lesions presents with technical challenges related to anatomical constrains and properties of the pancreatic parenchyma [108–110]. As a consequence of the adoption of EUS-guided RFA, with its minimally invasive nature, accessibility to all areas of pancreas, real-time visualization of the needle probe placement and other technical advances, the

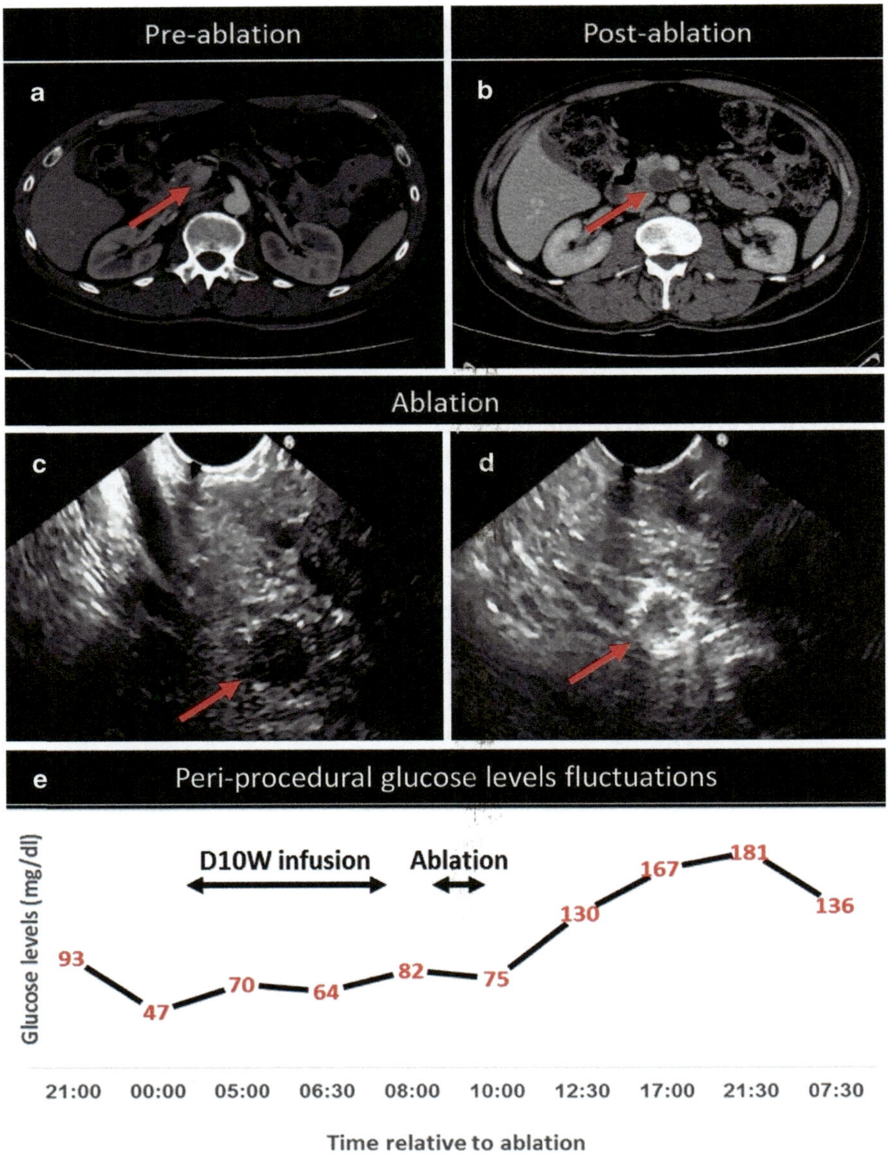

Fig. 12.1 Findings in insulinoma patient treated with EUS-RFA. (**a**) 3-phase CT examination (axial view), showing a contrast-enhanced lesion (12 mm in diameter) in the uncinate process of the pancreas (arrow); (**b**) Contrast-enhanced CT examination (axial view) 6 month after RFA. Complete ablation is reflected by the presence of a non-enhancing area at the ablation site (arrow); (**c**) Endoscopic ultrasound (EUS) examination confirming the hypoechoic tumor lesion (arrow); (**d**) EUS image of the lesion obtained during the RFA. The peripheral hyperechoic area at the ablation site reproduced the shape of the treated tumor (arrow); (**e**) Time frame of glucose level fluctuations in patient prior, during and post EUS-RFA procedure; D10W infusion = continuous 10% dextrose infusion; Ablation = EUS-RFA procedure

reported rates of complications from RFA application in the pancreas are relatively low compared to surgery [111–115].

Insulinomas may be the ideal candidates for ablation due to their indolent nature in most cases, younger age of patients, and possibility of earlier clinical detection in case of recurrence. It may be a valid first alternative to surgery, considering that in the case of failure, surgical resection can still be performed. Our experience in seven insulinoma patients with well-differentiated, small size lesions [WHO classification Grade 1; mean size 14.8 mm (range 12–19)] demonstrated successful ablation in all cases with a lasting resolution of hypoglycemic episodes at a mean follow-up of 9.7 months (*unpublished data*); (Fig. 12.1 demonstrates pre- and post EUS-RFA treatment findings in the index insulinoma patient).

Several other small series and case reports demonstrated successful treatment with EUS-RFA with rapid resolution of clinical signs, which contribute to the growing body of evidence of the safety and feasibility of the EUS-RFA procedure [111–115]. However, its role in management of insulinomas is yet to be established, requiring long-term follow-up and prospective controlled studies comparing ablation with surgery in terms of tumor response, complications, and disease-specific survival.

12.6.3 Medical Therapy

Dietary consultation is important to prevent prolonged periods of fasting, the development of hypoglycemia, and its associated symptoms. Self-monitoring of glucose levels is recommended to insulinoma patients in order to detect asymptomatic hypoglycemia and to prevent occurrence of hypoglycemic spells [13, 17]. The patients should be advised regarding everyday personal safety such as avoidance of driving, to prevent its possible consequences.

Medical management is reserved only for patients who are unable or unwilling to undergo cytoreductive treatment or for unresectable metastatic disease.

Continuous glucose infusion may be necessary in some patients, while waiting for surgery or for the effect of other treatments. Vitamin B1 supplementation is recommended for patients with severe recurrent hypoglycemia requiring large infusions of glucose, in order to prevent Wernicke's encephalopathy. In refractory cases, simultaneous administration of glucose and glucagon has been used, with only temporary beneficial effect. This shortcoming is associated with a further stimulation of insulin release by glucose and glucagon and later relapse of hypoglycemia [26].

Diazoxide is usually a first line drug for controlling insulin-mediated hypoglycemia; at a dosage of 50–300 mg/day (up to 600 mg/day), it achieves symptomatic control in 50–60% of the cases [116]. The effect is exerted by suppression of insulin secretion from the beta cells via stimulation of α-adrenergic receptors and inhibition of cyclic adenosine monophosphate phosphodiesterase resulting in glycogenolysis enhancement [117]. However, the disturbing side effects of diazoxide (e.g., fluid retention and edema, weight gain, nausea and digestive intolerance, renal impairment, skin rashes, and hirsutism) render its use to be limited. Verapamil and diphenylhydantoin have also been reported to be helpful in the control of hypoglycemia [118–120]. Glucocorticoids can be effective in refractory cases, by decreasing insulin secretion and increasing peripheral insulin resistance [121]. Albeit, their association with well-known adverse effects makes these drugs poor candidates for long-term use.

Somatostatin analogues (SSAs) inhibit insulin secretion mainly through their effect in $SSTR_{2A}$ and $SSTR_5$ subtypes. The short-acting formulation octreotide was found to control hypoglycemia in doses varied between 50 and 2000 μg/day (in quantities of 50 μg subcutaneously two or three times a day), while long-acting release octreotide administered in a dose of 30 mg every 28 days, and injected lanreotide dose is 120 mg every 28 days. This therapy was found effective in up to 50% of insulinoma-related hypoglycemia with a few side effects, mostly digestive intolerance with diarrhea and steatorrhea that can be managed by pancreatic enzymes supplementation [122]. It is noteworthy that SSA may have a paradoxical effect on insulin secretion via its action on other receptors involved in the suppression of growth hormone and glucagon secretion, thereby worsening hypoglycemia in some insulinoma patients [123, 124]. Thus, in hospital, short acting 100 μg octreotide test is indicated, before initiating long-term analogues therapy.

12.6.3.1 Specific Treatments for Patients with Malignant Insulinoma

Malignant insulinomas present complex therapeutic challenge, in terms of both the control of tumor progression and the control of symptomatic hypoglycemia. The course of the metastatic disease is very heterogeneous, with a reported 10-year survival of about 30% [4]. Some patients may present a very slow progression rate, whereas other patients present rapid tumor progression and poor survival rate.

Symptomatic treatment of metastatic insulinomas aims at achieving short-term control of the hypoglycemia while awaiting the effects of anti-tumor treatment or when anti-tumor treatments do not prove to be effective. All the medications used in benign insulinomas can be employed, but usually, a combination of several hyperglycemic drugs is needed. In malignant insulinomas with predominant $SSTR_5$ expression, pasireotide—a novel multireceptor ($SSTR_{1,2,3,5}$) somatostatin analogue—may be effective [125]. The observed hyperglycemia (79%) in treatment of Cushing's disease and acromegaly with pasireotide is a well-known side effect that is of benefit in insulinoma patients. The mechanism by which pasireotide causes hyperglycemia involves reduced insulin secretion and incretins response without altering peripheral tissue insulin sensitivity [126]. A clinical case was reported on a patient with malignant insulinoma and refractory hypoglycemia despite combination therapy of diazoxide and long-acting SSA that resulted in near resolution of hypoglycemic episodes with pasireotide treatment [127]. The anti-proliferative effect of pasireotide in NETs is currently assessed by several ongoing phase 1–2 trials.

Everolimus is another novel targeted biologic therapy that has been shown to improve progression-free survival of patients with well-differentiated progressive metastatic pancreatic NETs [128]. The drug antiproliferative effect is by inhibiting signaling of (PI3K)/Akt/mTOR pathway and also involved in glucose homeostasis. Long-term administration of everolimus may alter insulin secretion, as well as insulin-mediated peripheral glucose utilization and insulin-mediated suppression of hepatic glucose production, thereby resulting in normo- or hyperglycemia in most of the patients with malignant insulinomas [129–131]. A study in patients with malignant insulinomas clearly demonstrated that 11/12 patients (91%) experienced a complete symptomatic response on everolimus, despite failure of other previous therapeutic lines [132].

Since malignant insulinomas are rare, and there is no prospective study to date on this disease specifically, the therapeutic approach is as for other pancreatic neuroendocrine carcinomas. Whenever it is possible, surgery has to be considered, aiming at a total excision of all detectable lesions. However, as recurrence is frequent (about 60%), other treatments should be considered, such as chemoembolization of liver metastases, radiofrequency ablation, cytotoxic chemotherapy (traditionally with a combination of streptozotocin, doxorubicin and 5-fluoro-uracil; capecitabine and temozolomide, peptide receptor radionuclide therapy (PRRT, especially with ^{177}Lutetium-DOTATATE), or targeted therapies with tyrosine kinase inhibitors (sunitinib) or mTOR inhibitors (everolimus) [4, 133–140].

References

1. Service FJ, McMahon MM, O'Brien PC, Ballard DJ (1991) Functioning insulinoma—incidence, recurrence, and long-term survival of patients: a 60-year study. In: Mayo Clinic proceedings, vol. 66, No. 7. Elsevier, pp 711–719
2. Anderson CW, Bennett JJ (2016) Clinical presentation and diagnosis of pancreatic neuroendocrine tumors. Surg Oncol Clin 25(2):363–374
3. Placzkowski KA, Vella A, Thompson GB, Grant CS, Reading CC, Charboneau JW et al (2009) Secular trends in the presentation and management of functioning insulinoma at the Mayo Clinic, 1987–2007. J Clin Endocrinol Metabol 94(4):1069–1073
4. De Herder WW, Niederle B, Scoazec JY, Pauwels S, Klöppel G, Falconi M, Rindi G (2006) Well-differentiated pancreatic tumor/carcinoma: insulinoma. Neuroendocrinology 84(3):183–188
5. Mehrabi A, Fischer L, Hafezi M, Dirlewanger A, Grenacher L, Diener MK, Rahbari NN (2014) A systematic review of localization, surgical treatment options, and outcome of insulinoma. Pancreas 43(5):675–686
6. Thakker RV, Newey PJ, Walls GV, Bilezikian J, Dralle H, Ebeling PR, Brandi ML (2012) Clinical practice guidelines for multiple endocrine neoplasia type 1 (MEN1). J Clin Endocrinol Metabol 97(9):2990–3011
7. Service FJ (1995) Hypoglycemic disorders. N Engl J Med 332(17):1144–1152
8. Grant CS (2005) Insulinoma. Best Pract Res Clin Gastroenterol 19(5):783–798
9. Freeman R (2007) Hypoglycemia and the autonomic nervous system. In: Diabetic neuropathy. Humana Press, pp 379–388
10. Routh V (2010) Glucose sensing neurons in the ventromedial hypothalamus. Sensors 10(10):9002–9025
11. Halpin K, McDonough R, Alba P, Halpin J, Singh V, Yan Y (2016) Vague neuroglycopenic complaints camouflage diagnosis of adolescent insulinoma: a case report. Int J Pediatr Endocrinol 2016(1):14
12. Maestri M, Monzani F, Bonanni E, Di Coscio E, Cignoni F, Dardano A, Murri L (2010) Insulinoma presenting as idiopathic hypersomnia. Neurol Sci 31(3):349–352

13. Munir A, Choudhary P, Harrison B, Heller S, Newell-Price J (2008) Continuous glucose monitoring in patients with insulinoma. Clin Endocrinol 68(6):912–918
14. Tesfaye N, Seaquist ER (2010) Neuroendocrine responses to hypoglycemia. Ann N Y Acad Sci 1212(1):12–28
15. Diaz AG, Herrera J, López M, Puchulu FM, Ferraina P, Bruno OD (2008) Insulinoma associated with pregnancy. Fertil Steril 90(1):199-e1
16. Christiansen E, Vestergaard H (2008) Insulinoma in a third-trimester pregnant woman combined with pre-eclampsia: a case report and review of the diagnostic strategies. Gynecol Endocrinol 24(7):417–422
17. Service FJ (1999) Diagnostic approach to adults with hypoglycemic disorders. Endocrinol Metab Clin N Am 28(3):519–532
18. Service FJ, Natt N, Thompson GB, Grant CS, van Heerden JA, Andrews JC, Lloyd RV (1999) Noninsulinoma pancreatogenous hypoglycemia: a novel syndrome of hyperinsulinemic hypoglycemia in adults independent of mutations in Kir6. 2 and SUR1 genes. J Clin Endocrinol Metabol 84(5):1582–1589
19. Cryer PE, Axelrod L, Grossman AB, Heller SR, Montori VM, Seaquist ER, Service FJ (2009) Evaluation and management of adult hypoglycemic disorders: an Endocrine Society clinical practice guideline. J Clin Endocrinol Metabol 94(3):709–728
20. Kar P, Price P, Sawers S, Bhattacharya S, Reznek RH, Grossman AB (2006) Insulinomas may present with normoglycemia after prolonged fasting but glucose-stimulated hypoglycemia. J Clin Endocrinol Metabol 91(12):4733–4736
21. Vezzosi D, Bennet A, Fauvel J, Caron P (2007) Insulin, C-peptide and proinsulin for the biochemical diagnosis of hypoglycaemia related to endogenous hyperinsulinism. Eur J Endocrinol 157(1):75–83
22. Tohidi M, Arbab P, Ghasemi A (2017) Assay-dependent variability of serum insulin concentrations: a comparison of eight assays. Scand J Clin Lab Invest 77(2):122–129
23. Staten MA, Stern MP, Miller WG, Steffes MW, Campbell SE, Insulin Standardization Workgroup (2010) Insulin assay standardization: leading to measures of insulin sensitivity and secretion for practical clinical care. Diabetes Care 33(1):205–206
24. Vezzosi D, Bennet A, Fauvel J, Boulanger C, Tazi O, Louvet JP, Caron P (2003) Insulin levels measured with an insulin-specific assay in patients with fasting hypoglycaemia related to endogenous hyperinsulinism. Eur J Endocrinol 149(5):413–419
25. Basu A, Sheehan MT, Thompson GB, Service FJ (2002) Insulinoma in chronic renal failure: a case report. J Clin Endocrinol Metabol 87(11):4889–4891
26. Wiesli P, Schmid C, Perren A, Pfammatter T, Spinas GA, Keller U (2004) Hypoglycemia in response to glucose and glucagon in insulinoma patients with a negative prolonged fast: functional and morphological properties. J Endocrinol Investig 27(9):832–838
27. Soh A, Kek P (2010) Insulinoma in a patient with normal results from prolonged fast and glucagon-induced hypoglycemia. Endocr Pract 16(5):838–841
28. Falconi M, Eriksson B, Kaltsas G, Bartsch DK, Capdevila J, Caplin M, Reed N (2016) ENETS consensus guidelines update for the management of patients with functional pancreatic neuroendocrine tumors and non-functional pancreatic neuroendocrine tumors. Neuroendocrinology 103(2):153–171
29. Zagury L, Moreira RO, Guedes EP, Coutinho WF, Appolinario JC (2004) Insulinoma misdiagnosed as dumping syndrome after bariatric surgery. Obes Surg 14(1):120–123
30. Iida K, Ohara T, Hino Y, Nobuhara M, Ishida J, Chihara K (2010) Glucose-responsive insulinoma in a patient with postprandial hypoglycemia in the morning. Intern Med 49(19):2123–2127
31. Vue MH, Setter SM (2011) Drug-induced glucose alterations part 1: drug-induced hypoglycemia. Diabetes Spectr 24(3):171–177
32. Salem CB, Fathallah N, Hmouda H, Bouraoui K (2011) Drug-induced hypoglycaemia. Drug Saf 34(1):21–45
33. Elmas ÖN, Demir K, Soylu N, Çelik N, Özkan B (2014) Importance of insulin immunoassays in the diagnosis of factitious hypoglycemia. J Clin Res Pediatr Endocrinol 6(4):258

34. Parfitt C, Church D, Armston A, Couchman L, Evans C, Wark G, McDonald TJ (2015) Commercial insulin immunoassays fail to detect commonly prescribed insulin analogues. Clin Biochem 48(18):1354–1357
35. DeWitt CR, Heard K, Waksman JC (2007) Insulin & C-peptide levels in sulfonylurea-induced hypoglycemia: A systematic review. J Med Toxicol 3(3):107–118
36. Thompson GB, Service FJ, Andrews JC, Lloyd RV, Natt N, van Heerden JA, Grant CS (2000) Noninsulinoma pancreatogenous hypoglycemia syndrome: an update in 10 surgically treated patients. Surgery 128(6):937–945
37. Chen Y, Lopez-Hisijos NM, Chen H, Valluru N, Ding X (2015) Adult onset nesidioblastosis after gastric bypass surgery, a clinical and pathologic review. Am J Digest Dis 2(2):68–75
38. Lloyd RV, Osamura RY, Klöppel G, Rosai J et al (2017) WHO classification of tumours of endocrine organs, 4th edn. International Agency for Research on Cancer, Lyon, p 355
39. Sorbye H, Baudin E, Borbath I, Caplin M, Chen J, Cwikla JB, Welin S (2019) Unmet needs in high-grade gastroenteropancreatic neuroendocrine neoplasms (WHO G3). Neuroendocrinology 108(1):53–61
40. Rindi G, Klöppel G (2004) Endocrine tumors of the gut and pancreas tumor biology and classification. Neuroendocrinology 80(Suppl. 1):12–15
41. Gao H, Wang W, Xu H, Wu C, Jin W, Zhang S, Liu L (2019) Distinct clinicopathological and prognostic features of insulinoma with synchronous distant metastasis. Pancreatology 19:472
42. Vanderveen K, Grant C (2010) Insulinoma. In: Endocrine neoplasia. Springer, Boston, MA, pp 235–252
43. Nahmias A, Grozinsky-Glasberg S, Salmon A, Gross DJ (2015) Pancreatic neuroendocrine tumors with transformation to insulinoma: an unusual presentation of a rare disease. Endocrinol Diabetes Metab Case Rep 2015(1):150032
44. Sundin A, Arnold R, Baudin E, Cwikla JB, Eriksson B, Fanti S, Krenning E (2017) ENETS consensus guidelines for the standards of care in neuroendocrine tumors: radiological, nuclear medicine and hybrid imaging. Neuroendocrinology 105(3):212–244
45. Guettier JM, Kam A, Chang R, Skarulis MC, Cochran C, Alexander HR, Gorden P (2009) Localization of insulinomas to regions of the pancreas by intraarterial calcium stimulation: the NIH experience. J Clin Endocrinol Metabol 94(4):1074–1080
46. Pattison DA, Hicks RJ (2017) Molecular imaging in the investigation of hypoglycaemic syndromes and their management. Endocr Relat Cancer 24(6):R203–R221
47. Zhu L, Xue HD, Sun H, Wang X, He YL, Jin ZY, Zhao YP (2016) Isoattenuating insulinomas at biphasic contrast-enhanced CT: frequency, clinicopathologic features and perfusion characteristics. Eur Radiol 26(10):3697–3705
48. Lin XZ, Wu ZY, Tao R, Guo Y, Li JY, Zhang J, Chen KM (2012) Dual energy spectral CT imaging of insulinoma—value in preoperative diagnosis compared with conventional multidetector CT. Eur J Radiol 81(10):2487–2494
49. Gouya H, Vignaux O, Augui J, Dousset B, Palazzo L, Louvel A, Legmann P (2003) CT, endoscopic sonography, and a combined protocol for preoperative evaluation of pancreatic insulinomas. Am J Roentgenol 181(4):987–992
50. Zhu L, Xue H, Sun Z, Li P, Qian T, Xing X, Jin Z (2017) Prospective comparison of biphasic contrast-enhanced CT, volume perfusion CT, and 3 Tesla MRI with diffusion-weighted imaging for insulinoma detection. J Magn Reson Imaging 46(6):1648–1655
51. Thoeni RF, Mueller-Lisse UG, Chan R, Do NK, Shyn PB (2000) Detection of small, functional islet cell tumors in the pancreas: selection of MR imaging sequences for optimal sensitivity. Radiology 214(2):483–490
52. Wei J, Liu X, Wu J, Xu W, Gao W, Jiang K, Miao Y (2016) Diagnosis and surgical management of insulinomas in 33 consecutive patients at a single institution. Langenbeck's Arch Surg 401(7):1019–1025
53. Daneshvar K, Grenacher L, Mehrabi A, Kauczor HU, Hallscheidt P (2011) Preoperative tumor studies using MRI or CT in patients with clinically suspected insulinoma. Pancreatology 11(5):487–495

54. Zimmer T, Stölzel U, Bäder M, Koppenhagen K, Hamm B, Buhr H et al (1996) Endoscopic ultrasonography and somatostatin receptor scintigraphy in the preoperative localisation of insulinomas and gastrinomas. Gut 39(4):562–568
55. Pitre J, Soubrane O, Palazzo L, Chapuis Y (1996) Endoscopic ultrasonography for the preoperative localization of insulinomas. Pancreas 13(1):55–60
56. Zimmer T, Scherübl H, Faiss S, Stölzel U, Riecken EO, Wiedenmann B (2000) Endoscopic ultrasonography of neuroendocrine tumours. Digestion 62(Suppl. 1):45–50
57. Téllez-Ávila FI, Acosta-Villavicencio GY, Chan C, Hernández-Calleros J, Uscanga L, Valdovinos-Andraca F, Ramírez-Luna MÁ (2015) Diagnostic yield of endoscopic ultrasound in patients with hypoglicemia and insulinoma suspected. Endosc Ultrasound 4(1):52
58. Pongprasobchai S, Lertwattanarak R, Pausawasdi N, Prachayakul V (2013) Diagnosis and localization of insulinoma in Thai patients: performance of endoscopic ultrasonography compared to computed tomography and magnetic resonance imaging. J Med Assoc Thai = Chotmaihet thangphaet 96:S187–SS93
59. Joseph A, Kapoor N, Simon E, Chacko A, Thomas E, Eapen A et al (2013) Endoscopic ultrasonography-a sensitive tool in the preoperative localization of insulinoma. Endocr Pract 19(4):602–608
60. Varma V, Tariciotti L, Coldham C, Taniere P, Buckels JA, Bramhall SR (2011) Preoperative localisation and surgical management of insulinoma: single Centre experience. Dig Surg 28(1):63–73
61. Nikfarjam M, Warshaw AL, Axelrod L, Deshpande V, Thayer SP, Ferrone CR, Fernández-del Castillo C (2008) Improved contemporary surgical management of insulinomas: a 25-year experience at the Massachusetts General Hospital. Ann Surg 247(1):165
62. Sotoudehmanesh R, Hedayat A, Shirazian N, Shahraeeni S, Ainechi S, Zeinali F, Kolahdoozan S (2007) Endoscopic ultrasonography (EUS) in the localization of insulinoma. Endocrine 31(3):238–241
63. Kaczirek K, Ba-Ssalamah A, Schima W, Niederle B (2004) The importance of preoperative localisation procedures in organic hyperinsulinism—experience in 67 patients. Wien Klin Wochenschr 116(11–12):373
64. Ardengh JC, Rosenbaum P, Ganc AJ, Goldenberg A, Lobo EJ, Malheiros CA et al (2000) Role of EUS in the preoperative localization of insulinomas compared with spiral CT. Gastrointest Endosc 51(5):552–555
65. Schumacher B, Lübke HJ, Frieling T, Strohmeyer G, Starke AAR (1996) Prospective study on the detection of insulinomas by endoscopic ultrasonography. Endoscopy 28(03):273–276
66. De Angelis C, Carucci P, Repici A, Rizzetto M (1999) Endosonography in decision making and management of gastrointestinal endocrine tumors. Eur J Ultrasound 10(2–3):139–150
67. Huai JC, Zhang W, Niu HO, Su ZX, McNamara JJ (1998) Localization and surgical treatment of pancreatic insulinomas guided by intraoperative ultrasound. Am J Surg 175(1):18–21
68. Hiramoto JS, Feldstein VA, LaBerge JM, Norton JA (2001) Intraoperative ultrasound and preoperative localization detects all occult insulinomas. Arch Surg 136(9):1020–1026
69. Nakamura Y, Matsushita A, Katsuno A, Yamahatsu K, Sumiyoshi H, Mizuguchi Y, Uchida E (2015) Clinical outcomes of 15 consecutive patients who underwent laparoscopic insulinoma resection: the usefulness of monitoring intraoperative blood insulin during laparoscopic pancreatectomy. Asian J Endosc Surg 8(3):303–309
70. Li W, An L, Liu R, Yao K, Hu M, Zhao G et al (2011) Laparoscopic ultrasound enhances diagnosis and localization of insulinoma in pancreatic head and neck for laparoscopic surgery with satisfactory postsurgical outcomes. Ultrasound Med Biol 37(7):1017–1023
71. Wong M, Isa SM, Zahiah M, Azmi KN (2007) Intraoperative ultrasound with palpation is still superior to intra-arterial calcium stimulation test in localising insulinoma. World J Surg 31(3):586–592
72. Chung JC, Choi SH, Jo SH, Heo JS, Choi DW, Kim YI (2006) Localization and surgical treatment of the pancreatic insulinomas. ANZ J Surg 76(12):1051–1055

73. Grover AC, Skarulis M, Alexander HR, Pingpank JF, Javor ED, Chang R, Libutti SK (2005) A prospective evaluation of laparoscopic exploration with intraoperative ultrasound as a technique for localizing sporadic insulinomas. Surgery 138(6):1003–1008
74. Nockel P, Babic B, Millo C, Herscovitch P, Patel D, Nilubol N, Kebebew E (2016) Localization of insulinoma using 68Ga-DOTATATE PET/CT scan. J Clin Endocrinol Metabol 102(1):195–199
75. Prasad V, Sainz-Esteban A, Arsenic R, Plöckinger U, Denecke T, Pape UF, Blankenstein O (2016) Role of 68 Ga somatostatin receptor PET/CT in the detection of endogenous hyperinsulinaemic focus: an explorative study. Eur J Nucl Med Mol Imaging 43(9):1593–1600
76. Sadowski SM, Millo C, Cottle-Delisle C, Merkel R, Yang LA, Herscovitch P, Kebebew E (2015) Results of 68Gallium-DOTATATE PET/CT scanning in patients with multiple endocrine neoplasia Type 1. J Am Coll Surg 221(2):509–517
77. Wild D, Christ E, Caplin ME, Kurzawinski TR, Forrer F, Brändle M, Ell PJ (2011) Glucagon-like peptide-1 versus somatostatin receptor targeting reveals 2 distinct forms of malignant insulinomas. J Nucl Med 52(7):1073–1078
78. Sharma P, Arora S, Dhull VS, Naswa N, Kumar R, Ammini AC, Bal C (2015) Evaluation of 68 Ga-DOTANOC PET/CT imaging in a large exclusive population of pancreatic neuroendocrine tumors. Abdom Imaging 40(2):299–309
79. Reubi JC, Waser B (2003) Concomitant expression of several peptide receptors in neuroendocrine tumours: molecular basis for in vivo multireceptor tumour targeting. Eur J Nucl Med Mol Imaging 30(5):781–793
80. Luo Y, Pan Q, Yao S, Yu M, Wu W, Xue H, Chen X (2016) Glucagon-like peptide-1 receptor PET/CT with 68Ga-NOTA-exendin-4 for detecting localized insulinoma: a prospective cohort study. J Nucl Med 57(5):715–720
81. Antwi K, Fani M, Heye T, Nicolas G, Rottenburger C, Kaul F, Gloor B (2018) Comparison of glucagon-like peptide-1 receptor (GLP-1R) PET/CT, SPECT/CT and 3T MRI for the localisation of occult insulinomas: evaluation of diagnostic accuracy in a prospective crossover imaging study. Eur J Nucl Med Mol Imaging 45(13):2318–2327
82. Jackson JE (2005) Angiography and arterial stimulation venous sampling in the localization of pancreatic neuroendocrine tumours. Best Pract Res Clin Endocrinol Metab 19(2):229–239
83. Guettier JM, Kam A, Chang R et al (2009) Localization of insulinomas to regions of the pancreas by intraarterial calcium stimulation: the NIH experience. J Clin Endocrinol Metab 94(4):1074–1080
84. Wu Z, Su T, Wu D, Ding X, Wang Z, Huang W, Zhang H (2017) Arterial stimulation with simultaneous venous sampling for localizing insulinomas. J Interv Med 1(1):28–31
85. Morera J, Guillaume A, Courtheoux P, Palazzo L, Rod A, Joubert M, Reznik Y (2016) Preoperative localization of an insulinoma: selective arterial calcium stimulation test performance. J Endocrinol Investig 39(4):455–463
86. Partelli S, Bartsch DK, Capdevila J, Chen J, Knigge U, Niederle B, Reed N (2017) ENETS consensus guidelines for the standards of care in neuroendocrine tumours: surgery for small intestinal and pancreatic neuroendocrine tumours. Neuroendocrinology 105(3):255–265
87. Zhao YP, Zhan HX, Zhang TP, Cong L, Dai MH, Liao Q, Cai LX (2011) Surgical management of patients with insulinomas: result of 292 cases in a single institution. J Surg Oncol 103(2):169–174
88. Hirshberg B, Libutti SK, Alexander HR, Bartlett DL, Cochran C, Livi A et al (2002) Blind distal pancreatectomy for occult insulinoma, an inadvisable procedure. J Am Coll Surg 194(6):761–764
89. Hashimoto LA, Walsh RM (1999) Preoperative localization of insulinomas is not necessary. J Am Coll Surg 189(4):368–373
90. Ravi K, Britton BJ (2007) Surgical approach to insulinomas: are pre-operative localisation tests necessary? Ann R Coll Surg Engl 89(3):212–217
91. Antonakis PT, Ashrafian H, Martinez-Isla A (2015) Pancreatic insulinomas: laparoscopic management. World J Gastrointest Endosc 7(16):1197

92. Ayav A, Bresler L, Brunaud L, Boissel P (2005) Laparoscopic approach for solitary insulinoma: a multicentre study. Langenbeck's Arch Surg 390(2):134–140
93. Isla A, Arbuckle JD, Kekis PB, Lim A, Jackson JE, Todd JF, Lynn J (2009) Laparoscopic management of insulinomas. Br J Surg: Incorporating European Journal of Surgery and Swiss Surgery 96(2):185–190
94. Hu M, Zhao G, Luo Y, Liu R (2011) Laparoscopic versus open treatment for benign pancreatic insulinomas: an analysis of 89 cases. Surg Endosc 25(12):3831–3837
95. Roland CL, Lo CY, Miller BS, Holt S, Nwariaku FE (2008) Surgical approach and perioperative complications determine short-term outcomes in patients with insulinoma: results of a bi-institutional study. Ann Surg Oncol 15(12):3532–3537
96. Su AP, Ke NW, Zhang Y, Liu XB, Hu WM, Tian BL, Zhang ZD (2014) Is laparoscopic approach for pancreatic insulinomas safe? Results of a systematic review and meta-analysis. J Surg Res 186(1):126–134
97. Tsang YP, Lang BHH, Shek TWH (2016) Assessing the short-and long-term outcomes after resection of benign insulinoma. ANZ J Surg 86(9):706–710
98. Al-Kurd A, Chapchay K, Grozinsky-Glasberg S, Mazeh H (2014) Laparoscopic resection of pancreatic neuroendocrine tumors. World J Gastroenterol: WJG 20(17):4908
99. Lopez CL, Albers MB, Bollmann C, Manoharan J, Waldmann J, Fendrich V, Bartsch DK (2016) Minimally invasive versus open pancreatic surgery in patients with multiple endocrine neoplasia type 1. World J Surg 40(7):1729–1736
100. Rostambeigi N, Thompson GB (2009) What should be done in an operating room when an insulinoma cannot be found? Clin Endocrinol 70(4):512–515
101. Kivlen M, Li M, Schneider D, Chuter T, Jensen RT (2003) Morbidity and mortality of aggressive resection in patients with advanced neuroendocrine tumors. Arch Surg 138(8):859–866
102. Kaltsas G, Caplin M, Davies P, Ferone D, Garcia-Carbonero R, Grozinsky-Glasberg S et al (2017) ENETS consensus guidelines for the standards of care in neuroendocrine tumors: pre-and perioperative therapy in patients with neuroendocrine tumors. Neuroendocrinology 105(3):245–254
103. De Herder WW, van Schaik E, Kwekkeboom D, Feelders RA (2011) New therapeutic options for metastatic malignant insulinomas. Clin Endocrinol 75(3):277–284
104. Lakhtakia S, Seo DW (2017) Endoscopic ultrasonography-guided tumor ablation. Dig Endosc 29(4):486–494
105. Rossi S, Ravetta V, Rosa L, Ghittoni G, Viera FT, Garbagnati F et al (2011) Repeated radiofrequency ablation for management of patients with cirrhosis with small hepatocellular carcinomas: a long-term cohort study. Hepatology 53(1):136–147
106. Rossi S, Dore R, Cascina A, Vespro V, Garbagnati F, Rosa L et al (2006) Percutaneous computed tomography-guided radiofrequency thermal ablation of small unresectable lung tumours. Eur Respir J 27(3):556–563
107. Mohan H, Nicholson P, Winter DC, O'Shea D, O'Toole D, Geoghegan J, Cantwell CP (2015) Radiofrequency ablation for neuroendocrine liver metastases: a systematic review. J Vasc Interv Radiol 26(7):935–942
108. Goldberg SN, Mallery S, Gazelle GS, Brugge WR (1999) EUS-guided radiofrequency ablation in the pancreas: results in a porcine model. Gastrointest Endosc 50(3):392–401
109. Carrara S, Arcidiacono PG, Albarello L, Addis A, Enderle MD, Boemo C et al (2008) Endoscopic ultrasound-guided application of a new hybrid cryotherm probe in porcine pancreas: a preliminary study. Endoscopy 40(04):321–326
110. Kim HJ, Seo DW, Hassanuddin A, Kim SH, Chae HJ, Jang JW et al (2012) EUS-guided radiofrequency ablation of the porcine pancreas. Gastrointest Endosc 76(5):1039–1043
111. Lakhtakia S, Ramchandani M, Galasso D, Gupta R, Venugopal S, Kalpala R, Reddy DN (2016) EUS-guided radiofrequency ablation for management of pancreatic insulinoma by using a novel needle electrode (with videos). Gastrointest Endosc 83(1):234–239
112. Choi JH, Seo DW, Song TJ, Park DH, Lee SS, Lee SK, Kim MH (2018) Endoscopic ultrasound-guided radiofrequency ablation for management of benign solid pancreatic tumors. Endoscopy 50(11):1099–1104

113. Lamine F, Godat S, Marino L, Di GS, Gonzalez RE, Desmartines N, Pitteloud N (2018) A case of benign insulinoma successfully treated with endoscopic ultrasound guided radiofrequency ablation. In: 20th European Congress of Endocrinology, vol 56. BioScientifica
114. Thosani N, Sharma NR, Raijman I et al (2018) 483 safety and efficacy of endoscopic ultrasound guided radiofrequency ablation (Eus-Rfa) in the treatment of pancreatic lesions: a multi-center experience. Gastrointest Endosc 87(6):AB84
115. Waung JA, Todd JF, Keane MG, Pereira SP (2016) Successful management of a sporadic pancreatic insulinoma by endoscopic ultrasound-guided radiofrequency ablation. Endoscopy 48(S 01):E144–E145
116. Goode PN, Farndon JR, Anderson J, Johnston ID, Morte JA (1986) Diazoxide in the management of patients with insulinoma. World J Surg 10(4):586–591
117. Stabile BE (1997) Islet cell tumors. Gastroenterologist 5(3):213–232
118. Stehouwer CD, Lems WF, Fischer HR, Hackeng WH (1989) Malignant insulinoma: is combined treatment with verapamil and the long-acting somatostatin analogue octreotide (SMS 201-995) more effective than single therapy with either drug? Neth J Med 35(1–2):86–94
119. Cohen MS, Bower RH, Fidler SM, Johnsonbaugh RE, Sode J (1973) Inhibition of insulin release by diphenylhydantoin and diazoxide in a patient with benign insulinoma. Lancet 1(7793):40–41
120. Brodows RG, Campbell RG (1974) Control of refractory fasting hypoglycemia in a patient with suspected insulinoma with diphenylhydantoin. J Clin Endocrinol Metabol 38(1):159–161
121. Novotny J, Janku F, Mares P, Petruzelka L (2005) Symptomatic control of hypoglycaemia with prednisone in refractory metastatic pancreatic insulinoma. Support Care Cancer 13(9):760–762
122. Vezzosi D, Bennet A, Courbon F, Caron P (2008) Short-and long-term somatostatin analogue treatment in patients with hypoglycaemia related to endogenous hyperinsulinism. Clin Endocrinol 68(6):904–911
123. Caplin ME, Pavel M, Ćwikła JB, Phan AT, Raderer M, Sedláčková E et al (2014) Lanreotide in metastatic enteropancreatic neuroendocrine tumors. N Engl J Med 371(3):224–233
124. Behr TH, Arnold R, Wied M (2002) Somatostatin analogues in the treatment of endocrine tumours of the gastrointestinal tract. Expert Opin Pharmacother 3(6):643–656
125. Vitale G, Dicitore A, Sciammarella C, Di Molfetta S, Rubino M, Faggiano A, Colao A (2018) Pasireotide in the treatment of neuroendocrine tumors: A review of the literature. Endocr Relat Cancer 25(6):R351–R364
126. Henry RR, Ciaraldi TP, Armstrong D, Burke P, Ligueros-Saylan M, Mudaliar S (2013) Hyperglycemia associated with pasireotide: results from a mechanistic study in healthy volunteers. J Clin Endocrinol Metabol 98(8):3446–3453
127. Hendren NS, Panach K, Brown TJ, Peng L, Beg MS, Weissler J, Mirfakhraee S (2018) Pasireotide for the treatment of refractory hypoglycaemia from malignant insulinoma. Clin Endocrinol 88(2):341–343
128. Yao JC, Shah MH, Ito T, Bohas CL, Wolin EM, Van Cutsem E et al (2011) Everolimus for advanced pancreatic neuroendocrine tumors. N Engl J Med 364(6):514–523
129. Bourcier ME, Sherrod A, DiGuardo M, Vinik AI (2009) Successful control of intractable hypoglycemia using rapamycin in an 86-year-old man with a pancreatic insulin-secreting islet cell tumor and metastases. J Clin Endocrinol Metabol 94(9):3157–3162
130. Kulke MH, Bergsland EK, Yao JC (2009) Glycemic control in patients with insulinoma treated with everolimus. N Engl J Med 360(2):195–197
131. Di Paolo S, Teutonico A, Leogrande D, Capobianco C, Schena PF (2006) Chronic inhibition of mammalian target of rapamycin signaling downregulates insulin receptor substrates 1 and 2 and AKT activation: a crossroad between cancer and diabetes? J Am Soc Nephrol 17(8):2236–2244
132. Bernard V, Lombard-Bohas C, Taquet MC, Caroli-Bosc FX, Ruszniewski P, Niccoli P et al (2013) Efficacy of everolimus in patients with metastatic insulinoma and refractory hypoglycemia. Eur J Endocrinol 168(5):665–674

133. Roche A, Girish BV, de Baère T, Baudin E, Boige V, Elias D et al (2003) Trans-catheter arterial chemoembolization as first-line treatment for hepatic metastases from endocrine tumors. Eur Radiol 13(1):136–140
134. Berber E, Flesher N, Siperstein AE (2002) Laparoscopic radiofrequency ablation of neuroendocrine liver metastases. World J Surg 26(8):985–990
135. Moertel CG, Lefkopoulo M, Lipsitz S, Hahn RG, Klaassen D (1992) Streptozocin–doxorubicin, streptozocin–fluorouracil, or chlorozotocin in the treatment of advanced islet-cell carcinoma. N Engl J Med 326(8):519–523
136. Strosberg JR, Nasir A, Hodul P, Kvols L (2008) Biology and treatment of metastatic gastrointestinal neuroendocrine tumors. Gastrointest Cancer Res 2(3):113
137. Strosberg JR, Fine RL, Choi J, Nasir A, Coppola D, Chen DT et al (2011) First-line chemotherapy with capecitabine and temozolomide in patients with metastatic pancreatic endocrine carcinomas. Cancer 117(2):268–275
138. Kulke MH, Stuart K, Enzinger PC, Ryan DP, Clark JW, Muzikansky A et al (2006) Phase II study of temozolomide and thalidomide in patients with metastatic neuroendocrine tumors. J Clin Oncol 24(3):401–406
139. Ong GS, Henley DE, Hurley D, Turner JH, Claringbold PG, Fegan PG (2010) Therapies for the medical management of persistent hypoglycaemia in two cases of inoperable malignant insulinoma. Eur J Endocrinol 162(5):1001–1008
140. Raymond E, Dahan L, Raoul JL, Bang YJ, Borbath I, Lombard-Bohas C et al (2011) Sunitinib malate for the treatment of pancreatic neuroendocrine tumors. N Engl J Med 364(6):501–513

Gastrinoma

13

Jane K. Mills, Anthony J. Chambers, and Janice L. Pasieka

13.1 Introduction

Gastrinomas are rare tumors of the neuroendocrine system, occurring within the pancreas and duodenum. The annual incidence is estimated to be 0.5–1.5 per million of the population [1, 2]. Overproduction of gastrin by these tumors produces a sustained increase in gastric acid secretion, leading to clinical manifestations of complicated peptic ulcer disease known as the Zollinger–Ellison Syndrome (ZES). [3] Although most gastrinomas have an indolent growth pattern, over 60% are malignant and 25% demonstrate an aggressive behavior [4–6]. Most commonly, gastrinomas metastasize to regional lymph nodes and the liver, and it is this malignant potential which has become increasingly important since the introduction of effective medical therapy to control gastric acid secretion. Gastrinomas can occur sporadically or in a familial pattern as a component of the multiple endocrine neoplasia type 1 (MEN 1) syndrome [4, 7, 8]. There have been recent advances in nuclear medicine imaging to localize these tumors using ^{68}Gallium (^{68}Ga) isotope tracers with positron emission technology (PET). In addition, many targeted therapeutic options are now available. Given that the endocrinopathy associated with these tumors can be well-controlled medically, the role of surgical resection in the setting of advanced disease and in patients with MEN 1 syndrome is the subject of continued debate.

J. K. Mills
AAES Fellow, University of Calgary, Calgary, AB, Canada

A. J. Chambers
St Vincent's Hospital Sydney and University of New South Wales, Sydney, NSW, Australia
e-mail: anthony.chambers@svha.org.au

J. L. Pasieka (✉)
Clinical Professor of Surgery, Faculty of Medicine, Cumming School of Medicine and Tom Baker Cancer Centre, University of Calgary, Calgary, AB, Canada
e-mail: janice.pasieka@ahs.ca

S. Yalcin, K. Öberg (eds.), *Neuroendocrine Tumours*,
https://doi.org/10.1007/978-3-031-56968-5_13

13.2 History

The first case of a gastrinoma was described by Sailer in 1946, when he reported the case of a patient with a large pancreatic islet cell tumor without clinical or biochemical evidence of hyperinsulinemia [9]. At that time, insulinomas were the only recognized functional islet cell tumors, and although a duodenal ulcer was present, Sailer did not associate the two findings. It was not until Robert M. Zollinger and Edwin H. Ellison presented their experience of two cases before the American Surgical Association in 1955 that it became apparent a relationship existed [3]. The two cases presented by Zollinger were unique in that they presented with marked gastric hypersecretion, complicated refractory peptic ulcer disease, and non-insulin secreting islet cell tumors of the pancreas. During the discussion following their presentation, another seven cases with the same clinical manifestations were described. This clinical triad associated with gastrin-secreting tumors now bears the authors' names [10]. They concluded in their report that excessive amounts of a substance produced by the islet cell tumors was likely responsible for the increased gastric acid secretion in these patients.

The role of gastrin in the causation of ZES was first proposed by Gregory in 1960, who injected an extract derived from a pancreatic islet cell tumor from a patient with refractory peptic ulcer disease into an animal model and demonstrated a dramatic increase in gastric acid secretion, concluding that a "gastrin-like substance" was secreted by these tumors [11]. Gastrin was first isolated from antral mucosal cells by Gregory in 1964 and later found to be nearly identical in composition to an extracted hormone from a gastrinoma [12]. The development of a radioimmunoassay for the measurement of serum gastrin concentrations by McGuigan and Trudeau in 1968 enabled the diagnosis of gastrinoma and ZES to be made preoperatively [13]. However, elevated gastrin levels can also be seen in other conditions such including atrophic gastritis, gastric outlet obstruction, retained gastric antrum, post-vagotomy, G-cell hyperplasia, and the use of proton-pump inhibitors. In this way, the diagnosis of ZES cannot be made solely on the basis of an elevated serum gastrin level [14] (Table 13.1). It was recognized by Isenberg in 1972 that there was a paradoxical rise in gastrin with the administration of secretin in patients with suspected ZES allowing for a more specific delineation of the disease [15].

The initial experience of 260 cases of ZES laid the foundation for the current understanding and management of this disease at that time [4]. Based on the data collected in this registry, Ellison and Wilson recommended total gastrectomy as the definitive initial operation. The first report of a successful resection of gastrinoma to treat ZES was by Rawson in 1960, where a patient with peptic ulcer disease and hypersecretion of gastric acid underwent removal of a pancreatic islet cell tumor by Professor Stammers at the University of Birmingham [16]. The patient did not undergo gastrectomy or vagotomy yet had a complete relief of symptoms and a marked reduction of gastric acid secretion after resection of the tumor. Consequently, the recommendation from these authors was that surgical management be directed at "eradication of the tumor and its local metastases rather than total gastrectomy." [17]. Although it is now recognized that duodenal gastrinomas are fairly common,

Table 13.1 Causes of hypergastrinemia

Inappropriate hypergastrinemia—Gastric pH < 2
Gastrinoma/Zollinger–Ellison syndrome
Helicobacter pylori infection
Retained gastric antrum
Gastric outlet obstruction
Short bowel syndrome
Appropriate hypergastrinemia—Associated with hypochlorhydria
Pernicious anemia
Chronic atrophic gastritis
Vagotomy
Gastric acid suppressing medications (PPI, H2–antagonist)
Renal impairment

in some series as high as 80% [1, 9, 15], it was in 1961 when Oberhelman first reported the occurrence of duodenal gastrinomas in patients with ZES [18]. Since Oberhelman's publication, duodenal gastrinomas were described more frequently and subsequently changed the operative approach. Both NW Thompson and JA Norton recognized the necessity of performing a duodenotomy in sporadic gastrinoma patients when no pancreatic tumor was found [19–21].

Interestingly, in the discussion section of the paper by Oberhelman, Dr. Victor Richards said "the demonstration by Gregory that these tumours produce either gastrin or a gastrin-like substance has led many people to work experimentally on the concept of producing an antihormone. I do not know of any clinical experience, however, with the use of antigastrin in the management of these cases, but it is an idea that is worth thinking about for the future." A decade later, this idea would conceptually come to fruition with the development of H2-receptor antagonists followed by proton-pump inhibitors (PPIs) [10].

In 1953, Underdahl and coworkers published their experience at the Mayo Clinic of eight cases of multiple adenomas involving a combination of two or all three of the pituitary, parathyroid glands, or pancreas and a review of the literature. Parathyroid tumors were present in all, pituitary tumors in four and five had pancreatic islet cell tumors. They commented that the "multiplicity of tumors was a striking feature and occurred both in relation to the parathyroids and in relation to the pancreatic islets." [22]. It is interesting to note that two cases of the 14 reviewed, and two of their own eight cases, suffered from duodenal ulcers as well as one of their cases having had a peptic ulcer. In the following year, Wermer stated that "this complex clinical pathologic picture has now been seen so often that the possibility of mere coincidence can be dismissed." He went on to say that "we are dealing here with an example of dominant hereditary transmission and it appears probable that one single autosomal gene is responsible for the whole pathologic picture." [23].

From the five cases which he presented in his 1954 paper, he astutely observed that there were two instances of gastric ulcer and two of duodenal ulcers—a finding which he did not believe to be mere coincidence, but another manifestation of the abnormal gene. In the review article by Ellison and Wilson from 1964, they identified an association with other endocrine diseases in patients with ZES in 21% of cases [4]. We now recognize that MEN 1 syndrome is found in approximately 20–30% of patients with ZES [24, 25].

13.3 Clinical Features and Diagnosis

When ZES was first described, the gastrinomas were mainly pancreatic tumors and patients suffered from refractory peptic ulcer disease, vomiting, diarrhea, and weight loss (Table 13.2). Treatment was based on controlling the acid production (total gastrectomy) and resection of the pancreatic tumor if possible. Nowadays, gastrinomas are often small and up to 80% are in the duodenal wall. Symptoms are often those of peptic ulcer disease without diarrhea and weight loss, as PPI is very effective at controlling the gastric acid secretions. Delay in the diagnosis of ZES has increased as a result of the effective use of PPIs [6, 26–28].

Gastrinomas are rare tumors, occurring with an incidence of approximately 0.5–2 cases per million population per year [2, 24, 26, 29]. Gastrinomas occur more frequently in males, with a male to female ratio of 1.3–2:1 [2, 5, 27, 30]. Pancreatic gastrinomas make up approximately 15% of all pancreatic neuroendocrine tumors (PNETs). The tumor typically presents in late adulthood with a mean age at diagnosis between 41 and 54 years, earlier for patients with MEN 1 (33 years) [1, 26, 31, 32]. Historically, patients with gastrinoma were typically diagnosed late in the course of their disease with complications of severe refractory peptic ulcer disease. In the modern era with the widespread use of PPI therapy, a history of peptic ulceration is absent in 29% of patients at the time of diagnosis. Although patients with ZES may still present with more severe manifestations of peptic ulcer disease, the vast majority of ZES patients are indistinguishable from idiopathic peptic ulcer

Table 13.2 Clinical presentation of Zollinger–Ellison Syndrome

Symptom	Percentage of patients
Abdominal pain	78–94%
Peptic ulcer disease	74–96%
Duodenal ulcer	60–96%
Gastric ulcer	24%
Jejunal ulceration	29%
Bleeding	27–42%
Diarrhea	72%
Gastro-esophageal reflux	42%
Esophageal ulceration or stricture	4–6%
Weight loss	7–18%

disease [26]. As a result, many patients are initially treated with PPIs early in the course of their disease, leading to improvement or resolution of their symptoms, with the potential to develop metastatic disease before the diagnosis is established [1, 6, 26, 27]. Ellison reported an increase in the proportion of patients with gastrinoma presenting with more advanced disease between 1986 and 1998. Patients diagnosed before 1985 had an incidence of metastatic disease of 19% and a 5-year disease free survival (DFS) of 29% compared with an incidence of metastatic disease of 55% and 5-year DFS of 2% after 1986 [33].

ZES patients typically present with symptoms of abdominal pain (83%) and diarrhea (71%), including long-standing symptoms related to gastro-esophageal reflux and/or recurrent peptic ulcer disease (PUD) (Table 13.2). Only 11% of patients have a single symptom. Gastrinomas present less frequently with complications of PUD in the modern era. In 1964, 45% of patients presented with life-threatening bleeding from peptic ulceration, whereas in the National Institutes of Health report from 1999, only 24% presented with this complication [1, 4]. Up to 20–25% of gastrinoma occur in the setting of MEN 1. The diagnosis of ZES should be considered in patients with PUD who lack evidence of *H. pylori* infection, are refractory to standard medical treatment, have ulceration at unusual locations, or who have features suggestive of MEN 1 syndrome [6].

The diagnosis of gastrinoma is based on biochemical testing, demonstrating an elevation of fasting serum gastrin (FSG) level (>150 pg/mL) in the presence of raised gastric acid secretion [31]. In patients receiving acid suppressing therapy with H2-receptor antagonists or PPIs, FSG is secondarily raised by these medications and as such these should be discontinued prior to testing [6, 26, 34]. FSG can also be elevated in other disease states that must be differentiated from ZES (Table 13.1). Gastric secretory studies showing a basal acid output (BAO) of more than 15 mEq/h (more than 5 mEq/h in the presence of previous gastric resection) or a pH of less than 2 are the most commonly used criteria to determine acid hypersecretion [31]. Nasogastric tube aspiration and endoscopic acid sampling have both been used to estimate gastric pH. A recent innovation is an ingestible wireless pH sensor (SmartPill™, Covidien, USA) with similar results in measurement of gastric acid secretions [35, 36]. Many patients with gastrinoma have highly elevated gastrin levels, with 36% having levels more than ten times normal [37]. When the results of FSG and acid secretory studies are borderline or non-diagnostic in patients where a clinical suspicion for ZES exists, provocative testing of FSG after administration of intravenous secretin (2 mg/kg) or calcium is indicated. Because most of these patients are on PPIs, these drugs must be stopped a week prior to provocative testing. H2-receptor antagonists may not only be utilized for symptom control but also must be stopped 48 h before [26]. There is a risk for developing rebound hypersecretion following PPI withdrawal, and precautions should be considered [34]. The day of the secretin test is the ideal time to get a gastric pH and upper endoscopic ultrasound (EUS), to avoid having to withdrawal PPIs again at a later date. Following secretin injection, FSG increases from baseline levels within 2–3 min by more than 100 pg/mL in 94% of patients with gastrinoma and rises by more than 50% in 84% of cases [37]. Similarly, provocative testing after calcium infusion results in a rise in serum gastrin of more than 50% from baseline levels in 84% of cases [6]. Combining these two investigations leads to an increased sensitivity for confirming the diagnosis of gastrinoma. In an analysis of 293 ZES patients from the National Institutes of Health and 537 patients from the literature, an increase in serum gastrin after secretin stimulation to ≥120 pg/mL was considered diagnostic of gastrinoma (sensitivity 94%, specificity 100%), replacing the old criteria of >200 pg/mL [37].

Chromogranin-A (CgA), a protein contained within the secretory granules of neuroendocrine cells, is a non-specific marker for neuroendocrine tumors and is elevated in 90% of patients with gastrinoma [38]. CgA levels tend to correlate with those of serum gastrin; however, higher levels are not associated with an increased risk of advanced or metastatic disease. In a series of 72 patients with gastrinoma having serial measurements of gastrin and CgA, these markers did not have sufficient sensitivity to replace serial imaging for the detection of small but important changes in tumor burden [39].

13.4 Location of Primary Tumors

Although sporadic ZES was first described in association with PNETs, the primary tumor can be located in the duodenum in an equivalent proportion of cases and may also arise uncommonly from other sites [1, 5, 40]. In 90% of cases, the primary tumor can be localized within the "gastrinoma (Stabile's) triangle," a region encompassing the proximal duodenum and head of the pancreas [41]. This triangle is defined by (a) the junction of the cystic and common bile ducts (superiorly), (b) the junction of the second and third parts of the duodenum (inferiorly), and (c) the junction of the neck and body of the pancreas (medially).

Duodenal gastrinomas are small tumors arising within the submucosa and are found in the first and second parts of the duodenum in 83–92% of cases, and rarely distal to this [21, 32, 42] (Fig. 13.1a, b). The mean size ranges from 6 to 13 mm in diameter, and 49–80% of tumors are less than 10 mm in size, and for this reason, they are rarely seen on conventional cross-sectional imaging studies [5, 19, 42–44].

The pancreas is the site of gastrinoma in 17–55% of patients with sporadic ZES, and the tumor is located proximally in the head of the pancreas in 33–53% of cases [1, 5, 40, 45]. Gastrinoma is the second most common functional neuroendocrine tumor of the pancreas, accounting for 36% of these lesions [46, 47]. Pancreatic gastrinomas tend to be larger than their duodenal counterparts with a mean diameter of 27–32 mm [5, 42, 43, 45, 46]. Sporadic gastrinomas may uncommonly occur at multiple sites (11–16%), and pancreatic and duodenal gastrinomas may coexist in 9–11% of cases [5, 30]. In contrast, in patients with MEN 1 who have ZES, more than 75% will have multiple pancreatic and/or duodenal gastrinomas [48, 49].

Gastrinomas arising from sites other than the pancreas and duodenum are rare, accounting for only 6% of reported ZES cases [49]. Primary "ectopic" gastrinomas have been reported in the liver, biliary tree, ovary, kidney, heart, stomach, jejunum, and within the greater or lesser omentum [1, 6, 50, 51]. The entity of primary lymph node gastrinoma is controversial. This can be defined by the following conditions:

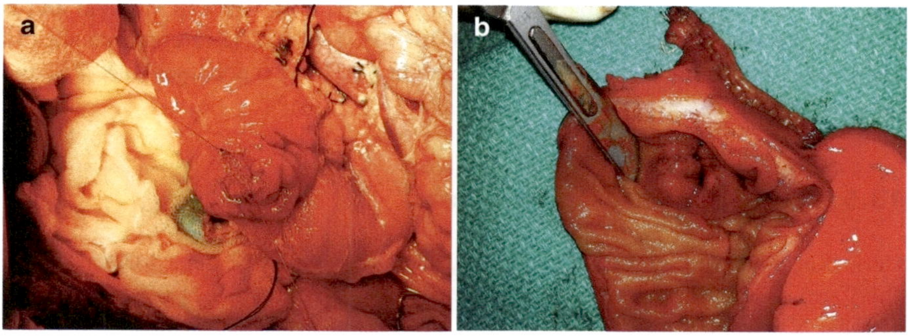

Fig. 13.1 Submucosal duodenal gastrinomas in Zollinger–Ellison syndrome. (**a**) This 5 mm gastrinoma in the second portion of the duodenum was locally excised from the submucosa. (**b**) Demonstrates a 10 mm gastrinoma found within the fourth part of the duodenum. The lesion was resected with a small bowel resection including the positive lymph nodes found in the adjacent mesentery

(a) removal of an involved lymph node in the absence of a gastrinoma primary found elsewhere and (b) normalization of FSG and secretin stimulation tests after excision [1]. In a large series from NIH, 26% of patients with ZES undergoing laparotomy had only involved lymph nodes removed without identification of a primary tumor, with subsequent normalization of serum gastrin post-operatively [40]. Whether these nodal lesions represent metastases from a small primary tumor that evaded detection at the time of initial operation or are a true primary remains controversial. However, in long-term follow-up from this NIH series, 69% of patients thought to have primary lymph node gastrinomas remained biochemical cured, leading these authors to conclude that lymph nodes can be the primary site of gastrinoma in 10% of patients with ZES [52]. Primary lymph node gastrinoma is thought to rarely occur in the context of ZES/MEN 1, with lymph node involvement most likely due to metastatic spread from an occult pancreatic or duodenal location [1, 53].

Metastatic disease affecting regional lymph nodes or the liver can be demonstrated in 52–69% of patients with gastrinoma on initial imaging studies or at the time of laparotomy [40, 54, 55]. Involvement of regional lymph nodes, particularly peri-pancreatic and peri-duodenal nodes, can be demonstrated in 40–75% of patients with duodenal gastrinoma and 50% with pancreatic tumors [6, 54, 56]. In contrast to metastatic liver disease, regional lymph node involvement alone has not been associated with a reduction in survival, with an overall 10-year survival approaching 100% [5, 56, 57].

Hepatic metastases are present in 8–22% of patients with gastrinoma at the time of initial assessment [54, 56, 57]. Several authors have found that pancreatic gastrinoma is more frequently associated with hepatic metastases than duodenal tumors (52% vs. 5%) [5, 56]. Larger primary tumors are associated with an increased risk of hepatic metastases. The risk of hepatic metastases for tumors smaller than 10 mm is 4%, for tumors 10–30 mm is 28%, and for tumors greater than 30 mm is 61% [56,

58]. The development of hepatic metastases significantly worsens survival and is associated with a 10-year survival rate of 26–30% [56, 57]. Less common sites of metastatic disease include peritoneal disease in 6%, bone metastases in 3–7%, and lung metastases in 2% [30, 59].

13.5 The Genetics of Gastrinomas

Germ-line mutation of the MEN 1 gene, a tumor suppressor gene located on the short arm of chromosome 11 (11q31), is responsible for the MEN 1 syndrome [7]. The MEN 1 gene codes for the nuclear protein *menin* which is involved in cell growth regulation. Twenty-five percent of gastrinomas are associated with the MEN 1 syndrome [1, 8]. Mutations of the MEN 1 gene are inherited in an autosomal dominant pattern, and between 36 and 42% of patients with this mutation will develop gastrinoma [48]. Mutation of the MEN 1 gene has also been implicated in the pathogenesis of sporadic gastrinoma. Mutations of this gene have been found between 17 and 58% of gastrinomas in patients who do not possess germ-line MEN 1 mutations or a family history of MEN 1-related tumors [60, 61]. It has been proposed that MEN 1 gene mutation is an early event in the pathogenesis of both sporadic and familial gastrinomas, with mutations occurring equally in both duodenal and pancreatic tumors [8]. The biological behavior of gastrinomas displaying MEN 1 gene mutation is similar to those where this mutation is not found, with no increased risk of metastatic disease or of recurrence after surgical resection [60, 61].

Several other genetic mechanisms are involved in the pathogenesis of gastrinoma in addition to mutations affecting the MEN 1 gene. Chromosomal deletions causing loss of heterozygosity of chromosomes 1q and 22q have also been identified in gastrinomas [62, 63]. Inactivation or deletion of the p16 tumor suppressor gene at chromosome 9p21, coding for the p16 protein involved in the regulation of cell growth and cell cycle inhibition, has also been demonstrated in 52% of gastrinomas [64]. Gene expression analysis using microarrays has identified numerous additional gene alterations in pancreatic neuroendocrine tumors including gastrinomas; however, none has been clearly implicated in their pathogenesis [6, 8, 58, 65].

13.6 Imaging

Cross-sectional imaging with computed tomography (CT) and magnetic resonance (MR), somatostatin receptor scintigraphy (SRS), positron emission tomography (PET), and endoscopic ultrasound (EUS) has all been utilized for the localization and staging of patients with ZES and to detect recurrent disease. Gastrinomas are hypervascular and therefore demonstrate a greater degree of enhancement than the normal pancreas [1]. Conventional cross-sectional imaging with CT and MR does not possess the resolution to detect duodenal primary tumors due to their small size but can detect pancreatic gastrinomas with a sensitivity of 54–71% [54, 66, 67]. Enlarged regional lymph nodes involved with metastatic disease may also be identified and at times in the clue to the site of the primary (Fig. 13.2). Hepatic metastases are best visualized utilizing a triple-phase CT imaging as NETs typically appear hyperintense in the arterial phase. On MR imaging, NET hepatic metastases are usually intermediate/high single intensity of T2-weighted images (Fig. 13.3). CT or MR enterography is gaining popularity in the investigation of small bowel neuroendocrine tumors and may have an increasing role in the detection of gastrinomas. CT enterography and enteroclysis have demonstrated a sensitivity between 86% and 100% in the detection of NETs in the bowel [68, 69] (Fig. 13.4a, b). Somatostatin receptors are expressed by 85–100% of gastrinomas, and for this reason SRS using Indium (^{111}In)-labeled octreotide has been utilized to detect primary gastrinomas and nodal or distant metastatic lesions [66] (Fig. 13.5). SRS has a sensitivity of 11–30% for the identification of duodenal lesions, 25–77% for pancreatic lesions, 72–82% for nodal metastases, and 67–100% for hepatic metastases from gastrinoma [1, 66, 70]. In a study of 122 patients with ZES by Termanini, SRS was positive for disease in 61% of patients, was the only imaging modality that localized the tumor in 12% of cases, and changed the management of 47% of cases [71]. In another study, SRS was able to detect primary tumors and metastatic lesions with a sensitivity superior to that of CT, MRI, and angiography combined, however was unable to identify 33% of primary tumors subsequently found at laparotomy [66]. In this study, the sensitivity of SRS varied with tumor size and location. SRS detected only 30% of gastrinoma size <10 mm, 64% of those between 11 and 20 mm, and 96% of those >20 mm. No duodenal tumors were successfully imaged on SRS. Combining SRS with single photon emission spectography (SPECT) can significantly improve detection rates (sensitivity and specificity 87.8% and 96.6%, respectively) and may alter management decisions in 14% of patients [35, 72–75].

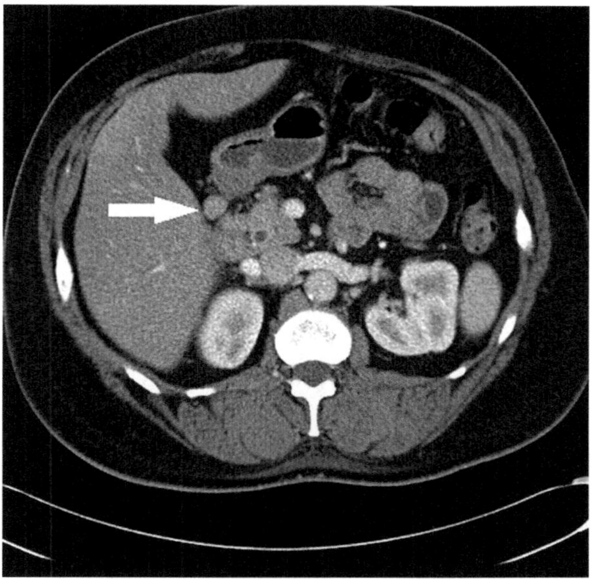

Fig. 13.2 Computed tomography arrow showing an enlarged peripancreatic lymph node. The primary 8 mm duodenal gastrinoma was not seen on this scan, yet the lymph node was the clue to the duodenal location of the primary

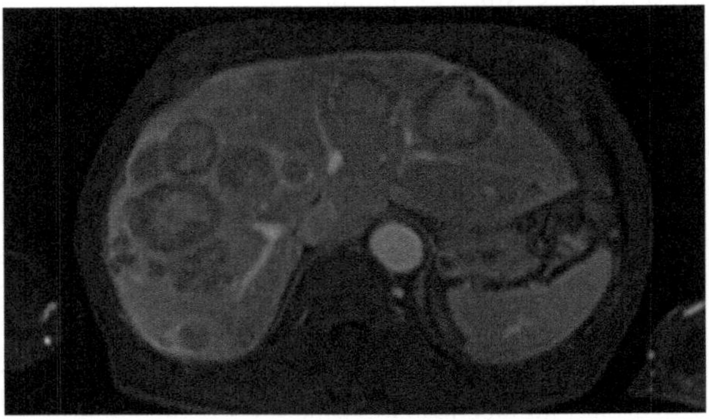

Fig. 13.3 MRI demonstrating metastatic liver disease in a patient with Zollinger–Ellison syndrome from a large pancreatic gastrinoma

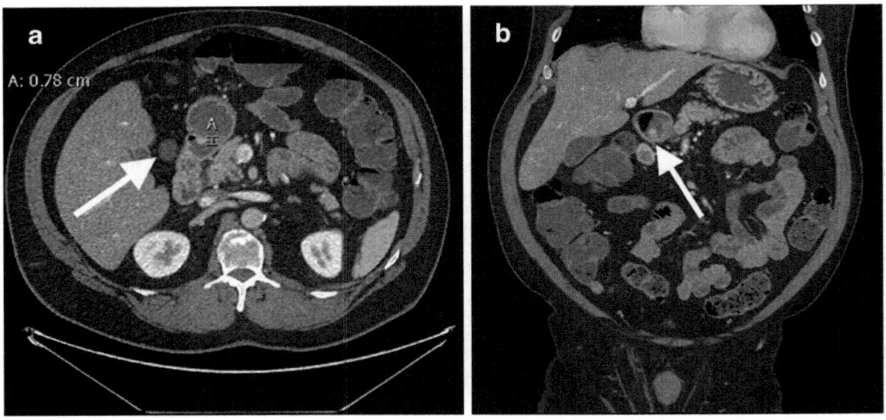

Fig. 13.4 (**a**) CT enterography demonstrating detection of 14x8x13 mm submucosal arterially enhancing nodule in inferior aspect of the distal pylorus/duodenal bulb consistent with the primary site of gastrinoma. (A) The arrow demonstrates a 2 cm biopsy proven metastatic periportal lymph node. (**b**) The coronal sections demonstrating the enhancing duodenal gastrinoma (arrow)

Whole-body positron emission tomography (PET) scans hold several advantages over SPECT technology with higher reported sensitivity, higher spatial image resolution, and reduced radiation exposure [76]. PET using 18-fluoro-deoxy-glucose (18-FDG) is a powerful modality for oncological imaging yet unfortunately does not accumulate in most well-differentiated neuroendocrine tumors including gastrinomas. Somatostatin receptor-targeted PET tracers using Gallium-68 (^{68}Ga) have demonstrated superior detection rates for localizing PNETs and other neuroendocrine tumors compared with 18-FDG PET, somatostatin receptor SPECT, CT, or MR [77]. For this reason, ^{68}Ga-PET/CT is now considered the imaging modality of choice to localize and correctly stage non-insulinoma PNETs including gastrinoma [78].

Several ^{68}Ga-labeled somatostatin receptor ligands are available, including ^{68}Ga-DOTATOC, ^{68}Ga-DOTATATE, and ^{68}Ga-DOTANOC. All ligands

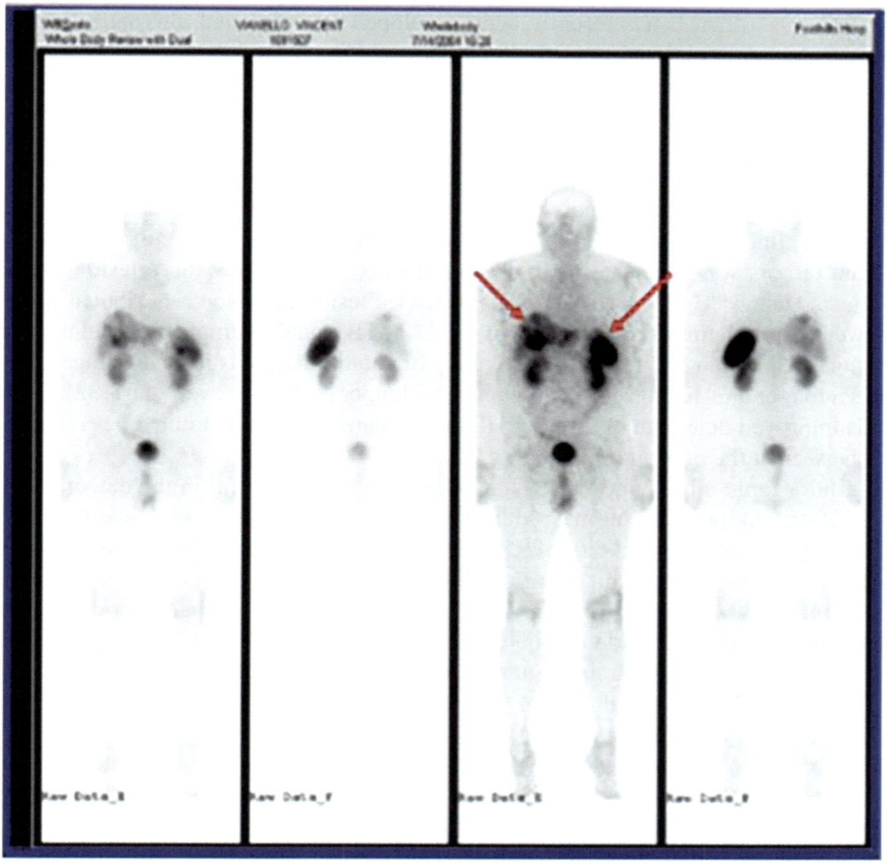

Fig. 13.5 Ga-68 Dotatate scan of metastatic tumours from a patient with Zollinger-Ellison Syndrome

demonstrate improved performance compared to ^{111}In-DTPA-octreotide. No single ^{68}Ga-labeled tracer has demonstrated superiority when compared head to head, and tracer choice is often determined by local availability [76, 77, 79, 80]. PET using ^{68}Gallium-labeled DOTATOC has been associated with a sensitivity of 97% and a specificity of 92% for the detection of neuroendocrine tumors and their metastases and is more accurate to detect bone metastases than CT or bone scintigraphy [81–83]. The addition of CT to PET improves diagnostic accuracy. A meta-analysis performed by Geijer and Breimer in 2013 analyzed over 2000 patients with neuroendocrine tumors. They reported a pooled sensitivity of 93% and a specificity of 96% [84]. Furthermore,^{68}Ga-labeled PET/CT scans have been demonstrated to alter management in as many as 40–60% of patients, illustrating the significant contribution this imaging modality has made to the treatment of ZES [35, 85, 86].

^{64}Cu-DOTATATE has recently been developed as a new and alternative somatostatin receptor radiotracer for PET imaging and has been demonstrated to have a superior diagnostic sensitivity (97%) and accuracy (97%) compared to ^{111}In-DTPA-octreotide (87% and 88%, respectively) [87]. In a recent study by Johnbeck and coworkers, 59 patients were examined comparing ^{64}Cu-DOTATATE and ^{68}Ga-DOTATOC PET/CT images. There were 701 lesions found concordantly with both imaging modalities, and 68 additional lesions were identified on only one of the modalities. Although patient-based sensitivity for the diagnosis of neuroendocrine tumors was the same for both radiotracers, significantly more lesions were detected using ^{64}Cu-DOTATATE. This increased lesion detection is attributed to the lower positron emission range of ^{64}Cu-DOTATATE, enabling improved spatial resolution. In addition, ^{64}Cu-DOTATATE may offer additional logistical advantages as it has a longer half-life (12.7 h), allowing for a longer shelf-life (over 24 h) [88]. How this improved detection of disease will be translated into patient outcomes remains to be seen at the present time.

Endoscopic ultrasound (EUS) has been shown to be useful in the detection of PNETs including gastrinomas, identifying even small lesions with a sensitivity of 75–100% and a specificity of 95% [89]. This technique also has the advantage of defining the relationship of primary tumors to pancreatic ductal and vascular structures, as well as facilitating fine needle biopsy (FNA) of pancreatic lesions. EUS has been shown to detect up to 91% of PNETs not seen on CT [89]. In addition, EUS-guided FNA is better able to diagnose PNETs compared with CT-guided FNA, particularly for lesions in the pancreatic head [90]. A recent study by van Asselt demonstrated the superiority of EUS for detecting pancreatic lesions over CT, MR, and SRS. EUS detected 101 lesions in 34 patients compared with CT, MRI, and SRS which detected only 32 lesions in 18 patients ($p < 0.001$) [35, 91]. EUS unfortunately is less sensitive (38–63%) in the detection of duodenal gastrinomas due to their small size, making its utility less effective in the localization of these tumors in sporadic ZES [35, 92]. In patients with MEN1, EUS is a useful surveillance tool for the follow-up of small non-functioning well-differentiated PNETs. It has been recommended that annual surveillance of the MEN 1 pancreas should be performed. A recent study by Kappelle and coworkers found that the growth of PNETs in patients with MEN 1 was slow (overall growth rate 0.1 mm/year), and therefore surveillance intervals may be safely extended [93].

Invasive testing involving arteriography or selective venous sampling has been utilized to assist in the localization of gastrinoma in patients where conventional CT, MR, SRS, and EUS all fail to localize the tumor. Selective angiography with secretin injection (SASI) involves cannulation of the right or left hepatic veins and sampling of gastrin levels from this location after intra-arterial injection of secretin or calcium into the gastroduodenal, hepatic, splenic, left gastric, and superior mesenteric arteries [94]. Secretin stimulates gastrin release from tumor present in the vascular distribution of the arterial injection, producing an increase in gastrin levels as measured in the hepatic veins. Utilizing the same principles, intravenous calcium injection has also proven to be effective in localizing the gastrinoma [95]. The proportion of patients with gastrinoma where the tumor can be "regionalized" by SASI varies from 71% to 89% [1].

In patients with negative imaging, an experienced surgeon becomes an invaluable localizing tool. Norton and coworkers were able to successfully identify the gastrinoma at the time of surgery in 57 of 58 patients who had negative preoperative imaging. These tumors were small (mean 8 mm) and found in the duodenum in 67% of cases, the pancreas in 17%, and thought to be primary gastrinomas occurring within lymph nodes in 10% [44]. Immediate biochemical cure was established in 35 patients (60%), with long-term biochemical cure (mean 9.4 years) in 27 (46%). In this way, if the tumor is unable to be localized using cross-sectional imaging studies, EUS, or angiographic techniques such as SASI, then surgical exploration in the hands of an experienced surgeon is indicated.

13.7 Staging of Gastrinomas

Gastrinomas are currently considered well-differentiated NETs and are therefore classified and staged accordingly. There are currently three staging systems proposed for these tumors: by the World Health Organization (WHO), European Neuroendocrine Tumour Society (ENETS), and the American Joint Committee on Cancer (AJCC) [96, 97]. Disease stage and classification have important implications in recommending treatment strategies and may have both prognostic and predictive values. Tumor grade is classified as low grade (G1), intermediate grade (G2), and high grade/poorly differentiated (G3) depending on proliferation, defined by mitotic rate and Ki-67. It is increasingly recognized that not all G3 tumors behave in a uniform fashion. Cell differentiation is now recognized as an important prognostic marker and may predict response to therapy. In addition, well-differentiated (G1/2) and poorly differentiated (G3) tumors have different etiologies and molecular profiles [98–100]. The WHO staging guidelines have recently been updated to reflect these changes [101]. In addition, molecular analysis has demonstrated certain genetic signatures are prognostic. Examples include chromosome instability, due to loss of genes including DAXX or ATRX, that has been associated with decreased overall survival [78, 102, 103].

The presence of liver metastases is one of the strongest prognostic factors in PNETs. Ten-year survival without liver metastases is 70–90%, whereas when liver disease is present, it is only 10–20% [24, 47]. The impact and extent of nodal involvement on prognosis, however, is more controversial [78]. Recent studies have demonstrated the number of lymph nodes resected, and the number of involved nodes has prognostic significance. Lymphadenectomy reduces persistent disease and improves survival and should be included in the initial operation for sporadic gastrinomas [78, 104, 105].

13.8 Management of Localized Sporadic Disease

With the introduction of effective medical therapy for the control of gastric acid hypersecretion in patients with ZES, the role of surgery in the management of patients with gastrinoma has shifted from the control of gastric acid secretion to the requirement for oncological resection of the primary tumor to prevent disease progression and metastatic spread [30, 33, 42, 47, 74, 106]. Surgical resection is the only modality capable of achieving cure in patients with ZES. Given the malignant potential of the primary tumor, surgery also has an important role in preventing the progression to metastatic disease. In their study comparing the long-term follow-up of 160 patients with ZES undergoing surgical resection of gastrinoma with 35 ZES patients managed non-operatively, Norton et al. found significantly fewer patients undergoing surgical resection developed hepatic metastases during long-term follow-up (5% vs. 29%) [40]. More importantly, this group demonstrated that surgery can increase survival. The 15-year disease-specific survival was 98% in the surgery group versus 74% in the non-operative group. In those patients who did not undergo surgery, 90% of deaths were secondary to progressive metastatic disease. Similarly Ellison et al. found that patients undergoing R0 resections had a significantly greater long-term survival than those who had incomplete resection of disease or who did not undergo surgery (10-year survival 85% vs. 30%) [40].

Surgical resection of the primary tumor and involved regional lymph nodes is curative in patients with gastrinoma that have not metastasized to distant sites. Inspection and palpation of the structures in the gastrinoma triangle are performed after Kocherization of the duodenum and can successfully detect 61–71% of primary gastrinomas [21, 42, 43]. Intraoperative ultrasound (IOS) has been shown to improve the ability to localize primary tumors of the pancreas and identify metastatic disease within the liver but is not more sensitive than palpation in the detection of duodenal primaries [19, 43]. Small primary tumors within the duodenum are best identified by inspection and palpation of the mucosal surface via a longitudinal duodenotomy of the second part of the duodenum and inversion of the mucosa [20, 21]. After introducing routine duodenotomy to the operative exploration of patients with ZES, Norton et al. demonstrated a significant improvement in the ability to localize the primary tumors from 76% to 98% of cases [19]. Routine duodenotomy also had significantly higher rates of long-term biochemical cure post-operatively, occurring in 52% of patients undergoing duodenotomy versus 26% of patients who did not.

Options for resection of the primary gastrinoma are dependent on the location and size of the tumor (Table 13.3). Most duodenal lesions are small and can be resected locally, either removing from the submucosa or with an elliptical resection of the full-thickness of the duodenal wall (Fig. 13.1). Lesions of the pancreas can be enucleated or formally resected depending on their size, relationship with the pancreatic duct and location within the gland. Lesions within the head of the pancreas smaller than 2 cm can be enucleated in most cases. Pancreaticoduodenectomy is required for large or locally invasive tumors of the head of the pancreas. Distal

Table 13.3 Surgical strategies for Zollinger–Ellison Syndrome

Clinical scenario	Strategy
Sporadic localized disease	
Pancreatic gastrinoma	
Size <3 cm	Enucleation (open or laparoscopic)
Size >3 cm	En-bloc resection
	Whipple or distal pancreatctomy + lymph node resection
Duodenal gastrinoma	
Solitary/small	Local resection + portal lymph node resection
Multiple +/−large +/−	Pancreaticoduodenectomy + portal node resection
Local invasion	
Metastatic gastrinoma	Consider surgical cytoreduction of hepatic metastases if >70–90% of tumor volume removable
	And/or
	Multimodality medical therapy: PPI, SSAs, PRRT, hepatic artery embolization, mTOR inhibitors, chemotherapy
ZES/MEN 1	
Biochemical or image detected <2 cm	Duodenotomy, 80% distal pancreatectomy & enucleation of pNETs—Head of pancreas + lymph nodes resection
	Or
	Duodenotomy, local resection of pNETs
	Consider lymph nodes resection
	Or
	Treat medically with PPIs
Image detected >2 cm	Duodenotomy and en-bloc pancreatic resection with regional lymph nodes

MEN1 multiple endocrine neoplasia type I, *mTOR* mammalian target of rapamycin, *pNET* pancreatic neuroendocrine tumor, *PPI* proton pump inhibitor, *SSA* somatostatin analogues, *ZES* Zollinger-Ellison syndrome, *PRRT* peptide receptor radionuclide therapy

pancreatectomy is the procedure of choice for the less common scenario where the gastrinoma is located in the body or tail of the gland [54, 107] (Fig. 13.6a, b).

Although not considered standard of care, intralesional injection with ethanol using EUS guidance has been used in small pancreatic neoplasms with some success [108–110]. In a series of eight patients with small pancreatic neoplasms (including 1 gastrinoma), complete response was seen in 6, persistent disease in 2, and recurrence in 1. The study authors concluded that EUS-guided ethanol ablation may be a potential treatment option for patients with small solid pancreatic neoplasms [110].

Metastatic involvement of regional lymph nodes can be demonstrated in 36–67% of patients with gastrinoma; therefore, resection of regional lymph node groups should occur at the time of resection of the primary tumor [47, 55, 57]. In a study of 41 patients with sporadic gastrinoma, Bartsch et al demonstrated systematic lymphadenectomy with excision of more than 10 lymph nodes resulted in a higher rate of biochemical cure and a trend toward prolonged disease-specific survival ($p = 0.06$), disease-free survival ($p = 0.120$), and reduced risk of death ($p = 0.037$), when

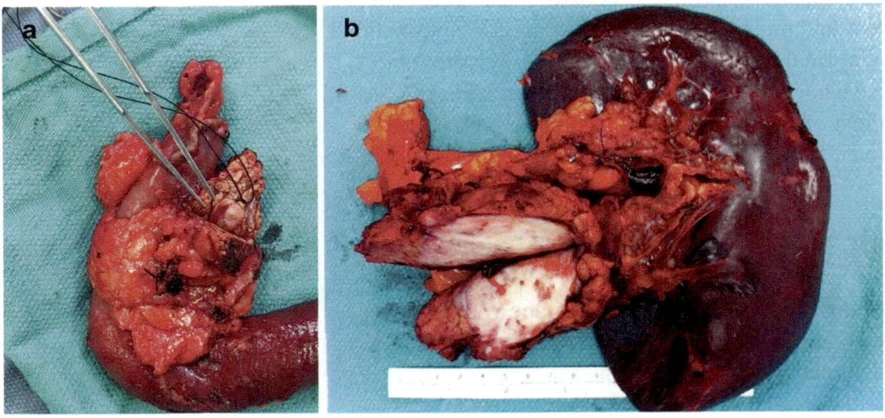

Fig. 13.6 (**a**) The surgical specimen following a pancreatoduodenectomy (Whipple procedure) for a 2.6 cm gastrinoma in the head of the pancreas (suture). This tumor was found to be a well-diffientiated neuroendocrine tumor with local invasion and negative lymph nodes. Biochemical cure at 1 year was obtained. (**b**) Surgical specimen following a distal pancreatectomy for a rare distal pancreas gastrinoma

compared to patients who did not undergo nodal dissection or where only selective lymphadenectomy was performed [111]. Therefore, it is recommended that peritumoural lymph node dissection should be routinely performed in patients with gastrinoma [78].

Laparoscopic and minimally invasive techniques have been successfully utilized for patients with NET, including gastrinoma. Although minimally invasive pancreatic surgery may be more technically challenging than open techniques, it has been successfully reported in the literature with good clinical outcomes for the resection of PNETs [106, 112]. Whether the gastrinoma is resected endoscopically, laparoscopically, or with an open procedure, it is paramount that adherence to the surgical principles outlined above is maintained.

Because primary tumors in ZES are usually small, tumor localization remains challenging in some patients, even despite recent advances and improvements in targeted molecular imaging. As a result, exploratory surgery to identify the primary lesion is sometimes required. In the open era of surgery duodenal palpation, duodenotomy and intraoperative ultrasound allows for the identification of more than 90% of gastrinomas [19]. However, in the era of laparoscopic surgery, tactile feedback is lacking. Fluorescence-guided surgery is an emerging technique as an intraoperative adjunct to define surgical anatomy, facilitate tumor localization, and to identify nodal disease and metastatic deposits in many tumor types [113–115]. Using this technique, a vital dye, Indocyanine green (ICG), is delivered intravenously during the procedure. ICG binds rapidly to serum proteins and is identified using near-infrared (NIR) fluorescence imaging (approximately 820 nm). ICG has been available since the 1950s and has been traditionally used for determining cardiac output, hepatic function, and ophthalmic perfusion [114]. It has a short half-life (150–180 s) and is metabolized by the liver. It is thought that ICG accumulates in neoplastic tissue due to neovascularization and increased permeability of tumor vasculature, and due to impaired clearance. NIR allows visualization of tissue uptake in real time and is capable of penetrating tissues more than 5 mm. In a recent case report by Muntean et al., ICG successfully identified a small (3 mm) submucosal tumor in the duodenum in a patient with ZES which facilitated local resection [116] (Fig. 13.7).

Biochemical cure following surgery for ZES is defined as a normal FSG and negative secretin/calcium stimulation test. Most large series report that initial biochemical cure after surgery is achieved in more than 60% of cases. Rates of biochemical cure however reduce over time, and this is maintained in only 23–50% of cases at 10 years [5, 40, 111]. Although recurrence after potentially curative surgery occurs commonly, disease-specific survival remains excellent with 15-year survival rates between 74% and 98% [5, 40, 111]. Natural history studies demonstrate that 25% of sporadic ZES patients have an aggressive clinical course [56, 57]. In one retrospective study, negative prognostic factors for disease-specific survival were pancreatic location, tumor size >2.5 cm, Ki-67 index >5%, preoperative FSG > 3000 pg/mL, and the presence of liver metastases [111]. Interestingly, sex, age, type of surgery, and presence of lymph nodes metastases had no influence on disease-free or disease-specific survival. Others have found female gender, ectopic ACTH production, and bone metastases also are negative prognostic factors [6, 57].

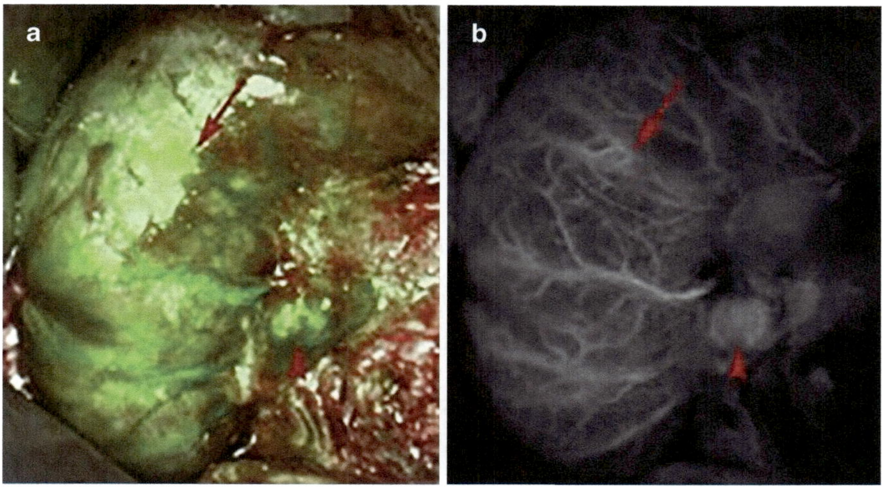

Fig. 13.7 Near infrared fluorescence visualization of the pancreatic head and duodenum 30 s after intravenous ICG injection. Color image with ICG overlay (**a**) and grayscale (**b**) A 92% signal is evident on the juxta-duodenal metastatic lymph node (arrowhead). Another 90% signal is visible on the duodenal wall, 2 cm cranial to the major duodenal papilla (arrow). Reproduced with permission V Muntean, A Tantau, S Strilciuc, MV Muntean, Intraoperative nearinfrared fluorescence visualization of the duodenal gastrinoma in a patient with Zollinger–Ellison syndrome, Surgery, 159, 1474–6, Elsevier, copyright 2016

13.9 Management of Advanced and Metastatic Disease

Both H2-receptor antagonists (H2RAs) and PPIs are highly effective and are the cornerstone of medical management of gastric hypersecretion of ZES. PPIs have been demonstrated to have an excellent safety profile, are well tolerated, and carry minimal long-term side effects. There is increasing evidence, however, that long-term use is not benign and may result in hypomagnesmia as well as vitamin B_{12} and calcium deficiency due to hypochlorhydria. Recent studies have demonstrated increased risk of bone fractures with long-term use [117–119]. PPIs and H2RAs are safe to use in pregnancy in ZES patients [24]. In addition, PPI use may be associated with proliferation of enterochromaffin-like cells (ECL cells) due to chronic hypergastrinemia. Animal models have demonstrated an increased risk of developing malignant gastric carcinoid tumors in this setting, and ECL cell hyperplasia is also seen in humans, although its clinical significance is yet to be qualified [24, 120, 121].

Novel agents targeting gastrin/CCK2 receptors have been developed. Netazepide (YF476) is a potent, highly selective antagonist of gastrin/CCK2 receptor with good bioavailability that suppresses gastric acid secretion. Animal models have shown Netazepide prevents ECL hyperplasia, reduces rebound acidity from PPI withdrawal, and prevents the growth and development of ECL tumors [122–125]. Although it has theoretical advantages to existing PPI treatment, its utilization in metastatic ZES remains to be seen.

13.9.1 Surgical Resection

Synchronous liver metastases are found in 20–30% of patients with ZES at the time of diagnosis. In addition, up to 40% of patients will develop disease recurrence following an R0 resection [1, 126, 127]. Medical therapy with PPI is highly effective in the control of gastric acid hypersecretion and for this reason the role of surgical palliative debulking for the control of the endocrinopathy is somewhat controversial. Due to the rarity of ZES, many of the therapies utilized for NETs have been performed on a heterogeneous group of patients, often with small numbers of gastrinomas. Data generated by clinical trials and many cohort studies on functioning and nonfunctioning metastatic NETs are extrapolated and applied to patients with ZES.

As a general principle, multi-modality cytoreduction, including radiofrequency ablation, cryotherapy, surgical resection, and liver-directed therapies for functional NETs, does appear to provide a palliative benefit in patients with endocrinopathies and may improve survival in carefully selected patients [126–132]. In a series of 213 ZES patients, hepatic metastases occurred in 32% of cases [131]. Of these cases, diffuse involvement of the liver precluded resection in 75%, whereas the remaining 19 patients had all gross disease within the liver resected. Patients undergoing resection of hepatic metastases had a 5-year survival rate of 85%, which was superior to those patients with hepatic disease who were not suitable for surgery. Although selection bias played a role in these results, others have also demonstrated a survival benefit associated with the aggressive surgical debulking of NET metastases [132–134]. A 2009 Cochrane Database review concluded that liver resection was the mainstay of survival-prolonging therapy for Stage IV NETs, although no randomized controlled trials were available [135]. More recently, a multi-institutional analysis of the surgical management of hepatic NET metastasis found a prolonged 5- and 10-year survival of 74% and 51%, respectively [130]. Although only 12 (4%) of these patients had ZES, patients with hormonally functioning NETs benefitted the most from surgery. When considering resection of metastatic disease, fluorescence and NIR imaging using ICG are emerging surgical techniques that may be used as an intraoperative adjunct to identify metastatic tumor deposits and ensure adequate margins are achieved [136]. Liver transplantation has been successfully used as a treatment modality in patients with refractory hormone-excess states where the metastatic disease is confined to the liver [25, 137, 138].

13.9.2 Ablative Therapies

Radiofrequency ablation (RFA) of liver metastases may be combined with surgical resection or performed percutaneously to target inaccessible lesions. It has been successfully used to control both tumor burden and patient symptoms. Several criteria for RFA have been proposed based on the number of lesions, size, anatomic location, and proximity to vital structures [25, 139, 140].

13.9.3 Embolization

Hepatic artery embolization (HAE), chemoembolization (HACE), and selective internal radiotherapy (SIRT) with ^{90}Y-labeled microspheres offer options for cytoreduction of bilobar disease not amenable to surgical resection or RFA. They are usually employed for unresectable oligometastatic deposits 3–5 cm in diameter [137]. Response rates after embolization vary between 50 and 96% depending upon the criteria utilized such as biochemical, radiographic, and symptomatic control [128]. Median duration of response extends up to 18 months (range 4–51) [128, 141–143]. Radioembolization of the hepatic artery using $^{90-}$Yttrium-bound resin (SIR-Spheres [Sirtex Medical LDT, New South Wales, Australia]) or glass microspheres (Theraspheres [MDS Nordion, Ottawa, Canada]) has been used in the treatment of hepatic NET metastases including gastrinomas. In a multicenter retrospective review of 148 NET patients undergoing radioembolization, Kennedy et al. found partial response rate of 61%, stable disease 23%, complete response 3%, and progression in 5% at 6 months [144]. King et al. found similar results in 34 NET patients treated with SIR-Spheres. Radiological response was seen in 50%, with symptomatic improvement occurring in 50% of cases at 6 months, with a median survival of 29.4 months [145]. More recently, a study by Barbier and colleagues demonstrated SIRT with ^{90}Y-labeled microspheres was safe and effective for patients with metastatic NETs even when patients had received prior peptide receptor radionuclide therapy. In 40 patients who underwent 54 SIRT procedures, tumor response was seen in 54% at 3 months and 34% at 20 months, with a median survival of 24.7 months. Unlike HAE and HACE, SIRT requires more vigorous patient selection and pre-procedural evaluation for hepatopulmonary shunts. It is recommended that no more than 20% of blood flow is diverted to the lung and some patients may require pre-procedural occlusion of these shunts to minimize extrahepatic delivery of Yttrium [146]. A recent study by Chen and colleagues compared outcomes in 155 patients with NET liver metastases after HACE, HAE, and SIRT. They found no significant differences in disease free survival between these modalities [147]. The timing of liver targeted therapies and utilization with systemic therapies is still unclear. A Phase III trial (NCT02724540) is currently being undertaken to compare clinical outcomes using these modalities [137].

13.9.4 Peptide Receptor Radioligand Therapy

Because more than 80% of NETs express somatostatin receptors, radiolabeled somatostatin analogues can be used therapeutically as targeted therapies in the treatment of metastatic disease. This therapy is known as peptide receptor radioligand therapy (PRRT). Initially, 111-Indium (^{111}In)-labeled octreotide was used, but despite frequent symptomatic responses (seen in 53% of cases), radiographic response was rare [148]. This agent has since been surpassed by more potent somatostatin analogues including DOTATOC, DOTATATE, and DOTANOC labeled with either ^{90}Y or ^{177}Lu [25, 137, 149]. Multiple studies have demonstrated the efficacy of PRRT in the treatment of unresectable low to intermediate grade metastatic NETs [25, 150, 151]. Treatment is usually given over four cycles and is usually well tolerated. Adverse effects include nausea, headache, myelosuppression, and hypocalcemia which are usually mild and reversible [152].

There is limited data in the effectiveness of PRRT in patients with gastrinoma, and much of the data has been extrapolated from a heterogeneous population of NETs. Kwekkeboom et al. presented data from a cohort of over 500 patients with NETs treated with ^{177}Lu-DOTATATE, including 12 patients with gastrinoma. They demonstrated a complete response in 2% and partial response in 38%. Median survival was 128 months, significantly longer than that of historical controls. Patients with gastrinoma had a delayed time to progression and improved overall survival [150]. In a separate retrospective study of 11 patients with gastrinomas treated with PRRT, this was associated with effective symptom control and a reduction of serum gastrin levels. Complete response occurred in one patient, partial response in 5, and stable disease in 5 [2, 153].

NETTER-1 (NCT01578230) is a landmark trial using PRRT to establish patient safety and therapeutic effectiveness in patients with progressive NETs. This prospective, phase III, randomized trial compared treatment with ^{177}Lu-DOTATATE plus long-acting octreotide (LAR) 30 mg against high dose (60 mg) LAR in 229 patients with progressive, non-resectable somatostatin receptor positive midgut NETs. Preliminary results have indicated significantly improved progression free survival (PFS) and a significantly higher response rate for patients treated with PRRT and LAR compared to patients receiving high-dose LAR alone ($p < 0.0001$). Although the time point has not yet been reached to perform a median overall survival analysis, these preliminary results suggest an improvement in overall survival for the arm that received PRRT [154]. How PRRT effects gastrinomas has yet to be demonstrated, but the efficacy of this therapy in small bowel NET may indicate a role for this therapy in the management of patients with ZES where unresectable metastatic disease is present.

13.9.5 Systemic Therapies

Medical treatment with somatostatin analogs (SSAs) including octreotide and lanreotide is utilized in metastatic gastrinoma to reduce both tumor gastrin production and for their anti-proliferate properties [58]. SSAs act via G-coupled membrane receptors to inhibit neuroendocrine function by modulating adenylate cyclase activity and calcium exchange. Somatostatin may also inhibit cell proliferation via MAP kinase pathways. In humans, there are five identified somatostatin receptor subtypes, designated sstr1,2,3,4, and 5. The SSAs octreotide and lanreotide bind with high affinity to sstr2A receptors, moderate affinity to sstr5 receptors, and low affinity to sstr3 receptors. Gastrinomas and their metastases strongly express sstr2. In fact, sstr2 was expressed in 100% of gastrinomas in a series of 33 patients by Kulaksiz and colleagues. In addition, sstr3 and sstr5 were expressed in 79% and 76% of gastrinomas, respectively. This high level of sstr expression in gastrinomas provides the rationale for the use of SSAs. Because of the effectiveness of PPIs in controlling clinical symptoms, SSAs are not usually recommended as the first line of therapy for symptom control. They are, however, currently indicated in patients with progressive low-grade metastatic gastrinomas [47, 155–157].

There is limited data on the efficacy of SSAs in ZES. Most data are extrapolated from series involving a mixture of NETs. There are small series supporting the use of SSAs in gastrinomas and ZES. The largest of these studies involved the prospective analysis of 15 patients with progressive metastatic gastrinoma treated with subcutaneous octreotide, including three patients with MEN 1. A radiological response was seen in 53% of cases and disease stabilization achieved in 47%. The mean duration of the clinical response was 25 months [158].

Systemic therapy with cytotoxic chemotherapy has traditionally been thought to have only a limited role in the management of disseminated metastatic gastrinoma. Recently however there has been a resurgence of interest in these treatments with a recognition that tumor biology may predict the response to systemic therapy. Tumor Ki67 levels appear to correlate with response rates. Patients with high Ki67 (>55%) demonstrate higher tumor response rates but have worse overall survival [99]. Previously, streptozotocin-based chemotherapy regimes were used for metastatic gastrinoma but were associated with significant toxicity. These have now largely been replaced by combinations of platinum-based agents and etoposide which have a better side effect profile [24, 155, 159]. Combination cisplatin and irinotecan has also shown similar efficacy in patients with metastatic NET, but to date has mainly been used to treat patients with small cell lung cancer [160, 161]. The combination of temzolamide and capecitabine also shows promising results in well-differentiated metastatic neuroendocrine tumors, with objective response rates of 43–70% and improved progression free survival of 12–18 months [162].

Several medical agents targeting growth factor receptors and related signaling pathways have recently been studied for the management of metastatic NET. Everolimus is an inhibitor of mammalian target of rapamycin (mTOR), a serine-threonine kinase involved in cell-cycle growth regulation, and apoptosis via the PI3K/AKT/mTOR signaling pathway. In the RADIANT-3 study, a prospective, double blind, randomized, placebo-controlled multicenter study examining 410 patients with low-to-intermediate grade pancreatic NET, patients were randomized to everolimus (10 mg/day) or placebo. Patients treated with everolimus demonstrated an improved progression free survival from 4.6 to 11 months [163]. Median overall survival was 44 months and associated with a survival benefit of 6.3 months; however, this was not statistically significant and the authors speculate this may be due to crossover of a large number of patients from the placebo to the treatment arm [164]. The RADIANT-4 study was a randomized, double-blind phase III, placebo-controlled study and examined 302 patients with advanced, progressive, well-differentiated nonfunctional neuroendocrine tumors of the lung or gastrointestinal tract. Patients were randomized to everolimus (10 mg/day) or placebo. Results demonstrated significantly improved progression free survival from 3.9 months on placebo to 11 months for treated patients. The treatment was found to be beneficially independent of the site of the primary NET (including GI and lung sites), and as a result, the US Food and Drug Administration (FDA) has approved the use of everolimus for the treatment of advanced or metastatic NET regardless of primary site [164].

Sunitinib is a tyrosine kinase inhibitor that inhibits vascular endothelial growth factor receptors (VEGFRs) and platelet-derived growth factor receptors (PDGFRs), both of which are expressed on pancreatic NETs. In a phase III multicenter, double-blinded, randomized, placebo-controlled trial, patients with low-to-intermediate grade progressive pancreatic NETs treated with sunitinib had improved progression-free survival (11.4 vs. 5.5 months), and increased overall survival compared with placebo [165]. As a result, TKIs have been approved by the FDA for patients with advanced and metastatic NET. Although adverse reactions are commonly seen during treatment with TKIs, most events are grade 1 or 2 toxicities.

Other anti-angiogenic agents including pazopanib and axitinib have been investigated for the treatment of metastatic NET. A phase II trial examining the combination of pazopanib with octreotide LAR in 32 patients with advanced pancreatic NET demonstrated an objective tumor response in 21% [166]. Bevacizumab is a monoclonal antibody that targets VEGF. Increased expression of VEGF in both gastrointestinal and pulmonary NET has been associated with poor outcomes [167]. Initial phase II trials of bevacizumab showed promising results; however, a phase III trial in 427 patients with advanced NET did not show an improvement in progression free survival compared with placebo [168, 169].

Combination therapies using these drugs have also been examined with some promising results in phase II trials. A trial of 56 patients with progressive pancreatic NET treated with a combination of bevacizumab and temsirolimus showed objective tumor response in 41% with a median progression-free survival of 13.2 months [170]. In another phase II trial, 150 patients were treated with either everolimus and octreotide or the combination of everolimus, bevacizumab, and octreotide. Treatment with the triple regime resulted in an objective tumor response in 31% and a small benefit in progression-free survival, but this did not meet statistical significance (14 months vs. 16.7 months; $p = 0.12$) These studies provide optimism for the systemic treatment of NETs; however, few trials have included significant numbers of patients with gastrinoma or ZES. In this way, the choice of drug and optimal sequence of therapeutic options for metastatic gastrinoma remains unanswered [47, 106, 171–173].

13.10 Management of ZES/MEN 1

The management of the gastrinomas occurring as part of MEN 1 syndrome remains controversial [5, 6, 8, 174, 175]. The role of surgery in the management of ZES in the context of MEN 1 is less clearly defined than for sporadic tumors. Patients with ZES/MEN 1 have better long-term survival rates yet lower rates of long-term cure after surgical resection compared with sporadic ZES cases, and treatment with PPI offers effective medical control of this condition [5, 6, 40].

ZES occurring in the context of MEN 1 displays important differences in biological behavior compared with sporadic gastrinomas. The mean age of onset of ZES in patients with MEN 1 is younger (34–42 years), and rare before the age of 24 years. The duodenum is the most common site of gastrinoma in patients with MEN 1, occurring in up to 88% of cases, with synchronous tumors of the duodenum and the pancreas occurring in 24%. ZES is the most common functional endocrinopathy in patients with MEN 1 (42–60%), followed by insulinoma (19%), vasoactive intestinal polypeptide producing tumors (4%), and non-functional NETs (35%) also occurring [8, 176]. The long-term survival of patients with ZES/MEN 1 is excellent, and there is evidence that gastrinomas occurring in the context of MEN 1 may have a lower malignant potential than sporadic tumors. Hepatic metastases are present in only 3–4% of MEN 1 patients with gastrinoma at the time of diagnosis but will develop in long-term follow-up in as many as 14–23% [177]. A number of studies have found that the long-term survival of patients with MEN 1 developing ZES is superior to that seen in sporadic forms of the tumor [8]. Utilizing the long-term prospective NIH database, Ito et al. found that the 30-year overall survival for ZES/MEN 1 was 85% and disease-related survival 88% [178]. Factors predicting a poorer prognosis were high serum gastrin levels, development of other endocrinopathies, the need for more than three parathyroid operations, high tumor mitotic count, and distant metastases [179, 180].

Since the introduction of effective medical therapy for control of gastric acid hypersecretion, patients with ZES/MEN 1 no longer die from complications of severe PUD, and long-term survival can be expected [177, 178, 181]. The rate of biochemical cure of ZES/MEN 1 is rare except when either a Whipple's procedure or total pancreaticoduodenectomy has been performed. Most of the pancreatic NET found in the MEN 1 pancreas are non-functioning. In ZES/MEN 1 most gastrinomas are found in the duodenum, and as such if surgery is undertaken a duodenotomy must be performed in search of these small lesions. Most surgeons who believe surgery is beneficial to the MEN 1 patient advocate the *Thompson procedure* [174, 175]. This involves a distal pancreatectomy, enucleation of NETs in the head of the pancreas, a duodenotomy and resection of any duodenal tumors, along with a lymph node dissection around the porta hepatis [101]. Unfortunately, long-term biochemical cure after this operation for ZES/MEN 1 patients is rarely achieved [54, 182]. Initially, postoperative normalization of FSG occurred in 68% of ZES/MEN 1 patients without hepatic metastases, but this rate falls to 33% with provocative testing with intravenous secretin, implying that most patients harbor microscopic foci of residual disease [182, 183]. Many of the original ZES/MEN 1 patients operated on by Thompson have had to undergo a completion Whipple operation [183]. A more focused approach to resection of pancreatic NETs, leaving a larger pancreatic remnant and enucleating lesions in the body of the gland, has been adopted by the University of Michigan due to the high incidence of recurrent disease and surgical challenges associated with completion Whipple procedures.

Since biochemical cure is rare after surgery in patients with ZES/MEN 1, and symptomatic control is easily achieved with PPIs, it has been argued that surgery is more important in reducing the risk of subsequent metastatic disease in these patients [175, 184]. Akerström et al. utilize both biochemical and EUS screening to identify patients early before the development of metastases [175]. Once the patient develops an endocrinopathy such as ZES, the risk of lymph node metastases is more than 50%. Therefore, these authors do not wait for anatomical imaging to demonstrate NETs. Thompson on the other hand suggested that surgery should be done when any tumor was visualized by cross-sectional imaging [185]. Others have taken a more conservative approach, utilizing surgical resection for tumors of more than 2–3 cm in size, citing the low risk of hepatic metastases with smaller tumors [177, 186, 187]. From the NIH database, Norton et al. demonstrated that patients with tumors less than 2.5 cm size can be safely monitored with a minimal risk of developing liver metastases or mortality [187]. Triponez et al. showed that the metastatic risk increased in MEN 1 patients for tumors >2 cm in size [186]. This data has recently been updated and confirmed that a watchful waiting strategy for patient with MEN 1 with pancreatic NET <2 cm is oncologically safe and avoids the risk of significant complications of major surgery [188–190]. Finally, in a study of 55 patients with MEN 1 and pancreatic NETs, Kouvaraki et al. found that patients who underwent surgical resection had a significantly higher 10-year survival compared with those who did not (81% vs. 34%) [191]. As there is an absence of randomized controlled data examining the role of surgery, the indications for surgical resection for patients with ZES/MEN 1 remains institution specific.

13.11 Summary

The management of ZES has evolved due to advances in diagnostic imaging, medical therapies, and improvements in surgical technique. Surgical resection is the procedure of choice for sporadic gastrinomas and has an important role in the ongoing management of selected patients with ZES/MEN 1 syndrome. As we move from the open era of surgery to minimally invasive endoscopic/robotic approaches, it is important to maintain the principles of localization and adequate loco-regional resection of these tumors. A multimodality approach to treatment of advanced and disseminated disease in patients with ZES is critical. These patients benefit from aggressive cytoreductive approaches to the metastatic disease with the addition of systemic therapies to control both tumor growth and the endocrinopathy.

References

1. Ellison EC, Johnson JA (2009) The Zollinger-Ellison syndrome: a comprehensive review of historical, scientific, and clinical considerations. Curr Probl Surg 46(1):13–06
2. Guarnotta V, Martini C, Davì MV, Pizza G, Colao A, Faggiano A (2017) The Zollinger-Ellison syndrome: is there a role for somatostatin analogues in the treatment of the gastrinoma? Endocrine 142:1–13
3. Zollinger RM, Ellison EH (1955) Primary peptic ulcerations of the jejunum associated with islet cell tumors of the pancreas. Ann Surg 142(4):709–723
4. Ellison EH, Wilson SD (1964) The Zollinger-Elison syndrome: re-appraisal and evaluation of 260 registered cases. Ann Surg 160:512–530
5. Ellison EC, Sparks J, Verducci JS, Johnson JA, Muscarella P, Bloomston M et al (2006) 50-year appraisal of gastrinoma: recommendations for staging and treatment. J Am Coll Surg 202(6):897–905
6. Osefo N, Ito T, Jensen RT (2009) Gastric acid hypersecretory states: recent insights and advances. Curr Gastroenterol Rep 11(6):433–441
7. Bartsch D, Kopp I, Bergenfelz A, Rieder H, Münch K, Jäger K et al (1998) MEN1 gene mutations in 12 MEN1 families and their associated tumors. Eur J Endocrinol 139(4):416–420
8. Jensen RT, Berna MJ, Bingham DB, Norton JA (2008) Inherited pancreatic endocrine tumor syndromes: advances in molecular pathogenesis, diagnosis, management, and controversies. Cancer 113(7 Suppl):1807–1843
9. Sailer S, Zinninger MM (1946) Massive islet cell tumor of the pancreas without hypoglycemia. Surg Gynecol Obstet 82:301–305
10. Yeung MJ, Pasieka JL (2009) Gastrinomas: a historical perspective. J Surg Oncol 100(5):425–433
11. Gregory RA, Tracy HJ, French JM, Sircus W (1960) Extraction of a gastrin-like substance from a pancreatic tumour in a case of Zollinger-Ellison syndrome. Lancet 1(7133):1045–1048
12. Gregory RA, Grossman MI, Tracy HJ, Bentley PH (1967) Nature of the gastric secretagogue in Zollinger-Ellison tumours. Lancet 2(7515):543–544
13. McGuigan JE, Trudeau WL (1968) Immunochemical measurement of elevated levels of gastrin in the serum of patients with pancreatic tumors of the Zollinger-Ellison variety. N Engl J Med 278(24):1308–1313
14. Murugesan SVM, Varro A, Pritchard DM (2009) Strategies to determine whether hypergastrinaemia is due to Zollinger-Ellison syndrome rather than a more common benign cause. Aliment Pharmacol Ther 29(10):1055–1068

15. Isenberg JI, Walsh JH, Passaro E, Moore EW, Grossman MI (1972) Unusual effect of secretin on serum gastrin, serum calcium, and gastric acid secretion in a patient with suspected Zollinger-Ellison syndrome. Gastroenterology 62(4):626–631
16. Rawson AB, England MT, Gillam GG, French JM, Stammers FA (1960) Zollinger-Ellison syndrome with diarrhoea and malabsorption. Observations on a patient before and after pancreatic islet-cell tumour removal with-out resort. Lancet 2(7142):131–134
17. Oberhelman HA, Nelsen TS (1964) Surgical consideration in the management of ulcerogenic tumors of the pancreas and duodenum. Am J Surg 108:132–141
18. Oberhelman HA, Nelsen TS, Johnson AN, Dragstedt LR (1961) Ulcerogenic tumors of the duodenum. Ann Surg 153(2):214–227
19. Norton JA, Alexander HR, Fraker DL, Venzon DJ, Gibril F, Jensen RT (2004) Does the use of routine duodenotomy (DUODX) affect rate of cure, development of liver metastases, or survival in patients with Zollinger-Ellison syndrome? Ann Surg 239(5):617–625. discussion626
20. Thompson NW, Vinik AI, Eckhauser FE (1989) Microgastrinomas of the duodenum. A cause of failed operations for the Zollinger-Ellison syndrome. Ann Surg 209(4):396–404
21. Thompson NW, Pasieka J, Fukuuchi A (1993) Duodenal gastrinomas, duodenotomy, and duodenal exploration in the surgical management of Zollinger-Ellison syndrome. World J Surg 17(4):455–462
22. Underdahl LO, Woolner LB, Black BM (1953) Multiple endocrine adenomas; report of 8 cases in which the parathyroids, pituitary and pancreatic islets were involved. J Clin Endocrinol Metab 13(1):20–47
23. Wermer P (1954) Genetic aspects of adenomatosis of endocrine glands. Am J Med 16(3):363–371
24. De Angelis C, Cortegoso Valdivia P, Venezia L, Bruno M, Pellicano R (2017) Diagnosis and management of Zollinger-Ellison syndrome in 2017. Minerva Endocrinol
25. Ito T, Lee L, Jensen RT (2016) Treatment of symptomatic neuroendocrine tumor syndromes: recent advances and controversies. Expert Opin Pharmacother 17(16):2191–2205
26. Metz DC (2012) Diagnosis of the Zollinger–Ellison syndrome. Clin Gastroenterol Hepatol 10(2):126–130
27. Roy PK, Venzon DJ, Shojamanesh H, Abou-Saif A, Peghini P, Doppman JL et al (2000) Zollinger-Ellison syndrome. Clinical presentation in 261 patients. Medicine (Baltimore) 79(6):379–411
28. Corleto VD, Annibale B, Gibril F, Angeletti S, Serrano J, Venzon DJ et al (2001) Does the widespread use of proton pump inhibitors mask, complicate and/or delay the diagnosis of Zollinger-Ellison syndrome? Aliment Pharmacol Ther 15(10):1555–1561
29. Yao JC, Eisner MP, Leary C, Dagohoy C, Phan A, Rashid A et al (2007) Population-based study of islet cell carcinoma. Ann Surg Oncol 14(12):3492–3500
30. Soga J, Yakuwa Y (1998) The gastrinoma/Zollinger-Ellison syndrome: statistical evaluation of a Japanese series of 359 cases. J Hepato-Biliary-Pancreat Surg 5(1):77–85
31. Roy PK, Venzon DJ, Feigenbaum KM, Koviack PD, Bashir S, Ojeaburu JV et al (2001) Gastric secretion in Zollinger-Ellison syndrome. Correlation with clinical expression, tumor extent and role in diagnosis-a prospective NIH study of 235 patients and a review of 984 cases in the literature. Medicine 80(3):189–222
32. Fendrich V, Langer P, Waldmann J, Bartsch DK, Rothmund M (2007) Management of sporadic and multiple endocrine neoplasia type 1 gastrinomas. Br J Surg 94(11):1331–1341
33. Ellison EC, Sparks J (2003) Zollinger-Ellison syndrome in the era of effective acid suppression: are we unknowingly growing tumors? Am J Surg 186(3):245–248
34. Ito T, Igarashi H, Jensen RT (2013) Zollinger-Ellison syndrome: recent advances and controversies. Curr Opin Gastroenterol 29(6):650–661
35. Mendelson AH, Donowitz M. Catching the zebra: clinical pearls and pitfalls for the successful diagnosis of Zollinger-Ellison syndrome. Dig Dis Sci 2017;62(9):2258–2265. 10 ed.
36. Weinstein DH, deRijke S, Chow CC, Foruraghi L, Zhao X, Wright EC et al (2013) A new method for determining gastric acid output using a wireless pH-sensing capsule. Aliment Pharmacol Ther 37(12):1198–1209. 5 ed.

37. Berna MJ, Hoffmann KM, Serrano J, Gibril F, Jensen RT (2006) Serum gastrin in Zollinger-Ellison syndrome: I. Prospective study of fasting serum gastrin in 309 patients from the National Institutes of Health and comparison with 2229 cases from the literature. Medicine 85(6):295–330
38. Vezzosi D, Walter T, Laplanche A, Raoul J-L, Dromain C, Ruszniewski P et al (2011) Chromogranin A measurement in metastatic well-differentiated gastroenteropancreatic neuroendocrine carcinoma: screening for false positives and a prospective follow-up study. Int J Biol Markers 26(2):94–101
39. Abou-Saif A, Gibril F, Ojeaburu JV, Bashir S, Entsuah LK, Asgharian B et al (2003) Prospective study of the ability of serial measurements of serum chromogranin a and gastrin to detect changes in tumor burden in patients with gastrinomas. Cancer 98(2):249–261
40. Norton JA, Fraker DL, Alexander HR, Gibril F, Liewehr DJ, Venzon DJ et al (2006) Surgery increases survival in patients with gastrinoma. Ann Surg 244(3):410–419
41. Stabile BE, Morrow DJ, Passaro E (1984) The gastrinoma triangle: operative implications. Am J Surg 147(1):25–31
42. Zogakis TG, Gibril F, Libutti SK, Norton JA, White DE, Jensen RT et al (2003) Management and outcome of patients with sporadic gastrinoma arising in the duodenum. Ann Surg 238(1):42–48
43. Sugg SL, Norton JA, Fraker DL, Metz DC, Pisegna JR, Fishbeyn V et al (1993) A prospective study of intraoperative methods to diagnose and resect duodenal gastrinomas. Ann Surg 218(2):138–144
44. Norton JA, Fraker DL, Alexander HR, Jensen RT (2012) Value of surgery in patients with negative imaging and sporadic Zollinger-Ellison syndrome. Ann Surg 256(3):509–517
45. Pipeleers-Marichal M, Donow C, Heitz PU, Klöppel G (1993) Pathologic aspects of gastrinomas in patients with Zollinger-Ellison syndrome with and without multiple endocrine neoplasia type I. World J Surg 17(4):481–488
46. Phan GQ, Yeo CJ, Hruban RH, Littemoe KD, Pitt HA, Cameron JL (1998) Surgical experience with pancreatic and peripancreatic neuroendocrine tumors: review of 125 patients. J Gastrointest Surg 2(5):473–482
47. Jensen RT, Cadiot G, Brandi ML, de Herder WW, Kaltsas G, Komminoth P, et al. (2012) ENETS Consensus Guidelines for the management of patients with digestive neuroendocrine neoplasms: functional pancreatic endocrine tumor syndromes; 98–119. https://doi.org/10.1111/jne.13249
48. Bartsch DK, Fendrich V, Langer P, Celik I, Kann PH, Rothmund M (2005) Outcome of duodenopancreatic resections in patients with multiple endocrine neoplasia type 1. Ann Surg 242(6):757–764. – discussion764–6
49. Wu PC, Alexander HR, Bartlett DL, Doppman JL, Fraker DL, Norton JA et al (1997) A prospective analysis of the frequency, location, and curability of ectopic (nonpancreaticoduodenal, nonnodal) gastrinoma. Surgery 122(6):1176–1182
50. Harvey A, Pasieka JL, Al-Bisher H, Dixon E (2012) Primary hepatic gastrinoma causing zollinger-ellison syndrome: a rare and challenging diagnosis. Cancers 4(1):130–140
51. Hirasawa K, Yamada M, Kitagawa M, Takehira Y, Tamakoshi K, Nakamura T et al (2000) Ovarian mucinous cystadenocarcinoma as a cause of Zollinger-Ellison syndrome: report of a case and review of the literature. Am J Gastroenterol 95(5):1348–1351
52. Norton JA, Alexander HR, Fraker DL, Venzon DJ, Gibril F, Jensen RT (2003) Possible primary lymph node gastrinoma: occurrence, natural history, and predictive factors: a prospective study. Ann Surg 237(5):650–657. –discussion657–9
53. Anlauf M, Enosawa T, Henopp T, Schmitt A, Gimm O, Brauckhoff M et al (2008) Primary lymph node gastrinoma or occult duodenal microgastrinoma with lymph node metastases in a MEN1 patient: the need for a systematic search for the primary tumor. Am J Surg Pathol 32(7):1101–1105
54. Norton JA, Fraker DL, Alexander HR, Venzon DJ, Doppman JL, Serrano J et al (1999) Surgery to cure the Zollinger-Ellison syndrome. N Engl J Med 341(9):635–644

55. Giovinazzo F, Butturini G, Monsellato D, Malleo G, Marchegiani G, Bassi C (2013) Lymph nodes metastasis and recurrences justify an aggressive treatment of gastrinoma. Updat Surg 65(1):19–24
56. Weber HC, Venzon DJ, Lin JT, Fishbein VA, Orbuch M, Strader DB et al (1995) Determinants of metastatic rate and survival in patients with Zollinger-Ellison syndrome: a prospective long-term study. Gastroenterology 108(6):1637–1649
57. Yu F, Venzon DJ, Serrano J, Goebel SU, Doppman JL, Gibril F et al (1999) Prospective study of the clinical course, prognostic factors, causes of death, and survival in patients with long-standing Zollinger-Ellison syndrome. J Clin Oncol 17(2):615–630
58. Metz DC, Jensen RT (2008) Gastrointestinal neuroendocrine tumors: pancreatic endocrine tumors. Gastroenterology 135(5):1469–1492
59. Gibril F, Doppman JL, Reynolds JC, Chen CC, Sutliff VE, Yu F et al (1998) Bone metastases in patients with gastrinomas: a prospective study of bone scanning, somatostatin receptor scanning, and magnetic resonance image in their detection, frequency, location, and effect of their detection on management. J Clin Oncol 16(3):1040–1053
60. Goebel SU, Heppner C, Burns AL, Marx SJ, Spiegel AM, Zhuang Z et al (2000) Genotype/phenotype correlation of multiple endocrine neoplasia type 1 gene mutations in sporadic gastrinomas. J Clin Endocrinol Metab 85(1):116–123
61. Kawamura J, Shimada Y, Komoto I, Okamoto H, Itami A, Doi R et al (2005) Multiple endocrine neoplasia type 1 gene mutations in sporadic gastrinomas in Japan. Oncol Rep 14(1):47–52
62. Wild A, Langer P, Celik I, Chaloupka B, Bartsch DK (2002) Chromosome 22q in pancreatic endocrine tumors: identification of a homozygous deletion and potential prognostic associations of allelic deletions. Eur J Endocrinol 147(4):507–513
63. Chen Y-J, Vortmeyer A, Zhuang Z, Gibril F, Jensen RT (2004) X-chromosome loss of heterozygosity frequently occurs in gastrinomas and is correlated with aggressive tumor growth. Cancer 100(7):1379–1387
64. Serrano J, Goebel SU, Peghini PL, Lubensky IA, Gibril F, Jensen RT (2000) Alterations in the p16INK4a/CDKN2A tumor suppressor gene in gastrinomas. J Clin Endocrinol Metab 85(11):4146–4156
65. Capelli P, Martignoni G, Pedica F, Falconi M, Antonello D, Malpeli G et al (2009) Endocrine neoplasms of the pancreas: pathologic and genetic features. Arch Pathol Lab Med 133(3):350–364
66. Alexander HR, Fraker DL, Norton JA, Bartlett DL, Tio L, Benjamin SB et al (1998) Prospective study of somatostatin receptor scintigraphy and its effect on operative outcome in patients with Zollinger-Ellison syndrome. Ann Surg 228(2):228–238
67. Gibril F, Reynolds JC, Doppman JL, Chen CC, Venzon DJ, Termanini B et al (1996) Somatostatin receptor scintigraphy: its sensitivity compared with that of other imaging methods in detecting primary and metastatic gastrinomas. A prospective study. Ann Intern Med 125(1):26–34
68. Soyer P, Dohan A, Eveno C, Dray X, Hamzi L, Hoeffel C et al (2013) Carcinoid tumors of the small-bowel: evaluation with 64-section CT-enteroclysis. Eur J Radiol 82(6):943–950
69. Kamaoui I, De-Luca V, Ficarelli S, Mennesson N, Lombard-Bohas C, Pilleul F (2010) Value of CT enteroclysis in suspected small-bowel carcinoid tumors. AJR Am J Roentgenol 194(3):629–633
70. Trudeau WL, McGuigan JE (1969) Effects of calcium on serum gastrin levels in the zollinger-Ellison syndrome. N Engl J Med 281(16):862–866
71. Termanini B, Gibril F, Reynolds JC, Doppman JL, Chen CC, Stewart CA et al (1997) Value of somatostatin receptor scintigraphy: a prospective study in gastrinoma of its effect on clinical management. Gastroenterology 112(2):335–347
72. Krausz Y, Keidar Z, Kogan I, Even-Sapir E, Bar-Shalom R, Engel A et al (2003) SPECT/CT hybrid imaging with 111In-pentetreotide in assessment of neuroendocrine tumours. Clin Endocrinol 59(5):565–573

73. Ruf J, Wedel von F, Furth C, Denecke T, Stelter L, Steffen IG et al (2016) Significance of a single-time-point somatostatin receptor SPECT/multiphase CT protocol in the diagnostic work-up of gastroenteropancreatic neuroendocrine neoplasms. J Nucl Med 57(2):180–185
74. Wong K-K, Gandhi A, Viglianti BL, Fig LM, Rubello D, Gross MD (2016) Endocrine radionuclide scintigraphy with fusion single photon emission computed tomography/computed tomography. World J Radiol 8(6):635–655
75. Sainz-Esteban A, Olmos R, González-Sagrado M, González ML, Ruiz MÁ, García-Talavera P et al (2015) Contribution of ^{111}In-pentetreotide SPECT/CT imaging to conventional somatostatin receptor scintigraphy in the detection of neuroendocrine tumours. Nucl Med Commun 36(3):251–259
76. Kjaer A, Knigge U (2015) Use of radioactive substances in diagnosis and treatment of neuroendocrine tumors. Scand J Gastroenterol 50(6):740–747
77. Wild D, Bomanji JB, Benkert P, Maecke H, Ell PJ, Reubi JC et al (2013) Comparison of 68Ga-DOTANOC and 68Ga-DOTATATE PET/CT within patients with gastroenteropancreatic neuroendocrine tumors. J Nucl Med 54(3):364–372
78. Falconi M, Eriksson B, Kaltsas G, Bartsch DK, Capdevila J, Caplin M, et al. (2016) ENETS consensus guidelines update for the management of patients with functional pancreatic neuroendocrine tumors and non-functional pancreatic neuroendocrine tumors. 153–71. https://doi.org/10.1111/jne.13318
79. Poeppel TD, Binse I, Petersenn S, Lahner H, Schott M, Antoch G et al (2011) 68Ga-DOTATOC versus 68Ga-DOTATATE PET/CT in functional imaging of neuroendocrine tumors. J Nucl Med 52(12):1864–1870
80. Kabasakal L, Demirci E, Ocak M, Decristoforo C, Araman A, Ozsoy Y et al (2012) Comparison of ^{68}Ga-DOTATATE and ^{68}Ga-DOTANOC PET/CT imaging in the same patient group with neuroendocrine tumours. Eur J Nucl Med Mol Imaging 39(8):1271–1277
81. Gabriel M, Decristoforo C, Kendler D, Dobrozemsky G, Heute D, Uprimny C et al (2007) 68Ga-DOTA-Tyr3-octreotide PET in neuroendocrine tumors: comparison with somatostatin receptor scintigraphy and CT. J Nucl Med 48(4):508–518
82. Frilling A, Sotiropoulos GC, Radtke A, Malago M, Bockisch A, Kuehl H et al (2010) The impact of 68Ga-DOTATOC positron emission tomography/computed tomography on the multimodal management of patients with neuroendocrine tumors. Ann Surg 252(5):850–856
83. Putzer D, Gabriel M, Henninger B, Kendler D, Uprimny C, Dobrozemsky G et al (2009) Bone metastases in patients with neuroendocrine tumor: 68Ga-DOTA-Tyr3-octreotide PET in comparison to CT and bone scintigraphy. J Nucl Med 50(8):1214–1221
84. Geijer H, Breimer LH (2013) Somatostatin receptor PET/CT in neuroendocrine tumours: update on systematic review and meta-analysis. Eur J Nucl Med Mol Imaging 40(11):1770–1780
85. Skoura E, Michopoulou S, Mohmaduvesh M, Panagiotidis E, Harbi Al M, Toumpanakis C et al (2016) The impact of 68Ga-DOTATATE PET/CT imaging on management of patients with neuroendocrine tumors: experience from a National Referral Center in the United Kingdom. J Nucl Med 57(1):34–40
86. Herrmann K, Czernin J, Wolin EM, Gupta P, Barrio M, Gutierrez A et al (2015) Impact of 68Ga-DOTATATE PET/CT on the management of neuroendocrine tumors: the referring physician's perspective. J Nucl Med 56(1):70–75
87. Pfeifer A, Knigge U, Binderup T, Mortensen J, Oturai P, Loft A et al (2015) 64Cu-DOTATATE PET for neuroendocrine tumors: a prospective head-to-head comparison with 111In-DTPA-octreotide in 112 patients. J Nucl Med 56(6):847–854
88. Johnbeck CB, Knigge U, Loft A, Berthelsen AK, Mortensen J, Oturai P et al (2017) Head-to-head comparison of (64)Cu-DOTATATE and (68)Ga-DOTATOC PET/CT: a prospective study of 59 patients with neuroendocrine tumors. J Nucl Med 58(3):451–457
89. Fusaroli P, Kypraios D, Caletti G, Eloubeidi MA (2012) Pancreatico-biliary endoscopic ultrasound: a systematic review of the levels of evidence, performance and outcomes. World J Gastroenterol 18(32):4243–4256

90. Wang J, Zhao S, Chen Y, Jia R, Zhang X (2017) Endoscopic ultrasound guided fine needle aspiration versus endoscopic ultrasound guided fine needle biopsy in sampling pancreatic masses: a meta-analysis. Medicine 96(28):e7452
91. van Asselt SJ, Brouwers AH, van Dullemen HM, van der Jagt EJ, Bongaerts AHH, Kema IP et al (2015) EUS is superior for detection of pancreatic lesions compared with standard imaging in patients with multiple endocrine neoplasia type 1. Gastrointest Endosc 81(1):159–167.e2
92. Norton JA, Jensen RT (2004) Resolved and unresolved controversies in the surgical management of patients with Zollinger-Ellison syndrome. Ann Surg 240(5):757–773
93. Kappelle WFW, Valk GD, Leenders M, Moons LMG, Bogte A, Siersema PD et al (2017) Growth rate of small pancreatic neuroendocrine tumors in multiple endocrine neoplasia type 1: results from an endoscopic ultrasound based cohort study. Endoscopy 49(1):27–34
94. Imamura M, Takahashi K (1993) Use of selective arterial secretin injection test to guide surgery in patients with Zollinger-Ellison syndrome. World J Surg 17(4):433–438
95. Wada M, Komoto I, Doi R, Imamura M (2002) Intravenous calcium injection test is a novel complementary procedure in differential diagnosis for gastrinoma. World J Surg 26(10):1291–1296
96. Klöppel G (2011) Classification and pathology of gastroenteropancreatic neuroendocrine neoplasms. Endocr Relat Cancer 18(Suppl 1):S1–S16
97. Kim JY, Hong S-M, Ro JY (2017) Recent updates on grading and classification of neuroendocrine tumors. Ann Diagn Pathol 29:11–16
98. Yachida S, Vakiani E, White CM, Zhong Y, Saunders T, Morgan R et al (2012) Small cell and large cell neuroendocrine carcinomas of the pancreas are genetically similar and distinct from well-differentiated pancreatic neuroendocrine tumors. Am J Surg Pathol 36(2):173–184
99. Sorbye H, Welin S, Langer SW, Vestermark LW, Holt N, Osterlund P et al (2013) Predictive and prognostic factors for treatment and survival in 305 patients with advanced gastrointestinal neuroendocrine carcinoma (WHO G3): the NORDIC NEC study. Ann Oncol 24(1):152–160
100. Tang LH, Untch BR, Reidy DL, O'Reilly E, Dhall D, Jih L, et al. Well-differentiated neuroendocrine tumors with a morphologically apparent high-grade component: a pathway distinct from poorly differentiated neuroendocrine carcinomas. Clin Cancer Res; 2016;22(4):1011–1017
101. Klöppel G, Anlauf M, Perren A (2007) Endocrine precursor lesions of gastroenteropancreatic neuroendocrine tumors. Endocr Pathol 18(3):150–155
102. Marinoni I, Kurrer AS, Vassella E, Dettmer M, Rudolph T, Banz V et al (2014) Loss of DAXX and ATRX are associated with chromosome instability and reduced survival of patients with pancreatic neuroendocrine tumors. Gastroenterology 146(2):453–455
103. Kruljac I, Pape U-F, ulrich-frank. (2017) The classification of neuroendocrine neoplasms: "neuroendocrine carcinomas" revisited—a 2017 update and future perspectives. Endocr Oncol Metabol 3(2):37–42
104. Krampitz GW, Norton JA, Poultsides GA, Visser BC, Sun L, Jensen RT (2012) Lymph nodes and survival in pancreatic neuroendocrine tumors. Arch Surg 147(9):820–819
105. Ito T, Igarashi H, Jensen RT (2012) Therapy of metastatic pancreatic neuroendocrine tumors (pNETs): recent insights and advances. J Gastroenterol 47(9):941–960
106. Howe JR, Merchant NB, Conrad C et al. (2020) The north american neuroendocrine tumor society consensus paper on the surgical management of pancreatic neuroendocrine tumors. Pancreas 49(1)
107. Sarmiento JM, Farnell MB, Que FG, Nagorney DM (2002) Pancreaticoduodenectomy for islet cell tumors of the head of the pancreas: long-term survival analysis. World J Surg 26(10):1267–1271
108. Jürgensen C, Schuppan D, Neser F, Ernstberger J, Junghans U, Stölzel U (2006) EUS-guided alcohol ablation of an insulinoma. Gastrointest Endosc 63(7):1059–1062
109. Levy MJ, Thompson GB, Topazian MD, Callstrom MR, Grant CS, Vella A (2012) US-guided ethanol ablation of insulinomas: a new treatment option. Gastrointest Endosc 75(1):200–206

110. Paik WH, Seo DW, Dhir V, Wang H-P (2016) Safety and efficacy of EUS-guided ethanol ablation for treating small solid pancreatic neoplasm. Medicine 95(4):e2538–e25e5
111. Bartsch DK, Waldmann J, Fendrich V, Boninsegna L, Lopez CL, Partelli S et al (2012) Impact of lymphadenectomy on survival after surgery for sporadic gastrinoma. Br J Surg 99(9):1234–1240
112. Al-Kurd A, Chapchay K, Grozinsky-Glasberg S, Mazeh H (2014) Laparoscopic resection of pancreatic neuroendocrine tumors. World J Gastroenterol 20(17):4908–4916
113. Vahrmeijer AL, Hutteman M, van der Vorst JR, van de Velde CJH, Frangioni JV (2013) Image-guided cancer surgery using near-infrared fluorescence. Nat Rev Clin Oncol 10(9):507–518
114. Boni L, David G, Mangano A, Dionigi G, Rausei S, Spampatti S et al (2015) Clinical applications of indocyanine green (ICG) enhanced fluorescence in laparoscopic surgery. Surg Endosc 29(7):2046–2055
115. Paiella S (2017) Is there a role for near-infrared technology in laparoscopic resection of pancreatic neuroendocrine tumors? Results of the COLPAN "colour-and-resect the pancreas" study. Surg Endosc 31(11):4478–4484
116. Muntean V, Tantau A, Strilciuc S, Muntean MV (2016) Intraoperative near-infrared fluorescence visualization of the duodenal gastrinoma in a patient with Zollinger-Ellison syndrome. Surgery 159(5):1474–1476
117. Reimer C (2013) Safety of long-term PPI therapy. Best Pract Res Clin Gastroenterol 27(3):443–454
118. Ito T, Jensen RT (2010) Association of long-term proton pump inhibitor therapy with bone fractures and effects on absorption of calcium, vitamin B12, iron, and magnesium. Curr Gastroenterol Rep 12(6):448–457
119. Freedberg DE, Kim LS, Yang Y-X (2017) The risks and benefits of long-term use of proton pump inhibitors: expert review and best practice advice from the American Gastroenterological Association. Gastroenterology 152(4):706–715
120. Jensen RT (2006) Consequences of long-term proton pump blockade: insights from studies of patients with gastrinomas. Basic Clin Pharmacol Toxicol 98(1):4–19. 2nd ed.
121. Song H, Zhu J, Lu D (2014) Long-term proton pump inhibitor (PPI) use and the development of gastric pre-malignant lesions. Song H, editor. Cochrane Database Syst Rev 35(12):CD010623
122. Boyce M, Dowen S, Turnbull G, van den Berg F, Zhao C-M, Chen D et al (2015) Effect of netazepide, a gastrin/CCK 2receptor antagonist, on gastric acid secretion and rabeprazole-induced hypergastrinaemia in healthy subjects. Br J Clin Pharmacol 79(5):744–755
123. Boyce M, Thomsen L. Gastric neuroendocrine tumors: prevalence in Europe, USA, and Japan, and rationale for treatment with a gastrin/CCK2 receptor antagonist. Scand J Gastroenterol 2015;50(5):550–559. 4 ed.
124. Kidd M, Siddique Z-L, Drozdov I, Gustafsson BI, Camp RL, Black JW et al (2010) The CCK(2) receptor antagonist, YF476, inhibits Mastomys ECL cell hyperplasia and gastric carcinoid tumor development. Regul Pept 162(1–3):52–60
125. Sato Y, Hashimoto S, Mizuno K-I, Takeuchi M, Terai S (2016) Management of gastric and duodenal neuroendocrine tumors. World J Gastroenterol 22(30):6817–6813
126. Maire F, Sauvanet A, Couvelard A, Rebours V, Vullierme MP, Lebtahi R et al (2012) Recurrence after surgical resection of gastrinoma: who, when, where and why? Eur J Gastroenterol Hepatol 24(4):368–374
127. Grobmyer SR, Hochwald SN (2010) Reoperative surgery for the Zollinger-Ellison syndrome. Adv Surg 44:327–346
128. Lewis MA, Hubbard J (2011) Multimodal liver-directed management of neuroendocrine hepatic metastases. Int J Hepatol 2011(4):452343–12
129. Karabulut K, Akyildiz HY, Lance C, Aucejo F, McLennan G, Agcaoglu O et al (2011) Multimodality treatment of neuroendocrine liver metastases. Surgery 150(2):316–325
130. Mayo SC, de Jong MC, Pulitano C, Clary BM, Reddy SK, Gamblin TC et al (2010) Surgical management of hepatic neuroendocrine tumor metastasis: results from an international multi-institutional analysis. Ann Surg Oncol 17(12):3129–3136

131. Norton JA, Doherty GM, Fraker DL, Alexander HR, Doppman JL, Venzon DJ et al (1998) Surgical treatment of localized gastrinoma within the liver: a prospective study. Surgery 124(6):1145–1152
132. Mayo SC, de Jong MC, Pawlik TM (2011) Surgical management and emerging therapies to prolong survival in metastatic neuroendocrine cancer. Ann Surg Oncol 18(Suppl 3):S220–S2S1
133. Touzios JG, Kiely JM, Pitt SC, Rilling WS, Quebbeman EJ, Wilson SD et al (2005) Neuroendocrine hepatic metastases: does aggressive management improve survival? Ann Surg 241(5):776–783. –discussion783–5
134. Sarmiento JM, Heywood G, Rubin J, Ilstrup DM, Nagorney DM, Que FG (2003) Surgical treatment of neuroendocrine metastases to the liver: a plea for resection to increase survival. J Am Coll Surg 197(1):29–37
135. Gurusamy KS, Ramamoorthy R, Sharma D, Davidson BR (2009) Liver resection versus other treatments for neuroendocrine tumours in patients with resectable liver metastases. Gurusamy KS, editor. Cochrane Database Syst Rev 32(2):CD007060
136. Barabino G, Porcheron J, Cottier M, Cuilleron M, Coutard J-G, Berger M et al (2016) Improving surgical resection of metastatic liver tumors with near-infrared optical-guided fluorescence imaging. Surg Innov 23(4):354–359
137. Cives M, Strosberg J (2017) Treatment strategies for metastatic neuroendocrine tumors of the gastrointestinal tract. Curr Treat Options Oncol 18(3):1–14
138. Fan ST, Le Treut YP, Mazzaferro V, Burroughs AK, Olausson M, Breitenstein S et al (2015) Liver transplantation for neuroendocrine tumour liver metastases. HPB J 17(1):23–28
139. Cazzato RL, Garnon J, Ramamurthy N, Tsoumakidou G, Imperiale A, Namer IJ et al (2016) 18F-FDOPA PET/CT-guided radiofrequency ablation of liver metastases from neuroendocrine tumours: technical note on a preliminary experience. 7 ed. Cardiovasc Intervent Radiol 39:1315–1321
140. Kennedy AS (2016) Hepatic-directed therapies in patients with neuroendocrine tumors. Hematol Oncol Clin North Am 30(1):193–207
141. Zappa M, Abdel-Rehim M, Hentic O, Vullierme MP, Ruszniewski P, Vilgrain V (2012) Liver-directed therapies in liver metastases from neuroendocrine tumors of the gastrointestinal tract. Target Oncol 7(2):107–116
142. John BJ, Davidson BR (2012) Treatment options for unresectable neuroendocrine liver metastases. Expert Rev Gastroenterol Hepatol 6(3):357–369
143. Gupta S, Yao JC, Ahrar K, Wallace MJ, Morello FA, Madoff DC et al (2003) Hepatic artery embolization and chemoembolization for treatment of patients with metastatic carcinoid tumors: the M.D. Anderson experience. Cancer J 9(4):261–267
144. Kennedy AS, Dezarn WA, McNeillie P, Coldwell D, Nutting C, Carter D et al (2008) Radioembolization for unresectable neuroendocrine hepatic metastases using resin 90Y-microspheres: early results in 148 patients. Am J Clin Oncol 31(3):271–279
145. King J, Quinn R, Glenn DM, Janssen J, Tong D, Liaw W et al (2008) Radioembolization with selective internal radiation microspheres for neuroendocrine liver metastases. Cancer 113(5):921–929
146. Lau W-Y, Kennedy AS, Kim YH, Lai HK, Lee R-C, Leung TWT et al (2012) Patient selection and activity planning guide for selective internal radiotherapy with yttrium-90 resin microspheres. Int J Radiat Oncol Biol Phys 82(1):401–407
147. Chen JX, Rose S, White SB, El-Haddad G, Fidelman N, Yarmohammadi H et al (2017) Embolotherapy for neuroendocrine tumor liver metastases: prognostic factors for hepatic progression-free survival and overall survival. Cardiovasc Intervent Radiol 40(1):69–80
148. De Jong M, Valkema R, Jamar F, Kvols LK, Kwekkeboom DJ, Breeman WAP et al (2002) Somatostatin receptor-targeted radionuclide therapy of tumors: preclinical and clinical findings. Semin Nucl Med 32(2):133–140
149. Frilling A, Modlin IM, Kidd M, Russell C, Breitenstein S, Salem R et al (2014) Recommendations for management of patients with neuroendocrine liver metastases. Lancet Oncol 15(1):e8–e21

150. Kwekkeboom DJ, Krenning EP (2016) Peptide receptor radionuclide therapy in the treatment of neuroendocrine tumors. Hematol Oncol Clin North Am 30(1):179–191
151. Cives M, Strosberg J (2017) Radionuclide therapy for neuroendocrine tumors. Curr Oncol Rep 19(2):9
152. Frilling A, Clift AK (2015) Therapeutic strategies for neuroendocrine liver metastases. Cancer 121(8):1172–1186
153. Grozinsky-Glasberg S, Barak D, Fraenkel M, Walter MA, Müeller-Brand J, Eckstein J et al (2010) Peptide receptor radioligand therapy is an effective treatment for the long-term stabilization of malignant gastrinomas. Cancer 117(7):1377–1385
154. Strosberg J, El-Haddad G, Wolin E, Hendifar A, Yao J, Chasen B et al (2017) Phase 3 trial of 177Lu-Dotatate for midgut neuroendocrine tumors. N Engl J Med 376(2):125–135
155. Pavel M, Baudin E, Couvelard A, Krenning E, Öberg K, Steinmüller T, et al. (2012) ENETS Consensus Guidelines for the management of patients with liver and other distant metastases from neuroendocrine neoplasms of foregut, midgut, hindgut, and unknown primary. 157–76. https://doi.org/10.1111/jne.13249
156. Delle Fave G, O'Toole D, Sundin A, Taal B, Ferolla P, Ramage JK, et al. (2016) ENETS consensus guidelines update for gastroduodenal neuroendocrine neoplasms. 119–24.
157. Lamberts SW, van der Lely AJ, De Herder WW, Hofland LJ (1996) Octreotide. Wood AJJ, editor. N Engl J Med 334(4):246–254
158. Shojamanesh H, Gibril F, Louie A, Ojeaburu JV, Bashir S, Abou-Saif A et al (2002) Prospective study of the antitumor efficacy of long-term octreotide treatment in patients with progressive metastatic gastrinoma. Cancer 94(2):331–343
159. Strosberg JR, Coppola D, Klimstra DS, Phan AT, Kulke MH, Wiseman GA et al (2010) The NANETS consensus guidelines for the diagnosis and management of poorly differentiated (high-grade) extrapulmonary neuroendocrine carcinomas. Pancreas 39:799–800
160. Ikeda M, Okuyama H, Takahashi H, Ohno I, Shimizu S, Mitsunaga S et al (2015) Chemotherapy for advanced poorly differentiated pancreatic neuroendocrine carcinoma. J Hepatobiliary Pancreat Sci 22(8):623–627. 4 ed.
161. Lara PN, Natale R, Crowley J, Lenz H-J, Redman MW, Carleton JE et al (2009) Phase III trial of irinotecan/cisplatin compared with etoposide/cisplatin in extensive-stage small-cell lung cancer: clinical and pharmacogenomic results from SWOG S0124. J Clin Oncol 27(15):2530–2535
162. Kotteas EA, Syrigos KN, Saif MW (2016) Profile of capecitabine/temozolomide combination in the treatment of well-differentiated neuroendocrine tumors. Onco Targets Ther 9:699–704
163. Yao JC, Shah MH, Ito T, Bohas CL, Wolin EM, Van Cutsem E et al (2011) Everolimus for advanced pancreatic neuroendocrine tumors. N Engl J Med 364(6):514–523
164. Yao JC, Fazio N, Singh S, Buzzoni R, Carnaghi C, Wolin E et al (2016) Everolimus for the treatment of advanced, non-functional neuroendocrine tumours of the lung or gastrointestinal tract (RADIANT-4): a randomised, placebo-controlled, phase 3 study. Lancet 387(10022):968–977
165. Raymond E, Dahan L, Raoul J-L, Bang Y-J, Borbath I, Lombard-Bohas C et al (2011) Sunitinib malate for the treatment of pancreatic neuroendocrine tumors. N Engl J Med 364(6):501–513
166. Phan AT, Halperin DM, Chan JA, Fogelman DR, Hess KR, Malinowski P et al (2015) Pazopanib and depot octreotide in advanced, well-differentiated neuroendocrine tumours: a multicentre, single-group, phase 2 study. Lancet Oncol 16(6):695–703
167. Zhang J, Jia Z, Li Q, Wang L, Rashid A, Zhu Z et al (2007) Elevated expression of vascular endothelial growth factor correlates with increased angiogenesis and decreased progression-free survival among patients with low-grade neuroendocrine tumors. Cancer 109(8):1478–1486
168. Yao JC, Phan A, Hoff PM, Chen HX, Charnsangavej C, Yeung S-CJ et al (2008) Targeting vascular endothelial growth factor in advanced carcinoid tumor: a random assignment phase II study of depot octreotide with bevacizumab and pegylated interferon alpha-2b. J Clin Oncol 26(8):1316–1323

169. Yao JC, Guthrie KA, Moran C, Strosberg JR, Kulke MH, Chan JA et al (2017) Phase III prospective randomized comparison trial of depot octreotide plus interferon alfa-2b versus depot octreotide plus bevacizumab in patients with advanced carcinoid tumors: SWOG S0518. J Clin Oncol 35(15):1695–1703
170. Hobday TJ, Qin R, Reidy-Lagunes D, Moore MJ, Strosberg J, Kaubisch A et al (2015) Multicenter phase II trial of temsirolimus and bevacizumab in pancreatic neuroendocrine tumors. J Clin Oncol 33(14):1551–1556
171. Yao JC, Lagunes DR, Kulke MH (2013) Targeted therapies in neuroendocrine tumors (NET): clinical trial challenges and lessons learned. Oncologist 18(5):525–532
172. Hammel P, Hentic O, Neuzillet C, Faivre S, Raymond E, Ruszniewski P (2012) New treatment options with cytotoxic agents in neuroendocrine tumours. Target Oncol 7(3):169–172
173. Raymond E, Dreyer C, Faivre S (2012) Targeting neuroendocrine tumor: mixing standard options with novel therapies. Target Oncol 7(3):151–152
174. Doherty GM, Thompson NW (2003) Multiple endocrine neoplasia type 1: duodenopancreatic tumours. J Intern Med 253(6):590–598
175. Akerström G, Stålberg P, Hellman P (2012) Surgical management of pancreatico-duodenal tumors in multiple endocrine neoplasia syndrome type 1. Clinics (Sao Paulo). Hospital das Clinicas da Faculdade de Medicina da Universidade de Sao Paulo 67(Suppl 1):173–178
176. Schimmack S, Svejda B, Lawrence B, Kidd M, Modlin IM (2011) The diversity and commonalities of gastroenteropancreatic neuroendocrine tumors. Langenbeck's Arch Surg 396(3):273–298
177. Gibril F, Jensen RT (2005) Advances in evaluation and management of gastrinoma in patients with Zollinger-Ellison syndrome. Curr Gastroenterol Rep 7(2):114–121
178. Ito T, Igarashi H, Uehara H, Berna MJ, Jensen RT (2013) Causes of death and prognostic factors in multiple endocrine neoplasia type 1: a prospective study: comparison of 106 MEN1/Zollinger-Ellison syndrome patients with 1613 literature MEN1 patients with or without pancreatic endocrine tumors. Medicine 92(3):135–181
179. Gibril F, Venzon DJ, Ojeaburu JV, Bashir S, Jensen RT (2001) Prospective study of the natural history of gastrinoma in patients with MEN1: definition of an aggressive and a nonaggressive form. J Clin Endocrinol Metab 86(11):5282–5293
180. Conemans EB, Brosens LAA, Raicu-Ionita GM, Pieterman CRC, de Herder WW, Dekkers OM et al (2017) Prognostic value of WHO grade in pancreatic neuro-endocrine tumors in multiple endocrine neoplasia type 1: results from the DutchMEN1 Study Group. Pancreatology 17(5):766–772
181. Wilson SD, Krzywda EA, Zhu Y-R, Yen TWF, Wang TS, Sugg SL et al (2008) The influence of surgery in MEN-1 syndrome: observations over 150 years. Surgery 144(4):695–701
182. Hausman MS, Thompson NW, Gauger PG, Doherty GM (2004) The surgical management of MEN-1 pancreatoduodenal neuroendocrine disease. Surgery 136(6):1205–1211
183. Gauger PG, Doherty GM, Broome JT, Miller BS, Thompson NW (2009) Completion pancreatectomy and duodenectomy for recurrent MEN-1 pancreaticoduodenal endocrine neoplasms. Surgery 146(4):801–806
184. Triponez F, Goudet P, Dosseh D, Cougard P, Bauters C, Murat A et al (2006) Is surgery beneficial for MEN1 patients with small (< or = 2 cm), nonfunctioning pancreaticoduodenal endocrine tumor? An analysis of 65 patients from the GTE. World J Surg 30(5):654–662
185. Thompson NW (1998) Current concepts in the surgical management of multiple endocrine neoplasia type 1 pancreatic-duodenal disease. Results in the treatment of 40 patients with Zollinger-Ellison syndrome, hypoglycaemia or both. J Intern Med 243(6):495–500
186. Triponez F, Dosseh D, Goudet P, Cougard P, Bauters C, Murat A et al (2006) Epidemiology data on 108 MEN 1 patients from the GTE with isolated nonfunctioning tumors of the pancreas. Ann Surg 243(2):265–272
187. Norton JA, Alexander HR, Fraker DL, Venzon DJ, Gibril F, Jensen RT (2001) Comparison of surgical results in patients with advanced and limited disease with multiple endocrine neoplasia type 1 and Zollinger-Ellison syndrome. Ann Surg 234(4):495–505. –discussion505–6

188. Nell S, Verkooijen HM, Pieterman CRC, de Herder WW, Hermus AR, Dekkers OM et al (2017) Management of MEN1 related nonfunctioning pancreatic NETs: a shifting paradigm: results from the Dutch MEN1 Study Group. Ann Surg 1
189. Triponez F, Sadowski SM, Pattou F, Cardot-Bauters C, Mirallié E, Le Bras M et al (2017) Long-term follow-up of MEN1 patients who do not have initial surgery for small ≤2 cm nonfunctioning pancreatic neuroendocrine tumors, an AFCE and GTE study: Association Francophone de Chirurgie Endocrinienne & Groupe d'Etude des Tumeurs endocrines. Ann Surg 1
190. van Leeuwaarde RS, de Laat JM, Pieterman CRC, Dreijerink K, Vriens MR, Valk GD (2017) The future: medical advances in MEN1 therapeutic approaches and management strategies. Endocr Relat Cancer 24(10):T179–TT93
191. Kouvaraki MA, Shapiro SE, Cote GJ, Lee JE, Yao JC, Waguespack SG et al (2006) Management of pancreatic endocrine tumors in multiple endocrine neoplasia type 1. World J Surg 30(5):643–653

VIPoma and PPoma

14

Laura Wuyts, Timon Vandamme, Willem Lybaert, and Marc Peeters

14.1 VIPoma

14.1.1 Epidemiology

Pancreatic neuroendocrine tumors (p-NETs) include tumors associated with a functional syndrome (functional p-NETs) and those not associated with a distinct clinical syndrome (non-functional p-NETs). Functional p-NETs give rise to clinical symptoms related to the secretion of specific hormones such as insulin, gastrin, VIP, glucagon, somatostatin, etc. These functional p-NETs derive their name from the hormone they secrete for example VIP-secreting tumors are called VIPomas. Although non-functional p-NETs frequently secrete pancreatic polypeptide, chromogranin A, neuron-specific enolase, human chorionic gonadotrophin subunits, calcitonin, neurotensin, or other peptides, they are considered to be non-functional tumors because they don't produce clinical symptoms. VIPomas account for less than 5% of all pancreatic NETs corresponding to an incidence of 0.01/100,000 yearly [1–3]. They are mostly located intrapancreatic in adults (95%) [4]. Rare extrapancreatic subtypes exist including VIPomas in the oesophagus, colon, jejunum, lung, liver, and retroperitoneum [2]. However, these subtypes are mainly

L. Wuyts
NETwerk and Department of Oncology, Antwerp University Hospital, Edegem, Belgium
e-mail: Laura.wuyts@emmaus.be

T. Vandamme · M. Peeters (✉)
NETwerk and Department of Oncology, Antwerp University Hospital, Edegem, Belgium

Center for Oncology Research (CORE), University of Antwerp, Antwerp, Belgium
e-mail: timon.vandamme@uantwerpen.be; marc.peeters@uza.be

W. Lybaert
NETwerk and Department of Oncology, Antwerp University Hospital, Edegem, Belgium

Department of Oncology, AZ Nikolaas, Sint Niklaas, Belgium
e-mail: Willem.lybaert@vitaz.be

S. Yalcin, K. Öberg (eds.), *Neuroendocrine Tumours*,
https://doi.org/10.1007/978-3-031-56968-5_14

present in children. In young age, they are mostly attributable to either ganglioneuromas or ganglioneuroblastomas, arising from neural crest tissue of the sympathetic ganglia, in mediastinum or peritoneum, which can also produce VIP [3, 4]. In addition, they may arise from the adrenal medulla, as pheochromocytomas can present with elevated VIP levels [1, 2, 4]. Pancreatic VIPomas are more likely to be malignant than neurogenic VIPomas (65% vs. 33%) and develop metastases in 56% vs. 29% [5].

In the pancreas, VIPomas usually arise from pancreatic islet cells as a unique sporadic tumors greater than 3 cm in diameter [1, 6]. The dimensions of VIPomas at diagnosis vary from 1.5 to 14.5 cm (median 5 cm) in a case series. The predominant location was the pancreatic tail (53.8%), followed by pancreatic head (30.8%) and pancreatic body (15.4%). Approximately 70–90% of VIPomas have metastatic potential, while 60–80% are already metastasized at the time of diagnosis [6]. Most common sites of metastasis are the liver, lymph nodes, bones, and kidney [4]. No sex predominance was noted in a series of 15 VIPomas by Angelousi et al. in 2019, and the mean age at diagnosis was 51 years [2]. A systematic review by Schizas et al. in 2019 with a total number of 65 patients of VIPomas in literature, described a median age of 54 years and a slight female predominance (35 females, 53.8% vs. 30 males, 46.2%) [6]. Pediatric VIP-producing tumors are mostly diagnosed in patients between the ages of 2 and 4 years [4]. .

14.1.2 Molecular Mechanisms

The majority of VIPomas occur as isolated sporadic, non-familial, tumors [7]. However, 5% of VIPomas arise in the context of the hereditary multiple endocrine neoplasia type 1 (MEN1) syndrome [2]. MEN1 is an autosomal dominant disorder characterized clinically by the combined occurrence of tumors of the parathyroids or p-NETs, bronchial NETs, pituitary and adrenal adenomas, and angiofibromas [7]. Patient may also develop other endocrine or non-endocrine tumors [8]. Approximately 30–70% of MEN1 patients will develop p-NETs, which are often multifocal [7]. MEN1 has a lifetime penetrance of nearly 100% [9]. It is the result of inactivating mutations of the putative tumor-suppressor *MEN1* gene located on chromosome 11q13.1 coding for menin [7, 8]. Physiological menin influences cell cycle regulation via increasing expression of CDKN2C/CDKN1B (suppresses cell cycle), suppressing the function of PI3K/mTOR pathway signaling, and promoting homologous DNA repair which targets double-strand breaks [10]. *MEN1* germline mutations are found in >90% of patients, consistent with whole or partial gene deletions, frameshift deletions or insertions, in-frame deletions or insertions, and splice site, missense, and nonsense mutations, and result in a functional deficiency of menin. MEN1 tumors will have somatic mutations as well as germline mutations, consistent with the Knudson two-hit hypothesis for the role of tumor suppressor genes in oncogenesis. In >90% of MEN1 tumors, the somatic abnormality is loss of heterozygosity (LOH), with the remaining 10% having intragenic deletions or point mutations. There is no clear genotype–phenotype correlation [8].

Other inheritable syndromes associated with p-NETs include von Hippel Lindau syndrome (VHL), MEN4, and rarely neurofibromatosis type 1 and tuberous sclerosis, caused by mutations in *VHL* gene, *CDKN1B, NF1*, and *TSC1* and *TSC2*, respectively. Gene products of the latter three play a role in PI3K/Akt/mTOR pathway. In approximately, 15% of sporadic p-NETs somatic mutations of genes associated with the mTOR pathway, involved in the regulation of cell proliferation and growth, have been found [11]. Sequencing of germline DNA of patients with p-NET led to identification of pathogenic mutations in cancer susceptibility genes in 10–16% of patients, including *MEN1, VHL, CDKN1B, APC, TSC2, MUTYH, CHEK2,* and *BRCA1*. This suggests a higher proportion of patients may have in fact inheritable disease [12].

Very little is known about the genetic constitution of sporadic, non-familial, VIPomas. However, recent studies in p-NETs using next-generation sequencing (NGS) techniques include a proportion of functional tumors. For instance, Scarpa et al. performed whole-genome sequencing on 102 p-NETs of which 13 tumors were functional, including one VIPoma. Results showed that 17% of sporadic p-NETs carried germline mutations also including DNA repair genes (e.g., MUTYH, CHEK2, BRCA2). Hence, the results of these studies could shed a light on the genetic makeup of VIPomas [13].

An initial study by Jiao et al., using exome sequencing of 10 sporadic p-NETs with screening of commonly mutated genes in a further sample of 58 p-NETs, showed that 44% of tumors demonstrated mutations in *MEN1*, and 43% had mutations in *DAXX* (encoding the death-domain-associated protein (DAXX) or *ATRX* (encoding transcriptional regulator ATRX; mutations in ATRX cause X-linked alpha-thalassaemia/mental retardation syndrome)). These results were later confirmed by Scarpa et al. in whole-genome sequencing results of sporadic 102 p-NET patient samples [13]. Mutations in *DAXX* or *ATRX* appeared mutually exclusive. DAXX functions as an apoptotic regulator and influences the intracellular distribution of the known tumor suppressor PTEN, whilst ATRX functions include chromatin remodeling. These mutations may promote chromosomal instability, and alternative telomere maintenance (i.e., via telomerase-independent mechanisms) compliant with later observations that 61% of p-NET display abnormal telomeres, all of which had *DAXX* or *ATRX* mutation. Clinical relevance of DAXX or ATRX loss was shown in a cohort of 321 individuals undergoing p-NET resection: alternative lengthening of telomeres and DAXX or ATRX loss was significantly associated with higher tumor grade, increased rate of lymph node metastases, and distant metastases [10]. DAXX/ATRX loss is considered a late event, although it still occurs before the development of metastatic disease and might be a driving factor in tumor metastasis [12].

Although different genes have been implicated in sporadic p-NET, further studies are needed. Routine use of NGS panels on p-NET tumor tissue is not currently recommended. NGS analysis might be of use in G3 p-NETs, as a small minority may harbor potential actionable alterations (e.g., NTRK fusions and microsatellite instability) [7].

14.1.3 Clinical Manifestations

The first description of watery diarrhea and hypokalemia in relation to a pancreatic islet cell tumor was by Priest and Alexander in 1957 [14]. In 1958, Verner and Morrison described two patients with diarrhea, hypokalemia, achlorhydria, and metabolic acidosis [15, 16]. For this syndrome, an acronym was used: WDHA (watery diarrhea, hypokalemia, achlorhydria) [17]. It was also defined as "pancreatic cholera," but this definition is not correct as VIPoma can have an extrapancreatic origin [1, 17]. The WDHA often precedes diagnosis by 3–4 years [2, 17]. Watery diarrhea is the most common clinical symptom (54.4%), and the classical triad of symptoms in 42.2% of patients [6]. The term VIPoma was suggested by the elevated plasma levels of the vasoactive intestinal polypeptide (VIP), which are associated with this kind of tumor. VIP is a 28-amino acid polypeptide that is distributed throughout the body and normally functions as a neurotransmitter. In the gut, it regulates the blood flow, smooth muscle activity, pancreatic and intestinal secretions and inhibits gastric acid production. Aside being present in enteric neurons, VIP is also distributed in neurons of the brain, spinal cord, lung, urogenital system, and other endocrine organs [18].

The elevated serum levels of VIP result in all segments of the intestine secreting Na^+, K^+, Cl^-, and HCO^{-3}, as well as water, thus accounting for the dehydration, hypokalemia, and acidosis associated with this syndrome. Other effects of excessive circulating VIP include inhibition of gastric acid secretion, bone resorption, glycogenolysis, and vasodilation leading, respectively, to the achlorhydria, hypercalcemia, hyperglycemia, and flushing often seen with these tumors [18].

The Verner–Morrison syndrome is characterized by sizeable diarrhea (6–8 l/day), which is watery and increasing. The diarrhea associated with VIPoma is a secretory diarrhea characterized by its persistence for 48–72 h after fasting [17]. The hydro-electrolytic disequilibrium is a consequence of diarrhea and includes hypokalemia, hypomagnesemia, hypovolemia, and metabolic acidosis. These events induce lethargy, muscular weakness, tetany, cardiac conduction disturbances, weight loss, abdominal pain, paralytic ileus, dyspepsia, and gallbladder hypotonia. Rhabdomyolysis and paralysis of the extremities secondary to hypokalemia have been described [2]. Flushing could be found in about 20% of VIPomas [17]. Children with VIP-producing tumors can present with failure to thrive and chronic diarrhea [4].

Other conditions may mimic the Verner–Morrison syndrome. Laxative abuse and the Zollinger–Ellison syndrome can have similar presentations. A careful medication history and a measurement of serum gastrin and serum VIP and quantifying gastric acid production are important in differentiating the diseases [6]. Small bowel ischemia, carcinoid syndrome, microscopic colitis, infectious enterocolitis, and bile salt malabsorption due to ileal resection are important differential diagnoses [4, 6]. Secretory diarrhea can also occur in Crohn's disease and short bowel syndrome. Munchausen syndrome (by proxy) needs to be ruled out. In children, rare inherited electrolyte transport defects like congenital chloride diarrhea and congenital sodium diarrhea may cause secretory diarrhea, which presents in early infancy [4].

14.1.4 Biochemical Indicators

Diagnosis is based on secretory diarrhea (>700 ml/day) and plasma VIP levels above 200 pg/ml [19]. Serum VIP level varies around 250–500 pg/ml in VIPoma with a median value of 636 pg/ml in a systematic review of 61 patients [2]. Fasting normal VIP values range between 150 and 170 pg/ml. The fecal osmotic gap is low, less than 50 mOsm/kg. It is important to note that functional hormonal biomarkers such as VIP, gastrin, etc. should only be measured selectively in p-NETs patients experiencing appropriate symptoms [7]. VIP levels are not always elevated between episodes of diarrhea, so a repeat measurement of VIP levels is important [6]. In children, catecholamine levels should also be measured [4]. Dehydration is common (45–95%), and electrolyte abnormalities of VIPoma consist of hypokalemia (70–100%), achlorhydria (35–76%), hypophosphatemia, hypomagnesemia, hyperglycemia (20–50%), and hypercalcemia (25–50%) [6]. Hypokalemia and hyperchloremic metabolic acidosis are a consequence of gastro-intestinal loss by secretory diarrhea and bicarbonate wasting. Achlorhydria is secondary to the direct gastric acid inhibitory effect of VIP. Hypercalcemia can be secondary to dehydration, co-incidental MEN1 syndrome with secreting parathyroid tumors, or secretion by the tumor of calcitrophic peptide. VIP stimulates glycogenolysis causing hyperglycemia [4].

Pancreatic islet cell tumors can secrete more than one hormone, as they may be comprised of more than one cell type. VIPomas have been noted to produce additional peptides including pancreatic polypeptide (PP), calcitonin, gastrin, neurotensin, gastric inhibitory peptide, serotonin, glucagon, insulin, somatostatin, growth hormone-releasing hormone, and peptide histidine–methionine [20]. Approximately 30% of the patients described in the literature had elevated blood levels of multiple hormones [4, 18].

14.1.5 Diagnosis

The diagnosis of functional p-NET requires clinical evidence of hormonal secretion and is not only determined by immunohistochemical results [3]. In the absence of radiologically visible tumor, an elevated VIP level (<500 pg/ml), and suggestive clinical symptoms, the diagnosis can be established [20]. Sensitivity of abdominal contrast-enhanced multiphasic computed tomography (CT) scans is greater than 80% for detecting intrapancreatic NETs. Pancreatic VIPoma's are mostly greater than 3 cm in diameter. CT is used for determining size, location, and organ of tumor origin and participation of adjacent structures, vessels, lymph nodes, and presence of calcification. Typical features are a hyperattenuating lesion on arterial phase followed by an obscure mass on venous phase. Calcifications may be present. VIPomas are highly vascularized tumors rich in cells and fibrous tissue, the latter of which is poorly supplied and as a consequence contrast is retained within the lesion. Magnetic resonance imaging (MRI) has a sensitivity of 85%, is useful for indeterminate lesions, has a higher sensitivity for the detection of liver metastases, and is superior to CT for the evaluation of p-NETs [3]. It is also useful for the assessment of

VIP-producing spinal tumors [6]. Abdominal ultrasound can be used for follow-up, can be valuable in some patients in whom liver metastases are better visualized by US than CT, and for biopsy of new or rapidly growing lesions. Endoscopic ultrasound (EUS), with fine needle aspiration or preferable core biopsy, can determine the local extent of disease and is useful for follow-up in selected patients (T and N staging), and also in patients with MEN1 [3]. The sensitivity of EUS is 86% and specificity 92% and is the optimal imaging method for small p-NETs [21].

Occasionally findings may be aspecific and require additional imaging modalities [2]. Over 90% of p-NETs (including non-functional p-NETs) express subtypes of somatostatin receptors with the level of expression changing in relation to type, origin, and grade of the tumor [2, 6]. Given the high expression of somatostatin receptors in VIPomas in more than 80%, somatostatin receptor imaging may be particularly useful in extrapancreatic VIPomas, within the sympathetic chain or for visualizing occult metastases [2, 5]. Somatostatin receptor scintigraphy using radiolabeled somatostatin analogues (SSA) can detect small, occult metastases intra- and extra-abdominally. Due to its better sensitivity, lower radiation dose, and shorter duration, a FDA-approved somastostatin PET imaging technique with 68-Ga DOTATATE injection as a radioactive diagnostic agent is replacing the Indium-111-labeled DTPA (Octreoscan®) somatostatin receptor scintigraphy [3]. Sensitivity of PET-CT 68-Ga DOTATATE is 97% for the detection of VIPomas. 68-Ga DOTATATE PET may reveal bone and lymph node metastases not visualized on somatostatin receptor scintigraphy or CT [3].

Although imaging characteristics can be highly suggestive of p-NET, a biopsy is needed to confirm the diagnosis. Histological examination of VIPoma shows molecular patterns, such as solid, acinar, or trabecular tissue architecture with scant mitoses. The cells are cytologically bland, with a modest amount of cytoplasm and round nuclei without visible nucleoli. Few mitotic figures can be found [20]. Immunohistological analysis of specimens in a systematic review of 61 patients in literature described positivity to chromogranin A and synaptophysin in all cases [6]. About 90% of VIPomas are immunoreactive with VIP immunohistochemical stain [20]. p-NETs should be graded according to the 2019 World Health Organization (WHO) classification of Digestive System Tumors [22]. The current WHO classification of 2019 includes three grades (G1, G2, and G3) for NETs, with Ki-67 proliferation index and mitotic count incorporated. NECs are no longer graded, as they are recognized to be uniformly high grade by definition. Important to note that well-differentiated NETs may be high grade (G3 in the WHO grading system, defined as having a mitotic rate >20 per 2 mm^2 or Ki67 > 20%), but these neoplasms remain well-differentiated genetically and distinct from poorly differentiated NECs [7].

14.1.6 Treatment Options

Most VIPoma's (50–70%) tend to grow insidiously at a slow rate. According to a systematic review of 61 patients, overall five-year survival of patients with pancreatic VIPoma is 67.7%, recurrence rate 40.4%, and median disease-free interval

16 months [6]. Overall prognosis depends on symptom control, grading (Ki-67 labeling and mitotic index), tumor growth rate, differentiation, and extent of metastatic disease [2, 19]. In different case series, Ki-67 varies from 1–17% to 40% at mainly metastatic sites [2]. Before any curative or palliative treatment is started, the life-threatening hydro-electrolytic disorders must be corrected by aggressive replacement of fluids and electrolytes [4, 5]. Treatment options are summarized in Fig. 14.1.

Surgery is considered the gold standard for treatment of localized VIPoma and resectable metastases and is the only potentially curative treatment, resulting in curation in 40% of patients with non-metastatic disease. Concurrent treatment with short-acting octreotide, a SSA, can improve preoperative electrolyte management [6]. Surgery can be considered in the setting of metastatic disease as a debulking procedure or even with the intent of curation when resection of all metastasis is possible [23]. Patients with curative surgery are described to have a 5-year survival of 80%. In a review of 15 patients, 66% of patients that underwent curative surgery had complete and immediate post-surgery resolution of symptoms such as diarrhea and increase in body weight [2]. The most commonly applied surgical procedure is a distal pancreatectomy with or without splenectomy, due to the pancreatic tail being the predominant pancreatic location [4, 6].

The medical treatment of VIPoma when curative surgery is not possible is mainly directed to symptom control caused by excessive VIP levels and to prolong

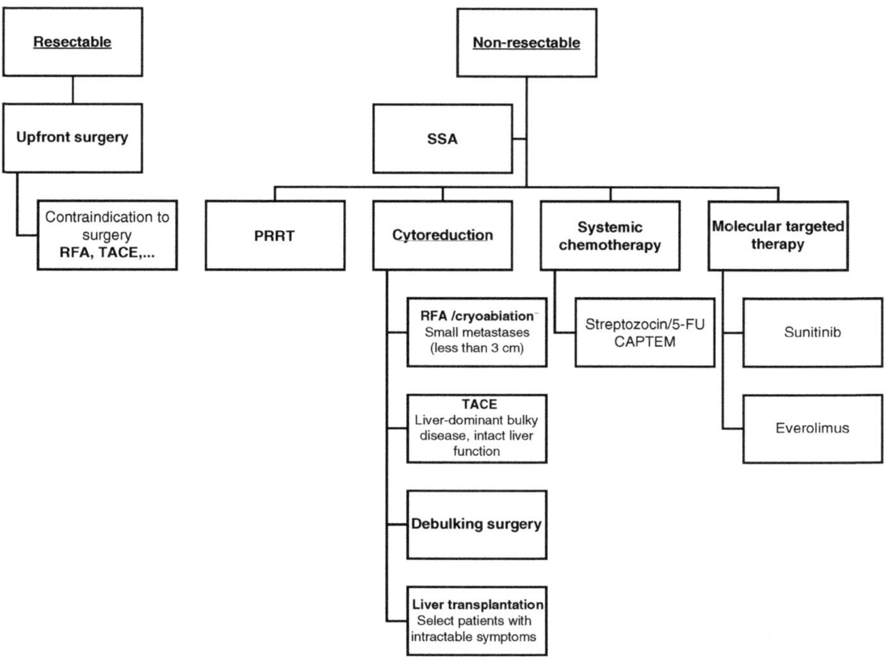

Fig. 14.1 Therapeutic options and treatment algorithm for VIPomas

progression-free survival (PFS). Long-acting SSA like octreotide and lanreotide imitate the effect of somatostatin on G-coupled receptors of cell membrane and reduce secretion of VIP, thereby controlling symptoms and inhibit tumor growth [4, 6]. Octreotide is started at 50–100 mcg subcutaneous every 8 h and titrated for symptom control. Long-acting forms of octreotide are started at a dose of 30 mg intramuscularly monthly, while the dose of long-acting lanreotide is 120 mg monthly [4]. SSA's achieved prompt improvement of diarrhea in more than half of patients with VIPomas, and in 60–80% a reduction in VIP levels is observed [3, 6]. Symptomatic relief is not always a consequence of a reduction in circulating hormone levels, indicating that SSA may have direct effects on the peripheral target organ. SSA's can exert anti-proliferative effects on p-NETs [2]. SSA have shown to have tumor-stabilizing effects in 50–60% of non-functioning p-NETs [24]. In gastro-enteropancreatic NET, the CLARINET study showed a hazard reduction of 42% for progression when patients without functional syndrome received lanreotide in comparison to placebo [7]. In VIPoma, a case series by Angelousi et al. in 2019 showed a PFS of 24.5 months [2].

Interferon-α treatment may help control symptoms of hormone excess in functional low-proliferating tumors, it has however been less well studied than the use of SSA [3]. Glucocorticoids, loperamide, and opiated can also be used for symptom control [2, 6].

A patient with advanced disease can become refractory to the effect of medical therapy (SSA and/or interferon, etc.), resulting in a state of uncontrolled hormone excess. If refractory symptomatic disease develops, various anti-tumor therapies including systemic treatment, liver directed therapies (embolization, transarterial (chemo) embolization (TACE), radiofrequent ablation (RFA), radiolabeled microspheres), peptide receptor radionuclide treatment (PRRT), or cytoreductive surgery, can be considered which are reported to improve symptomatic control in many patients. With these different modalities, symptoms improve in 40–80% of patients [3]. Cytoreductive surgery includes palliative debulking of the primary tumor. This treatment achieves a tumor bulk reduction, the improvement of hormone-mediated symptoms, and the prevention of local and systemic tumor effects. A complete resection of the primary tumor improves the prognosis greatly [2, 6, 23].

Systemic treatment options should be considered in patients with >50–75% hepatic tumor burden [7]. Systemic chemotherapy can be used in patients with large, bulky tumors, or extrahepatic metastases. Chemotherapy with streptozotocin and fluorouracil is described in the literature to result in objective responses in progressive or symptomatic unresectable VIPomas in 1 out of 4 patients. In case series, chemotherapy was administered in 33% of patients and showed a median PFS of 30 months. However, adverse reactions and toxicity related to chemotherapy were reported [2]. The Eastern Cooperative Oncology Group 2211 trial compared temozolomide monotherapy with capetitabine/temozolomide (CAPTEM) combination in 144 patients with progressive low- and intermediate-grade p-NETs. Median PFS with temozolomide alone of 14.4 months improved to 22.7 months with the CAPTEM combination (HR, 0.58; $p = 0.02$) [25]. A recent case report described a metastatic insulin co-secreting VIPoma with complete response 2 years after starting treatment with capecitabine and temozolomide in combination with SSA [26].

Molecular-targeted therapy with agents like sunitinib, a tyrosine kinase inhibitor and everolimus, an mTOR inhibitor, are approved for treatment of advanced, well-differentiated pancreatic NET including VIPomas [27, 28]. Sunitinib may exert a specific antisecretory effect in addition to controlling tumor growth [2]. Data in literature about therapy with sunitinib is scarce. When administered with SSA in metastatic VIPomas which were already treated with TACE and debulking surgery previously, sustained relief of symptoms and stable disease was described in for 7 months in one patient and 4 years in the other [29]. Partial response and progression-free survival of 13 months during treatment with sunitinib were seen in one patient, which was refractory to SSA [30]. In a case series by Angelousi et al. in 2019, sunitinib led to amelioration of diarrhea and hypokalemia in two patients (33%) and six patients who received sunitinib had a median PFS of 11.5 months with poor control of symptoms in four out of six patients. Of note is that the molecular-targeted therapy was co-administered with TACE in three cases and in five cases with SSA. In the RADIANT-3 study of 410 patients with progressing low- and intermediate-grade p-NETs median PFS improved from 4.6 months on placebo to 11.0 months with everolimus. Objective response rate was 5%. There was a trend to improved overall survival (OS) with a median of 37.7 months on placebo vs. 44.0 months on everolimus [7, 31]. In a case series, everolimus had little effect on VIPoma symptoms, when administered to one patient in first-line and to six patients after sunitinib treatment [2].

Cytoreduction can also be achieved with cytoreductive techniques such as TACE or radioembolization. RFA or cryoablation is the treatment modality of choice in case of small metastases (less than 3 cm) [4]. In 3 out of 15 patients with VIPoma, RFA was used for patients with persistent symptoms and progressive disease as first- and second-line treatment, co-administered with SSA and sunitinib in one case. All patients had resolution of diarrhea and hypokalemia. Median PFS was 40 months [2].

In case of liver-dominant, bulky disease and intact liver function, TACE is a valid choice. In p-NETs, there is an associated ~50% response rate [7]. Three out of five patients with liver metastasis had TACE as second and third line of treatment with improvement of symptoms along with a median PFS of 17 months. In one patient, both SSA and sunitinib were associated to TACE [2].

A retrospective study of PRRT in 34 patients with metastatic functioning p-NET (WHO grade 1 or 2) included five VIPomas. All patients were treated with four cycles of 177Lu-DOTATATE. Mean PFS after PRRT was 18.1 months. A partial or complete response was observed in 59% of patients, while disease control rate was 78% (67% in VIPomas). About 71% of patients with uncontrolled symptoms experienced a reduction of symptoms and a decrease of more than 80% of circulating hormone levels was observed [32]. A decrease in diarrhea was seen in four (80%) patients with VIPoma. One out of five patients with VIPoma stopped after three cycles because of clinical progression (severe diarrhea causing dehydration). Antidiarrheicals should be prescribed as needed, and in severe cases IV fluids and electrolyte administration are required. A hormonal crisis occurred in three patients (9%), and subacute hematological toxicity (grade 3 or 4) occurred in four patients (12%). Symptomatic response was highly associated with radiological response [32]. In a case series of 15 patients with VIPoma, six received PRRT. Five patients had resolution of symptoms, and one patient required concomitant use of SSAs. Median PFS was 26.5 months [2]. PRRT seems to be most efficacious second-line treatment in refractory VIPoma syndrome, despite maximum doses of SSA [2, 32]. There are many case reports in literature of liver transplantation in patients with intractable symptomatic disease with multiple liver metastases [5].

ENETs guidelines suggest that patients with aggressive and rapidly growing tumors in follow-up schedules should have follow-up with imaging and serum VIP level every 3 months, and patients with stable or slowly growing tumors every 6–12 months [3]. ESMO guidelines suggest in R0/R1-resected NET G1–2, imaging should be performed every 3–6 months. Follow-up should be lifelong, staging intervals may however be extended to 1–2 years with increasing length of follow up [21]. Continued measurement of a specific hormone, before and after therapeutic intervention, in conjunction with radiologic testing, can help determine tumor progression, recurrence, and response to therapy [7]. Patients with hereditary diseases such as MEN1, VHL, and NF type 1 should be followed according to the organ of the primary tumor [3]. National Comprehensive Cancer Network (NCCN) guidelines, post-resection surveillance included history and physical examination, multiphasic CT or MRI and serum VIP level in the initial 3–12-month period. After 1 year, the interval can be increased to every 6–12 months [4].

14.2 PPoma

PPoma belongs to non-functioning NETs and are not associated with a clinical syndrome. Non-functional tumors account for 50–60% of all p-NETs. They are clinically silent. The endocrine part of the pancreas is constituted of clusters of cells, the islets of Langerhans. Within these there are four types of cells (alpha, beta, delta, and PP). The PP cells, less than 2% of the exocrine pancreas, produce the pancreatic polypeptide. It is in inhibitory peptide for the exocrine pancreas and reduces the release of somatostatin. The PP cells are situated mainly in the endocrine pancreas, although these cells tend to be also spread throughout the exocrine pancreas [9]. Ninety percent of the cells are situated in the head of the pancreas [33]. It consists of 36 aminoacids, it contrasts gallbladder contraction being a cholecystokinin antagonist, suppressor of pancreatic secretion, and simulant of gastric secretion. Secretion is increased after protein meal, fasting, exercise, and acute hypoglycemia. It is diminished by somatostatin and intravenous glucose. PP secretion can also be found in other p-NETs (for instance, 75% of VIPomas and 25% of gastrinoma secrete PP), in multiple endocrine neoplasias (MENs) and in other intestinal and bronchial tumors [9].

PPoma is extremely rare, representing less than 1% of non-functional NET [9, 33]. They are diagnosed between the fifth and sixth decades of life and are mostly metastatic when diagnosed (90%). The predominant site of metastases is the liver. They are usually incidentally diagnosed or as a consequence of compressive symptoms, such as most frequently enlargement of the liver, obstruction of the pancreatic duct, or jaundice secondary to its location in the pancreatic head. Furthermore, abdominal pain, palpable mass, diabetes mellitus and weight loss, gastrointestinal bleeding and watery diarrhea (only in case of very high PP levels) [9].

PPomas may occur in 20–40% of patients with MEN and can be found in VHL disease. The syndrome is characterized by inactivating mutations of the VHL gene (3p25) encoding the elongin protein [13].

To date no histological features have been identified to distinguish PPomas from other pancreatic NETs. In fact, they show all the typical neuroendocrine characteristics. Neurosecretory granules can be identified in electron microscopy of immunohistochemical studies can be positive for PP chromogranin, synaptophysin, specific neural enolase, or PGP 95 (protein of the product gene 9.5). A cut-off of more than 50% of tumor cells expressing PP was established to classify a tumor PPoma, since this peptide could be also expressed by other islet cell tumors. Biochemical abnormalities include abnormal serum concentrations of chromogranin A (60–100%), pancreatic polypeptide (PP 25–70%; also reported as growth inhibiting factor, GIF, or human pancreatic polypeptide, hPP) and pancreastatin. In healthy individuals, PP is lower than 300 pg/ml. The finding of high PP levels is not sufficient for PPoma diagnosis. In fact, it is also elevated in other NETs (25–70%) and in non-neoplastic patients including patients with chronic pancreatitis, kidney failure, diabetes, hypoglycemia, duodenal ulcers, alcoholism, advanced age, and medication use (erythromycin, cisapride, laxative abuse) [34]. The association of high basal plasma PP levels with highly vascularized tumors on CT scan should increase the suspicion of PPoma. Novel markers such as transcriptomic analysis, circulating tumor cells, and cell-free tumor DNA are investigational; therefore, more studies are required prior to incorporation into daily practice [7]. Subtype 2 of 5 known somatostatin receptor subtypes is found in PPoma. Octreotide conjugated to indium-111-labeled DTPA has a high affinity for somatostatin receptors (mainly subtypes 2 and 5) expressed in several neuroectodermal lineage tumors [9]. PET-CT with ^{68}Ga-DOTATATE is superior to somatostatin receptor imaging with higher sensitivity, spatial resolution, identification of more lesions, less radiation and shorter investigation time, and is preferred in staging and follow-up [3].

Staging must be performed by contrast-enhanced multiphasic CT. MRI of the liver is particularly useful for detecting liver metastases. Upper digestive endoscopy with ultrasonography can be used to detect small lesions, for which a needle biopsy is possible. The somatostatin receptor imaging in combination with CT and MRI imaging has improved detection of primary and metastatic lesions and is useful to select patients suited for PRRT [35]. In patients with MEN1, ultrasound of parathyroid glands should be performed as 90–97% of patients with MEN1 syndrome have primary hyperparathyroidism. Bone scintigraphy can be performed in case of suspected bone metastases. Plasma chromogranin levels are increased in 80% of cases, regardless of a functional tumor or not-functioning tumor. Elevation may anticipate tumor growth detected by imaging. Calcium, serum phosphorus, and, in case of abnormal calcium levels, parathyroid hormone, and urinary calcium should be performed at least once at diagnosis according to NANETS Guidelines. Especially in patients younger than 50 years, testing for MEN1 should be considered [7].

The ENETS scores are used in Europe, in the United States of America the AJCC/UICC system is used. The definitions of T stages for pancreatic tumors are different in these two systems. The pathologist should report the used classification for TNM stage [35]. Disease stage by TNM classification and tumor grade are the two major independent prognostic parameters that should always be assessed [21].

The relative five-year survival rate is 8% for all combined stages of PPoma. For the 9% of patients who are diagnoses with localized disease, the five-year survival rate is 29%. The five-year survival rate of 90% of patients with PPoma, being diagnosed at an advanced stage, is 3% [9].

As PPoma is biologically inactive, its diagnosis is usually late, when it has already become metastatic and of greater dimensions. Curative surgery is only possible in 10% of PPomas. A maximum of tumor mass should be attempted to be resected with preservation of pancreatic function. An embolization of the hepatic artery can be performed in patients who are not candidates for surgery. Chemoembolization, the combination of cytotoxic chemotherapy and local ischemia, provides symptom and tumor growth control in 90% of cases with a five-year survival of approximately 40% and median survival of 32 weeks.

Cytoreductive surgery, with preferably resection of 90% of tumor volume, can be performed to alleviate symptoms. Liver metastases resection with palliative intent can lead to long-term symptom relief and increased survival by 3–4 times [9].

Radiofrequency ablation (RFA) or cryoablation is suitable for solitary small liver lesions (<3–5 cm in size). RFA provides 70–80% symptomatic responses with sustained symptom control for up to 1 year. A role for the SSA lanreotide in controlling tumor progression has been demonstrated in p-NET in the CLARINET trial [36].

In progressive metastatic disease, systemic chemotherapy can be used. Streptozocin, doxorubicin, 5-fluorouracil, capecitabine, and temozolomide are used, with modest responses. Combination of streptozocin and doxorubicin has an objective response of 65% with a mean duration of response of 20 months. Temozolomide has shown a radiological response rate of 45%, comparable to dacarbazine and streptozocin. Chemotherapy should be initiated when the disesase show significant and rapid progression [9, 37, 38]. Molecular-targeted therapy such as sunitinib (PFS of 33 weeks, response rate of 17%) and everolimus are other therapeutic options in progressive PPoma [9].

Uptake at somatostatin receptor imaging and homogeneity of uptake should be specified to evaluate patient eligibility for PRRT [3]. In patients with octreotide hypercaptation (an uptake greater than that of the hepatic parenchyma), PRRT is possible [9]. PRRT with ^{177}Lu-DOTATATE produces good tumor response rates for patients with grade 1–2 GEP-NETs and bronchial NETs in study of 1200 patients with PRRT since the year 2000. The side effects are limited and most often reversible on short term. Severe long-term toxicities are acute leukemia or MDS (2% of patients). The PFS for pancreatic NETs with radiologic progression at baseline after therapy with ^{177}Lu-DOTATATE was 31 months, which is longer than with the currently available molecular-targeted therapies [39].

References

1. Song S, Shi R, Li B, Liu Y (2009) Diagnosis and treatment of pancreatic vasoactive intestinal peptide endocrine tumours. Pancreas 38(7):811–814. https://doi.org/10.1097/MPA.0b013e3181b2bc7c
2. Angelousi A, Koffas A, Grozinsky-Glasberg S et al (2019) Diagnostic and management challenges in vasoactive intestinal peptide secreting Tumours: a series of 15 patients. Pancreas 48(7):934–942. https://doi.org/10.1097/MPA.0000000000001347
3. Knigge U, Capdevila J, Bartsch DK et al (2017) ENETS consensus recommendations for the standards of Care in Neuroendocrine Neoplasms: follow-up and documentation. Neuroendocrinology 105(3):310–319. https://doi.org/10.1159/00045815
4. Sandhu S, Jialal I (2020) ViPoma. In: StatPearls. StatPearls Publishing, Treasure Island, FL
5. Siddappa PK, Vege SS (2019) Vasoactive intestinal peptide-secreting Tumours, a review. Pancreas 45:1119–1125
6. Schizas D, Mastoraki A, Bagias G et al (2019) Clinicopathological data and treatment modalities for pancreatic vipomas: a systematic review. J BUON 24(2):415–423
7. Halfdanarson TR, Strosberg JR, Tang L et al (2020) The north American neuroendocrine tumour society consensus guidelines for surveillance and medical Management of Pancreatic Neuroendocrine Tumours. Pancreas 49(7):863–881. https://doi.org/10.1097/MPA.0000000000001597
8. Frost M, Lines KE, Thakker RV (2018) Current and emerging therapies for PNETs in patients with or without MEN1. Nat Rev Endocrinol 14(4):216–227. https://doi.org/10.1038/nrendo.2018.3
9. Ligiero Braga T, Santos-Oliveira R (2018) PPoma review: epidemiology, Aetiopathogenesis, prognosis and treatment. Diseases 6(1):8. https://doi.org/10.3390/diseases6010008
10. Clift AK, Kidd M, Bodei L et al (2020) Neuroendocrine neoplasms of the small bowel and pancreas. Neuroendocrinology 110(6):444–476. https://doi.org/10.1159/000503721
11. Jiao Y, Shi C, Edil BH et al (2011) DAXX/ATRX, MEN1, and mTOR pathway genes are frequently altered in pancreatic neuroendocrine tumours. Science 331(6021):1199–1203. https://doi.org/10.1126/science.1200609
12. Boons G, Vandamme T (2019) Clinical applications of (epi)genetics in gastroenteropancreatic neuroendocrine neoplasms: moving towards liquid biopsies. Rev Endocr Metab Disord. https://doi.org/10.1007/s11154-019-09508-w
13. Scarpa A, Chang DK, Nones K et al (2017) Whole-genome landscape of pancreatic neuroendocrine tumours. Nature 543(7643):65–71. https://doi.org/10.1038/nature21063
14. Priest WM, Alexander MK (1957) Islet cell tumour of the pancreas with peptic ulceration, diarrhea and hypokalemia. Lancet 273:1145–1147
15. Verner JV, Morrison AB (1958) Islet cell tumour and a syndrome of refractory watery diarrhea and hypokalemia. Am J Med 25:374–380
16. Verner JV, Morrison AB (1974) Endocrine pancreatic islet disease with diarrhea. Report of a case due to diffuse hyperplasia of nonbeta islet tissue with a review of 54 additional cases. Arch Intern Med 133:492–499
17. Vinik A (2017) Vasoactive intestinal peptide tumour (VIPoma). In: Feingold KR, Anawalt B, Boyce A et al (eds) Endotext. MDText.com, Inc., South Dartmouth, MA
18. Ghaferi AA, Chojnacki KA, Long WD, Cameron JL, Yeo CJ (2008) Pancreatic VIPomas: subject review and one institutional experience. J Gastrointest Surg 12(2):382–393. https://doi.org/10.1007/s11605-007-0177-0
19. Strosberg J, Gardner N, Kvols L (2009) Survival and prognostic factor analysis in patients with metastatic pancreatic endocrine carcinomas. Pancreas 38:255–228
20. Guilmette JM, Nosé V (2019) Neoplasms of the neuroendocrine pancreas: an update in the classification, definition, and molecular genetic advances. Adv Anat Pathol 26(1):13–30. https://doi.org/10.1097/PAP.0000000000000201
21. Pavel M, Öberg K, Falconi M, Krenning EP, Sundin A, Perren A, Berruti A (2020) Gastroenteropancreatic neuroendocrine neoplasms: ESMO clinical practice guidelines for diagnosis, treatment and follow-up. Ann Oncol 31(7):844–860

22. Klimstra DS (2019) Classification of neuroendocrine neoplasms of the digestive system. In: WHO classification of Tumours editorial board. Digestive system tumours, 5th edn. International Agency for Research on Cancer, Lyon, pp 16–19
23. Frilling A, Li J, Malamutmann E, Schmid KW, Bockisch A, Broelsch CE (2009) Treatment of liver metastases from neuroendocrine tumours in relation to the extent of hepatic disease. Br J Surg 96(2):175–184. https://doi.org/10.1002/bjs.6468
24. Rinke A, Müller HH, Schade-Brittinger C et al (2009) Placebo-controlled, double-blind, prospective, randomized study on the effect of octreotide LAR in the control of tumour growth in patients with metastatic neuroendocrine midgut tumours: a report from the PROMID study group. J Clin Oncol 27(28):4656–4663. https://doi.org/10.1200/JCO.2009.22.8510
25. Kunz PL, Catalano PJ, Nimeiri H et al (2018) A randomized study of temozolomide or temozolomide and capecitabine in patients with advanced pancreatic neuroendocrine tumours: a trial of the ECOG-ACRIN cancer research group (E2211). J Clin Oncol 36(15):4004
26. Marques B, Monteiro AR, Martins RG, Couto J, Rodrigues F, Ribeiro J (2020) Metastatic VIPoma, Cosecreting insulin, with complete response to Lanreotide, Capecitabine, and Temozolomide. Pancreas 49(3):e19–e20. https://doi.org/10.1097/MPA.0000000000001514
27. Yao JC, Shah MH, Ito T et al (2011) Everolimus for advanced pancreatic neuroendocrine tumours. N Engl J Med 364(6):514–523. https://doi.org/10.1056/NEJMoa1009290
28. Raymond E, Kulke MH, Qin S et al (2018) Efficacy and safety of Sunitinib in patients with well-differentiated pancreatic neuroendocrine Tumours. Neuroendocrinology 107(3):237–245. https://doi.org/10.1159/000491999
29. de Mestier L, Walter T, Brixi H, Lombard-Bohas C, Cadiot G (2015) Sunitinib achieved fast and sustained control of VIPoma symptoms. Eur J Endocrinol 172(1):K1–K3. https://doi.org/10.1530/EJE-14-0682
30. Bourcier ME, Vinik AI (2013) Sunitinib for the treatment of metastatic paraganglioma and vasoactive intestinal polypeptide-producing tumour (VIPoma). Pancreas 42(2):348–352. https://doi.org/10.1097/MPA.0b013e31825c53fa
31. Yao JC, Pavel M, Lombard-Bohas C et al (2016) Everolimus for the treatment of advanced pancreatic neuroendocrine Tumours: overall survival and circulating biomarkers from the randomized, phase III RADIANT-3 study. J Clin Oncol 34(32):3906–3913. https://doi.org/10.1200/JCO.2016.68.0702
32. Zandee WT, Brabander T, Blažević A et al (2019) Symptomatic and radiological response to 177Lu-DOTATATE for the treatment of functioning pancreatic neuroendocrine Tumours. J Clin Endocrinol Metab 104(4):1336–1344. https://doi.org/10.1210/jc.2018-01991
33. Ilić I, Katić V, Randjelović P, Stojanović N, Antovic A, Ilić R (2019) Pancreatic polypeptide-secreting tumour of the proximal pancreas (PPoma)-ultra rare pancreatic tumour: clinically malign, histologically benign. Medicina (Kaunas) 55(9):523. https://doi.org/10.3390/medicina55090523
34. Modlin IM, Tang LH (1997) Approaches to the diagnosis of gut neuroendocrine tumours: the last word (today). Gastroenterology 112(2):583–590. https://doi.org/10.1053/gast.1997.v112.pm9024313
35. Falconi M et al (2016) ENETS consensus guidelines update for the Management of Patients with functional pancreatic neuroendocrine Tumours and non-functional pancreatic neuroendocrine Tumours. Neuroendocrinology 103:153–171
36. Caplin ME, Pavel M, Jaroslaw CB et al (2014) Lanreotide in metastatic Enteropancreatic neuroendocrine tumors. N Engl J Med 371:224–233. https://doi.org/10.1056/NEJMoa1316158
37. Gonzalez MA, Biswas S, Clifton L, Corrie PG (2003) Treatment of neuroendocrine tumours with infusional 5-fluorouracil, folinic acid and streptozocin. Br J Cancer 89(3):455–456. https://doi.org/10.1038/sj.bjc.6601167
38. Ramanathan RK, Cnaan A, Hahn RG, Carbone PP, Haller DG (2001) Phase II trial of dacarbazine (DTIC) in advanced pancreatic islet cell carcinoma. Study of the eastern cooperative oncology group-E6282. Ann Oncol 12(8):1139–1143. https://doi.org/10.1023/a:1011632713360
39. Brabander T, van der Zwan WA, Teunissen JJM et al (2017) Long-term efficacy, survival, and safety of [177Lu-DOTA0,Tyr3]octreotate in patients with Gastroenteropancreatic and bronchial neuroendocrine Tumours. Clin Cancer Res 23(16):4617–4624. https://doi.org/10.1158/1078-0432.CCR-16-2743

15 Glucagonoma

Suayib Yalcin, Cenk Sokmensuer, and Ece Esin

15.1 Introduction

Glucagonomas are neuroendocrine tumors of the pancreas (PNET) originating from alpha islet cell, which synthesize and secrete glucagon or other peptides derived from the preproglucagon gene. These tumors are associated with a well-described glucagonoma syndrome characterized by hyperglucagonemia, skin rash, glucose intolerance, hypoalbuminemia, weight loss, and anemia [1].

15.2 History

The glucagonoma syndrome was first reported by Becker et al in a patient with skin rash associated with pancreatic tumor in 1942 [2]. However, the syndrome initially was not attributed to hypersecretion of glucagon until McGavran et al. reported the first case of a patient with the glucagonoma syndrome, who had elevated plasma immunoreactive glucagon level, diabetes mellitus, skin rash, and PNET in 1966 [3]. In 1974, Mallinson et al. reported the association of skin rash with hyperglucagonoma, describing nine cases with clinical glucagonoma syndrome consisted of dermatitis, diabetes mellitus, unexplained weight loss, hypoaminoacidemia, anemia, and a glucagon-producing tumor of pancreas [4]. In 1984, Wilkinson described necrolytic migratory erythema (NME) for the skin rash associated with pancreatic tumors [5].

S. Yalcin (✉)
Department of Medical Oncology, Hacettepe University Cancer Institute, Ankara, Turkey

C. Sokmensuer
Department of Pathology, Hacettepe University, Ankara, Turkey

E. Esin
Department of Medical Oncology, Bayindir Söğütözü Hospital, Ankara, Turkey

S. Yalcin, K. Öberg (eds.), *Neuroendocrine Tumours*,
https://doi.org/10.1007/978-3-031-56968-5_15

15.3 Epidemiology

Representing around 1% of all PNETs, the incidence of glucagonoma is about 1 in 20 million [6]. Patients usually present between the ages 19 and 72 years, typically around 50 s. No glucagonama case has been reported in children, yet [7]. Although, initially a female tendency was suggested in the incidence [6], in the most recent series an even distribution among men and women has been reported [7]. No race predilection is known for glucagonoma either. Most glucagonomas are sporadic tumors whilst up to 20% of cases may be associated with multiple endocrine neoplasia syndrome 1 (MEN1).

15.4 Molecular Pathogenesis

The molecular pathogenesis of glucagonomas is still largely unknown. Glucagonomas may be associated with the MEN-1 characterized by a family history of pituitary, pancreatic islet cell, or parathyroid tumors in 3% of the cases, and glucagonoma is associated with 13% of MEN-1 related tumors. The malignant progression of glucagonoma may be associated with complex genetic mechanisms, but no specific molecular markers of malignancy have been defined with certainty so far [8].

15.5 Histopathology

Histologically glucagonomas are classified as well-differentiated functioning PNETs since these tumors demonstrate the typical morphological characteristics of other PNETs. Glucagonomas usually present as encapsulated firm nodules varying in size from several mms up to 25 cm (Fig. 15.1) [1, 7]. The majority of glucagonomas are 5–10 cm large in size at the time of diagnosis. The tail of pancreas is predominantly involved. In one study, slightly more than 50% of glucagonomas

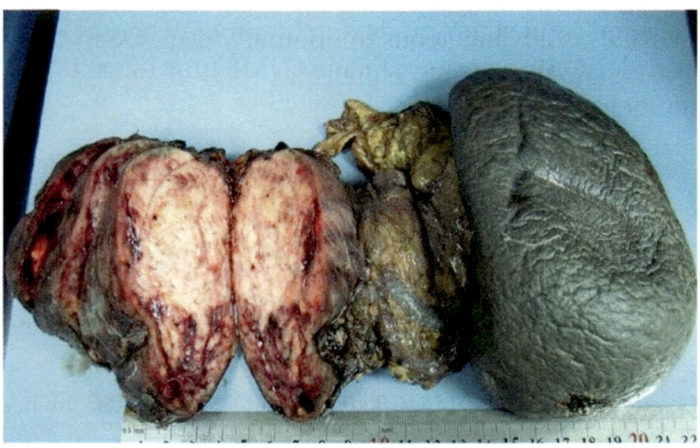

Fig. 15.1 An example of a firm encapsulated glucagonoma nodule

occurred in the tail and 80% in another study. However in the largest study, 22% of glucagonomas were in the head region of pancreas, 14% in the body, and 51% in the pancreatic tail. Most glucagonomas are within the pancreas; however, two glucagonomas with the clinical syndrome were found in the proximal duodenum and kidney. Glucagonomas usually occur as a single tumor; although, 10–12% patients have been reported as multicentric tumors or diffuse lesions thoroughout the pancreas.

Immunocytochemical and histologic studies show typical findings of NETs. The tumors consist of cords and nests of well-differentiated islet cells (Fig. 15.2). Despite their benign histologic appearance and slow growth rate such as low mitotic index and uncommon nuclear atypia, most glucagonomas are malignant with high metastatic potential. About 60% of glucagonomas were reported as malignant and 51.4% of all malignant glucagonomas were metastatic at the time of diagnosis.

Glucagon is usually detectable within the tumor cells by immunoperoxidase staining, and glucagon mRNA maybe detected by in situ hybridization. Glucagonomas are often mixed with pancreatic polypeptide-containing cells, or less often with insulin- or somatostatin-containing cells. Characteristic alpha cell granules may be seen on electron microscopy. Alpha cell tumors can be divided into two distinct types. Those associated with the glucagonoma syndrome are usually solitary and large, with undescriptive microscopic pattern, atypical granules ultrastructurally, few cells positive for glucagon immunohistochemically. These ultrastructural and immunohistochemical aberrations may be the result of abnormalities in the biosynthesis and secretion of glucagon, sometimes with alternative production of the

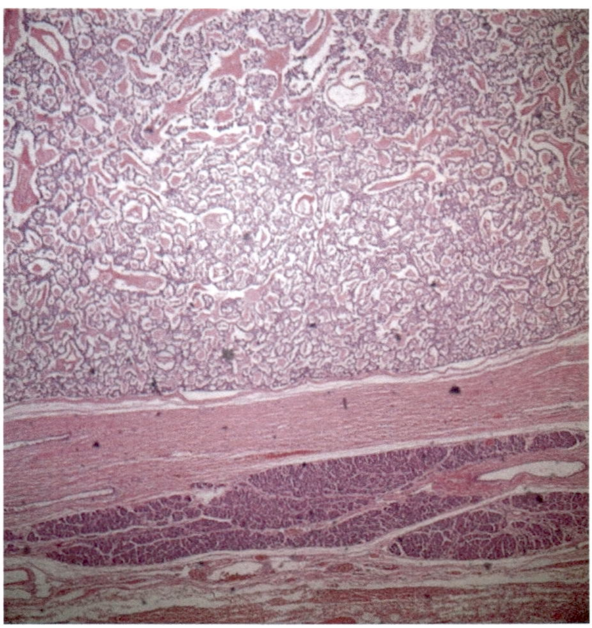

Fig. 15.2 Well-differentiated islet cells with cords and nests

related precursor peptides glycentin and oxyntomodulin. The α cell tumors that are not associated with the glucagonoma syndrome are often multiple and small, have gyriform pattern of growth, are strongly immunoreactive for glucagon, exhibit typical α cell granules ultrastructurally, and are nearly always benign. In one series of 1366 autopsy cases, the frequency of adenomas was reported to be 0.8%, and all contained glucagon-producing cells and argyrophilia can be demonstrated with Grimelius technique [7, 9–12]. In contrast, detection of atypical granules is typical in patients with tumors associated with hyperglucagonoma syndrome.

Skin biopsies are not diagnostic. The histopathology of necrolytic migratory erithema changes can be numerous as much as the clinical presentation. Typical histological findings include epidermal necrosis, parakeratotic hyperkeratosis, irregular epidermal hyperplasia, papillary dermal angiodysplasia, subcorneal pustules, and suppurative folliculitis. None of these findings indicate a pathognomonic finding, in contrast histologically and clinically it is similar to the rash of zinc deficiency, acrodermatitis enteropathica. In its classic form, early lesions demonstrate superficial spongiosis or necrosis with subcorneal and midepidermal bullae. Fusiform keratinocytes with pycnotic nuclei are often with mononuclear inflammatory infiltrates. This characteristic histologic pattern is best seen in an early lesions. The most specific feature on skin histological examination is necrolysis of the upper epidermis with vacuolated keratinocytes, leading to focal or confluent necrosis, but this histopathologic feature may be seen in other deficiency states like pellagra, necrolytic acral erythema, or zinc deficiency [9].

15.6 Pathophysiology

The etiology and pathogenesis of clinicopathologic characteristics of glucagonoma syndrome have not been enlightened yet. But the pathophysiology of glucagonoma syndrome is probably related to the known actions of glucagon. Glucagon stimulates glycogenolysis, gluconeogenesis, ketogenesis, lipolysis, and insulin secretion; alters intestinal secretion; and inhibits pancreatic and gastric secretion and gut motility. Hyperglycemia in the glucagonoma syndrome results from the increased glycogenolysis and gluconeogenesis. Because glucagon increases secretion of insulin, which prevents lipolysis and maintains normal free fatty acid concentrations, ketonemia usually does not develop.

Venous thromboembolism, NME, and angular cheilitis were observed in patients treated with continuous intravenous glucagon for refractary tumor-induced hypoglycemia. This observation indicates that glucagon may have a direct, causative role in diabetico-dermatogenic syndrome (DDS) [13]. Normalization of glucagon concentrations by surgery results in a rapid disappearance of the skin rash. Further evidence for the role of preproglucagon-derived peptides in the pathogenesis of necrolytic migratory erythema comes from its rare association with other diseases, notebly hepatic cirrhosis and coeliac disease. The patient with coeliac disease had marked elevation of circulating enteroglucagon levels. In those patients with cirrhosis, glucagon values were not invariably elevated, but hepatocellular dysfunction may result in increased levels of other preproglucagon-derived peptides, such as enteroglucagon. In one case of cirrhosis, the rash was successfully treated with fatty acid and zinc supplementation. However, it is not clearly established that the skin rash is associated with hyperglucagonemia since numerous patients have been given large doses of glucagon for long periods did not develop skin rash. Hypoaminoacidemia, nutritional lack of zinc and fatty acids, or hepatocellular dysfunction are all considered as possible triggering factors of NME. Hyperglucagonemia provokes multiple nutrient and vitamin B deficiencies, which in turn are the probable cause of this typical skin disorder [14].

15.7 Clinical Features

NME and mild diabetes are the predominant signs of the glucagonoma syndrome. The incidence of this DDS was reported to be as 57.2% [14]. Glucagonomas predominantly metastasize to the liver and adjacent lymph nodes, less frequently to the vertebra, ovary, peritoneum, and adrenals. Unlike carcinoid syndrome, liver metastases are not a prerequisite for the clinical syndrome to occur. The rash may occasionally appear prior to the onset of systemic symptoms. Although rash can be the only symptom, most patients with rash usually also have weight loss, diarrhea, sore mouth, weakness, mental status changes, or diabetes mellitus.

The characteristic feature of the glucagonoma syndrome is the rash, which is called as NME. It occurs in 90% of the cases and is usually the presenting feature. The rash exibits a 7- to 14-day sequence of erythema, blister, secondary breakdown, infection, healing, and hyperpigmentation. The initial manifestation of the rash is well-demarcated symmetrical areas of erythema (an annular or arciform erythema) at interriginous and periorificial sites, usually in groins, which migrates principally to the limbs, buttocks, and perineum. These lesions may become vesicopustular or bullous and coalesce, eroding and encrusting may occur. The rash may be mildly pruritic and occasionally painful. The extent and severity of lesions may wax and wane. The healing process commences after 10–15 days, lesions clearing centripetally to leave endurated and hyperpigmented areas, which are usually permanent. The rash remits and relapses unpredictably and this has made it difficult to assess treatment efficacy. On the basis of this morphology, differential diagnosis includes pemphigus foliaceus, pemphigoid, vasculitis, psoriasis, herpes, seborrheic or contact dermatitis, eczema, pellegra, zinc deficiency (inherited acrodermatits enteropathica or acquired), extensive candidiasis, or even chemical burn. Usually necrolytic migratory erythema rapidly disappears after successful surgical removal of the glucagon-secreting tumor. Although this eruption is a very specific cutaneous marker for underlying glucagonoma, in a few affected patients no evidence of associated malignant disease has been found. Glucagon itself may act directly on the skin to cause the rash, perhaps by increasing arachiodonic acid levels, which it does in human keratinocyte cultures. The rapid response of the rash to octreotide, before changes in circulating amino acids or glucagon, suggests a direct action on the skin, consistent with the inhibition of hormone action. Topical application of zinc or oral supplementation has been reported to improve the rash, although circulating zinc levels are normal in patients with glucagonoma.

In addition to skin rash, the disease may affect the mucous membranes. Angular stomatitis, cheilitis, and atrophic glosittis with a beefy red tongue occur almost invariably. Blepharitis, vulvovaginitis, and urethritis accompanied by dysuria are frequent features. Mucosal lesions are associated with the cutaneous rash in about 70% of patients. Glossitis or angular stomatitis was reported to occur in 34–68% of patients. Nail and scalp involvement may result in onycholysis and alopecia. Some patients develop nail dystrophy with brittleness and crumbling.

Amino acid levels are frequently diminished in the serum of patients with glucagonoma. Glucagon, acting on the liver, increases both amino acid oxidation and gluconeogenesis from amino acid substrates [11]. The intensity of hypoaminoacidemia may vary with the intensity of the disease. Glucagon stimulates sustained gluconeogenesis, which depletes the glycogenic amino acids, particularly alanin, serine, and glycine, and hepatic proteolysis with the conversion of amino acid nitrogen to urea nitrogen, which depletes all amino acids. It has been postulated that this results in an increase in protein degradation, depleting epidermal protein, and ultimately resulting in skin necrosis. Amino acid deficiency is a frequent finding in the glucagonoma syndrome, in two large series incidence was reported as 26% and 60%. Plasma concentrations of amino acids are frequently less than 25% of normal, with glycogenic amino acids most affected, whereas branch-chain amino acids are reportedly less affected. Hypoaminoacidemia may be clinically important because it may be the cause of NME; in one patient, amino acid infusion led to an improvement in the characteristic rash [15]. Intravenous amino acid infusion, although not correcting hypoaminoacidemia, has been reported to ameliorate the rash, but oral amino acid supplementation is ineffective. Similarly a high protein diet, despite normalizing plasma amino acids and nitrogen balance, may have no effect on the rash. If glucagonoma-induced hypoaminoacidemia is corrected, the dermatitis may improve without changing plasma glucagon levels. The occurrence of the rash in patients without suppressed amino acid levels casts further doubt on a casual association. Resolution of rash, however, has been reported after simple hydration with glucose and saline; therefore, it is not established that either hypoaminoacidemia or zinc deficiency is causative in all patients [7, 9–11].

Glucose intolerance is usually mild and non-ketotic since beta cell function is preserved and insulin secretion is normal. Diabetes mellitus occurs in 75–95% of patients with glucagonoma [16]. Diabetes usually precedes skin rash (and diagnosis) by years, in one study with an average time of 5 years. The hyperglycemia due to glucagonoma may be mild or moderate (median glycated hemoglobin level of 9.8% in one series [16]), is easily controlled by diet, oral agents, or insulin. In another report, 42% of patients required oral hyperglycemic agents and 24% insulin. There is little correlation between the plasma glucagon levels and the degree of glucose intolerance. This probably reflects variability in beta (β) cell insulin secretion, which may be influenced by loss of β cells as a result of tumor growth. Other factors may include insulin gene expression in glucagonoma cells, secretion of biologically inactive forms of immunoreactive glucagon by the tumor, depletion of glycogen stores, and down regulation of glucagon receptors. Various treatments have resulted in changes in plasma glucagon concentrations that did not correlate with subsequent changes in blood glucose levels. In cases where infusion of a somatostatin analog decreased plasma glucagon levels in patients with glucagonoma no effect on plasma glucose level was observed. Furthermore, tumor resection and normalization of blood glucagon may not result in normalization of the glucose tolerance in all of the patients. In some cases, the removal of glucagonoma improved glucose tolerance. It has been suggested that the development of diabetes or glucose intolerance depends to a large degree on the patient's insulin reserve. If the latter is intact, enhanced insulin release may compensate for the hyperglucagenemia and increased hepatic glucose production. Otherwise diabetes mellitus or glucose intolerance may develop.

Unrelenting weight loss affects the majority of cases (56–96% of patients), usually despite a good appetite. Weight loss may be profound. A number of observations suggest that the weight loss is a unique aspect of the syndrome. It is seen even in patients with small tumor without metastatic spread. Weight loss is prominent in patients with small tumor as well as in those with metastatic tumor, suggesting that cachexia is a consequence of the catabolic actions of glucagon. This is supported by a study in which a patient's weight loss was reversed after being given long-acting somatostatin analog, octreotide, which reduced the plasma glucagon level to a near-normal range. The main cause is probably the organ protein catabolism, which occurs in response to the depletion of amino acids. If the weight loss exceeds 50% of body weight, it can be fatal. It is not seen early in other pancreatic endocrine tumors, unless malabsorption is present. It is suggested that the anorectic effects of glucagonoma are due to the production of a novel substance by the glucagonoma and not due to glucagon per se because other transplanted glucagonomas producing similar levels of plasma glucagon elevation do not cause anorexia.

Nonspecific abdominal pain has been reported in approximately 12% of patients. The elevation of preproglucagon-derived peptides would be anticipated to affect gastrointestinal function. Enteroglucagon has been proposed as a humoral mediator of intestinal adaptation in response to injury. It appears to have a trophic action on intestinal mucosa, elevated levels causing villous hypertrophy. Three patients have been described with an enteroglucagonoma, in whom the principal clinical finding was giant villous hypertrophy. Large molecular weight forms of glucagon inhibit gastrointestinal smooth muscle, resulting in constipation. Diarrhea is reported in 14–15% of patients, occasionally with severe steatorrhea, and occurs far more commonly than constipation (15% versus 4% in one study). The etiology of the diarrhea remains unclear. Jejunal biopsies have been reported to be normal or it may show hypertrophic folds. It remains possible that other hormones secreted by the tumor could be contributing to the development of diarrhea. Rarely, nausea and vomiting occur, possibly as a result of local tumor effects.

A normochromic, normocytic anemia is common, being present in up to 90% of patients in some series. It is probably due to the anemia of chronic disease, but a direct effect of glucagon on erythropoiesis has also been suggested [17]. The anemia is usually mild with a mean hemoglobin concentration of 9.4 g/dl, but occasionally the hemoglobin may fall as low as 4 g/dl. Serum iron, B_{12}, and serum folat concentrations usually are normal, anemia does not respond to therapy with any of these agents. It does respond to resection of the tumor, however. Further evidence of anemia related to glucagon excess is that the prolonged therapy with a long-acting glucagon preparation decreased erythropoiesis in rats and mice.

Other abnormal laboratory findings in patients with glucagonoma are renal glycosuria and hypocholesterolemia. Renal glycosuria may occur early and may represent a direct renal effect of glucagon. Hypocholesterolemia was reported in 80% of cases.

Neuropsychiatric symptoms may be underdiagnosed. Neurologic symptoms associated with glucagonoma include ataxia, dementia, and proximal muscle weakness. Depression is the most commonly reported abnormality, patients may suffer from severe depression or other psychotic syndromes. The demonstration of glucagon gene expression in central nervous system may provide an explanation for these manifestations. Paraneoplastic syndromes, notebly optic atrophy, have also been attributed to this syndrome.

A late feature of the disease is widespread venous thrombosis and pulmonary embolism which is resistant to conventional anticoagulant therapy [18]. In one series, venous thrombosis (VT) occurred in 24% of patients and pulmonary emboli (PTE) in 12%. Glucagon is not known to affect coagulation parameters; and the pathophysiological process of the thromboembolic events in glucagonoma has not been elucidated, yet. Secretion of factor X, which is synthesized in α cells and is found in higher concentration in glucagonomas, may explain this complication. Venous thrombosis and PTE can frequently be a contributing factor to the patient's death; therefore, it should be carefully sought. This association with thromboembolism appears to be unique among endocrine tumors. A single case of reversible dilated cardiomyopathy associated with a glucagonoma has been reported [19].

In glucagonoma patients associated with MEN 1 syndrome, the characteristic syndrome associated with sporadic tumors is often absent, and in particular necrolytic migratory erythema rarely occurs [7, 9–11].

15.8 Diagnosis

Glucagonoma is often diagnosed relatively late in the course of the disease since many of the symptoms are nonspecific. NME is the most important manifestation which leads to the diagnosis of glucagonoma but it is not pathognomonic. With recognition of NME, further diagnostic work-up should be done.

Glucagonoma is usually suspected in patients with chronic dermatitis or unexplained and therapy-resistant dermatitis, elevated sedimentation rates associated with glucose intolerance, thromboembolic phenomena, or the MEN I syndrome. Diagnosis rests on demonstrating a pathological elevation of the plasma glucagon concentration.

Once the syndrome has been recognized or suspected, the diagnosis is easily made by demonstrating increased plasma glucagon levels. Plasma glucagon level is usually elevated 10–20 fold, up to 70% of immunoreactive glucagon may be biologically inactive. In most laboratories, the upper limit of normal for fasting glucagon concentration using antibody 30 K of Unger is 150–200 pg/ml. In one large review of glucagonomas, the plasma glucagon level was 200–500 pg/ml in only two patients, in four it was between 500 and 1000 pg/ml, and in 52 it was >1000 pg/ml. These results are in close agreement with another study in which the mean plasma glucagon concentrations was 2110 ± 334 pg/ml with a range of 550–6600 pg/ml, and with a 0% being <500 pg/ml, 30% being 500–1000 pg/ml, and the remainder >1000 pg/ml in 73 cases. In some cases, glucagon levels remain in the "physiologically elevated" range even in patients with NME. Hence, a serum glucagon concentration below 500 pg/mL does not exclude a glucagonoma.

Hyperglucagonemia has been reported to occur in chronic renal insufficiency and hepatic insufficiency which reduce clearance of increased glucagon, diabetic ketoacidosis, prolonged starvation, acute pancreatitis, acromegaly, hypercortisolism, septicemia, severe burns, severe stress (trauma, exercise), familial hyperglucagonemia, and with some drugs (danazol and oral contraceptives). There has been one case of a familial hyperglucagonemia, with autosomal dominant inheritance, in which there were no sequelae attributable to the elevated glucagon levels. Plasma glucagon level in these conditions does not exceed 500 pg/ml. A plasma glucagon concentration of >1000 pg/ml has therefore been suggested as diagnostic of glucagonoma. The one reported exception to this is in a patient with severe liver disease after portocaval anastomosis, in whom plasma level of glucagon was 1000 pg/ml. Because a necrolytic migratory erythematosus-like rash has been reported in this patient with severe hepatic disease, diagnostic confusion could occasionally result. However, in one review of 13 cases, no overlap in plasma glucagon levels was found between patients with cirrhosis or any other of the aforementioned conditions and values seen in patients with glucagonoma. Glucagon levels are highest in patients with NME and DM.

Provocative testing with tolbutamid, secretin, a mixed or carbohydrate-rich meal, or arginine is of little additional value in the evaluation of patients with suspected glucagonoma. Other biochemical abnormalities associated with the syndrome are impaired glucose tolerance and hypoaminoacidemia.

Blood investigations reveal anemia, hypoaminoacidemia, hypoalbuminemia, and hypocholestrolemia as the most common disorders. Hypoaminoacidemia occurs in most patients and, as originally pointed out by Mallinson and collegues, the levels may vary with the intensity of the disease [4].

Diabetes mellitus and glucose intolerance are among the most frequent findings in patients with the glucagonoma syndrome. Because of the effect of glucagon on glucose regulation, diabetes mellitus might be expected to be a constant feature of glucagonoma syndrome, but it is not uniformly present. Diabetes mellitus or even glucose intolerance is a much less constant feature of the syndrome than is hypoaminoacidemia.

Pancreatic polypeptide (PP) and chromogranin A are frequently elevated in glucagonoma syndrome. Most neuroendocrine tumors produce and secrete general tumor markers and circulating neuroendocrine tumor markers, such as CgA, PP, serum neuron-specific enolase, human chorionic gonadotrophin, and subunit of glucoprotein hormones. Pancreatic polypeptide and CgA can be used for screening purposes in patients without distinct clinical hormone-related symptoms. Chromogranin A, although its precise function is not yet established, has been shown to be a very sensitive and specific serum marker for various types of neuroendocrine tumors. At the moment, CgA is considered to be the best general neuroendocrine serum or plasma marker available for both diagnosis and therapeutic evaluation. Chromagranin A level increased in 50–100% of patients with various endocrine tumors. Chromogranin A serum or plasma levels reflect tumor load, and it may be an independent marker of prognosis in patients with midgut carcinoids [20].

Radiological abnormalities of the small bowel, such as thickening of mucosal folds, villous hypertrophy, and delayed gastric emptying may be demonstrated on abdominal computed tomography scanning or barium examination.

Histological specimens show the characteristic features of neuroendocrine tumors and immunocytochemistry can confirm the presence of immunoreactive glucagon. Most of the neuroendocrine tumors are immunostained positively for CgA, synaptophysin, and neuron-specific enolase.

15.9 Tumor Localization and Diagnosis

Because the most glucagonomas are malignant, it is important to attempt to localize the primary tumor and surgically resect if it has not already metastasized or to establish the presence of metastases so that unnecessary surgery can be avoided. However, careful assessment of the extent of the tumor is indicated even in patients with extensive disease because aggressive surgical resection and tumor reduction may alleviate the debilitating effects of hyperglucagonemia. At the time of diagnosis, over 50% of glucagonomas will be metastasized, and most primary tumors will be greater than 3 cm, with tumors up to 35 cm in diameter reported. Thus localization of these tumors rarely presents a problem and abdominal CT scanning is usually adequate for this purpose. The initial procedure of choice should be computed tomography since CT will detect 95% of primary pancreatic endocrine tumors more than 3 cm in diameter and 95% of metastatic pancreatic endocrine tumors in the liver. CT is particularly useful for assessing local spread. Intravenous contrast enhances the detection of smaller lesions, especially when images are obtained during the arterial phase. In addition, arterial phase and portal venous phase sequences can be used to maximize the conspicuity of liver metastases compared to the surrounding normal liver parenchyma. In liver metastasis, magnetic resonance imaging may be considered more specific to CT.

For some patients especially those with smaller primary tumors, CT or ultrasonography may not localize the tumor, and then selective angiography or EUS is the procedure of choice, depending on expertise of institution. Endoscopic ultrasound can detect pancreatic tumors as small as 2–3 mm, provide accurate information on the local extent of disease, and allow transmucosal needle biopsy of pancreatic lesions. The experience with selective venous sampling for localization of glucagonomas is much more limited than for insulinomas or gastrinomas. In the largest single-center experience reported to date, 82 patients underwent a total examination by EUS. One hundred tumors were visualized in 54 different patients, in 38 of cases no tumor was found in pancreas by EUS. On the basis of results of surgery, EUS correctly localized pancreatic tumor in 50 of 54 patients (93%). Only one of them was glucagonoma. These results may support the use of EUS as a primary diagnostic modality in the evaluation and in the management of patients with P-NET [21].

Peptide receptor scintigraphy has been developed successfully for visualization of somatostatin receptors on neuroendocrine tumors. After the intravenous administration of ^{111}In-diethylenetriamine penta-aceticacid octreotide (Octreoscan), the primary tumors and the previously unrecognized metastases of most carcinoids, islet cell tumors, paragangliomas, pheochromocytomas, medullary thyroid cancers, and small cell lung carcinoma can be visualized. In one study, 38 patients with suspected pancreatic neuroendocrine tumors were evaluated by Octreoscan SPET (OCTSPET). SPET studies were acquired at 4 and 24 h after the injection of octreoscan. The OCTOSPET results were positive in 18 of 19 patients (10 gasrinomas, 5 insulinomas, 1 neuroendocrine tumor, 1 glucagonoma, and 1 carcinoid) and false negative in one insulinoma. These data indicate that Octreoscan represents an excellent tool for the diagnosis of pancreatic neuroendocrine tumors [22].

Angiography is highly specific since the vascularity of P-NETs are high. Although angiography is considered to be gold standard, it is invasive. Angiography is now performed almost exclusively for embolization and/or infusion of chemotherapy via the hepatic artery.

Tumor calcification and cystic degeneration are common findings of glucagonomas which reflect an indolent course of the disease. However, most of the cystic neoplasms of pancreas are nonfunctioning glucagon-producing neuroendocrine tumors instead of glucagonoma.

Somatostatin receptor scintigraphy (SRS) using the indium-111 labeled somatostatin analog, pentetreotide, is the best method for evaluating the extent of metastatic disease, and, to date, all glucagonomas have been somatostatin-receptor positive. Such an evaluation is most crucial in patients being considered for hepatic transplantation but may also be of value in deciding on therapeutic modalities and assessing the response to treatment [7, 10, 11].

Several positron emission tomography (PET) tracers have been developed for functional imaging such as dihydroxy-phenyl-alanine (18F-DOPA); 11-C-hydroxytrytophan (11-C-HTP); Ga-69-DOTA-D-Phe-Tyr-Octreotide (gallium-Ga-68-DOTATOC); and Ga-68-DOTA-Phe-Tyr-Octreotate (Ga-68-DOTATATE). These PET tracers have been found more sensitive than conventional SRS.

After the detection of primary tumor, needle biopsy is needed to confirm the diagnosis. EUS-guided biopsy or in the case of liver metastasis, CT-guided biopsy are the preferred methods. Immunohistochemical staining is required to confirm the presence of glucagon in the tumor cells. The secretion of glucagon in tumor cells is heterogenous therefore occasionally the needle biopsy specimen may yield negative results for glucagon staining.

15.10 Staging

The prevalence of metastatic disease at the time of diagnosis varies from series to series, ranging from 50% to 100% [16, 18]. Liver is the most common site for metastasis, regional lymph nodes, bone, adrenal gland, kidney, and lung following it. American Joint Committee on Cancer (AJCC)/ International Union Against Cancer (UICC) TNM staging is also proper for Pancreatic NETs (Table 15.1) [23]. Survival rates according to stages are summarized in Table 15.2 [24].

Table 15.1 TNM staging for exocrine and endocrine tumors of pancreas

Primary tumor (T stage)		Lymph nodes, regional (N stage)		Distant Metastasis (M stage)	
Tx	Cannot be assessed	Nx	Cannot be assessed	M0	No distant metastasis
T0	No evidence of primary tumor	N0	No metastasis	M1	Distant metastasis
Tis	Carcinoma in situ: PanInIII	N1	Lymph node metastasis		
T1	Limited to the pancreas, <2 cm				
T2	>2 cm but limited to pancreas				
T3	Tumor extended from pancreas but no involvement of celiac axis, or SMA				
T4	Unresectable, Celiac axis or SMA involvement				

SMA Superior mesenteric artery

Table 15.2 Five- and ten-year survival rates for resected pancreatic neuroendocrine tumor patients

Stage		Observed survival 5-year (%)	Observed survival 10-year (%)	Median survival (months)
T1N0M0	Stage 1A	61.0	46.0	112
T2N0M0	Stage 1B			
T3N0M0	Stage IIA	52.0	28.8	63
T1N1M0 T2N1M0 T3N1M0	Stage IIB			
T4 any N M0	Stage III	41.4	18.5	46
Any T any N M1	Stage IV	15.5	5.1	14

15.11 Treatment

Initial management consists of supportive care and treatment of glucose intolerance/diabetes. Patient with malnutrition may need intervention to reverse the catabolic events. Intermittent aminoacid infusions have been observed for long-term resolution of NME but not otherwise a response in tumor growth or other symptoms.

Surgery is the only curative therapeutic option. The cure potential is as low as 5%. The exact percentage of cases that can be cured by surgical resection is unknown. Glucagonomas are usually diagnosed at later stages; therefore, the probability of surgical resection is probably less than 20%. In one large review of 92 cases with glucagonoma, only 16 of the malignant cases were treated by surgical resection alone. Postoperatively, only seven patients had normal plasma glucagon levels. Recurrence with elevated plasma glucagon level was reported in a number of patients after R0 resection. Even if R0 resection is amenable there will be an eventual recurrence. However despite the recurrence of disease, an extended disease-free interval may be achieved. In another study, 125 patients with NET, who underwent surgery, were investigated. Only two (3%) patients had glucagonoma. The most common operative procedures were; 50 pancreaticoduodenectomies (40%), 39 distal pancreatectomies (31%), and 21 tumor enucleations (17%). Nine synchronous hepatic resections were performed for metastases. Of the evaluable patients, 46 (43%) had postoperative complications, the most common of which were pancreatic fistula (16%), wound infection (15%), and delayed gastric emptying (8%). There were three in-hospital deaths. The most favorable outcomes for neuroendocrine tumors were observed in patients with benign functional tumors and in those with completely resected malignant pancreatic NETs [25].

Cure can be achieved for malignant disease if tumor metastases are confined to the liver and the patient is a candidate for hepatic transplantation. Cytoreductive surgery may be appropriate as palliative therapy to reduce hyperglucagonemia if there are well-circumscribed metastases amenable to enucleation. However, this can be more complicated by venous thrombosis, hypercatabolic state, and anemia. Total parenteral nutrition and blood transfusions are often required preoperatively. As a result of these factors, medical options are usually preferred for palliative therapy for metastatic disease. Control of liver metastases by metastasectomy, cryoablation, RFA, or chemoembolization may be feasible. Hepatic artery embolization involves occlusion of hepatic artery collaterals to glucagonoma metastases in the liver, the portal vein maintaining supply to the normal liver. There is usually dramatic symptomatic relief following embolization and the procedure can be repeated at 6–9 month intervals. The response rates associated with embolization or chemoembolization, as measured either by decrease in hormonal secretion or by radiographic regression, are generally greater than 50%. However, the necrotic tumor load and the remaining low amount of healthy liver tissue may be poorly tolerated in frail patients.

Another approach for liver-predominant metastatic disease is radiofrequency ablation and cryoablation. They can be applied alone or in conjuction with surgical removal. Long-term efficacy of both of these procedures remains uncertain.

Recent studies suggest that conventional contraindications to surgical resection, such as superior mesenteric vein invasion and nodal or distant metastases, should be redefined in patients with advanced neuroendocrine tumors. These patients will benefit from extensive surgical debulking in combination with adjuvant medical treatments, such as somatostatin analogues. This combination may result in enhanced survival rates compared with either procedure alone.

The morbidity associated with glucagonomas results principally from the hormonal syndrome. The effects of tumor bulk rarely become apperant until the patient is in a terminal condition. Initial treatment should be directed to control symptoms, restoring nutritional status, and controlling the hyperglycemia. Thus palliative medical therapy aims to reduce hormone levels either by reducing tumor bulk or by inhibiting the release of hormone. Cytotoxic chemotherapy or hepatic embolization may be used to reduce tumor bulk while the somatostatin analog, octreotide, both inhibits hormone levels and antagonizes hormone action.

The glucagonoma patients suffer from a prolonged catabolic state due to the effects of glucagon in liver. Hence, nutritional support is an integral component of treatment. Total parenteral nutrition should be considered preoperatively in potentially operable patients to decrease the perioperative morbidity.

In patients with widely metastatic disease in whom surgical debulking is not possible, various chemotherapeutic agents are frequently used. The conventional chemotherapy for glucagonomas and pancreatic endocrine tumors is 5-flourouracil and streptozocin. For patients with a glucagonoma, the response rate, measured by 50% reduction in plasma glucagon levels, is about 70–80%, with remission often lasting a year, although no effect on overall survival has been observed. An alternative chemotherapeutic agent is dacarbazine which has been reported to be particularly successful in patients with glucagonoma, with a biochemical response sustained for over a year in all patients. The modest efficacy of cytotoxic treatments has prompted the development of new treatment strategies.

Recently, orally active alkyating agent temozolomide has been found to be effective on P-NETs. Progress in the understanding of pathophysiology of pancreatic NETs has revealed the importance of growth factors and their receptors (vascular endothelial growth factor receptor-VEGFR) and the involvement of the Mammalian Target of Rapamycin (mTOR) in pancreatic neuroendocrine tumorigenesis [26–28]. Many of the growth factor receptors function as thyrosine kinases. Two molecularly targeted agents, an oral tyrosine kinase inhibitor (TKI) sunitib and an inhibitor of mammalian target of rapamycin (mTOR), have been approved in treatment of metastatic P-NETs.

Sunitinib is a small molecule TKI with multimodal inhibition on TKs. In a phase II trial, sunitinib was given to 109 advanced stage P-NETS [29]. Glucagonoma was presented by four cases in study group. Eighteen percent of patients had a partial response and 68% had a stable disease. Median time to tumor progression was 7.7 months. Continuous 37.5 mg daily administration of sunitinib was tested in a phase III trial [30]. Accrual was stopped prematurely due to efficacy of sunitinib in treatment arm. Median PFS was significantly longer with sunitinib (11.4 vs 5.5 months). Although a small number of patients were glucagonoma, sunitinib treatment may be considered for advanced stage diseases in which symptomatology is not much prominent and visceral crises do not exist. Side effects may include hypertension, proteinuria, and other forms of renal toxicity, arterial thromboembolism, left ventricular dysfunction, and clinical heart failure, thyroid dysfunction, bleeding, myelosuppression, hand–foot skin reaction, delayed wound healing, hepatotoxicity, and muscle wasting.

Everolimus activity is explored in many phase II and III trials in P-NET [31]. In RADIANT-3 trial, everolimus monotherapy was tested [32]. Everolimus was associated with a significant prolongation in median PFS (11.0 vs 4.6 months, hazard ratio [HR] for progression 0.35, 95% CI 0.27–0.45). There were confirmed objective partial responses in 5% versus 2% of the placebo group. The most common grade 3 or 4 drug-related adverse events were stomatitis (7%), anemia (6%), and hyperglycemia (5%). The rates of grade 3 or 4 hyperglycemia were similar in those with glucagonoma versus those without glucagonoma (9.1 vs 7.8%). However the safety of everolimus should be tested in glucagonoma patients further.

PNETs are generally considered to be radioresistant. However, some anecdotal reports have showed that in some patients local control and symptom control can be achieved by external beam radiotherapy [33–36].

Somatostatin and its long-acting analogs (Octreotide and Lanreotide) have been introduced for the treatment of endocrine tumors of the gastrointestinal tract. Somatostatin analogs have been shown to effectively control symptoms resulting from excessive hormone release in patients with carcinoid, Verner–Morrison syndrome, and glucagonoma syndromes. This beneficial effect is due to the presence of somatostatin receptors in high density in the majority of these tumors. Lanreotide is as effective as octreotide and also available in depot form. Long-term studies have shown that somatostatin analogs are safe. The most serious adverse effect is the developement of gallstones. The antiproliferative potency of somatostatin and its analogs in vitro, in experimental tumor models prompted a number of studies in patients with metastatic endocrine tumors that are generally unresponsive to conventional chemotherapeutic protocols. Promid and Clarinet studies now clearly showed the antiproliferative potency of somatostatin analogs in patients with neuroendocrine tumors. Therefore, octreotide is now the first-line therapy for the glucagonoma syndrome. Octreotide dose ranges from 150 to 1500 μg daily. Therapy is generally initiated with short-acting octreotide 50 mcg subcutaneously three times a day [16]. The dose is increased gradually as needed to control symptoms. The patient is then rapidly transitioned to a long-acting formulation. The duration of response ranges from 2 months to 3.5 years. It is particularly effective against the NME, with resolution usually occuring within a week, independently of changes in plasma amino acids or glucagon. According to various reviews, the rash improved with octreotide treatment in 54–90% of patients, complete remission of rash occurs in up to 30%. The effect is prolonged at least 6 months and frequency of recurrence is further reduced thereafter. Octreotide is less effective at reversing weight loss and has an inconsistent effect on diabetic control, perhaps reflecting inhibition of secretion of other hormones, such as insulin. It generally improves abdominal pain and diarrhea. Plasma glucagon levels decrease in from 80% to 90% of patients, but the normal range can be reached in from 10% to 20% of patients with octreotide treatment. It is not known whether octreotide has any effect on the tendency to develop VT. The combination of chemotherapy or hepatic embolization with octreotide may delay the development of octreotide resistance, which usually develops after a mean of 2 years of therapy.

Octreotide long-acting repeteable (LAR) is a new somatostatin anolog whose activity lasts 28 days. It appears to have good therapeutic efficacy, tolerability, and safety in the treatment of neuroendocrine tumors. Its effects are similar to those of octreotide and lanreotide. However, because it only needs to be administered once every 28 days, it is preferable in clinical practice [37].

Interferon-alpha (IFN-α) is another effective agnets that can be used in treatment. IFN induces tumor stabilization in 20–40%, improves symptom control in 40–50%, and objective tumor regression in 15%. However, its efficacy is concealed by high toxicity. Adverse effects like myelosupression, mental changes like depression, and alterations of thyroid functions result in detrimental effects in quality of life of patients.

Combination treatment with SA and IFN may be an option for SA-resistant patients; however, the superiority of combination is not proven yet.

Simple measures to amelioriate the NME such as topical and oral zinc and a high-protein diet, although unproven, are worth to try. Acetylsalicilic acid may be usuful in preventing thromboembolic disease, but conventional anticoagulants are ineffective. If diabetic control cannot be achieved with diet alone, insulin should be used.

Radioligand therapy based on ^{111}Indium, ^{90}Yttrium, and ^{177}Lutetium coupled to somatostatin analogs via bifunctional cheletors is currently under investigation with promising data concerning long-lasting control of symptoms and tumor growth from Phase I studies [38].

15.12 Prognosis and Follow-Up

The prognosis for patients with glucagonoma is unpredictable. Glucagonomas are slow growing tumors but due to this indolent behaviour most patients present late in the course of the disease. The 10-year survival rate in patients with DDS was 51.6% in those with metastases and 64.3% in those without metastases ($P < 0.001$) [14]. Once metastasis occurs, cure can be rarely achieved. However, with more advanced knowledge about the disease, better supportive care, better management of complications, and with the implemantation of new therapeutic modalities, prolonged survival is expected. The median survival from diagnosis is about 3 years, according to recent reports more patients are living longer, an average of 4.9 years after the diagnosis of metastasis.

A postsurgical prognostic system has been proposed upon a series of 3851 patients (75 of them were glucagonoma) [24]. Age at the diagnosis, tumor grade, and presence of metastasis are the most important predictive factors. Scoring allows patients to be categorized into three groups: Prognostic score 1 (raw score of 0), Prognostic score 2 (raw score 1–2), and Prognostic score 3 (raw score ≥3). The expected 5-year survival rates are 77%, 51%, and 36%, respectively.

Postsurgically (R0 resection) patients can be followed 3–6 months period with history and physical examination, serum glucagon, and CT/MRI. Exacerbations of the rash is a surrogate marker in long term. Those patients in remission should be seen at least yearly, when a gut hormone screen should be performed, since up to 10% of tumors will be associated with secondary hormone syndromes. In long term patients should be followed with history and physical examination with tumor markers every 6–12 months for years 1–3, and as clinically indicated thereafter. Imaging studies are recommended as clinically indicated.

References

1. Solcia EKG, Sobin LH (2000) World Health Organization international histological classification of tumors: histological typing of endocrine tumors, 2nd edn. Springer-Verlag, Berlin, pp 56–58
2. Becker ER (1942) The Iowa Academy of Science. Science 95:651–652
3. McGavran MH, Unger RH, Recant L et al (1966) A glucagon-secreting alpha-cell carcinoma of the pancreas. N Engl J Med 274:1408–1413
4. Mallinson CN, Bloom SR, Warin AP et al (1974) A glucagonoma syndrome. Lancet 2:1–5
5. Wilkinson DS (1984) [Necrolytic migratory erythema: glucagonoma syndrome. Clinical and histological aspects]. Ann Med Interne (Paris) 135:654–657
6. Kufe DWPR, Weichselbaum RR, Bast RC, Gansler TS, Holland JF, Frei E (2003) Cancer medicine, 4th edn. BC Decker, Hamilton, pp 1289–1290
7. Sheaves RJP, Wass JAH (1997) Clinical endocrine oncology, 1st edn. Blackwell Science, Oxford, pp 380–382
8. Furlan D, Cerutti R, Uccella S et al (2004) Different molecular profiles characterize well-differentiated endocrine tumors and poorly differentiated endocrine carcinomas of the gastroenteropancreatic tract. Clin Cancer Res 10:947–957
9. De Groot LJ, Jameson JL: Endocrinology (ed 4). Philadelphia W B Saunders, 2001 pp. 2506
10. Yamada TAD, Owyang C, Powell DW, Silverstein EF (2003) Textbook of gastroenterology, 4th edn. Lippincott Williams and Wilkins, Philadelphia, pp 2115–2117
11. Sleisenger MHFJ (2002) Gastrointestinal diseases. WB: Saunders Company, Philadelphia, pp 994–997
12. Mosby JR (2004) Surgical pathology. Wiley, London, pp 1088–1089
13. Case CC, Vassilopoulou-Sellin R (2003) Reproduction of features of the glucagonoma syndrome with continuous intravenous glucagon infusion as therapy for tumor-induced hypoglycemia. Endocr Pract 9:22–25
14. Soga J, Yakuwa Y (1998) Glucagonomas/diabetico-dermatogenic syndrome (DDS): a statistical evaluation of 407 reported cases. J Hepato-Biliary-Pancreat Surg 5:312–319
15. Alexander EK, Robinson M, Staniec M et al (2002) Peripheral amino acid and fatty acid infusion for the treatment of necrolytic migratory erythema in the glucagonoma syndrome. Clin Endocrinol 57:827–831
16. Wermers RA, Fatourechi V, Wynne AG et al (1996) The glucagonoma syndrome. Clinical and pathologic features in 21 patients. Medicine (Baltimore) 75:53–63

17. Boden G (1989) Glucagonomas and insulinomas. Gastroenterol Clin N Am 18:831–845
18. Stacpoole PW (1981) The glucagonoma syndrome: clinical features, diagnosis, and treatment. Endocr Rev 2:347–361
19. Chang-Chretien K, Chew JT, Judge DP (2004) Reversible dilated cardiomyopathy associated with glucagonoma. Heart 90:e44
20. Eriksson B, Oberg K, Stridsberg M (2000) Tumor markers in neuroendocrine tumors. Digestion 62(Suppl 1):33–38
21. Anderson MA, Carpenter S, Thompson NW et al (2000) Endoscopic ultrasound is highly accurate and directs management in patients with neuroendocrine tumors of the pancreas. Am J Gastroenterol 95:2271–2277
22. Briganti V, Matteini M, Ferri P et al (2001) Octreoscan SPET evaluation in the diagnosis of pancreas neuroendocrine tumors. Cancer Biother Radiopharm 16:515–524
23. Edge SB, Byrd DR, Compton CC, Fritz AG, Greene FL, Trotti A (2010) AJCC cancer staging handbook, 7th edn. Springer
24. Bilimoria KY, Bentrem DJ, Merkow RP et al (2007) Application of the pancreatic adenocarcinoma staging system to pancreatic neuroendocrine tumors. J Am Coll Surg 205:558–563
25. Phan GQ, Yeo CJ, Hruban RH et al (1998) Surgical experience with pancreatic and peripancreatic neuroendocrine tumors: review of 125 patients. J Gastrointest Surg 2:473–482
26. Oberg K, Casanovas O, Castano JP et al (2013) Molecular pathogenesis of neuroendocrine tumors: implications for current and future therapeutic approaches. Clin Cancer Res 19:2842–2849
27. Missiaglia E, Dalai I, Barbi S et al (2010) Pancreatic endocrine tumors: expression profiling evidences a role for AKT-mTOR pathway. J Clin Oncol 28:245–255
28. Zhang J, Francois R, Iyer R et al (2013) Current understanding of the molecular biology of pancreatic neuroendocrine tumors. J Natl Cancer Inst 105:1005–1017
29. Kulke MH, Lenz HJ, Meropol NJ et al (2008) Activity of sunitinib in patients with advanced neuroendocrine tumors. J Clin Oncol 26:3403–3410
30. Raymond E, Dahan L, Raoul JL et al (2011) Sunitinib malate for the treatment of pancreatic neuroendocrine tumors. N Engl J Med 364:501–513
31. Yao JC, Lombard-Bohas C, Baudin E et al (2010) Daily oral everolimus activity in patients with metastatic pancreatic neuroendocrine tumors after failure of cytotoxic chemotherapy: a phase II trial. J Clin Oncol 28:69–76
32. Yao JC, Shah MH, Ito T et al (2011) Everolimus for advanced pancreatic neuroendocrine tumors. N Engl J Med 364:514–523
33. Contessa JN, Griffith KA, Wolff E et al (2009) Radiotherapy for pancreatic neuroendocrine tumors. Int J Radiat Oncol Biol Phys 75:1196–1200
34. Strosberg J, Hoffe S, Gardner N et al (2007) Effective treatment of locally advanced endocrine tumors of the pancreas with chemoradiotherapy. Neuroendocrinology 85:216–220
35. Tennvall J, Ljungberg O, Ahren B et al (1992) Radiotherapy for unresectable endocrine pancreatic carcinomas. Eur J Surg Oncol 18:73–76
36. Torrisi JR, Treat J, Zeman R et al (1987) Radiotherapy in the management of pancreatic islet cell tumors. Cancer 60:1226–1231
37. Tomassetti P, Migliori M, Corinaldesi R et al (2000) Treatment of gastroenteropancreatic neuroendocrine tumours with octreotide LAR. Aliment Pharmacol Ther 14:557–560
38. Arnold R, Wied M, Behr TH (2002) Somatostatin analogues in the treatment of endocrine tumors of the gastrointestinal tract. Expert Opin Pharmacother 3:643–656

Somatostatinoma

16

James Matthew Lloyd Williamson

16.1 Introduction

Somatostatinomas are rare neuroendocrine tumours (NETs) that arise in the pancreas or duodenum. They are the fifth most common pancreatoduodenal NET (after insulinomas, non-functioning tumours, gastrinomas and VIPomas), with an incidence of 1 in 40 million [1–3]. They tend to be non-functioning, although they are rarely active and can produce a spectrum of symptoms called 'somatostatinoma syndrome' (see subsection below) [4–6]. A degree of discord exists regarding the functional component of a somatostatinoma; some clinicians argue a 'syndrome' of clinical symptoms must be present for the diagnosis of somatostatinoma, others that the diagnosis is purely immunohistochemical [7]. As most of these tumours are biochemically inert, they are either detected incidentally or by causing mass-effect pressure symptoms, and most will have metastasised by the time of diagnosis [6, 8, 9].

There is little to distinguish somatostatinomas from other pancreatoduodenal NETs on radiological imaging or preoperative histology, but the presence of strong and diffuse positive somatostatin staining on immunohistochemistry is diagnostic [4]. Thus, many somatostatinomas are only diagnosed post-operatively when the histopathologist has had access to the resected specimen [6]. Like most NETs, operative resection even in the presence of metastases is recommended, with somatostatin analogues and chemotherapy reserved for patients not amenable to operation [10]. A variety of techniques exist for the management of metastases, with operative resection being advocated when suitable [7, 10–12]. Outcomes tend to much be more favourable than for an associated adenocarcinoma of the pancreas or duodenum, largely due to the indolent nature of these tumours.

J. M. L. Williamson (✉)
Department of Upper GI Surgery, The Great Western Hospital,
Swindon, Wiltshire, UK
e-mail: james.williamson5@nhs.net

S. Yalcin, K. Öberg (eds.), *Neuroendocrine Tumours*,
https://doi.org/10.1007/978-3-031-56968-5_16

16.2 Incidence

Somatostatinoma was first described in 1977 [1] and since then approximately eight cases per year have been reported [2]. The suggested incidence of 1 in 40 million may increase with improved understanding and diagnosis of the tumour [1, 2]. They are the fifth most common NET in the pancreas [4], while in the duodenum they account for 15% of all NETs [13]. Patients typically present between the ages of 40 and 60 years of age, and there is a possible slight female predominance [6, 14, 15]. There are no known environmental risk factors [3]. Somatostatinomas can either be functioning or non-functioning, with less than 10% of cases thought to be associated with somatostatinoma syndrome, although some tumours may be intermittently biochemically active [16].

16.3 Location

Somatostatinomas tend to be solitary and almost exclusively confined to the pancreas or duodenum, presumably reflecting the high concentration of delta-cells in these organs [3, 6, 14]. Between 50% and 60% of somatostatinomas originate in the pancreas, where there is a preference for the head of the gland (50%), followed by the tail (25%) and then diffuse infiltration of the gland (25%) [6, 10, 13]. Of the remaining extrapancreatic lesions, approximately 50% originate in the duodenum and 50% precisely at the ampulla; less than 1% arise from the jejunum. Isolated cases in the colon and rectum have been reported as well as the stomach, bile duct, cystic duct, rectum, and ovaries [6, 17–21].

Somatostatinomas are associated with malignancy rates of up to 78%, while 70–92% have metastatic disease at presentation [6, 8, 9]. Rates of malignancy and metastasis are highest for pancreatic tumours [22, 23]. The liver is most commonly involved, followed by regional lymph nodes and then bony deposits [6]. The presence of metastatic disease is thought to be a consequence of late diagnosis and does not appear to be dependent upon the tissue of origin [6].

16.4 Associations

Most somatostatinomas are sporadic, but there are well-known associations with MEN (multiple endocrine neoplasia) type 1 and neurofibromatosis type 1 (NF1), also known as von Recklinghausen disease. Less than 1% of somatostatinomas are associated with MEN, however; this percentage being lower than for other pancreatoduodenal NETs [24]. Duodenal somatostatinomas are associated with NF1 in up to 50% of patients, but there is less of a clear-cut association for pancreatic tumours [9, 14]. NF1 patients have an inherited mutation of the NF1 gene on chromosome 17q11, which codes for the protein neurofibromin. Somatostatinomas diagnosed in the presence of NF1 are thought to have a lower risk of metastases at presentation. There is a well-recognised association between NF1, duodenal somatostatinomas and phaeochromocytomas, so that the presence of an adrenal lesion should be sought in this group of patients [3, 15, 25].

There have been occasional case reports of somatostatinomas in combination with conditions including von Hippel–Lindau disease [26, 27], tuberous sclerosis [28] and gastrointestinal stromal tumours [29–32].

16.5 Biochemistry

16.5.1 Somatostatin

Somatostatin is also known as growth hormone-inhibiting hormone (GHIH), somatotropin release-inhibiting factor (SRIF) or somatotropin release-inhibiting hormone. It is a small cyclic peptide derived from proteolytic processing of two larger molecules (prepro-somatostatin and pro-somatostatin) [14]. Somatostatin is secreted from exocrine cells in the gastrointestinal (GI) tract and from delta cells of the pancreas under physiological conditions. It has two active forms, somatostatinoma-14 and somatostain-28 (consisting of 14 and 28 amino acids, respectively) [33].

Somatostatin has a general inhibitory effect up on the gastrointestinal tract. It affects gastrointestinal motility (increasing gastrointestinal transit time and intestinal mobility), gastric acid production (inhibiting basal and prostaglandin-stimulated gastric acid secretion), pancreatic enzyme secretion, bile secretion and colonic fluid secretion [19, 33]. As a result of these actions, there is decreased absorption of nutrients within the small bowel, including a delay in the uptake of fat and calcium from the gut [19]. Somatostatin also inhibits the secretion of pancreatic and intestinal hormones such as insulin, glucagon, secretin and vasoactive intestinal polypeptide. Some of these actions are thought to occur via paracrine modulation and a reduction in splanchnic perfusion [3].

Somatostatin may also control cell proliferation both in normal tissues and NETs [33]. Somatostatin analogues (such as octreotide, octreotate, edotreotide and lanreotide) can be used in a variety of clinical contexts, including the palliation of vomiting, symptomatic control in neuroendocrine and thyroid tumours and prevention of complications following pancreatic surgery.

16.5.2 Somatostatin Receptors

The physiological effects of somatostatin are mediated by a family of seven G-protein-coupled transmembrane receptors; five subtypes exist ($SST_{1\text{-}5}$), each being coded by its relevant gene (SSTR1-5) [33, 34]. Most cells within the body express somatostatin receptors in various concentrations [35]. Of note, SSTR1 is expressed in its highest concentrations in the jejunum (and stomach), and SSTR3 is expressed in its highest concentrations in pancreatic islet cells [36]. The expression of somatostatin receptors by a tumour does not necessarily indicate that it is functional, but it can influence patient management [8, 9]. Approximately 80% of NETs express somatostatin receptors [10].

Tumours that express SST2 and SSTR5 are associated with a better outcome than those that do not [36]. In addition, tumour expression of receptors can be useful for both diagnostic and treatment purposes (see below): Somatostatin receptor scintigraphy (SRS) relies on this expression for the accurate location of both primary tumours and metastatic deposits [6, 35, 37]. Somatostatin analogues (e.g. octreotide, octreotate, edotreotide and lanreotide) can be used to control symptoms and inhibit cell growth [5, 7, 10, 38], while radionuclide therapy (via radiolabelled somatostatin analogues) can be used to deliver targeted radiotherapy to the tumour [4, 39, 40].

16.6 Pathology

Immunohistochemistry is the diagnostic investigation of choice for somatostatinomas as it reveals characteristic immunoreactivity for somatostatin [3, 13]. Management and survival of somatostatinomas is based on pathological findings, the Ki-67 index and the TNM (tumour, node, metastases) staging. All pathology reports from NETs should include a minimum data set of tumour site, immunohistochemical staining, grade (mitotic rate and Ki-67 index), presence of non-ischaemic tumour necrosis and presence of other pathological components (e.g. non-neuroendocrine components) [41].

16.6.1 Macroscopic

Macroscopic examination of a somatostatinoma reveals a round lesion which is well demarcated [13]. Lesions are typically solitary and measure 1–5 cm in diameter [3]. There is nothing to distinguish these tumours from other pancreatoduodenal NETs on macroscopic appearance.

16.6.2 Microscopic

Most somatostatinomas show typical features of a NET on histological examination: they tend to be well differentiated and show a glandular pattern (Fig. 16.1a) [3, 6, 13]. Some somatostatinomas show a mixed picture, with separate zones of well differentiated and anaplastic cells. The differentiated areas have cells arranged in lobular or acinar patterns, which are separated by fibrovascular stroma. The less well-differentiated areas have cells interrupted by fibrous septa [6].

Psammoma bodies (round collections of calcium that arise after infarction and calcification) may be present in somatostatinomas. They are circular in appearance and are laminar, acellular and basophilic on histological examination. Psammomas are more commonly found in duodenal lesions (49–68%) [23] and may be

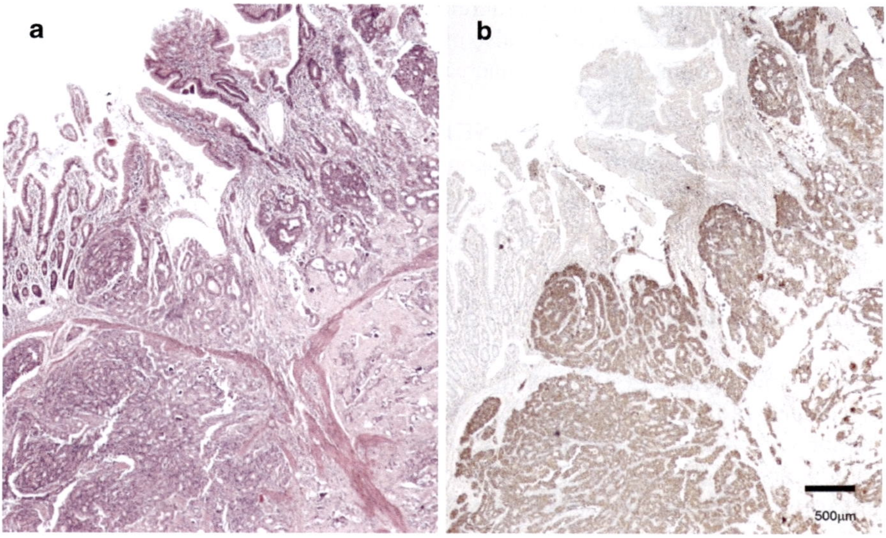

Fig. 16.1 Microscopic appearances of ampullary somatostatinoma. (**a**) Haematoxylin and eosin staining (left) and (**b**) strongly positive immunostaining with somatostatin (right). (Image kindly reproduced from the Annals of the Royal College of Surgeons of England)

associated with neurofibromatosis [13]. In contrast, pancreatic somatostatinomas do not consistently exhibit psammoma bodies [23].

16.6.3 Differentiation

Tumour differentiation—the extent of resemblance to normal cellular architecture—plays a role in assessing of how aggressive a NET is [42]. Most somatostatinomas are well-differentiated and have a uniform cellular pattern consistent with the organ of origin. Cells produce abundant neurosecretory granules and may also be arranged in nesting, trabecular or gyriform patterns [13, 42]. Poorly differentiated somatostatinomas less closely resemble non-neoplastic cells and have a more sheet-like or diffuse structural arrangement, with irregular nuclei and less cytoplasmic granularity.

16.6.4 Immunohistochemistry

Most NETs reveal some positivity for somatostatin immunohistochemistry due to the presence of somatostatin receptors. Somatostatinomas show diffuse positive immunoreactivity for somatostatin, and this expression is characteristic (Fig. 16.1b) [3, 6, 13]. The immunoexpression is related to the differentiation of the tumour, with well-differentiated somatostatinomas revealing strong immunoreactivity for somatostatin staining and poorly differentiated tumours showing less immunoreactivity [42]. Somatostatinomas will also often stain positive for synaptophysin, chromogranin A, insulin, glucagon, pancreatic polypeptide and vasoactive intestinal peptide [23].

The absence of staining for other NET hormones (vasoactive intestinal polypeptide (VIP), gastrin, insulin and glucagon) also confirms the diagnosis. In addition, there may be immunoexpression of general neuroendocrine markers such as chromogranin A and synaptophysin [42].

16.6.5 Grading

Although no grading system can fully predict the behaviour of somatostatinoma, an estimate of the biological aggressiveness of NET can provide significant information on prognosis [42]. Biological activity can be assessed by cellular mitotic activity and the Ki-67 index (to estimate the growth fraction of a cellular population). Both of these measures assess tumour proliferative rate; mitotic activity requires counting the number of mitoses seen over a microscopic field, whereas the Ki-67 index provides a percentage of cells reacting to labelling with MIB1 antibody [42, 43]. These measures are broadly equivalent in assessing grading but can sometimes give conflicting information (in which case the more aggressive score is adopted) [42]. If limited amounts of tissue are available (e.g. following biopsy), a mitotic index may not be possible to perform as it requires counting 40–50 high-power microscopic fields (more than most biopsy samples contain). In these cases, Ki67 staining provides a more accurate assessment of proliferative rate [42].

Histological grading for pancreatoduodenal NETs ranges is either low (G1), intermediate (G2) or high (G3) (Table 16.1). Low-grade NETs are relatively indolent, while intermediate grade tumours have a less predictable, moderately aggressive course [42]. Somatostatinomas that are either G1 or G2 tend to be well-differentiated NETs, while G3 tumours are poorly differentiated [42, 43].

Table 16.1 Grading system for foregut neuroendocrine tumours [40, 41]

Grade	Mitotic count (10 HPF)	Ki-67 index (%)
Low-grade G1	<2	≤2
Intermediate grade G2	2–20	3–20
High-grade G3	>30	>20

10 HPF: high power field = 2 mm^2, at least 40 fields (at 40× magnification) evaluated in areas of highest mitotic density. Ki-67 index: labelling with MIB1 antibody; % of 2000 tumour cells in areas of highest nuclear labelling

16.7 Staging

A number of different staging systems exist to classify the extent of tumour spread for NETs, and while the criteria for assessment vary between each method the underlying basic data are similar [42]. The TNM staging system is becoming the most widespread method for assessment; it reveals the extent of invasion into the organ of origin and regional or distant spread (Table 16.2) [42, 43].

Table 16.2 TNM classification for pancreatoduodenal neuroendocrine tumours

TNM grade	Duodenum/ampulla/proximal jejunum	Pancreas
Tx	Primary tumour cannot be assessed	Primary tumour cannot be assessed
T0	No evidence of primary tumour	In situ tumour/dysplasia
T1	Tumour invades lamina propria or submucosa and size ≤1 cm	Tumour invades lamina propria or submucosa for ≤1 cm
T2	Tumour invades muscularis propria or size ≥1 cm	Tumour invades muscularis propria or subserosa for ≥1 cm
T3	Tumour invades pancreas of retroperitoneum	Tumour penetrates serosa
T4	Tumour invades peritoneum or other organs	Tumour invades adjacent structures
Nx	Regional lymph nodes cannot be assessed	Regional lymph nodes cannot be assessed
N0	No regional lymph node metastasis	No regional lymph node metastasis
N1	Regional lymph node metastasis	Regional lymph node metastasis present
Mx	Distant metastases cannot be assessed	Distant metastases cannot be assessed
M0	No distant metastases	No distant metastases
M1	Distant metastases	Distant metastases

Adapted from Rindi et al. [43]

T primary tumour (add (m) for multiple tumours), *N* regional lymph nodes, *M* distant metastases. M1 specific sites as defined according to Sobin and Wittekind [44]

16.8 Presentation

The functionality of the somatostatinoma greatly influences presentation. Non-functional tumours, which are not associated with somatostatinoma syndrome, tend to present with local mass effects, though many are detected incidentally. Symptoms are non-specific but include upper abdominal pain, abdominal swelling and mass, jaundice, weight loss, nausea and vomiting [3]. Some patients will present with tumour burden from metastatic disease. Often non-functioning tumours are detected incidentally during investigation of non-specific gastrointestinal symptoms in the same manner as other gastroduodenal NETs. Some NETs have presented with upper GI bleeding, and it is possible that somatostatinomas could manifest with these symptoms [45].

16.8.1 Somatostatinoma Syndrome

Functioning tumours are rare and cause somatostatinoma syndrome as a result of overexpression of somatostatin. This syndrome comprises of diarrhoea (secondary to decreased pancreatic enzyme and bicarbonate secretion), steatorrhoea and diabetes (resulting from insulin inhibition), gallstones (from cholecystokinin inhibition) and hypochlorhydria [4–6, 19, 46]. Some authors argue that this syndrome must be present for a secure diagnosis of somatostatinoma [7]. Functioning tumours are likely to present earlier than non-functioning tumours, given their symptomatology and subsequent investigation.

16.9 Investigation

Although radiology provides the mainstay of investigation, it will only reveal the presence of a pancreatoduodenal NET rather than a definitive diagnosis of a somatostatinoma [3]. Nuclear medicine and endoscopic assessment play an increasingly important role in the management of this group of tumours. Biochemical assessment may also reveal the presence of a NET and may diagnostic for somatostatinoma. Definitive diagnosis tends to come from tissue diagnosis and immunohistochemistry (either biopsy or pathological specimen).

16.9.1 Biochemical and Haematological Assessment

Patients with pancreatoduodenal NETs should be investigated with both standard and specific blood tests. Routine full blood count, liver function tests, urea and electrolytes and clotting screen should be performed to check for any derangement in organ function: significant hepatic metastases may result in derangement in liver function. Blood glucose should also be measured for signs of diabetes, either due to somatostatin syndrome or to pancreatic dysfunction secondary to tumour invasion.

These tests should also be used as a work-up for further management, both in terms of radiological investigation and suitability for operative intervention.

Chromogranin A and pancreatic polypeptide are non-specific markers for pancreatoduodenal NETs; elevated levels are found in 50–80% of tumours, including somatostatinomas [24]. Chromogranin A is a protein contained within the neurosecretory vesicles of NETs, and elevated levels may reflect metastatic disease or a high Ki-67 index [47, 48]. However, the specificity of Chromogranin A is limited by a high false positive rate: stress conditions, liver and renal disorders and proton pump inhibitors can all give rise to elevated chromogranin A levels [47, 48]. Serum Chromogranin A is generally used for the surveillance of patients with any NETs as it can be used to monitor the patient's response to treatment and to detect signs of disease recurrence [10, 48].

Elevated plasma somatostatin levels (SLI) are strongly indicative of somatostatinoma, but these findings they are rarely found [5, 7]. Only 70% of documented somatostatinomas reported within the literature had their plasma SLI levels measured [49]. Pancreatic somatostatinomas tend to have higher SLI concentrations (up to 50 times normal) compared to intestinal somatostatinomas in which the concentration is often normal [6]. Patients with high plasma levels of somatostatin are thought to present earlier than those with normal levels [4]. Plasma SLI levels decrease following operative resection and therefore measurement of these levels can be used for surveillance and to detect any evidence of recurrence (or disease progression) [49].

16.10 Radiological Imaging

Accurate imaging of the primary tumour and the extent of disease is vital in all stages of management of somatostatinomas. Imaging should provide the location and extent of the primary tumour and assist in determining whether operative intervention should be performed, either curative resection or debulking. In addition, local invasion and the presence of metastases should be sought for investigation. Functional somatostatinomas may be harder to identify than tumours without somatostatinoma syndrome, as they are likely to be smaller at initial presentation.

Conventional imaging provides the mainstay of initial investigation. Computed tomography (CT), ultrasound scanning and magnetic resonance imaging (MRI) can all be employed to assist diagnosis, with selective use of small bowel series (barium or gastrografin) (Fig. 16.2) and angiography (Fig. 16.3) [3]. Dual-phase, thin-slice CT (Fig. 16.4) is the usual first-line investigation; detection rates are proportional to the size of the lesion, with an overall sensitivity of 73% [50]. Somatostatinomas are isodense (and thus not visible on unenhanced CT), but intravenous contrast will reveal a characteristic hypervascular lesion [51]. Typically lesions are 5 cm in diameter at presentation [41]. More than 70% of lesions greater than 3 cm in size can be identified, but only 40–50% of lesions measuring less than 1 cm are detected [10, 50, 52]. Thus, small somatostatinomas and hepatic metastases may be missed. Dual-phase CT and MRI have equivalent

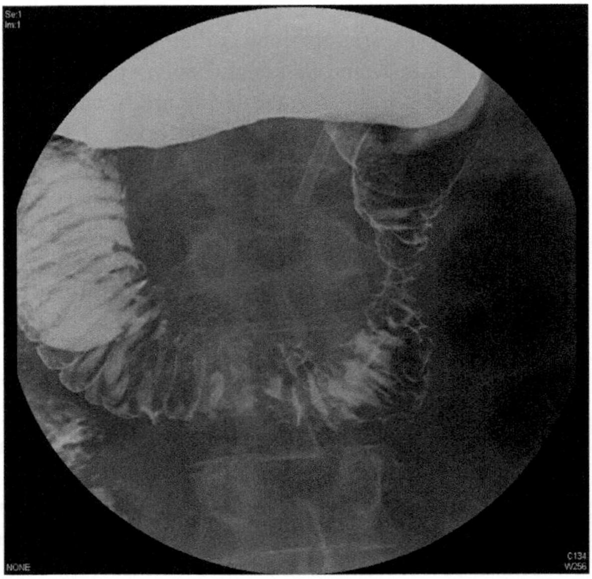

Fig. 16.2 Small bowel Gastrograffin study showing constricting duodenal lesion (subsequently confirmed as somatostatinoma)

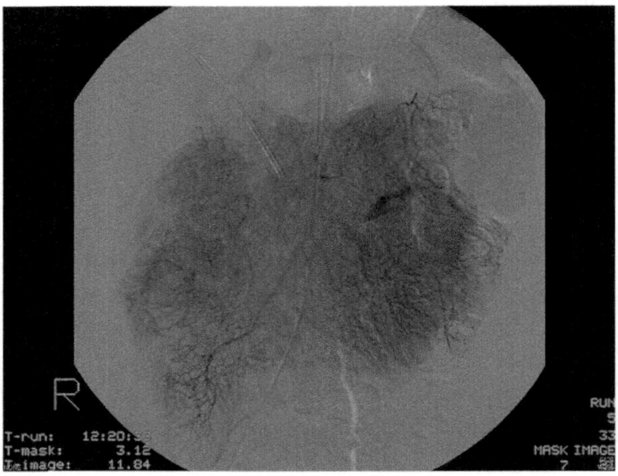

Fig. 16.3 Visceral angiography of patient with duodenal somatostatinoma. Increased tumour 'blush' noted to right-hand side of image, but no gross vascular invasion present (patient subsequently underwent successful pylorus-preserving proximal pancreatoduodenectomy)

sensitivities for the detection of NETs; CT is thought to be better for detection of peritoneal and mesenteric disease than MRI, which is more sensitive for detecting liver and bony metastases [6, 53].

Transabdominal ultrasound is not used routinely because it has a low sensitivity (9–64%) for pancreatic lesions [10, 52]. Angiography may reveal a characteristic

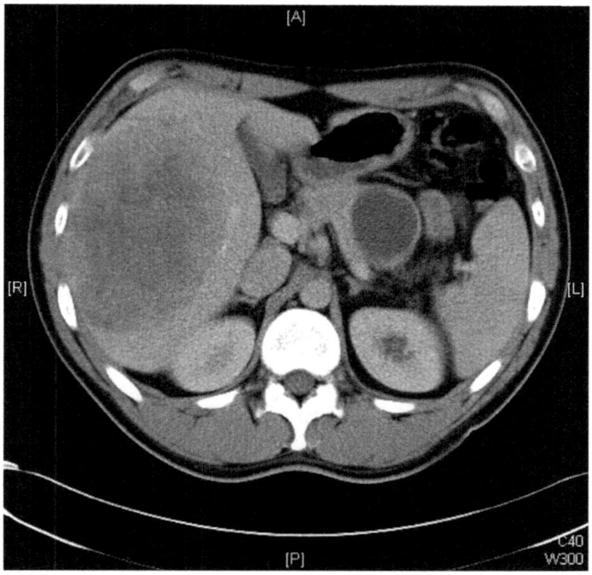

Fig. 16.4 Computed tomography showing the presence of a large pancreatic primary somatostatin and hepatic metastases

tumour blush and can be combined with selective visceral cannulation and assessment of hormonal gradients. These techniques have now been largely superseded by other imaging modalities, notably CT.

16.11 Nuclear Medicine Imaging

16.11.1 Somatostatin Receptor Scintigraphy

The overexpression of somatostatin receptors (particularly subtypes SSTR 2 and 5) by more than 80% of pancreatoduodenal NETs has allowed the development of somatostatin receptor scintigraphy (SRS) [37, 54, 55]. A number of different radiolabelled somatostatin analogues will bind to the receptors with high affinity. One of the agents most widely used worldwide for SRS is ^{111}IN-DTPA-octreotide (Octreoscan), which has an overall sensitivity of 80–90% [6, 10, 24, 37, 56]. SRS allows whole body scanning, which is invaluable in detecting metastases (especially at unexpected locations), but it does not provide information on tumour size or resectability [4, 6]. After the radiolabelled agent is injected into the patient, scans are generally performed at either 4–6 h or at 24 h. With earlier scans, lesions may be obscured by a relatively high background activity. Delayed scans provide better contrast (due to lower background activity) but can result in false-positive results secondary to physiological bowel activity [6].

16.11.2 SPECT (Somatostatin Receptor Scintigraphy Combined with Computed Tomography)

SPECT is more sensitive than conventional imaging for detection of both the primary somatostatinoma and its metastases [37, 57]. Seventy percent of primary lesions and more than 90% of distant disease can be detected with SPECT [37, 57]. It has the additional advantage over conventional imaging that it can provide whole body scanning at one time, and it alters patient management in up to 47% of patients [7, 37]. False-positive localisations can occur in up to 12% of patients, but this figure can be reduced to 3% when findings are corroborated with clinical assessment [7, 10, 37, 39].

16.11.3 Positron Emission Tomography

Positron emission tomography (PET) scanning (Fig. 16.5) has greater sensitivity than either SRS or conventional cross-sectional imaging [10]. As a result, this new technique is becoming increasingly employed for the detection of all pancreatoduodenal NETs, including somatostatinomas [3, 58]. Two main agents are used: ^{11}C-5-HTP or 68gallium-labelled somatostatin analogues. These agents rely on the fact that all grades of NETs express well-differentiated somatostatin receptors on their surface, which allows uptake of radiolabelled somatostatin analogues. Clearly defined foci of uptake of PET (away from areas of physiological uptake) should be considered as representing a NET [56]. Grade 3 pNETs are characterised by high metabolism and intake of glucose [47].

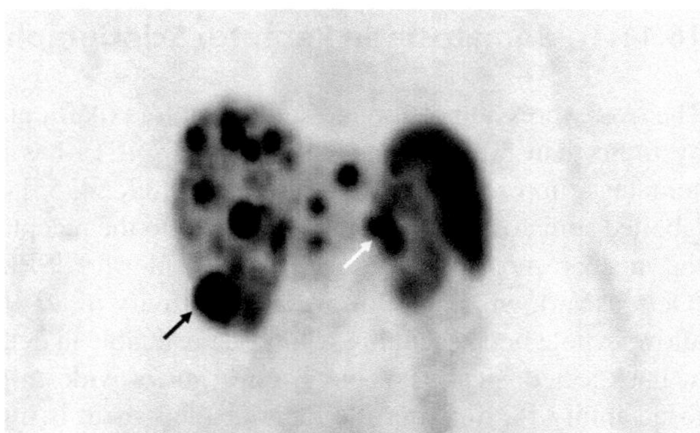

Fig. 16.5 PET scan showing extensive hepatic metastases as well as uptake in the inferior pole of the right kidney (black arrow) and the pancreatic primary tumour (white arrow). (Image kindly reproduced from the Annals of the Royal College of Surgeons of England)

16.12 Endoscopic

Endoscopy allows direct visualisation of the upper gastrointestinal tract and can help diagnose gastroduodenal lesions. It should be combined with concurrent endoscopic ultrasound, which can detect lesions as small as 0.5 cm [59]. Endoscopic ultrasound is more effective at localising tumours in the pancreas than the duodenum, although the tail of the gland can be inaccessible [7, 60]. Fine needle aspirates can be taken, which can be useful in providing cytological assessment of suspect lesions.

16.13 Intraoperative Techniques

Both intraoperative ultrasonography and endoscopic transillumination are recommended to assist in detection of small lesions not appreciated on conventional imaging [7, 10]. In addition, they can be used to help plan the route of resection and enucleation of lesions [4]. However, these techniques may fall out of routine use with the increasing availability and sensitivity of nuclear imaging.

16.14 Management

The overall 5-year survival rate in pancreatic and periampullary somatostatinoma is 60–100% with localised disease or 15–60% in metastatic disease [15, 61]. Large size (>3 cm), poor differentiation and lymph node involvement are poor prognostic markers. Tumours that are hormonally inactive (non-functioning), which predominate, have a worse prognosis than functioning somatostatinomas.

Operative resection, when feasible, is recommended for all pancreatoduodenal NETs, including somatostatinomas. Curative resection is the aim of intervention, but in the presence of liver metastases either complete resection or debulking of primary tumour is recommended. Medical management, in the form of chemotherapy, somatostatinoma analogues or radionuleotide therapy, plays an important role in controlling both symptoms and tumour growth, but it is not considered as a first-line intervention.

16.15 Medical

16.15.1 Somatostatin Analogues

Somatostatin analogues such as octreotide, octreotate, edotreotide and lanreotide, help control the symptoms of pancreatoduodenal NETs [5, 7]. These analogues act on somatostatin receptors and stimulate the inhibitory effects of somatostatin.

Long-acting depot forms of these analogues allow monthly injection therapy, which increases patient convenience and therefore compliance [10]. Long-term treatment may be associated with symptomatic breakthrough, in which case a stronger or more frequent doses may be required; in some cases, a treatment 'holiday' is required before recommencing the analogue [10]. These analogues have mild side effects in up to half of all patients, including flatulence, diarrhoea/steatorrhoea, nausea, gallstones and glucose intolerance [5, 7]. The addition of α-interferon therapy may help control symptoms if first-line intervention is inadequate [24].

In addition to symptomatic relief, somatostatin analogues are thought to have tumourostatic effect in 40–80% of patients but have not been shown to cause tumour regression [7, 10, 39]. This stabilisation of disease has increased progression-free survival for midgut neuroendocrine tumours [4, 62].

16.15.2 Anti-Angiogenic Agents

The recent development of anti-angiogenic agents (including Sunitinib, a multitarget tyrosine tyrosine kinanse inhibitor) has led to novel strategies for treating NETs. Sunitinib (37.5 mg) appears to improve medial progression free survival (versus placebo) in a recent study of 171 patients with advanced pancreatic NETs (11.4 vs 5.5 months), with relatively few side effects (neutropenia and hypertension in 12% and 10% of patients, respectively) [63].

16.15.3 Immunosuppression

Everolimus, an oral inhibitor or mammalian target of rapamycin (mTOR), has shown anti-tumoural effects in both a phase II and phase III trial (RADIANT-2 and RADIANT-3) of 410 patients with grade 1 and grade 2 pNETs; median progression survival rates of 11 months versus 4.6 months (placebo) have been reported [64, 65]. Further research is required to define the optimal role for immunosuppressants in pNETs therapy.

16.15.4 Traditional Oncological Treatments (Chemotherapy and Radiotherapy)

Generally, pancreatoduodenal NETs do not respond well to oncological agents, because they are slow-growing and thus have an inherent resistance to therapies targeted at rapidly dividing cells. Nevertheless, chemotherapy and radiotherapy are frequently employed for disease that is not amenable to operative resection. A number of different chemotherapeutic regimes have been employed, with an overall objective response rate of 10–45% [4]. Chemotherapeutic agents include streptozotocin, doxorubicin, 5-FU, temozolomide, dacarbazine and chlorozotocin; streptozotocin is thought to be the best therapy with response rates as high as 70% [3, 4]. However, these regimes result appreciable toxicity. Complete tumour response to any therapy is rare and all drugs are associated with side effects that may make the regime intolerable. Trans-arterial chemoembolization (TACE) can also be successfully employed for the treatment of hepatic metastases (see below).

Systemic radiotherapy is not usually suitable for patients with somatostatinomas (or any pancreatoduodenal NETs) due to the location of the primary tumour and associated lymphatic spread. Its use is not supported in the literature except for providing symptom relief for bony metastases [4].

16.15.5 Radionuclide Therapy (Peptide Receptor Radionuclide Therapy [PRRT])

Radionuclide therapy is a novel technique that is being increasingly utilised for the treatment of inoperable or metastatic pancreatoduodenal NETs [40, 66]. This therapy delivers targeted local radionuleotides that release γ-radiation or β-radiation to the tissues, thus decreasing overall radiation exposure to the patient [39, 40]. The exact dosage of radiation needs to be calculated to ensure that sensitive organs, for example kidneys and bone marrow, do not suffer irreversible damage [40]. PRRT is generally well tolerated with manageable toxicity; studies of combination of PRRT in combination with other therapies are currently taking place [47].

The overexpression of somatostatin receptors by most NETs, particularly somatostatinomas, makes targeted peptide receptor radionuclide therapy (PRRT) particularly appealing. Radiolabelled somatostatin analogues with attached radionuclides of ^{177}lutrium, ^{90}ytrium or ^{111}indium can be used to target pancreatoduodenal NETS. No randomised controlled studies exist, but several studies have reported favourable response rates [4, 39, 66]. Of all the agents commercially available [^{177}Lu-DOTA^{0},Tyr3], octreotate (DOTATATE) has showed a complete response rate in 2% patients, a partial response in 32% and stabilisation of disease in 34% [66]. Overall, median survival rates with DOTATATE of more than 40 months have been reported.

16.16 Operative

Operative resection of the primary tumour, even in the presence of metastases, is recommended for all pancreatoduodenal NETs unless the patient has [10]:

1. Another medical condition limiting life expectancy or increasing surgical risk
2. Diffuse metastatic liver disease
3. One of the inherited PNET syndromes

This strategy is governed, in part, by better outcomes of operative resection and the traditionally poor outcomes associated with non-operative interventions. When curative resection cannot be performed, surgical debulking of the primary tumour is advocated; hepatic resection of metastatic disease is also advocated when possible, although there are a number of alternatives to hepatectomy (see below). Any resection should be combined with cholecystectomy because of the likelihood of gallstone formation with increasing somatostatin levels (with associated cholecystokinin inhibition) postoperatively [4].

16.16.1 Curative Resection

Any patient without metastatic disease should be considered for curative resection of the tumour. Unfortunately with up to 90% of patients presenting with metastatic disease, curative resections are not that common particularly when sensitive whole body scanning, in the form of SRS or PET, is now commonplace [6, 8, 9]. When possible, somatostatinomas should be locally excised or enucleated, with major resections reserved for more extensive disease in patients who are fit enough to tolerate the operation [7, 10, 24]. As somatostatinomas are located in the periampullary duodenum or pancreatic head, a pylorus-preserving pancreatoduodenectomy or Whipple's procedure is the most common resection, although total pancreatoduodenectomy may occasionally be required for multiple tumours or bulky tumours in the pancreatic neck [3]. Ampullary lesions can be resected en-bloc with a pancreatoduodenecomty, but small lesions (<2 cm) can be considered for local resection with ampullectomy or via an endoscopic enucleation if they are small (≤5 mm) as they are likely to be confined to the papilla [67–69].

Well-defined and localised intrapancreatic lesions can be resected laparoscopically, but most somatostatinomas are approached by laparotomy. An extensive abdominal exploration has traditionally been recommended to search for lymph node metastases, although this may not be required given the sensitivity of SRS and PET [7, 10, 24].

16.16.2 Palliative Resection

By definition, tumours that have metastasised cannot undergo curative resection, but resection of the primary tumour even in the presence of hepatic metastases is advocated [3, 10]. There are many options for the management of hepatic metastases (see below) that can improve patient survival and alter the natural history of the disease process [70]. A recent systematic review has shown a trend towards improved survival post resection of primary lesion in the presence of metastases, although it is unknown whether this is a true reflection or simply that patients in the operative group are healthier than those not deemed for surgery, that is a positive selection bias for treatment in patients with better overall performance status [12]. Regardless of the underlying mechanism, a 30% improvement in 5-year survival in patients undergoing resection has been reported [12].

Thus all patients should be considered for operative intervention if complete (or near-complete) resection of hepatic metastases can be achieved [70]. Resection of the primary tumour should be undertaken in the same manner as outlined above and it can be combined with concurrent resection of metastatic disease.

16.16.3 Debulking of Primary Tumour

Operative tumour debulking, to remove at least 90% of primary tumour volume, is only possible in 5–15% of patients [7, 10, 71, 72]. Although there is little evidence to suggest that cytoreductive surgery improves symptoms and survival, it is generally advocated especially since other interventions have low efficacy [4, 7, 71–73]. Some studies have shown that debulking can improve symptoms associated with 'tumour mass, that is pain and vomiting, with up to half of patients reporting benefit for a mean duration of 39 months, compared to best combination chemotherapy offering a median survival of 26 months [73, 74].

16.17 Management of Liver Metastases

Given that most non-functioning somatostatinomas are indolent and present with metastatic deposits, aggressive management of these liver lesions is advocated; hepatectomy should be considered in all cases and can be performed in isolation or combined with other hepatic intervention (see below). Patients who are deemed unresectable, either due to co-morbidities or diffuse hepatic involvement, may be managed with targeted tissue destruction.

16.17.1 Resection of Liver Metastases

Aggressive resection of liver metastatases is associated with better long-term outcomes compared with non-operative intervention, such as hepatic artery embolisation (HAE), radiofrequency ablation or radioactive octreotide [3]. Five-year survival rates of 76% have been reported following hepatectomy, compared with 50% for HAE and 26% for medical therapy [73]. Complete resection of hepatic metastases improves survival threefold compared with incomplete resection [75]. For young, otherwise healthy patients, liver transplantation for widespread hepatic metastatic infiltration should be considered, especially if the patient's symptoms cannot be managed by other therapies [10]. However, the role of transplantation is unclear due to the absence of defined selection criteria and lack of data regarding long-term outcomes [76, 77].

16.17.2 Non-Operative Management of Liver Metastases

Several hepatic interventions exist for the management of metastatic disease, but no randomised studies exist comparing the efficacy of any procedure either against each other or against resection [4, 11]. Non-operative intervention is recommended for palliation in patients who are unsuitable for surgical resection provided they have an otherwise preserved performance status, with disease confined to the liver and a patent portal vein [10, 11]. These techniques are considered particularly relevant for patients with hormone excess who cannot be controlled by any other means [11]. Non-operative strategies include gel foam embolisation, transhepatic arterial chemoebolisation (TACE), hepatic artery embolisation (HAE) with radioactive mircospheres, percutaneous alcohol ablation, radiofrequency ablation and cryoablation.

The rationale for TACE is that metastatic tumour cells are thought to derive more than 90% of their oxygenation and nutrition from the hepatic artery [b]. Response rates following TACE are generally greater than 50% and are measured by radiographic regression and/or a decrease in serum hormones [11]. No data exist showing superiority of any one of the TACE techniques (bland embolisation, chemoembolisation, embolisation with chemotherapy beads and embolisation using radioisotopes) compared with each other. RFA and cryoablation are recommended only in selected patients who have low-volume disease [10, 11]. All these techniques can be performed either intraoperatively (either combined with resection of primary metastatic disease, or during separate laparoscopy) or via a percutaneous approach [10].

16.18 Surveillance

Like most pancreatoduodenal NETs, somatostatinoma has an indolent course compared with pancreatic adenocarcinoma. These tumours therefore generally have a longer overall survival even if untreated [4]. The natural history of the disease is not fully understood and, as such, there are no guidelines for prognosis or surveillance of disease. Generally, patient surveillance is advocated, especially when operative resection has occurred. Patients should have their chromogranin A, pancreatic polypeptide and plasma somatostatin levels monitored in addition to periodic cross-sectional imaging of the abdomen [10, 48, 49]. Some clinicians advocate yearly postoperative SRS studies to detect signs of disease recurrence [10].

16.18.1 Tumour Recurrence or Progression

No established guidelines exist for the management of patients with progressive or recurrent disease. Options include reoperation (including debulking for symptom relief from space-occupying lesions or hormonal effects) and systemic chemotherapy. Therapy should be based on the individual's characteristics, site of recurrence and prior therapy [4].

16.19 Conclusion

Somatostatinomas are rare neuroendocrine tumours that arise in the pancreas or peripancreatic duodenum. They are a fascinating group of tumours that are poorly understood and relatively unpredictable. These tumours are relatively indolent and present late, often with metastatic disease. Although there is some dispute as to whether functional activity (somatostatinoma syndrome) is required for diagnosis, most tumours are diagnosed histologically on diffuse positive immunoreactivity to somatostatin. An increased awareness of this group of tumours and improved imaging (particularly in the form of SRS and PET scanning) is thought to be related to an increasing incidence of disease.

Operative resection provides the mainstay of treatment for both primary lesions and metastatic disease, with somatostatin analogues, chemotherapy and radionulceotide therapy considered second-line intervention. No randomised control trials for the management of somatostatinomas exist to guide treatment, owing to their rarity and the difficulty with correct pre-operative. Survival is generally good and certainly much better than for an equivalent pancreatoduodenal adenocarcinoma.

Acknowledgements Annals of the Royal College of Surgeons (image rights).

Funding Nil

Disclosures Nil

References

1. Ganda OP, Weir GC, Soeldner JS, Legg MA, Chick WL, Patel YC, Ebeid AM, Gabbay KH, Reichlin S (1977) "Somatostatinoma": a somatostatin-containing tumor of the endocrine pancreas. N Engl J Med 296:963–967
2. House MG, Yeo CJ, Schulick RD (2002) Periampullary pancreatic somatostatinoma. Ann Surg Oncol 9:869–874
3. Williamson JML, Thorn CC, Spalding D, Williamson RCN (2011) Pancreatic and peripancreatic somatostatinomas. Ann R Coll Surg Engl 93:356–360
4. Ellison TA, Edil BH (2012) The current management of pancreatic neuroendocrine tumours. Adv Surg 46:283–296
5. O'Toole D, Salazar R, Falconi M, Kaltsas G, Couvelard A, de Herder WW, Hyrdel R, Nikou G, Krenning E, Vullierme MP, Caplin M, Jensen R, Eriksson B, Frascati Consensus Conference, European Neuroendocrine Tumor Society (2006) Rare functioning pancreatic endocrine tumors. Neuroendocrinol 84:189–195
6. Vinik AI, Woltering EA, Warner RRP, Caplin M, O'Dorisio TM, Wiseman GA, Coppola D, Go VLW (2010) NANETS guidelines: NANETS consensus guidelines for the diagnosis of neuroendocrine tumor. Pancreas 39:713–734
7. Metz DE, Jensen RT (2008) Gastrointestinal neuroendocrine tumors: pancreatic endocrine tumors. Gastroenterol 135:1469–1492
8. Vinik AI, Strodel WE, Eckhauser FE, Moattari AR, Lloyd R (1987) Somatostatinomas, PPomas, neurotensinomas. Semin Oncol 14:263–281
9. Doherty GM (2005) Rare endocrine tumours of the GI tract. Best Pract Res Clin Gastroenterol 19:807–817
10. Kulke MH, Anthony LB, Bushnell DL, de Herder WW, Goldsmith SJ, Klimstra DS, Marx SJ, Pasieka JL, Pommier RF, Yao JC, Jensen RT (2010) NANETS treatment guidelines: well-differentiated neuroendocrine tumors of the stomach and pancreas. Pancreas 39:735–752
11. Steinmuller T, Kianmanesh R, Falconi M et al (2008) Consensus guidelines for the management of patients with liver metastases from digestive (neuro)endocrine tumours: foregut, midgut, hindgut and unknown primary. Neuroendocrinol 87:47–62
12. Capurso G, Bettini R, Rinzivillo M, Boninsegna L, Delle Fave G, Falconi M (2011) Role of resection of the primary pancreatic neuroendocrine tumour only in patients with unresectable metastatic liver disease: a systemic review. Neuroendorcinol 93:223–229

13. Klöppel G (2007) Tumour biology and histopatholgy of neuroendocrine tumours. Best Pract Res Clin Endocrinol Metabol 21:15–31
14. Mao C, Shah A, Hanson DJ, Howard JM (1995) Von Recklinghausen's disease associated with duodenal somatostatinoma: contrast of duodenal versus pancreatic somatostatinomas. J Surg Oncol 59:67–73
15. Soga J, Yakuwa Y (1999) Somatostatinoma/inhibitory syndrome: a statistical evaluation of 173 reported cases as compared to other pancreatic endocrinomas. J Exp Clin Cancer Res 18:13–22
16. Mozell E, Stenzel P, Woltering EA, Rosch J, O'Dorisio TM (1990) Functional endocrine tumors of the pancreas: clinical presentation, diagnosis, and treatment. Curr Probl Surg 27(6):301–386
17. Ectors N (1999) Pancreatic endocrine tumors: diagnostic pitfalls. Hepato-Gastroenterol 46:679–690
18. Harris GJ, Tio F, Cruz AB Jr (1987) Somatostatinoma: a case report and review of the literature. J Surg Oncol 36:8–16
19. Greggersen G, Holst JJ, Trankjaer A, Stadil F, Mogensen AM (2002) Somatostatin producing teratoma, causing rapidly alternating extreme hyperglycemia and hypoglycaemia, and ovarin somatostatinoma. Metabolism 51:1180–1183
20. Goodman ZD, Albores-Saavedra J, Lundblad DM (1984) Somatostatinoma of the cystic duct. Cancer 53:498–502
21. Kitagawa M, Hayakawa T, Kondo T, Shibata T, Sakai Y, Ono H, Kiriyama S, Yokoi T (1989) Somatostatinoma of the rectum. Am J Gastroenterol 84:1452–1455
22. Moayedoddin B, Booya F, Wermers RA, Lloyd RV, Rubin J, Thompson GB, Fatourechi V (2006) Spectrum of malignant somatostain-producing neuroendocrine tumors. Endocr Pract 12:394–400
23. Garbrecht N, Anlauf M, Schmitt A et al (2008) Somatostatin-producing neuroendocrine tumors of the duodenum and pancreas: incidence, types, biological behaviour, association with inherited syndromes, and functional activity. Endocr Relat Cancer 15:229–241
24. Oberg K, Eriksson B (2005) Endocrine tumours of the pancreas. Best Pract Res Clin Gastroenterol 19:753–781
25. Cappelli C, Agosti B, Braga M, Cumetti D, Gandossi E, Rizzoni D, Agabiti RE (2004) Von Recklinghausen's neurofibromatosis associated with duodenal somatostatinoma. A case report and review of the literature. Minerva Endocrinol 29:19–24
26. Karasawa Y, Sakaguchi M, Minami S, Kitano K, Kawa S, Aoki Y, Itoh N, Sakurai A, Miyazaki M, Watanabe T, Akimoto M, Arakura N, Kiyosawa K (2001) Duodenal somatostatinoma and erythrocytosis in a patient with von Hippel-Lindau disease type 2A. Intern Med 40:38–43
27. Maki M, Kaneko Y, Ohta Y, Nakamura T, Machinami R, Kurokawa K (1995) Somatostatinoma of the pancreas associated with von Hippel-Lindau disease. Intern Med 34:661–665
28. Sreenarasimhaiah J, Armstrong LA, Tang SJ, Barnett C (2009) Pancreatic somatostatinoma and tuberous sclerosis: an exceedingly rare association. Gastrointest Endosc 69:379–381
29. Barahona-Garrido J, Aguirre-Gutiérrez R, Gutiérrez-Manjarrez JI, Tellez-Avila FI, López-Arce G, Fomperoza-Torres A, Criales S, Sánchez-Cortés E, Sarti HM, Yamamoto-Furusho JK (2009) Association of GIST and somatostatinoma in a patient with type-1 neurofibromatosis: is there a common pathway? Am J Gastroenterol 104:797–799
30. Sakorafas GH, Giannopoulos GA, Parasi A, Konstantoudakis G, Tzanakis N, Stergiopoulos S, Peros G (2008) Large somatostatin-producing endocrine carcinoma of the ampulla of vater in association with GIST in a patient with von Recklinghausen's disease. Case report and review of the literature. JOP 9:633–639
31. Tewai N, Rollins K, Gandhi N, Kaye PV, Lobo DN (2014) Mixed periampullary adenocarcinoma and somatostainoma with small bowel gastrointestinal tumour in neurofibromatosis type 1. JOP (Online) 28:600–603
32. Juergens KU, Weckesser BO, Wormanns D (2006) Duodenal somatostatinoma and gastrointestinal stromal tumor associated with neurofibromatosis type 1: diagnosis with PET/CT. Am J Roentgenol 187:W223–W234
33. de Herder WW, Hofland LJ, van der Lely AJ, Lamberts SWJ (2003) Somatostain receptors in gastroenteropancreatic neuroendocrine tumours. Endocr Relat Cancer 10:451–458

34. Yamada Y, Stoffel M, Espinosa R 3rd, Xiang KS, Seino M, Seino S, Le Beau MM, Bell GI (1993) Human somatostatin receptor genes: localization to human chromosomes 14, 17, and 22 and identification of simple tandem repeat polymorphisms. Genomics 15:449–452
35. Volante M, Bozzalla-Cassione F, Papotti M (2004) Somatostain receptors and their interest in diagnostic pathology. Endocr Pathol 15:275–292
36. Corleto VD, Falconi M, Panzuto F et al (2009) Somatostain receptor subtypes 2 and 5 are associated with better survival in well-differentiated endocrine carcinomas. Neuroendocrinology 82:223–230
37. Gibril F, Jensen R (2004) Diagnostic uses of radiololabelled somatostain-receptor analogues in gastroenteropancreatic endocrine tumors. Dig Liver Dis 36:S106–S120
38. Capurso G, Panzuto F, Delle FG (2010) Clinical relevance of the expression of somatostain receptors in digestive endocrine tumours. Dig Liver Dis 42:173–174
39. Gibril F, Jensen RT (2004) Diagnostic use of radiolabelled somatostain receptor analogues in gastroenteropancreatic endocrine tumours. Dig Liver Dis 36:S106–S120
40. Kam BLR, Teunissen JJM, Krenning EP, de Herder WW, Khan S, van Vilet EI, Kwekkeboom DJ (2012) Lutetium-labelled peptides for therapy of neuroendocrine tumours. Eur J Nucl Med Mol Imaging 39:S103–S112
41. Klimstra DS, Modlin IR, Adsay NV et al (2010) Pathological reporting of neuroendocrine tumors: application of the Delphic consensus process to the development of a minimum pathology data set. Am J Surg Pathol 34:300–313
42. NANETS Guidelines (2010) The pathological classification of neuroendocrine tumors: a review of nomenclature, grading, and staging systems. Pancreas 39:707–712
43. Anon (2006) TNM staging of foregut (neuro)endocrine tumours: a consensus proposal including a grading system. Virchows Archives 449:395–401
44. Sorbin LH, Wittekind C (eds) (2002) TNM classification of malignant tumours. Wiley-Liss, New York
45. Xu B, Wang Y, Li X, Lin J (2017) Nonfunctional pancreatic neuroendocrine tumour masked as anemia. Medicine 96:e7441
46. Ito T, Igarashia H, Jensen RT (2012) Pancreatic neuroendocrine tumours: clinical features, diagnosies and medical treatment: advances. Best Pract Res Clin Gastroenterol 26:737–781
47. Orditura M, Petrillo Am Venriglia J, Diana A, Maddalena Laterza M, Fabozzi A, Savastano B, Franzese E, Conzo G, Santini L, Ciardiello F, De Vita F (2016) Pancreatic neuroendocrine tumors: nosography, management and treatment. Int J Surg 28(S1):S156–S162
48. Paik WH, Ryu JK, Song BJ, Kim J, Park JK, Kim Y-T, Yoon YB (2013) Clinical usefulness of plasma chromogranin A in pancreatic neuroendocrine neoplasm. J Korean Med Sci 28:750–754
49. Konomi K, Chijiiwa K, Katsuta T, Yamaguchi K (1990) Pancreatic somatostatinoma: a case report and review of the literature. J Surg Oncol 43:259–265
50. Manta R, Nardi E, Pagano N, Ricci C, Sica M, Castellani D, Bertani H, Piccoli M, Mullineris B, Tringali A, Marini F, Germani U, Vilanacci V, Casadei R, Mutignani M, Conigliaro R, Bassotti G, Zullo A (2016) Pre-operative diagnosis of pancreatic neuroendocrine tumours with endoscopic ultrasonography and computed tomography in a large series. JGLD 3:317–321
51. King CM, Reznek RH, Dacie JE, Wass JA (1994) Imaging islet cell tumours. Clin Radiol 49:295–303
52. Rockall AG, Reznek RH (2007) Imaging of neuroendocrine tumours (CT/MR/US). Best Pract Res Clin Endocrinol Metabol 21:43–68
53. Debray MP, Geoffroy O, Laissy JP, Lebtahi R, Sibermann-Hoffman O, Henry-Feugeas MC, Cadiot G, Mignon M, Schouman-Claeys E (2001) Imaging appearances of metastases from neuroendocrine tumours of the pancreas. Br J Radiol 74:1065–1070
54. Angeletti S, Corleto VD, Schillaci O, Marignani M, Annibale B, Moretti A, Silecchia G, Scopinaro F, Basso N, Bordi C, Delle FG (1998) Use of the somatostatin analogue octreotide to localise and manage somatostatin-producing tumours. Gut 42:792–794
55. Reubi JC (1995) Neuropeptide receptors in health and disease: the molecular basis for in vivo imaging. J Nucl Med 36:825–835
56. Termanini B, Gibril F, Reynolds JC, Doppman JL, Chen CC, Stewart CA, Sutliff VE, Jensen RT (1997) Value of somatostatin receptor scintigraphy: a prospective study in gastrinoma of its effect on clinical management. Gastroenterology 112:335–347

57. Krenning EP, Kwekkeboom DJ, Oei HY, de Jong RJ, Dop FJ, Reubi JC, Lamberts SW (1994) Somatostatin-receptor scintigraphy in gastroenteropancreatic tumors. An overview of European results. Annal New York Acad Sci 733:416–424
58. Bodei L, Ambrosini V, Herrmann K, Modlin I (2017. (in press)) Current concepts in 68Ga-DOTATATE new imaging: interpretation, biodistribution, dosimetry and molecular strategies. J Nucl Med 58:1718
59. O'Grady HL, Conlon KC (2008) Pancreatic neuroendocrine tumours. Eur J Surg Oncol 34:424–432
60. McClean AM, Fairclough PD (2005) Endoscopic ultrasound in the localisation of pancreatic islet cell tumours. Best Pract Res Clin Endocrinol Metabol 19:177–193
61. O'Brien TD, Chejfec G, Prinz RA (1993) Clinical features of duodenal somatostatinomas. Surgery 114:1144–1147
62. Saif MW (2011) Pancreatic neoplasm in 2011: an update. JOP 12:316–321
63. Raymond E, Dahan L, Raoul JL, Bang Y-J, Borbath I, Lombard-Bohas CL, Valle J, Metrzoks P, Smith D, Vinik A, Chen J-S, Hörsch D, Hammel P, Wiedenmann B, Cutsem EV, Patyna S, Ray D, Blanckmeister C, Chao R, Ruszniewski P (2011) Sunitinib malate for the treatment of pancreatic neuroendocrine tumors. N Engl Med J 364:501–513
64. Pavel ME, Hainsworth JD, Baudin E, Peeters M, Hörsch D, Winkler RE, Klimovsky J, Lebwohl D, Jehl V, Wolin EM, Öberg K, Van Cutsem E, Yao JC (2011) Everolimus plus octreotide long-acting repeatable for the treatment of advanced neuroendocrine tumours associated with carcinoid syndrome (RADIANT-2): a randomised placebo-controlled, phase 3 study. Lancet 378:2005–2012
65. Yao JC, Shah MH, Ito T, Bohas CL, Wolin EM, Cutsem EV, Hobday TJ, Okusaka T, Capdevila J, de Vries EGE, Tomassetti P, Pavel ME, Hoosen S, Haas T, Lincy J, Lebwohl D, Öberg K, RAD001 in Advanced Neuroendocrine Tumors, Third Trial (RADIANT-3) Study Group (2011) Everolimus for advanced pancreatic neuroendocrine tumors. N Engl Med J 364:514–523
66. Kwekkeboom DJ, de Herder WW, Kam BL et al (2008) Treatment with the radiolabelled somatostain analog [^{177}Lu-DOTA^{0},Tyr3]octreotate: toxicity, efficacy and survival. J Clin Oncol 26:2124–2130
67. Mahajan SK, Mahajan LA, Malangoni MA, Jain S (1996) Somatostatinoma of the ampulla of Vater. Gastrointest Endosc 44:612–614
68. Hiroaki S, Takeyuki M, Shigeki W, Tomonori I, Yuichi I, Katsuhiko Y (2010) Pedunculated early ampullary carcinoma treated by ampullectomy: report of a case. J Gastrointest Cancer 41:138–140
69. Bassan M, Bourke M (2012) Endoscopic ampullectomy: a practical guide. J Interv Gastroenterol 2:23–30
70. Chamberlain RS, Canes D, Brown KT, Saltz L, Jarnagin W, Fong Y, Blumgart LH (2000) Hepatic neuroendocrine metastases: does intervention alter outcome? J Am Coll Surg 4:432–445
71. Norton JA (2005) Endocrine tumours of the gastrointestinal tract. Surgical treatment of neuroendocrine metastases. Best Pract Clin Res Gastroenterol 19:577–583
72. Que FG, Sarmiento JM, Nogorney DM (2006) Hepatic surgery for metastatic gastrointestinal tumours. Adv Exp Med Bio 574:43–56
73. Chamberlain RS, Canes D, Brown KT, Saltz L, Jarnagin W, Fong Y, Blumgart LH (2000) Hepatic neuroendocrine metastases: does intervention alter outcomes? J Am Coll Surg 190:432–445
74. Moretel CG, Lefkopoulo M, Lipsitz S, Hagn RG, Klaassen D (1992) Streptozocin-doxorubicin, streptozocin-fluorouracil or chlorozotocin in the treatment of advanced islet-cell carcinoma. N Engl J Med 326:519–523
75. Chen H, Hardacre JM, Uzar A, Cameron JL, Choti MA (1998) Isolated liver metastases from neuroendocrine tumors: does resection prolong survival? J Am Coll Surg 187:88–92; discussion 92–93
76. Olausson M, Friman S, Herlenius G, Cahlin C, Nilsson O, Jansson S, Wängberg B, Ahlman H (2007) Orthotopic liver or multivisceral transplantation as a treatment of metastatic neuroendocrine tumors. Liver Transpl 13:327–333
77. Mazzaferro V, Pulvirenti A, Coppa J (2007) Neuroendocrine tumors metastatic to the liver: how to select patients for liver transplantation? J Hepatol 47:460–466

Less Common Types of Pancreatic Neuroendocrine Tumors

17

Deniz Can Guven and Suayib Yalcin

17.1 Introduction

Neuroendocrine tumors are a rare group of heterogeneous disorders with a wide range of clinical behavior. They are located most commonly in the intestines and pancreas followed by rather rare locations including bronchi, thymus, etc. Pancreatic neuroendocrine tumors (pNETs) roughly divided into non-functional and functional tumors. Although non-functional pNETs are more common partly due to increased rate of incidental detection with modern imaging techniques, functional pNETs are more well known due to specific clinical syndromes. Gastrinomas and insulinomas are more frequent members of the functional pNET family with typical features of Zollinger–Ellison's syndrome (ZES) and hypoglycemia episodes, respectively. The other functional pNETs are very rare and include both the pNETs with well-known clinical syndromes like VIPoma and glucagonoma and also the pNETs with possible clinical syndromes; although, causality cannot be established due to the low number of reported cases. These possible rare functional pNETs can secrete many substances such as calcitonin, renin, and insulin-like growth factor (Table 17.1) [4].

Rare functional pNETs represent less than 10% of pNETs. Mostly, they are diagnosed as WHO Group 2 tumors and affect the patients in the fifth decade. A significant percentage of cases are metastatic to the liver (40–90%). Their clinical behavior is very heterogenous with a changing disease course such as malignant tumors showing a slow growth or malignant behavior in a previously benign lesion. They can also be associated with familial genetic syndromes leading by MEN1. In MEN1 syndrome, the reported frequency glucagonomas and VIPomas are around 3% and GRHomas, somatostatinomas are around 1%. Another well-known association is the presence of up to 10% somatostatinoma in neurofibromatosis type 1; however, almost all of these tumors are non-functional. There is a 10% risk of pNET in von

D. C. Guven · S. Yalcin (✉)
Department of Medical Oncology, Hacettepe University Cancer Institute, Ankara, Turkey
e-mail: syalcin@hacettepe.edu.tr

S. Yalcin, K. Öberg (eds.), *Neuroendocrine Tumours*,
https://doi.org/10.1007/978-3-031-56968-5_17

Table 17.1 Rare pancreatic neuroendocrine tumors [1–3]

Name	Biologically active secreted peptide(s)	Incidence (new cases/10^6 population/year)	Tumor location	Main symptoms/signs
VIPoma	Vasoactive intestinal peptide	0.05–0.2	Pancreas (90%, adult), other (10%)	Diarrhea (90–100%) Hypokalemic (80–100%) Dehydration (83%)
Glucagonoma	Glucagon	0.01–0.1	Pancreas (100%)	Rash Glucose intolerance Weight loss Depression Thrombosis
GHRHoma	Growth hormone-releasing hormone	Unknown	Pancreas (30%) Lung (54%) Jejunum (7%) Other (13%)	Acromegaly (100%)
Calcitoninoma	Calcitonin	Rare	Pancreas	Watery diarrhea (51%) Abdominal pain (35%)
ACTHoma	ACTH	Rare	Pancreas (4–16% all ectopic Cushing's syndrome)	Cushing's syndrome (100%)
P-NET causing hypercalcemia (PTHrPoma)	PTHrpP	Rare	Pancreas	Hypercalcemia
P-NET secreting renin	Renin	Rare	Pancreas	Hypertension
P-NET secreting luteinizing hormone	Luteinizing hormone	Rare	Pancreas	Anovulation virilization (female)/reduced libido (male)
P-NET secreting erythropoietin	Erythropoietin	Rare	Pancreas	Polycythemia
P-NET secreting insulin-like growth factor 2	Insulin-like growth factor II	Rare	Pancreas	Hypoglycemia
P-NET secreting CCK (CCKoma)	CCK	Rare	Pancreas	Diarrhea Ulcer disease Weight loss Cholelithiasis
P-NET secreting GLP-1	GLP-1	Rare	Pancreas	Hypoglycemia

VIP Vasoactive intestinal peptide, *PTHrP* parathyroid hormone-related peptide

Hippel Lindau disease but the vast majority of these cases are also non-functional. Tuberous sclerosis is another inherited disorder with around 20 reported cases of accompanying pNET [1, 2, 5, 6].

In this chapter, we will discuss the general clinical features, diagnosis, and treatments of rare functional pNETs and discuss some distinct clinical syndromes related with rare functional pNETs.

17.2 Specific Clinical Rare Functional pNET Syndromes

17.2.1 GRHoma

Ectopic growth hormone-releasing hormone (GHRH) secretion due to neuroendocrine tumors is a rare clinical syndrome with less than 100 reported cases. Acromegaly develops in all cases and the clinical picture is similar to the somatotroph adenoma. In a systematic review of 74 reported cases, the median age was 39 and there was a slight male predominance. The primary tumor located most commonly in the lung followed by the pancreas. The association with MEN-1 mutations was striking in the pNETs (19 of 25 cases) and should be investigated in these patients. The GHRH plasmatic measurement was used for a good specificity. The surgical approach is preferred if the curative resection is deemed feasible, while the somatostatin analogs can control the symptoms of hypersecretion in other cases. Although the disease was detected rather late as evidenced by the metastatic disease at diagnosis in 50% cases, the overall prognosis was good [7, 8].

17.2.2 ACTHoma

Ectopic adrenocorticotropic hormone (ACTH) producing pNETs are rare neoplasms. Cushing syndrome is the main clinical feature and is seen in almost all cases while adrenal hyperplasia accompanies in more than 80% of cases. There is a strong female predominance (2/1) with more than 75% stage IV cases [9]. pNETs are among the most common (15%) causes of ectopic ACTH production and should always be kept in mind in cases of Cushing syndrome. After the demonstration of cortisol excess with increased 24-h urinary free cortisol levels and unsuppressed serum cortisol after 1 mg overnight dexamethasone suppression test (DST), the cause of Cushing syndrome should be diagnosed with the help of overnight 8 mg DST and inferior petrosal sinus sampling. The lack of central-peripheral ACTH gradient in petrosal sinus sampling is suggestive of the ectopic ACTH syndrome and should be followed with imaging for the primary tumor [10]. Recently, Gallium-68-Dota derivatives positron emission tomography/computed tomography (PET-CT) started to be used more frequently and increased sensitivity for primary tumor detection [11]. While the surgery was used both for the definitive diagnosis and symptom palliation, adrenalectomy was required for palliation of Cushingoid syndromes like the systemic treatments [10]. The prognosis is generally poor with less than 40% of cases living more than 5 years [9].

17.2.3 pNET Causing Hypercalcemia (PTHrPoma)

The secretion of the parathyroid hormone-related peptide (PTHrP) is the main mechanism of humoral hypercalcemia of malignancy (HHM). Lung and breast cancer are the most common causes of HHM, while pNETs could be a rare cause of HHM [12]. It is a very rare NET with around 10 reported cases in the literature. The underlying pNET is of low grade in most cases and diagnosis is possible with the combination of imaging and the increased PTHrP levels. After the control of hypercalcemia with hydration, biphosphonates, and diuretics, somatostatin analogs are the mainstay of treatment for the prevention of hypercalcemia episodes [12–14].

17.2.4 Ghrelinoma

Ghrelin is a 28 amino acid peptide releasing mainly from the stomach. The main functions of ghrelin are the growth hormone secretion and regulation of energy balance with appetite secretion [15]. Interestingly, the expression of ghrelin mRNA and protein had recently been identified in pancreatic neuroendocrine tumors [16]. However, the ghrelinoma secondary to pNETs is very rare with only a handful of reported cases. In these cases, the clinical picture was non-specific and there were no signs of acromegaly or increased appetite. More than 10 times increased serum ghrelin levels were used for the diagnosis. All three cases were diagnosed with the advanced stage and treated with systemic agents with poor outcomes in two of three cases (deceased in the 5th, 28th, and 56th month after diagnosis) [17–19].

17.2.5 Calcitoninoma

Increased calcitonin secretion is among the main features of medullary thyroid carcinoma [20]. Rarely, increased levels of calcitonin could be secondary to pNETs. There are less than 50 reported cases of calcitoninoma in the literature. In a systematic review of 37 calcitoninoma cases, most patients presented in the fifth or sixth decade, and 60% of cases were metastatic. The mean calcitonin levels were strikingly elevated (89.2 folds upper levels of normal). The main symptoms were watery diarrhea, abdominal pain, and weight loss. The VIP levels were increased in some cases with diarrhea; however, diarrhea without VIP elevation was possible. The therapeutic options are similar to other pNETs with octreotide and conventional chemotherapy [21]. Ondansetron reported being useful for the control of watery diarrhea [22].

17.2.6 Serotoninoma

Pancreatic neuroendocrine tumors causing carcinoid syndrome due to secretion of serotonin and tachykinins are extremely rare and comprise the 1–2% of pNETs. The diagnosis is based on the elevation of serotonin in the serum and/or elevation of

5-hydroxy indol acetyl acid in the urine in a patient with pNET and the absence of another elevated dominant hormone. The typical clinic picture is the episodic flushing and accompanying diarrhea and weight loss. Most of the cases present in the advanced stages with frequent liver metastases. Somatostatin analogs are the mainstay of therapy for symptom control [23].

17.2.7 Other Rare Functional pNETs

There are many other pNETs associated with specific clinical syndromes. However, the causality couldn't be confirmed due to a low number (≤5) of cases. Among these syndromes, pNETs secreting cholecystokinin (CCKoma) is important due to the possibility of confusion with ZES due to the very similar clinical picture [24, 25]. Similarly, pNETs secreting insulin-like growth factor 2 [26] and glucagon-like peptide 1 present with hypoglycemia [27] and could be confused with insulinoma (Table 17.1).

17.3 Clinical Features and Prognosis

Clinical features of rare functional pNETs are mostly related to tumor extent and secreted substances (Table 17.1). Most of the tumors have already metastasized at the time of diagnoses (40–90%) due to a rather indolent course in the early diseases and the non-specific nature of most symptoms. Although the data is scarce, the 5-year survival of patients with advanced disease is estimated to be around 30–50% [1]. Most of the survival/prognostic data on the functional pNETs come from retrospective studies and the subgroup analyses of recent pNET studies. These studies demonstrate survival is related to the extent and growth rate of the tumor, tumor Ki67 percentage, and also the presence of various molecular features (chromosome 7q gain and chromosomal instability) [28, 29].

The typical clinical syndromes are usually seen in the later stages of the disease which makes the possibility of early diagnoses due to symptoms not possible. This explains the lack of better survival rates compared to non-functional tumors. These symptoms can be troublesome and may require the use of somatostatin analogs and local treatments to the liver for the control of the symptoms [30].

17.4 Diagnosis

The diagnosis of functional pNETs requires the demonstration of an inappropriate elevation of the specific serum hormonal marker combined with clinical/laboratory evidence of oversecretion of the appropriate hormone. Chromogranin A may be helpful for monitoring the disease's course but does not establish the diagnosis. All biochemical tests should be performed at the first patient visit.

Histopathological examination is the mainstay of the diagnosis after the suspicion from biochemistry and imaging studies. In biopsy, functional pNETs show common NET phenotypic characteristics. So, they show immunoreactivity to pan neuroendocrine markers, chromogranin A, and synaptophysin and should be performed in all cases. Mitotic index and Ki67 index are also needed for treatment selection and prognosis estimation. WHO TNM classification is used for the staging.

Baseline imaging studies are essential to plan surgery, to localize the primary tumor, to determine the extent of the disease, and to assess response to treatments. For imaging procedure, the previous baseline recommendation is to perform a multidetector CT and SRS-SPECT at minimum. However, this recommendation was changed in the ENETS 2016 guideline after the demonstration of the higher sensitivity of positron emission tomography with CT (PET/CT) with Ga68-labeled somatostatin analogs for pNET localization. In various studies on pNETs, the sensitivity varied from 86% to 100% and the specificity from 79% to 100% for all pNETs except insulinomas. Ga68-labeled somatostatin analogs have also been shown to change the management in a significant percentage of patients, and therefore, they should generally be used as the imaging modality in patients with non-insulinoma pNETs [1, 2].

17.5 Surgery

Surgery is the only treatment modality with the potential to cure. Attempted curative resection is still recommended for all patients with rare functional pNETs if the resection of all metastases seems attainable considering the long disease-free intervals with liver surgery in patients with limited liver metastases [3].

Debulking surgery with or without radiofrequency ablation (RFA) can also be performed for symptom palliation in symptomatic patients if the tumor resection of more than 90% seems to be resectable. RFA can also be used for symptom control for the oligometastatic disease if the largest lesion is <5 cm [31].

Due to the usually large size of the tumor and the high prevalence of liver metastases in rare functional pNETs, pancreatic resection and lymphadenectomy with laparotomy are the procedure of choice for curative surgery. Laparoscopic resection is not recommended except small insulinomas because of the need for lymphadenectomy and careful inspection for invasion/metastases. The location and the size of the tumor are important for the selection between the enucleation and local resection or the Whipple procedure. Intraoperative ultrasonography may be used for the localization of lesions in the pancreas and the liver when the preoperative imaging results are unequivocal [3, 32].

17.6 Medical Treatment

The data on the medical treatment of rare functional pNETs are scarce and the recommendations are mostly based on the studies including all pNET patients.

Somatostatin analogs are the mainstay of treatment as an effective option in the control of symptoms, especially in VIPomas, GRHomas, glucagonomas, and in some cases of somatostatinomas. In patients with Cushing's syndrome, adrenal-blocking agents (ketoconazole, metyrapone) are usually used before adrenalectomy. If somatostatin analogs fail in the control of hormone production, interferon-α with or without somatostatin analogs may be effective for controlling the symptoms. Promising results with the multiligand somatostatin receptor antagonist pasireotide had recently been presented and expected to affect clinical practice [1, 33, 34].

If refractory symptoms develop, various anti-tumor therapies including liver-directed therapies (embolization, chemoembolization, RFA), peptide radioreceptor treatment (PRRT), or cytoreductive surgery may be used for the symptomatic control in many patients and reported to be effective in around the 40–80% of patients. The presence of a strong expression of sstr2 in somatostatin receptor imaging is necessary for the use of PPRT [2].

Everolimus and sunitinib are therapeutic options in patients with advanced pNETs both for the first and the later lines of treatment. In grade 3 tumor (neuroendocrine carcinomas) and progressive cases, chemotherapy is the treatment of choice [1, 31].

17.7 Follow-Up

Follow-up for patients with rare functional pNETs should be at 3- to 9-month intervals. In patients with no evidence of residual disease, detailed biochemical assessment should be initially performed without further imaging. When the biochemical tests are negative, further tests are not usually required. For patients with residual disease, biochemical markers coupled with imaging studies should be performed [1, 2].

References

1. Jensen RT, Cadiot G, Brandi ML et al (2012) ENETS Consensus Guidelines for the management of patients with digestive neuroendocrine neoplasms: functional pancreatic endocrine tumor syndromes. Neuroendocrinology 95:98–119
2. Falconi M, Eriksson B, Kaltsas G et al (2016) ENETS Consensus Guidelines Update for the management of patients with functional pancreatic neuroendocrine tumors and non-functional pancreatic neuroendocrine tumors. Neuroendocrinology 103:153–171
3. Metz DC, Jensen RT (2008) Gastrointestinal neuroendocrine tumors: pancreatic endocrine tumors. Gastroenterology 135:1469–1492
4. Oronsky B, Ma PC, Morgensztern D, Carter CA (2017) Nothing but NET: a review of neuroendocrine tumors and carcinomas. Neoplasia 19:991–1002
5. Larson AM, Hedgire SS, Deshpande V et al (2012) Pancreatic neuroendocrine tumors in patients with tuberous sclerosis complex. Clin Genet 82:558–563
6. Jensen RT, Berna MJ, Bingham DB, Norton JA (2008) Inherited pancreatic endocrine tumor syndromes: advances in molecular pathogenesis, diagnosis, management, and controversies. Cancer 113:1807–1843
7. Borson-Chazot F, Garby L, Raverot G et al (2012) Acromegaly induced by ectopic secretion of GHRH: a review 30 years after GHRH discovery. Ann Endocrinol 73:497–502

8. Ghazi AA, Amirbaigloo A, Dezfooli AA et al (2013) Ectopic acromegaly due to growth hormone releasing hormone. Endocrine 43:293–302
9. Maragliano R, Vanoli A, Albarello L et al (2015) ACTH-secreting pancreatic neoplasms associated with Cushing syndrome: clinicopathologic study of 11 cases and review of the literature. Am J Surg Pathol 39:374
10. Maria Vittoria D, Elisa C, Serena P et al (2017) Prognostic factors in ectopic Cushing's syndrome due to neuroendocrine tumors: a multicenter study. Eur J Endocrinol 176:453–461
11. Varlamov E, Hinojosa-Amaya JM, Stack M, Fleseriu M (2019) Diagnostic utility of gallium-68-somatostatin receptor PET/CT in ectopic ACTH-secreting tumors: a systematic literature review and single-center clinical experience. Pituitary 22:445–455
12. Srirajaskanthan R, McStay M, Toumpanakis C et al (2009) Parathyroid hormone-related peptide-secreting pancreatic neuroendocrine tumours: case series and literature review. Neuroendocrinology 89:48–55
13. Shah RH, Martinez D (2013) Pancreatic neuroendocrine tumor associated with humoral hypercalcemia of malignancy and carcinoid tumor: a case report and review of the literature. Pancreas 42:549–551
14. Clemens P, Gregor M, Lamberts R (2001) Pancreatic neuroendocrine tumor with extensive vascularisation and parathyroid hormone-related protein (PTHrP)—associated hypercalcemia of malignancy. Exp Clin Endocrinol Diabetes 109:378–385
15. Vinik A, Hughes MS, Feliberti E et al (2018) Carcinoid tumors. In: Endotext [Internet]. MDText.com, Inc
16. Papotti M, Cassoni P, Volante M et al (2001) Ghrelin-producing endocrine tumors of the stomach and intestine. J Clin Endocrinol Metab 86:5052–5059
17. Chauhan A, Ramirez RA, Stevens MA et al (2015) Transition of a pancreatic neuroendocrine tumor from ghrelinoma to insulinoma: a case report. J Gastrointest Oncol 6:E34–E36
18. Corbetta S, Peracchi M, Cappiello V et al (2003) Circulating ghrelin levels in patients with pancreatic and gastrointestinal neuroendocrine tumors: identification of one pancreatic ghrelinoma. J Clin Endocrinol Metabol 88:3117–3120
19. Thomas W, Laurence C, Valérie H et al (2009) Major hyperghrelinemia in advanced well-differentiated neuroendocrine carcinomas: report of three cases. Eur J Endocrinol 161:639–645
20. Uccella S, Blank A, Maragliano R et al (2017) Calcitonin-producing neuroendocrine neoplasms of the pancreas: clinicopathological study of 25 cases and review of the literature. Endocr Pathol 28:351–361
21. Schneider R, Waldmann J, Swaid Z et al (2011) Calcitonin-secreting pancreatic endocrine tumors: systematic analysis of a rare tumor entity. Pancreas 40:213–221
22. Vlaemynck K, De Man M, De Man K et al (2020) Neuroendocrine tumor with diarrhea: not always the usual suspects—a case report of metastatic calcitoninoma with literature review. Acta Clin Belg 76:1–5
23. Tsoukalas N, Chatzellis E, Rontogianni D et al (2017) Pancreatic carcinoids (serotonin-producing pancreatic neuroendocrine neoplasms): report of 5 cases and review of the literature. Medicine 96:e6201–e6201
24. Rehfeld JF, Federspiel B, Bardram L (2013) A neuroendocrine tumor syndrome from cholecystokinin secretion. N Engl J Med 368:1165–1166
25. Rehfeld JF, Federspiel B, Agersnap M et al (2016) The uncovering and characterization of a CCKoma syndrome in enteropancreatic neuroendocrine tumor patients. Scand J Gastroenterol 51:1172–1178
26. Modica R, Di Sarno A, Colao A, Faggiano A (2016) Pancreatic neuroendocrine tumor with hypoglycemia and elevated insulin-like growth factor II: a case report. J Cancer Metasta Treat 2:345–347
27. Roberts RE, Zhao M, Whitelaw BC et al (2012) GLP-1 and glucagon secretion from a pancreatic neuroendocrine tumor causing diabetes and hyperinsulinemic hypoglycemia. J Clin Endocrinol Metabol 97:3039–3045
28. Jonkers YMH, Claessen SMH, Perren A et al (2007) DNA copy number status is a powerful predictor of poor survival in endocrine pancreatic tumor patients. Endocr Relat Cancer 14:769–779

29. Ekeblad S, Skogseid B, Dunder K et al (2008) Prognostic factors and survival in 324 patients with pancreatic endocrine tumor treated at a single institution. Clin Cancer Res 14:7798
30. de Celis R, Ferrari AC, Glasberg J, Riechelmann RP (2018) Carcinoid syndrome: update on the pathophysiology and treatment. Clinics (Sao Paulo) 73:e490s
31. Öberg K, Knigge U, Kwekkeboom D et al (2012) Neuroendocrine gastro-entero-pancreatic tumors: ESMO Clinical Practice Guidelines for diagnosis, treatment and follow-up. Ann Oncol 23:vii124-vii130
32. Tamburrino D, Spoletini G, Partelli S et al (2016) Surgical management of neuroendocrine tumors. Best Pract Res Clin Endocrinol Metab 30:93–102
33. Wolin EM, Jarzab B, Eriksson B et al (2015) Phase III study of pasireotide long-acting release in patients with metastatic neuroendocrine tumors and carcinoid symptoms refractory to available somatostatin analogues. Drug Des Devel Ther 9:5075–5086
34. Torniai M, Scortichini L, Tronconi F et al (2019) Systemic treatment for lung carcinoids: from bench to bedside. Clin Transl Med 8:22–22

Non-Functioning Pancreatic Neuroendocrine Tumors

18

Nicola Fazio and Anna Koumarianou

Abbreviations

5FU	5-Fluorouracil
ALT	Alternative lengthening of telomeres
ATRX	Alpha thalassemia/mental retardation syndrome X-linked
DAXX	Death domain-associated protein
Dox	Doxorubicin
ENETS	European Neuroendocrine Tumor Society
G	Differentiation grade
HACE	Hepatic arterial chemoembolization
HAE	Hepatic arterial embolization
HIF1a	Hypoxia-inducible factor 1a
IHC	Immunohistochemistry
LAR	Long-acting release
MEN1	Multiple endocrine neoplasia type 1
mTOR	Mammalian target of rapamycin
NF-panNETs	Non-functioning pancreatic neuroendocrine tumors
OS	Overall survival
PD	Progressive disease
PFS	Progression-free surviva
PR	Partial responses
PRRT	Peptide receptor radionuclide therapy

N. Fazio
Division of Gastrointestinal Medical Oncology and Neuroendocrine Tumors, European Institute of Oncology, IEO, IRCCS, Milan, Italy
e-mail: nicola.fazio@ieo.it

A. Koumarianou (✉)
Hematology Oncology Unit, Fourth Department of Internal Medicine, 'Attikon' University Hospital, National and Kapodistrian University of Athens, Athens, Greece

S. Yalcin, K. Öberg (eds.), *Neuroendocrine Tumours*,
https://doi.org/10.1007/978-3-031-56968-5_18

RFA	Radiofrequency ablation
RR	Response rate
SD	Stable disease
SSA	Somatostatin analogues
SSTR	Somatostatin receptors
STZ	Streptozotocin
TMZ	Temozolomide
TSC	Tuberous sclerosis complex
TTP	Time to progression
VHL	Von Hippel–Lindau

18.1 Epidemiology and Genetics

Pancreatic neuroendocrine tumors (panNETs), in general, include a heterogeneous group of malignant diseases exhibiting unique clinical and biological features [1–3]. They can range from indolent to highly aggressive and when unresectable have no curative therapy. The term non-functioning (NF) describes the lack of a specific clinical syndrome related with hormone oversecretion. This does not necessarily mean that no peptide or amine production takes place. A clinically undefined syndrome in panNETs may well be associated with positive immunohistochemistry (IHC) for hormonal production, indicating that the quantity secreted is small or biologically inactive (e.g. pancreatic polypeptide) or simply accumulated in the cytoplasm rather than released in the intercellular compartment [4]. Recently, the European Neuroendocrine Tumor Society (ENETS) held working sessions composed of members of the advisory board and other neuroendocrine neoplasm (NEN) experts to attempt to identify unmet needs in patients with panNETs [5].

A SEER-database analysis reported that panNETs have an annual incidence of 0.48 per 100,000 persons [6]. In the same study, it was indicated that panNETS had the worse median OS of 3.6 years compared to other NET primaries including lung. Global European high-quality epidemiologic data on Neuroendocrine Neoplasms (NEN) are lacking. A recent Registry study has been initiated to include patients with NEN from as many as possible Eurpean countries [7].

Non-functioning panNETs can present with symptoms due to mass-effect, including obstruction, bleeding, abdominal pain, vomiting and jaundice or systemic ones as anorexia and weight loss [8, 9]. More than 50% of NF-panNET patients who initially present with localized disease will develop liver metastasis after resection of their primary tumor [10]. The survival of patients with NF-panNETs was found to be similar to that of the functioning counterpart; an interesting finding given that the lack of clinical syndrome was thought to be associated with a more aggressive biology [11]. In accordance, a recent SEER database U.S. analysis indicated that NF-panNETs were associated with somewhat higher mortality than functioning within the first few years after diagnosis, no major differences were observed long term [12].

The molecular basis of NF-panNET tumorigenesis is not well understood and although 90% of cases are sporadic a minority may be included in the context of important genetic syndromes such as Multiple Endocrine Neoplasia type 1 (MEN1), von Hippel-Lindau (VHL) disease and tuberous sclerosis complex (TSC) syndrome [13].

MEN1 syndrome is associated with many neoplasms, most commonly pituitary adenoma, parathyroid adenoma and pancreatic islet cell tumor. Menin is a predominantly nuclear protein that has a role in transcriptional regulation, genome stability, cell division, and proliferation. At least 1336 mutations have been reported in the menin chromosomal region 11q13 [14]. Menin has been found to epigenetically suppress Hedgehog signaling, a proproliferative and oncogenic pathway and to downregulate AKT and its kinase activity that in turn induces proliferation and anti-apoptotic signaling [15, 16].

In the context of MEN1 syndrome, NF-panNETs occur typically within a field of numerous pancreatic microadenomas and a prospective study indicated their frequency to be approximately 55% [17]. Pancreatic NETs arising in the context of MEN1 syndrome are usually non-functioning [18]. With respect to the time of clinical onset, a study in children with MEN1 syndrome has shown that they may have asymptomatic NF-panNETs well before the age of 20 years [19].

VHL disease is a very rare autosomal dominant inherited syndrome characterized by inactivating mutations of the VHL gene that resides on chromosome 3p25-26. The VHL gene encodes, by alternative splicing, two proteins (pVHL) with as main role the inactivation of hypoxia-inducible factor 1a (HIF1a) [20]. Loss of heterozygosity of VHL leads to the upregulation of HIF1a and other angiogenic factors such as VEGF resulting in the proliferation of vascular tissue and the development of retinal and cerebellar hemangioblastomas, renal cell carcinoma, pheochromocytoma and NF-panNETs [21].

Tuberous sclerosis complex is a very rare hereditary autosomal dominant syndrome that involves two genes located on 9q34 (TSC1) and 16p13.3 (TSC2) encoding for hamartin and tuberin, respectively. In the normal cell, hamartin and tuberin form a heterodimer complex that inhibits the mammalian target of rapamycin (mTOR) pathway and thus cell growth and proliferation [22]. Patients with deficiency in these proteins develop widespread hamartomas in several organs, including the brain, heart, skin, eyes, kidney, lung and liver but also neurological disorders and NF-panNETs [23, 24]. Most features of tuberous sclerosis become evident in childhood at 3 years of age, limiting their usefulness for early diagnosis.

18.2 Molecular Biology of Sporadic NF-panNETs

The genetic background of sporadic panNETs is complex. Many studies support that panNETs have different deregulated cellular mechanisms when compared to other NETs, or related with different grades of disease and presence or absence of a syndrome [25–27].

Functioning panNETs compared with normal pancreas and NF-panNETs showed several differences at gene expression level including decreased protein expression of TSC2 and PTEN and increased expression of somatostatin receptor type (sstr) 2 [25]. PTEN was one of the first reported proteomic alteration observed in panNETs and it was found to be mutated or abnormally localized in the cytoplasm instead of the nucleus [28]. Mutations in chromosome 11 involving menin are also observed in 8–26% of NF-panNETs [18].

Except the well-studied genetic mutations, several newer studies support the role of epigenetics in the pathogenesis of neoplastic diseases. Epigenetics are potentially modifiable/reversible factors by environmental conditions or even heritable changes in gene expression caused by several other factors other than mutations of DNA sequence such as DNA methylation, histone alterations and miRNAs. Some of these recognized changes have been observed in sporadic NF-panNETs and mainly include the inactivated pathway of menin that has been linked to H3 histone variation [29, 30]. Histone variants cause post-translational modifications (histone code) and are one of the reasons of silencing genes that are not found mutated.

Another important pathway in the pathogenesis of the tumors is telomere preservation that is under the control of several enzymatic processes and is gradually decreasing in size in normal cells and is responsible for the cellular senescence. This pathway is commonly found deranged in tumor cells. Telomere maintenance is indispensable for cellular immortalization and tumors achieve that either by activation of telomerase or by activation of the alternative lengthening of telomeres (ALT). In a pivotal study of 149 genes, 16 tumours were found mutated in panNETs a much lower incidence than in adenocarcinomas. Three main groups were identified (a) MEN1 in 44%, (b) death domain-associated protein (DAXX)/alpha thalassemia/mental retardation syndrome X-linked (ATRX) in 45%, and (c) TSC2, PTEN and PIK3CA genes involved in the mTOR pathway in 14%. The DAXX and ATRX are both required for Histone 3.3 incorporation in telomeres. When ATRX/DAXX are mutated the ALT pathway becomes activated [24]. In 19/19 patients with mutated ATRX or DAXX, ALT was positive as determined by fluorescence in situ hybridization. Six out of 20 ALT positive without ATRX or DAXX mutations had lost nuclear expression of ATRX or DAXX nuclear protein by IHC indicating an error in another point of the telomere pathway. Nevertheless, ALT and MEN1 positive patients had a superior survival, and mutations of the mTOR pathway may be used as predictive factors of response to treatment with everolimus [24].

A different study in well-differentiated panNETs showed DAXX and ATRX loss in 45% of cases, whereas p53 and Rb immunolabelling were maintained [31].

A more recent study characterized the genomic alterations by whole-exome and targeted panel sequencing of 225 patients enrolled in three RADIANT phase 3 clinical trials [32]. All NET displayed broad copy number aberrations involving multiple chromosomes but panNETs displayed the highest average mutation rates (1.16/Mb). Most importantly, the presence of chromosomal instability was associated with a trend towards longer survival.

18.3 Classification and Staging

The currently valid histopatologic diagnosis of panNET is based on the WHO 2019 classification and, depending on the differentiation grade and Ki-67, divides panNETs into neuroendocrine tumors G1, G2, G3 and neuroendocrine carcinomas who are G3 by definition [33]. Pancreatic NET G3 are considered a molecularly, radiologically and prognostically distinct entity compared to panNEC and panNET G1/G2. A main challenge in G3 is the identification of the best treatment algorithm that will take into consideration the unique characteristics of such patients.

Staging involves a site-specific tumor–node–metastasis (TNM) classification according to the recommendations of the American Joint Cancer Committee (AJCC) (Table 18.1). Current staging is based on the TNM eighth edition [34]. The WHO

Table 18.1 TNM staging of pancreatic neuroendocrine neoplasms according to the TNM eighth edition of AJCC Cancer Staging Manual

AJCC 2017 TNM	
T classification	
Pancreatic neuroendocrine tumors	Pancreatic neuroendocrine carcinomas
T1: Tumor limited to the pancreas, <2 cm	T1: Limited to the pancreas, ≤2 cm in greatest dimension
T2: Tumor limited to the pancreas, 2–4 cm	T2: Limited to the pancreas, 2–4 cm
T3: Tumor limited to the pancreas, >4 cm; or tumor invading the duodenum or common bile duct	T3: Limited to the pancreas, >4 cm
T4: Tumor invading adjacent organs (stomach, spleen, colon, adrenal gland) or the wall of large vessels (celiac axis or the superior mesenteric artery)	T4: Tumor invading the wall of large vessels (celiac axis or the superior mesenteric artery or common hepatic artery), regardless of size
N classification	
N0: No regional lymph node involvement	N0: No regional lymph node metastasis
N1: Regional lymph node involvement	N1: Metastasis in one to three regional lymph nodes
	N2: Metastasis in four or more regional lymph nodes
M classification	
M0: No distant metastasis	M0: No distant metastasis
M1a: Metastases confined to the liver	M1: Distant metastasis
M1b: Metastases in at least one extrahepatic site (e.g. lung, ovary, nonregional lymph node, peritoneum, bone)	
M1c: Both hepatic and extrahepatic metastases	
Stage classification	
I: T1N0M0	IA: T1N0M0
II: T2-3N0M0	IB: T2N0M0
III: T4N0M0	IIA: T3N0M0
III: T1-4N1M0	IIB: T1-T3N1M0
IV: T1-4N0-1M1	III: T1-3N2M0
	III: T4N0-2M0
	IV: T14N0-2M1

AJCC American Joint Committee on Cancer, *NA* Not Applicable

2019 classification and TNM staging aim to standardize pathology reporting and staging procedures across the different countries and ultimately to enable meaningful patient stratification into prognostic and treatment groups. As this is a rare disease, it is crucial to be able to collect the information and deduct conclusions that are significant for patient management.

18.4 Prognostic and Predictive Factors

Over the past few years, a few studies have identified certain clinical parameters that may contribute to the formation of an accurate prognostic assessment, which is of paramount importance for therapeutic decision-making. The most prognostically important pathological factors are the presence of angioinvasion as well as the proliferation index [35, 36]. With respect to the latter, Ki-67 labelling index emerges as an independent predictor of survival using a cut-off value of 5% in both functioning and NF-panNETs [37]. Together with G3 histology and the proliferative index Ki-67, with an increasing risk of progression of 2% for each increasing Ki-67 unit, are the major factors to predict tumor progression [38]. One Italian study evaluating prognostic factors in NF-panNETs including 180 patients support that the evaluation of nodal metastasis and weight loss should be included along with liver metastasis, Ki-67 index and grade of differentiation [8]. One of the largest studies in the literature evaluating 2158 NF-panNETs showed that systemic metastases, local, vascular/lymphatic invasion and grade are more powerful indicators of outcome with tumor grade influencing survival more than distant metastases [9].

It is well established that radical surgery is the only chance for cure in NF-panNETs, with a 5-year survival rate of 93% [8]. Nevertheless, the surgical choice is the direct result of the disease stage at diagnosis, a well-established prognostic factor in all tumors.

With respect to predictive factors and response to chemotherapy, this was found to be related to Ki-67 > 10%, the performance status and age <60 years [39]. Additionally, a confirmatory study showed that both a Ki-67 labelling index >5% and the lymph node ratio (number of lymph nodes with metastases/total number of resected lymph nodes) in resected panNETs are powerful predictors of recurrence and support their investigation in relation to adjuvant treatment in the context of clinical trials [40].

18.5 Therapies

18.5.1 Surgical Therapy

Surgical resection remains the cornerstone therapy and the only approach that may cure patients with G1 and G2 panNETs. With respect to G3 tumors, surgery is rarely curative but offers a significant long-term palliation in highly selected patients [41, 42].

Over the last decade, novel and less invasive pancreatic surgical approaches have been developed and depending on clinical scenarios are applied in patients with panNETs [43]. These involve mainly partial pancreatectomies or tumor enucleation that may also be performed laparoscopicaly [41]. Generally, typical and atypical pancreatic resections are intended for different sites, and sizes of panNETs and the decision should be ideally based on previous histological confirmation by endoscopic ultrasound. Tumor enucleation has been proposed in well-demarcated, less than 2 cm and benign or uncertain behaviour lesions [44]. Centrally located lesions of the pancreatic head require pancreaticoduodenectomy, while lesions of the body and tail may be handled with a left pancreatectomy with or without spleen preservation. Middle pancreatectomy is usually performed for small tumors of the pancreatic body, while enucleation is considered when the main pancreatic duct can be preserved.

The role of surgical resection of the primary panNET in the presence of inoperable metastases is controversial. In a 2158 NF-panNETs patient from the SEER-database, it was shown that removal of the primary tumor significantly prolonged survival in the entire cohort (median 1.2 vs. 8.4 years; $p < 0.001$) even among those with metastasic disease (median 1.0 vs. 4.8 years; $p < 0.001$) [9]. On the other hand, a systematic review of small studies specifically investigating the role of surgery in this scenario was inconclusive supporting the need of a prospective randomized trial [45]. Furthermore, no survival difference was seen between enucleation and more aggressive resection of the primary tumor (median 10.2 vs 9.2 years, $p = 0.456$) [9].

Commonly, typical pancreatectomies are associated with a high rate of perioperative complications as well as exocrine and endocrine insufficiency [46]. Atypical resections, on the other hand, are associated with a decreased long-term endocrine/exocrine impairment but with a high incidence of pancreatic fistulas, a disturbing but ultimately a manageable complication [47, 48].

Whichever the type of resection, for a more than 2-cm suspicious lesion it is imperative to perform a wide excision with clear margins and to remove draining lymphnodes for proper TNM assessment, particularly in cases with G2 and G3 panNETs. Controversial is the management of tumors 1–2 cm and those found incidentally as several studies have shown that these may be malignant and have lymph nodal metastases [49–51]. It is recommended that depending on each case either to close monitor or to remove with draining lymphnodes.

A retrospective, single-center study, comparing laparoscopic versus open distal pancreatectomy for NF-panNET indicated similar oncologic outcomes, but laparoscopic pancreatectomy was associated with a shorter hospital stay [52].

18.5.1.1 Surgical Therapy of Patients with NF-panNETs in the Context of MEN1

MEN1 syndrome represents a difficult challenge for surgeons mainly because it is associated with eterochronous and multifocal NF-panNETs. Prophylactic pancreatectomies could remove all premalignant lesions prior to malignant conversion but are not an accepted approach. It is, therefore, of utmost importance to carefully monitoring of these patients for the early diagnosis and surgical excision of any arising tumors with malignant potential [53]. Based on previous evidence, the European Neuroendocrine Tumor Society (ENETS) recommends operating MEN1-related NF-panNETs with a diameter of more than 2 cm, with a yearly size increment in diameter of more than 0.5 cm or with metastases [54, 55]. The management of NF-panNETs of less than 2 cm is debated as they may also have an aggressive biology but they usually are microadenomas and have a more indolent behavior and their management is close monitoring.

A recent North American Neuroendocrine Tumor Society consensus paper on the surgical management of pancreatic neuroendocrine tumors recommended that the decision to observe or resect an asymptomatic panNET 1–2 cm in size be individualized based on age, comorbidities, tumor growth over time, estimated risk of symptom development, details of imaging, grade, the extent of surgical resection required, the patient's wishes and access to long-term follow-up [56]. ENETs has a prospective study underway, the 'ASPEN study', to evaluate the management of asymptomatic sporadic, NF-panNENs ≤2 cm.

Overall, the refinement and personalization of surgical procedures in NF-panNETs have resulted in improved long-term survival in patients with locally advanced and metastatic disease, as well as shorter hospital stays and comparable long-term outcomes in patients with limited disease treated minimally invasively. There are still controversies related to issues of surgical treatment of panNETs, such as to what extent enucleation, lymph node sampling and vascular reconstruction are beneficial for the oncologic outcome particularly in MEN1 patients and in tumors 1–2 cm in diameter. It is expected that endoscopic ultrasound-guided biopsies will shed light on all these gray zones [57]. In addition, endoscopic ultrasound-guided radiofrequency ablation of panNETs was recently proposed as a minimally invasive, safe and technically feasible procedure for selected patients [58].

18.5.2 Medical Therapies

During the past decade, advances in therapeutics have introduced novel exciting agents in the treatment of panNETs that have shown to improve the survival of patients. Some interesting combinations including triplets of chemotherapy, radiopeptides or targeted agents have recently been exploited in this rapidly evolving field (Table 18.2).

18.5.2.1 Somatostatin Analogues

The clinical application of long acting somatostatin analogues (SSAs) has changed dramatically the quality of life and prognosis of patients with NETs [68]. Their benefit was initially thought to be related to their antisecretory effect as they were shown to relieve patients from troubling clinical syndromes related to the peptide secretion. Altogether, SSAs have been shown to be well tolerated and safe in all available forms as patients may experience only mild and infrequent side effects such as abdominal pain, steatorrhea and cholelithiasis [26, 27]. This last effect is due to the inhibitory effects of octreotide on gallbladder contractility and, although it requires follow-up attention, which is rarely of clinical significance.

Table 18.2 List of mainstream clinical studies in pancreatic neuroendocrine tumors

Drugs	N Pts	Ki-67	SSTR+	PR %	PFS*/ TTP** months	Study Type	Author
STZ/ ADM/5FU	84	NR	NR	34	9*	Retrospective	Kouvaraki et al. [59]
TMZ	36	NR	NR	14	7**	Retrospective	Ekeblad et al. [60]
STZ/ CDDP/5FU	49	25	39	38	9**	Retrospective	Turner et al. [61]
TMZ/ XELODA	30	NR	NR	70	18*	Retrospective	Strosberg et al. [62]
TMZ/BEV	15	<20%	NR	33	14.3*	Phase II	Chan et al. [63]
PRRT (Lu)	91	NR	91	43	40*	Retrospective	Kwekkeboom et al. [64]
PRRT(Lu)	52	NR	52	29	29*	Phase II	Sansovini et al. [65]
Sunitinib	86	36	NR	7	11.4*	Phase III	Raymond et al. [66]
Placebo	85	36		0	5.5*		
Everolimus	207	NR	NR	5	11*	Phase III	Yao et al. [67]
Placebo	203				4.6*		

*: time in months for *PFS*
**: time in months for *TTP*
STZ Streptozotocin, *ADM* Adriamycin, *TMZ* Temozolomide, *XELOX* Xeloda/oxaliplatin, *CDDP* Cisplatin, *5FU* 5-Fluorouracil, *BEV* Bevacizumab, *PRRT* Peptide receptor radionuclide therapy, *Lu* Lutetium, *SSTR* Somatostatin receptors, *PR* Partial response, *TTP* Time to progression, *PFS* Progression free Survival, *NR* Not reported

From the advent of the first SSA, an improved survival has been shown in NET patients and although a clear gain could be seen by the fact that patients' quality of life was improved together with their symptoms, it was not clear whether there was also an antiproliferative effect. Several groups have reported a possible anti-proliferative action from SSA, by induction of apoptosis [69–71], although significant tumour shrinkage has been reported to occur in <5% of cases [68]. Initial in vitro studies suggested a number of direct and indirect mechanisms of such an effect. Direct mechanisms involve the activation of somatostatin receptors (SSRs) leading to modulation of intracellular signaling transduction such as the activation of MAP-kinase pathway [72]. Indirect antiproliferative effects are exerted through activation of SSRs on endothelial cells and monocytes leading to blocking of tumor angiogenesis [73, 74]. A randomized Phase III double-blind trial testing lanreotide Autogel versus placebo in advanced NF well-differentiated enteropancreatic NETs (The CLARINET Study) was associated with significantly prolonged progression-free survival among patients with tumors of grade 1 or 2 and Ki-67 < 10% [75]. This study added evidence on the efficacy of SSAs in NF-NETs, particularly in patients with Ki-67 = 5–10%, panNETs, hindgut or unknown primary as monotherapy. The extension study CLARINET open-label extension (OLE) study provided evidence on the good safety profile of long-term use of lanreotide Autogel as patients in the treatment arm of the core and OLE trial received a median (range) of 40.0 (26.0–74.3) months [76]. A possible therapeutic option for a minor response would be to increase the dose of SSA. CLARINET FORTE, a phase II study in patients with pancreatic and midgut NETs who had progressed on standard-dose lanreotide 120 mg (once every 28 days), tested the toxicity and effectiveness of lanreotide 120 mg once every 14 days [77]. Evaluated clinical responses in panNETs according to RECIST included 66.7% SD and 31.3% PD. Although the mPFS for all panNETs was 5.6 months, the mPFS for patients with Ki67 ≤ 10% was 8.0 months whereas for patients with Ki67 > 10% was only 2.8 months. Treatment-related side effects observed by doubling the dose were typical for SSA, mostly gastrointestinal and grade 1 (16 patients) and 2 (4 patients).

SSAs are included as standards of care in the guidelines for the first-line treatment of advanced NF panNET by the relevant societies such as ESMO and ENETS [78, 79].

18.5.2.2 Interferon

Early studies had shown that interferon-alpha (IFN-α) has antiproliferative, antisecretory, antiangiogenic and antiapoptotic effects [80–82]. A possible positive immunomodulatory effect on T cell and natural killer cell activity was also suggested [83–85], but it has not been confirmed since by later studies. Interferon-α may be used as monotherapy or in combination with SSAs, as antisecretory and antiproliferative treatment, with variable response rates (RRs). There has been biochemical response in 40–60% of patients, symptomatic improvement in 40–70% of patients and significant tumor shrinkage in a median of 10–15% of patients [84–87]. Side-effects of IFN-α are significant and include flu-like syndrome, chronic fatigue, depression, weight loss, polyneuropathy, myositis, thrombocytopenia, anaemia, leukopenia and autoantibodies in 15% of patients (autoimmune hepatitis/thyroiditis, psoriasis, systemic lupus erythematosus syndrome with antinuclear factors and parietal cell antibodies with pernicious anemia; [84, 85, 88]. There are no studies employing IFN monotherapy or in combination with SSA in NF-panNETs. A prospective randomized study showed a significantly reduced risk of tumour progression during follow-up in patients with midgut carcinoid tumours metastatic to the liver receiving octreotide and IFN-α as compared to single agent octreotide [89]. A randomized phase III study comprised three arms to compare lanreotide, IFN and Lanreotide plus IFN [90]. All arms had equivalent results with respect to symptom control and survival. The combination arm showed a trend of better survival but was more toxic. Another randomized trial comparing octreotide to octreotide/IFN-α showed no survival advantage between the two arms [91]. It is hypothesized that the difference in the results lies on the heterogeneity of the disease and further larger trials are required. At present we do not have enough statistical evidence for an upfront use of the combination of IFN-α and SSA in patients with NETs, but we have some clinical evidence coming from non-randomized studies and the sub-analysis of randomized trials that would justify the sequential use of the two drugs or the combination after progression to single-agent therapy [92]. Head-to-head comparisons of octreotide/IFN-α to other biological combinations has not been performed yet. A randomized phase III trial is currently recruiting patients in order to compare the efficacy of octreotide/IFN-α2b and octreotide/bevacizumab in metastatic or locally advanced, high-risk NETs (Clinical Trials Link: http://clinicaltrials.gov/show/NCT00569127). This trial was based on a previous phase II study showing better PFS and objective responses of octreotide/bevacizumab compared to octreotide/PEG-IFN [93].

18.5.2.3 Targeted Therapies

The more thorough understanding of signaling pathways implicated in tumor cell proliferation and angiogenesis underlining the pathogenesis of NETs has prompted the application of small molecules targeting these pathways such as everolimus and sunitinib.

Everolimus (Afinitor®, Novartis Pharmaceuticals)

Based on preliminary observations, a phase II clinical trial conducted by J. Yao at the MD Anderson Cancer Center studied everolimus, an oral inhibitor of mTOR, and octreotide LAR in advanced low-grade neuroendocrine caricnomas [93]. A total of 60 evaluable patients were treated in two cohorts; patients received either everolimus at 5 or 10 mg/day. Out of the 60 treated patients, 30 had carcinoid and 30 islet cell tumours. Sixty-five percent of the patients were in progression at the time of study entry. Overall, 12 (20%) patients were reported to have partial response (PR; 4 carcinoids and 8 islet cell tumours, respectively), 43 (72%) had stable disease (SD; 25 in carcinoids and 18 in islet cell, respectively) and 5 (8%) had progressive disease (PD; 1 in carcinoids and 4 in islet cell, respectively). Overall median progression free survival (PFS) was 59 weeks (64 weeks in carcinoids and 50 in islet cell tumours, respectively). Median OS was not reached, with a 2-year survival rate of 78%. The combination of everolimus and octreotide LAR 30 mg appears to have been well tolerated. The most common toxicity reported was mucositis. Grade 3/4 toxicities observed included anemia, thrombocytopenia, aphthous ulcer, diarrhea, edema, fatigue, hypoglycemia, nausea, pain and rash.

Another phase II open-label, parallel group study was conducted in patients with advanced panNETs. Patients received either everolimus 10 mg daily as monotherapy (stratum 1; $n = 115$) or everolimus 10 mg daily in combination with ≤ 30 mg octreotide LAR q 28 days (stratum 2; $n = 45$), based on prior octreotide LAR treatment [94]. In stratum 1, there were 11 PRs (9.6%), 78 patients with SD (67.8%) and 16 patients with PD (13.9%); median progression-free survival was 9.7 months. In stratum 2, there were two PRs (4.4%), 36 patients (80%) with SD and no patients with PD; median PFS was 16.7 months.

On the basis of a Phase III trial, the RADIANT-3 [67] showing that everolimus significantly prolonged PFS compared with placebo in advanced panNET; everolimus was approved by the FDA and EMA authorities for patients with progressing advanced well/moderately differentiated panNETs. The RADIANT-3 involved 410 patients with advanced well-moderately differentiated, radiologically progressing, panNETs receiving 10 mg everolimus daily continuously or placebo. The results of this study showed prolongation of PFS from 4.6 months in the placebo arm to 11.4 months in the everolimus arm. Grade 1–2 toxicity including stomatitis or aphthous ulceration (64%), diarrhea (34%), fatigue (31%) and infections (23%)

primarily of the upper respiratory tract was mainly observed [67]. Other adverse events include non-infectious pneumonitis and laboratory abnormalities such as anemia, neutropenia, thrombocytopenia, hypercholesterolemia hypertriglyceridemia and hyperglycemia [67].

Another study investigating safety and tolerability of pasireotide LAR in combination with everolimus in patients with advanced NETs showed promising antitumor activity and is further being investigated [95]. Evidence accumulates on the beneficial role of combining the SSA octreotide 30 mg LAR with everolimus in NF-panNETS although comparative studies are not available [96, 97]. Cooperate 2, a randomized phase II, comparative study of everolimus with pasireotide, a different SSA targeting multiple somatostatin receptors, versus everolimus single agent was not associated with the improvement in PFS compared with everolimus alone in this study [98].

Sunitib (Sutent®, Pfeizer Pharmaceuticals)

Sunitinb is an oral multi-tyrosine kinases inhibitor that has demonstrated both antiangiogenic and antiproliferative activity by blocking a range of signaling pathways and receptors such as VEGFR-1 to VEGFR-3, stem cell factor receptor, platelet-derived growth factor receptor (PDGFR)- and PDGFR-β, RET, colony-stimulating factor-1 receptor and fetal liver tyrosine kinase receptor 3 (FLT-3) [99]. It was originally approved for the treatment of advanced renal cell carcinoma (RCC) and gastrointestinal stromal tumor (GIST) refractory to imatinib treatment. Sunitinib was granted authorization for the treatment of advanced well-differentiated progressing panNETs. The exact mechanism underlining the antiproliferative effect of sunitinib is unknown. However, in a NET mouse model, sunitinib has shown an antiangiogenic effect by inhibiting pericytes that support endothelial cell function [100]. This is most probably achieved by the targeting of PDGFR-β, expressed on pericytes, that drives recruitment and maturation of vessels [101]. The efficacy of sunitinib has been demonstrated in two major clinical studies. The first was a Phase II study involving 109 patients with advanced NETs where sunitinib was administered at 50 mg daily for 4 of every 6 weeks [102]. Of 61 patients with panNETs, 16.7% had an objective RR and 68% a prolonged period of SD. The median time to tumour progression was 7.7 months.

The second was a multinational, randomized, double-blind, placebo-controlled phase III trial comparing sunitinib and best supportive care with placebo and best supportive care. This study recruited patients with advanced well-differentiated panNETs, and sunitinib was delivered at 37.5 mg continuous daily dose [66]. The study was discontinued early as the monitoring committee observed more deaths in the placebo group and a statistically significant difference in progression-free survival (PFS) favoring sunitinib by 6 months [66]. The most frequent adverse events in the sunitinib group were diarrhea (59%), nausea (44.6%), vomiting (33.7%), asthenia (33.7%) and fatigue (32.5%). As it results from previous studies, the proactive assessment of other sunitinib-related side effects, such as anorexia, oral changes, hand-foot syndrome and other skin toxicity, thyroid dysfunction, myelotoxicity, hypertension, cardiotoxicity and thromboembolic events, is critical to ensure optimal treatment benefit by allowing appropriate drug dosing and prolonged treatment periods [103, 104]. Additionally, the objective RR observed in the Phase III study was low as it regarded only 9.3% in the sunitinib group. It is important to identify those patients who may benefit by sunitinib therapy.

Due to the early termination of the phase III study, a phase IV was committed by the FDA to confirm the efficacy and safety of sunitinib in advanced/metastatic, WD, unresectable panNETs. Sixty-one treatment-naive and 45 previously treated patients received sunitinib 37.5 mg/day continuously. Median treatment duration was 11.7 months. Investigator-assessed median PFS per RECIST was similar in the two subgroups with a 95% confidence interval [CI] of 13.2 and 13.0 months in treatment-naive and previously treated patients, respectively. A total ORR per RECIST of 24.5% was observed, without significant difference between the two subgroups [105]. A combined analysis of the phase III and IV study confirmed a low ORR at 16.7% and a HR of 0.303 [106].

A post-hoc pharmacogenomic analysis was performed in a subgroup of patients included in the phase IV study to evaluate potential associations between clinical outcomes and single nucleotide polymorphisms (SNPs) in genes involved in angiogenesis, protein transport or inflammatory response. SNPs are the most common type of genetic variation, that are stable single-base substitutions present in >1% of a population [107]. No significant correlation was observed between SNPs including ABCB1, VEGFA, VEGFR 2/KDR, VEGFR1 and clinical outcome, such as PFS or OS. However, a significant correlation was observed, regarding the heterozygous genotype G/A of IL1B rs16944, with a higher overall tumor response rate versus the homozygous genotype G/G (46.4 vs 4.5%, OR: 18.2, 95% CI: 2.2–809.3; $p = 0.001$) [108].

Furthermore, a significant positive correlation with VEGFR-3 SNPs and OS was reported in a Spanish study of 43 panNET patients receiving SUN [109].

Comparison of sunitinib to everolimus in the context of a prospective comparative phase III study is not available. A recent retrospective, multicenter European study including 92 NETS, indicated that PFS at first-line everolimus was longer than sunitinib (31 months vs 9 months) in the whole cohort and the subset of 57 panNENs, mostly NF ($p < 0.0001$) [110]. In the same study, treatment with sunitinib and prior chemotherapy was negative predictors for PFS at first line in multivariable and also confirmed at multi-state modelling analyses. Discontinuation rate due to SEs was 20/85 for everolimus versus 4/41 for sunitinib ($p = 0.065$). Based on these findings, and until reliable predictors of response become available, everolimus may be preferable to sunitinib when initiating targeted therapy in progressive NF-PNENs.

The increased awareness of the different biology of NET G3 tumors have risen important issues on the treatment of this subgroup of tumors. The optimal first-line management in NET G3 and sequencing therapies remains a challenge awaiting future trials taking into consideration the unique characteristics of this category. Everolimus and sunitinib have been evaluated in advanced panNETs G3 considering that tumor morphology rather than proliferation index was the inclusion criterion for the regulatory trials. Furthermore, an interesting report indicated specific activity of everolimus and sunitinib in panNET G3 [111]. Guidelines and recommendations suggest that clinicians should manage NET G3 in a different manner than the NEC G3 even considering therapeutic options usually discussed in the G2 [79, 112].

Finally, as newer tyrosine kinase inhibitors, such as cabozantinib, lenvatinib, pazopanib, surufatinib are completing investigation in panNETs the role of another TKI following sunitinib failure remains to be elucidated [113].

Belzutifan

Patients with von Hippel–Lindau (VHL) disease have a higher incidence of panNET and other tumors owing to a rare autosomal dominant hereditary disorder associated with VHL gene inactivation and constitutive activation of the transcription factor hypoxia-inducible factor 2α (HIF-2α). Belzutifan is an oral inhibitor of HIF-2α, that at a dose of 120 mg once daily was associated with 77% objective response rates in patients with VHL-related panNETs [114]. Adverse events were generally grade 1 or 2 and included mainly anemia, fatigue, headache and dizziness. Grade 3–5 adverse events of any cause were reported in 20 patients (33%). Grade 3 events were considered to be treatment-related in nine patients (15%). Belzutifan received approval by FDA in August 2021 and at the time of writing this chapter was being considered for approval also by EMA [115].

Surufatinib

Surufatinib, a novel TKI, was designed to improve clinical outcomes by the simultaneous targeting of neoangiogenesis and immune evasion and through the inhibition of VEGF, fibroblast growth factor and macrophage colony-stimulating factor 1 pathways [116]. In the SANET-p phase III clinical trial in panNETs, carried out in China, a preplanned interim analysis (at 70% of the planned PFS events) by blinded independent image review committee indicated a statistically significant superior PFS of 13.9 months (95% CI 11.0–24.9) in the surufatinib group versus 4·6 months (3.6–7.4) in the placebo group (HR 0.34, 95% CI 0·21–0.55; $p < 0{\cdot}0001$). The drug has been approved in China and received FDA fast track designation of the drug in April 2020. However, at full review of the file in May 2022, FDA requested clinical evidence from a multiregional randomized clinical trial.

Lenvatinib

Lenvatinib is an oral multikinase inhibitor that targets VEGFR1, 2, and 3, PDGFRα, Fibroblast growth factor receptor (FGFR), and the KIT and RET tyrosine kinases. A phase II clinical trial (TALENT) tested lenvatinib 24 mg once daily in patients with grade 1–2 GEP NETs with documented tumor progression after treatment with a targeted agent (panNET) or somatostatin analogs (GI-NET) [117]. The observed response rate was 44.2% and the median duration of response was 19.9 months in the panNET group. Although 93.7% of patients required dose reductions or interruptions, the study reported one of the highest centrally confirmed response to date with a multikinase inhibitor in panNETs.

18.5.2.4 Chemotherapy

Systemic chemotherapy is indicated in G3 panNET and in panNEC [118]. Over the last three decades, the applied cytotoxic agents for panNETs included DNA damaging agents such as the antimetabolite 5-Fluorouracil (5FU), the alkylating agents streptozotocin (STZ), dacarbazine (DTIC) and temozolomide (TMZ), the topoisomerase inhibitors doxorubicin (Dox) and etoposide and the DNA crosslinker platinum derivative, such as cisplatin (CDDP), carboplatin (CBDCA) and oxaliplatin. Single-agent chemotherapy has not shown any real benefit [119] and the newer chemotherapy regimens based on the combination of these active drugs show low RRs, which set the need to improve the results of the medical treatment of these malignancies [39]. One of the first tested combinations was STZ/5FU in 1970s and remained a standard treatment until now [120, 121]. Until today, there have been no phase III trials in panNET comparing chemotherapy to best supportive care or placebo. In the field of panNETs, there have been two Phase III trials; one comparing STZ to STZ/5FU that found no difference between the two arms [119] and a second one comparing Chlorozotocin, STZ/5FU and STZ/Dox showing a statistically significant benefit in the last arm [122]. During the past decade, there have been few chemotherapy studies in advanced well and moderately differentiated NETs with encouraging results: (a) with STZ and Dox [123], (b) STZ, 5FU and Dox [59] (c) 5FU, Epirubicin and Dacarbazine [124] and (d) a study with STZ, 5FU and Cisplatin [61]. The very high response rates reported in the first studies with STZ-based chemotherapy were criticized since they derived in part from the historical use of non-standard response criteria. Furthermore, STZ-related toxicity and not manageable schedule limited its use and prompted to newer and better manageable agents like TMZ.

Chemotherapy has heterogeneous results in NET patients mainly due to the large variability of biological features among the disease subgroups. For example, chemotherapy in functioning advanced NETs has limited efficacy with a RR of 15% [125], whereas NF-panNETs have a RR of 30–40% although with significant toxicity [60, 126].

One of the earliest observations regarding these tumours was that the differentiation grade represents one of the most important predictive markers of response to chemotherapy. Patients with metastatic disease of well and moderately differentiated NF-panNETs are expected to respond better to STZ-based and targeted therapy, whereas those of high-grade NF-panNETs with Ki-67 labelling index above 20% are likely to benefit from platinum-based combination chemotherapy.

More specifically, an early report from Mayo clinic suggested that anaplastic NETs independently of the primary site location are responsive to combination chemotherapy including etoposide and cisplatin [127]. Overall, the population with anaplastic disease had an overall RR of 67%, a median time to progression (TTP) of 8 months and a median survival of 19 months. Although toxicity of this regimen was severe with vomiting, leucopenia, thrombocytopenia, anemia, alopecia and neuropathy, the efficacy of this regimen remains unsurpassed by any other treatment until today as there is no unequivocal evidence of survival improvement. Newer studies confirm that for the poorly differentiated NETs, the most effective combination chemotherapy remains cisplatin with etoposide [128]. A more recent multicentre and retrospective study including 113 patients with poorly dedifferentiated extra-pulmonary lung NETs indicated that the combination is active, effective and well tolerated [129].

Similarly, to the grade of differentiation, growing evidence suggests that a careful evaluation of the mitotic index and the Ki-67 assessment can provide further information on the overall prognosis and the degree of response to systemic cytotoxic treatment. Interestingly, it has been reported that gastroenteropancreatic carcinomas with Ki-67 < 55% had a lower RR to platinum-based chemotherapy while having a better prognosis compared with those having Ki-67 > 55% [130]. As a result, it was proposed that patients with Ki-67 < 55% may respond to different chemotherapy schedules such as TMZ but this needs to be further investigated in the context of a clinical trial [131].

Temozolomide has been investigated as a monotherapy or in combination with other drugs (capecitabine, bevacizumab, thalidomide, everolimus) in low- and intermediate-grade NENs showing significant tumor responses in panNENs but has also been evaluated in G3 tumors [132]. An interesting combination chemotherapy is CAPTEM, an oral regimen with capecitabine and TMZ that has been shown to exert high activity and low toxicity both in well-differentiated [62] and poorly differentiated neuroendocrine tumors [133]. A more recent study indicated that patients with panNENs seem to benefit more in absolute survival rates compared to other NEN primaries or UPO NENs [134]. However, a larger study comparing this regiment with STZ-based therapy or TMZ monotherapy is missing.

Another phase II trial testing the combination of irinotecan and cisplatin followed by octreotide LAR maintenance (IPO-NEC study) including patients with high-grade GEP-NET and high-grade GEP-NEC resulted in 0% and 51.4% response rates, respectively [135].

Based on the findings of a study assessing retrospectively the triplet Capecitabine, STZ and CDDP, the National Cancer Research Network approved NET01 a randomized phase II study comparing two chemotherapy regimens, Capecitabine/STZ and Capecitabine/STZ/Cisplatin in unresectable metastatic NETs of the foregut and pancreas and NETs of unknown primary site [61].

Another interesting approach with promising efficacy is the combination of targeted agents with oral TMZ chemotherapy. One such doublet is TMZ and the anti-angiogenic agent bevacizumab that has been explored in two different TMZ schedules; a standard [63] and a low continous dose [136]. A second doublet is TMZ with everolimus that has been tested in 40 patients with panNETs and shown to achieve a PR in 40% and a PFS of 15.4 months [137]. However further studies evaluating the efficacy of these combination therapies compared to TMZ alone are warranted.

18.5.2.5 Immunotherapy

With the advent of cancer immunotherapy era, phase I/II clinical trials of immune checkpoint inhibitors such as programmed cell death-ligand 1 (PD-L1) inhibitors, programmed cell death-1 (PD-1) inhibitors and cytotoxic T-lymphocyte antigen 4 inhibitors have been reported in the NET field [138]. The phase 2 KEYNOTE-158 trial, investigated pembrolizumab in GEPNETs, reported partial response in three patients with panNET [139]. Similarly, the anti-PD1 antibody spartalizumab reported an ORR of 3% in panNET [140]. The multicenter phase II clinical trial CA209–538 clinical trial testing nivolumab and ipilimumab in panNETs reported a 43% of patients experiencing an ORR [141]. Testing of MSI, TMB and PD-1/PD-L1 expression is not well established in the field of NETs, as they differ according to tumour types but it may provide the opportunity to treat selected patients with immunotherapy [142].

18.5.3 Peptide Receptor Radionuclide Therapy

Peptide receptor radionuclide therapy (PRRT) is a targeted radiation therapy involving an intravenously administered radiolabelled somatostatin analogue designed to bind on type 2 SSTR overexpressed on panNET cells and deliver a direct and a bystander lethal effect.

Accumulating clinical experience has indicated that this therapy achieves significant clinical survival benefit and improved quality of life with a usually manageable toxicity in patients with G1–2 NETs overexpressing SSTRs [143]. A committee of international experts under the auspices of the International Atomic Energy Agency, in cooperation with the European Association of Nuclear Medicine and the American Society of Nuclear Medicine and Molecular Imaging have published the PRRT eligibility requirements such as disease inoperability and high SSTR expression determined by functional studies such as ^{111}In-pentetreotide (OctreoScan) or SPECT/PET with ^{68}Ga-labelled SSA [144].

Lutetium is a lower energy beta-emitting radionuclide. The therapeutic use of lutetium-177 (177Lu) has shown better results in advanced gastroenteropancreatic and bronchial neuroendocrine tumors when compared with other available therapies. NETTER-1 was a randomized, controlled trial that evaluated the efficacy and safety of 177Lu-DOTATE in patients with advanced, progressive, somatostatin-receptor–positive midgut neuroendocrine tumors and showed a remarkable progression-free survival of 65.2% at 20 months [145]. This clinical trial provided evidence that 177Lu-DOTATE was associated with significant improvement of patients' quality of life [145, 146]. In January 2018, the Food Drug and Authority (FDA) approved ^{177}Lu-Dotatate for use in gastroenteropancreatic neuroendocrine tumors (GEP-NETs). Randomized studies of PRRT in NF-panNETs are lacking but comparisons among different single-arm studies have shown that the median response duration for Lutetium-labeled compounds is 40 months that compare favourably with other treatments for advanced disease [143].

In one of the largest retrospective PRRT studies including 504 patients of whom 310 GEP NET treated with ^{177}Lu-DOTATE median overall survival from treatment initiation was 46 months [64]. In the same cohort, 72 were NF-panNETs of whom 4 achieved complete response (6%), 26 PR (36%), 13 minor response (18%) and 19 SD (26%). Of the four patients who originally had inoperable locally advanced disease and achieved complete response, three were successfully operated 6–12 months following treatment completion, suggesting a possible role of PRRT also in the neoadjuvant setting [64].

In another study, evaluating ^{177}Lu-DOTATE in 52 G1-G2 panNET patients of whom 46 were NF-panNETs a statistically significant prolongation of survival was observed in patients receiving a total dose of 27.8 GBq as compared to those receiving 18.5 GBq due to kidney or bone marrow low reserve [65]. In the same study, the disease control rate was reported to be 81% including a CR of 12%, a PR of 27% and a SD of 46% [65]. The same group published another study indicating that FDG PET evaluation prior to PRRT is useful for predicting response to ^{177}Lu-DOTATE in patients with G1-G2 advanced panNETs [147]. A more recent retrospective study included 112 patients with NF-panNETs indicated high disease control rate at 85%, a PFS of 30 months and an OS of 69 months [148]. Finally, evidence from a prospective, phase 2 study including 29 patients with NF-panNETs indicated a disease control rate at 90% and a PFS of 27 months [149].

A comprehensive review on PRRT treatment of patients with panNETs describing the responses from several studies and safety issues, mainly short- and long-term hematologic toxicity, was recently published [150]. One important issue is the long-term development of myelodysplastic syndrome and leukemia particularly in patients treated also with chemotherapy, a common approach in panNETS. PRRT was approved for all GEP NETs, including panNETs G1 and G2; however, its positioning in the therapies sequencing of panNETs was not defined and it needs further investigation.

18.5.4 Liver-Directed Treatments

Liver-directed treatments include surgery, radiofrequency ablation, laser-induced thermotherapy or selective hepatic transcatheter arterial embolization, chemoembolization and selective internal radiation therapy (SIRT). There are no prospective comparative studies investigating the efficacy of the cytoreductive approaches, but several retrospective studies have validated their individual role in G1 and G2 NETs. The choice of any of these options depends on patient and tumor characteristics such as performance status (PS), comorbidities, number and size of metastases as well as the availability of the specific approach. Based on available evidence and the most recent ESMO guidelines, a surgical approach is indicated in selected patients affected by metastatic panNETs after having carefully evaluated the tumour grading, distribution of liver metastases and primary site [79]. Upfront surgery should be excluded in the presence of extraabdominal metastases and high-grade panNENs [79]. It seems reasonable to consider the presence of an advanced panNEC G3 as an absolute contraindication for surgery, whereas panNET G3 should not be excluded a priori [79]. More specifically, surgical resection should be attempted in the presence of resectable or potentially resectable liver metastases, mainly for panNETs with Ki-67 $\leq$ 10% or slow tumor growth [151]. On the other hand, the role of palliative resection is controversial when multiple, unresectable liver metastases are present. As a general guidance, primary site and presence of symptoms are important factors to be considered before planning a possible palliative surgical resection. In patients with liver metastases who are ineligible for complete surgical resection, vascular and ablative locoregional modalities can be considered as an alternative to surgery [79]. Locoregional treatments can also be considered as an alternative therapy to liver metastasectomy in patients with resectable liver metastases combining resection and radiofrequency ablation may provide the opportunity to achieve complete tumour removal, allowing more limited resections when otherwise more extensive hepatectomies could compromise residual liver function [79].

Here in is described the experience gained in NF-panNETs.

18.5.4.1 Surgical and Ablative Liver-Directed Treatments

There are no prospective trials investigating the role of surgical resection in patients with advanced or metastatic NF-panNETs and information mainly comes from retrospective analysis of patients treated individualy and not according to a specific protocol. One of the first studies from MD Anderson in 163 NF-panNETs indicated that patients with advanced disease who underwent a potentially curative resection had an improved survival [10]. A large retrospective SEER study including 2158 NF-panNET patients indicated that those treated with resection of either the primary tumor or distant metastatic site had increased survival compared to those who were not operated [9]. In a retrospective study from Mayo clinic including 72 NF-panNETs patients with liver metastases indicated that surgical debulking of more that 90% of tumor load leads to a similar patient prognosis when compared to completly resected patients [11]. In the same study, patients achieved a median overall survival of 55.2 months and a 5-year overall survival of 59.9% that compare very favorably with historical survival data of patients with untreated liver metastasis (median survival 27 months; 5-year survival of 29%) [11].

Radiofrequency ablation (RFA) is a procedure that can be applied during standard surgery, laparoscopically or percutaneously through an image-guided procedure, with probes that deliver a lethal hit by extreme heat directly in the lesion of interest. There are no prospective studies assessing RFA in a patient population diagnosed selectively with NF-panNETs. In one of the largest prospective trial including 54 patients with liver metastases of NET, RFA performed laparoscopically with ultrasound guidance reported a median overall survival of 11.0 years, a median post-diagnosis of hepatic metastases survival time of 5.5 years and a medical of 3.9 years post-first RFA [152].

18.5.4.2 Intravascular Treatments: Embolization and Chemoembolization

Hepatic arterial embolization (HAE) and chemoembolization (HACE) are two alternative therapeutic options for liver metastases of G1 and G2 tumors, not amenable to surgical resection, that have shown efficacy but have never been compared in NF-panNETs. HAE and HACE are delivered through percutaneous incanulation of the femoral artery and when into the relevant hepatic vascular territory an agent such as polyvinyl alcohol in HAE or a chemotherapeutic agent with lipiodol in HACE is injected in the engaged vessel to provoke stasis and ischemia in the downstream tissues. Regarding these procedures, several questions remain unanswered such as whether combining chemotherapy and which drug (5-FU, Dox and mitomycin C) adds to the overall benefit of embolization, which are the appropriate dosage intervals and the timing of the procedure evaluation [54]. Both procedures are safe but are contraindicated in patients with portal vein thrombosis, borderline liver function and previous Whipple procedure [153]. The most common side effect is the so-called 'postembolization syndrome' that includes abdominal pain, fever, nausea, vomiting and elevated liver enzymes that usually respond to symptomatic treatment and lasts for 3 days [154]. More severe side effects such as pancreatitis, liver and renal failure, sepsis, myocardial infarction that may be responsible for increased 30-day mortality rate and support the application of these methods only in high-volume centres [154].

A small prospective study compared 12 midgut NET patients receiveing HACE to 14 patients receiving HAC and found equal tumor control in 95% of cases and similar 2-year PFS [155].

From the published literature, it is noted that both procedures result in 50–90% tumor marker responses and 30–50% in imaging response; this smaller response in imaging is due to the difficulty in assessing necrosis caused by embolization by RECIST criteria [153].

18.5.4.3 Radioembolization

Radioembolization employes either biodegradable resin-based (SIR-Spheres; Sirtex Medical Limited, New South Wales, Australia) or non-biodegradable glass-based (Theraspheres; MDS Nordion, Ottawa, ON, Canada) microspheres labelled with Yttrium-90 (Y-90). Most studies in NETs evaluate resin microsphere radioembolization and there have been none analyzing only NF-panNETs. In one of the largest studies, 184 patients treated with ^{90}Y resin microspheres in 10 centres reported a very low toxicity profile mainly fatigue (6.5%), a high disease response (CR in 2.7%, PR in 60.5%, SD in 22.7%) and a median survival of 70 months [156].

Radioembolization with Y-labeled spheres is still considered investigational although several small studies in NET patients with liver metastases show high RRs [153]. Nevertheless, a randomized trial comparing HAE and ^{90}Yttrium-labelled microspheres is urgently needed.

18.6 Follow-Up

The role of surveillance after a radical resection for panNETs is to evaluate the results of treatment and to identify early relapse for curative treatment. According to the recent ENETS guidelines, follow-up investigations should include clinical symptom monitoring, biochemical parameters and conventional and SSTR imaging [79]. In patients with R0/R1-resected panNET G1 and NET G2 with low Ki-67 (<5%), it is recommended that imaging is carried out every 6 months (CT or MRI), in panNET G2 (Ki-67 > 5%) every 3 months and in panNEC G3 every 2–3 months [79]. Similar staging intervals apply to advanced disease. Follow-up should be life-long, although the staging intervals can be extended to 1–2 years with increasing length of follow-up (>5 years), except in G3 NEN, where shorter intervals should be kept [54, 79, 153].

Depending on each patient, the follow-up program includes clinical examination and routine investigations with full blood count, biochemistry, biomarkers (CgA or NSE) and imaging (ultrasound, CT or MRI) [69, 157, 158]. If chromogranin A is not elevated NSE may be found abnormal and used as an alternative biomarker [153]. Other imaging procedures include endoscopy, endoscopic ultrasound, octreotide scintigraphy and PET imaging with different tracer bound compounds such as 68Ga-DOTA-TOC/-NOC/–TATE or ^{18}FDG [153, 157] are recommended every 18–24 months [153].

In the case of a patient with rapid tumor progression, it may become necessary to perform new CT- or ultrasound-guided biopsies of the metastases in order to evaluate whether the proliferative activity has changed [153].

18.7 Clinical Trials

Eagerly awaited are the results of the following clinical trials that are in progress or recently concluded

1. Evaluating bevacizumab in combination with FOLFIRI after the failure of platinum-etoposide regimen in patients with advanced poorly differentiated neuroendocrine carcinoma: The PRODIGE 41-BEVANEC randomized phase II study (NCT02820857).
2. A phase II study from Stanford University. NCT01525082 Capecitabine, temozolomide and bevacizumab for metastatic or unresectable pancreatic neuroendocrine tumors.
3. A phase I/II study from Northwestern University, USA. NCT01465659 Temozolomide and pazopanib hydrochloride in treating patients with advanced pancreatic neuroendocrine tumors that cannot be removed by surgery.
4. A phase II study of carfilzomib for the treatment of patients with advanced neuroendocrine cancers NCT02318784.
5. Antitumor efficacy of peptide receptor radionuclide therapy with ^{177}Lutetium-octreotate randomized versus sunitinib in unresectable progressive well-differentiated neuroendocrine pancreatic tumor: First randomized phase II. (OCCLURANDOM) NCT02230176.
6. Study of CVM-1118 for patients with advanced neuroendocrine tumors NCT03600233.
7. Randomized, double-blinded phase III study of cabozantinib versus placebo in patients with advanced neuroendocrine tumors after progression on everolimus (CABINET).

8. A randomized phase II study of temozolomide or temozolomide and capecitabine in patients with advanced pancreatic neuroendocrine tumors NCT01824875.
9. Assessment of the efficacy of bevacizumab in combination with folfiri as second-line treatment in patients suffering from an advanced inoperable poorly differentiated neuroendocrine carcinoma of an unknown or gastroentero-pancreatic primary cancer (BEVANEC) NCT02820857.
10. Cisplatin, carboplatin and etoposide or temozolomide and capecitabine in treating patients with neuroendocrine carcinoma of the gastrointestinal tract or pancreas that is metastatic or cannot be removed by surgery NCT02595424.
11. Study of efficacy and safety of PDR001 in patients with advanced or metastatic, well-differentiated, non-functional neuroendocrine tumors of pancreatic, gastrointestinal (GI), or thoracic origin or poorly differentiated gastroenteropancreatic neuroendocrine carcinoma (GEP-NEC) NCT02955069.
12. Liposomal irinotecan, fluorouracil and leucovorin in treating patients with refractory advanced high-grade neuroendocrine cancer of gastrointestinal, unknown, or pancreatic origin. NCT03736720.
13. Sapanisertib in treating patients with metastatic or refractory pancreatic neuroendocrine tumor that cannot be removed by surgery NCT02893930.
14. VEGFR/PDGFR dual kinase inhibitor X-82 and everolimus for treating patients with pancreatic neuroendocrine tumors NCT01784861.

18.8 Conclusions

Pancreatic neuroendocrine tumors are relatively rare and heterogeneous malignancies, with an increasing incidence. Around three decades after the approval of streptozotocin, two biological agents, everolimus and sunitinib, showed a clinical and statistical benefit in terms of PFS and they have been approved for patients with progressing advanced well/moderately differentiated panNETs. However, the prognosis of poorly differentiated panNETs remains dismal even when treated with chemotherapy. A vital challenge remains the recognition of key molecular pathways for the development of targeted therapies that could improve the prognosis of these patients.

References

1. Panzuto F, Nasoni S, Falconi M, Corleto VD, Capurso G, Cassetta S, Di Fonzo M, Tornatore V, Milione M, Angeletti S, Cattaruzza MS, Ziparo V, Bordi C, Pederzoli P, Delle Fave G (2005) Prognostic factors and survival in endocrine tumor patients: comparison between gastrointestinal and pancreatic localization. Endocr Relat Cancer 12(4):1083–1092
2. Tsoli M, Chatzellis E, Koumarianou A, Kolomodi D, Kaltsas G (2019) Current best practice in the management of neuroendocrine tumors. Ther Adv Endocrinol Metab 10:2042018818804698
3. Zikusoka MN, Kidd M, Eick G, Latich I, Modlin IM (2005) The molecular genetics of gastroenteropancreatic neuroendocrine tumors. Cancer 104(11):2292–2309

4. Liu TH, Zhu Y, Cui QC, Cai LX, Ye SF, Zhong SX, Jia HP (1992) Nonfunctioning pancreatic endocrine tumors. An immunohistochemical and electron microscopic analysis of 26 cases. Pathol Res Pract 188(1–2):191–198
5. Jensen RT, Bodei L, Capdevila J, Couvelard A, Falconi M, Glasberg S, Kloppel G, Lamberts S, Peeters M, Rindi G, Rinke A, Rothmund M, Sundin A, Welin S, Fazio N (2019) Unmet needs in functional and nonfunctional pancreatic neuroendocrine neoplasms. Neuroendocrinology 108(1):26–36
6. Dasari A, Shen C, Halperin D, Zhao B, Zhou S, Xu Y, Shih T, Yao JC (2017) Trends in the incidence, prevalence, and survival outcomes in patients with neuroendocrine tumors in the United States. JAMA Oncol 3(10):1335–1342
7. Borbath I, Bikmukhametov D, Maasberg S, Garcia-Carbonero R, Jiménez-Fonseca P, Castaño A, Kollar A, Sedlackova E, Barkmanova J, Kos-Kudla B, Handkiewicz-Junak D, G K, Koumarianou A, Falconi M, Oberg KE, Wiedenmann B, Holger F, Ruediger L, UF P, Verslype C (2018) Assessing prognosis of neuroendocrine neoplasms: results of a collaborative multinational effort including over 10.000 European patients—the ENETS registry. J Clin Oncol 36(15_suppl):4095–4095
8. Bettini R, Boninsegna L, Mantovani W, Capelli P, Bassi C, Pederzoli P, Delle Fave GF, Panzuto F, Scarpa A, Falconi M (2008) Prognostic factors at diagnosis and value of WHO classification in a mono-institutional series of 180 non-functioning pancreatic endocrine tumours. Ann Oncol 19(5):903–908
9. Franko J, Feng W, Yip L, Genovese E, Moser AJ (2010) Non-functional neuroendocrine carcinoma of the pancreas: incidence, tumor biology, and outcomes in 2, 158 patients. J Gastrointest Surg 14(3):541–548
10. Solorzano CC, Lee JE, Pisters PW, Vauthey JN, Ayers GD, Jean ME, Gagel RF, Ajani JA, Wolff RA, Evans DB (2001) Nonfunctioning islet cell carcinoma of the pancreas: survival results in a contemporary series of 163 patients. Surgery 130(6):1078–1085
11. Cusati D, Zhang L, Harmsen WS, Hu A, Farnell MB, Nagorney DM, Donohue JH, Que FG, Reid-Lombardo KM, Kendrick ML (2012) Metastatic nonfunctioning pancreatic neuroendocrine carcinoma to liver: surgical treatment and outcomes. J Am Coll Surg 215(1):117-124; discussion 124-115
12. Brooks JC, Shavelle RM, Vavra-Musser KN (2019) Life expectancy in pancreatic neuroendocrine cancer. Clin Res Hepatol Gastroenterol 43(1):88–97
13. Capurso G, Festa S, Valente R, Piciucchi M, Panzuto F, Jensen RT, Delle Fave G (2012) Molecular pathology and genetics of pancreatic endocrine tumours. J Mol Endocrinol 49(1):R37–R50
14. Lemos MC, Thakker RV (2008) Multiple endocrine neoplasia type 1 (MEN1): analysis of 1336 mutations reported in the first decade following identification of the gene. Hum Mutat 29(1):22–32
15. Gurung B, Feng Z, Iwamoto DV, Thiel A, Jin G, Fan CM, Ng JM, Curran T, Hua X (2013) Menin epigenetically represses Hedgehog signaling in MEN1 tumor syndrome. Cancer Res 73(8):2650–2658
16. Wang Y, Ozawa A, Zaman S, Prasad NB, Chandrasekharappa SC, Agarwal SK, Marx SJ (2011) The tumor suppressor protein menin inhibits AKT activation by regulating its cellular localization. Cancer Res 71(2):371–382
17. Thomas-Marques L, Murat A, Delemer B, Penfornis A, Cardot-Bauters C, Baudin E, Niccoli-Sire P, Levoir D, Choplin Hdu B, Chabre O, Jovenin N, Cadiot G (2006) Prospective endoscopic ultrasonographic evaluation of the frequency of nonfunctioning pancreaticoduodenal endocrine tumors in patients with multiple endocrine neoplasia type 1. Am J Gastroenterol 101(2):266–273
18. Moore PS, Missiaglia E, Antonello D, Zamo A, Zamboni G, Corleto V, Falconi M, Scarpa A (2001) Role of disease-causing genes in sporadic pancreatic endocrine tumors: MEN1 and VHL. Genes Chromosomes Cancer 32(2):177–181
19. Newey PJ, Jeyabalan J, Walls GV, Christie PT, Gleeson FV, Gould S, Johnson PR, Phillips RR, Ryan FJ, Shine B, Bowl MR, Thakker RV (2009) Asymptomatic children with multiple

endocrine neoplasia type 1 mutations may harbor nonfunctioning pancreatic neuroendocrine tumors. J Clin Endocrinol Metab 94(10):3640–3646
20. Jensen RT, Berna MJ, Bingham DB, Norton JA (2008) Inherited pancreatic endocrine tumor syndromes: advances in molecular pathogenesis, diagnosis, management, and controversies. Cancer 113(7 Suppl):1807–1843
21. Corcos O, Couvelard A, Giraud S, Vullierme MP, Dermot OT, Rebours V, Stievenart JL, Penfornis A, Niccoli-Sire P, Baudin E, Sauvanet A, Levy P, Ruszniewski P, Richard S, Hammel P (2008) Endocrine pancreatic tumors in von Hippel-Lindau disease: clinical, histological, and genetic features. Pancreas 37(1):85–93
22. Tee AR, Fingar DC, Manning BD, Kwiatkowski DJ, Cantley LC, Blenis J (2002) Tuberous sclerosis complex-1 and -2 gene products function together to inhibit mammalian target of rapamycin (mTOR)-mediated downstream signaling. Proc Natl Acad Sci USA 99(21):13571–13576
23. Curatolo P, Bombardieri R, Jozwiak S (2008) Tuberous sclerosis. Lancet 372(9639):657–668
24. Jiao Y, Shi C, Edil BH, de Wilde RF, Klimstra DS, Maitra A, Schulick RD, Tang LH, Wolfgang CL, Choti MA, Velculescu VE, Diaz LA Jr, Vogelstein B, Kinzler KW, Hruban RH, Papadopoulos N (2011) DAXX/ATRX, MEN1, and mTOR pathway genes are frequently altered in pancreatic neuroendocrine tumors. Science 331(6021):1199–1203
25. Missiaglia E, Dalai I, Barbi S, Beghelli S, Falconi M, della Peruta M, Piemonti L, Capurso G, Di Florio A, DelleFave G, Pederzoli P, Croce CM, Scarpa A (2010) Pancreatic endocrine tumors: expression profiling evidences a role for AKT-mTOR pathway. J Clin Oncol 28(2):245–255
26. Oberg K (2009) Genetics and molecular pathology of neuroendocrine gastrointestinal and pancreatic tumors (gastroenteropancreatic neuroendocrine tumors). Curr Opin Endocrinol Diabetes Obes 16(1):72–78
27. Oberg K (2009) Somatostatin analog octreotide LAR in gastro-entero-pancreatic tumors. Expert Rev Anticancer Ther 9(5):557–566
28. Perren A, Komminoth P, Saremaslani P, Matter C, Feurer S, Lees JA, Heitz PU, Eng C (2000) Mutation and expression analyses reveal differential subcellular compartmentalization of PTEN in endocrine pancreatic tumors compared to normal islet cells. Am J Pathol 157(4):1097–1103
29. Hessman O, Lindberg D, Skogseid B, Carling T, Hellman P, Rastad J, Akerstrom G, Westin G (1998) Mutation of the multiple endocrine neoplasia type 1 gene in nonfamilial, malignant tumors of the endocrine pancreas. Cancer Res 58(3):377–379
30. Larsson C (2013) Epigenetic aspects on therapy development for gastroenteropancreatic neuroendocrine tumors. Neuroendocrinology 97(1):19–25
31. Yachida S, Vakiani E, White CM, Zhong Y, Saunders T, Morgan R, de Wilde RF, Maitra A, Hicks J, Demarzo AM, Shi C, Sharma R, Laheru D, Edil BH, Wolfgang CL, Schulick RD, Hruban RH, Tang LH, Klimstra DS, Iacobuzio-Donahue CA (2012) Small cell and large cell neuroendocrine carcinomas of the pancreas are genetically similar and distinct from well-differentiated pancreatic neuroendocrine tumors. Am J Surg Pathol 36(2):173–184
32. Yao J, Garg A, Chen D, Capdevila J, Engstrom P, Pommier R, Van Cutsem E, Singh S, Fazio N, He W, Riester M, Patel P, Voi M, Morrissey M, Pavel M, Kulke MH (2019) Genomic profiling of NETs: a comprehensive analysis of the RADIANT trials. Endocr Relat Cancer 26(4):391–403
33. Rindi G, Klimstra DS, Abedi-Ardekani B, Asa SL, Bosman FT, Brambilla E, Busam KJ, de Krijger RR, Dietel M, El-Naggar AK, Fernandez-Cuesta L, Kloppel G, McCluggage WG, Moch H, Ohgaki H, Rakha EA, Reed NS, Rous BA, Sasano H, Scarpa A, Scoazec JY, Travis WD, Tallini G, Trouillas J, van Krieken JH, Cree IA (2018) A common classification framework for neuroendocrine neoplasms: an International Agency for Research on Cancer (IARC) and World Health Organization (WHO) expert consensus proposal. Mod Pathol 31(12):1770–1786
34. Amin M, Edge S, Greene F, Byrd D, Brookland R, Washington M, Gershenwald J, Compton C, Hess K, Sullivan DC, Jessup JM, Brierley JD, Gaspar LE, Schilsky RL, Balch CM (2017)

AJCC cancer staging manual, 8th edn. Springer International Publishing: American Joint Commission on Cancer, Chicago
35. La Rosa S, Sessa F, Capella C, Riva C, Leone BE, Klersy C, Rindi G, Solcia E (1996) Prognostic criteria in nonfunctioning pancreatic endocrine tumours. Virchows Arch 429(6):323–333
36. Pelosi G, Bresaola E, Bogina G, Pasini F, Rodella S, Castelli P, Iacono C, Serio G, Zamboni G (1996) Endocrine tumors of the pancreas: Ki-67 immunoreactivity on paraffin sections is an independent predictor for malignancy: a comparative study with proliferating-cell nuclear antigen and progesterone receptor protein immunostaining, mitotic index, and other clinicopathologic variables. Hum Pathol 27(11):1124–1134
37. Scarpa A, Mantovani W, Capelli P, Beghelli S, Boninsegna L, Bettini R, Panzuto F, Pederzoli P, Fave G d, Falconi M (2010) Pancreatic endocrine tumors: improved TNM staging and histopathological grading permit a clinically efficient prognostic stratification of patients. Mod Pathol 23(6):824–833
38. Panzuto F, Boninsegna L, Fazio N, Campana D, Pia Brizzi M, Capurso G, Scarpa A, De Braud F, Dogliotti L, Tomassetti P, Delle Fave G, Falconi M (2011) Metastatic and locally advanced pancreatic endocrine carcinomas: analysis of factors associated with disease progression. J Clin Oncol 29(17):2372–2377
39. Vilar E, Salazar R, Perez-Garcia J, Cortes J, Oberg K, Tabernero J (2007) Chemotherapy and role of the proliferation marker Ki-67 in digestive neuroendocrine tumors. Endocr Relat Cancer 14(2):221–232
40. Boninsegna L, Panzuto F, Partelli S, Capelli P, Delle Fave G, Bettini R, Pederzoli P, Scarpa A, Falconi M (2012) Malignant pancreatic neuroendocrine tumour: lymph node ratio and Ki67 are predictors of recurrence after curative resections. Eur J Cancer 48(11):1608–1615
41. Fernandez-Cruz L, Blanco L, Cosa R, Rendon H (2008) Is laparoscopic resection adequate in patients with neuroendocrine pancreatic tumors? World J Surg 32(5):904–917
42. Merola E, Falconi M, Rinke A, Staettner S, Krendl F, Partelli S, Andreasi V, Gress TM, Pascher A, Arsenic R, Doglioni C, Kaemmerer D, Wiedenmann B, Pavel ME (2020) Radical intended surgery for highly selected stage IV neuroendocrine neoplasms G3. Am J Surg 220:284
43. Haugvik SP, Labori KJ, Edwin B, Mathisen O, Gladhaug IP (2012) Surgical treatment of sporadic pancreatic neuroendocrine tumors: a state of the art review. Sci World J 2012:357475
44. Falconi M, Zerbi A, Crippa S, Balzano G, Boninsegna L, Capitanio V, Bassi C, Di Carlo V, Pederzoli P (2010) Parenchyma-preserving resections for small nonfunctioning pancreatic endocrine tumors. Ann Surg Oncol 17(6):1621–1627
45. Capurso G, Bettini R, Rinzivillo M, Boninsegna L, Delle Fave G, Falconi M (2011) Role of resection of the primary pancreatic neuroendocrine tumour only in patients with unresectable metastatic liver disease: a systematic review. Neuroendocrinology 93(4):223–229
46. Smith JK, Ng SC, Hill JS, Simons JP, Arous EJ, Shah SA, Tseng JF, McDade TP (2010) Complications after pancreatectomy for neuroendocrine tumors: a national study. J Surg Res 163(1):63–68
47. Aranha GV, Shoup M (2005) Nonstandard pancreatic resections for unusual lesions. Am J Surg 189(2):223–228
48. Falconi M, Mantovani W, Crippa S, Mascetta G, Salvia R, Pederzoli P (2008) Pancreatic insufficiency after different resections for benign tumours. Br J Surg 95(1):85–91
49. Ferrone CR, Tang LH, Tomlinson J, Gonen M, Hochwald SN, Brennan MF, Klimstra DS, Allen PJ (2007) Determining prognosis in patients with pancreatic endocrine neoplasms: can the WHO classification system be simplified? J Clin Oncol 25(35):5609–5615
50. Haynes AB, Deshpande V, Ingkakul T, Vagefi PA, Szymonifka J, Thayer SP, Ferrone CR, Wargo JA, Warshaw AL, Fernandez-del Castillo C (2011) Implications of incidentally discovered, nonfunctioning pancreatic endocrine tumors: short-term and long-term patient outcomes. Arch Surg 146(5):534–538
51. Parekh JR, Wang SC, Bergsland EK, Venook AP, Warren RS, Kim GE, Nakakura EK (2012) Lymph node sampling rates and predictors of nodal metastasis in pancreatic neuroendocrine tumor resections: the UCSF experience with 149 patients. Pancreas 41(6):840–844

52. Han SH, Han IW, Heo JS, Choi SH, Choi DW, Han S, You YH (2018) Laparoscopic versus open distal pancreatectomy for nonfunctioning pancreatic neuroendocrine tumors: a large single-center study. Surg Endosc 32(1):443–449
53. Kouvaraki MA, Solorzano CC, Shapiro SE, Yao JC, Perrier ND, Lee JE, Evans DB (2005) Surgical treatment of non-functioning pancreatic islet cell tumors. J Surg Oncol 89(3):170–185
54. Falconi M, Bartsch DK, Eriksson B, Kloppel G, Lopes JM, O'Connor JM, Salazar R, Taal BG, Vullierme MP, O'Toole D (2012) ENETS Consensus Guidelines for the management of patients with digestive neuroendocrine neoplasms of the digestive system: well-differentiated pancreatic non-functioning tumors. Neuroendocrinology 95(2):120–134
55. Triponez F, Goudet P, Dosseh D, Cougard P, Bauters C, Murat A, Cadiot G, Niccoli-Sire P, Calender A, Proye CA (2006) Is surgery beneficial for MEN1 patients with small (< or = 2 cm), nonfunctioning pancreaticoduodenal endocrine tumor? An analysis of 65 patients from the GTE. World J Surg 30(5):654–662. discussion 663–654
56. Howe JR, Merchant NB, Conrad C, Keutgen XM, Hallet J, Drebin JA, Minter RM, Lairmore TC, Tseng JF, Zeh HJ, Libutti SK, Singh G, Lee JE, Hope TA, Kim MK, Menda Y, Halfdanarson TR, Chan JA, Pommier RF (2020) The North American neuroendocrine tumor society consensus paper on the surgical management of pancreatic neuroendocrine tumors. Pancreas 49(1):1–33
57. Scherubl H, Cadiot G (2017) Early gastroenteropancreatic neuroendocrine tumors: endoscopic therapy and surveillance. Visc Med 33(5):332–338
58. Oleinikov K, Dancour A, Epshtein J, Benson A, Mazeh H, Tal I, Matalon S, Benbassat CA, Livovsky DM, Goldin E, Gross DJ, Jacob H, Grozinsky-Glasberg S (2019) Endoscopic ultrasound-guided radiofrequency ablation: a new therapeutic approach for pancreatic neuroendocrine tumors. J Clin Endocrinol Metab 104(7):2637–2647
59. Kouvaraki MA, Ajani JA, Hoff P, Wolff R, Evans DB, Lozano R, Yao JC (2004) Fluorouracil, doxorubicin, and streptozocin in the treatment of patients with locally advanced and metastatic pancreatic endocrine carcinomas. J Clin Oncol 22(23):4762–4771
60. Ekeblad S, Sundin A, Janson ET, Welin S, Granberg D, Kindmark H, Dunder K, Kozlovacki G, Orlefors H, Sigurd M, Oberg K, Eriksson B, Skogseid B (2007) Temozolomide as monotherapy is effective in treatment of advanced malignant neuroendocrine tumors. Clin Cancer Res 13(10):2986–2991
61. Turner NC, Strauss SJ, Sarker D, Gillmore R, Kirkwood A, Hackshaw A, Papadopoulou A, Bell J, Kayani I, Toumpanakis C, Grillo F, Mayer A, Hochhauser D, Begent RH, Caplin ME, Meyer T (2010) Chemotherapy with 5-fluorouracil, cisplatin and streptozocin for neuroendocrine tumours. Br J Cancer 102(7):1106–1112
62. Strosberg JR, Fine RL, Choi J, Nasir A, Coppola D, Chen DT, Helm J, Kvols L (2011) First-line chemotherapy with capecitabine and temozolomide in patients with metastatic pancreatic endocrine carcinomas. Cancer 117(2):268–275
63. Chan JA, Stuart K, Earle CC, Clark JW, Bhargava P, Miksad R, Blaszkowsky L, Enzinger PC, Meyerhardt JA, Zheng H, Fuchs CS, Kulke MH (2012) Prospective study of bevacizumab plus temozolomide in patients with advanced neuroendocrine tumors. J Clin Oncol 30(24):2963–2968
64. Kwekkeboom DJ, de Herder WW, Kam BL, van Eijck CH, van Essen M, Kooij PP, Feelders RA, van Aken MO, Krenning EP (2008) Treatment with the radiolabeled somatostatin analog [177 Lu-DOTA 0,Tyr3]octreotate: toxicity, efficacy, and survival. J Clin Oncol 26(13):2124–2130
65. Sansovini M, Severi S, Ambrosetti A, Monti M, Nanni O, Sarnelli A, Bodei L, Garaboldi L, Bartolomei M, Paganelli G (2013) Treatment with the radiolabelled somatostatin analog Lu-DOTATATE for advanced pancreatic neuroendocrine tumors. Neuroendocrinology 97(4):347–354
66. Raymond E, Dahan L, Raoul JL, Bang YJ, Borbath I, Lombard-Bohas C, Valle J, Metrakos P, Smith D, Vinik A, Chen JS, Horsch D, Hammel P, Wiedenmann B, Van Cutsem E, Patyna S, Lu DR, Blanckmeister C, Chao R, Ruszniewski P (2011) Sunitinib malate for the treatment of pancreatic neuroendocrine tumors. N Engl J Med 364(6):501–513

67. Yao JC, Shah MH, Ito T, Bohas CL, Wolin EM, Van Cutsem E, Hobday TJ, Okusaka T, Capdevila J, de Vries EG, Tomassetti P, Pavel ME, Hoosen S, Haas T, Lincy J, Lebwohl D, Oberg K (2011) Everolimus for advanced pancreatic neuroendocrine tumors. N Engl J Med 364(6):514–523
68. Oberg K (2001) Established clinical use of octreotide and lanreotide in oncology. Chemotherapy 47(Suppl 2):40–53
69. Aparicio T, Ducreux M, Baudin E, Sabourin JC, De Baere T, Mitry E, Schlumberger M, Rougier P (2001) Antitumour activity of somatostatin analogues in progressive metastatic neuroendocrine tumours. Eur J Cancer 37(8):1014–1019
70. Ducreux M, Ruszniewski P, Chayvialle JA, Blumberg J, Cloarec D, Michel H, Raymond JM, Dupas JL, Gouerou H, Jian R, Genestin E, Hammel P, Rougier P (2000) The antitumoral effect of the long-acting somatostatin analog lanreotide in neuroendocrine tumors. Am J Gastroenterol 95(11):3276–3281
71. Imam H, Eriksson B, Lukinius A, Janson ET, Lindgren PG, Wilander E, Oberg K (1997) Induction of apoptosis in neuroendocrine tumors of the digestive system during treatment with somatostatin analogs. Acta Oncol 36(6):607–614
72. Yoshitomi H, Fujii Y, Miyazaki M, Nakajima N, Inagaki N, Seino S (1997) Involvement of MAP kinase and c-fos signaling in the inhibition of cell growth by somatostatin. Am J Phys 272(5 Pt 1):E769–E774
73. Danesi R, Agen C, Benelli U, Paolo AD, Nardini D, Bocci G, Basolo F, Campagni A, Tacca MD (1997) Inhibition of experimental angiogenesis by the somatostatin analogue octreotide acetate (SMS 201-995). Clin Cancer Res 3(2):265–272
74. Koizumi M, Onda M, Tanaka N, Seya T, Yamada T, Takahashi Y (2002) Antiangiogenic effect of octreotide inhibits the growth of human rectal neuroendocrine carcinoma. Digestion 65(4):200–206
75. Caplin ME, Pavel M, Cwikla JB, Phan AT, Raderer M, Sedlackova E, Cadiot G, Wolin EM, Capdevila J, Wall L, Rindi G, Langley A, Martinez S, Blumberg J, Ruszniewski P, CLARINET Investigators (2014) Lanreotide in metastatic enteropancreatic neuroendocrine tumors. N Engl J Med 371(3):224–233
76. Caplin ME, Pavel M, Cwikla JB, Phan AT, Raderer M, Sedlackova E, Cadiot G, Wolin EM, Capdevila J, Wall L, Rindi G, Langley A, Martinez S, Gomez-Panzani E, Ruszniewski P, CLARINET Investigators (2016) Anti-tumour effects of lanreotide for pancreatic and intestinal neuroendocrine tumours: the CLARINET open-label extension study. Endocr Relat Cancer 23(3):191–199
77. Pavel M, Cwikla JB, Lombard-Bohas C, Borbath I, Shah T, Pape UF, Capdevila J, Panzuto F, Truong Thanh XM, Houchard A, Ruszniewski P (2021) Efficacy and safety of high-dose lanreotide autogel in patients with progressive pancreatic or midgut neuroendocrine tumours: CLARINET FORTE phase 2 study results. Eur J Cancer 157:403–414
78. Pavel M, O'Toole D, Costa F, Capdevila J, Gross D, Kianmanesh R, Krenning E, Knigge U, Salazar R, Pape UF, Oberg K, Vienna Consensus Conference participants (2016) ENETS Consensus Guidelines update for the management of distant metastatic disease of intestinal, pancreatic, bronchial neuroendocrine neoplasms (NEN) and NEN of unknown primary site. Neuroendocrinology 103(2):172–185
79. Pavel M, Oberg K, Falconi M, Krenning E, Sundin A, Perren A, Berruti A, Committee EG (2020) Gastroenteropancreatic neuroendocrine neoplasms: ESMO Clinical Practice Guidelines for diagnosis, treatment and follow-up. Ann Oncol 31:844
80. Detjen KM, Welzel M, Farwig K, Brembeck FH, Kaiser A, Riecken EO, Wiedenmann B, Rosewicz S (2000) Molecular mechanism of interferon alfa-mediated growth inhibition in human neuroendocrine tumor cells. Gastroenterology 118(4):735–748
81. Oberg K (1992) The action of interferon alpha on human carcinoid tumours. Semin Cancer Biol 3(1):35–41
82. von Marschall Z, Scholz A, Cramer T, Schafer G, Schirner M, Oberg K, Wiedenmann B, Hocker M, Rosewicz S (2003) Effects of interferon alpha on vascular endothelial growth factor gene transcription and tumor angiogenesis. J Natl Cancer Inst 95(6):437–448

83. Funa K, Alm GV, Ronnblom L, Oberg K (1983) Evaluation of the natural killer cell-interferon system in patients with mid-gut carcinoid tumours treated with leucocyte interferon. Clin Exp Immunol 53(3):716–724
84. Oberg K (1996) Biological aspects of neuroendocrine gastro-enteropancreatic tumours. Digestion 57(Suppl 1):42–44
85. Oberg K (1996) Interferon-alpha versus somatostatin or the combination of both in gastro-enteropancreatic tumours. Digestion 57(Suppl 1):81–83
86. Oberg K, Funa K, Alm G (1983) Effects of leukocyte interferon on clinical symptoms and hormone levels in patients with mid-gut carcinoid tumors and carcinoid syndrome. N Engl J Med 309(3):129–133
87. Frank M, Klose KJ, Wied M, Ishaque N, Schade-Brittinger C, Arnold R (1999) Combination therapy with octreotide and alpha-interferon: effect on tumor growth in metastatic endocrine gastroenteropancreatic tumors. Am J Gastroenterol 94(5):1381–1387
88. Oberg K, Kvols L, Caplin M, Delle Fave G, de Herder W, Rindi G, Ruszniewski P, Woltering EA, Wiedenmann B (2004) Consensus report on the use of somatostatin analogs for the management of neuroendocrine tumors of the gastroenteropancreatic system. Ann Oncol 15(6):966–973
89. Kolby L, Persson G, Franzen S, Ahren B (2003) Randomized clinical trial of the effect of interferon alpha on survival in patients with disseminated midgut carcinoid tumours. Br J Surg 90(6):687–693
90. Faiss S, Pape UF, Bohmig M, Dorffel Y, Mansmann U, Golder W, Riecken EO, Wiedenmann B (2003) Prospective, randomized, multicenter trial on the antiproliferative effect of lanreotide, interferon alfa, and their combination for therapy of metastatic neuroendocrine gastroenteropancreatic tumors—the International Lanreotide and Interferon Alfa Study Group. J Clin Oncol 21(14):2689–2696
91. Arnold R, Rinke A, Klose KJ, Muller HH, Wied M, Zamzow K, Schmidt C, Schade-Brittinger C, Barth P, Moll R, Koller M, Unterhalt M, Hiddemann W, Schmidt-Lauber M, Pavel M, Arnold CN (2005) Octreotide versus octreotide plus interferon-alpha in endocrine gastroenteropancreatic tumors: a randomized trial. Clin Gastroenterol Hepatol 3(8):761–771
92. Fazio N, de Braud F, Delle Fave G, Oberg K (2007) Interferon-alpha and somatostatin analog in patients with gastroenteropancreatic neuroendocrine carcinoma: single agent or combination? Ann Oncol 18(1):13–19
93. Yao JC, Phan AT, Chang DZ, Wolff RA, Hess K, Gupta S, Jacobs C, Mares JE, Landgraf AN, Rashid A, Meric-Bernstam F (2008) Efficacy of RAD001 (everolimus) and octreotide LAR in advanced low- to intermediate-grade neuroendocrine tumors: results of a phase II study. J Clin Oncol 26(26):4311–4318
94. Yao JC, Lombard-Bohas C, Baudin E, Kvols LK, Rougier P, Ruszniewski P, Hoosen S, St Peter J, Haas T, Lebwohl D, Van Cutsem E, Kulke MH, Hobday TJ, O'Dorisio TM, Shah MH, Cadiot G, Luppi G, Posey JA, Wiedenmann B (2010) Daily oral everolimus activity in patients with metastatic pancreatic neuroendocrine tumors after failure of cytotoxic chemotherapy: a phase II trial. J Clin Oncol 28(1):69–76
95. Chan JA, Ryan DP, Zhu AX, Abrams TA, Wolpin BM, Malinowski P, Regan EM, Fuchs CS, Kulke MH (2012) Phase I study of pasireotide (SOM 230) and everolimus (RAD001) in advanced neuroendocrine tumors. Endocr Relat Cancer 19(5):615–623
96. Bajetta E, Catena L, Fazio N, Pusceddu S, Biondani P, Blanco G, Ricci S, Aieta M, Pucci F, Valente M, Bianco N, Mauri CM, Spada F (2014) Everolimus in combination with octreotide long-acting repeatable in a first-line setting for patients with neuroendocrine tumors: an ITMO group study. Cancer 120(16):2457–2463
97. Koumarianou A, Pectasides D, Koliou GA, Dionysopoulos D, Kolomodi D, Poulios C, Skondra M, Sgouros J, Pentheroudakis G, Kaltsas G, Fountzilas G (2020) Efficacy and safety of first-line everolimus therapy alone or in combination with octreotide in gastroenteropancreatic neuroendocrine tumors. A Hellenic Cooperative Oncology Group (HeCOG) Study. Biology (Basel) 9(3):51

98. Kulke MH, Ruszniewski P, Van Cutsem E, Lombard-Bohas C, Valle JW, De Herder WW, Pavel M, Degtyarev E, Brase JC, Bubuteishvili-Pacaud L, Voi M, Salazar R, Borbath I, Fazio N, Smith D, Capdevila J, Riechelmann RP, Yao JC (2017) A randomized, open-label, phase 2 study of everolimus in combination with pasireotide LAR or everolimus alone in advanced, well-differentiated, progressive pancreatic neuroendocrine tumors: COOPERATE-2 trial. Ann Oncol 28(6):1309–1315
99. Faivre S, Delbaldo C, Vera K, Robert C, Lozahic S, Lassau N, Bello C, Deprimo S, Brega N, Massimini G, Armand JP, Scigalla P, Raymond E (2006) Safety, pharmacokinetic, and antitumor activity of SU11248, a novel oral multitarget tyrosine kinase inhibitor, in patients with cancer. J Clin Oncol 24(1):25–35
100. Paez-Ribes M, Allen E, Hudock J, Takeda T, Okuyama H, Vinals F, Inoue M, Bergers G, Hanahan D, Casanovas O (2009) Antiangiogenic therapy elicits malignant progression of tumors to increased local invasion and distant metastasis. Cancer Cell 15(3):220–231
101. Bergers G, Song S, Meyer-Morse N, Bergsland E, Hanahan D (2003) Benefits of targeting both pericytes and endothelial cells in the tumor vasculature with kinase inhibitors. J Clin Invest 111(9):1287–1295
102. Kulke MH, Lenz HJ, Meropol NJ, Posey J, Ryan DP, Picus J, Bergsland E, Stuart K, Tye L, Huang X, Li JZ, Baum CM, Fuchs CS (2008) Activity of sunitinib in patients with advanced neuroendocrine tumors. J Clin Oncol 26(20):3403–3410
103. Kollmannsberger C, Bjarnason G, Burnett P, Creel P, Davis M, Dawson N, Feldman D, George S, Hershman J, Lechner T, Potter A, Raymond E, Treister N, Wood L, Wu S, Bukowski R (2011) Sunitinib in metastatic renal cell carcinoma: recommendations for management of noncardiovascular toxicities. Oncologist 16(5):543–553
104. Vaklavas C, Lenihan D, Kurzrock R, Tsimberidou AM (2010) Anti-vascular endothelial growth factor therapies and cardiovascular toxicity: what are the important clinical markers to target? Oncologist 15(2):130–141
105. Ito T, Tori M, Hashigaki S, Kimura N, Sato K, Ohki E, Sawaki A, Okusaka T (2019) Efficacy and safety of sunitinib in Japanese patients with progressive, advanced/metastatic, well-differentiated, unresectable pancreatic neuroendocrine tumors: final analyses from a Phase II study. Jpn J Clin Oncol 49(4):354–360
106. Fazio N, Kulke M, Rosbrook B, Fernandez K, Raymond E (2021) Updated efficacy and safety outcomes for patients with well-differentiated pancreatic neuroendocrine tumors treated with sunitinib. Target Oncol 16(1):27–35
107. Beuselinck B, Lambrechts D, Van Brussel T, Wolter P, Cardinaels N, Joniau S, Lerut E, Karadimou A, Couchy G, Sebe P, Ravaud A, Zerbib M, Caty A, Paridaens R, Schoffski P, Verkarre V, Berger J, Patard JJ, Zucman-Rossi J, Oudard S (2014) Efflux pump ABCB1 single nucleotide polymorphisms and dose reductions in patients with metastatic renal cell carcinoma treated with sunitinib. Acta Oncol 53(10):1413–1422
108. Fazio N, Martini JF, Croitoru AE, Schenker M, Li S, Rosbrook B, Fernandez K, Tomasek J, Thiis-Evensen E, Kulke M, Raymond E (2019) Pharmacogenomic analyses of sunitinib in patients with pancreatic neuroendocrine tumors. Future Oncol 15(17):1997–2007
109. Jimenez-Fonseca P, Martin MN, Carmona-Bayonas A, Calvo A, Fernandez-Mateos J, Redrado M, Capdevila J, Lago NM, Lacasta A, Munarriz J, Segura A, Fuster J, Baron F, Llanos M, Serrano R, Castillo A, Cruz Hernandez JJ, Grande E (2018) Biomarkers and polymorphisms in pancreatic neuroendocrine tumors treated with sunitinib. Oncotarget 9(97):36894–36905
110. Daskalakis K, Tsoli M, Angelousi A, Kassi E, Alexandraki KI, Kolomodi D, Kaltsas G, Koumarianou A (2019) Anti-tumour activity of everolimus and sunitinib in neuroendocrine neoplasms. Endocr Connect 8(6):641–653
111. Panzuto F, Rinzivillo M, Spada F, Antonuzzo L, Ibrahim T, Campana D, Fazio N, Delle Fave G (2017) Everolimus in pancreatic neuroendocrine carcinomas G3. Pancreas 46(3):302–305
112. Garcia-Carbonero R, Sorbye H, Baudin E, Raymond E, Wiedenmann B, Niederle B, Sedlackova E, Toumpanakis C, Anlauf M, Cwikla JB, Caplin M, O'Toole D, Perren A, Vienna Consensus Conference participants (2016) ENETS consensus guidelines for high-

grade gastroenteropancreatic neuroendocrine tumors and neuroendocrine carcinomas. Neuroendocrinology 103(2):186–194
113. Fazio N, Cella CA, Del Re M, Laffi A, Rubino M, Zagami P, Spada F (2019) Pharmacodynamics, clinical findings and approval status of current and emerging tyrosine-kinase inhibitors for pancreatic neuroendocrine tumors. Expert Opin Drug Metab Toxicol 15(12):993–1004
114. Jonasch E, Donskov F, Iliopoulos O, Rathmell WK, Narayan VK, Maughan BL, Oudard S, Else T, Maranchie JK, Welsh SJ, Thamake S, Park EK, Perini RF, Linehan WM, Srinivasan R, Investigators MK (2021) Belzutifan for renal cell carcinoma in von Hippel-Lindau disease. N Engl J Med 385(22):2036–2046
115. Deeks ED (2021) Belzutifan: first approval. Drugs 81(16):1921–1927
116. Koumarianou A, Kaltsas G (2021) Surufatinib—a novel oral agent for neuroendocrine tumours. Nat Rev Endocrinol 17(1):9–10
117. Capdevila J, Fazio N, Lopez C, Teule A, Valle JW, Tafuto S, Custodio A, Reed N, Raderer M, Grande E, Garcia-Carbonero R, Jimenez-Fonseca P, Hernando J, Bongiovanni A, Spada F, Alonso V, Antonuzzo L, Spallanzani A, Berruti A, La Casta A, Sevilla I, Kump P, Giuffrida D, Merino X, Trejo L, Gajate P, Matos I, Lamarca A, Ibrahim T (2021) Lenvatinib in patients with advanced grade 1/2 pancreatic and gastrointestinal neuroendocrine tumors: results of the phase II TALENT trial (GETNE1509). J Clin Oncol 39(20):2304–2312
118. Garcia-Carbonero R, Rinke A, Valle JW, Fazio N, Caplin M, Gorbounova V, Connor JO, Eriksson B, Sorbye H, Kulke M, Chen J, Falkerby J, Costa F, de Herder W, Lombard-Bohas C, Pavel M, Antibes Consensus Conference participants (2017) ENETS consensus guidelines for the standards of care in neuroendocrine neoplasms. Systemic therapy 2: chemotherapy. Neuroendocrinology 105(3):281–294
119. Moertel CG, Hanley JA, Johnson LA (1980) Streptozocin alone compared with streptozocin plus fluorouracil in the treatment of advanced islet-cell carcinoma. N Engl J Med 303(21):1189–1194
120. Capdevila J, Ducreux M, Garcia Carbonero R, Grande E, Halfdanarson T, Pavel M, Tafuto S, Welin S, Valenti V, Salazar R (2022) Streptozotocin. 1982-2022: forty years from the FDA's approval to treat pancreatic neuroendocrine tumors. Neuroendocrinology 112:1155
121. Moertel CG, Engstrom P, Lavin PT, Gelber RD, Carbone PP (1979) Chemotherapy of gastric and pancreatic carcinoma: a controlled evaluation of combinations of 5-fluorouracil with nitrosoureas and "lactones". Surgery 85(5):509–513
122. Moertel CG, Lefkopoulo M, Lipsitz S, Hahn RG, Klaassen D (1992) Streptozocin-doxorubicin, streptozocin-fluorouracil or chlorozotocin in the treatment of advanced islet-cell carcinoma. N Engl J Med 326(8):519–523
123. Delaunoit T, Ducreux M, Boige V, Dromain C, Sabourin JC, Duvillard P, Schlumberger M, de Baere T, Rougier P, Ruffie P, Elias D, Lasser P, Baudin E (2004) The doxorubicin-streptozotocin combination for the treatment of advanced well-differentiated pancreatic endocrine carcinoma; a judicious option? Eur J Cancer 40(4):515–520
124. Walter T, Bruneton D, Cassier PA, Hervieu V, Pilleul F, Scoazec JY, Chayvialle JA, Lombard-Bohas C (2010) Evaluation of the combination 5-fluorouracil, dacarbazine, and epirubicin in patients with advanced well-differentiated neuroendocrine tumors. Clin Colorectal Cancer 9(4):248–254
125. Sun W, Lipsitz S, Catalano P, Mailliard JA, Haller DG (2005) Phase II/III study of doxorubicin with fluorouracil compared with streptozocin with fluorouracil or dacarbazine in the treatment of advanced carcinoid tumors: Eastern Cooperative Oncology Group Study E1281. J Clin Oncol 23(22):4897–4904
126. Modlin IM, Latich I, Kidd M, Zikusoka M, Eick G (2006) Therapeutic options for gastrointestinal carcinoids. Clin Gastroenterol Hepatol 4(5):526–547
127. Moertel CG, Kvols LK, O'Connell MJ, Rubin J (1991) Treatment of neuroendocrine carcinomas with combined etoposide and cisplatin. Evidence of major therapeutic activity in the anaplastic variants of these neoplasms. Cancer 68(2):227–232

128. Iwasa S, Morizane C, Okusaka T, Ueno H, Ikeda M, Kondo S, Tanaka T, Nakachi K, Mitsunaga S, Kojima Y, Hagihara A, Hiraoka N (2010) Cisplatin and etoposide as first-line chemotherapy for poorly differentiated neuroendocrine carcinoma of the hepatobiliary tract and pancreas. Jpn J Clin Oncol 40(4):313–318
129. Frizziero M, Spada F, Lamarca A, Kordatou Z, Barriuso J, Nuttall C, McNamara MG, Hubner RA, Mansoor W, Manoharan P, Fazio N, Valle JW (2019) Carboplatin in combination with oral or intravenous etoposide for extra-pulmonary, poorly-differentiated neuroendocrine carcinomas. Neuroendocrinology 109(2):100–112
130. Sorbye H, Welin S, Langer SW, Vestermark LW, Holt N, Osterlund P, Dueland S, Hofsli E, Guren MG, Ohrling K, Birkemeyer E, Thiis-Evensen E, Biagini M, Gronbaek H, Soveri LM, Olsen IH, Federspiel B, Assmus J, Janson ET, Knigge U (2013) Predictive and prognostic factors for treatment and survival in 305 patients with advanced gastrointestinal neuroendocrine carcinoma (WHO G3): the NORDIC NEC study. Ann Oncol 24(1):152–160
131. Koumarianou A, Chatzellis E, Boutzios G, Tsavaris N, Kaltsas G (2013) Current concepts in the diagnosis and management of poorly differentiated gastrointestinal neuroendocrine carcinomas. Endokrynol Pol 64(1):60–72
132. Koumarianou A, Kaltsas G, Kulke MH, Oberg K, Strosberg JR, Spada F, Galdy S, Barberis M, Fumagalli C, Berruti A, Fazio N (2015) Temozolomide in advanced neuroendocrine neoplasms: pharmacological and clinical aspects. Neuroendocrinology 101(4):274–288
133. Welin S, Sorbye H, Sebjornsen S, Knappskog S, Busch C, Oberg K (2011) Clinical effect of temozolomide-based chemotherapy in poorly differentiated endocrine carcinoma after progression on first-line chemotherapy. Cancer 117(20):4617–4622
134. Chatzellis E, Angelousi A, Daskalakis K, Tsoli M, Alexandraki KI, Wachuła E, Meirovitz A, Maimon O, Grozinsky-Glasberg S, Gross D, Kos-Kudła B, Koumarianou A, Kaltsas G (2019) Activity and safety of standard and prolonged capecitabine/temozolomide administration in patients with advanced neuroendocrine neoplasms. Neuroendocrinology 109(4):333–345
135. Li J, Lu M, Lu Z, Li Z, Liu Y, Yang L, Li J, Zhang X, Zhou J, Wang X, Gong J, Gao J, Li Y, Shen L (2017) Irinotecan plus cisplatin followed by octreotide long-acting release maintenance treatment in advanced gastroenteropancreatic neuroendocrine carcinoma: IPO-NEC study. Oncotarget 8(15):25669–25678
136. Koumarianou A, Antoniou S, Kanakis G, Economopoulos N, Rontogianni D, Ntavatzikos A, Tsavaris N, Pectasides D, Dimitriadis G, Kaltsas G (2012) Combination treatment with metronomic temozolomide, bevacizumab and long-acting octreotide for malignant neuroendocrine tumours. Endocr Relat Cancer 19(1):L1–L4
137. Chan JA, Blaszkowsky L, Stuart K, Zhu AX, Allen J, Wadlow R, Ryan DP, Meyerhardt J, Gonzalez M, Regan E, Zheng H, Kulke MH (2013) A prospective, phase 1/2 study of everolimus and temozolomide in patients with advanced pancreatic neuroendocrine tumor. Cancer 119:3212
138. Kole C, Charalampakis N, Vailas M, Tolia M, Sotiropoulou M, Tsakatikas S, Kouris NI, Tsoli M, Koumarianou A, Karamouzis MV, Schizas D (2022) Immunotherapy for gastroenteropancreatic neuroendocrine neoplasms (GEP-NENs): a 2021 update. Cancer Immunol Immunother 71(4):761–768
139. Strosberg J, Mizuno N, Doi T, Grande E, Delord JP, Shapira-Frommer R, Bergsland E, Shah M, Fakih M, Takahashi S, Piha-Paul SA, O'Neil B, Thomas S, Lolkema MP, Chen M, Ibrahim N, Norwood K, Hadoux J (2020) Efficacy and safety of pembrolizumab in previously treated advanced neuroendocrine tumors: results from the phase II KEYNOTE-158 study. Clin Cancer Res 26(9):2124–2130
140. Yao JC, Strosberg J, Fazio N, Pavel ME, Bergsland E, Ruszniewski P, Halperin DM, Li D, Tafuto S, Raj N, Campana D, Hijioka S, Raderer M, Guimbaud R, Gajate P, Pusceddu S, Reising A, Degtyarev E, Shilkrut M, Eddy S, Singh S (2021) Spartalizumab in metastatic, well/poorly-differentiated neuroendocrine neoplasms. Endocr Relat Cancer:ERC-20-0382
141. Klein O, Kee D, Markman B, Michael M, Underhill C, Carlino MS, Jackett L, Lum C, Scott C, Nagrial A, Behren A, So JY, Palmer J, Cebon J (2020) Immunotherapy of ipilimumab

and nivolumab in patients with advanced neuroendocrine tumors: a subgroup analysis of the CA209-538 clinical trial for rare cancers. Clin Cancer Res 26(17):4454–4459
142. Luchini C, Bibeau F, Ligtenberg MJL, Singh N, Nottegar A, Bosse T, Miller R, Riaz N, Douillard JY, Andre F, Scarpa A (2019) ESMO recommendations on microsatellite instability testing for immunotherapy in cancer, and its relationship with PD-1/PD-L1 expression and tumour mutational burden: a systematic review-based approach. Ann Oncol 30(8):1232–1243
143. Kwekkeboom DJ, de Herder WW, Krenning EP (2011) Somatostatin receptor-targeted radionuclide therapy in patients with gastroenteropancreatic neuroendocrine tumors. Endocrinol Metab Clin N Am 40(1):173–185. ix
144. Zaknun JJ, Bodei L, Mueller-Brand J, Pavel ME, Baum RP, Horsch D, O'Dorisio MS, O'Dorisiol TM, Howe JR, Cremonesi M, Kwekkeboom DJ (2013) The joint IAEA, EANM, and SNMMI practical guidance on peptide receptor radionuclide therapy (PRRNT) in neuroendocrine tumours. Eur J Nucl Med Mol Imaging 40(5):800–816
145. Strosberg J, El-Haddad G, Wolin E, Hendifar A, Yao J, Chasen B, Mittra E, Kunz PL, Kulke MH, Jacene H, Bushnell D, O'Dorisio TM, Baum RP, Kulkarni HR, Caplin M, Lebtahi R, Hobday T, Delpassand E, Van Cutsem E, Benson A, Srirajaskanthan R, Pavel M, Mora J, Berlin J, Grande E, Reed N, Seregni E, Oberg K, Lopera Sierra M, Santoro P, Thevenet T, Erion JL, Ruszniewski P, Kwekkeboom D, Krenning E, NETTER-1 Trial Investigators (2017) Phase 3 trial of (177)Lu-Dotatate for midgut neuroendocrine tumors. N Engl J Med 376(2):125–135
146. Strosberg J, Wolin E, Chasen B, Kulke M, Bushnell D, Caplin M, Baum RP, Kunz P, Hobday T, Hendifar A, Oberg K, Sierra ML, Thevenet T, Margalet I, Ruszniewski P, Krenning E, NETTER-1 Study Group (2018) Health-related quality of life in patients with progressive midgut neuroendocrine tumors treated with (177)Lu-Dotatate in the phase III NETTER-1 trial. J Clin Oncol 36(25):2578–2584
147. Severi S, Nanni O, Bodei L, Sansovini M, Ianniello A, Nicoletti S, Scarpi E, Matteucci F, Gilardi L, Paganelli G (2013) Role of 18FDG PET/CT in patients treated with 177Lu-DOTATATE for advanced differentiated neuroendocrine tumours. Eur J Nucl Med Mol Imaging 40(6):881–888
148. Brabander T, van der Zwan WA, Teunissen JJM, Kam BLR, Feelders RA, de Herder WW, van Eijck CHJ, Franssen GJH, Krenning EP, Kwekkeboom DJ (2017) Long-term efficacy, survival, and safety of [(177)Lu-DOTA(0),Tyr(3)]octreotate in patients with gastroenteropancreatic and bronchial neuroendocrine tumors. Clin Cancer Res 23(16):4617–4624
149. Garske-Roman U, Sandstrom M, Fross Baron K, Lundin L, Hellman P, Welin S, Johansson S, Khan T, Lundqvist H, Eriksson B, Sundin A, Granberg D (2018) Prospective observational study of (177)Lu-DOTA-octreotate therapy in 200 patients with advanced metastasized neuroendocrine tumours (NETs): feasibility and impact of a dosimetry-guided study protocol on outcome and toxicity. Eur J Nucl Med Mol Imaging 45(6):970–988
150. Ramage J, Naraev BG, Halfdanarson TR (2018) Peptide receptor radionuclide therapy for patients with advanced pancreatic neuroendocrine tumors. Semin Oncol 45(4):236–248
151. Frilling A, Li J, Malamutmann E, Schmid KW, Bockisch A, Broelsch CE (2009) Treatment of liver metastases from neuroendocrine tumours in relation to the extent of hepatic disease. Br J Surg 96(2):175–184
152. Mazzaglia PJ, Berber E, Milas M, Siperstein AE (2007) Laparoscopic radiofrequency ablation of neuroendocrine liver metastases: a 10-year experience evaluating predictors of survival. Surgery 142(1):10–19
153. Oberg K, Knigge U, Kwekkeboom D, Perren A (2012) Neuroendocrine gastro-entero-pancreatic tumors: ESMO Clinical Practice Guidelines for diagnosis, treatment and follow-up. Ann Oncol 23 Suppl 7:vii124-130
154. Lee E, Leon Pachter H, Sarpel U (2012) Hepatic arterial embolization for the treatment of metastatic neuroendocrine tumors. Int J Hepatol 2012:471203

155. Maire F, Lombard-Bohas C, O'Toole D, Vullierme MP, Rebours V, Couvelard A, Pelletier AL, Zappa M, Pilleul F, Hentic O, Hammel P, Ruszniewski P (2012) Hepatic arterial embolization versus chemoembolization in the treatment of liver metastases from well-differentiated midgut endocrine tumors: a prospective randomized study. Neuroendocrinology 96(4):294–300
156. Kennedy AS, McNeillie P, Dezarn WA, Nutting C, Sangro B, Wertman D, Garafalo M, Liu D, Coldwell D, Savin M, Jakobs T, Rose S, Warner R, Carter D, Sapareto S, Nag S, Gulec S, Calkins A, Gates VL, Salem R (2009) Treatment parameters and outcome in 680 treatments of internal radiation with resin 90Y-microspheres for unresectable hepatic tumors. Int J Radiat Oncol Biol Phys 74(5):1494–1500
157. Arnold R, Chen YJ, Costa F, Falconi M, Gross D, Grossman AB, Hyrdel R, Kos-Kudla B, Salazar R, Plockinger U (2009) ENETS consensus guidelines for the standards of care in neuroendocrine tumors: follow-up and documentation. Neuroendocrinology 90(2):227–233
158. Nehar D, Lombard-Bohas C, Olivieri S, Claustrat B, Chayvialle JA, Penes MC, Sassolas G, Borson-Chazot F (2004) Interest of chromogranin A for diagnosis and follow-up of endocrine tumours. Clin Endocrinol 60(5):644–652

High-Grade Gastroenteropancreatic Neuroendocrine Neoplasms (WHO 3)

19

Halfdan Sorbye

19.1 Background

Extrapulmonary neuroendocrine carcinoma (EP-NEC) has been found in most organs, but the most common sites are the gastrointestinal tract, cervix uteri, urogenital tract, and breast [1]. No primary site can be identified in up to 30% of cases. NEN G3 have a much higher proliferation rate than well-differentiated neuroendocrine tumors (G1-G2), by definition the proliferation rate (Ki67) is above 20% [2]. In devising treatment strategies for EP-NEC, many authors refer to the extensive literature surrounding high-grade neuroendocrine carcinoma of the lung. Several series have however questioned the rationale for this and pointed out many differences between pulmonary small-cell carcinoma and extra-pulmonary small-cell neuroendocrine carcinoma (EP-SCNEC). EP-SCNEC has less smoking history, a much lower frequency of brain metastases, a better survival, and survival is site-specific that is gynaecologic and head and neck cancers have better outcomes than GI primaries [1, 3]. Furthermore, there are molecular differences. GEP NEC seems to have a lower rate of TP53 and alteration RB1 than small-cell lung cancer and other genes were more frequently altered [4]. Half of small-cell pancreatic NEC has a KRAS mutation, in contrast to small-cell lung cancer where KRAS mutations are rarely found [5, 6]. Small-cell lung cancer has further a 90% RB1 loss compared to 60% in pancreatic small-cell NEC. Studies reporting results from mainly pulmonary NEC, or EP-NEC studies with mixed primary will therefore not be included in this chapter.

Clinical data on GEP NEN have been sparse, and for the new subgroup of NET G3 even less data exist. There has been a lack of epidemiological, clinical, and treatment data and little has been known on possible prognostic and predictive factors. Most studies are hampered by a center bias, operability, and resulting availability of histological materials; therefore, all studies show a bias toward resected tumors.

H. Sorbye (✉)
Department of Oncology, Haukeland University Hospital, Bergen, Norway
e-mail: halfdan.sorbye@helse-bergen.no

S. Yalcin, K. Öberg (eds.), *Neuroendocrine Tumours*,
https://doi.org/10.1007/978-3-031-56968-5_19

Recently, however, several studies with novel treatment data on such patients have been published.

19.2 Epidemiology

Gastroenteropancreatic primary neoplasms account for 35% of all NEC outside the lung [1]. They can originate anywhere in the gastrointestinal (GI) tract but are mainly located in the esophagus, pancreas, and large bowel [1, 7, 8]. A primary tumor of uncertain origin will usually be considered GI if the metastatic load is dominating in liver and abdomen [7, 8]. Poorly differentiated neuroendocrine neoplasms account for about 20% of malignant digestive neuroendocrine neoplasms [9]. Data from the SEER database show that the median survival for GEP NEN G3 was 34 months with localized disease, 14–16 months with regional disease, and 5 months with distant disease [1, 10]. Five-year survival is 42% in localized disease, 26% in regional disease, and 5% with advanced disease, depending on primary tumor site and seems better for large-cell GEP NEN G3 [1, 11]. Survival of patients with GEP NET G3 is significantly better than of patients with GEP NEC [12–15]. Median survival for metastatic patients was 41 months for GEP NET G3 vs 17 months for non-small cell GEP NEC [13]. Other studies do unfortunately not separate according to stage, and present OS data combining all stages although the majorities are stage IV patients. In one study, survival for GEP NET G3 was 99 months vs 19 months for GEP NEC [14]. For pancreatic primaries, median OS was 42–75 months compared to pancreatic NEC with a median OS of 8.5–13 months [5, 16–18]. A recent proposal not included in the 2017 WHO classification was to separate the NEN G3 into three groups based on morphology and Ki67 [12]. In a high-grade GEP-NEN population of 136 patients, median survival was 43.6 months for NET G3, 24.5 months for NEC with a Ki67 21–55%, and only 5.3 months for NEC cases with a Ki67 ≥ 55%. In the EUROCARE study, 5-year survival rates for poorly differentiated NEC varied between 6% and 11% according to European region [9]. The number of patients with NEC seems to be increasing [7, 11, 19], probably due to better pathology work-up. In the SEER database, 5-year survival for localized disease (Stage II) depended on the primary site; for colorectal, stomach, and pancreas primaries 5-year survival is 46–55%, compared to 25–33% for anal and esophageal primaries [1]. Five-year survival for regional disease (Stage III) was 22–30% for colorectal, stomach, and pancreas primaries compared to 9–15% for anal and esophageal primaries.

19.3 Diagnosis

19.3.1 Histology

A gastroenteropancreatic NEC has been defined as a poorly differentiated, high-grade malign cancer composed of small cells or large to intermediate cells. The

European Neuroendocrine Tumor Society (ENETS) recommends that a pathology report on GEP NEN G3 should report morphology concerning both differentiation (well or poorly differentiated) and small-cell vs large-cell as well as proliferation rate as an absolute Ki67 value in hot spots [20]. These tumors may contain different tumor components, often a mixture of neuroendocrine and adenocarcinoma parts can be seen. Up to 40% of NEC contains elements of non-NEC, usually adenocarcinoma. If the neoplasm consists of a neuroendocrine component and a gland-forming component both exceeding 30%, the new 2017 WHO classification defines it as a mixed neuroendocrine-non-neuroendocrine neoplasm (MiNEN) [21–23]. No differences in clinical features, Ki67 level, or survival were seen between NEC and high-grade MiNEN [24]. The terms poorly differentiated high-grade neuroendocrine tumors and neuroendocrine carcinoma have been used synonymously. However, recently data show that among large-cell NEN G3 there are neoplasms that are well-differentiated neoplasm with much longer survival than in poorly differentiated NEC but less response to platinum-based chemotherapy [5, 13, 14, 16, 25]. These tumors are now defined as NET G3 and are mainly located in the pancreas [21]. In NEC, Ki67 is usually much higher than 20% as median Ki67 is 70–80% [8, 14]. Ki67 is usually lower in NET G3. For pancreatic primaries, median Ki67 has been reported in pancreatic NET G3 to be 29–47% (range 21–80%), compared to pancreatic NEC with a median Ki67 of 70–80% (range 21–100%) [5, 16, 26]. Unfortunately, the Ki-67 value alone cannot distinguish between NET G3 and NEC, as the Ki67 value overlaps among NET G3 and NEC especially in the area of 30–50% although a Ki67 > 60% is rare for NET G3 [8, 14, 16] (Fig. 19.1).

Poorly differentiated NEC less closely resembles non-neoplastic neuroendocrine cells, having a more diffuse or sheet-like architecture, irregular nuclei, and less cytoplasmic granularity. There are two distinct histologic entities: small-cell and large-cell NEC (Fig. 19.2). Small-cell carcinomas are composed of small- to medium-sized round to oval cells with scant cytoplasm and hyperchromatic nuclei with indistinct nucleoli. The large-cell subtype is composed of large cells with vesicular nuclei showing prominent nucleoli and abundant eosinophilic cytoplasm.

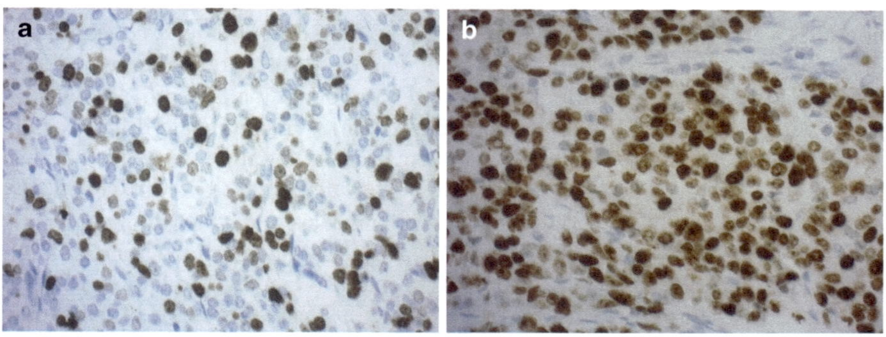

Fig. 19.1 (**a**) Well-differentiated pancreatic NET G3 with a Ki67 index of 30%. (**b**) Poorly differentiated colon NEC with a Ki67 index of 90%

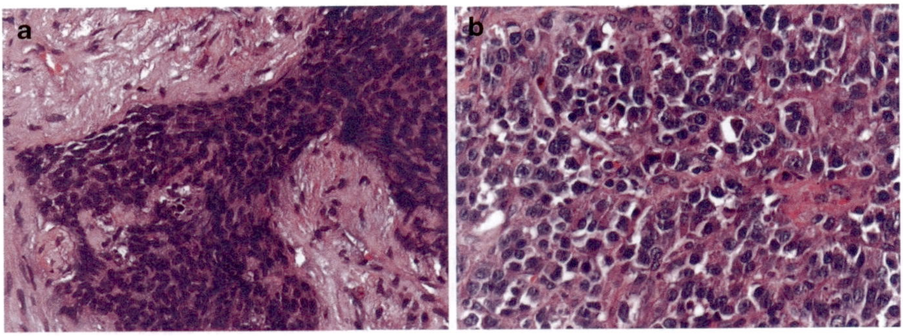

Fig. 19.2 (**a**) Small-cell NEC from pancreas (**b**) Large-cell NEC from colon

In both cases, the tumor cells grow in sheets often with large confluent areas of necrosis. Perineural and vascular invasions are frequently observed. In contrast, high-grade well-differentiated NET more closely resemble non-neoplastic neuroendocrine cells, with characteristic "organoid" arrangements of the tumor cells, with solid/nesting, trabecular, gyriform, or sometimes glandular patterns. The cells are relatively uniform, and they have round to oval nuclei, coarsely stippled chromatin, and finely granular cytoplasm. However, classification based on morphological differentiation alone is challenging in many cases [16]. Immunohistochemical staining may also be helpful for differentiating NEC from NET G3. For example, PanNET G3 show loss of DAXX and ATRX in roughly one-half of cases, similar to PanNET G1 and G2 tumors, whereas loss of RB1 or abnormality of TP53 expression supports a diagnosis of PanNEC G3 [5, 16, 25]. These results indicate that NET G3 seem to develop from an initial NET G1-G2 in contrast to NEC [17]. Large-cell NEC is morphologically distinguished from small-cell NEC by cytological features of a non-small-cell carcinoma, including large cell size, low nuclear to cytoplasm volume ratio, coarse chromatin, and frequent nucleoli. There is small-cell histological preponderance in the squamous GI tract (esophagus and anus) and large-cell carcinomas in the glandular parts [1]. Awareness of the latter is essential, as these tumors often are indistinguishable from poorly differentiated non-NET carcinomas. In a study on 87 high-grade GI tract tumors, no significant difference in survival was detected among small-cell, mixed, and large-cell subtypes, nor were there any differences between tumors of the upper GI tract versus the lower GI tract [27]. There are conflicting results on significant differences in survival, but response to chemotherapy seems similar based on these histological subtypes [1, 7, 11, 27, 28]. In pancreatic NEC, small-cell NEC was genetically similar to large-cell NEC, and these genetic changes were distinct from pancreatic NET [29]. No difference was seen in RB1 or KRAS mutations concerning small-cell vs large-cell pancreatic NEC [5]. NEC is characterized by immunohistochemical markers of neuroendocrine differentiation with synaptophysin, neuron-specific enolase, chromogranin A (CgA), and CD56 being the primary stains. Several pathologists advocate for routine staining with synaptophysin and CgA for all tumors initially classified as poorly differentiated gastrointestinal adenocarcinoma.

Usually synaptophysin immunohistochemistry staining is positive, whereas staining for CgA may be negative.

19.3.2 Diagnostic Procedures

FDG-PET is usually positive in NEC and could be of prognostic value [30]. FDG-PET may be especially indicated for patients with apparently localized disease, to locate possible metastatic disease and avoid unnecessary surgery. However, most NET G3 also seem to have a positive FDG-PET, in one study 9/12 (75%) NET G3 cases were positive compared to 56/64 (88%) GEP-NEC cases [14]. The relevance of tumor markers in NEN G3 is uncertain, although CgA was elevated in two-third of 188 patients with advanced GI-NEC disease [7]. The relevance of somatostatin receptor imaging (SRI) in NEN G3 patients is uncertain. GEP NET G3 usually have a high uptake on SRI; however, also NEC shows an uptake as recently shown in 20–40% of cases [8, 31, 32]. The benefit of peptide receptor radionuclide therapy (PRRT) in NEC patients with a high uptake on SRI is unknown. A recent retrospective study reported promising data on 29 GEP NEN G3 patients treated with PRRT [33]. SRI may therefore be considered if the patient has a NET G3 or a Ki67 < 55%, as PRRT may be a later treatment option. Routine measurement of U-5HIAA does not seem meaningful, as hormone-related symptoms are rare and U-5HIAA elevated in few patients [7]. Several baseline laboratory abnormalities seem to be correlated with poor survival in NEC; elevated levels of platelets, white blood cell count, lactate dehydrogenase (LDH), alkaline phosphatase, and C-reactive protein (CRP) [7, 8, 34]. It is increasingly recognized that variations in outcome are not solely determined by the characteristics of the tumor but also by host-response factors. Markers of a systemic host inflammatory response, for example elevated platelets and leucocytes, have a prognostic value in a variety of common solid tumors [35]. LDH may be a biomarker for hypoxia and highly angiogenetic tumors, and high LDH-5 is directly related to an upregulated HIF pathway and linked with an aggressive tumor phenotype [36].

19.4 Treatment

Treatment of this very aggressive disease remains a challenge for clinicians. NEN G3 are frequently characterized by a high proclivity for metastatic dissemination even in patients with clinically localized tumors. Extensive disease is almost invariably treated by systemic chemotherapy. In contrast, the treatment approach for limited disease, a potentially curable condition, is presently neither consistent nor uniform. Many patients with local or locoregional disease can be cured [1]. Therefore, chemotherapy combined with surgery or in some cases, radiation should be the initial consideration in such patients. Adjuvant or neoadjuvant chemotherapy is usually given with cisplatin/carboplatin and etoposide, based on the effect seen in metastatic setting.

19.4.1 Surgery

Treatment recommendations for patients with apparently localized disease are not based on prospective data, and supporting evidence from heterogeneous retrospective studies is limited. There is relative consensus that surgery alone is rarely curative and that patients with limited disease should receive multi-modality-based therapy. Surgery as part of the treatment can be curative in patients even with regional lymph node disease [18, 37–42]. Five-year survival depends on primary site but can be as high as 55% for localized disease (Stage II) and 30% for regional disease (Stage III) [1]. Surgery as part of the treatment should therefore be considered for all localized and regional GEP NEN patients with exceptions for esophageal primaries. Several small series confirm poor results after surgical treatment of esophageal NEC, especially for stage III disease where chemoradiation seems better [43, 44]. Some authors suggest that a sequence of neoadjuvant chemotherapy followed by definitive surgery seems appropriate. Potential advantages to a neoadjuvant approach include earlier treatment of micrometastatic disease, better compliance to treatment, determination of responsiveness to chemotherapy, and avoidance of unnecessary surgery for patients with early systemic disease progression. It has been suggested that NET G3 patients should receive the same approach to surgery of the primary and metastatic disease as patients with NET G2 [18, 45]. In contrast, debulking surgery and surgery for liver metastasis are not recommended for NEC patients [46–49]. A recent retrospective study however indicates that very selected NEC patients may benefit from metastatic liver surgery [50].

19.4.2 Postoperative Adjuvant Chemotherapy

Although there are no studies examining postoperative adjuvant chemotherapy in NEC, their aggressive behavior warrants consideration of adjuvant therapy in most cases. The North American Neuroendocrine Tumor Society (NANETS) and ENETS both recommend 4–6 cycles of cisplatin or carboplatin and etoposide as adjuvant therapy for resected patients [48, 51]. As rapid recurrence often occurs after surgery, postoperative radiological staging with FDG-PET should be performed before initiation of adjuvant chemotherapy. A new and unanswered question is whether NET G3 patients should receive adjuvant chemotherapy or should be treated as NET G2 patients without any adjuvant therapy as recommended in a recent review [45].

19.4.3 Palliative Chemotherapy

Advanced GEP-NEC is an aggressive disease where rapid referral to an oncologist is necessary, some advocate referral within a week. Patients should be referred for possible treatment before the performance status (PS) deteriorates to the extent that the patient is no longer fit to receive chemotherapy. Median survival in 53 patients not given chemotherapy was only 1 month after diagnosis of advanced disease [7].

Patients not receiving palliative chemotherapy were older, had a worse PS, and less positive SRI, less intense CgA staining, and more often elevated white blood cell count and CRP. The very short median survival for patients not receiving chemotherapy indicates that the benefit from palliative chemotherapy is probably substantial.

19.4.3.1 First-Line Chemotherapy

Guidelines for advanced GEP NEN G3 advocate the use of platinum-based chemotherapy combined with etoposide as first-line treatment [48, 51, 52]. Three recent large retrospective studies show quite similar results on first-line treatment with cisplatin/carboplatin and etoposide (Fig. 19.3). They show a response rate of 30–50%, median progression free survival (PFS) of 4–6 months, and a median OS of 11–16 months [7, 8, 14]. In all studies as many as one-third of patients have an immediate disease progression at first evaluation, indicating no benefit at all of platinum-based therapy. Although treatment with cisplatin/etoposide often induces initial tumor reduction, progressive disease usually occurs rapidly in most cases (Fig. 19.4). Poor performance status, high tumor burden, liver metastases, high proliferation rate, and elevated lactate dehydrogenase are usually baseline negative prognostic factors for survival in metastatic patients [7, 8, 12, 34, 53]. RB1 loss may predict response to platinum-based chemotherapy in pancreatic NEC patients [5]. In the Nordic NEC study, no differences in outcomes were seen comparing patients treated with cisplatin-based versus carboplatin-based treatment, which has led to more frequent use of carboplatin due to its better tolerability for the patients [7]. In the Nordic study, cases with Ki67 < 55% had a significantly longer survival; however, no data separation between NEC and NET G3 has yet been published. Several studies have shown that a Ki67 proliferation rate in the lower range (<60%) may predict less benefit from chemotherapy with platinum-etoposide, although further validation is necessary [7, 31, 54, 55]. In 258 patients with poorly differentiated

	Chemo	No	Diff	RR%	PD %	PFS	mOS
Sorbye et al Cancer 2013[7]	Cisplatin or carboplatin + etoposide	252	?	31	36	4 m	11 m
Yamaguchi et al Cancer Sci 2014[53]	Cisplatin + irinotecan or etoposide	258	Poor?	50/27		5.2 m	11.5 m
Heetfeld et al Endo Rel Cancer 2015[14]	Platinum/ etoposide	113	Poor	35	27	5 m	16.4 m Stage mix
Walter et al Eur J Can 2017[8]	Platinum/ etoposide	152	Poor	50	27	6.2 m	11.6 m

Fig. 19.3 Recent large retrospective first-line chemotherapy studies in metastatic high-grade gastroenteropancreatic neuroendocrine neoplasms (G3). *Diff* differentiation, *RR* response rate, *PD* progressive disease as best response, *PFS* progression-free survival, *mOS* median survival

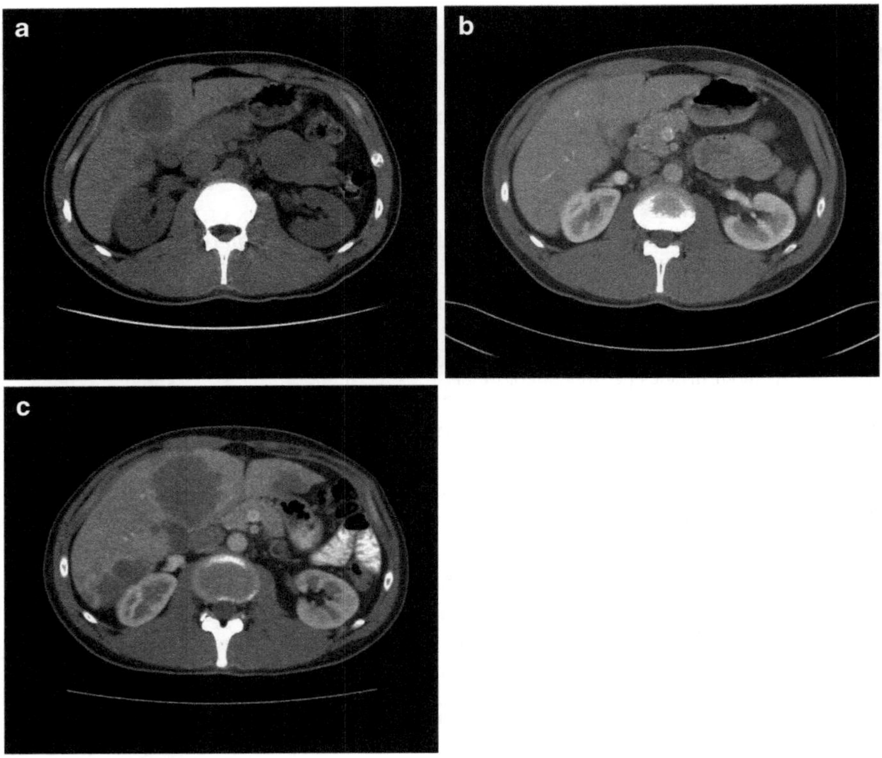

Fig. 19.4 (**a**–**c**) Baseline (**a**) and partial response after 6 months of cisplatin/etoposide treatment (**b**), but massive progression of disease after a 2-month treatment break (**c**) in a 39-year-old patient with primary rectal NEC

GEP NEC, response rate and survival were numerically better for irinotecan/etoposide compared to cisplatin/etoposide, but the treatment regimen was not an independent predictive factor for survival [53]. Recent studies have shown that temozolomide-based schedules and FOLFOX are the most promising first line chemotherapy schedules for metastatic NET G3.

Most chemotherapy studies are a mixture of NET G3 and NEC, and specific data on the NET G3 subgroup are scarce and based on a very small number of patients. The optimal first-line palliative treatment for patients with metastatic NET G3 is therefore unclear [45]. Several recent retrospective studies suggest relatively low response rates to platinum/etoposide regimens in patients with a NET G3 [5, 13, 14]. It has been suggested that NET G3 may benefit from medical treatments used in NET G2, and temozolomide/capecitabine is frequently used but larger prospective data are lacking [14].

19.4.3.2 Second-Line Chemotherapy

After first-line treatment, no further standard therapy has been established in GI-NEC. Re-introduction of cisplatin/carboplatin and etoposide after a treatment break resulted in a response rate of 15% and another 27% achieved SD [7]. These data indicate that retreatment with cisplatin/carboplatin and etoposide is a valid option, as 42% had a re-stabilization of the disease.

Not much has been known about the possible benefit from second-line treatment; however, recently several small retrospective studies have been published suggesting that GEP NEC patients can benefit from further lines of chemotherapy after failure of platinum/etoposide treatment. Temozolomide-based chemotherapy resulted in a 33% response rate and a PFS of 6 months, and most benefits seem to be for patients with a Ki67 < 60% [31]. Irinotecan- and oxaliplatin-based chemotherapy may benefit as second-line treatments with response rates of 16–31% and PFS of 2.3–6.2 months [32, 55]. A recent retrospective study with FOLFIRI or FOLFOX resulted however in a very short median PFS (<3 months) and OS (<6 months) [8].

For NET G3 little data are available. Everolimus was given to 15 patients with pancreatic NET G3 with Ki67 ≤ 55% (median 30%), mainly after first-line treatment [56]. Results were promising with median PFS 6 months and OS 28 months after everolimus initiation and 40% had disease stabilization for at least 12 months. If a NET G3 shifts into a more aggressive course, many will try platinum-based chemotherapy; however frequently without great success. Depending on first line treatment, temozolomide-based schedules and FOLFOX are used as second-line treatments for metastatic NET G3.

19.4.4 Other Treatments

Somatostatin analogs have an anti-proliferative effect in NET G1-2 where Ki-67 is typically 2–10%. There are no data supporting the use of somatostatin analogs in NEC. PRRT is regularly used for G1-G2 NET tumors with a high uptake of SRI. The benefit of PRRT in patients with a higher proliferation rate is unknown. A recent retrospective study reported data on 29 GEP NEN G3 patients treated with PRRT where the majority had failed prior chemotherapy [33]. Primary tumor was located in the pancreas in 17/28 cases and 22 cases had a Ki67 < 55%. The results were promising with PFS of 9 months and OS of 21 months. The median PFS and OS for patients with Ki67 ≤ 55% was 12 and 41 months, compared to 4 and 7 months if Ki67 was >55%. As most of these patients in this study had a Ki67 < 55% and a primary tumor in the pancreas, many of these cases might have been NET G3. Palliative external beam radiation may be useful, especially for painful bone metastasis.

Immunotherapy studies have shown limited benefit in NEN G3.

References

1. Dasari A, Mehta K, Byers LA, Sorbye H, Yao JC (2017) Comparative study of lung and extra-pulmonary poorly differentiated neuroendocrine carcinomas: a SEER database analysis of 162,983 cases. Cancer 124:807. https://doi.org/10.1002/cncr.31124. (Epub ahead of print)
2. Bosman FTCF, Hruban RH, Theise ND (2010) WHO classification of tumours of the digestive system, 4th edn. IARC Press, Lyon
3. Brennan SM, Gregory DL, Stillie A, Herschtal A, Mac Manus M, Ball DL (2010) Should extra-pulmonary small cell cancer be managed like small cell lung cancer? Cancer 116(4):888–895
4. Bergsland EK, Roy R, Stephens P, Ross JS, Bailey M, Olshen A (2016) Genomic profiling to distinguish poorly differentiated neuroendocrine carcinomas: a new clinicopathologic entity. ASCO Meeting Abstr 34:4020
5. Hijioka S, Hosoda W, Matsuo K, Ueno M, Furukawa M, Yoshitomi H et al (2017) Rb loss and *KRAS* mutation are predictors of the response to platinum-based chemotherapy in pancreatic neuroendocrine neoplasm with grade 3: a Japanese Multicenter Pancreatic NEN-G3 Study. Clin Cancer Res 23(16):4625–4632
6. George J, Lim JS, Jang SJ, Cun Y, Ozretic L, Kong G et al (2015) Comprehensive genomic profiles of small cell lung cancer. Nature 524(7563):47–53
7. Sorbye H, Welin S, Langer SW, Vestermark LW, Holt N, Osterlund P et al (2013) Predictive and prognostic factors for treatment and survival in 305 patients with advanced gastrointestinal neuroendocrine carcinoma (WHO G3): the NORDIC NEC study. ESMO 24(1):152–160
8. Walter T, Tougeron D, Baudin E, Le Malicot K, Lecomte T, Malka D et al (2017) Poorly differentiated gastro-entero-pancreatic neuroendocrine carcinomas: are they really heterogeneous? Insights from the FFCD-GTE national cohort. Eur J Cancer 79:158–165
9. Lepage C, Ciccolallo L, De Angelis R, Bouvier AM, Faivre J, Gatta G et al (2010) European disparities in malignant digestive endocrine tumours survival. Int J Cancer 126(12):2928–2934
10. Sorbye H, Strosberg J, Baudin E, Klimstra DS, Yao JC (2014) Gastroenteropancreatic high-grade neuroendocrine carcinoma. Cancer 120(18):2814–2823
11. Korse CM, Taal BG, van Velthuysen ML, Visser O (2013) Incidence and survival of neuroendocrine tumours in The Netherlands according to histological grade: experience of two decades of cancer registry. Eur J Cancer 49(8):1975–1983
12. Milione M, Maisonneuve P, Spada F, Pellegrinelli A, Spaggiari P, Albarello L et al (2017) The clinicopathologic heterogeneity of grade 3 gastroenteropancreatic neuroendocrine neoplasms: morphological differentiation and proliferation identify different prognostic categories. Neuroendocrinology 104(1):85–93
13. Velayoudom-Cephise FL, Duvillard P, Foucan L, Hadoux J, Chougnet CN, Leboulleux S et al (2013) Are G3 ENETS neuroendocrine neoplasms heterogeneous? Endocr Relat Cancer 20(5):649–657
14. Heetfeld M, Chougnet CN, Olsen IH, Rinke A, Borbath I, Crespo G et al (2015) Characteristics and treatment of patients with G3 gastroenteropancreatic neuroendocrine neoplasms. Endocr Relat Cancer 22(4):657–664
15. Basturk O, Yang Z, Tang LH, Hruban RH, Adsay V, McCall CM et al (2015) The high-grade (WHO G3) pancreatic neuroendocrine tumor category is morphologically and biologically heterogenous and includes both well differentiated and poorly differentiated neoplasms. Am J Surg Pathol 39(5):683–690
16. Tang LH, Basturk O, Sue JJ, Klimstra DS (2016) A practical approach to the classification of WHO Grade 3 (G3) Well-differentiated Neuroendocrine Tumor (WD-NET) and Poorly Differentiated Neuroendocrine Carcinoma (PD-NEC) of the Pancreas. Am J Surg Pathol 40(9):1192–1202
17. Tang LH, Untch BR, Reidy DL, O'Reilly E, Dhall D, Jih L et al (2016) Well-differentiated neuroendocrine tumors with a morphologically apparent high-grade component: a pathway distinct from poorly differentiated neuroendocrine carcinomas. Clin Cancer Res 22(4):1011–1017

18. Crippa S, Partelli S, Bassi C, Berardi R, Capelli P, Scarpa A et al (2016) Long-term outcomes and prognostic factors in neuroendocrine carcinomas of the pancreas: morphology matters. Surgery 159(3):862–871
19. Dasari A, Shen C, Halperin D, Zhao B, Zhou S, Xu Y et al (2017) Trends in the incidence, prevalence, and survival outcomes in patients with neuroendocrine tumors in the United States. JAMA Oncol 3(10):1335–1342
20. Perren A, Couvelard A, Scoazec JY, Costa F, Borbath I, Delle Fave G et al (2017) ENETS consensus guidelines for the standards of care in neuroendocrine tumors: pathology: diagnosis and prognostic stratification. Neuroendocrinology 105(3):196–200
21. Klöppel GCA, Hruban RH, Klimstra DS, Komminoth P, Osamura RY, Perren A, Rindi G (2017) Neoplasms of the neuroendocrine pancreas, 4th edn. IARC Press, Lyon
22. de Mestier L, Cros J, Neuzillet C, Hentic O, Egal A, Muller N et al (2017) Digestive system mixed neuroendocrine-non-neuroendocrine neoplasms. Neuroendocrinology 105:412
23. La Rosa S, Sessa F, Uccella S (2016) Mixed Neuroendocrine-Nonneuroendocrine Neoplasms (MiNENs): unifying the concept of a heterogeneous group of neoplasms. Endocr Pathol 27(4):284–311
24. La Rosa S, Marando A, Furlan D, Sahnane N, Capella C (2012) Colorectal poorly differentiated neuroendocrine carcinomas and mixed adenoneuroendocrine carcinomas: insights into the diagnostic immunophenotype, assessment of methylation profile, and search for prognostic markers. Am J Surg Pathol 36(4):601–611
25. Konukiewitz B, Schlitter AM, Jesinghaus M, Pfister D, Steiger K, Segler A et al (2017) Somatostatin receptor expression related to TP53 and RB1 alterations in pancreatic and extrapancreatic neuroendocrine neoplasms with a Ki67-index above 20%. Mod Pathol 30(4):587–598
26. Raj N, Valentino E, Capanu M, Tang LH, Basturk O, Untch BR et al (2017) Treatment response and outcomes of grade 3 pancreatic neuroendocrine neoplasms based on morphology: well differentiated versus poorly differentiated. Pancreas 46(3):296–301
27. Shia J, Tang LH, Weiser MR, Brenner B, Adsay NV, Stelow EB et al (2008) Is nonsmall cell type high-grade neuroendocrine carcinoma of the tubular gastrointestinal tract a distinct disease entity? Am J Surg Pathol 32(5):719–731
28. Bernick PE, Klimstra DS, Shia J, Minsky B, Saltz L, Shi W et al (2004) Neuroendocrine carcinomas of the colon and rectum. Dis Colon Rectum 47(2):163–169
29. Yachida S, Vakiani E, White CM, Zhong Y, Saunders T, Morgan R et al (2012) Small cell and large cell neuroendocrine carcinomas of the pancreas are genetically similar and distinct from well-differentiated pancreatic neuroendocrine tumors. Am J Surg Pathol 36(2):173–184
30. Binderup T, Knigge U, Loft A, Federspiel B, Kjaer A (2010) 18F-fluorodeoxyglucose positron emission tomography predicts survival of patients with neuroendocrine tumors. Clin Cancer Res 16(3):978–985
31. Welin S, Sorbye H, Sebjornsen S, Knappskog S, Busch C, Oberg K (2011) Clinical effect of temozolomide-based chemotherapy in poorly differentiated endocrine carcinoma after progression on first-line chemotherapy. Cancer 117(20):4617–4622
32. Hentic O, Hammel P, Couvelard A, Rebours V, Zappa M, Palazzo M et al (2012) FOLFIRI regimen: an effective second-line chemotherapy after failure of etoposide-platinum combination in patients with neuroendocrine carcinomas grade 3. Endocr Relat Cancer 19(6):751–757
33. Thang SP, Lung MS, Kong G, Hofman MS, Callahan J, Michael M et al (2017) Peptide receptor radionuclide therapy (PRRT) in European Neuroendocrine Tumour Society (ENETS) grade 3 (G3) neuroendocrine neoplasia (NEN)—a single-institution retrospective analysis. Eur J Nucl Med Mol Imaging 45:262
34. Lamarca A, Walter T, Pavel M, Borbath I, Freis P, Nunez B et al (2017) Design and validation of the GI-NEC score to prognosticate overall survival in patients with high-grade gastrointestinal neuroendocrine carcinomas. J Natl Cancer Inst 109(5):djw277
35. Maltoni M, Caraceni A, Brunelli C, Broeckaert B, Christakis N, Eychmueller S et al (2005) Prognostic factors in advanced cancer patients: evidence-based clinical recommendations—

study by the Steering Committee of the European Association for Palliative Care. J Clin Oncol 23(25):6240–6248
36. Koukourakis MI, Giatromanolaki A, Simopoulos C, Polychronidis A, Sivridis E (2005) Lactate dehydrogenase 5 (LDH5) relates to up-regulated hypoxia inducible factor pathway and metastasis in colorectal cancer. Clin Exp Metastasis 22(1):25–30
37. Haugvik SP, Janson ET, Osterlund P, Langer SW, Falk RS, Labori KJ et al (2016) Surgical treatment as a principle for patients with high-grade pancreatic neuroendocrine carcinoma: a Nordic Multicenter Comparative Study. Ann Surg Oncol 23(5):1721–1728
38. Shafqat H, Ali S, Salhab M, Olszewski AJ (2015) Survival of patients with neuroendocrine carcinoma of the colon and rectum: a population-based analysis. Dis Colon Rectum 58(3):294–303
39. Mosquera C, Koutlas NJ, Fitzgerald TL (2016) Localized high-grade gastroenteropancreatic neuroendocrine tumors: defining prognostic and therapeutic factors for a disease of increasing clinical significance. EJSO 42(10):1471–1477
40. Shen C, Chen H, Chen H, Yin Y, Han L, Chen J et al (2016) Surgical treatment and prognosis of gastric neuroendocrine neoplasms: a single-center experience. BMC Gastroenterol 16:111
41. Ishida M, Sekine S, Fukagawa T, Ohashi M, Morita S, Taniguchi H et al (2013) Neuroendocrine carcinoma of the stomach: morphologic and immunohistochemical characteristics and prognosis. Am J Surg Pathol 37(7):949–959
42. Xie JW, Sun YQ, Feng CY, Zheng CH, Li P, Wang JB et al (2016) Evaluation of clinicopathological factors related to the prognosis of gastric neuroendocrine carcinoma. EJSO 42(10):1464–1470
43. Meng MB, Zaorsky NG, Jiang C, Tian LJ, Wang HH, Liu CL et al (2013) Radiotherapy and chemotherapy are associated with improved outcomes over surgery and chemotherapy in the management of limited-stage small cell esophageal carcinoma. Radiother Oncol 106(3):317–322
44. Deng HY, Ni PZ, Wang YC, Wang WP, Chen LQ (2016) Neuroendocrine carcinoma of the esophagus: clinical characteristics and prognostic evaluation of 49 cases with surgical resection. J Thorac Dis 8(6):1250–1256
45. Coriat R, Walter T, Terris B, Couvelard A, Ruszniewski P (2016) Gastroenteropancreatic well-differentiated grade 3 neuroendocrine tumors: review and position statement. Oncologist 21(10):1191–1199
46. Oberg K, Knigge U, Kwekkeboom D, Perren A, Group EGW (2012) Neuroendocrine gastro-entero-pancreatic tumors: ESMO Clinical Practice Guidelines for diagnosis, treatment and follow-up. Eur Soc Med Oncol 23(Suppl 7):vii124–vii130
47. Pavel M, O'Toole D, Costa F, Capdevila J, Gross D, Kianmanesh R et al (2016) ENETS Consensus Guidelines Update for the management of distant metastatic disease of intestinal, pancreatic, bronchial neuroendocrine neoplasms (NEN) and NEN of unknown primary site. Neuroendocrinology 103(2):172–185
48. Strosberg JR, Coppola D, Klimstra DS, Phan AT, Kulke MH, Wiseman GA et al (2010) The NANETS consensus guidelines for the diagnosis and management of poorly differentiated (high-grade) extrapulmonary neuroendocrine carcinomas. Pancreas 39(6):799–800
49. Frilling A, Modlin IM, Kidd M, Russell C, Breitenstein S, Salem R et al (2014) Recommendations for management of patients with neuroendocrine liver metastases. Lancet Oncol 15(1):e8–e21
50. Galleberg RB, Knigge U, Tiensuu Janson E, Vestermark LW, Haugvik SP, Ladekarl M et al (2017) Results after surgical treatment of liver metastases in patients with high-grade gastroenteropancreatic neuroendocrine carcinomas. EJSO 43(9):1682–1689
51. Garcia-Carbonero R, Sorbye H, Baudin E, Raymond E, Wiedenmann B, Niederle B et al (2016) ENETS consensus guidelines for high-grade gastroenteropancreatic neuroendocrine tumors and neuroendocrine carcinomas. Neuroendocrinology 103(2):186–194
52. Janson ET, Sorbye H, Welin S, Federspiel B, Gronbaek H, Hellman P et al (2014) Nordic guidelines 2014 for diagnosis and treatment of gastroenteropancreatic neuroendocrine neoplasms. Acta Oncol 53(10):1284–1297

53. Yamaguchi T, Machida N, Morizane C, Kasuga A, Takahashi H, Sudo K et al (2014) Multicenter retrospective analysis of systemic chemotherapy for advanced neuroendocrine carcinoma of the digestive system. Cancer Sci 105(9):1176–1181
54. Olsen IH, Knigge U, Federspiel B, Hansen CP, Skov A, Kjaer A et al (2014) Topotecan monotherapy in heavily pretreated patients with progressive advanced stage neuroendocrine carcinomas. J Cancer 5(8):628–632
55. Hadoux J, Malka D, Planchard D, Scoazec JY, Caramella C, Guigay J et al (2015) Post-first-line FOLFOX chemotherapy for grade 3 neuroendocrine carcinoma. Endocr Relat Cancer 22(3):289–298
56. Panzuto F, Rinzivillo M, Spada F, Antonuzzo L, Ibrahim T, Campana D et al (2017) Everolimus in pancreatic neuroendocrine carcinomas G3. Pancreas 46(3):302–305

Small Intestinal, Colorectal, and Appendicular Neuroendocrine Tumors

20

Lowell B. Anthony, Garima Gupta, and Aman Chauhan

20.1 Introduction

Intestinal neuroendocrine tumors (NETs) arise from the diffuse endocrine system present throughout its submucosal lining. These tumor cells are typically well-differentiated, slow growing, store various peptides and amino acids that, when secreted, can give rise to specific clinical syndromes. As tumor detection techniques, awareness, and education increase, the annual incidence has risen more than sixfold over four decades [1, 2]. With advancements in molecular biology, procedural techniques, medical therapeutics and imaging, clinical management has grown more complex with patients typically seen by multi-specialty teams focused on the unique characteristics of NETs. From the first recognition of the Kulchitsky cell being responsible for the synthesis, storage, and release of serotonin to the current state of theranostics and precision medicine, survival outcomes have improved. The epidemiology, biology, natural history, clinical presentation, and management of these intestinally derived well-differentiated malignancies are the focus of this review. Finally, the authors will address some current limitations, impact of the COVID-19 pandemic on NET patient care, and opportunities for the future.

20.2 Epidemiology

Though GI NETs constitute a small percentage of all malignancies, jejuno-ileal primaries are the most common small bowel malignancy, and over the last 30 years, the incidence has risen [1, 3–5]. The prevalence of GI NETs is only second to colorectal cancer and has increased eightfold over two decades [1]. It is conjectured that changes in the classification, greater awareness, increased use of screening

L. B. Anthony (✉) · G. Gupta · A. Chauhan
Division of Medical Oncology, University of Kentucky, Lexington, KY, USA
e-mail: lowell.anthony@uky.edu; kbschaberg@ucdavis.edu

S. Yalcin, K. Öberg (eds.), *Neuroendocrine Tumours*,
https://doi.org/10.1007/978-3-031-56968-5_20

procedures and imaging studies account for this rising incidence. NETs' natural history coupled with earlier detection and more therapeutic options may explain the increasing prevalence [6]. GI NETs typically arise in an older population with a median age of 66 years at the time of diagnosis, a slight male dominance (52.4%) and are more common in Caucasians (80.4%) [7]. Stage IV disease is common at the time of initial assessment as GI NETs follow an indolent course, and despite delays in diagnosis, survival outcomes exceed that of other malignancies [8, 9].

20.3 Classification

In 2019, the World Health Organization (WHO) updated the digestive system's tumor classification (Table 20.1) [10]. Even though histopathological classification remains the gold standard, neuroendocrine neoplasms (NENs) are divided into NETs and neuroendocrine carcinomas (NECs) based on their molecular phenotypes. MEN1, DAXX, and ATRX define well-differentiated NETs, while NECs are defined by TP53 and RB1 mutations. For appendiceal goblet cell adenocarcinomas, the neuroendocrine component is now recognized as being minor [10, 11].

In addition to pathological classification, NETs are clinically classified as functional (syndromic) or nonfunctional (non-syndromic) depending upon their secretory characteristics. Specific clinical symptoms such as flushing, secretory diarrhea, and wheezing arise from the release of bioactive amines and peptides by the tumors, while nonspecific symptoms including anorexia, fatigue, pain, and weight loss are more reflective of anatomical tumor location and/or disease bulk. These clinical

Table 20.1 WHO (2019) classification and grading criteria for neuroendocrine neoplasms of the gastrointestinal tract and hepatopancreatobiliary organs [10]

Terminology	Differentiation	Grade	Ki-67 index[a]	Mitotic rates[b]
NET, Grade 1	Well-differentiated (WD)	Low	<3%	<2
NET, Grade 2		Intermediate	3–20%	2–20
NET, Grade 3		High	>20%	>20
NEC, small-cell type (SCNEC)	Poorly differentiated (PD)	High	>20%	>20
NEC, large-cell (LCNEC)			>20%	>20
MiNEN[c]	Well (WD) or poorly (PD) differentiated	Variable	Variable	Variable

WHO World Health Organization, *NET* neuroendocrine tumor, *NEC* neuroendocrine carcinoma, *SCNEC* small-cell neuroendocrine carcinoma, *LCNEC* large-cell neuroendocrine carcinoma, *MiNEN* mixed neuroendocrine–non-neuroendocrine neoplasm

[a]Ki-67 proliferation index percentages are determined by counting at least 500 cells in the regions of highest labeling (hot-spots) which are identified at scanning magnification; the final grade is based on whichever of the two proliferation indexes places the neoplasm in the higher-grade category

[b]Mitotic rates reflect the number of mitoses/2 mm^2 determined by counting in 50 fields of 0.2 mm^2 (i.e., in a total area of 10 mm^2)

[c]For MiNENs, both the NE and non-NE components are PD; the NE component usually has proliferative indices in the same range as other NECs; however, one or both components may be well-differentiated; when possible, each component is graded individually

symptoms coupled with the biology in defining some of the hallmark features of NETs that include (a) delay in diagnosis, (b) misdiagnosis, (c) advanced disease (Stages III and IV) at the time of diagnosis, and (d) fibrosis [12–15].

Clinical classification also includes recognizing specific phenotypes described by their dominant metastatic site(s) such as liver, lymph node, bone, or mixed. Examples of integrating pathological and clinical classifications into medical decision-making are shown in Fig. 20.1a where disease bulk is also included. The heterogeneity of NETs is present not only in the biology as defined pathologically

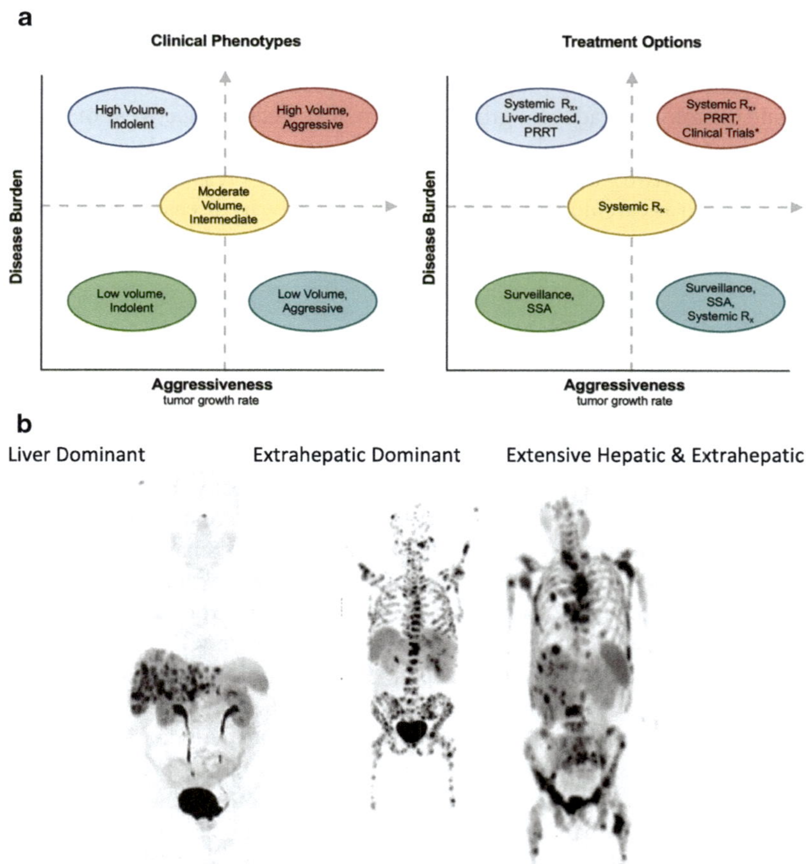

Fig. 20.1 (**a**) Clinical assessment and decision-making in Stage IV NETs. Managing advanced disease includes recognizing the many distinct clinical phenotypes, being aware of the natural history of each, and selecting the appropriate care pathway. As patient performance status ranges from an ECOG 0 to 4, treatment options include observation, surgical debulking, somatostatin analogs, locoregional procedures, molecularly targeted agents, cytotoxic chemotherapy, radiation, and clinical trials. After localizing all sites of disease and estimating tumor burden, the biology of the disease coupled with the patient's comorbidities will determine the appropriate order of interventions to optimally achieve the highest quality of life while increasing overall survival. *While clinical trials are broadly endorsed as treatment options, this cohort represents a high unmet medical need. (**b**) Clinical classification of Stage IV NETs using somatostatin receptor scintigraphy with ^{64}Cu- or ^{68}Ga-dotatate

but also clinically with somatostatin receptor imaging identifying the three dominant clinical phenotypes: (1) hepatic dominant, (2) extrahepatic dominant, and (3) mixed hepatic and extrahepatic (Fig. 20.1b).

20.4 Classification and Staging

In 2019, the WHO grading classification for GI NETs was updated (Table 20.1). The TNM staging system for NETs was first proposed by ENETs in 2006 and by the AJCC 4 years later [16, 17]. The eighth AJCC TNM staging system edition staged NETs according to primary site as their natural history varies significantly [18–21]. For jejunal and ileal NETs, a minimum of eight lymph nodes are to be examined for accurate pathologic staging [22, 23]. Prognostic predictors include tumor stage, primary site, histologic grade and growth pattern, age, gender, race, year of diagnosis, elevated neuron-specific enolase (NSE), primary resection, complete resection, and doubling of the Ki-67 index over time [7, 24–30]. The presence of paraneoplastic conditions such as carcinoid syndrome and carcinoid heart disease portends a poorer prognosis though is not part of the classification systems [31–34].

20.4.1 Biology of NETs

Even though NETs are predominantly derived from the enterochromaffin cells (EC) of the gastroenteropancreatic and bronchopulmonary systems and have endocrine and neural markers in common, heterogeneity best describes their biology [35]. As NETs comprise many diseases because of this heterogeneity that includes the primary site, genetic mutations, hormonal secretions, symptoms, familial incidence, receptor expression, growth characteristics, and metastatic behavior, their biology is complex. Common aspects of NETs such as the high overexpression of G protein-coupled membrane peptide hormone receptors including somatostatin, glucagon-like peptide-1 (GLP-1), and gastric inhibitory polypeptide (GIP) are offset by the variable expression of these same receptors [36–41]. NETs' cell surface and intracellular transporter proteins also include norepinephrine, dopamine, and glucose, as they were previously referred to as "APUDomas" (amine peptide uptake and decarboxylation) [42–45]. NETs also overexpress a wide variety of proangiogenic molecules that include vascular endothelial growth factor, platelet-derived growth factor, fibroblast growth factor, semaphorins, and angiopoietins resulting in their being among some of the most vascularized malignancies [46–51]. An important commonality within NETs includes the presence of altered mammalian target of rapamycin signaling that comprises a major therapeutic pathway [52, 53].

Areas of NET biology under investigation include the immune and tumor microenvironments (TME) that consist of complex interactions between the circulation, cellular stromal elements, and molecular mediators that communicate between and within the cells resulting in growth stimulatory, inhibitory, or cytotoxic effects [54]. The characterization of these interactions between the immune system and the TME by these mediators not only has basic physiologic implications but therapeutic ones as well [55, 56].

20.5 Biomarkers

NET biomarkers include those that are tissue based, e.g., Ki-67 index, microRNAs, genetic and epigenetic alterations, and those that are circulating (blood) and image derived (Table 20.2). Some biomarkers are incorporated into the pathologic diagnostic criteria (Ki-67), while others define the functional/secretory status and are useful in clinical staging and management. A conceptual framework is proposed by a working group as no "perfect" biomarker exists for screening, diagnosis, follow-up monitoring, and estimating tumor burden along with predictive and prognostic characteristics [57]. While nomograms can integrate these variables for a specific patient and are externally validated, prospective validation remains [58–61].

Because neuroendocrine neoplasms have the potential of secreting a spectrum of bioactive and inactive products including amino acids, peptides, growth factors, and biotranscripts, these biomarkers can support the diagnosis but are generally

Table 20.2 Biomarkers of intestinal NETs

Biomarker	Description	Comments
Circulating		
Chromogranin A (CGA)	50kD glycoprotein present in NE and neuronal dense core granules; co-secreted with amines and peptides	Extensively evaluated with varying assays across disease states; high false-positive rates with PPIs and many disease states (CAG, RF, CHF, LF)
Pancreastatin	Peptide subunit of CGA	Not elevated with PPIs; limited studies
Gastrin	Peptide hormone stimulating acid secretion	May be elevated in duodenal NETs
Neuron-specific enolase (NSE)	Glycolytic enzyme	Elevated in more aggressive tumors
Serotonin (5-HT)	Amine secreted by NET cell	Useful in diagnosis
5-HIAA	Serotonin metabolite	24-hr urinary measurement of serotonin production; less variable than blood serotonin
NETest	Algorithm using multiple mRNA transcripts	Useful in detecting recurrence following surgery and predicting response to RPT; not tested in prospective clinical trials
Imaging		
CT	Anatomical imaging	Requires IV contrast to accurately define tumor measurement(s)
MRI	Anatomical imaging	Useful in planning surgical procedures
^{68}Ga or ^{64}Cu-dotatate PET/CT	Physiologic imaging	Useful in whole-body tumor localization and quantitation
^{123}I-MIBG SPECT	Physiologic imaging	Possible role in somatostatin receptor-negative tumors

insufficient to definitively diagnose a disease without a tissue sample because of specificity and sensitivity issues [62–65]. Biomarkers do have relevance with medical decision-making in the standard of care of NET patients [64, 66]; however, until more data are available, biomarkers remain as secondary or exploratory endpoints in clinical research protocols.

There are a few circulating NET-specific biomarkers that have either predictive and/or prognostic characteristics. Emerging new biomarkers are being identified and under investigation with human progastrin having potential therapeutic value [62, 67–69].

20.5.1 Serotonin (5-HT)

Serotonin discovery, biochemistry, and physiology occurred in parallel with the clinical recognition of the carcinoid syndrome and carcinoid heart disease [70–72]. Cloning of the two NET relevant receptor systems, serotonin, and somatostatin proceeded simultaneously as well [73, 74]. Dietary tryptophan (TP) is converted to serotonin or 5-hydroxytryptamine in two enzymatic reactions [75]. The rate-limiting step occurs initially with the conversion of tryptophan to 5-hydroxytryptophan (5-HTP) by the enzyme, tryptophan hydroxylase (TPH) existing in two isoforms [76]. Decarboxylation of 5-HTP by aromatic amino acid decarboxylase results in 5-HT. Serotonin, secreted by the intestinal enterochromaffin cells, is both a hormone and a neurotransmitter in the gut and brain and is stored in platelets [77, 78]. Serotonin, despite being vasoconstrictive, is not responsible for the flushing symptoms of carcinoid syndrome but is a main mediator of the diarrhea and mesenteric/cardiac fibrosis [79–82]. Serial serotonin levels as a tumor marker have limited usefulness as it does not reflect total serotonin production [83]. More recent serotonin whole blood assays are more reliable and reproducible as platelet release during collection/storage is minimized; however, more data are necessary before circulating serotonin can be established as a valuable tumor biomarker [84].

5-HT does not cross the blood–brain barrier, resulting in two distinct compartments anatomically and functionally separate: the central nervous system (CNS) and the extra-CNS [85]. As TPH1, expressed in the enterochromaffin (EC) cells, is responsible for the conversion of TP to 5-HT in the extra-CNS compartment, TPH2, mainly expressed in the central and enteric nervous systems, converts TP to 5-HT in the CNS and the enteric nerve plexus [86, 87]. Defining the biochemistry and physiology of serotonin impacts both oncologic (telotristat ethyl) and psychiatric (SSRIs) therapeutics.

20.5.2 5-HIAA

Serotonin is metabolized in two steps by monoamine oxidase and aldehyde dehydroxylase to 5-hydroxyindole-3-acetaldehyde (5-HIAL) and 5-hydroxyindole acetic acid (5-HIAA), respectively, with the latter measured in the serum or urine as a meaningful biomarker [88–91]. In carcinoid syndrome, the overall sensitivity and specificity of urinary 5-HIAA are in the range of 70 and 90%, respectively [92, 93]. Even though urinary 5-HIAA was one of the first diagnostic biomarker in NETs, its usefulness as a prognostic marker is less established. In some series, elevated urinary 5-HIAA significantly correlates with overall survival [94, 95]; however, other investigators using multivariate analysis did not show any significant correlation [33, 96].

20.5.3 Chromogranin A (CGA)

CGA, a 49 kDa acidic glycoprotein present in secretory granules, is co-released with amine and peptide hormones [97]. CGA acts as a precursor to other bioactive substances including vasostatin-1, angiostatin, chromostatin, catestatin, serpinin, and pancreastatin and may be a useful tumor marker, especially if there is a rapid rise during management including surveillance post-surgery [98–100]. The CGA system is complex and occupies a role in the cardiovascular, immunometabolic, cancer regulation and as a prognostic and predictive biomarker [101–105]. CGA levels are subject to variability related to concomitant medications, food intake, disease states including chronic atrophic gastritis, cardiac, hepatic, and renal insufficiencies, and other confounding conditions [63, 106, 107]. Serial CGA measurements are considered routine in NET management as supported by practice guidelines but still need cautious interpretation [66, 108–110].

20.5.4 Pancreastatin

A potentially more useful biomarker is pancreastatin, a subunit of CgA. Pancreastatin levels offer additional insight into CGA elevations that commonly occur reflexly with proton pump inhibitors. NET was ruled out in patients taking PPIs and who had an elevated CGA but a normal pancreastatin level [111]. Detecting the presence of liver metastases in small intestinal NETs with elevated pancreastatin levels had greater sensitivity and specificity than CGA in an observational study [112]. Pancreastatin as a prognostic biomarker was studied in a retrospective analysis of 176 resected GEPNETs patients of which 62% had metastatic disease. CGA and pancreastatin were measured pre- and post-operatively (post-op). Elevated baseline levels of both pancreastatin and CgA were associated with decreased progression-free survival (PFS) and overall survival (OS); however, with a multivariate analysis, only pancreastatin had prognostic significance. Normalization of high pancreastatin levels post-op predicted an improved PFS but not OS [113]. Others have shown that it was the rate of change of pancreastatin levels, or its velocity, that is associated with a worse prognosis [114, 115]. Pancreastatin was a marker of treatment response and a predictor of overall survival in 122 liver-predominant metastatic NETs patients undergoing transarterial chemoembolization (TACE) [116, 117]. Pancreastatin levels are closely monitored in some centers; however, assay availability globally inhibits its universal adoption [64, 68].

20.5.5 Neurokinin A (NKA)

NKA, a tachykinin, and other tachykinins such as substance P, are elevated in intestinal NETs patients [82, 84]. These tachykinins, stored and secreted by NETs, increase intestinal motility and vasodilation and are mediators in the carcinoid syndrome [118, 119]. Monitoring NKA blood levels is more practical than the less stable substance P. NKA is an independent prognostic biomarker that predicts survival in response to hormonal and surgical treatment [96, 120, 121].

20.5.6 Neuron-Specific Enolase (NSE)

NSE, an enzyme expressed by cells of neuronal origin, is commonly elevated in high-grade NETs and neuroendocrine carcinoma [122]. Its elevation in NETs correlates with an aggressive biology [28]. Approximately, 1 in 5 ileal NETs will have NSE elevation with prognostic significance [123, 124]. NSE was a poor prognostic marker in patients with pNETs as an early decrease in NSE with everolimus treatment correlated with a longer PFS, despite a normal CGA [125]. NSE may be a useful biomarker in patients with Grade 2 or 3 disease, low SUV on somatostatin receptor scintigraphy, significant uptake on FDG-PET imaging, or change in differentiation.

20.5.7 Circulating Biotranscripts

Measuring circulating biotranscripts—liquid biopsy—in NETs is now possible but not widely integrated into clinical practice. The NETest, available from Wren Laboratories, Branford, CT, in the USA and Sarah Cannon Molecular Diagnostics (HCA), London, in Europe, is a blood mRNA-based assay measuring 51 NET marker gene expressions using q-PCR [126]. The NETest outperformed CGA measurement as a diagnostic marker; however, a large independent validation study found that the NETest was not useful as a screening test for GEPNETs because of its low specificity [127–129]. The NETest's sensitivity over CgA is significant (93 vs. 56%; $p < 0.001$) and its usefulness in detecting residual post-surgery is established and can predict response to peptide receptor radiotherapy [128, 130, 131]. A recent meta-analysis provided a systemic literature review of 10 papers meeting inclusion criteria [132]. The NETest's diagnostic accuracy is 95–96% and 84.5–85.5% distinguishes stable from progressive disease. As an interventional/response monitoring test, the NETest had an accuracy of 93.7–97.4% [132]. The NETest results may be useful for select patients; however, like CGA, NETest results alone should not guide management decisions. Integration of the NETest into prospective clinical trials as either a secondary response indicator or as an exploratory biomarker coupled with guidance from the United States National Cancer Co-operative Network (NCCN) and/or other published guidelines will be anticipated before a more generalized adoption of the NETest into routine clinical decision-making.

MiRNAs, short RNA sequences that regulate gene expression post-transcriptionally, are tumor-type specific and can be measured in tumor tissue samples and blood [133–135]. MiRNAs profiling in small intestinal NETs has correlated high levels of circulating miR-22-3p and miR-21-5p, and low levels of miR-150-5p were prognostic for survival (HR 0.47, 95% CI 0.27–0.82) [136]. The biologic function, biomarker usefulness, and potential therapeutic targets of miRNAs in small intestinal NETs remain undefined.

20.5.8 Intestinal Nets

20.5.8.1 Duodenal Neuroendocrine Tumors

Duodenal NETs (d-NETs), considered foregut derived, are frequently found incidentally at the time of endoscopy, represent 2–3% of all GI NETs, are more common in males, and have a median age of diagnosis of 65 years of age [137–140]. The four types of d-NETs are the more proximal ones (gastrinomas and non-functioning), the ampullary or per-ampullary somatostatinomas, and the peri-ampullary gangliocytic paragangliomas [137]. The presenting symptoms of gastrinomas include recurrent/refractory peptic ulcer disease, chronic diarrhea, and gastroesophageal reflux [141]. Somatostatinomas can present with vague symptoms of nausea, abdominal pain, obstructive jaundice, weight loss, and rarely the somatostatinoma syndrome [142]. For gangliocytic paragangliomas and non-functioning d-NETs, symptoms may be absent or associated with nausea, emesis, and in some cases, anemia and gastrointestinal bleeding [143].

Once there is a tissue diagnosis, fasting diagnostic workup after endoscopy/EUS-FNA would include biomarkers such as gastrin, CGA, somatostatin, and anatomical/physiological imaging with IV contrasted CT or MRI and Cu-64 or Ga-68 dotatate PET/CT scanning to complete the clinical staging. Assessment of acid production and secretion suppression test is specific to gastrinomas.

Once staging is completed, therapy is dependent upon size and extent of disease. For those <1 cm and can be mucosally resected, EMR in advanced endoscopy centers is an option. Other potentially curative modalities include surgical resection or enucleation depending upon tumor size and location. Transduodenal excision for 1–2 cm tumors and Whipple's surgery with local lymph node resection for tumors >2 cm [144]. For advanced stage disease, systemic treatment options may follow that for pancreatic NETs more than intestinal NETs. This approach includes somatostatin analogs (lanreotide, octreotide), cytotoxic agents (capecitabine, temozolomide), targeted agents (everolimus, sunitinib, pazopanib), locoregional therapies (hepatic artery embolotherapy with or without chemotherapy), cytoreductive surgery, and radiopharmaceutical therapy with Lu-177 dotatate.

20.5.8.2 Jejunal and Ileal Neuroendocrine Tumors

Intestinal NETs, classically referred to as "midgut carcinoids" were among the first to be described pathologically with uncertainty regarding their malignant characteristics [145–147]. Jejunal and ileal NETs are typically well-differentiated (mostly

Grade 1), argentaffin-positive, substance P-containing, and serotonin-producing EC-cell tumors. With hepatic or nodal metastases bioactive products, e.g., serotonin, substance P, tachykinins, etc., may be released directly into the systemic circulation producing the symptoms of carcinoid syndrome: flushing, secretory diarrhea, and in some cases, wheezing. Ileal NETs occur predominantly in the terminal ileum where there is a greater density of EC-cells [148].

This subgroup of intestinal NETs occurs slightly more in men (52.4%) with an average age of 66 at the time of diagnosis [7]. The biologic tendency for jejunal/ileal NETs to metastasize is variable. Their typical pattern of metastatic spread is to lymph nodes and the liver. Even with the presence of nodal and hepatic metastases, patients may be completely asymptomatic.

The early symptoms of jejunal/ileal NETs are typically nonspecific, vague, and mistaken for more common diseases. Symptoms associated with the primary tumor include intermittent and crescendo episodes of nausea with or without emesis from the partial small bowel obstruction. Primary tumors are submucosal, grow concentrically resulting in luminal narrowing, and are associated with a local fibrotic reaction that can cause ischemia or "intestinal angina" and bleeding. Intermittent crampy abdominal pain, weight loss, fatigue, abdominal distention, explosive watery diarrhea, flushing, nausea, and emesis may present for an extended period before diagnosis [149–151]. At the time of diagnosis, ileal NETs may be greater than 2 cm in diameter and have metastasized to regional lymph nodes. Multifocality occurs as many as 40% of cases [148].

20.5.8.3 Colonic and Rectal Neuroendocrine Tumors

Most colorectal NETs are rectal with some arising in the cecum [149]. Rectal NETs account for ~25% of all GI NETs but fewer than 1% of all rectal neoplasms [152]. Most rectal NETs have L-cell differentiation, a mean age at diagnosis of 56 years vs. 66 years for colonic NETs. There is no specific gender predilection for colorectal NETs; however, rectal NETs occur more commonly in blacks [152, 153]. Presenting symptoms of colonic NETs include abdominal pain and weight loss, while more than half of rectal NETs patients are asymptomatic. Rectal NETs are diagnosed by routine rectal examinations or screening endoscopies [154]. Symptoms of rectal NETs may include bleeding, pain, and constipation. Metastatic disease from colonic NETs may produce carcinoid syndrome, whereas metastatic disease from rectal NETs usually does not [155, 156].

20.5.8.4 Appendicular Neuroendocrine Tumors

The appendix as a distinct primary was recognized early in the pathologic description of NETs and is now ranked as the third most common site of GI NETs [157–160]. Among all appendicular neoplasms, aNETs account for up to 60% of the cases [161–164], with SEER database reporting a lower prevalence due to only including malignant carcinoids [159]. Compared to other GI NETs, aNETs are diagnosed at a younger age of 32–42 years [165–167]. A higher incidence among females has been shown in some [168–170] but not all studies [157, 166], possibly attributed to a high rate of gynecological laparoscopies performed in females [170].

While majority of aNETs are diagnosed at a lower stage with an indolent course and favorable overall survival, a minority with advanced stage and distant metastasis have poor prognosis [7, 167]. Overall, aNETs have been shown to have better overall survival rates compared to other GI NETs [1]. Goblet cell carcinomas are mixed adenoneuroendocrine on histology with distinctive clinical course and are not covered under aNETs.

There are no specific symptoms associated with aNETs and most are incidental discoveries post-appendectomy [170]. When symptoms are present, they are frequently indistinguishable from acute appendicitis [171]. Since most tumors are located at the tip of the appendix, luminal obstruction is uncommon [170, 172–174]. Some patients, especially those with extensive local disease or metastasis, may experience nonspecific right lower quadrant abdominal pain from luminal or bowel obstruction [172, 173]. Carcinoid syndrome when rarely seen is associated with metastatic aNETs [174]. Even more rare is Cushing's syndrome, which has only been reported in a few cases [175, 176].

Since a majority of aNETs are small and confined to the distal third of the appendix, they may elude radiological detection [170, 177, 178]. Anatomical imaging with either CT or MRI with institution-specific protocols remains first-line modalities [179]. Tumors located at the base may cause obstruction and present as appendicitis on imaging [177]. Diagnostic colonoscopy is not recommended as it will only detect tumors invading the cecum, which is an uncommon phenomenon [179, 180]. Functional imaging including both SRS and PET scans using ^{68}Ga-labeled somatostatin analogues in combination with anatomical imaging should be considered in patients with risk factors or suspicion for metastatic disease [179].

Histopathological diagnosis and characterization of aNETs require: (1) immunostaining for synaptophysin and CgA and (2) determination of the proliferative potential using the mitotic rate per 10 HPF and Ki-67 index for WHO grading. Other biomarkers, including secretoneurin, *catestatin*, *beta-catenin,* and *CDX2* have been studied but are not included in the guidelines [181]. The pathologist must comment on the size, location within the appendix, lymphovascular involvement, extent of invasion into the mesoappendix (if present), and infiltration of peritoneum and other neighboring structures [179]. These features are key in determining the TNM stage and formulating an optimal treatment plan for the patient.

The histopathological factors impact on the malignant potential as well as the TNM staging. The majority of aNETs, up to 80%, are located at the tip of the appendix, followed by the body and then the base [170, 171, 174, 182]. Theoretically, there is a higher risk of incomplete resection with basal aNETs, which in turns results in recurrence, metastasis, and poor prognosis for patients. However, this has not been reliably illustrated in studies and remains an area of controversy [174, 179].

aNET size is a key factor in determining the risk of local and distant metastasis [170, 183]. While most studies have shown that aNETs measuring ≤1 cm pose negligible risk for metastasis [170, 182, 183], some others have disputed this finding, suggesting a potential risk of up to 15% [167, 174, 184]. aNETs measuring ≥2 cm, although rare, represent the group with highest risk of metastasis [170, 174, 182–184]. In one study, 24 out of 28 (86%) patients with aNET size >2 cm showed evidence of lymph node metastasis [184]. aNETs measuring between 1 and 2 cm, especially those measuring ≥1.5 cm, are the most challenging to manage due to conflicting data, with studies showing a significant variation in metastatic risk, from 0 to up to 47% [170, 174, 183, 184].

The mesoappendix refers to the peritoneal fold connecting the ileum to the appendix. When there is extension of the aNET into this structure, it is referred to as mesoappendiceal infiltration (MI). Extent of MI, either < or >3 mm, is used as one of the features, besides size, to differentiate between T2 and T3 stages of the ENETS guidelines, respectively [179]. Studies have questioned this recommendation as there is not sufficient evidence to suggest its role as an independent predictor of malignant potential [181, 185]. The use of MI for aNETs was first suggested in 1979, where investigators also showed a correlation between tumor size and extent of MI [186]. Another study showed significant association between MI and metastasis in patients with tumors measuring <2 cm [187]. In a more recent study, 5 out of 13 patients with aNET size ≥1 cm and ≤2 cm and MI extension of <3 cm had lymph node metastasis [174].

Management of aNETs depends on the stage with surgical options including a simple appendectomy or a right-sided hemicolectomy (RHC) (Fig. 20.2). For aNETs measuring ≤1 cm, a simple appendectomy is usually curative [179, 184, 185]. In special circumstances when the tumor is located at the base of the appendix or when there is evidence of extensive MI, complete resection should be considered [179]. aNETs measuring >1 but ≤2 cm are challenging to manage due to conflicting data. Therefore, it is crucial to recognize other factors such as the location, presence, and extent on MI, WHO grade, and lymphovascular invasion. When one or

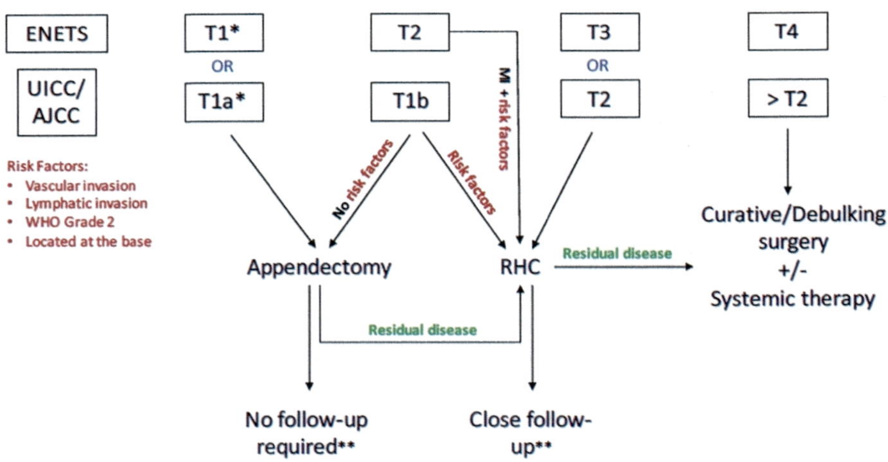

Fig. 20.2 Treatment and follow-up algorithm for aNETs. * For ENETS T1 or UICC/AJCC T1a aNETs, a more extensive surgical approach may be considered when tumors are located at the base of the appendix or when there is extensive MI. ** For tumors measuring ≤2 cm with risk factors, follow-up should be considered. ENETS guidelines recommend follow-up at 6 months, 12 months, and then yearly. This schedule is not validated and may be tailored on a case-to-case basis

more of these factors are present, a more aggressive surgical approach is reasonable. Some investigators have labeled this as the "gray zone," and guidelines recommend discussing the risks of an incomplete resection with a simple appendectomy versus the perioperative morbidity and mortality associated with a more extensive surgical approach, before making a joint decision [174, 179, 185].

20.6 Imaging

Net imaging combines anatomy with physiology. Historically, CT and MRI scanning formed the basis of tumor imaging and replaced the physical exam in measuring response to treatment. Scintigraphy was introduced in 1994 with the FDA approval of In-111 pentetreotide. Invasive imaging with endoscopic ultrasound with aspiration biopsy offers the potential for pathologic diagnosis.

20.6.1 Computed Tomography (CT)

Contrast-enhanced multiphasic CT scanning is noninvasive and useful in surveillance and monitoring response to therapy. Limitations of CT scanning include size and site of primary. Tumors less than 1 cm in size may be nonvisualized and with superficial NETs such as rectal, endoscopy is preferred. The challenge with CT imaging of intestinal NETs with liver metastases is optimizing conspicuity. As over 80% of these tumors are hypervascular, they appear isodense with the normal hepatic parenchyma. Administering iodinated contrast intravenously allows for greater visualization of liver NET metastases; however, 6–20% are hypovascular [188, 189]. The personalization of CT scanning includes ordering the optimal phase of IV contrast for each patient to obtain adequate "conspicuity" and thus allowing for meaningful comparisons between time intervals.

CT localization of intestinal primaries is limited as the size of appendiceal, jejunal, and ileal primaries are frequently small. Improving detection includes ordering a helical, multiphasic CT scan with neutral oral contrast and multiplanar reformations [188]. Frequently accompanying small intestinal NETs are mesenteric masses with desmoplastic fibrosis. The classic CT appearance is a mass with "spokes" radiating into the mesenteric fat. Retraction of the bowel with tethering and angulation is not uncommon. The mass may be calcified but often is not. Sclerosing mesenteritis has a similar appearance and can be mistaken for a NET [190]. Colonic primaries tend to be greater than 2 cm, involve the cecum, ascending colon, invade the terminal ileum, and have a similar appearance to adenocarcinoma on CT scans [191].

20.6.2 Magnetic Resonance Imaging (MRI)

MRI is the most sensitive imaging method for the detection of NET hepatic metastases [192]. Such detail of hepatic involvement is potentially useful in diagnosing and surgical planning though MRI significantly still underestimates the total tumor burden as many lesions' size remains below the threshold for detection [193]. Early arterial phase imaging combined with fast spin-echo T2-weighted images is the optimal MRI scanning protocol to detect small hepatic metastases in one study of 64 patients. The choice of contrast agent can also affect findings. Gadoxetate disodium contrast agent (Eovist) compared to gadopentetate dimeglumine provided a higher contrast-to-noise ratio and interobserver agreement of tumor sizes [194].

20.6.3 Endoscopy

Upper and lower endoscopy can detect a primary NET and its incidental discovery accounts, at least in part, for the increased incidence of NETs over the last three decades. The diagnosis and management of rectal NETs incorporate endoscopy as the primary tool for potential therapy with endoscopic mucosal resection feasible in small tumors and for surveillance [154]. MR- and CT-enterography can detect primary jejunal or ileal tumors but can require sedation and is potentially performed to avoid a more invasive procedure [195, 196].

Capsule endoscopy (CE) provides an alternative method to other endoscopic procedures for the evaluation of occult NET primaries [197]. The risk of capsule retention limits it role in NET evaluation, especially as other imaging modalities, such as dotatate PET scanning has emerged [198]. CE's usefulness is more in the diagnostic work-up by a gastroenterologist rather than incorporating it into metastatic disease evaluation solely to detect a primary site [199].

20.6.4 Somatostatin Receptor Imaging

The expression of somatostatin receptors (SRS) is a defining characteristic of well-differentiated neuroendocrine tumors [200]. As the molecular visualization of these receptors was made possible using in vitro autoradiographic techniques, the in vivo equivalent was also achieved with radiolabeled octreotide [201]. In 1994, In-111 pentetreotide (OctreoScan™) became FDA approved and the preferred imaging modality until 2016 when PET technology using Ga-68 dotatate (Netspot™) replaced it [202]. Being generator (germanium-68/gallium-68) dependent, Ga-68 dotatate scanning was limited to institutions physically close to the generator as Ga-68's half-life is 68 min. Cyclotron produced Cu-64 dotatate's (Detectnet™) FDA approval in 2020 allows all sites with PET technology to integrate SRS imaging as the preferred modality [203].

SRS imaging coupled with anatomical scanning is a critical portion of NET patient assessment and present/future care planning. Identifying all sites of disease, the "relative" expression of the somatostatin receptor, correlating with pathologic and clinical information, comprises the initial dataset to build a comprehensive care plan. Scintigraphic imaging encompasses more "whole-body" than CT/MRI scanning that is usually limited to specific body regions; thus, SRS imaging is more likely to detect progressive disease in occult sites but unable to accurately provide tumor measurements without an accompanying "diagnostic" CT/MRI scan using IV contrast. Ordering SRS imaging simultaneously with diagnostic CT/MRI scans is frequently met with insurance denial in the United States as third-party payers interpret these imaging modalities as repetitive rather than complementary.

20.6.5 Bone Scintigraphy

Bone is a common site after liver, lymph node, peritoneal/pelvic implants for NET metastases that, historically, went undetected [204]. Bone scintigraphy using ^{99}mTc-MDP has high sensitivity in identifying NET bone metastases [205]. With SRS receptor imaging, the usefulness of dedicated bone scintigraphy is less now, than historically, but may continue to assist in some cases, diagnostically [206].

20.7 Treatment

Neuroendocrine tumor patient management is multi-disciplinary incorporating pathologists, radiologists, surgeons, and multiple medical specialties (see Fig. 20.3). In-depth review and discussions at multi-disciplinary tumor boards allow for a comprehensive care plan development for initial and potential subsequent lines of therapy to accomplish either curative or palliative goals. Identifying clinical trial opportunities is also considered.

Clinical decision-making is aligned with patient stage and grade (Fig. 20.4a). Functional status at the time of diagnosis of patients with somatostatin receptor subtype 2 positive metastatic intestinal G1/G2 disease is an early indication for SMSA initiation (Fig. 20.4b).

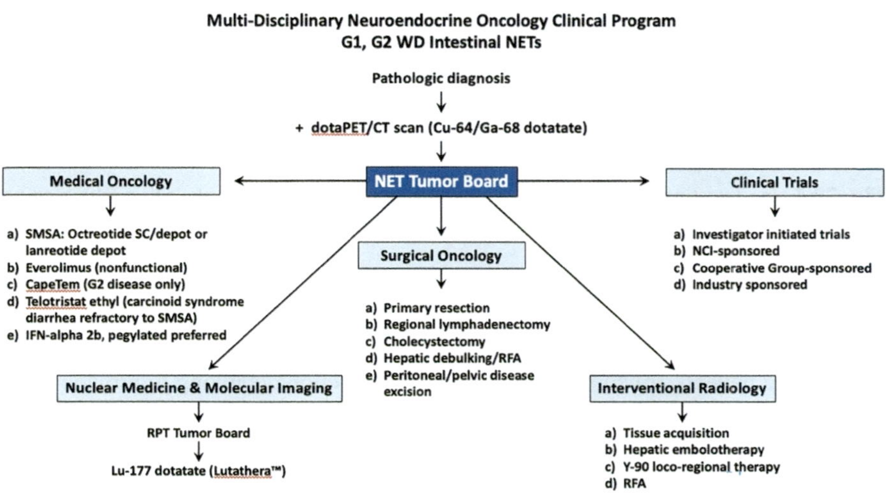

Fig. 20.3 Multi-disciplinary neuroendocrine oncology clinical program

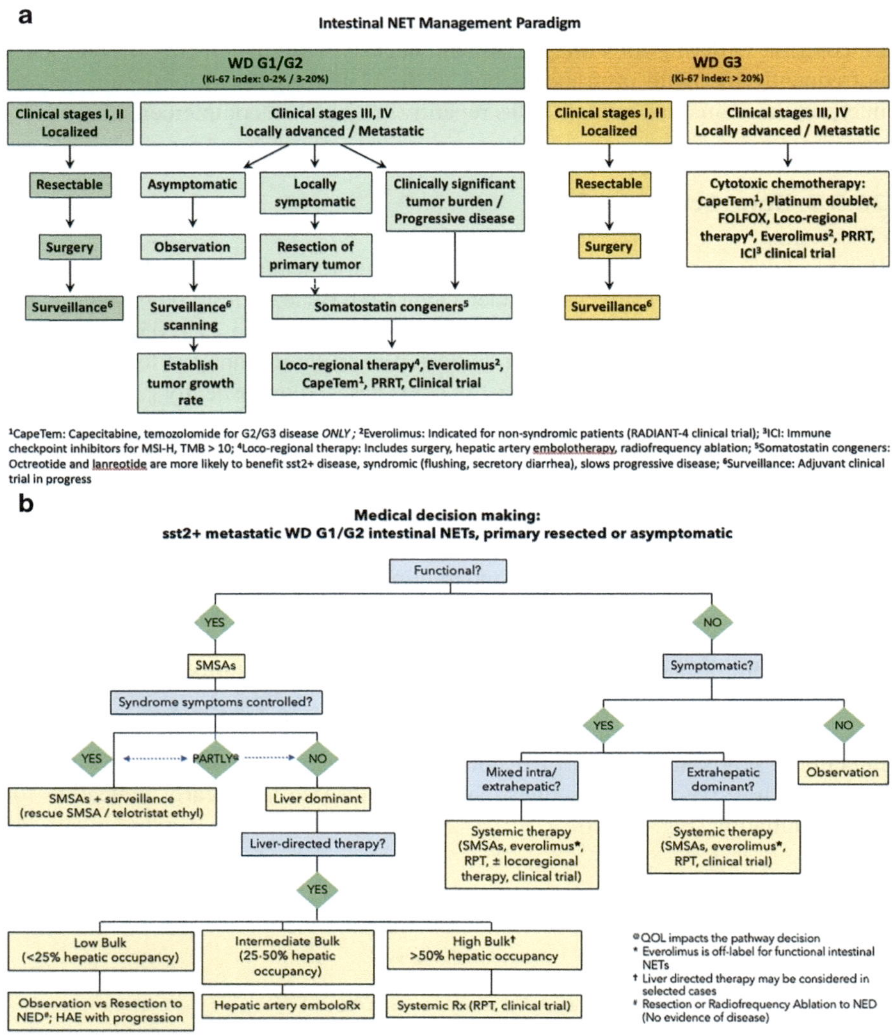

Fig. 20.4 (**a**) Intestinal neuroendocrine tumor management paradigm algorithm. (**b**) Medical decision-making in a common subgroup of metastatic intestinal neuroendocrine tumors

20.7.1 Localized and Locoregional Disease

20.7.1.1 Surgery

Early-stage patients are considered for surgical resection/debulking to provide relief of symptoms, pathologic staging, and potential cure. Jejunal, ileal, cecal, and colonic primaries may have laparoscopic-assisted surgical options to maximize the recovery time. Rectal primaries may have a more aggressive biologic behavior than previously thought requiring treatment decisions to be more individually based [155, 207–209].

20.7.1.2 Minimally Invasive Endoscopic Interventions

Minimally invasive endoscopic techniques are recommended treatment options in duodenal and rectal NETs that go beyond the simple polypectomy that typically has a high recurrence rate [155, 210]. Several techniques, including endoscopic mucosal resection (EMR), band-assisted EMR (band-EMR), endoscopic submucosal dissection (ESD), and over-the-scope clip-assisted endoscopic full-thickness resection (EFTR), have been studied; however, the best technique for endoscopic duodenal NET resection remains unclear [211]. These procedures require advanced endoscopic training, thus limited to large tertiary referral centers. The band ligation-assisted endoscopic mucosal resection may be the optimal treatment for broad base duodenal carcinoid tumors [212]. A disadvantage of EMR alone is that it can have a higher frequency of compromised margins requiring another resection. Even though the recurrence is low with ESD, perforation and bleeding risks are greater [213].

Rectal NETs ≤10 mm are best managed endoscopically as they are typically nonmalignant; however, the optimal resection technique also remains uncertain. ESD has a higher complete resection rate but is accompanied by higher complication risks including perforation. Additional studies are needed to compare, prospectively, the various endoscopic and surgical techniques to determine the optimal management of rectal NETs [154, 214].

20.7.1.3 Hepatic Artery Embolotherapy

The hepatic dual blood supply allows for the safe targeting of metastatic disease with regional arterial therapies delivered directly into a segmental, lobar, or whole liver distribution using angiographic catheters. Devascularizing hepatic disease with particle embolization alone (bland) or particles in combination with chemotherapy is effective in controlling symptoms, lowering biomarkers and debulking disease. A recent meta-analysis of non-randomized retrospective reports concluded that outcomes were similar between transarterial bland embolization (TAE) and transarterial chemoembolization (TACE); however, the latter is more toxic [215]. An expected adverse event with hepatic tumor infarction is the "post-embolization syndrome" or the onset of symptoms including malaise, fever, pain, nausea, and anorexia. The severity and duration of the syndrome are related to the amount of disease devascularized and individual patient factors. A prospective randomized embolization multicenter clinical trial for NET liver metastases (RETNET) is in progress and statistically powered to detect a significant difference between the two techniques (TAE vs. TACE) [216]. Combining systemic therapy with embolotherapy is emerging as only one retrospective series has continued antineoplastic therapy concomitantly with hepatic artery bland embolization [217].

Yttrium-90 radioembolization can induce complete responses rates but overall survival is not significantly different to that achieved with either bland or TACE and may cause cirrhosis with bilobar radiation as a long-term adverse effect [218–221].

20.7.1.4 Metastatic Disease

Somatostatin and Its Congeners

Somatostatin congeners or analogs (SMSAs) are first-line therapy in metastatic functional NETs to control symptoms and for disease control in functional and non-functional NETs. Somatostatin's discovery in 1973 resulted in its first therapeutic use a year later [222, 223]. The presence of somatostatin receptors on well-differentiated NETs, especially subtypes 2 and 5, focused the development of ligands for these receptors [224]. The early challenge was to develop peptides that were stable to circulating peptidases and dipeptidases that limited native somatostatin's biological half-life to only 2 min. The substitution of naturally occurring L-tryptophan and L-phenylalanine amino acids for their respective D-isomers not only maintained somatostatin's biologic activity but also increased the congener's half-life to 120 min by slowing its enzymatic degradation [225].

The effectiveness of SMSAs in inhibiting the secretion of biogenic amines and other vasoactive mediators resulting in either complete or partial control of carcinoid syndrome (flushing and/or secretory diarrhea) in 40–90% of patients resulted in octreotide's FDA approval with only physician-held Investigational New Drug (IND) Application in 1988 [226–229]. Octreotide (100–500 μg) subcutaneously administered 2–3 times per day was the standard of care until the monthly intramuscular microencapsulated formation (octreotide long-acting repeatable, 10, 20, 30 mg) was FDA approved 11 years later [229, 230]. The addition of lanreotide's monthly depot formulations (60, 90, 120 mg) was FDA approved in 2014 as an antineoplastic agent and 3 years later for carcinoid syndrome control [231–233]. As these depot formulations do not control symptoms for the entire 30-day period, immediate release octreotide is prescribed for "breakthrough" symptoms [230, 234].

SMSAs slow gut motility, inhibit intestinal secretory function, and decrease pancreatic exocrine function [229, 235]. Nausea from the decreased motility may result with initial dosing that usually resolves within a week. A test dose of 50–100 μg of immediate release octreotide is recommended prior to depot administration. For a small number of patients who may be allergic or intolerant to the glucose star polymer, D,L-lactic and glycolic acids copolymer (similar to that in absorbable suture material), the immediate release formulation of octreotide or lanreotide depot are options. Hyperglycemia, steatorrhea, gallstones are additional potential adverse effects of the SMSAs with rare hypoglycemia reported [236].

SMSA dose selection is based on the extent of disease and the severity of symptoms. Dose titration with either subcutaneous or intramuscular formulations may improve symptom control without worsening adverse effects, in most cases [237, 238]. Above-labeled SMSA doses are frequently prescribed for symptom and sometimes for disease control [239].

Everolimus

The mammalian target of rapamycin (mTOR), a serine/threonine kinase, regulates cellular processes including growth, proliferation, and protein synthesis. Inhibiting mTOR with everolimus improves PFS by 7 months when compared to placebo in intestinal NETs without carcinoid syndrome [240]. An earlier trial, RADIANT-2, in functional GEPNETs reported 5.1 months increase in PFS in the combination of everolimus and octreotide LAR group when compared to octreotide LAR alone but the hazard ratio (HR) between the groups was not statistically significant [241]. Everolimus is considered second-line therapy in progressive nonfunctional intestinal NETs (RADIANT-4) and first-line therapy in SSTR-negative disease [240, 242]. Real world data shows that the adverse effects of everolimus are increased when everolimus therapy follows PRRT and/or cytotoxic chemotherapy [243]. In addition, pneumonitis is significantly greater when everolimus follows PRRT and/or cytotoxic chemotherapy [244]. Clinical trials evaluating everolimus in combination with chemotherapy, molecularly targeted therapy, PRRT, and radiotherapy are in progress.

Telotristat Ethyl (TE)

The management of SMSA refractory secretory diarrhea includes inhibiting serotonin synthesis with TE, an orally administered 5-hydroxytryptophan inhibitor. The rate-limiting step in serotonin metabolism is the initial enzymatic conversion from tryptophan to 5-hydroxytryptophan [245]. TE selectively inhibits only 1 of the 2 tryptophan hydroxylase isoforms, thus not significantly impacting CNS serotonin [246]. Phase 3 registrational clinical trials comparing 2 doses of TE (500 mg and 250 mg every 8 h) to placebo demonstrated that TE not only significantly reduced mean daily bowel movement frequency but also urinary 5-HIAA levels without inducing significant mood disturbances at the FDA approved 250 mg every 8 h dose [247–249].

Serotonin pathways are implicated in tumor progression [250]. Preclinical data suggests some tumors may be significantly inhibited by blocking serotonin [251, 252]. Survival of metastatic NET TE-treated patients may be greater than that prior to TE but further clinical trials are necessary to firmly establish [253].

As lowering serotonin systemic exposure may also be important in delaying or preventing carcinoid heart disease, a prospective trial is in progress to offer future guidance [254]. With serotonin not implicated as a mediator of carcinoid flushing [79], TE is not considered effective nor indicated in controlling SMSA refractory flushing.

Interferons

Interferon alfa (IFNa) is an option for controlling refractory carcinoid syndrome symptoms [255]. The interferons exert their antitumor effects by stimulating T cells, promoting apoptosis, inhibiting angiogenesis, and inducing cell cycle arrest. A prospective study of IFNa-2a while demonstrating a transient effectiveness in reducing flushing and diarrheal symptoms, its toxicity outweighed any benefits [256]. In retrospective series, low doses (3–5 million units up to 3–5 times weekly) of IFNa-2b reduce flushing and diarrhea in 40–50% of SMSA refractory patients and induce a 10% response rate [257, 258]. A Southwest Oncology Group phase III study (S0518) randomized NET patients with progressive disease to either IFNa-2b five million units 3 times/week or bevacizumab. IFNa-2b resulted in a 4% objective tumor response [259]. Pegylated formulations of INFa are better tolerated but not approved in the United States [260]. Despite the effectiveness of the interferons in NETs, the lack of insurance support for the weekly pegylated formulations and the high incidence of adverse effects with daily or multiple times/week administration (i.e., fatigue, depression, chills, low grade fever, muscle aches) limit their use to refractory NETs.

Cytotoxic Chemotherapy

Prior to the development of molecularly targeted agents, cytotoxic chemotherapy was extensively investigated. In metastatic WD small bowel NET, non-radiologically measured response rates as per physical exams in streptozocin-based chemotherapy in combination with 5-fluorouracil vs. cyclophosphamide were reported as 44% and 37%, respectively, with no significant differences in median overall survival calculated from the time of diagnosis of "unresectable malignant disease" between the two arms [261]. Doxorubicin and dacarbazine (DTIC) were also investigated alone and with streptozotocin/5-FU/cyclophosphamide in varying combinations with response rates ranging from 16% to 33% and median survivals ranging between 10.8 and 20 months [262–265].

As the pathologic classification evolved in NETs, WD G2 and G3 subtypes with higher proliferative indices, cytotoxic chemotherapy has a role, especially when tumor growth is <6–12 months, bulky disease, or dedifferentiation to a more aggressive histology. A Ki-67 proliferative index ranging from 3 to 20% suggests tumor sensitivity to capecitabine/temozolomide (CapeTem) combination therapy though intestinal primaries comprised only 19% of the 79 patients [266]. A retrospective review of 32 small intestinal NET patients, 5 of 6 "high-grade" patients responded to a capecitabine/temozolomide regimen with only 1 of 23 "low/intermediate-grade" disease with a response [267]. Of the 9 reported studies of CapeTem in 231 patients, intestinal NETs were too few to offer future guidance [268]. CapeTem's most common adverse events include thrombocytopenia, lymphopenia, and palmar-plantar erythrodysesthesia. Nausea is usually worse during the 5 days of temozolomide and well controlled by antiemetics. The role of CapeTem remains unclear and is considered not active in WD G1 intestinal NETs. Recommending CapeTem for WD G2 disease intestinal NET is patient dependent with regard to disease bulk, tumor growth rate, and symptoms.

Radiopharmaceutical Therapy (RPT) (Open Source)

^{177}Lutetium (^{177}Lu)-Dotatate

^{177}Lu-dotatate (peptide receptor radioligand therapy or PRRT) is a radiolabeled somatostatin congener that delivers targeted beta-radiation to somatostatin receptor-expressing tumors. Early studies of radiolabeled somatostatin congeners demonstrated significant control of progressive disease and symptoms in NET patients who were refractory to octreotide [269, 270]. Two hundred and twenty-nine patients with progressive small intestinal NETs were randomized in a prospective multicenter phase 3 registrational Neuroendocrine Tumors Therapy trial (NETTER-1) between ^{177}Lu-dotatate with standard dose (30 mg) octreotide vs. high dose (60 mg) octreotide LAR. The primary endpoint, PFS, favored ^{177}Lu-dotatate (median not reached vs. 8.5 months, HR = 0.21; 95% CI 0.13–0.32) with response rates of 18% and 3%, respectively [271]. Quality of life was improved in approximately 75% of patients receiving ^{177}Lu-dotatate [272]. In a large retrospective study, a subset analysis ($N = 360$ of 1214) demonstrated that the PFS compared favorably to other therapeutic options with a 16% objective response rate with no long-term hepatic or renal failure over a 15-year period. These 2 studies provided the data for FDA approval of ^{177}Lu-dotatate in 2018 for GEPNETs patients [273]. Patient selection guidelines, workflow, and consideration for therapy in selected subgroups with hepatic or renal insufficiency are available [274–278].

Iobenguane I-131 (^{131}I-Meta-Iodobenzylguanidine or ^{131}I-MIBG)

RPT may remain an off-label option in sst2 negative NETs patients if there is uptake on a diagnostic ^{123}I-MIBG scan, a guanethidine derivative structurally like noradrenaline [279–284]. The catecholamine transporter complex incorporates MIBG into the cytoplasmic neurosecretory vesicles with a sensitivity between 50 and 61% in intestinal NETs [283, 285]. A Duke University Medical Center retrospective study of all Stage IV WD intestinal NETs patients ($N = 98$) treated with ^{131}I-MIBG between 1986 and 2001 suggested improved survival that was predicted by clinical responses but not by hormonal or radiographic responses. Cumulative doses >400 mCi resulted in significantly better survival than those receiving <400 mCi (4.69 years vs. 1.86 years, respectively, with $p = 0.05$). Five-year overall survival was 42% [286]. Another retrospective review study demonstrated symptomatic improvement and disease stabilization with 11.1 GBq (300 mCi) dose fractions of ^{131}I-MIBG treatment in a subgroup of 20 of 31 patients who were metastatic small intestinal NETs. The median OS was 47 months (95% CI 32–62) with a median PFS of 34 months (95% CI 13–55) [287].

External Beam Radiation Therapy (Closed Source)

Well-differentiated NETs are considered relatively radiation resistant secondary to its low mitotic index, though some series have suggested otherwise [288–291]. Responses to fractionated radiation range from 63% for brain ($N = 8$) to 88–92% for bone ($N = 8$) and spinal cord ($N = 11$) metastases, respectively. Median survival for those patients with brain metastases was 4 months. Radiation to patients with liver ($N = 10$) and extrahepatic disease ($N = 7$) had median overall survivals of 3 and 23 months, respectively [292]. Quality of life improved in those patients receiving external beam for metastatic bone disease as 88% ($N = 8$) had improvement in pain with a median survival of 13 months. For those patients with epidural metastases ($N = 13$), 77% maintained in-field control until their death [292]. Carcinoid syndrome patients are considered resistant to hepatic radiation [290, 293].

The grade of the tumor may account, at least in part, for the variance observed in radiation sensitivity as the pathology in these earlier series was not graded in accordance with the more recent WHO classification [10, 163]. Though intestinal primaries (9%) accounted for low percentage of patients ($N = 45$) reported, open-source radiation continues to a have role for local disease control independent of tumor grade [294]. Other series report few patients with intestinal primaries (2 of 19 treated over a 16 years) but recommend external beam radiation for palliation [295].

Over the last three decades, the tolerability to radiotherapy has improved with "beam shaping" technology such as intensity modulated radiation therapy (IMRT) and stereotactic techniques (SBRT/SRS—stereotactic body radiation therapy/stereotactic radiosurgery). There remains a scarcity of data guiding the use of external beam radiation in intestinal G1/G2 tumors as more experience is in other NET primary sites [296]. Palliative radiation for bone metastases remains the most common use in intestinal NETs for closed source radiation.

20.7.1.5 Surgery

Resecting asymptomatic primaries in the setting of advanced disease is generally recommended in the absence of level I–III evidentiary data [2]. Most studies supporting primary tumor resection in this patient population are small series at single tertiary referral centers [27, 297]; however, review of larger databases (California Cancer Registry, Medicare-SEER, NCDB) confirmed a survival advantage [26, 29, 298].

Surgical debulking of Grade IV NET patients is accompanied by improved survival. The amount of hepatic debulking is not well defined but those patients who underwent >70% hepatic cytoreduction benefitted more than those who had less (overall survival of 134 vs. 38 months, respectively) [299]. Concomitant hepatic debulking with primary resection at the time of initial presentation can be done without increased major morbidity [299–302]. For patients with asymptomatic primaries and hepatic bulk <75%, hepatic cytoreduction neoadjuvantly is a frequent approach at the University of Kentucky [217].

20.7.1.6 Immunotherapy

Malignant neoplasms can hijack immune cell-intrinsic checkpoints and thus evade host defenses. As NETs are typically indolent with a low proliferation rate and mutational burden, inhibitors of immune checkpoints, at least as single agents, would not be predicted to be highly active. A phase II study of spartalizumab, a humanized anti-programmed death protein 1 (PD-1) monoclonal antibody, was evaluated in metastatic well-differentiated Grades 1 and 2 NET patients. The study enrolled 32 intestinal NETs and demonstrated an overall response rate of 3.1%, well below the preset >10% threshold to detect efficacy [303]. Additional studies are needed to define any role of immune mediators in NET management.

20.8 Carcinoid Syndrome

Presenting symptoms are generally attributable to the presence of a well-differentiated (low or intermediate grade) NET metastatic to the liver, are commonly present for years prior to diagnosis, and occur in 20% of patients at the time of diagnosis [34]. Carcinoid syndrome symptoms are typically flushing and/or diarrhea in most cases with a smaller group experiencing wheezing that worsens during a flush [304, 305]. Arthralgia, peptic ulceration, and skin hyperpigmentation can also be present. As early symptoms are vague and nonspecific, misdiagnosis and a delay in diagnosis result in most patients presenting with advanced disease [306]. Provocative factors for flushing include ethanol, emotional upsets, exercise, eating, epinephrine, and pentagastrin [83, 307]. The Valsalva maneuver, hepatic palpation during the physical exam, breast compression during mammography, hepatic embolization or resection may also provoke symptoms and even crises in some circumstances [308–310].

With "hot flashes" being an early symptom in peri-menopausal females, confusion with pathologic "flushing" is common despite distinct differences between the two symptoms and their mechanisms. Menopausal "hot flashes" are typically "whole body," diaphoretic, and sensitive to estrogen therapy. The clinical history assists in distinguishing between these two symptoms which can co-exist in the same patient. Carcinoid syndrome flushing is usually facial, neck, and upper chest and may be accompanied by palmar and plantar erythema. Carcinoid syndrome flushing is usually a dry flush lasting from a few seconds to a few minutes for those primaries arising in the luminal intestinal tract vs. "atypical flushing" lasting 30 min to hours for those primaries originating in the bronchopulmonary system.

Carcinoid diarrhea is typically secretory in nature, may be nocturnal, and not respond to fasting. Weight loss, dehydration, malaise, electrolyte disturbances, and cramping can occur with their severity correlated with tumor bulk. Other manifestations of carcinoid syndrome may be a facial rash mimicking rosacea, cardiac valvular disease (tricuspid insufficiency, pulmonic stenosis), wheezing, and malaise.

Flushing, asthma, and secretory diarrheal symptoms require immediate control by octreotide with most patients responding within a few days to 1–2 weeks (see Fig. 20.1) [311]. The severity of symptoms will determine which octreotide formulation and route of administration are optimal. The subcutaneous route is satisfactory for most patients to control symptoms quickly with eventual conversion, usually within 2–4 weeks, to the intramuscular or depot monthly formulation, octreotide long-acting repeatable (LAR) [230]. Subcutaneous octreotide should be continued for 2 weeks after the initial intramuscular LAR injection as therapeutic levels are achieved. Breakthrough symptoms that occur after conversion to LAR are more common during the week prior to the recurring intramuscular injection and may require subcutaneous dosing depending upon their severity and duration.

Following octreotide initiation, the clinician can focus on other individual factors that may contribute to symptomatology and disease morbidity such as bowel obstruction, high tumor bulk, or concomitant illnesses such as irritable or inflammatory bowel disease, hypertension, dumping symptoms from bowel surgery, bile acid colitis, and malabsorptive syndromes. As a mesenteric desmoplastic process is common with intestinal NETs, chronic abdominal pain and recurrent bowel obstructions may limit quality of life.

As the SMSAs form the backbone of carcinoid syndrome management, it is common for refractory symptoms to eventually develop. Higher dose SMSAs, locoregional tumor debulking, inhibition of serotonin synthesis with telotristat ethyl, and radionuclide therapy may be options. Cytotoxic chemotherapy and everolimus do not significantly induce a response [312].

20.9 Carcinoid Crisis

NET patients are at risk for carcinoid crises defined as the sudden onset of hemodynamic instability usually accompanied by worsening of carcinoid syndrome symptoms. Carcinoid crisis may develop spontaneously or at the time of an invasive procedure as it can be provoked by physical and/or emotional stressors [313, 314]. Carcinoid crisis has occurred with abdominal examinations, hepatic embolotherapy, and procedures including transesophageal echocardiography, percutaneous biopsy, colonoscopy, mammography, and at the time of anesthesia induction [310, 315–319]. The intraoperative occurrence of carcinoid crisis increases postoperative complications [320, 321].

The complex products NETs synthesize, store, and potentially release include serotonin, histamine, bradykinin, tachykinin, kallikrein, and others. The sudden systemic release of these products may be, at least in part, responsible for the sudden cardiovascular instability and the worsening of carcinoid syndrome symptoms. Preventing its occurrence at the time of an "at-risk" procedure/operation is recommended using octreotide, though optimal dosing is not well defined [322–327]. Suppressing release of vasomediators with octreotide may not be enough to prevent intraoperative carcinoid crisis [328].

Carcinoid syndrome symptoms that are unremitting can be life-threatening and should be considered an oncologic emergency. Volume, electrolyte replacement, octreotide, and correcting the metabolic acidosis while improving any diarrheal symptoms are required to reverse clinical deterioration [329, 330]. Identifying and treating the precipitating event such as sepsis, bleeding, or a viral illness is critical in controlling the crisis. Corticosteroids, antibiotics, and infusional octreotide are additional options to consider in the acute care setting [331, 332].

20.9.1 Carcinoid Crisis Prophylaxis

For carcinoid syndrome patients undergoing general anesthesia or an invasive procedure such as embolization, decreasing the risk of carcinoid crises with supplemental octreotide is recommended [323, 333]. The risk for crisis is greater in the more symptomatic patient with greater disease bulk. Resuscitative intraoperative techniques for treating hypotension are unique in that symptoms are generally refractory to fluid resuscitation alone. Adding calcium and/or catecholamines, including low-dose dopamine, may only worsen the deterioration by provoking the additional release of tumor mediators (tachykinins). The blood pressure should be supported by infusion of colloid and octreotide (300–500 μg IV) given immediately [323, 329]. A continuous IV drip of octreotide may be necessary for an indefinite postoperative period. For patients at high risk of carcinoid crisis (significant hepatic tumor involvement and/or history of difficult to control syndrome symptoms), an IV octreotide drip may be initiated prophylactically preoperatively.

There are no guidelines for supplementing patients receiving monthly octreotide LAR. One approach is to schedule an elective procedure within 1–2 weeks after an intramuscular (IM) injection and to provide supplemental continuous infusion of octreotide for the high-risk patient undergoing general anesthesia or any stressful procedure. As octreotide's therapeutic index is wide, the risks are minimal with higher blood levels associated with greater somatostatin receptor occupancy [237].

20.10 Carcinoid Heart Disease

Carcinoid heart disease (CHD) or Hedinger's syndrome involves activation of valvular interstitial cells and infiltration by myofibroblasts resulting in a fibrous, plaque-like endocardial thickening, shortened chordae tendineae, and tricuspid/pulmonic valve cusps immobility [72, 334]. The resulting tricuspid regurgitation and/or pulmonic stenosis is associated with bilateral lower extremity edema, dyspnea, and elevated serum transaminases from the higher hepatic pressures. Echocardiographically confirmed carcinoid heart disease occurred in approximately two-thirds of patients with histologically proven intestinal NETs in the pre-somatostatin era [80]. The incidence of carcinoid heart disease is less in the post-somatostatin era with increased awareness, monitoring NT-proBNP and 5-HIAA levels, and with the increased availability of medical, surgical, and interventional radiologic procedures [335].

Managing carcinoid heart disease includes surveilling with transthoracic and transesophageal echocardiography, controlling carcinoid syndrome with somatostatin congeners, restricting salt and water, using compression stockings, leg elevation, and the monitoring of electrolytes, fluid balance, and weight coupled with the timing of potential surgical intervention. Diuretics can improve lower extremity edema while lowering left-sided cardiac output and lessen fatigue and dyspnea [336, 337]. Lowering serum serotonin levels by inhibiting tryptophan hydroxylase in preventing or managing CHD is not established and is being investigated [338]. The use of bioprosthetic valves over mechanical ones avoids chronic warfarin risks. Minimizing cardiac hepatopathy while maximizing cardiopulmonary function are the major goals in diagnosing and controlling carcinoid heart disease.

20.10.1 NETs Management During the COVID-19 Pandemic

The coronavirus pandemic impacted many aspects of NET healthcare from delaying diagnoses, restricting the timing and number of elective surgical, endoscopic, radioisotopic treatment infusions, and interventional radiologic procedures to increasing the fear of viral infection during monthly SMS depot injections. The Italian Association for NETs reported that the pandemic reduced the number of newly diagnosed cases of NETs and the number of surgical procedures while delaying peptide receptor radiotherapy infusions [339]. In a German center, there were delays in diagnostic procedures with a minority of physicians witnessing a major impact of the pandemic on NET patient medical care [340]. Additional experiences within specialized centers are documented [341, 342]. Specific guidelines are offered to optimize NET management during the pandemic [342, 343].

The COVID-19 pandemic accelerated the integration of telemedicine into routine medical care. Self-administration of octreotide subcutaneously combined with telemedicine offered patients options to effectively control their carcinoid symptoms while allowing physician supervision and reducing COVID-19 exposure simultaneously [344].

20.11 Conclusion and Future Perspective

Well-differentiated intestinal NETs represent a panoply of tumors with future challenges being earlier diagnosis, improved molecularly targeted therapies, and gaining further insights into NET biology. Additional understanding of the genetic and epigenetic alterations, the microenvironment, de novo and acquired resistance, cell adhesion molecules such as CDH17, and the host immune response remain existing areas of research [55, 345–350]. With outcomes that have significantly improved over the last 30 years with the introduction of the somatostatin congeners, expectations are such that survival should continue to improve in the precision medicine era. Treatment options include surgery, surveillance, somatostatin congeners, mTOR inhibition, locoregional therapies, and RPT. The optimal ordering of treatment remains undetermined but generally includes prescribing hormonal therapies earlier as both control of carcinoid syndrome and delaying progression are achieved. The use and sequencing of locoregional therapies, mTOR inhibitors, and RPT may vary between treatment centers as current guidelines identify these options but not their sequencing [351, 352].

Molecular transcripts have the potential for making an earlier and more specific diagnosis than other biomarkers to date [132]. Other exploratory biomarkers may have not only diagnostic value but also therapeutic implications [353]. Improved biomarker surveillance combined with more sensitive scanning techniques should further improve outcomes in patients at high risk for recurrence or a genetic predisposition. With the increasing number of active therapies for metastatic disease, effective adjuvant and potentially neoadjuvant therapies should be realized within the next decade. As a capecitabine and temozolomide adjuvant treatment protocol is in progress for pancreatic NETs, a similar regimen appears to be effective for G2 intestinal NETs [354]. Neoadjuvant treatment in bulky G1 intestinal NETs has potential as locoregional therapies become more effective and may be combined with intraoperative procedures at the time of primary tumor resection.

Improving RPT outcomes in Stage IV intestinal NETs is under investigation [355, 356]. These approaches include the use of DNA repair inhibitors, immunotherapies, tyrosine kinase inhibitors, anti-angiogenics, novel RPT agents, and radiation sensitizers [357–364]. Within the next decade, RPT should expand to include numerous alpha-emitters along with other beta-emitting isotopes and targets other than somatostatin [365–367]. Locally delivering RPT to sites of disease such as intra-hepatic may provide equal efficacy and less systemic radiation exposure, more fractions, and improved outcomes when compared to the current 4 dose systemic treatment strategy.

The intensity of translational research efforts in NETs over the last two decades is impressive. Multiple large global prospective randomized clinical trials in this rare disease were completed and redefined the standard of care. It is with this partnership between industry, academia, and government that further advances in the next two decades will meet, if not exceed, what has been accomplished to date.

Disclosure Statement The authors have nothing to disclose.

References

1. Dasari A, Shen C, Halperin D et al (2017) Trends in the incidence, prevalence, and survival outcomes in patients with neuroendocrine tumors in the United States. JAMA Oncol 3(10):1335–1342
2. Howe JR, Cardona K, Fraker DL et al (2017) The surgical management of small bowel neuroendocrine tumors: consensus guidelines of the north American Neuroendocrine Tumor Society. Pancreas 46(6):715–731
3. Fraenkel M, Kim M, Faggiano A et al (2014) Incidence of gastroenteropancreatic neuroendocrine tumours: a systematic review of the literature. Endocr Relat Cancer 21(3):R153–R163
4. Tsikitis VL, Wertheim BC, Guerrero MA (2012) Trends of incidence and survival of gastrointestinal neuroendocrine tumors in the United States: a seer analysis. J Cancer 3:292–302
5. Moertel CG (1987) Karnofsky memorial lecture. An odyssey in the land of small tumors. J Clin Oncol 5(10):1502–1522
6. Chauhan A, Yu Q, Ray N et al (2018) Global burden of neuroendocrine tumors and changing incidence in Kentucky. Oncotarget 9(27):19245–19254
7. Yao JC, Hassan M, Phan A et al (2008) One hundred years after "carcinoid": epidemiology of and prognostic factors for neuroendocrine tumors in 35,825 cases in the United States. J Clin Oncol 26(18):3063–3072
8. Vinik AI, Chaya C (2016) Clinical presentation and diagnosis of neuroendocrine tumors. Hematol Oncol Clin North Am 30(1):21–48
9. DiSario JA, Burt RW, Vargas H et al (1994) Small bowel cancer: epidemiological and clinical characteristics from a population-based registry. Am J Gastroenterol 89(5):699–701
10. Nagtegaal ID, Odze RD, Klimstra D et al (2020) The 2019 WHO classification of tumours of the digestive system. Histopathology 76(2):182–188
11. Rindi G, Klimstra DS, Abedi-Ardekani B et al (2018) A common classification framework for neuroendocrine neoplasms: an International Agency for Research on Cancer (IARC) and World Health Organization (WHO) expert consensus proposal. Mod Pathol 31(12):1770–1786
12. Perry RR, Vinik AI (1996) Endocrine tumors of the gastrointestinal tract. Annu Rev Med 47:57–68
13. Hallet J, Davis LE, Mahar AL et al (2019) Patterns of symptoms burden in neuroendocrine tumors: a population-based analysis of prospective patient-reported outcomes. Oncologist 24(10):1384–1394
14. Pasieka JL (2009) Carcinoid tumors. Surg Clin North Am 89(5):1123–1137
15. Rodriguez Laval V, Pavel M, Steffen IG et al (2018) Mesenteric fibrosis in midgut neuroendocrine tumors: functionality and radiological features. Neuroendocrinology 106(2):139–147

16. Rindi G, Kloppel G, Alhman H et al (2006) TNM staging of foregut (neuro)endocrine tumors: a consensus proposal including a grading system. Virchows Arch 449(4):395–401
17. Edge SBBD, Compton CC, Fritz AG, Greene FL, Trotti A (eds) (2010) AJCC cancer staging handbook, 7th edn, pp 183–187
18. Shi CH, Woltering E, Deyer DT, Amin MB et al (2017) Neuroendocrine tumors of the colon and rectum. In: AJCC cancer staging manual, 8th edn, pp 395–406
19. Woltering EA, Bergsland EK, Beyer DT et al (2016) Neuroendocrine tumors of the duodenum and ampulla of Vater. In: AJCC cancer staging manual, pp 361–373
20. Woltering EA, Bergsland E, Beyer DT, Amin MB et al (2017) Neuroendocrine tumors of the jejunum and ileum. In: AJCC cancer staging manual, vol eds, 8th edn, pp 389–394
21. Bergsland E, Woltering E, Rindi G et al (2016) Neuroendocrine tumors of the duodenum and ampulla of Vater. In: AJCC cancer staging manual, 8th edn, pp 361–373
22. Zaidi MY, Lopez-Aguiar AG, Dillhoff M et al (2019) Prognostic role of lymph node positivity and number of lymph nodes needed for accurately staging small-bowel neuroendocrine tumors. JAMA Surg 154(2):134–140
23. College_of_American_Pathologists_(CPA) (2020) Protocol for the examination of specimens from patients with neuroendocrine tumors (carcinoid tumors) of the jejunum and ileum. College of American Pathologists, Northfield, IL
24. Landerholm K, Zar N, Andersson RE et al (2011) Survival and prognostic factors in patients with small bowel carcinoid tumour. Br J Surg 98(11):1617–1624
25. Johnson LA, Lavin P, Moertel CG et al (1983) Carcinoids: the association of histologic growth pattern and survival. Cancer 51(5):882–889
26. Tsilimigras DI, Hyer JM, Paredes AZ et al (2021) Resection of primary gastrointestinal neuroendocrine tumor among patients with non-resected metastases is associated with improved survival: a SEER-Medicare analysis. J Gastrointest Surg 25(9):2368–2376
27. Givi B, Pommier SJ, Thompson AK et al (2006) Operative resection of primary carcinoid neoplasms in patients with liver metastases yields significantly better survival. Surgery 140(6):891–897. discussion 897–898
28. van Adrichem RC, Kamp K, Vandamme T et al (2016) Serum neuron-specific enolase level is an independent predictor of overall survival in patients with gastroenteropancreatic neuroendocrine tumors. Ann Oncol 27(4):746–747
29. Lewis A, Raoof M, Ituarte PHG et al (2019) Resection of the primary gastrointestinal neuroendocrine tumor improves survival with or without liver treatment. Ann Surg 270(6):1131–1137
30. Holmager P, Langer SW, Federspiel B et al (2021) Increase of Ki-67 index and influence on mortality in patients with neuroendocrine neoplasms. J Neuroendocrinol 33(9):e13018
31. Zuetenhorst JM, Bonfrer JM, Korse CM et al (2003) Carcinoid heart disease: the role of urinary 5-hydroxyindoleacetic acid excretion and plasma levels of atrial natriuretic peptide, transforming growth factor-beta and fibroblast growth factor. Cancer 97(7):1609–1615
32. Pellikka PA, Tajik AJ, Khandheria BK et al (1993) Carcinoid heart disease. Clinical and echocardiographic spectrum in 74 patients. Circulation 87(4):1188–1196
33. Janson ET, Holmberg L, Stridsberg M et al (1997) Carcinoid tumors: analysis of prognostic factors and survival in 301 patients from a referral center. Ann Oncol 8(7):685–690
34. Halperin DM, Shen C, Dasari A et al (2017) Frequency of carcinoid syndrome at neuroendocrine tumour diagnosis: a population-based study. Lancet Oncol 18(4):525–534
35. Pedraza-Arevalo S, Gahete MD, Alors-Perez E et al (2018) Multilayered heterogeneity as an intrinsic hallmark of neuroendocrine tumors. Rev Endocr Metab Disord 19(2):179–192
36. Reubi JC, Krenning E, Lamberts SW et al (1993) In vitro detection of somatostatin receptors in human tumors. Digestion 54(Suppl 1):76–83
37. Reubi JC, Laissue J, Waser B et al (1994) Expression of somatostatin receptors in normal, inflamed, and neoplastic human gastrointestinal tissues. Ann N Y Acad Sci 733:122–137
38. Reubi JC, Waser B (2003) Concomitant expression of several peptide receptors in neuroendocrine tumours: molecular basis for in vivo multireceptor tumour targeting. Eur J Nucl Med Mol Imaging 30(5):781–793

39. Korner M, Stockli M, Waser B et al (2007) GLP-1 receptor expression in human tumors and human normal tissues: potential for in vivo targeting. J Nucl Med 48(5):736–743
40. Waser B, Rehmann R, Sanchez C et al (2012) Glucose-dependent insulinotropic polypeptide receptors in most gastroenteropancreatic and bronchial neuroendocrine tumors. J Clin Endocrinol Metab 97(2):482–488
41. Reubi JC, Kvols LK, Waser B et al (1990) Detection of somatostatin receptors in surgical and percutaneous needle biopsy samples of carcinoids and islet cell carcinomas. Cancer Res 50(18):5969–5977
42. Friesen SR (1976) APUD tumors of the gastrointestinal tract. Curr Probl Cancer 1(4):1–51
43. Kolby L, Bernhardt P, Levin-Jakobsen AM et al (2003) Uptake of meta-iodobenzylguanidine in neuroendocrine tumours is mediated by vesicular monoamine transporters. Br J Cancer 89(7):1383–1388
44. Hoegerle S, Altehoefer C, Ghanem N et al (2001) Whole-body 18F dopa PET for detection of gastrointestinal carcinoid tumors. Radiology 220(2):373–380
45. Song YS, Lee WW, Chung JH et al (2008) Correlation between FDG uptake and glucose transporter type 1 expression in neuroendocrine tumors of the lung. Lung Cancer 61(1):54–60
46. Terris B, Scoazec JY, Rubbia L et al (1998) Expression of vascular endothelial growth factor in digestive neuroendocrine tumours. Histopathology 32(2):133–138
47. Funa K, Ahgren A (1997) Characterization of platelet-derived growth factor (PDGF) action on a mouse neuroblastoma cell line, NB41, by introduction of an antisense PDGF beta-receptor RNA. Cell Growth Differ 8(8):861–869
48. Serra S, Zheng L, Hassan M et al (2012) The FGFR4-G388R single-nucleotide polymorphism alters pancreatic neuroendocrine tumor progression and response to mTOR inhibition therapy. Cancer Res 72(22):5683–5691
49. Bollard J, Massoma P, Vercherat C et al (2015) The axon guidance molecule semaphorin 3F is a negative regulator of tumor progression and proliferation in ileal neuroendocrine tumors. Oncotarget 6(34):36731–36745
50. Detjen KM, Rieke S, Deters A et al (2010) Angiopoietin-2 promotes disease progression of neuroendocrine tumors. Clin Cancer Res 16(2):420–429
51. Scoazec JY (2013) Angiogenesis in neuroendocrine tumors: therapeutic applications. Neuroendocrinology 97(1):45–56
52. Wiederrecht GJ, Sabers CJ, Brunn GJ et al (1995) Mechanism of action of rapamycin: new insights into the regulation of G1-phase progression in eukaryotic cells. Prog Cell Cycle Res 1:53–71
53. Yao JC, Phan AT, Chang DZ et al (2008) Efficacy of RAD001 (everolimus) and octreotide LAR in advanced low- to intermediate-grade neuroendocrine tumors: results of a phase II study. J Clin Oncol 26(26):4311–4318
54. da Silva A, Bowden M, Zhang S et al (2018) Characterization of the neuroendocrine tumor immune microenvironment. Pancreas 47(9):1123–1129
55. Cives M, Pelle E, Quaresmini D et al (2019) The tumor microenvironment in neuroendocrine tumors: biology and therapeutic implications. Neuroendocrinology 109(2):83–99
56. de Hosson LD, Takkenkamp TJ, Kats-Ugurlu G et al (2020) Neuroendocrine tumours and their microenvironment. Cancer Immunol Immunother 69(8):1449–1459
57. Biomarkers Definitions Working Group (2001) Biomarkers and surrogate endpoints: preferred definitions and conceptual framework. Clin Pharmacol Ther 69(3):89–95
58. Liang W, Yang P, Huang R et al (2019) A combined nomogram model to preoperatively predict histologic grade in pancreatic neuroendocrine tumors. Clin Cancer Res 25(2):584–594
59. Ellison TA, Wolfgang CL, Shi C et al (2014) A single institution's 26-year experience with nonfunctional pancreatic neuroendocrine tumors: a validation of current staging systems and a new prognostic nomogram. Ann Surg 259(2):204–212
60. Pulvirenti A, Javed AA, Landoni L et al (2019) Multi-institutional development and external validation of a nomogram to predict recurrence after curative resection of pancreatic neuroendocrine tumors. Ann Surg 274:1051

61. Fang C, Wang W, Feng X et al (2017) Nomogram individually predicts the overall survival of patients with gastroenteropancreatic neuroendocrine neoplasms. Br J Cancer 117(10):1544–1550
62. Herrera-Martinez AD, Hofland LJ, Galvez Moreno MA et al (2019) Neuroendocrine neoplasms: current and potential diagnostic, predictive and prognostic markers. Endocr Relat Cancer 26(3):R157–R179
63. Sansone A, Lauretta R, Vottari S et al (2019) Specific and non-specific biomarkers in neuroendocrine gastroenteropancreatic tumors. Cancers (Basel) 11(8):1113
64. Oberg K, Couvelard A, Delle Fave G et al (2017) ENETS consensus guidelines for standard of care in neuroendocrine tumours: biochemical markers. Neuroendocrinology 105(3):201–211
65. Aluri V, Dillon JS (2017) Biochemical testing in neuroendocrine tumors. Endocrinol Metab Clin North Am 46(3):669–677
66. Shah MH, Goldner WS, Halfdanarson TR et al (2018) NCCN guidelines insights: neuroendocrine and adrenal tumors, version 2.2018. J Natl Compr Canc Netw 16(6):693–702
67. Korse CM, Taal BG, Bonfrer JMG et al (2011) An elevated progastrin-releasing peptide level in patients with well-differentiated neuroendocrine tumours indicates a primary tumour in the lung and predicts a shorter survival. Ann Oncol 22(12):2625–2630
68. Chan DL, Clarke SJ, Diakos CI et al (2017) Prognostic and predictive biomarkers in neuroendocrine tumours. Crit Rev Oncol Hematol 113:268–282
69. Chauhan A, Prieur A, Kolesar J et al (2022) hPG80 (Circulating Progastrin), a novel blood-based biomarker for detection of poorly differentiated neuroendocrine carcinoma and well differentiated neuroendocrine tumors. Cancers (Basel) 14(4):863
70. Erspamer V, Asero B (1952) Identification of enteramine, the specific hormone of the enterochromaffin cell system, as 5-hydroxytryptamine. Nature 169(4306):800–801
71. Rapport MM, Green AA, Page IH (1948) Serum vasoconstrictor, serotonin; isolation and characterization. J Biol Chem 176(3):1243–1251
72. Thorson A, Biorck G, Bjorkman G et al (1954) Malignant carcinoid of the small intestine with metastases to the liver, valvular disease of the right side of the heart (pulmonary stenosis and tricuspid regurgitation without septal defects), peripheral vasomotor symptoms, bronchoconstriction, and an unusual type of cyanosis; a clinical and pathologic syndrome. Am Heart J 47(5):795–817
73. Plassat JL, Amlaiky N, Hen R (1993) Molecular cloning of a mammalian serotonin receptor that activates adenylate cyclase. Mol Pharmacol 44(2):229–236
74. Yamada Y, Post SR, Wang K et al (1992) Cloning and functional characterization of a family of human and mouse somatostatin receptors expressed in brain, gastrointestinal tract, and kidney. Proc Natl Acad Sci U S A 89(1):251–255
75. Bender DA (1983) Biochemistry of tryptophan in health and disease. Mol Aspects Med 6(2):101–197
76. Coulson WF, Wardle E, Jepson JB (1968) Phenylalanine hydroxylase activity towards two substrates simultaneously: enhancement of inhibition by phenylalanine, tryptophan and their derivatives. Biochim Biophys Acta 167(1):99–109
77. Banskota S, Ghia JE, Khan WI (2019) Serotonin in the gut: blessing or a curse. Biochimie 161:56–64
78. De Ponti F (2004) Pharmacology of serotonin: what a clinician should know. Gut 53(10):1520–1535
79. Oates JA, Melmon K, Sjoerdsma A et al (1964) Release of a Kinin peptide in the carcinoid syndrome. Lancet 1(7332):514–517
80. Lundin L, Norheim I, Landelius J et al (1988) Carcinoid heart disease: relationship of circulating vasoactive substances to ultrasound-detectable cardiac abnormalities. Circulation 77(2):264–269
81. Gustafsson BI, Tommeras K, Nordrum I et al (2005) Long-term serotonin administration induces heart valve disease in rats. Circulation 111(12):1517–1522

82. Norheim I, Theodorsson-Norheim E, Brodin E et al (1986) Tachykinins in carcinoid tumors: their use as a tumor marker and possible role in the carcinoid flush*. J Clin Endocrinol Metabol 63(3):605–612
83. Feldman JM, O'Dorisio TM (1986) Role of neuropeptides and serotonin in the diagnosis of carcinoid tumors. Am J Med 81(6B):41–48
84. Ardill JE, O'Dorisio TM (2010) Circulating biomarkers in neuroendocrine tumors of the enteropancreatic tract: application to diagnosis, monitoring disease, and as prognostic indicators. Endocrinol Metab Clin North Am 39(4):777–790
85. Martin AM, Young RL, Leong L et al (2017) The diverse metabolic roles of peripheral serotonin. Endocrinology 158(5):1049–1063
86. Côté F, Thévenot E, Fligny C et al (2003) Disruption of the nonneuronal tph1 gene demonstrates the importance of peripheral serotonin in cardiac function. Proc Natl Acad Sci 100(23):13525–13530
87. Zhang X, Beaulieu J-M, Sotnikova TD et al (2004) Tryptophan hydroxylase-2 controls brain serotonin synthesis. Science 305(5681):217–217
88. Tormey WP, FitzGerald RJ (1995) The clinical and laboratory correlates of an increased urinary 5-hydroxyindoleacetic acid. Postgrad Med J 71(839):542–545
89. Tellez MR, Mamikunian G, O'Dorisio TM et al (2013) A single fasting plasma 5-HIAA value correlates with 24-hour urinary 5-HIAA values and other biomarkers in midgut neuroendocrine tumors (NETs). Pancreas 42(3):405–410
90. Becker A, Schalin-Jäntti C, Itkonen O (2021) Comparison of serum and urinary 5-Hydroxyindoleacetic acid as biomarker for neuroendocrine neoplasms. J Endocr Soc 5(8):bvab106
91. Carling RS, Degg TJ, Allen KR et al (2002) Evaluation of whole blood serotonin and plasma and urine 5-hydroxyindole acetic acid in diagnosis of carcinoid disease. Ann Clin Biochem 39(Pt 6):577–582
92. Meijer WG, Kema IP, Volmer M et al (2000) Discriminating capacity of indole markers in the diagnosis of carcinoid tumors. Clin Chem 46(10):1588–1596
93. Feldman JM (1986) Urinary serotonin in the diagnosis of carcinoid tumors. Clin Chem 32(5):840–844
94. van der Horst-Schrivers AN, Post WJ, Kema IP et al (2007) Persistent low urinary excretion of 5-HIAA is a marker for favourable survival during follow-up in patients with disseminated midgut carcinoid tumours. Eur J Cancer 43(18):2651–2657
95. Formica V, Wotherspoon A, Cunningham D et al (2007) The prognostic role of WHO classification, urinary 5-hydroxyindoleacetic acid and liver function tests in metastatic neuroendocrine carcinomas of the gastroenteropancreatic tract. Br J Cancer 96(8):1178–1182
96. Turner GB, Johnston BT, McCance DR et al (2006) Circulating markers of prognosis and response to treatment in patients with midgut carcinoid tumours. Gut 55(11):1586–1591
97. O'Connor DT, Deftos LJ (1986) Secretion of chromogranin a by peptide-producing endocrine neoplasms. N Engl J Med 314(18):1145–1151
98. Nobels FR, Kwekkeboom DJ, Coopmans W et al (1997) Chromogranin a as serum marker for neuroendocrine neoplasia: comparison with neuron-specific enolase and the alpha-subunit of glycoprotein hormones. J Clin Endocrinol Metab 82(8):2622–2628
99. Winkler H, Fischer-Colbrie R (1992) The chromogranins a and B: the first 25 years and future perspectives. Neuroscience 49(3):497–528
100. Welin S, Stridsberg M, Cunningham J et al (2009) Elevated plasma chromogranin a is the first indication of recurrence in radically operated midgut carcinoid tumors. Neuroendocrinology 89(3):302–307
101. Mahata SK, Corti A (2019) Chromogranin A and its fragments in cardiovascular, immunometabolic, and cancer regulation. Ann N Y Acad Sci 1455(1):34–58
102. Papantoniou D, Gronberg M, Landerholm K et al (2021) Assessment of hormonal levels as prognostic markers and of their optimal cut-offs in small intestinal neuroendocrine tumours grade 2. Endocrine 72(3):893–904

103. Dam G, Gronbaek H, Sorbye H et al (2020) Prospective study of chromogranin a as a predictor of progression in patients with pancreatic, small-intestinal, and unknown primary neuroendocrine tumors. Neuroendocrinology 110(3–4):217–224
104. Fuksiewicz M, Kowalska M, Kolasinska-Cwikla A et al (2018) Prognostic value of chromogranin a in patients with GET/NEN in the pancreas and the small intestine. Endocr Connect 7(6):803–810
105. Rogowski W, Wachula E, Lewczuk A et al (2017) Baseline chromogranin a and its dynamics are prognostic markers in gastroenteropancreatic neuroendocrine tumors. Future Oncol 13(12):1069–1079
106. Modlin IM, Gustafsson BI, Moss SF et al (2010) Chromogranin A—biological function and clinical utility in neuro endocrine tumor disease. Ann Surg Oncol 17(9):2427–2443
107. Campana D, Nori F, Piscitelli L et al (2007) Chromogranin a: is it a useful marker of neuroendocrine tumors? J Clin Oncol 25(15):1967–1973
108. Ardill JE, Erikkson B (2003) The importance of the measurement of circulating markers in patients with neuroendocrine tumours of the pancreas and gut. Endocr Relat Cancer 10(4):459–462
109. Singh S, Law C (2012) Chromogranin a: a sensitive biomarker for the detection and post-treatment monitoring of gastroenteropancreatic neuroendocrine tumors. Expert Rev Gastroenterol Hepatol 6(3):313–334
110. Bajetta E, Ferrari L, Martinetti A et al (1999) Chromogranin a, neuron specific enolase, carcinoembryonic antigen, and hydroxyindole acetic acid evaluation in patients with neuroendocrine tumors. Cancer 86(5):858–865
111. Raines D, Chester M, Diebold AE et al (2012) A prospective evaluation of the effect of chronic proton pump inhibitor use on plasma biomarker levels in humans. Pancreas 41(4):508–511
112. Khan TM, Garg M, Warner RR et al (2016) Elevated serum Pancreastatin is an indicator of hepatic metastasis in patients with small bowel neuroendocrine tumors. Pancreas 45(7):1032–1035
113. Sherman SK, Maxwell JE, O'Dorisio MS et al (2014) Pancreastatin predicts survival in neuroendocrine tumors. Ann Surg Oncol 21(9):2971–2980
114. Stronge RL, Turner GB, Johnston BT et al (2008) A rapid rise in circulating pancreastatin in response to somatostatin analogue therapy is associated with poor survival in patients with neuroendocrine tumours. Ann Clin Biochem 45(Pt 6):560–566
115. O'Dorisio TM, Krutzik SR, Woltering EA et al (2010) Development of a highly sensitive and specific carboxy-terminal human pancreastatin assay to monitor neuroendocrine tumor behavior. Pancreas 39(5):611–616
116. Desai DC, O'Dorisio TM, Schirmer WJ et al (2001) Serum pancreastatin levels predict response to hepatic artery chemoembolization and somatostatin analogue therapy in metastatic neuroendocrine tumors. Regul Pept 96(3):113–117
117. Bloomston M, Al-Saif O, Klemanski D et al (2007) Hepatic artery chemoembolization in 122 patients with metastatic carcinoid tumor: lessons learned. J Gastrointest Surg 11(3):264–271
118. Severini C, Improta G, Falconieri-Erspamer G et al (2002) The tachykinin peptide family. Pharmacol Rev 54(2):285–322
119. Bishop AE, Hamid QA, Adams C et al (1989) Expression of tachykinins by ileal and lung carcinoid tumors assessed by combined in situ hybridization, immunocytochemistry, and radioimmunoassay. Cancer 63(6):1129–1137
120. Woltering EA, Voros BA, Thiagarajan R et al (2018) Plasma neurokinin A levels predict survival in well-differentiated neuroendocrine tumors of the small bowel. Pancreas 47(7):843–848
121. Diebold AE, Boudreaux JP, Wang YZ et al (2012) Neurokinin A levels predict survival in patients with stage IV well differentiated small bowel neuroendocrine neoplasms. Surgery 152(6):1172–1176
122. Carney D, Ihde D, Cohen M et al (1982) Serum neuron-specific enolase: a marker for disease extent and response to therapy of small-CELL lung cancer. Lancet 319(8272):583–585

123. Baudin E, Gigliotti A, Ducreux M et al (1998) Neuron-specific enolase and chromogranin a as markers of neuroendocrine tumours. Br J Cancer 78(8):1102–1107
124. Oberg K (2011) Circulating biomarkers in gastroenteropancreatic neuroendocrine tumours. Endocr Relat Cancer 18(Suppl 1):S17–S25
125. Yao JC, Lombard-Bohas C, Baudin E et al (2010) Daily oral everolimus activity in patients with metastatic pancreatic neuroendocrine tumors after failure of cytotoxic chemotherapy: a phase II trial. J Clin Oncol 28(1):69–76
126. Modlin IM, Drozdov I, Kidd M (2013) The identification of gut neuroendocrine tumor disease by multiple synchronous transcript analysis in blood. PLoS One 8(5):e63364
127. Modlin IM, Kidd M, Bodei L et al (2015) The clinical utility of a novel blood-based multi-transcriptome assay for the diagnosis of neuroendocrine tumors of the gastrointestinal tract. Am J Gastroenterol 110(8):1223–1232
128. van Treijen MJC, Korse CM, van Leeuwaarde RS et al (2018) Blood transcript profiling for the detection of neuroendocrine tumors: results of a large independent validation study. Front Endocrinol (Lausanne) 9:740
129. Modlin IM, Kidd M, Malczewska A et al (2018) The NETest: the clinical utility of multigene blood analysis in the diagnosis and Management of Neuroendocrine Tumors. Endocrinol Metab Clin North Am 47(3):485–504
130. Filosso PL, Kidd M, Roffinella M et al (2017) The utility of blood neuroendocrine gene transcript measurement in the diagnosis of bronchopulmonary neuroendocrine tumours and as a tool to evaluate surgical resection and disease progression†. Eur J Cardiothorac Surg 53(3):631–639
131. Modlin IM, Kidd M, Oberg K et al (2021) Early identification of residual disease after neuroendocrine tumor resection using a liquid biopsy multigenomic mRNA signature (NETest). Ann Surg Oncol 28:7506
132. Oberg K, Califano A, Strosberg JR et al (2020) A meta-analysis of the accuracy of a neuroendocrine tumor mRNA genomic biomarker (NETest) in blood. Ann Oncol 31(2):202–212
133. Lu J, Getz G, Miska EA et al (2005) MicroRNA expression profiles classify human cancers. Nature 435(7043):834–838
134. Li SC, Essaghir A, Martijn C et al (2013) Global microRNA profiling of well-differentiated small intestinal neuroendocrine tumors. Mod Pathol 26(5):685–696
135. Ruebel K, Leontovich AA, Stilling GA et al (2010) MicroRNA expression in ileal carcinoid tumors: downregulation of microRNA-133a with tumor progression. Mod Pathol 23(3):367–375
136. Bowden M, Zhou CW, Zhang S et al (2017) Profiling of metastatic small intestine neuroendocrine tumors reveals characteristic miRNAs detectable in plasma. Oncotarget 8(33):54331–54344
137. Hoffmann KM, Furukawa M, Jensen RT (2005) Duodenal neuroendocrine tumors: classification, functional syndromes, diagnosis and medical treatment. Best Pract Res Clin Gastroenterol 19(5):675–697
138. Klimstra DS, Modlin IR, Coppola D et al (2010) The pathologic classification of neuroendocrine tumors: a review of nomenclature, grading, and staging systems. Pancreas 39(6):707–712
139. Shah CP, Mramba LK, Bishnoi R et al (2019) Survival trends of metastatic small intestinal neuroendocrine tumor: a population-based analysis of SEER database. J Gastrointest Oncol 10(5):869–877
140. Lipinski M, Rydzewska G, Foltyn W et al (2017) Gastroduodenal neuroendocrine neoplasms, including gastrinoma—management guidelines (recommended by the polish network of neuroendocrine tumours). Endokrynol Pol 68(2):138–153
141. Jensen RT (2004) Gastrinomas: advances in diagnosis and management. Neuroendocrinology 80(Suppl 1):23–27
142. Krejs GJ, Orci L, Conlon JM et al (1979) Somatostatinoma syndrome. Biochemical, morphologic and clinical features. N Engl J Med 301(6):285–292

143. Okubo Y, Wakayama M, Nemoto T et al (2011) Literature survey on epidemiology and pathology of gangliocytic paraganglioma. BMC Cancer 11:187
144. Tran CG, Sherman SK, Suraju MO et al (2022) Management of duodenal neuroendocrine tumors: surgical versus endoscopic mucosal resection. Ann Surg Oncol 29(1):75–84
145. Langhans T (1867) Ueber einen Drüsenpolyp im ileum. Arch Pathol Anat Phys Klin Med 38(4):559–560
146. Oberndorfer S (1907) Karzinoide tumoren des dunndarms. Frankfurt Z Path 1:426–432
147. Lubarsch O (1888) Ueber den primären Krebs des Ileum nebst Bemerkungen über das gleichzeitige Vorkommen von Krebs und Tuberculose. Arch Pathol Anat Phys Klin Med 111(2):280–317
148. Kloppel G (2007) Tumour biology and histopathology of neuroendocrine tumours. Best Pract Res Clin Endocrinol Metab 21(1):15–31
149. Levy AD, Sobin LH (2007) From the archives of the AFIP: gastrointestinal carcinoids: imaging features with clinicopathologic comparison. Radiographics 27(1):237–257
150. Sweeney JF, Rosemurgy AS (1997) Carcinoid tumors of the gut. Cancer Control 4(1):18–24
151. Akerstrom G, Hellman P, Hessman O et al (2005) Management of midgut carcinoids. J Surg Oncol 89(3):161–169
152. Modlin IM, Lye KD, Kidd M (2003) A 5-decade analysis of 13,715 carcinoid tumors. Cancer 97:934
153. Modlin IM, Sandor A (1997) An analysis of 8305 cases of carcinoid tumors. Cancer 79:813
154. Chablaney S, Zator ZA, Kumta NA (2017) Diagnosis and management of rectal neuroendocrine tumors. Clin Endosc 50(6):530–536
155. Anthony LB, Strosberg JR, Klimstra DS et al (2010) The NANETS consensus guidelines for the diagnosis and management of gastrointestinal neuroendocrine tumors (nets): well-differentiated nets of the distal colon and rectum. Pancreas 39(6):767–774
156. Jetmore AB, Ray JE, Gathright JB Jr et al (1992) Rectal carcinoids: the most frequent carcinoid tumor. Dis Colon Rectum 35(8):717–725
157. Landry CS, Woodall C, Scoggins CR et al (2008) Analysis of 900 appendiceal carcinoid tumors for a proposed predictive staging system. Arch Surg 143(7):664–670. discussion 670
158. Maggard MA, O'Connell JB, Ko CY (2004) Updated population-based review of carcinoid tumors. Ann Surg 240(1):117–122
159. McCusker ME, Cote TR, Clegg LX et al (2002) Primary malignant neoplasms of the appendix: a population-based study from the surveillance, epidemiology and end-results program, 1973-1998. Cancer 94(12):3307–3312
160. Beger A (1882) Ein Fall von Krebs des Wurmfortsatzes. Berl Klin Wochenschr 41:616–618
161. Connor SJ, Hanna GB, Frizelle FA (1998) Appendiceal tumors: retrospective clinicopathologic analysis of appendiceal tumors from 7,970 appendectomies. Dis Colon Rectum 41(1):75–80
162. Coskun H, Bostanci O, Dilege ME et al (2006) Carcinoid tumors of appendix: treatment and outcome. Ulus Travma Acil Cerrahi Derg 12(2):150–154
163. Niederle MB, Hackl M, Kaserer K et al (2010) Gastroenteropancreatic neuroendocrine tumours: the current incidence and staging based on the WHO and European neuroendocrine tumour society classification: an analysis based on prospectively collected parameters. Endocr Relat Cancer 17(4):909–918
164. Schmutzer KJ, Bayar M, Zaki AE et al (1975) Tumors of the appendix. Dis Colon Rectum 18(4):324–331
165. Benedix F, Reimer A, Gastinger I et al (2010) Primary appendiceal carcinoma—epidemiology, surgery and survival: results of a German Multi-Center Study. Eur J Surg Oncol 36(8):763–771
166. Hemminki K, Li X (2001) Incidence trends and risk factors of carcinoid tumors: a nationwide epidemiologic study from Sweden. Cancer 92(8):2204–2210
167. Hsu C, Rashid A, Xing Y et al (2013) Varying malignant potential of appendiceal neuroendocrine tumors: importance of histologic subtype. J Surg Oncol 107(2):136–143

168. Sadot E, Keidar A, Shapiro R et al (2013) Laparoscopic accuracy in prediction of appendiceal pathology: oncologic and inflammatory aspects. Am J Surg 206(5):805–809
169. Shaib WL, Goodman M, Chen Z et al (2017) Incidence and survival of appendiceal mucinous neoplasms: a SEER analysis. Am J Clin Oncol 40(6):569–573
170. Moertel CG, Weiland LH, Nagorney DM et al (1987) Carcinoid tumor of the appendix: treatment and prognosis. N Engl J Med 317(27):1699–1701
171. Roggo A, Wood WC, Ottinger LW (1993) Carcinoid tumors of the appendix. Ann Surg 217(4):385–390
172. Goede AC, Caplin ME, Winslet MC (2003) Carcinoid tumour of the appendix. Br J Surg 90(11):1317–1322
173. O'Donnell ME, Badger SA, Beattie GC et al (2007) Malignant neoplasms of the appendix. Int J Colorectal Dis 22(10):1239–1248
174. Grozinsky-Glasberg S, Alexandraki KI, Barak D et al (2013) Current size criteria for the management of neuroendocrine tumors of the appendix: are they valid? Clinical experience and review of the literature. Neuroendocrinology 98(1):31–37
175. Grossman AB, Kelly P, Rockall A et al (2006) Cushing's syndrome caused by an occult source: difficulties in diagnosis and management. Nat Clin Pract Endocrinol Metab 2(11):642–647
176. Perakakis N, Laubner K, Keck T et al (2011) Ectopic ACTH-syndrome due to a neuroendocrine tumour of the appendix. Exp Clin Endocrinol Diabetes 119(9):525–529
177. Pickhardt PJ, Levy AD, Rohrmann CA Jr et al (2003) Primary neoplasms of the appendix: radiologic spectrum of disease with pathologic correlation. Radiographics 23(3):645–662
178. Wallace S, Ajani JA, Charnsangavej C et al (1996) Carcinoid tumors: imaging procedures and interventional radiology. World J Surg 20(2):147–156
179. Pape UF, Niederle B, Costa F et al (2016) ENETS consensus guidelines for neuroendocrine neoplasms of the appendix (excluding goblet Cell carcinomas). Neuroendocrinology 103(2):144–152
180. Pape UF, Perren A, Niederle B et al (2012) ENETS consensus guidelines for the management of patients with neuroendocrine neoplasms from the jejuno-ileum and the appendix including goblet cell carcinomas. Neuroendocrinology 95(2):135–156
181. Alexandraki KI, Kaltsas GA, Grozinsky-Glasberg S et al (2016) Appendiceal neuroendocrine neoplasms: diagnosis and management. Endocr Relat Cancer 23(1):R27–R41
182. Fornaro R, Frascio M, Sticchi C et al (2007) Appendectomy or right hemicolectomy in the treatment of appendiceal carcinoid tumors? Tumori 93(6):587–590
183. Anderson JR, Wilson BG (1985) Carcinoid tumours of the appendix. Br J Surg 72(7):545–546
184. Mullen JT, Savarese DM (2011) Carcinoid tumors of the appendix: a population-based study. J Surg Oncol 104(1):41–44
185. Alexandraki KI, Griniatsos J, Bramis KI et al (2011) Clinical value of right hemicolectomy for appendiceal carcinoids using pathologic criteria. J Endocrinol Invest 34(4):255–259
186. Syracuse DC, Perzin KH, Price JB et al (1979) Carcinoid tumors of the appendix. Mesoappendiceal extension and nodal metastases. Ann Surg 190(1):58–63
187. MacGillivray DC, Heaton RB, Rushin JM et al (1992) Distant metastasis from a carcinoid tumor of the appendix less than one centimeter in size. Surgery 111(4):466–471
188. Ganeshan D, Bhosale P, Yang T et al (2013) Imaging features of carcinoid tumors of the gastrointestinal tract. Am J Roentgenol 201(4):773–786
189. Paulson EK, McDermott VG, Keogan MT et al (1998) Carcinoid metastases to the liver: role of triple-phase helical CT. Radiology 206(1):143–150
190. Horton KM, Lawler LP, Fishman EK (2003) CT findings in sclerosing mesenteritis (panniculitis): spectrum of disease. Radiographics 23(6):1561–1567
191. Ballantyne GH, Savoca PE, Flannery JT et al (1992) Incidence and mortality of carcinoids of the colon. Data from the Connecticut Tumor Registry. Cancer 69(10):2400–2405
192. Dromain C, de Baere T, Lumbroso J et al (2005) Detection of liver metastases from endocrine tumors: a prospective comparison of somatostatin receptor scintigraphy, computed tomography, and magnetic resonance imaging. J Clin Oncol 23(1):70–78

193. Elias D, Lefevre JH, Duvillard P et al (2010) Hepatic metastases from neuroendocrine tumors with a "thin slice" pathological examination: they are many more than you think .... Ann Surg 251(2):307–310
194. Morse B, Jeong D, Thomas K et al (2017) Magnetic resonance imaging of neuroendocrine tumor hepatic metastases: does hepatobiliary phase imaging improve lesion conspicuity and Interobserver agreement of lesion measurements? Pancreas 46(9):1219–1224
195. Paulsen SR, Huprich JE, Fletcher JG et al (2006) CT enterography as a diagnostic tool in evaluating small bowel disorders: review of clinical experience with over 700 cases. Radiographics 26(3):641–657. discussion 657–662
196. Dohan A, El Fattach H, Barat M et al (2016) Neuroendocrine tumors of the small bowel: evaluation with MR-enterography. Clin Imaging 40(3):541–547
197. Khapra AP, Warner RRP, Lewis B (2005) The capsule identifies obscure primary carcinoids in the small intestine: 221. Am J Gastroenterol 100:S95
198. Cheifetz AS, Kornbluth AA, Legnani PE et al (2004) Incidence and outcome of the retained video capsule endoscope (CE) in Crohn's disease (CD): 807. Am J Gastroenterol 99:S262
199. Enns RA, Hookey L, Armstrong D et al (2017) Clinical practice guidelines for the use of video capsule endoscopy. Gastroenterology 152(3):497–514
200. Reubi JC, Maurer R, von Werder K et al (1987) Somatostatin receptors in human endocrine tumors. Cancer Res 47(2):551–558
201. Lamberts SW, Hofland LJ, van Koetsveld PM et al (1990) Parallel in vivo and in vitro detection of functional somatostatin receptors in human endocrine pancreatic tumors: consequences with regard to diagnosis, localization, and therapy. J Clin Endocrinol Metab 71(3):566–574
202. Krenning EP, Kwekkeboom DJ, Oei HY et al (1994) Somatostatin-receptor scintigraphy in gastroenteropancreatic tumors. An overview of European results. Ann N Y Acad Sci 733:416–424
203. Johnbeck CB, Knigge U, Loft A et al (2017) Head-to-head comparison of (64)cu-DOTATATE and (68)Ga-DOTATOC PET/CT: a prospective study of 59 patients with neuroendocrine tumors. J Nucl Med 58(3):451–457
204. Ross EM, Roberts WC (1985) The carcinoid syndrome: comparison of 21 necropsy subjects with carcinoid heart disease to 15 necropsy subjects without carcinoid heart disease. Am J Med 79(3):339–354
205. Meijer WG, van der Veer E, Jager PL et al (2003) Bone metastases in carcinoid tumors: clinical features, imaging characteristics, and markers of bone metabolism. J Nucl Med 44(2):184–191
206. Putzer D, Gabriel M, Henninger B et al (2009) Bone metastases in patients with neuroendocrine tumor: 68Ga-DOTA-Tyr3-octreotide PET in comparison to CT and bone scintigraphy. J Nucl Med 50(8):1214–1221
207. Wang YZ, Diebold A, Boudreaux P et al (2014) Surgical treatment options for rectal carcinoid cancer: local versus low radical excision. Am Surg 80(1):31–35
208. Okubo Y, Kasajima R, Suzuki M et al (2017) Risk factors associated with the progression and metastases of hindgut neuroendocrine tumors: a retrospective study. BMC Cancer 17(1):769
209. Weinstock B, Ward SC, Harpaz N et al (2013) Clinical and prognostic features of rectal neuroendocrine tumors. Neuroendocrinology 98(3):180–187
210. Scherübl H, Jensen RT, Cadiot G et al (2011) Management of early gastrointestinal neuroendocrine neoplasms. World J Gastrointest Endosc 3(7):133–139
211. Yoon JY, Kumta NA, Kim MK (2021) The role of endoscopy in small bowel neuroendocrine tumors. Clin Endosc 54(6):818–824
212. Park SB, Kang DH, Choi CW et al (2018) Clinical outcomes of ligation-assisted endoscopic resection for duodenal neuroendocrine tumors. Medicine (Baltimore) 97(18):e0533
213. Brito HP, Torres IT, Turke KC et al (2021) Comparison of endoscopic resection techniques for duodenal neuroendocrine tumors: systematic review. Endosc Int Open 9(8):e1214–e1221
214. de Mestier L, Lorenzo D, Fine C et al (2019) Endoscopic, transanal, laparoscopic, and transabdominal management of rectal neuroendocrine tumors. Best Pract Res Clin Endocrinol Metab 33(5):101293

215. Tai E, Kennedy S, Farrell A et al (2020) Comparison of transarterial bland and chemoembolization for neuroendocrine tumours: a systematic review and meta-analysis. Curr Oncol 27(6):e537–e546
216. Chen JX, Wileyto EP, Soulen MC (2018) Randomized embolization trial for NeuroEndocrine tumor metastases to the liver (RETNET): study protocol for a randomized controlled trial. Trials 19(1):390
217. Anthony LB, Chauhan A, Wu J et al (2019) Antitumor efficacy of concurrent everolimus with hepatic transarterial bland embolization (evero-embo) in patients with metastatic well differentiated neuroendocrine tumor (NET). J Clin Oncol 37(15_suppl):4115–4115
218. Memon K, Lewandowski RJ, Mulcahy MF et al (2012) Radioembolization for neuroendocrine liver metastases: safety, imaging, and long-term outcomes. Int J Radiat Oncol Biol Phys 83(3):887–894
219. King J, Quinn R, Glenn DM et al (2008) Radioembolization with selective internal radiation microspheres for neuroendocrine liver metastases. Cancer 113(5):921–929
220. Rhee TK (2008) 90Y Radioembolization for metastatic neuroendocrine liver tumors: preliminary results from a multi-institutional experience. Ann Surg 247:1029
221. Currie BM, Nadolski G, Mondschein J et al (2020) Chronic hepatotoxicity in patients with metastatic neuroendocrine tumor: transarterial chemoembolization versus transarterial radioembolization. J Vasc Interv Radiol 31(10):1627–1635
222. Brazeau P, Vale W, Burgus R et al (1973) Hypothalamic polypeptide that inhibits the secretion of immunoreactive pituitary growth hormone. Science 179(4068):77–79
223. Yen SS, Siler TM, DeVane GW (1974) Effect of somatostatin in patients with acromegaly: suppression of growth hormone, prolactin, insulin and glucose levels. N Engl J Med 290(17):935–938
224. Reubi JC, Krenning E, Lamberts SW et al (1990) Somatostatin receptors in malignant tissues. J Steroid Biochem Mol Biol 37(6):1073–1077
225. Bauer W, Briner U, Doepfner W et al (1982) SMS 201-995: a very potent and selective octapeptide analogue of somatostatin with prolonged action. Life Sci 31(11):1133–1140
226. Kvols LK, Moertel CG, O'Connell MJ et al (1986) Treatment of the malignant carcinoid syndrome. Evaluation of a long-acting somatostatin analogue. N Engl J Med 315(11):663–666
227. Reichlin S (1983) Somatostatin (second of two parts). N Engl J Med 309(25):1556–1563
228. Reichlin S (1983) Somatostatin. N Engl J Med 309(24):1495–1501
229. Lamberts SW, van der Lely AJ, de Herder WW et al (1996) Octreotide. N Engl J Med 334(4):246–254
230. Rubin J, Ajani J, Schirmer W et al (1999) Octreotide acetate long-acting formulation versus open-label subcutaneous octreotide acetate in malignant carcinoid syndrome. J Clin Oncol 17(2):600–606
231. Caplin ME, Pavel M, Cwikla JB et al (2014) Lanreotide in metastatic enteropancreatic neuroendocrine tumors. N Engl J Med 371(3):224–233
232. Scherubl H, Wiedenmann B, Riecken EO et al (1994) Treatment of the carcinoid syndrome with a depot formulation of the somatostatin analogue lanreotide. Eur J Cancer 30A(10):1590–1591
233. Vinik AI, Wolin EM, Liyanage N et al (2016) Evaluation of Lanreotide depot/autogel efficacy and safety as a carcinoid syndrome treatment (elect): a randomized, double-blind, placebo-controlled trial. Endocr Pract 22(9):1068–1080
234. Anthony LB, O'Dorisio TM (2021) Opportunities to improve symptom control with somatostatin congeners in GEP-NETs: a review of key issues. Oncologist 26(7):e1171–e1178
235. Saif MW, Larson H, Kaley K et al (2010) Chronic octreotide therapy can induce pancreatic insufficiency: a common but under-recognized adverse effect. Expert Opin Drug Saf 9(6):867–873
236. Tomassetti P, Migliori M, Gullo L (1998) Slow-release lanreotide treatment in endocrine gastrointestinal tumors. Am J Gastroenterol 93(9):1468–1471
237. Anthony L, Johnson D, Hande K et al (1993) Somatostatin analogue phase I trials in neuroendocrine neoplasms. Acta Oncol 32(2):217–223

238. Faiss S, Rath U, Mansmann U et al (1999) Ultra-high-dose lanreotide treatment in patients with metastatic neuroendocrine gastroenteropancreatic tumors. Digestion 60(5): 469–476
239. Broder MS, Beenhouwer D, Strosberg JR et al (2015) Gastrointestinal neuroendocrine tumors treated with high dose octreotide-LAR: a systematic literature review. World J Gastroenterol 21(6):1945–1955
240. Yao JC, Fazio N, Singh S et al (2016) Everolimus for the treatment of advanced, non-functional neuroendocrine tumours of the lung or gastrointestinal tract (RADIANT-4): a randomised, placebo-controlled, phase 3 study. Lancet 387(10022):968–977
241. Pavel ME, Hainsworth JD, Baudin E et al (2011) Everolimus plus octreotide long-acting repeatable for the treatment of advanced neuroendocrine tumours associated with carcinoid syndrome (RADIANT-2): a randomised, placebo-controlled, phase 3 study. Lancet 378(9808):2005–2012
242. Strosberg JR, Halfdanarson TR, Bellizzi AM et al (2017) The north American neuroendocrine tumor society consensus guidelines for surveillance and medical management of midgut neuroendocrine tumors. Pancreas 46(6):707–714
243. Panzuto F, Rinzivillo M, Fazio N et al (2014) Real-world study of everolimus in advanced progressive neuroendocrine tumors. Oncologist 19(9):966–974
244. Taboada RG, Riechelmann RP, Mauro C et al (2022) Everolimus-induced pneumonitis in patients with neuroendocrine neoplasms: real-world study on risk factors and outcomes. Oncologist 27(2):97–103
245. Grenett HE, Ledley FD, Reed LL et al (1987) Full-length cDNA for rabbit tryptophan hydroxylase: functional domains and evolution of aromatic amino acid hydroxylases. Proc Natl Acad Sci U S A 84(16):5530–5534
246. Walther DJ, Peter JU, Bashammakh S et al (2003) Synthesis of serotonin by a second tryptophan hydroxylase isoform. Science 299(5603):76
247. Kulke MH, Horsch D, Caplin ME et al (2017) Telotristat ethyl, a tryptophan hydroxylase inhibitor for the treatment of carcinoid syndrome. J Clin Oncol 35(1):14–23
248. Pavel M, Horsch D, Caplin M et al (2015) Telotristat etiprate for carcinoid syndrome: a single-arm, multicenter trial. J Clin Endocrinol Metab 100(4):1511–1519
249. Pavel M, Gross DJ, Benavent M et al (2018) Telotristat ethyl in carcinoid syndrome: safety and efficacy in the TELECAST phase 3 trial. Endocr Relat Cancer 25(3):309–322
250. Sarrouilhe D, Mesnil M (2019) Serotonin and human cancer: a critical view. Biochimie 161:46–50
251. Drozdov I, Kidd M, Gustafsson BI et al (2009) Autoregulatory effects of serotonin on proliferation and signaling pathways in lung and small intestine neuroendocrine tumor cell lines. Cancer 115(21):4934–4945
252. Alpini G, Invernizzi P, Gaudio E et al (2008) Serotonin metabolism is dysregulated in cholangiocarcinoma, which has implications for tumor growth. Cancer Res 68(22):9184–9193
253. Morse MA, Liu E, Joish VN et al (2020) Antiproliferative effects of Telotristat ethyl in patients with neuroendocrine tumors: the TELEACE real-world chart review study. Cancer Manag Res 12:6607–6614
254. Anderson MD (2021) Telotristat ethyl for the treatment of carcinoid heart disease in patients with metastatic neuroendocrine tumor. Clinical trial NCT04810091 Sponsor. MD Anderson Cancer Center, Houston, TX
255. Oberg K, Funa K, Alm G (1983) Effects of leukocyte interferon on clinical symptoms and hormone levels in patients with mid-gut carcinoid tumors and carcinoid syndrome. N Engl J Med 309(3):129–133
256. Moertel CG, Rubin J, Kvols LK (1989) Therapy of metastatic carcinoid tumor and the malignant carcinoid syndrome with recombinant leukocyte a interferon. J Clin Oncol 7(7):865–868
257. Frank M, Klose KJ, Wied M et al (1999) Combination therapy with octreotide and alpha-interferon: effect on tumor growth in metastatic endocrine gastroenteropancreatic tumors. Am J Gastroenterol 94(5):1381–1387

258. Oberg K (1996) Interferon-alpha versus somatostatin or the combination of both in gastroenteropancreatic tumours. Digestion 57(Suppl 1):81–83
259. Yao JC, Guthrie KA, Moran C et al (2017) Phase III prospective randomized comparison trial of depot octreotide plus interferon alfa-2b versus depot octreotide plus bevacizumab in patients with advanced carcinoid tumors: SWOG S0518. J Clin Oncol 35(15):1695–1703
260. Pavel ME, Baum U, Hahn EG et al (2006) Efficacy and tolerability of pegylated IFN-alpha in patients with neuroendocrine gastroenteropancreatic carcinomas. J Interferon Cytokine Res 26(1):8–13
261. Moertel CG, Hanley JA (1979) Combination chemotherapy trials in metastatic carcinoid tumor and the malignant carcinoid syndrome. Cancer Clin Trials 2(4):327–334
262. Engstrom PF, Lavin PT, Moertel CG et al (1984) Streptozocin plus fluorouracil versus doxorubicin therapy for metastatic carcinoid tumor. J Clin Oncol 2(11):1255–1259
263. Bukowski RM, Johnson KG, Peterson RF et al (1987) A phase II trial of combination chemotherapy in patients with metastatic carcinoid tumors. A Southwest Oncology Group Study. Cancer 60(12):2891–2895
264. Bukowski RM, Tangen CM, Peterson RF et al (1994) Phase II trial of dimethyltriazenoimidazole carboxamide in patients with metastatic carcinoid. A Southwest Oncology Group study. Cancer 73(5):1505–1508
265. Sun W, Lipsitz S, Catalano P et al (2005) Phase II/III study of doxorubicin with fluorouracil compared with streptozocin with fluorouracil or dacarbazine in the treatment of advanced carcinoid tumors: eastern cooperative oncology group study E1281. J Clin Oncol 23(22):4897–4904
266. Chatzellis E, Angelousi A, Daskalakis K et al (2019) Activity and safety of standard and prolonged Capecitabine/Temozolomide administration in patients with advanced neuroendocrine neoplasms. Neuroendocrinology 109(4):333–345
267. Al-Toubah T, Morse B, Strosberg J (2022) Efficacy of Capecitabine and Temozolomide in small bowel (midgut) neuroendocrine tumors. Curr Oncol 29(2):510–515
268. Kotteas EA, Syrigos KN, Saif MW (2016) Profile of capecitabine/temozolomide combination in the treatment of well-differentiated neuroendocrine tumors. Onco Targets Ther 9:699–704
269. Bushnell DL Jr, O'Dorisio TM, O'Dorisio MS et al (2010) 90Y-edotreotide for metastatic carcinoid refractory to octreotide. J Clin Oncol 28(10):1652–1659
270. Anthony LB, Woltering EA, Espenan GD et al (2002) Indium-111-pentetreotide prolongs survival in gastroenteropancreatic malignancies. Semin Nucl Med 32(2):123–132
271. Strosberg J, El-Haddad G, Wolin E (2017) Phase 3 trial of 177Lu-DOTATATE for midgut neuroendocrine tumors. N Engl J Med 376:376
272. Strosberg J, Wolin E, Chasen B et al (2018) Health-related quality of life in patients with progressive midgut neuroendocrine tumors treated with (177)Lu-Dotatate in the phase III NETTER-1 trial. J Clin Oncol 36(25):2578–2584
273. Brabander T, van der Zwan WA, Teunissen JJM et al (2017) Long-term efficacy, survival, and safety of [(177)Lu-DOTA(0),Tyr(3)]octreotate in patients with gastroenteropancreatic and bronchial neuroendocrine tumors. Clin Cancer Res 23(16):4617–4624
274. Hope TA, Abbott A, Colucci K et al (2019) NANETS/SNMMI procedure standard for somatostatin receptor-based peptide receptor radionuclide therapy with (177)Lu-DOTATATE. J Nucl Med 60(7):937–943
275. Hope TA, Bodei L, Chan JA et al (2020) NANETS/SNMMI consensus statement on patient selection and appropriate use of (177)Lu-DOTATATE peptide receptor radionuclide therapy. J Nucl Med 61(2):222–227
276. Burkett BJ, Dundar A, Young JR et al (2021) How we do it: a multidisciplinary approach to (177)Lu DOTATATE peptide receptor radionuclide therapy. Radiology 298(2):261–274
277. Pavel M, Valle JW, Eriksson B et al (2017) ENETS consensus guidelines for the standards of care in neuroendocrine neoplasms: systemic therapy—biotherapy and novel targeted agents. Neuroendocrinology 105(3):266–280
278. Mittra ES (2018) Neuroendocrine tumor therapy: (177)Lu-DOTATATE. AJR Am J Roentgenol 211(2):278–285

279. Wafelman AR, Hoefnagel CA, Maessen HJ et al (1997) Renal excretion of iodine-131 labelled meta-iodobenzylguanidine and metabolites after therapeutic doses in patients suffering from different neural crest-derived tumours. Eur J Nucl Med 24(5):544–552
280. Pryma DA, Chin BB, Noto RB et al (2019) Efficacy and safety of high-specific-activity (131) I-MIBG therapy in patients with advanced pheochromocytoma or paraganglioma. J Nucl Med 60(5):623–630
281. Abdullaeva S, Botkin C, Frye S et al (2019) Examining ultratrace iobenguage I-131 for use in patients with malignant pheochromocytoma/paraganglioma or metastatic carcinoid. J Nucl Med 60:2046
282. Mukherjee JJ, Kaltsas GA, Islam N et al (2001) Treatment of metastatic carcinoid tumours, phaeochromocytoma, paraganglioma and medullary carcinoma of the thyroid with (131) I-meta-iodobenzylguanidine [(131)I-mIBG]. Clin Endocrinol (Oxf) 55(1):47–60
283. Feldman JM, Blinder RA, Lucas KJ et al (1986) Iodine-131 metaiodobenzylguanidine scintigraphy of carcinoid tumors. J Nucl Med 27(11):1691–1696
284. Bomanji JB, Wong W, Gaze MN et al (2003) Treatment of neuroendocrine tumours in adults with 131I-MIBG therapy. Clin Oncol (R Coll Radiol) 15(4):193–198
285. Kaltsas G, Korbonits M, Heintz E et al (2001) Comparison of somatostatin analog and meta-iodobenzylguanidine radionuclides in the diagnosis and localization of advanced neuroendocrine tumors. J Clin Endocrinol Metab 86(2):895–902
286. Safford SD, Coleman RE, Gockerman JP et al (2004) Iodine-131 metaiodobenzylguanidine treatment for metastatic carcinoid. Results in 98 patients. Cancer 101(9):1987–1993
287. Ezziddin S, Sabet A, Logvinski T et al (2013) Long-term outcome and toxicity after dose-intensified treatment with 131I-MIBG for advanced metastatic carcinoid tumors. J Nucl Med 54(12):2032–2038
288. Gaitan-Gaitan A, Rider WD, Bush RS (1975) Carcinoid tumor-cure by irradiation. Int J Radiat Oncol Biol Phys 1(1–2):9–13
289. Keane TJ, Rider WD, Harwood AR et al (1981) Whole abdominal radiation in the management of metastatic gastrointestinal carcinoid tumor. Int J Radiat Oncol Biol Phys 7(11):1519–1521
290. Moertel CG (1983) Treatment of the carcinoid tumor and the malignant carcinoid syndrome. J Clin Oncol 1(11):727–740
291. Divine RD, Anderson RL, Ossoinig KC (1982) Metastatic carcinoid unresponsive to radiation therapy presenting as a lacrimal fossa mass. Ophthalmology 89(5):516–520
292. Schupak KD, Wallner KE (1991) The role of radiation therapy in the treatment of locally unresectable or metastatic carcinoid tumors. Int J Radiat Oncol Biol Phys 20(3):489–495
293. Samlowski WE, Eyre HJ, Sause WT (1986) Evaluation of the response of unresectable carcinoid tumors to radiotherapy. Int J Radiat Oncol Biol Phys 12(3):301–305
294. Chen KS, Lawhn-Heath C, Behr S et al (2021) Outcomes after high-dose radiation in the management of neuroendocrine neoplasms. PLoS One 16(6):e0252574
295. Carter J, Aggarwal S, Radish K et al (2016) Effectiveness of radiation therapy for low-to intermediate-grade neuroendocrine tumors. Int J Radiat Oncol Biol Phys 96(2):E202–E203
296. Chan DL, Thompson R, Lam M et al (2018) External beam radiotherapy in the treatment of gastroenteropancreatic neuroendocrine tumours: a systematic review. Clin Oncol (R Coll Radiol) 30(7):400–408
297. Keutgen XM, Nilubol N, Glanville J et al (2016) Resection of primary tumor site is associated with prolonged survival in metastatic nonfunctioning pancreatic neuroendocrine tumors. Surgery 159(1):311–318
298. Tierney JF, Chivukula SV, Wang X et al (2019) Resection of primary tumor may prolong survival in metastatic gastroenteropancreatic neuroendocrine tumors. Surgery 165(3):644–651
299. Scott AT, Breheny PJ, Keck KJ et al (2019) Effective cytoreduction can be achieved in patients with numerous neuroendocrine tumor liver metastases (NETLMs). Surgery 165(1):166–175
300. Sarmiento JM, Heywood G, Rubin J et al (2003) Surgical treatment of neuroendocrine metastases to the liver: a plea for resection to increase survival. J Am Coll Surg 197(1):29–37

301. Que FG, Nagorney DM, Batts KP et al (1995) Hepatic resection for metastatic neuroendocrine carcinomas. Am J Surg 169(1):36–42. discussion 42–33
302. Maxwell JE, Sherman SK, O'Dorisio TM et al (2016) Liver-directed surgery of neuroendocrine metastases: what is the optimal strategy? Surgery 159(1):320–333
303. Yao JC, Strosberg J, Fazio N et al (2021) Spartalizumab in metastatic, well/poorly differentiated neuroendocrine neoplasms. Endocr Relat Cancer 28(3):161–172
304. Creutzfeldt W (1994) Historical background and natural history of carcinoids. Digestion 55(Suppl 3):3–10
305. Grahame-Smith DG (1968) The carcinoid syndrome. Am J Cardiol 21(3):376–385
306. Vinik A, Moattari AR (1989) Use of somatostatin analog in management of carcinoid syndrome. Dig Dis Sci 34(3 Suppl):14S–27S
307. Frolich JC, Bloomgarden ZT, Oates JA et al (1978) The carcinoid flush. Provocation by pentagastrin and inhibition by somatostatin. N Engl J Med 299(19):1055–1057
308. Kharrat HA, Taubin H (2003) Carcinoid crisis induced by external manipulation of liver metastasis. J Clin Gastroenterol 36(1):87–88
309. Muralidhar V, Sharma A (1996) Carcinoid crisis during a partial hepatic resection; lack of essential drugs: a cause for concern in the tropics. Trop Gastroenterol 17(1):26–29
310. Ozgen A, Demirkazik FB, Arat A et al (2001) Carcinoid crisis provoked by mammographic compression of metastatic carcinoid tumour of the breast. Clin Radiol 56(3):250–251
311. Kvols LK (1986) Metastatic carcinoid tumors and the carcinoid syndrome. A selective review of chemotherapy and hormonal therapy. Am J Med 81(6B):49–55
312. Hofland J, Herrera-Martinez AD, Zandee WT et al (2019) Management of carcinoid syndrome: a systematic review and meta-analysis. Endocr Relat Cancer 26(3):R145–R156
313. Kahil ME, Brown H, Fred HL (1964) The carcinoid crisis. Arch Intern Med 114:26–28
314. Ito T, Lee L, Jensen RT (2018) Carcinoid-syndrome: recent advances, current status and controversies. Curr Opin Endocrinol Diabetes Obes 25(1):22–35
315. Magabe PC, Bloom AL (2014) Sudden death from carcinoid crisis during image-guided biopsy of a lung mass. J Vasc Interv Radiol 25(3):484–487
316. Morrisroe K, Sim IW, McLachlan K et al (2012) Carcinoid crisis induced by repeated abdominal examination. Intern Med J 42(3):342–344
317. Janssen M, Salm EF, Breburda CS et al (2000) Carcinoid crisis during transesophageal echocardiography. Intensive Care Med 26(2):254
318. Fujie S, Zhou W, Fann P et al (2010) Carcinoid crisis 24 hours after bland embolization: a case report. Biosci Trends 4(3):143–144
319. Bissonnette RT, Gibney RG, Berry BR et al (1990) Fatal carcinoid crisis after percutaneous fine-needle biopsy of hepatic metastasis: case report and literature review. Radiology 174(3 Pt 1):751–752
320. Massimino K, Harrskog O, Pommier S et al (2013) Octreotide LAR and bolus octreotide are insufficient for preventing intraoperative complications in carcinoid patients. J Surg Oncol 107(8):842–846
321. Kwon DH, Paciorek A, Mulvey CK et al (2019) Periprocedural management of patients undergoing liver resection or embolotherapy for neuroendocrine tumor metastases. Pancreas 48(4):496–503
322. Marsh HM, Martin JK Jr, Kvols LK et al (1987) Carcinoid crisis during anesthesia: successful treatment with a somatostatin analogue. Anesthesiology 66(1):89–91
323. Parris WC, Oates JA, Kambam J et al (1988) Pre-treatment with somatostatin in the anaesthetic management of a patient with carcinoid syndrome. Can J Anaesth 35(4):413–416
324. Kinney MA, Warner ME, Nagorney DM et al (2001) Perianaesthetic risks and outcomes of abdominal surgery for metastatic carcinoid tumours. Br J Anaesth 87(3):447–452
325. Woltering EA, Wright AE, Stevens MA et al (2016) Development of effective prophylaxis against intraoperative carcinoid crisis. J Clin Anesth 32:189–193
326. Phan AT, Oberg K, Choi J et al (2010) NANETS consensus guideline for the diagnosis and management of neuroendocrine tumors: well-differentiated neuroendocrine tumors of the thorax (includes lung and thymus). Pancreas 39(6):784–798

327. Boudreaux JP, Klimstra DS, Hassan MM et al (2010) The NANETS consensus guideline for the diagnosis and management of neuroendocrine tumors: well-differentiated neuroendocrine tumors of the jejunum, ileum, appendix, and cecum. Pancreas 39(6):753–766
328. Condron ME, Pommier SJ, Pommier RF (2016) Continuous infusion of octreotide combined with perioperative octreotide bolus does not prevent intraoperative carcinoid crisis. Surgery 159(1):358–365
329. Castillo JG, Filsoufi F, Adams DH et al (2008) Management of patients undergoing multivalvular surgery for carcinoid heart disease: the role of the anaesthetist. Br J Anaesth 101(5):618–626
330. Kvols LK, Martin JK, Marsh HM et al (1985) Rapid reversal of carcinoid crisis with a somatostatin analogue. N Engl J Med 313(19):1229–1230
331. Boudreaux JP, Putty B, Frey DJ et al (2005) Surgical treatment of advanced-stage carcinoid tumors: lessons learned. Ann Surg 241:839–845
332. Bonomi P, Hovey C, Dainauskas JR et al (1979) Management of carcinoid syndrome. Med Pediatr Oncol 6(1):77–83
333. Vaughan DJ, Brunner MD (1997) Anesthesia for patients with carcinoid syndrome. Int Anesthesiol Clin 35(4):129–142
334. Thorson A, Nordenfelt O (1959) Development of valvular lesions in metastatic carcinoid disease. Br Heart J 21(2):243–248
335. Anthony L, Vinik AI (2011) Evaluating the characteristics and the management of patients with neuroendocrine tumors receiving octreotide LAR during a 6-year period. Pancreas 40(7):987–994
336. Luis SA, Pellikka PA (2016) Carcinoid heart disease: diagnosis and management. Best Pract Res Clin Endocrinol Metab 30(1):149–158
337. Bober B, Saracyn M, Kołodziej M et al (2020) Carcinoid heart disease: how to diagnose and treat in 2020? Clin Med Insights Cardiol 14:1179546820968101
338. NCI-2021–00852 (2021) TELEHEART: Telotristat ethyl in a heart biomarker study. clinicaltrials.gov
339. Panzuto F, Maccauro M, Campana D et al (2021) Impact of the SARS-CoV2 pandemic dissemination on the management of neuroendocrine neoplasia in Italy: a report from the Italian Association for Neuroendocrine Tumors (Itanet). J Endocrinol Invest 44(5):989–994
340. Krug S, Garbe J, Konig S et al (2020) Professional assessment of the impact of COVID-19 on handling NET patients. J Clin Med 9(11)
341. Ramirez RA, Bren-Mattison Y, Thiagarajan R et al (2020) A neuroendocrine tumor specialty Center in new Orleans' (NOLANETS) response to patient care during the COVID-19 pandemic. Oncologist 25(7):548–551
342. Rodriguez-Freixinos V, Capdevila J, Pavel M et al (2021) Practical recommendations for the management of patients with gastroenteropancreatic and thoracic (carcinoid) neuroendocrine neoplasms in the COVID-19 era. Eur J Cancer 144:200–214
343. Bergsland EK, Halperin DM, Dillon JS et al (2020) North American neuroendocrine tumor society guide for neuroendocrine tumor patient health care providers during COVID-19. Pancreas 49(6):723–728
344. Rakshit SL, Kendi A, Sonbol M, Starr J, Hobday T, Leventakos K, Halfdanarson T (2021) COVID-19 in patients with neuroendocrine tumors (NETs): the Mayo Clinic experience. J Neuroendocrinol 33:77
345. Mafficini A, Scarpa A (2019) Genetics and epigenetics of gastroenteropancreatic neuroendocrine neoplasms. Endocr Rev 40(2):506–536
346. Cives M, Strosberg J, Al Diffalha S et al (2019) Analysis of the immune landscape of small bowel neuroendocrine tumors. Endocr Relat Cancer 26(1):119–130
347. Sciammarella C, Luce A, Riccardi F et al (2020) Lanreotide induces cytokine modulation in intestinal neuroendocrine tumors and overcomes resistance to everolimus. Front Oncol 10:1047

348. Katz SC, Donkor C, Glasgow K et al (2010) T cell infiltrate and outcome following resection of intermediate-grade primary neuroendocrine tumours and liver metastases. HPB 12(10):674–683
349. Karpathakis A, Dibra H, Pipinikas C et al (2017) Progressive epigenetic dysregulation in neuroendocrine tumour liver metastases. Endocr Relat Cancer 24(2):L21–L25
350. Feng Z, He X, Zhang X et al (2022) Potent suppression of neuroendocrine tumors and gastrointestinal cancers by CDH17CAR T cells without toxicity to normal tissues. Nat Cancer 3:581
351. National Comprehensive Cancer Network (2021) NCCN guidelines version 3.2021 neuroendocrine tumors of the gastrointestinal tract (well-differentiated grade 1/2), lung, and thymus. National Cancer Institute, Bethesda, MD
352. Pavel M, Oberg K, Falconi M et al (2020) Gastroenteropancreatic neuroendocrine neoplasms: ESMO clinical practice guidelines for diagnosis, treatment and follow-up. Ann Oncol 31(7):844–860
353. Chauhan A, Prieur A, Kolesar J et al (2021) Abstract 735: hPG₈₀ (circulating progastrin), a novel blood-based biomarker for detection of poorly differentiated neuroendocrine carcinoma and well differentiated neuroendocrine tumors. Cancer Res 81(13 Supplement):735–735
354. Al-Toubah T, Pelle E, Valone T et al (2021) Efficacy and toxicity analysis of Capecitabine and Temozolomide in neuroendocrine neoplasms. J Natl Compr Canc Netw 20:1–8
355. Cives M, Pelle E, Strosberg J (2020) Emerging treatment options for gastroenteropancreatic neuroendocrine tumors. J Clin Med 9(11):3655
356. Das S, Dasari A (2021) Novel therapeutics for patients with well-differentiated gastroenteropancreatic neuroendocrine tumors. Therapeut Adv Med Oncol 13:17588359211018047
357. Chow Z, Johnson J, Chauhan A et al (2021) PI3K/mTOR dual inhibitor PF-04691502 is a schedule-dependent radiosensitizer for gastroenteropancreatic neuroendocrine tumors. Cells 10(5)
358. Bergsland EK, Mahoney MR, Asmis TR et al (2019) Prospective randomized phase II trial of pazopanib versus placebo in patients with progressive carcinoid tumors (CARC) (Alliance A021202). J Clin Oncol 37(15_suppl):4005–4005
359. Navalkissoor S, Grossman A (2019) Targeted alpha particle therapy for neuroendocrine tumours: the next generation of peptide receptor radionuclide therapy. Neuroendocrinology 108(3):256–264
360. Adant S, Shah GM, Beauregard JM (2020) Combination treatments to enhance peptide receptor radionuclide therapy of neuroendocrine tumours. Eur J Nucl Med Mol Imaging 47(4):907–921
361. Goedegebuure RSA, de Klerk LK, Bass AJ et al (2018) Combining radiotherapy with anti-angiogenic therapy and immunotherapy; a therapeutic triad for cancer? Front Immunol 9:3107
362. Ballal S, Yadav MP, Damle NA et al (2017) Concomitant 177Lu-DOTATATE and Capecitabine therapy in patients with advanced neuroendocrine tumors: a long-term-outcome, toxicity, survival, and quality-of-life study. Clin Nucl Med 42(11):e457–e466
363. Ballal S, Yadav MP, Bal C et al (2020) Broadening horizons with (225)ac-DOTATATE targeted alpha therapy for gastroenteropancreatic neuroendocrine tumour patients stable or refractory to (177)Lu-DOTATATE PRRT: first clinical experience on the efficacy and safety. Eur J Nucl Med Mol Imaging 47(4):934–946
364. Reidy-Lagunes D, Pandit-Taskar N, O'Donoghue JA et al (2019) Phase I trial of well-differentiated neuroendocrine tumors (NETs) with radiolabeled Somatostatin antagonist (177)Lu-Satoreotide Tetraxetan. Clin Cancer Res 25(23):6939–6947
365. Kaemmerer D, Träger T, Hoffmeister M et al (2015) Inverse expression of somatostatin and CXCR4 chemokine receptors in gastroenteropancreatic neuroendocrine neoplasms of different malignancy. Oncotarget 6(29):27566–27579
366. Sgouros G, Bodei L, McDevitt MR et al (2020) Radiopharmaceutical therapy in cancer: clinical advances and challenges. Nat Rev Drug Discov 19(9):589–608
367. Kanduluru AK, Low PS (2017) Development of a ligand-targeted therapeutic agent for Neurokinin-1 receptor expressing cancers. Mol Pharm 14(11):3859–3865

The Multiple Endocrine Neoplasia Syndromes

21

Kira Oleinikov, David J. Gross, and Simona Grozinsky-Glasberg

21.1 Introduction

The term multiple endocrine neoplasia (MEN) refers to hereditary neoplastic disorders involving more than one endocrine organ. Main syndrome subtypes are recognized, according to the involvement of specific endocrine glands: the MEN type 1 (MEN1); the MEN type 2A (MEN2A), and the MEN type 2B (MEN2B). All these forms either may be inherited in an autosomal dominant manner or may occur de novo [1]. The frequency of each of these syndromes is estimated at around 1 in 30,000, being characterized by complete penetrance but with variable expression [2]. The recent progress in our knowledge of both the molecular and the clinical phenotype of these syndromes has improved the clinical management of the patients [3]. On the one hand, the MEN1 gene, a tumor suppressor gene responsible for MEN1 syndrome development, is involved in the regulation of several cell functions (e.g., DNA replication and repair and transcriptional machinery). On the other hand, the RET proto-oncogene encodes for a receptor tyrosine kinase protein whose expression is fundamental for appropriate migration, development, and differentiation of neuroendocrine cells originating from neural crest [4]. Currently, DNA testing allows the early identification of germline mutations in presymptomatic mutant gene carriers in the MEN syndromes [5]. Consequently, early identification of the MEN-associated neoplasms improves the outcome and the quality of life for affected subjects [6].

K. Oleinikov · D. J. Gross · S. Grozinsky-Glasberg (✉)
Neuroendocrine Tumor Unit, ENETS Center of Excellence, Division of Medicine, Hadassah-Hebrew University Medical Center, Jerusalem, Israel
e-mail: gross@vms.huji.ac.il; simonag@hadassah.org.il

S. Yalcin, K. Öberg (eds.), *Neuroendocrine Tumours*,
https://doi.org/10.1007/978-3-031-56968-5_21

21.2 Multiple Endocrine Neoplasia Type 1 (MEN1, Wermer's Syndrome)

MEN1 is a rare hereditary endocrine cancer syndrome involving the occurrence in the same patient of tumors of the parathyroid glands, the anterior pituitary, and the pancreatic islet cells. Whereas firstly described in the early twentieth century, it was not until 1954 when Wermer described a familial occurrence in which a father and four of the nine offspring were affected [7]. The disease was initially described as a multiple endocrine adenomatosis, and it has subsequently become known as multiple endocrine neoplasia type 1 (MEN1).

Patients with MEN1 characteristically have tumors of the parathyroid glands (1HPT) (~95%), the anterior pituitary (~30%), and the pancreatic islets (~40%) (major criteria for diagnosis); less commonly, they may have some other endocrine (adrenal cortical adenomas and more rarely carcinoma, thyroid tumors, usually follicular adenomas, neuroendocrine tumors involving organs other than the pancreas such as duodenal gastrinoma and gastric, thymic, and bronchial carcinoids) [5, 8]. Non-endocrine neoplasms can also occur—visceral and cutaneous lipomas, meningiomas, facial angiofibromas, and collagenomas (minor criteria for diagnosis) [9–15]. The phenotype of MEN1 is extremely diverse, with over 20 different combinations of endocrine and non-endocrine manifestations described to date. MEN1 should be suspected in patients with an endocrinopathy of two of the three pathognomonic/major affected organs, or with an endocrinopathy of one of these organs plus two minor manifestations or with a first-degree relative affected by MEN1 syndrome [16].

The overall estimated incidence of MEN1 is 0.25%; estimated incidences are 1–18% in primary hyperparathyroidism, 16–38% in gastrinomas (pancreatic neuroendocrine tumors secreting gastrin), and <3% in pituitary tumors. The reported age range is 5– 81 years; however, 80% of patients develop clinical manifestations of the disorder by the fifth decade [17].

21.2.1 MEN1: Associated Primary Hyperparathyroidism (PHPT) (Table 21.1)

21.2.1.1 Clinical Features and Diagnosis

PHPT is the most common and frequently the earliest manifestation in MEN-1 mutation carriers, and occurs in ~95% of cases [9, 13, 18]. The PHPT in MEN1, as compared to the sporadic form, has an earlier age of onset (20–25 years, compared to 55–60 years), exhibits an equal male-to-female ratio (compared to a female preponderance in sporadic PHPT), and involves all 4 parathyroid glands (diffuse hyperplasia or multiple adenomas), rather than a single one (solitary adenomas) [8, 9]. Noteworthy is the increased frequency of supernumerary (up to 20%) and ectopic parathyroid glands in MEN 1 patients, usually localized within the thyroid gland, in the anterior mediastinum/thymus or exceptionally in the pericardium [19, 20].

Table 21.1 Clinical manifestations in MEN1

MEN1	Organ involved		Specific tumor (prevalence by 40 years)	Clinical presentation
	Parathyroid disease (95%)		Diffuse hyperplasia	Symptoms related to hypercalcemia or hypercalciuria
			Adenoma, multiple	
	NETs	PNETs (30–80%)	Gastrinomas (>50%)	ZES, diarrhea, abdominal pain
			Insulinomas (10–30%)	Whipple triad
			Glucagonomas (~3%)	Necrolytic migratory erythema, weight loss, anemia, stomatitis
			VIPomas (extremely rare)	Verner-Morrison syndrome
			NF PNETs (20–100%)	Asymptomatic, but with malignant potential
			Somatostatinomas (extremely rare)	Somatostatinomas syndrome, rare
			Other (e.g., GHRH-secreting)	Rare, increased GH and IGF1 levels
		Foregut NETs (2–10%)	Thymic, gastric, bronchial NETs	Organ specific
	Pituitary tumors (40%)		Prolactinomas (20%)	Oligomenorrhea, galactorrhea, infertility in woman; impotence and infertility in men
			Other: ACTH, TSH, GH + PRL, GH, NF (each 2–9%)	Hormone-dependent
	Other endocrine manifestations		Benign adrenocortical tumors (73%)	Most non-functioning
			Adrenocortical carcinoma (13%)	Hormone-dependent
			Pheochromocytomas (<1%)	Rarely described, mainly asymptomatic
			Thyroid adenomas, goiter and carcinoma (25%)	Usually incidental finding
	CNS-tumors		Ependymomas, schwannomas, meningiomas (1%)	Mainly asymptomatic
	Cutaneous manifestations		Multiple subcutaneous lipomas (33%); visceral, pleural, or retroperitoneal lipomas (rare)	

NETs, neuroendocrine tumors; *PNETs*, pancreatic neuroendocrine tumors; *ZES*, Zollinger-Ellison syndrome; *VIPomas*, vasointestinal polypeptide secreting tumors; *NF PNETs*, non-functioning pancreatic neuroendocrine tumors; *GHRH*, growth hormone releasing hormone; *IGF1*, insulin growth factor 1; *ACTH*, adrenocortical hormone; *TSH*, thyroid stimulating hormone; *PRL*, prolactin; *NF*, non-functioning; *CNS*, central nervous system

PHPT is a progressive disease in MEN1: whereas asymptomatic hypercalcemia is the most common manifestation, patients may present with symptoms (e.g., fatigue, weakness, polydipsia, polyuria, myalgias, or abdominal pain), or signs (nephrolithiasis or osteitis fibrosa cystica) related to the progressive increase in serum and/or urinary calcium and disease duration.

A major clinical manifestations of MEN1-associated PHPT is progressing demineralization with severe osteopenia (*T* score <−2.0) in ~44% of patients with uncontrolled disease, by the age of 35 [21]. Recurrent kidney stones are less frequently described in MEN1 families, and it is unusual for these patients to develop chronic renal failure as result of nephrolithiasis [22, 23].

The diagnosis of PHPT is based upon demonstrating elevated serum levels of calcium and parathyroid hormone (PTH). Mild hypercalcemia with normal/increased range serum PTH concentration can usually be detected during the second decade of life [24]. Total serum calcium concentration corrected for albumin level is considered the screening test for PHPT in MEN1 [25]. Noteworthy, identifying the "subclinical" stage of hyperparathyroidism has not been considered essential until recently when an increased cardiovascular risk has been reported in patients with mild normocalcemic hyperparathyroidism [26]. However, the performance of serum PTH measurement as a screening test remains controversial. Diagnosis of hyperparathyroidism requires levels of PTH inappropriately high for the concomitant calcium levels. At present, different kits for assessment of PTH are available. Second generation of kits, measuring concentrations of the so-called "intact PTH" (iPTH), are in general usage [27]. Genetic testing is recommended in specific patient populations: (1) multiple gland involvement (coexistence of other tumors characteristic for MEN1); (2) a first-degree relative of a MEN1 mutation carrier with or without clinical symptoms associated with MEN1. Furthermore, mutational analysis should be considered in an individual with primary hyperparathyroidism before age of 30 years or with a multiglandular parathyroid disease [28, 29].

21.2.1.2 Treatment of MEN1-Associated PHPT

In contrast to single gland-resection in sporadic cases, a more complex surgical approach, including total parathyroidectomy and thymectomy with autotransplantation of parathyroid tissue, or excision of 3.5 parathyroid glands, are indicated for PHPT in MEN1 [19, 28–31]. Moreover, postoperative hypoparathyroidism and higher rates of recurrent or persistent disease are more frequent in MEN1-associated PHPT than in the sporadic form of the disease [28, 29]. Recurrences (rate >50% at 12 years) usually located in preserved/residual parathyroid tissue, and is strongly influenced by the surgeon's experience and the possibility to perform intraoperative PTH determinations [28–32]. Intraoperative PTH assessment is mandatory in these patients to confirm the removal of all functional parathyroid tissue before parathyroid autotransplantation [30].

In MEN1 patients with preclinical/eucalcemic PHPT, the approach is still uncertain: early parathyroidectomy is recommended by some experts to control even mild hyperparathyroidism and to prevent the progressive decline of bone mineral density and the increased risk for kidney stones [33, 34].

In MEN1-associated PHPT patients in whom surgery is not possible or ineffective, medical treatment with calcimimetic drugs has emerged as an effective, though expensive, option [35, 36]. Cinacalcet therapy is well tolerated by most of the patients; rarely, gastrointestinal side effects may induce discontinuation of the therapy [36, 37]. Interestingly, the administration of the somatostatin analog octreotide-LAR controlled hypercalcemia and hypercalciuria in two-thirds of patients with MEN1-related PHP, this effect being most probably mediated by the octreotide-LAR binding to somatostatin receptors on parathyroid tumor cells in patients with MEN1-related PHP [38].

21.2.2 MEN1-Associated Pancreatic Islet Cell Neuroendocrine Tumors (PNETs)

Pancreatic and duodenal neuroendocrine tumors represent the second most frequent manifestation in MEN1 (occurring in 30–80% of cases) and continue to be the primary cause of tumor-related death in these patients [10, 28, 29]. In contrast with the sporadic PNETs, MEN1-related PNETs are characterized by an early onset, multifocality, variable biological behavior; both the histology and the size of the tumor are predictors of the malignant potential [5, 39–41]. Some of these tumors secrete gastrin, insulin, glucagon, vasoactive intestinal polypeptide (VIP) etc., and are associated with distinct clinical syndromes, whereas most PNETs are clinically silent tumors (nonfunctioning, secreting pancreatic polypeptide, PP) [5]. Given that MEN1-associated PNETs are usually multiple and of possible malignant behavior, their timely diagnosis and management are of major importance.

21.2.2.1 Gastrinomas

Clinical Manifestations and Diagnosis

Gastrin-secreting tumors (gastrinomas) are the most frequently functioning duodenopancreatic NETs in patients with MEN1 (>50%), and ~20% of patients with gastrinomas will have MEN1 [42–44]. Gastrinomas occur more often in patients with MEN1 who are older than 30 years, are associated with marked gastric acid secretion, recurrent and severe peptic ulcerations (the Zollinger Ellison Syndrome, ZES), which may perforate, and are usually metastatic at diagnosis [45, 46]. These features are responsible for the major morbidity (peptic ulcer disease, diarrhea and steatorrhea, cachexia, and abdominal pain) and mortality associated with MEN1 [47, 48].

In contrast to the sporadic gastrinomas that occur predominantly in the pancreas, in MEN1 most of these tumors develop in the proximal duodenum [49]. Gastrinomas are usually small (<5 mm) and multiple, growing slowly deep into the mucosa, and metastasizing frequently to the peri-pancreatic lymph nodes and further to the liver [50]. Pancreatic gastrinomas or other extra-pancreatic, extra-duodenal (e.g., ovary, liver, bile duct, pylorus, spleen, mesentery), and extra-abdominal (e.g., cardiac intraventricular septum) locations in MEN-1 patients are extremely rare [51, 52].

When found in the pancreas, it may be difficult to distinguish gastrinomas from concomitant nonfunctioning PNETs [43, 53].

The diagnosis is established by demonstration of an increased fasting serum gastrin concentration (found to be elevated in 90–98% of ZES patients) after stopping antisecretory drugs (proton pump inhibitors, PPIs, at least 1 week; histamine receptors 2, H2R, for at least 2 days) [54], in association with increased basal gastric acid secretion (gastric pH <2) [52, 55]. However, stopping antisecretory drugs in ZES patients is often impossible due to severe symptoms of peptic disease and diarrhea and may be hazardous—due to possible perforation or bleeding. Occasionally, iv provocative tests with either secretin (2 U/kg) or calcium infusion (4 mg Ca^{2+}/kg•h for 3 h) are required to distinguish patients with ZES from other patients with hypergastrinemia (e.g., those with antral G-cell hyperplasia) [50]. In two-thirds of patients with ZES, fasting serum gastrin levels overlap with values seen in other conditions. In these patients, gastrin provocative tests are needed to establish the diagnosis of ZES [56]. For unknown reasons, secretin stimulates the release of gastrin by gastrinoma cells, and therefore patients with these tumors have a dramatic rise in serum gastrin in response to a secretin infusion. In contrast, normal gastric G cells are inhibited by secretin, and therefore serum gastrin concentrations do not rise in patients with other causes of hypergastrinemia. The secretin stimulation test is performed by administering 0.4 μg of secretin per kg body weight (RepliGen Corporation, Waltham, MA) intravenously over 1 min; a baseline serum gastrin is measured twice before the secretin is administered and classically 2, 5, 10, 15, and 20 min later. An increase of ≥120 pg/mL in gastrin levels is highly suggestive of gastrinoma [56].

In some patients with MEN1 the diagnosis of ZES may be difficult, as it doesn't appear to develop in the absence of primary hyperparathyroidism, whereas hypergastrinemia has also been reported to be associated with hypercalcemia [54]. Moreover, successful treatment of MEN1-associated PHPT with restoration of normocalcemia is known to ameliorate clinical symptoms and biochemical abnormalities in ~20% of MEN1 patients with ZES [44].

Tumor localization and determination of the tumor extent are essential to the proper management of MEN1-gastrinomas: endoscopic ultrasonography, CT, MRI, selective abdominal angiography, and mainly somatostatin-receptor scintigraphy/^{68}Ga-DOTA-TATE/-TOC/-NOC PET-CT are very helpful in localizing the tumor [53, 57]. Moreover, the combination of intra-arterial calcium injections with hepatic venous gastrin sampling has been shown to regionalize the gastrinomas [58]. Importantly, these tumors are often occult to conventional exploration, and their detection requires duodenotomy and meticulous evaluation of the mucosa by eversion and direct palpation [59].

Management of MEN1-Associated Gastrinomas

Control of Gastric Hypersecretion

The management of patients with ZES is directed toward reducing basal acid output to less than 10 mmol/L, and includes acute and long-term control of gastric acid hypersecretion by parietal cell H^+-K^+-adenosine triphosphatase (proton pump) inhibitors, PPIs (omeprazole, lansoprazole, pantoprazole, rabeprazole, and esomeprazole), starting a dose equivalent to 60 mg/day of omeprazole [54]; the dosage should be increased to b.i.d. in patients with severe gastro-esophageal reflux disease (GERD) symptoms, previous Billroth II or gastroenterostomies, or with hypercalcemia with MEN1 [52]. Long-term PPI treatment is safe and without loss of efficacy; no gastric carcinoid development associated with PPIs-induced hypergastrinemia was demonstrated in humans [52]. Some patients may also require additional treatment with the histamine H2 receptor antagonists, cimetidine, or ranitidine [5].

Surgical Management of Gastrinoma

In patients with MEN1 and ZES, correction of the PHPT by parathyroidectomy can significantly decrease basal acid output, fasting gastrin level, and increase sensitivity to gastric antisecretory drugs [60]. The role of surgery in the treatment of gastrinoma in MEN1/ZES patients is controversial as these patients usually have multiple duodenal tumors with frequent lymph node metastases and cannot be cured [61, 62]. In addition, they usually have concomitant nonfunctional PNETs. As development of liver metastases, associated with a poor prognosis, is more frequent in the presence of large tumors, exploration is recommended whenever a PNET of >2 cm is found [62]. Surgical resection of duodenal MEN1-associated gastrinomas, based on preoperative and intraoperative (e.g., transillumination of the duodenum) tumor regionalization may be considered in specialized centers. Due to increased morbidity and potential mortality after extensive resections, the surgical excision has to be individualized based on preoperative findings, patient history (e.g., preexisting diabetes), and preference [63]. Interestingly, the presence of regional lymph node metastases in 50–60% of patients with MEN1-related duodenal gastrinomas is not usually associated with decreased survival [60].

Management of Metastatic MEN1-Gastrinoma

Long-acting somatostatin analogues (SSAs) in combination with PPIs are recommended as initial therapy [52, 64]. The main effect of these SSAs is a tumoristatic effect, with disease stabilization observed in ~40 to 70% of patients, whereas decrease in tumor size (partial response) is reported in only 10–20% of patients [65]; these agents are particularly effective in slower-growing PNETs [66]. Embolization of liver metastases, PRRT, or removal of all resectable tumor have been occasionally successful in patients with disseminated MEN1-gastrinomas [67, 68].

21.2.2.2 Insulinomas

Clinical Manifestations and Diagnosis

Insulinomas represent between 10% and 30% of all MEN1-related PNETs, and rarely (in 10% of patients with MEN1), they may coexist with a gastrinoma or with other nonfunctioning PNETs at the time of diagnosis, in the same patient [9, 69]. In MEN1 patients, insulinomas occur more often at an age younger than 40 year (in many patients even younger than 20 years and some as young as 5 years), in contrast to the sporadic insulinomas patients in whom the disease occurs usually after the age of 40 year [9, 70]. Insulinoma is the first manifestation of MEN1 in 10% of patients, whereas ~4% of patients with insulinomas will have MEN1 [5, 67]. The clinical presentation, biochemical of MEN1-related insulinomas, as well as the treatment of these patients are similar to those in sporadic insulinomas patients. However, the localization of insulinoma may be difficult in cases that coexist with other nonfunctioning PNETs at the time of diagnosis. In these cases, new adjunct modalities for localization such as ^{68}Ga-DOTA-exendin-4 PET/CT may be helpful, since insulinomas express glucagon-like peptide 1 (GLP1) receptors more than SSTR. More invasive techniques, such as selective angiography with intra-arterial calcium stimulation for insulin levels are addressed in detail in Chap. 12 of the present textbook [71, 72].

21.2.2.3 Glucagonomas

Clinical Manifestations and Diagnosis

Glucagon-secreting pancreatic tumors occur in fewer than 3% of patients with MEN1 [5, 50], are highly malignant and frequently are localized at the tail of the pancreas [5, 73]. Importantly, in MEN1-associated glucagonomas, the characteristic clinical manifestations (such as the necrolytic migratory erythema, weight loss, anemia, or stomatitis) [74, 75] may be absent, and the tumor may be detected in a completely asymptomatic patient with MEN1 undergoing routine pancreatic imaging, or detected by glucose intolerance and concomitant increase in glucagon levels [76, 77].

Management of MEN1-Associated Glucagonomas

Surgical removal is the treatment of choice. However, up to 80% of glucagonomas patients have metastatic disease at the time of diagnosis [78], and therefore systemic therapy using SSAs, PRRT, or hepatic artery embolization have been useful in some patients [64, 79–82].

21.2.2.4 VIPomas

Clinical Manifestations and Diagnosis

The VIP secreting tumors (VIPomas) are very rare in MEN1, occur commonly in the tail of the pancreas, and produce a clinical syndrome (Verner-Morrison syndrome) with watery diarrhea, hypokalemia, and achlorhydria (WDHA) [81, 83]. The diagnosis requires excluding laxative and diuretic abuse, demonstration of a large fasting stool volume (0.5–1 L/day) during a fast and an elevated serum VIP concentration [50].

Management of MEN1-Associated VIPomas

Surgical excision of VIPomas is the main therapeutic intervention in these patients, with a curative purpose. However, in patients with unresectable or metastatic tumors, systemic treatment with SSAs, corticosteroids, indomethacin, metoclopramide, lithium carbonate, and hepatic artery embolization has been used with varying efficacy [63, 84].

21.2.2.5 Nonfunctioning PNETs (NF PNETS)

Clinical Manifestations and Diagnosis

NF PNETs represent a heterogeneous group of tumors being increasingly identified as the result of increasing sensitivity of radiological screening methods [40, 41, 85]. Importantly, NF PNETs have been reported to occur in young asymptomatic patients who are even less than 15 year of age. NF PNETs are not associated with a hormonal syndrome and may be associated with minor elevation of specific pancreatic hormones (e.g., pancreatic polypeptide) but without clinical symptoms [84].

Identification of NF PNETs is of outmost importance, as they are the most common NETs occurring in the MEN1 setting, they have a well-recognized malignant potential, are associated with a worse prognosis, and are the commonest cause of death in MEN1 patients [47, 55, 86, 87]. In the absence of specific clinical and biochemical abnormalities, the diagnosis of NF PNETs may be delayed, and therefore radiological screening for entero-pancreatic NET in MEN1 is mandatory and should begin at the age of 10 year [84].

Endoscopic ultrasound (EUS) currently offers the most sensitive screening procedure to localize PNETs especially if they are multiple. In addition, it permits better evaluation of their proximity to vital structures (pancreatic duct, splenic vessels), enabling the operator to take biopsies [86, 88]. Furthermore, the contrast-enhanced harmonic technology combined with EUS allows real-time perfusion imaging without Doppler-related artifacts and has improved the diagnostic yield of EUS-guided fine needle aspiration (EUS-FNA) for very small lesions [89, 90].

Management of MEN1-Associated NF PNETs

Surgical Therapy of MEN1-NF PNETs

The treatment approach for asymptomatic NF PNETs is controversial. To date, treatment decision is based on tumor size, as the risk of metastases is thought to be higher in patients with larger tumors [89, 90]. Some reports suggest that early and aggressive surgery might reduce the risks for malignant progression [91]. However, other studies have not confirmed this association [45, 92]. The latest clinical guidelines argue against surgical resection for NF PNETs that are ≤2 cm in size, due to post-surgery short- and long-term complications, and the evidence in the literature of survival rates up to 100% at a 15 of follow-up [84, 93, 94]. For tumors size less than 1 cm, surgical resection should be considered for tumors with a size doubling time of a 3- to 6-month interval [63]. However, there are many factors influencing the decision on surgery in these patients, such as the increased morbidity of pancreatic surgery (as complications such as diabetes mellitus, steatorrhea, dumping syndromes, are not uncommon) [84], the possible presence of occult metastatic disease at the time of initial diagnosis, and the high risk for disease recurrence in the remnant pancreatic tissue after surgery [93–95].

Medical Therapy of MEN1-NF PNETs

PNETs cells may express different kinase receptors, such as tyrosine kinase receptors (TK-R)-vascular endothelial growth factor receptors (VEGF-R), and platelet-derived growth factor receptors (PDGF-R), whereas some exhibit over-activation of the mammalian target of rapamycin (mTOR) signaling pathway, which stimulates cell proliferation and angiogenesis. Recently, systemic therapy with tyrosine kinase receptor inhibitors (TKI; sunitinib maleate) or with mTOR inhibitors (mTORi; everolimus) were reported as significantly increasing time to tumor progression in patients with locally progressive or metastatic PNETs [96, 97]. Moreover, all the other treatment modalities considered for functioning PNETs such as chemotherapy (the classic streptozotocin and 5-FU combination), or the new combination of temozolomide-capecitabine, SSAs, peptide receptor radioligand therapy (PRRT), hepatic artery chemoembolization, radio-frequency ablation etc. may be individually used in treating patients with metastatic NF PNETs [98–102].

21.2.2.6 Other PNETs

Rare PNETs ectopically secreting growth hormone-releasing hormone (GHRH), have been reported in some patients with MEN1 [67, 103]. They may occur in the lungs, pancreas or small intestine, and should be suspected when elevated levels of growth hormone (GH) and GHRH are found in the serum of the patient or when the patient has clinical acromegaly.

About 0.65% of MEN1-related PNET may produce somatostatin and are defined as somatostatinomas, rare tumors which are usually non-functioning or, in 10% of cases, associated with a clinical syndrome of hyperglycemia, cholelithiasis, low acid output, steatorrhea, diarrhea, abdominal pain, anemia, and weight loss (the somatostatinoma syndrome) [73, 104].

Surgical removal is the treatment of choice for these rare tumors.

21.2.3 MEN1-Associated Pituitary Tumors

Patients affected by the MEN1 syndrome display a high incidence (~42%) of pituitary adenomas [105–107], which may occur as early as 5 years of age and as late as the ninth decade, and have been reported to occur more frequently in women than men [105]. The molecular pathways involved in their development seem different from the sporadic tumors [108–110]; approximately 40% of patients with MEN1 have pituitary adenomas and 17% present with a pituitary tumor [111].

All types of adenomas can be found in MEN1 patients with a predominance of prolactinoma and macroadenoma (i.e., diameter greater than 1 cm) compared to a control population. Acromegaly is seen in 9% of cases and has a greater female preponderance in MEN-1 than in sporadic disease [107]. Nonsecreting adenomas, thyroid-stimulating hormone (TSH)-secreting and adrenocorticotropic hormone (ACTH)-secreting adenomas do occur MEN1 patients, in decreasing frequency [107]. Interestingly, plurihormonal expression is frequently observed in MEN1-associated pituitary tumors compared with sporadic pituitary tumors [107]. The

MEN1 tumors seem to have a more aggressive behavior, to be more invasive (with infiltration of tumor cells into surrounding normal pituitary tissue) and more resistant to treatment, therefore requiring a long and careful life follow-up [108, 112]. However, no increased prevalence of pituitary carcinoma is observed in MEN1. These tumors may occur in the pediatric population and may be the first and only manifestation of MEN1 for some years [108, 113].

21.2.3.1 Clinical Manifestations and Diagnosis

Clinical manifestations of MEN1-associated pituitary tumors are similar to those in sporadic pituitary tumors [105]. They depend on the hormone secreted e.g., symptoms of increased prolactin, such as oligomenorrhea, galactorrhea, infertility in woman, impotence and infertility in men; symptoms of acromegaly due to increased GH/IGF-I secretion; symptoms of Cushing's disease due to increased cortisol secretion; etc) and on the size of the tumor. Enlarging pituitary tumors may compress adjacent structures such as the optic chiasm or normal pituitary tissue and may cause visual disturbances, and/or hypopituitarism [108].

In a MEN1 patient, periodic biochemical monitoring, including measurement of serum prolactin and IGF-I levels, as well as MRI of the pituitary, are indicated, and further hypothalamic-pituitary hormonal testing should be performed in patients with abnormal results [63, 85].

21.2.3.2 Treatment of MEN1-Related Pituitary Tumors

Treatment of these tumors is similar to the one in patients with sporadic tumors and includes medical therapy (specifically dopamine agonists for prolactinoma, or somatostatin analogs for GH-secreting adenoma together with surgical excision) and, if feasible, surgical excision, e.g., selective transsphenoidal tumor resection, with adjuvant radiotherapy in case of residual unresectable tumor tissue [107]. Noteworthy, as result of the aggressive tumor behavior, MEN1 patients with pituitary tumors are less responsive to medical or surgical therapy, with a hormone normalization rate of 42% compared with 90% in patients with sporadic tumors, after therapy [105, 112, 114].

21.2.4 Other MEN1-Associated Tumors

MEN1 patients frequently develop tumors involving tissues other than the parathyroid glands, pancreas, and pituitary gland, such as neuroendocrine tumors (carcinoids), adrenal cortical tumors, thyroid tumors, facial angiofibromas, collagenomas, lipomatous tumors, and meningiomas [115, 116].

21.2.4.1 MEN1-Related Neuroendocrine Tumors (NETs)

Extrapancreatic NETs occur in ~3% of MEN1 patients, with the lungs, gastrointestinal tract, or thymus being more frequent sites of origin. In MEN1 patients these tumors may be gender-related, with a women predominance for lung NETs, and a male predominance for thymic NETs, cigarette smokers have an increased risk for developing thymic tumors; moreover, there are no hormonal or biochemical abnormalities consistently reported in MEN1 patients with thymic or lung NETs [67, 117, 118]. Importantly, MEN1-associated thymic NETs seem to be particularly aggressive, with a median survival time of approximately 9.5 year and with 70% of patients dying as a direct result of the tumor [118].

Screening for these NETs is of major importance and their diagnosis depends on the imaging method used and the skills of the radiologist; contrast-enhanced CT is a sensitive method, whereas somatostatin-receptor scintigraphy may be useful, although there is still insufficient evidence to recommend its routine use [1, 118]. The current guidelines for the early detection of MEN1-related thymic and lung NETs recommend the use CT or MRI imaging every 1–2 years [1]. Noteworthy, thymic NETs have occurred also after prophylactic thymectomy, suggesting that surveillance imaging is still required even after tumor excision [119].

Type II gastric NETs are associated with MEN1 and the Zollinger-Ellison syndrome, are usually multiple and smaller than 1.5 cm, and may be detected incidentally during endoscopy in these patients [119].

Surgical excision is the treatment of choice. For unresectable or metastatic disease, treatment with somatostatin analogs, such as octreotide or lanreotide, has resulted in improvement in symptoms and tumor regression [119]. In addition, chemotherapeutic agents (e.g., capecitabine, temozolomide) or radiotherapy may be used in patients with aggressive tumors [120].

21.2.4.2 MEN1-Related Adrenal Tumors

Adrenocortical tumors occur in up to 73% of the patients with MEN1 [85, 121–123], and include adenomas, hyperplasia, cysts, or carcinomas. Most are nonfunctioning [123], whereas functional tumors are reported to occur in less than 10% of patients, with primary hyperaldosteronism and ACTH-independent Cushing's syndrome most commonly reported [121]. Pheochromocytomas are rarely described in MEN1 patients, whereas adrenocortical carcinoma is reported to occur in up to 13% of MEN1 patients, in parallel with a tumor size of more than 1 cm [121].

Biochemical investigation (e.g., plasma renin and aldosterone concentrations, low-dose dexamethasone suppression test or 24 urine collection for free cortisol, urinary catecholamines and metanephrines, or plasma metanephrines) should be performed as routine for adrenal tumors. It is recommended that MEN1 patients with adrenal tumors should undergo an annual imaging screening (CT or MRI) of the adrenal glands [1, 121, 123].

The treatment of MEN1-related adrenal tumors is similar to that for tumors occurring in the sporadic context. Surgical excision is recommended for adrenal tumors that are more than 4 cm in diameter, or less than 4 cm but with suspicious radiological features, or for tumors with significant growth over a 6-month interval [123].

21.2.4.3 MEN1-Related Breast Cancer

A recent study from the Dutch MEN1 registry demonstrated that females with MEN 1 appeared to have a 2–3 times higher chance of breast cancer at 10 years earlier age compared to the general population [124]. In comparison to the findings in sporadic breast cancer, female MEN1 patients have an increased risk to develop mostly luminal-type breast cancer. The proliferative role of menin mutations is consistent with its function as a regulator of ESR1 gene expression and as co-activator of estrogen receptor alpha (ERα), a critical driver in approximately 70% of sporadic breast cancer cases [125]. Therefore, it was suggested to start screening in MEN1 female patients from the age of 40 years biennially [126].

21.2.4.4 MEN1-Related Central Nervous System (CNS)-Tumors

Different CNS tumors have been reported in MEN1 patients, including ependymomas, schwannomas, and meningiomas. The majority of meningiomas are asymptomatic, and do not enlarge. Their follow-up and treatment are similar to that occurring in non-MEN1 patients [127].

21.2.4.5 MEN1-Related Thyroid Tumors

Thyroid adenomas, nodular goiter, and thyroid carcinoma have all been reported in more than 25% of MEN1 patients. However, the occurrence of thyroid abnormalities in these patients may be incidental, as these disorders are also frequent in the general population. The treatment of MEN1-related thyroid tumors is similar to that for sporadic cases [50].

21.2.4.6 MEN1-Related Cutaneous Manifestations

Multiple subcutaneous lipomas are reported in more than 33% of MEN1 patients. Rarely, visceral, pleural, or retroperitoneal lipomas may also occur [50]. They are usually treated conservatively but may be excised for cosmetic reasons. Facial angiofibromas and collagenomas may occur in up to 88% of MEN1 patients. Usually, no treatment is required [128].

21.2.5 Genetic Testing and Screening in MEN1

21.2.5.1 MEN1 Gene

The MEN1 gene is located on chromosome 11q13 and consists of 10 exons, which encode menin, a 610-amino acid protein [129, 130], and a tumor suppressor that regulates transcription, genome stability, cell division, and proliferation [67, 131]. Inheritance of a germline MEN1 mutation predisposes an individual to develop a tumor that arises after an additional somatic mutation of the normal allele, which may be a point mutation or a deletion, leading to loss of heterozygosity (LOH) in the tumor DNA (the Knudson two-hit hypothesis) [67].

21.2.5.2 MEN1 Germline Mutations

Over 1336 mutations of the MEN1gene have been characterized in the first decade following identification of the gene [67]. About 75% of the MEN1 germline mutations are inactivating, consistent with those expected in a tumor-suppressor gene. There are nine sites in the MEN1 gene accounting for over 20% of all the germ-line mutations [67]. Noteworthy, it appears that there is no clear-cut correlation between MEN1 mutations and MEN1 clinical manifestations. The apparent lack of genotype/phenotype correlation, together with the wide diversity of mutations in the 1830-bp coding region of the MEN1 gene, renders mutational analysis more difficult [77, 131]. Importantly, more than 10% of MEN1 germline mutations arise de novo [131]. Up to 25% of MEN1 patients may not harbor germline mutations in the MEN1 gene coding region, probably related to whole or partial gene deletions, or mutations in the promoter or untranslated regions [131, 132]. Phenocopies may mimic MEN1 either by occurrence of a single sporadic endocrine tumor in a patient with familial MEN1, or occurrence of two endocrine abnormalities associated with different etiologies. Phenocopies arose in >5% of MEN1 families and awareness of them is important in the clinical management of MEN1 and other hereditary disorders [133].

21.2.5.3 MEN1 Gene Polymorphisms

A gene is said to be polymorphic if more than one allele occupies that gene's locus within a population [134]. Twenty-four different polymorphisms of the MEN1 gene have been reported [131]. The recognition of these polymorphisms is important as they may occasionally help in families without any MEN1 mutation identified [63].

21.2.5.4 MEN1 Tumor Somatic Mutations

More than 90% of the tumors originating in MEN1 patients exhibit LOH on 11q13, consistent with Knudson's two-hit (second-hit) hypothesis [131]. Beside the LOH mechanism, the second hit hypothesis may result also from intragenic deletions and point mutations.

In clinical practice, the mutational analysis of tumor DNA to identify somatic mutations adds little value as LOH involving chromosome 11q13 in the MEN1 location has been observed in up to 50% of sporadic endocrine tumors [131, 135].

21.2.5.5 MEN1 Variants

In rare families with MEN1 variants, only some of MEN1 characteristic clinical manifestations may be observed. Familial isolated hyperparathyroidism (FIHP) is a condition characterized by the development of parathyroid tumors as the sole endocrinopathy, being reported to date in more than 40 FIHP families with germline mutations in MEN1, CDC73, GCM2, and CaSR genes [131, 132]. Another MEN1 variant is the $\text{MEN1}_{\text{burin}}$ or prolactinomas variant, characterized by a high occurrence of prolactinomas and a low occurrence of gastrinomas [136–138] as a result of nonsense mutations (Tyr312Stop and Arg460Stop) [139].

21.2.5.6 MEN1 Mutational Analysis in Clinical Practice

MEN1 mutational analysis is important for the confirmation of the clinical diagnosis, the identification of family members who require screening for tumor detection and appropriate treatment, as well as for the identification of the 50% of family members who do not harbor the familial germline MEN1 mutation and can therefore be reassured [50].

MEN1 mutational analysis should be performed in the following circumstances [1, 28, 140, 141]:

- in an index case with ≥2 classic MEN1-associated endocrine tumors (i.e., parathyroid, pancreatic, or pituitary tumors);
- in an asymptomatic first-degree relative of a known MEN1 mutation carrier;
- in a first-degree relative of an MEN1 mutation carrier having symptoms, signs, biochemical, or radiological evidence for one or more MEN1-associated tumors;
- in patients with suspicious or atypical MEN1, including individuals with parathyroid adenomas diagnosed before the age of 30 years;
- in patients with multiglandular parathyroid disease, gastrinoma, or multiple pancreatic NETs at any age;
- in individuals who have two or more MEN1-associated tumors not part of the classical triad of parathyroid, pancreatic islet, and anterior pituitary tumors;
- in individuals presenting at an early age with a single, apparently sporadic MEN1-associated tumor.

21.2.5.7 MEN1 Tumors Identification

As MEN1 syndrome is associated with a complex spectrum of clinical, diagnostic, and therapeutic aspects, it is recommended for these patients and their families to be followed by teams with expertise in the management of MEN1, including an endocrinologist experienced in MEN syndromes [1, 50]. As the MEN1 gene mutation appears to be non-penetrant in individuals younger than 5 year, but with a >50% penetrance by 20 year of age and >95% by 40 year, a timely biochemical and imaging screening in asymptomatic members of MEN1 families is imperative, as earlier diagnosis and treatment may reduce the morbidity and mortality related to these tumors [5, 39, 67, 142].

PHPT-induced hypercalcemia is usually the first manifestation in about 85% of MEN1 patients and therefore has become an easy biochemical screening investigation. In addition, hyperprolactinemia, usually asymptomatic, may represent the first manifestation in approximately 15% of patients and may be easily detected [67]. PNETs may be detected in asymptomatic individuals by measuring fasting plasma concentrations of gastrin, pancreatic polypeptide, glucagon, and chromogranin A, and by abdominal imaging [143, 144].

The latest guidelines suggest that mutant MEN1 gene carriers should undergo biochemical screening (including evaluation of serum calcium, PTH, gastrin, insulin with a fasting glucose, glucagon, VIP, pancreatic polypeptide, chromogranin A, prolactin, and IGF-I) annually [1]. Baseline pituitary and abdominal imaging (e.g., MRI or CT) should be performed and then repeated at 1–3 years interval, as well as imaging for thymic and bronchial carcinoids using CT or MRI every 1–2 years. Screening should possibly commence in early childhood (e.g., by the age of 5 years for insulinoma), and should be repeated throughout life [1].

21.3 Multiple Endocrine Neoplasia Type 2 (MEN2, Sipple Syndrome)

Type 2 multiple endocrine neoplasia (MEN2) is a rare familial cancer syndrome caused by mutations in the RET proto-oncogene. The association between thyroid cancer and pheochromocytoma was first described by Sipple in 1961 [145]. In 1965, the thyroid cancer occurring in association with pheochromocytoma was defined as medullary thyroid carcinoma (MTC), characterized by stromal amyloid. Since 1968, the familial constellation of MTC in conjunction with pheochromocytoma and parathyroid hyperplasia was recognized as MEN2. Although patients with mucosal neuromas were already identified, the distinction between MEN2A and MEN2B subtypes was only in 1975 [146]. MEN2 is an autosomal dominant syndrome classified into main two variants: MEN2A and MEN2B [147]. All variants of MEN2 show a high penetrance for MTC, which is diagnosed in as much as 90% of MEN2 carriers (as a palpable thyroid nodule or an increase in blood calcitonin levels) [147, 148]. In 1985 the proto-oncogene RET (*RE*-arranged during *T*ransfection) was discovered by Takahashi and associates [146]. All MEN2 subtypes are caused by germline mutations in the RET proto-oncogene, specifically with selected RET codon mutations [149, 150].

21.3.1 The Clinical Presentation of MEN2 Syndromes (Table 21.2)

21.3.1.1 Clinical Presentation of MEN2A

The classical MEN2A subtype is characterized by the development of MTC in 90% of adult gene carriers, unilateral or bilateral pheochromocytoma in 50%, and multigland parathyroid adenoma/hyperplasia with primary hyperparathyroidism (PHPT) in 20–30% [151–153]. The classical MEN2A accounts for over 95% of MEN2, and may present as rare variants including familial MTC (FMTC), MEN2A with cutaneous lichen amyloidosis, and MEN2A with Hirschsprung's disease with variable penetrance for pheochromocytomas and PHPT [152, 154–158].

MEN2A-Related MTC

Constitutive activation of the mutated RET tyrosine kinase receptor is thought to be the main driver (primary hit) that gives rise to parafollicular or C cells neoplastic hyperplasia [159, 160]. Multifocal C cell hyperplasia (CCH) is the precursor lesion to hereditary MTC, and the age of transformation from CCH to microscopic MTC varies with different germline RET mutations and subsequent somatic mutations (second hits) [161, 162]. MTC is generally the first manifestation of MEN2A, and the patients typically present with a neck mass or neck pain, usually before age 35 years, with cervical lymph node metastases in up to 70% [163, 164]. Diarrhea, the most frequent systemic manifestation (~30% of patients with advanced MTC), occurs in affected individuals with a higher plasma calcitonin concentration and implies a poor prognosis [165]. Approximately 10% of MTC patients have flushing often induced by alcohol ingestion, calcium infusion, or pentagastrin injection

Table 21.2 Clinical manifestations in MEN2

MEN2	MEN2A (95%)	Organ involved	Specific tumor/ manifestation (prevalence by 40 years)	Clinical presentation
	MEN2A (95%)	Thyroid	MTC (90%)	Neck mass or neck pain, diarrhea, flushing
	MEN2A (95%)	Adrenal	Pheochromocytomas (50%)	Subtle symptoms, usually bilateral
	MEN2A (95%)	Parathyroid	Multi-gland adenoma/ hyperplasia (20–30%)	Usually asymptomatic
	MEN2A (95%)	Skin	CLA	Pruritic, lichenoid skin lesion in the upper portion of the back
	MEN2A (95%)	MEN2A-genetically related	HSCR	Bowel enlargement and constipation/obstipation
	MEN2A (95%)	MEN2A-genetically related	PTC	Concomitant PTC and MTC
	FMTC	Thyroid	MTC (100%)	≥4 individuals with MTC in the same family in the absence of pheochromocytoma or parathyroid adenoma/hyperplasia
	MEN2B (5%)	Thyroid	MTC (90%)	Very aggressive, usually metastatic
	MEN2B (5%)	Adrenal	Pheochromocytomas (50%)	Usually multiple/bilateral (50%)
	MEN2B (5%)	Other	Mucosal neuromas, frequent	Tongue, palate, or pharynx; eyelid
	MEN2B (5%)	Other	Ocular signs, frequent	Inability of to cry tears; thickened corneal nerves; ptosis; eyelid eversion
	MEN2B (5%)	Other	Diffuse ganglioneuromatosis of the GIT (40%)	Abdominal distension, megacolon, constipation, or diarrhea
	MEN2B (5%)	Other	Marfanoid habitus (75%)	Associated with kyphoscoliosis or lordosis, joint laxity, decreased subcutaneous fat, proximal muscle wasting, weakness

FMTC, familial medullary thyroid carcinoma; *MTC*, medullary thyroid carcinomas; *CLA*, cutaneous lichen amyloidosis; *HD*, Hirschsprung disease; *PTC*, papillary thyroid carcinoma; *GIT*, gastrointestinal tract

[166]. All individuals with an MTC-predisposing mutation who have not undergone prophylactic thyroidectomy demonstrate biochemical evidence of MTC by age 35 years [148]. Metastatic spread may occur locally (to the central, lateral, cervical, and mediastinal lymph nodes) or distantly (to the lungs, liver, or bones) [167].

MEN2A-Related Pheochromocytomas

Pheochromocytomas usually present concomitantly or after MTC, however, they may be the presenting symptom in up to 27% of individuals with MEN2A [168–170]. MEN2-related pheochromocytomas are usually diagnosed earlier, have subtler symptoms, and are more likely to be bilateral than sporadic tumors [171, 172]. Pheochromocytomas in MEN2 patients entail a distinct biochemical phenotype in that they consistently produce epinephrine (or epinephrine and norepinephrine) [173]. Malignant transformation was reported in ~4% of cases [174].

MEN2A-Related Primary Hyperparathyroidism (PHPT)

MEN2A-related PHPT is usually mild, being diagnosed many years after the diagnosis of MTC, with an average age of onset ~38 years [175]. Most individuals are asymptomatic; however, hypercalciuria with renal calculi may occur. In case of longstanding or under-diagnosed disease, hypercalcemia-related symptoms may develop and become severe, in parallel with disease progression [176].

MEN2A-Related Cutaneous Lichen Amyloidosis (CLA)

Pruritic CLA, a lichenoid skin lesion usually located over the upper portion of the back, corresponding to dermatomes T2-T6, has been reported in a small number of families with MEN2A carrying codon 634 mutations [177, 178].

FMTC

FMTC is historically diagnosed in families with four or more cases of MTC in the absence of pheochromocytoma or parathyroid adenoma/hyperplasia. Because *RET* accounts for all clinical subtypes of MEN2, FMTC may be viewed as MEN2A with reduced organ-specific penetrance [154, 155]. The age of onset of FMTC is later, and the penetrance of MTC is lower than what is observed in MEN2A and MEN2B [179, 180].

MEN2A-Related Hirschsprung Disease (HD)

HD is a genetic disorder characterized by aganglionosis of the gut, likely due to absent gut ganglia, and typically resulting in bowel enlargement and constipation/obstipation in neonates [181].

Two to five percent of patients with HD have MEN2A. Conversely, HD occurs in approximately 7% of patients with MEN2A [182, 183]. The RET mutations in patients with MEN2A and HD are point mutations involving codons in exon 10: 609, 611, 618, and codon 620 [184, 185]. Interestingly, the RET mutations associated with HD are "loss of function," while the RET mutations associated with MEN2A are "gain of function." This seemingly paradoxical occurrence may be explained by constitutive activation of RET that is sufficient to trigger neoplastic transformation of the C-cells and adrenal chromaffin cells, but still insufficient to generate a trophic response in the precursor neurons [186, 187].

21.3.1.2 Clinical Presentation of MEN2B

MEN2B comprises approximately 5% of cases of MEN2 and it is the most aggressive variant of MEN2 syndrome, characterized by MTC and pheochromocytoma, together with typical facies, ophtalmologic abnormalities, marfanoid habitus, skeletal malformations, mucosal (lips and tongue), and aerodigestive ganglioneuromatosis, but not PHPT [188, 189].

MEN2B-Related MTC

MEN2B-related MTC is the most aggressive form of MTC in all affected individuals and may appear as macroscopic disease and nodal metastases as early as the first year of life. Before intervention with early prophylactic thyroidectomy, the average age of death in individuals with MEN2B was 21 years [190].

MEN2B-Related Pheochromocytomas

Pheochromocytomas occur in 50% of individuals with MEN2B; approximately half are multiple and often bilateral [191]. Most commonly these patients complain of palpitations, anxiety spells, or headaches early in their disease, however in many patients whose tumors were found by family screening there are no symptoms. Hypertension spells may not be noted until a crisis is induced by an operation or delivery [192].

MEN2B-Related Other Clinical Presentations

- ***Mucosal neuromas*** may be identified in early childhood in MEN2B carriers, and develop on the anterior dorsal surface of the tongue, palate, or pharynx, together with a distinctive facial appearance (Fig. 21.1). The lips become prominent (or "blubbery") over time as a result of submucosal nodules present on the vermilion border of the lips. Eyelids neuromas may cause thickening and even eversion of the upper eyelid margins [193].
- ***Ophthalmologic Manifestations of MEN2B***

Children with MEN2B have the inability to cry tears, and this is an important clinical symptom for early diagnosis preceding the development of metastatic MTC [194]. Other ocular signs develop during childhood and include prominent thickened corneal nerves (seen by slit lamp examination) [195, 196], eyelid neuromas, lid margin eversion or thickening, subconjunctival neuromas, or ptosis [197–199]. There are usually no fundal findings on examination, but in patients presenting already with MTC, choroidal metastases have been observed [200].

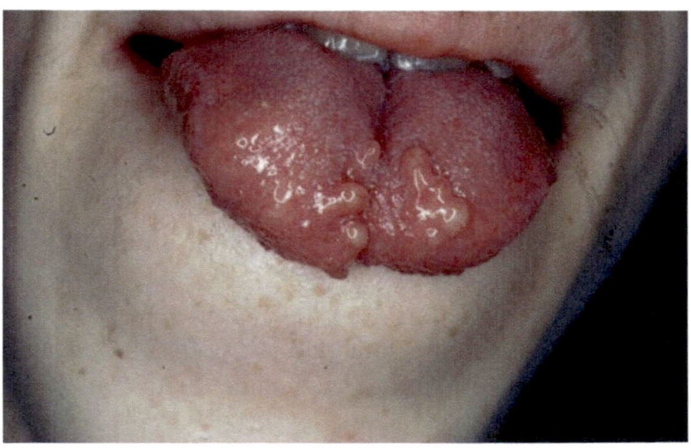

Fig. 21.1 MEN 2B-associated oral mucosal neuromas

- ***Diffuse ganglioneuromatosis of the aerodigestive tract*** is reported in ~40% of affected individuals, and it is associated with early childhood symptoms of aganglionic megacolon [201].
- ***Marfanoid habitus***, often with kyphoscoliosis or lordosis, joint laxity, decreased subcutaneous fat, proximal muscle wasting, and weakness can also be seen in ~75% of affected individuals [202].

21.3.1.3 The Diagnosis of MEN2 Syndromes Manifestations

MTC Diagnosis

Serum calcitonin values (basal or stimulated by pentagastrin, calcium, or both) are nearly always elevated in MTC, being a specific and sensitive marker [203]. Serum calcitonin levels closely correlate with the disease burden and elevation after surgery suggests persistent or recurrent disease [204]. Importantly, biochemical detection and surgical resection of asymptomatic disease results in better clinical outcomes and increases chances for cure postoperatively. Reference levels for basal calcitonin vary across laboratories, and usually levels of <10 pg/mL for adult males and <5 pg/mL for adult females are typically considered normal. Noticeably, biochemical cure is possible when pre-operative basal calcitonin levels are below 100 pg/mL and thus is considered an operative "window of opportunity" for the preemptive procedure [205, 206]. Preoperative calcitonin testing may be useful for assessing CCH (C-Cell hyperplasia) or tumor spread and should be considered when deciding the extent of surgery for MEN 2A MTC [207].

Pheochromocytoma Diagnosis

In MEN2 the pheochromocytomas are predominantly benign and are usually multicentric, bilateral, and confined to the adrenal gland. The tumors may be associated with diffuse nodular adrenal medullary hyperplasia, particularly in patients with RET mutations in codons 918 and 634 [172, 208–210]. Pheochromocytoma should be suspected whenever elevated levels of catecholamines and/or their metabolites are demonstrated in plasma or 24-h urine collections [172, 211]. Noteworthy, in MEN2, pheochromocytomas consistently produce epinephrine or epinephrine and norepinephrine [211]. Computed tomography (CT) is conventional localizing modality whenever a pheochromocytoma is suspected clinically or biochemically [212] ^{18}F-DOPA PET/CT is sensitive functional imaging modality in the localization of pheochromocytomas, in addition to being useful imaging modality for advanced MTC ^{18}F-3,4-Dihydroxyphenylalanine (DOPA) is the radio-labeled analog of DOPA, a precursor of dopamine and catecholamines, taken up by a neutral-amino acid-transporter (LAT1), is used for further tumor localization and staging and is probably the most promising PET alternative to ^{123}I-MIBG [212].

PHPT Diagnosis

The PHPT in patients with classical MEN2A is usually mild and asymptomatic. A RET codon 634 mutation is associated with a moderate penetrance of PHPT (up to

30%), and codons 609, 611, 618, and 620 are associated with a penetrance between 2% and 12% [172].

The diagnosis of PHPT is made when simultaneously elevated serum concentrations of calcium and elevated or high-normal parathyroid hormone are demonstrated on biochemical screening. For adenoma localization, either pre- or postoperatively (in case of recurrence/persistence), localizing studies with ^{99}mTc-sestamibi scintigraphy or four-dimensional single photon emission CT may be used [213].

21.3.1.4 Management of MEN2-Manifestations

MEN2-Related MTC Treatment

The main therapeutic approach is surgery; successful excision is dependent upon the adequacy and timing of the initial operation [214–217, 218]. Surgery for MTC should be performed, if possible, before the age of the possible malignant progression [219]. If the basal or stimulated calcitonin values are elevated, a minimum surgical approach should include total thyroidectomy with central lymph node dissection [220]. Total thyroidectomy with central and complete bilateral neck dissection should be performed routinely in all patients with hereditary MTC, even in those with small thyroid tumors—a contralateral neck dissection may be avoided only in sporadic MTC patients with unilateral involvement of the thyroid gland in the absence of central and ipsilateral neck involvement [220]. If after the primary thyroid surgery the basal (or stimulated) plasma calcitonin levels are high, it is important to define the extent of the residual disease; if there is no evidence of distant spread and local disease is found, then reoperation is recommended [221–223]. Surgical intervention is not indicated if distant metastases are found unless the patient develops respiratory symptoms or secretory diarrhea, for which tumor debulking may help [224]. For systemic disease, standard chemotherapeutic regimens have not proven beneficial, have considerable toxicity and are therefore not recommended [205, 225, 226], whereas the benefit of external beam irradiation therapy is controversial [227]. Several kinase inhibitors (including axitinib, cabozantinib, lenvatinib, motesanib, pazopanib, sorafenib, sunitinib, and vandetanib) have been evaluated in phase I,II clinical trials, and two of these drugs, vandetanib, and cabozantinib, have completed phase III clinical trials. Vandetanib (300 mg/day) prolonged median progression-free survival (PFS) from 19 months in the placebo arm to a predicted median of 31 months in the vandetanib arm and was therefore approved by the FDA in April 2011 and by the EMEA in February 2012 [228, 229]. Cabozantinib (175 mg/day) prolonged PFS prolongation from 4 to 11 months and was approved by the FDA in November 2012 [230]. However, since toxicity of these drugs is significant, with dose reduction or treatment withdrawal in a significant proportion of patients, and the lack of evidence for a higher treatment efficacy at an earlier disease stage nor survival benefit, these treatments should be initiated only in patients with documented tumor progression [231].

MEN2-Related Pheochromocytomas Treatment

Pheochromocytomas are usually removed by adrenalectomy, which may be performed by laparoscopy [232]. Before operation, anti-hypertensive treatment should be instituted with initial α-adrenergic blockade and if tachycardia ensues β-adrenergic receptor blockade can be added [172, 233]. Because of an increased risk of adrenal insufficiency after bilateral adrenalectomy, most experts recommend to date unilateral adrenalectomy in unilateral tumors and cortical-sparing adrenal surgery with close monitoring of the remnant tissue in persons with one remaining adrenal gland or bilateral pheochromocytoma [168].

The presence of pheochromocytoma has to be excluded in any individual with MTC or MEN2 before any surgery, as patients with undiagnosed tumors may die from an uncontrolled hypertensive crisis peri-operatively [234]. If detected, pheochromocytoma excision should precede any other surgical intervention to avoid an intraoperative crisis [235].

MEN2-Related Primary Hyperparathyroidism (PHPT) Treatment

Once the biochemical diagnosis of PHPT is confirmed in a MEN2 patient, the indications for surgical excision are similar to those in patients with sporadic PHPT and include symptomatic or marked hypercalcemia, nephrolithiasis, major hypercalciuria, and evidence of bone loss [236]. The presence/absence of pheochromocytoma should be established before the parathyroid surgery in order to avoid a life-threatening pheochromocytoma crisis.

One of the important concerns in the management of MEN2-related PHP is the ability to identify single versus multiple gland disease, and subsequently decide on the appropriated surgical procedure in order to prevent recurrences. Initially, treatment of MEN2-related PHPT included subtotal parathyroidectomy or total parathyroidectomy with forearm autograft [175]. However, it appears that sporadic PHPT, MEN1-, and MEN2A-related PHPT are three distinct entities as is reflected preoperatively by differences in gender, age at diagnosis, and calcium and PTH levels; MEN2A patients are very similar to sporadic PHPT with respect to operative approach and findings [237]. Minimally invasive procedure is the treatment of choice for both, with low rates of persistent and recurrent PHPT and a low complication rate. The percentage of multiglandular disease and recurrences is significantly higher in MEN1 patients, demonstrating the need for a different approach [237].

Individuals with PHPT who have undergone prior thyroidectomy should have preoperative localization with excision of the localized hypertrophied parathyroid glands and forearm autotransplantation. Therapy with medications to control PHPT should be considered in individuals with a high risk of surgical mortality, limited life expectancy, or persistent or recurrent PHPT after one or more surgical attempts [175].

21.3.1.5 Molecular Genetic Testing for MEN2 Patients

MEN2 is associated with activating mutations in the RET proto-oncogene, and therefore RET molecular genetic testing is indicated in all individuals with a clinical diagnosis of MTC, of MEN 2 or primary CCH [5].

It is recommended that all MTC patients, those with clinical/family suspicion for MEN2 and presumed sporadic MTC, should undergo initial RET analysis for exons 10 (codons 609, 611, 618, and 620), exon 11 (codons 630 and 634), and exons 8, 13–16, as ~98% of MEN2A patients have a mutation in exon 10 or 11 [154, 205], ~95% of FMTC patients have a mutation in exons 10, 11, and 13–16 [238].

In case of MEN2B phenotype, mutation analysis for RET codon M918T (exon 16) should be performed, and if negative, the RET codon A883F (exon 15) should be evaluated [154]. Importantly, if exon-specific testing is negative, then sequencing of the entire RET coding region should be completed in the settings of MEN2 phenotype and expected genotype [154].

MEN2 Genotype-Phenotype Correlation

MEN2 RET genotype-phenotype correlations were the first to be found in inherited neoplasia syndromes [154], and the gain-of-function mutations affected several hotspot codons (the great majority mutating cysteine residues in exons 10 and 11) [154].

The American Thyroid Association Guidelines Task Force has classified common RET mutations based on their risk for aggressive MTC. The risk classification is recommended to guide the decision for the age of prophylactic thyroidectomy or when to begin biochemical screening for pheochromocytoma and hyperparathyroidism [154]. The "highest risk" (ATA-HST)—exon 16, mutation M918T; "high risk" (ATA-H)—exon 11, mutations C634R/G/R/S/W/Y and exon 15, mutation A883F; "moderate risk" (ATA-MOD)—exon 8 (codon 533), exon 10 (codons 609, 611, 618, 620), exon 11 (codons 630, 631, 666), exon 13 (codons 768, 790), exon 14 (codon 804), exon 15 (codons 891, 912) [154].

Classical MEN2A is the most common MEN2A variant and in 95% of patients RET germline mutations occur in codons 609, 611, 618, or 620 of exon 10 or codon 634 of exon 11 [154]. Notably, RET mutations C634R/G/R/S/W/Y are highly penetrant and aggressive (ATA-H) [1, 239]. Twenty-five percent of FMTC kindreds harbor a mutation in codon 634 (commonly p.C634Y) [238].

RET germline M918T mutations, categorized as "highest risk" by current ATA guidelines (ATA-HST) are associated with MEN2B [154]. About 75% of MEN2B cases are diagnosed in affected patients who have de novo RET mutations, while 25% of cases occur in families with previous or current manifestations of MEN2B. Approximately 95% of patients with MEN2B have RET germline mutations in exon 16 (codon M918T). Fewer than 5% have RET germline mutations in exon 15 (codon A883F) [240].

Mutations involving the cysteine codons 609, 618, and 620 in exon 10 of RET are associated with MEN2A or FMTC together with HD [241]. Mutations at codons 768, 804, and 891 that were initially only associated with FMTC have subsequently been found in rare families with MEN2A [242–244].

Phenotypic expression of mutations at codon 804 has been shown to be highly variable, even within the same family: some individuals have MTC at age 5 years and fatal metastatic MTC at age 12 years, whereas other individuals have been shown to have normal thyroid histology at age 27 years, normal biochemical screening at age 40 years, and no clinical evidence of MTC at age 86 years [245–247]. Interestingly, it was suggested that in addition to their association with MTC, mutations in codons 790 or 804 may be associated with PTC [187].

21.3.1.6 Prevention of MEN2-Related Primary Manifestations

Prophylactic thyroidectomy, a major preventive measure for all age groups of carriers of a germline RET mutation [163, 205], is a reasonably safe decision when performed by experienced surgeons. The timing of the surgery is recommended to be guided by the codon position of the RET mutation [154, 205]. Thyroidectomy before progression to invasive MTC may allow thyroidectomy with sparing of lymph nodes [248]. In children in the ATA-HST category (M918T mutation) surgery should be performed in the first year of life, with or without central lymph node dissection based on presence of suspicious lymph nodes and localization of parathyroid glands [154]. Children in the ATA-H category should have a surgery performed at age 5 years or earlier if the serum calcitonin levels are above 40 pg/mL. Children in the ATA-MOD category should be surveilled by a physical examination, US of the neck, and measurement of serum calcitonin levels beginning at 5 years of age. The timing of a surgery should be based on the detection of an elevated serum calcitonin level [154].

Importantly, caution should be used in interpreting calcitonin results for children younger than 3 years, and mainly in children younger than 6 months [205].

21.3.1.7 MEN2 Patients Surveillance

Medullary Thyroid Carcinoma

Recurrent disease is expected in as much as 50% of MTC patients following total thyroidectomy and neck dissections [163] and therefore, continued monitoring for residual or recurrent MTC is indicated for life. The screening protocol for MTC includes an annual measurement of serum calcitonin; a more frequent follow-up (3–6 months) is recommended for those with residual disease, and should include biochemical analysis for calcitonin, together with appropriate imaging (neck ultrasound, high-resolution CT or complementary functional imaging) in case of elevated tumor markers [5].

Pheochromocytoma

Screening for children in the ATA-H and ATA-HST categories should begin by age 11 years and in children in the ATA-MOD category by age 16 years [154]. Screening includes measurement of free plasma metanephrines and normetanephrines or 24-h urinary metanephrines and normetanephrines. Adrenal imaging is indicated in patients with positive biochemical results [154].

If the initial screening for pheochromocytoma is negative, then annual biochemical screening is recommended. Women with MEN 2 should be screened for pheochromocytoma before a planned pregnancy [154].

PHPT

Annual serum calcium and parathyroid hormone concentrations are recommended for at-risk individuals who have not had parathyroidectomy [249]. In MEN 2A, screening should begin at age 11 years for individuals in the ATA-H category and at age 16 years for patients in the ATA-MOD category. The HPTH predominantly occurs in patients with exon 11 RET codon mutations, and less frequently in patients with exon 10 RET codon mutations [154].

References

1. Thakker RV (2014) Multiple endocrine neoplasia type 1 (MEN1) and type 4 (MEN4). Mol Cell Endocrinol 386(1–2):2–15
2. Thakker RV (1998) Multiple endocrine neoplasia—syndromes of the twentieth century. J Clin Endocrinol Metabol 83(8):2617–2620
3. Falchetti A, Marini F, Tonelli F, Brandi ML (2005) Lessons from genes mutated in multiple endocrine neoplasia (MEN) syndromes. Ann Endocrinol (Paris) 66(3):195–205
4. Kouvaraki MA, Shapiro SE, Perrier ND et al (2005) RET proto-oncogene: a review and update of genotype-phenotype correlations in hereditary medullary thyroid cancer and associated endocrine tumors. Thyroid 15(6):531–544
5. Brandi ML, Gagel RF, Angeli A et al (2001) Guidelines for diagnosis and therapy of MEN type 1 and type 2. J Clin Endocrinol Metab 86(12):5658–5671
6. Carling T (2005) Multiple endocrine neoplasia syndrome: genetic basis for clinical management. Curr Opin Oncol 17(1):7–12
7. Wermer P (1954) Genetic aspects of adenomatosis of endocrine glands. Am J Med 16(3):363–371
8. Thakker RV (2000) Multiple endocrine neoplasia type 1. Endocrinol Metab Clin N Am 29(3):541–567
9. Trump D, Farren B, Wooding C et al (1996) Clinical studies of multiple endocrine neoplasia type 1 (MEN1). QJM 89(9):653–669
10. Grama D, Skogseid B, Wilander E et al (1992) Pancreatic tumors in multiple endocrine neoplasia type 1: clinical presentation and surgical treatment. World J Surg 16(4):611–618; discussion 18–9
11. Skogseid B, Larsson C, Lindgren PG et al (1992) Clinical and genetic features of adrenocortical lesions in multiple endocrine neoplasia type 1. J Clin Endocrinol Metab 75(1):76–81
12. Duh QY, Hybarger CP, Geist R et al (1987) Carcinoids associated with multiple endocrine neoplasia syndromes. Am J Surg 154(1):142–148
13. Marx SJ, Vinik AI, Santen RJ, Floyd JC Jr, Mills JL, Green J III. (1986) Multiple endocrine neoplasia type I: assessment of laboratory tests to screen for the gene in a large kindred. Medicine (Baltimore) 65(4):226–241
14. Brandi ML, Aurbach GD, Fitzpatrick LA et al (1986) Parathyroid mitogenic activity in plasma from patients with familial multiple endocrine neoplasia type 1. N Engl J Med 314(20):1287–1293
15. Darling TN, Skarulis MC, Steinberg SM, Marx SJ, Spiegel AM, Turner M (1997) Multiple facial angiofibromas and collagenomas in patients with multiple endocrine neoplasia type 1. Arch Dermatol 133(7):853–857
16. Asgharian B, Turner ML, Gibril F, Entsuah LK, Serrano J, Jensen RT (2004) Cutaneous tumors in patients with multiple endocrine neoplasm type 1 (MEN1) and gastrinomas: prospective study of frequency and development of criteria with high sensitivity and specificity for MEN1. J Clin Endocrinol Metab 89(11):5328–5336
17. Thakker RV (2001) Multiple endocrine neoplasia. Horm Res 56(Suppl 1):67–72

18. Hannan FM, Nesbit MA, Christie PT et al (2008) Familial isolated primary hyperparathyroidism caused by mutations of the MEN1 gene. Nat Clin Pract Endocrinol Metab 4(1):53–58
19. Kivlen MH, Bartlett DL, Libutti SK et al (2001) Reoperation for hyperparathyroidism in multiple endocrine neoplasia type 1. Surgery 130(6):991–998
20. Agha A, Carpenter R, Bhattacharya S, Edmonson SJ, Carlsen E, Monson JP (2007) Parathyroid carcinoma in multiple endocrine neoplasia type 1 (MEN1) syndrome: two case reports of an unrecognised entity. J Endocrinol Investig 30(2):145–149
21. Burgess JR, David R, Greenaway TM, Parameswaran V, Shepherd JJ (1999) Osteoporosis in multiple endocrine neoplasia type 1: severity, clinical significance, relationship to primary hyperparathyroidism, and response to parathyroidectomy. Arch Surg 134(10):1119–1123
22. Molino C, Fabbian F, Russo G et al (2007) [MEN type 1 and chronic renal failure: a rarely reported association]. G Ital Nefrol 24(1):79–82
23. Satoh A, Iigaya T (2002) Multiple endocrine neoplasia type 1 with pyonephrosis. Int J Urol 9(7):402–404
24. Burgess JR, Greenaway TM, Shepherd JJ (1998) Expression of the MEN-1 gene in a large kindred with multiple endocrine neoplasia type 1. J Intern Med 243(6):465–470
25. Benson L, Ljunghall S, Akerstrom G, Oberg K (1987) Hyperparathyroidism presenting as the first lesion in multiple endocrine neoplasia type 1. Am J Med 82(4):731–737
26. Hagstrom E, Lundgren E, Rastad J, Hellman P (2006) Metabolic abnormalities in patients with normocalcemic hyperparathyroidism detected at a population-based screening. Eur J Endocrinol 155(1):33–39
27. Sukovaty RL, Lee JW, Fox J et al (2006) Quantification of recombinant human parathyroid hormone (rhPTH(1-84)) in human plasma by immunoassay: commercial kit evaluation and validation to support pharmacokinetic studies. J Pharm Biomed Anal 42(2):261–271
28. Thakker RV, Newey PJ, Walls GV, Bilezikian J, Dralle H, Ebeling PR, Melmed S, Sakurai A, Tonelli F, Brandi ML (2012) Clinical practice guidelines for multiple endocrine neoplasia type 1 (MEN1). J Clin Endocrinol Metab 97(9):2990–3011
29. Tonelli F, Marcucci T, Giudici F, Falchetti A, Brandi ML (2009) Surgical approach in hereditary hyperparathyroidism. Endocr J 56(7):827–841
30. Pandian TK, Buckarma EH, Farley DR (2016) Parathyroid surgery in multiple endocrine neoplasia type 1. In: Hyperparathyroidism. Springer, Cham, pp 75–85
31. Akerstrom G, Stalberg P (2009) Surgical management of MEN-1 and -2: state of the art. Surg Clin North Am 89(5):1047–1068
32. Salmeron MD, Gonzalez JM, Sancho Insenser J et al (2010) Causes and treatment of recurrent hyperparathyroidism after subtotal parathyroidectomy in the presence of multiple endocrine neoplasia 1. World J Surg 34(6):1325–1331
33. Burgess J (2010) How should the patient with multiple endocrine neoplasia type 1 (MEN 1) be followed? Clin Endocrinol 72(1):13–16
34. Norton JA, Venzon DJ, Berna MJ et al (2008) Prospective study of surgery for primary hyperparathyroidism (HPT) in multiple endocrine neoplasia-type 1 and Zollinger-Ellison syndrome: long-term outcome of a more virulent form of HPT. Ann Surg 247(3):501–510
35. Peacock M, Bilezikian JP, Klassen PS, Guo MD, Turner SA, Shoback D (2005) Cinacalcet hydrochloride maintains long-term normocalcemia in patients with primary hyperparathyroidism. J Clin Endocrinol Metab 90(1):135–141
36. Wada M, Furuya Y, Sakiyama J et al (1997) The calcimimetic compound NPS R-568 suppresses parathyroid cell proliferation in rats with renal insufficiency. Control of parathyroid cell growth via a calcium receptor. J Clin Invest 100(12):2977–2983
37. Moyes VJ, Monson JP, Chew SL, Akker SA (2010) Clinical use of cinacalcet in MEN1 hyperparathyroidism. Int J Endocrinol 2010:906163
38. Faggiano A, Tavares LB, Tauchmanova L et al (2008) Effect of treatment with depot somatostatin analogue octreotide on primary hyperparathyroidism (PHP) in multiple endocrine neoplasia type 1 (MEN1) patients. Clin Endocrinol 69(5):756–762

39. Machens A, Schaaf L, Karges W et al (2007) Age-related penetrance of endocrine tumours in multiple endocrine neoplasia type 1 (MEN1): a multicentre study of 258 gene carriers. Clin Endocrinol 67(4):613–622
40. Newey PJ, Jeyabalan J, Walls GV et al (2009) Asymptomatic children with multiple endocrine neoplasia type 1 mutations may harbor nonfunctioning pancreatic neuroendocrine tumors. J Clin Endocrinol Metab 94(10):3640–3646
41. Triponez F, Dosseh D, Goudet P et al (2006) Epidemiology data on 108 MEN 1 patients from the GTE with isolated nonfunctioning tumors of the pancreas. Ann Surg 243(2):265–272
42. Anlauf M, Garbrecht N, Henopp T et al (2006) Sporadic versus hereditary gastrinomas of the duodenum and pancreas: distinct clinico-pathological and epidemiological features. World J Gastroenterol 12(34):5440–5446
43. Epelboym I, Mazeh H (2014) Zollinger-Ellison syndrome: classical considerations and current controversies. Oncologist 19(1):44–50
44. Gibril F, Schumann M, Pace A, Jensen RT (2004) Multiple endocrine neoplasia type 1 and Zollinger-Ellison syndrome: a prospective study of 107 cases and comparison with 1009 cases from the literature. Medicine (Baltimore) 83(1):43–83
45. Lowney JK, Frisella MM, Lairmore TC, Doherty GM (1998) Pancreatic islet cell tumor metastasis in multiple endocrine neoplasia type 1: correlation with primary tumor size. Surgery 124(6):1043–1048, discussion 48–9
46. Yu F, Venzon DJ, Serrano J et al (1999) Prospective study of the clinical course, prognostic factors, causes of death, and survival in patients with long-standing Zollinger-Ellison syndrome. J Clin Oncol 17(2):615–630
47. Goudet P, Murat A, Binquet C et al (2010) Risk factors and causes of death in MEN1 disease. A GTE (Groupe d'Etude des Tumeurs Endocrines) cohort study among 758 patients. World J Surg 34(2):249–255
48. Geerdink EA, Van der Luijt RB, Lips CJ (2003) Do patients with multiple endocrine neoplasia syndrome type 1 benefit from periodical screening? Eur J Endocrinol 149(6):577–582
49. Pipeleers-Marichal M, Donow C, Heitz PU, Kloppel G (1993) Pathologic aspects of gastrinomas in patients with Zollinger-Ellison syndrome with and without multiple endocrine neoplasia type I. World J Surg 17(4):481–488
50. Thakker RV (2012) Multiple endocrine neoplasia type 1. Indian J Endocrinol Metab 16(Suppl 2):S272–S274
51. Anlauf M, Perren A, Kloppel G (2007) [Gastrin cell hyperplasia associated with duodenal MEN1-related gastrinomas: histopathology and genetics]. Verh Dtsch Ges Pathol 91:320–329
52. Jensen RT (2004) Gastrinomas: advances in diagnosis and management. Neuroendocrinology 80(Suppl 1):23–27
53. Imamura M, Komoto I, Ota S et al (2011) Biochemically curative surgery for gastrinoma in multiple endocrine neoplasia type 1 patients. World J Gastroenterol 17(10):1343–1353
54. Roy PK, Venzon DJ, Feigenbaum KM et al (2001) Gastric secretion in Zollinger-Ellison syndrome. Correlation with clinical expression, tumor extent and role in diagnosis—a prospective NIH study of 235 patients and a review of 984 cases in the literature. Medicine (Baltimore) 80(3):189–222
55. Dean PG, van Heerden JA, Farley DR et al (2000) Are patients with multiple endocrine neoplasia type I prone to premature death? World J Surg 24(11):1437–1441
56. Berna MJ, Hoffmann KM, Long SH, Serrano J, Gibril F, Jensen RT (2006) Serum gastrin in Zollinger-Ellison syndrome: II. Prospective study of gastrin provocative testing in 293 patients from the National Institutes of Health and comparison with 537 cases from the literature. Evaluation of diagnostic criteria, proposal of new criteria, and correlations with clinical and tumoral features. Medicine (Baltimore) 85(6):331–364
57. Gibril F, Reynolds JC, Doppman JL et al (1996) Somatostatin receptor scintigraphy: its sensitivity compared with that of other imaging methods in detecting primary and metastatic gastrinomas. A prospective study. Ann Intern Med 125(1):26–34
58. Turner JJ, Wren AM, Jackson JE, Thakker RV, Meeran K (2002) Localization of gastrinomas by selective intra-arterial calcium injection. Clin Endocrinol 57(6):821–825

59. Thompson NW, Pasieka J, Fukuuchi A (1993) Duodenal gastrinomas, duodenotomy, and duodenal exploration in the surgical management of Zollinger-Ellison syndrome. World J Surg 17(4):455–462
60. Jensen RT (1998) Management of the Zollinger-Ellison syndrome in patients with multiple endocrine neoplasia type 1. J Intern Med 243(6):477–488
61. Norton JA, Fraker DL, Alexander HR et al (1999) Surgery to cure the Zollinger-Ellison syndrome. N Engl J Med 341(9):635–644
62. Norton JA, Alexander HR, Fraker DL, Venzon DJ, Gibril F, Jensen RT (2004) Does the use of routine duodenotomy (DUODX) affect rate of cure, development of liver metastases, or survival in patients with Zollinger-Ellison syndrome? Ann Surg 239(5):617–625; discussion 26
63. Marini F, Giusti F, Tonelli F, Brandi ML (2018) When parathyroidectomy should be indicated or postponed in adolescents with MEN1-related primary hyperparathyroidism. Front Endocrinol 9:597
64. Grozinsky-Glasberg S, Shimon I, Korbonits M, Grossman AB (2008) Somatostatin analogues in the control of neuroendocrine tumours: efficacy and mechanisms. Endocr Relat Cancer 15(3):701–720
65. Arnold R, Wied M, Behr TH (2002) Somatostatin analogues in the treatment of endocrine tumors of the gastrointestinal tract. Expert Opin Pharmacother 3(6):643–656
66. Shojamanesh H, Gibril F, Louie A et al (2002) Prospective study of the antitumor efficacy of long-term octreotide treatment in patients with progressive metastatic gastrinoma. Cancer 94(2):331–343
67. Thakker RV (2010) Multiple endocrine neoplasia type 1 (MEN1). Best Pract Res Clin Endocrinol Metab 24(3):355–370
68. Grozinsky-Glasberg S, Barak D, Fraenkel M et al (2011) Peptide receptor radioligand therapy is an effective treatment for the long-term stabilization of malignant gastrinomas. Cancer 117(7):1377–1385
69. Vasen HF, Lamers CB, Lips CJ (1989) Screening for the multiple endocrine neoplasia syndrome type I. A study of 11 kindreds in The Netherlands. Arch Intern Med 149(12):2717–2722
70. Fabbri HC, Mello MP, Soardi FC et al (2010) Long-term follow-up of an 8-year-old boy with insulinoma as the first manifestation of a familial form of multiple endocrine neoplasia type 1. Arq Bras Endocrinol Metabol 54(8):754–760
71. Giudici F, Nesi G, Brandi ML, Tonelli F (2012) Surgical management of insulinomas in multiple endocrine neoplasia type 1. Pancreas 41(4):547–553
72. Langer P, Kann PH, Fendrich V et al (2004) Prospective evaluation of imaging procedures for the detection of pancreaticoduodenal endocrine tumors in patients with multiple endocrine neoplasia type 1. World J Surg 28(12):1317–1322
73. Levy-Bohbot N, Merle C, Goudet P et al (2004) Prevalence, characteristics and prognosis of MEN 1-associated glucagonomas, VIPomas, and somatostatinomas: study from the GTE (Groupe des Tumeurs Endocrines) registry. Gastroenterol Clin Biol 28(11):1075–1081
74. Zhang M, Xu X, Shen Y, Hu ZH, Wu LM, Zheng SS (2004) Clinical experience in diagnosis and treatment of glucagonoma syndrome. Hepatobiliary Pancreat Dis Int 3(3):473–475
75. van Beek AP, de Haas ER, van Vloten WA, Lips CJ, Roijers JF, Canninga-van Dijk MR (2004) The glucagonoma syndrome and necrolytic migratory erythema: a clinical review. Eur J Endocrinol 151(5):531–537
76. Yamazaki M, Suzuki S, Kosugi S et al (2012) Delay in the diagnosis of multiple endocrine neoplasia type 1: typical symptoms are frequently overlooked. Endocr J 59(9):797–807
77. Sakurai A, Suzuki S, Kosugi S et al (2012) Multiple endocrine neoplasia type 1 in Japan: establishment and analysis of a multicentre database. Clin Endocrinol 76(4):533–539
78. Soga J, Yakuwa Y (1998) Glucagonomas/diabetico-dermatogenic syndrome (DDS): a statistical evaluation of 407 reported cases. J Hepato-Biliary-Pancreat Surg 5(3):312–319
79. Kindmark H, Sundin A, Granberg D et al (2007) Endocrine pancreatic tumors with glucagon hypersecretion: a retrospective study of 23 cases during 20 years. Med Oncol 24(3):330–337
80. Wermers RA, Fatourechi V, Wynne AG, Kvols LK, Lloyd RV (1996) The glucagonoma syndrome. Clinical and pathologic features in 21 patients. Medicine (Baltimore) 75(2):53–63

81. O'Toole D, Salazar R, Falconi M et al (2006) Rare functioning pancreatic endocrine tumors. Neuroendocrinology 84(3):189–195
82. Eldor R, Glaser B, Fraenkel M, Doviner V, Salmon A, Gross DJ (2011) Glucagonoma and the glucagonoma syndrome—cumulative experience with an elusive endocrine tumour. Clin Endocrinol 74(5):593–598
83. Brown CH, Crile G Jr (1964) Pancreatic adenoma with intractable diarrhea, hypokalemia, and hypercalcemia. JAMA 190:30–34
84. Falconi M, Eriksson B, Kaltsas G, Bartsch DK, Capdevila J, Caplin M, Kos-Kudla B, Kwekkeboom D, Rindi G, Klöppel G, Reed N (2016) ENETS consensus guidelines update for the management of patients with functional pancreatic neuroendocrine tumors and non-functional pancreatic neuroendocrine tumors. Neuroendocrinology 103(2):153–171
85. Scarsbrook AF, Thakker RV, Wass JA, Gleeson FV, Phillips RR (2006) Multiple endocrine neoplasia: spectrum of radiologic appearances and discussion of a multitechnique imaging approach. Radiographics 26(2):433–451
86. Tamagno G, Scherer V, Caimo A, Bergmann SR, Kann PH (2018) Endoscopic ultrasound features of multiple endocrine neoplasia type 1-related versus sporadic pancreatic neuroendocrine tumors: a single-center retrospective study. Digestion 98(2):112–118
87. Doherty GM, Olson JA, Frisella MM, Lairmore TC, Wells SA Jr, Norton JA (1998) Lethality of multiple endocrine neoplasia type I. World J Surg 22(6):581–586; discussion 86–7
88. Kann PH, Balakina E, Ivan D et al (2006) Natural course of small, asymptomatic neuroendocrine pancreatic tumours in multiple endocrine neoplasia type 1: an endoscopic ultrasound imaging study. Endocr Relat Cancer 13(4):1195–1202
89. Kann PH (2018) Is endoscopic ultrasonography more sensitive than magnetic resonance imaging in detecting and localizing pancreatic neuroendocrine tumors? Rev Endocr Metab Disord 19(2):133–137
90. Sadowski SM, Triponez F (2015) Management of pancreatic neuroendocrine tumors in patients with MEN 1. Gland Surg 4(1):63
91. Akerstrom G, Hessman O, Hellman P, Skogseid B (2005) Pancreatic tumours as part of the MEN-1 syndrome. Best Pract Res Clin Gastroenterol 19(5):819–830
92. Bartsch DK, Fendrich V, Langer P, Celik I, Kann PH, Rothmund M (2005) Outcome of duodenopancreatic resections in patients with multiple endocrine neoplasia type 1. Ann Surg 242(6):757–764, discussion 64–6
93. Partelli S, Tamburrino D, Lopez C, Albers M, Milanetto AC, Pasquali C, Manzoni M, Toumpanakis C, Fusai G, Bartsch D, Falconi M (2016) Active surveillance versus surgery of nonfunctioning pancreatic neuroendocrine neoplasms ≤2 cm in MEN1 patients. Neuroendocrinology 103(6):779–786
94. Sadot E, Reidy-Lagunes DL, Tang LH, Do RK, Gonen M, D'Angelica MI, DeMatteo RP, Kingham TP, Koerkamp BG, Untch BR, Brennan MF (2016) Observation versus resection for small asymptomatic pancreatic neuroendocrine tumors: a matched case–control study. Ann Surg Oncol 23(4):1361–1370
95. Anlauf M, Schlenger R, Perren A et al (2006) Microadenomatosis of the endocrine pancreas in patients with and without the multiple endocrine neoplasia type 1 syndrome. Am J Surg Pathol 30(5):560–574
96. Yao JC, Shah MH, Ito T et al (2011) Everolimus for advanced pancreatic neuroendocrine tumors. N Engl J Med 364(6):514–523
97. Raymond E, Dahan L, Raoul JL et al (2011) Sunitinib malate for the treatment of pancreatic neuroendocrine tumors. N Engl J Med 364(6):501–513
98. Oleinikov K, Dancour A, Epshtein J, Benson A, Mazeh H, Tal I, Matalon S, Benbassat CA, Livovsky DM, Goldin E, Gross DJ (2019) Endoscopic ultrasound-guided radiofrequency ablation: a new therapeutic approach for pancreatic neuroendocrine tumors. J Clin Endocrinol Metabol 104(7):2637–2647
99. Koumarianou A, Antoniou S, Kanakis G et al (2012) Combination treatment with metronomic temozolomide, bevacizumab and long-acting octreotide for malignant neuroendocrine tumours. Endocr Relat Cancer 19(1):L1–L4

100. Kulke MH, Bendell J, Kvols L, Picus J, Pommier R, Yao J (2011) Evolving diagnostic and treatment strategies for pancreatic neuroendocrine tumors. J Hematol Oncol 4:29
101. Grozinsky-Glasberg S, Grossman AB, Korbonits M (2008) The role of somatostatin analogues in the treatment of neuroendocrine tumours. Mol Cell Endocrinol 286(1–2):238–250
102. Welin S, Sorbye H, Sebjornsen S, Knappskog S, Busch C, Oberg K (2011) Clinical effect of temozolomide-based chemotherapy in poorly differentiated endocrine carcinoma after progression on first-line chemotherapy. Cancer 117(20):4617–4622
103. Sano T, Yamasaki R, Saito H et al (1987) Growth hormone-releasing hormone (GHRH)-secreting pancreatic tumor in a patient with multiple endocrine neoplasia type I. Am J Surg Pathol 11(10):810–819
104. Kloppel G, Anlauf M (2005) Epidemiology, tumour biology and histopathological classification of neuroendocrine tumours of the gastrointestinal tract. Best Pract Res Clin Gastroenterol 19(4):507–517
105. Trouillas J, Labat-Moleur F, Sturm N et al (2008) Pituitary tumors and hyperplasia in multiple endocrine neoplasia type 1 syndrome (MEN1): a case-control study in a series of 77 patients versus 2509 non-MEN1 patients. Am J Surg Pathol 32(4):534–543
106. Melmed S (2011) Pathogenesis of pituitary tumors. Nat Rev Endocrinol 7(5):257–266
107. Verges B, Boureille F, Goudet P et al (2002) Pituitary disease in MEN type 1 (MEN1): data from the France-Belgium MEN1 multicenter study. J Clin Endocrinol Metab 87(2):457–465
108. Delemer B (2012) MEN1 and pituitary adenomas. Ann Endocrinol (Paris) 73(2):59–61
109. Biondi CA, Gartside MG, Waring P et al (2004) Conditional inactivation of the MEN1 gene leads to pancreatic and pituitary tumorigenesis but does not affect normal development of these tissues. Mol Cell Biol 24(8):3125–3131
110. Bertolino P, Tong WM, Galendo D, Wang ZQ, Zhang CX (2003) Heterozygous Men1 mutant mice develop a range of endocrine tumors mimicking multiple endocrine neoplasia type 1. Mol Endocrinol 17(9):1880–1892
111. Beckers A, Daly AF (2007) The clinical, pathological, and genetic features of familial isolated pituitary adenomas. Eur J Endocrinol 157(4):371–382
112. Beckers A, Betea D, Valdes Socin H, Stevenaert A (2003) The treatment of sporadic versus MEN1-related pituitary adenomas. J Intern Med 253(6):599–605
113. Tichomirowa MA, Lee M, Barlier A et al (2012) Cyclin-dependent kinase inhibitor 1B (CDKN1B) gene variants in AIP mutation-negative familial isolated pituitary adenoma kindreds. Endocr Relat Cancer 19(3):233–241
114. Burgess JR, Shepherd JJ, Parameswaran V, Hoffman L, Greenaway TM (1996) Spectrum of pituitary disease in multiple endocrine neoplasia type 1 (MEN 1): clinical, biochemical, and radiological features of pituitary disease in a large MEN 1 kindred. J Clin Endocrinol Metab 81(7):2642–2646
115. Vortmeyer AO, Lubensky IA, Skarulis M et al (1999) Multiple endocrine neoplasia type 1: atypical presentation, clinical course, and genetic analysis of multiple tumors. Mod Pathol 12(9):919–924
116. Chandrasekharappa SC, Teh BT (2001) Clinical and molecular aspects of multiple endocrine neoplasia type 1. Front Horm Res 28:50–80
117. Goudet P, Bonithon-Kopp C, Murat A et al (2011) Gender-related differences in MEN1 lesion occurrence and diagnosis: a cohort study of 734 cases from the Groupe d'etude des Tumeurs Endocrines. Eur J Endocrinol 165(1):97–105
118. Goudet P, Murat A, Cardot-Bauters C et al (2009) Thymic neuroendocrine tumors in multiple endocrine neoplasia type 1: a comparative study on 21 cases among a series of 761 MEN1 from the GTE (Groupe des Tumeurs Endocrines). World J Surg 33(6):1197–1207
119. Berna MJ, Annibale B, Marignani M et al (2008) A prospective study of gastric carcinoids and enterochromaffin-like cell changes in multiple endocrine neoplasia type 1 and Zollinger-Ellison syndrome: identification of risk factors. J Clin Endocrinol Metab 93(5):1582–1591
120. Girard N, Ruffini E, Marx A, Faivre-Finn C, Peters S (2015) Thymic epithelial tumours: ESMO clinical practice guidelines for diagnosis, treatment and follow-up. Ann Oncol 26(Suppl 5):v40–v55

121. Gatta-Cherifi B, Chabre O, Murat A et al (2012) Adrenal involvement in MEN1. Analysis of 715 cases from the Groupe d'etude des Tumeurs Endocrines database. Eur J Endocrinol 166(2):269–279
122. Schaefer S, Shipotko M, Meyer S et al (2008) Natural course of small adrenal lesions in multiple endocrine neoplasia type 1: an endoscopic ultrasound imaging study. Eur J Endocrinol 158(5):699–704
123. Langer P, Cupisti K, Bartsch DK et al (2002) Adrenal involvement in multiple endocrine neoplasia type 1. World J Surg 26(8):891–896
124. Dreijerink KM, Goudet P, Burgess JR, Valk GD (2014) Breast-cancer predisposition in multiple endocrine neoplasia type 1. N Engl J Med 371(6):583–584
125. Dreijerink KM, Groner AC, Vos ES, Font-Tello A, Gu L, Chi D, Reyes J, Cook J, Lim E, Lin CY, De Laat W (2017) Enhancer-mediated oncogenic function of the menin tumor suppressor in breast cancer. Cell Rep 18(10):2359–2372
126. Van Leeuwaarde RS, Dreijerink KM, Ausems MG, Beijers HJ, Dekkers OM, De Herder WW, van der Horst-Schrivers AN, Drent ML, Bisschop PH, Havekes B, Peeters PH (2017) MEN1-dependent breast cancer: indication for early screening? Results from the Dutch MEN1 Study Group. J Clin Endocrinol Metabol 102(6):2083–2090
127. Asgharian B, Chen YJ, Patronas NJ et al (2004) Meningiomas may be a component tumor of multiple endocrine neoplasia type 1. Clin Cancer Res 10(3):869–880
128. Vidal A, Iglesias MJ, Fernandez B, Fonseca E, Cordido F (2008) Cutaneous lesions associated to multiple endocrine neoplasia syndrome type 1. J Eur Acad Dermatol Venereol 22(7):835–838
129. Lemmens I, Van de Ven WJ, Kas K et al (1997) Identification of the multiple endocrine neoplasia type 1 (MEN1) gene. The European Consortium on MEN1. Hum Mol Genet 6(7):1177–1183
130. Chandrasekharappa SC, Guru SC, Manickam P et al (1997) Positional cloning of the gene for multiple endocrine neoplasia-type 1. Science 276(5311):404–407
131. Cristina EV, Alberto F (2018) Management of familial hyperparathyroidism syndromes: MEN1, MEN2, MEN4, HPT-jaw tumour, familial isolated hyperparathyroidism, FHH, and neonatal severe hyperparathyroidism. Best Pract Res Clin Endocrinol Metab 32:861
132. Marx SJ (2019) New concepts about familial isolated hyperparathyroidism. J Clin Endocrinol Metabol 104:4058
133. Turner JJ, Christie PT, Pearce SH, Turnpenny PD, Thakker RV (2010) Diagnostic challenges due to phenocopies: lessons from multiple endocrine neoplasia type1 (MEN1). Hum Mutat 31(1):E1089–E1101
134. Karges W, Jostarndt K, Maier S et al (2000) Multiple endocrine neoplasia type 1 (MEN1) gene mutations in a subset of patients with sporadic and familial primary hyperparathyroidism target the coding sequence but spare the promoter region. J Endocrinol 166(1):1–9
135. Jiao Y, Shi C, Edil BH et al (2011) DAXX/ATRX, MEN1, and mTOR pathway genes are frequently altered in pancreatic neuroendocrine tumors. Science 331(6021):1199–1203
136. Agarwal SK, Ozawa A, Mateo CM, Marx SJ (2009) The MEN1 gene and pituitary tumours. Horm Res 71(Suppl 2):131–138
137. Olufemi SE, Green JS, Manickam P et al (1998) Common ancestral mutation in the MEN1 gene is likely responsible for the prolactinoma variant of MEN1 (MEN1Burin) in four kindreds from Newfoundland. Hum Mutat 11(4):264–269
138. Hao W, Skarulis MC, Simonds WF et al (2004) Multiple endocrine neoplasia type 1 variant with frequent prolactinoma and rare gastrinoma. J Clin Endocrinol Metab 89(8):3776–3784
139. Burgess JR, Nord B, David R et al (2000) Phenotype and phenocopy: the relationship between genotype and clinical phenotype in a single large family with multiple endocrine neoplasia type 1 (MEN 1). Clin Endocrinol 53(2):205–211
140. Newey PJ, Thakker RV (2011) Role of multiple endocrine neoplasia type 1 mutational analysis in clinical practice. Endocr Pract 17(Suppl 3):8–17
141. Langer P, Wild A, Hall A, Celik I, Rothmund M, Bartsch DK (2003) Prevalence of multiple endocrine neoplasia type 1 in young patients with apparently sporadic primary hyperparathyroidism or pancreaticoduodenal endocrine tumours. Br J Surg 90(12):1599–1603

142. Stratakis CA, Schussheim DH, Freedman SM et al (2000) Pituitary macroadenoma in a 5-year-old: an early expression of multiple endocrine neoplasia type 1. J Clin Endocrinol Metab 85(12):4776–4780
143. Skogseid B, Eriksson B, Lundqvist G et al (1991) Multiple endocrine neoplasia type 1: a 10-year prospective screening study in four kindreds. J Clin Endocrinol Metab 73(2):281–287
144. Skogseid B, Larsson C, Oberg K (1991) Genetic and clinical characteristics of multiple endocrine neoplasia type 1. Acta Oncol 30(4):485–488
145. Keiser HR, Beaven MA, Doppman J, Wells S Jr, Buja LM (1973) Sipple's syndrome: medullary thyroid carcinoma, pheochromocytoma, and parathyroid disease. Studies in a large family. NIH conference. Ann Intern Med 78(4):561–579
146. Carney JA (2005) Familial multiple endocrine neoplasia: the first 100 years. Am J Surg Pathol 29(2):254–274
147. Easton DF, Ponder MA, Cummings T et al (1989) The clinical and screening age-at-onset distribution for the MEN-2 syndrome. Am J Hum Genet 44(2):208–215
148. Ponder BA, Ponder MA, Coffey R et al (1988) Risk estimation and screening in families of patients with medullary thyroid carcinoma. Lancet 1(8582):397–401
149. Mulligan LM, Eng C, Healey CS et al (1994) Specific mutations of the RET proto-oncogene are related to disease phenotype in MEN 2A and FMTC. Nat Genet 6(1):70–74
150. Frank-Raue K, Hoppner W, Frilling A et al (1996) Mutations of the ret protooncogene in German multiple endocrine neoplasia families: relation between genotype and phenotype. German Medullary Thyroid Carcinoma Study Group. J Clin Endocrinol Metab 81(5):1780–1783
151. Steiner AL, Goodman AD, Powers SR (1968) Study of a kindred with pheochromocytoma, medullary thyroid carcinoma, hyperparathyroidism and Cushing's disease: multiple endocrine neoplasia, type 2. Medicine (Baltimore) 47(5):371–409
152. Melvin KE, Tashjian AH Jr, Miller HH (1972) Studies in familial (medullary) thyroid carcinoma. Recent Prog Horm Res 28:399–470
153. Gagel RF, Tashjian AH Jr, Cummings T et al (1988) The clinical outcome of prospective screening for multiple endocrine neoplasia type 2a. An 18-year experience. N Engl J Med 318(8):478–484
154. Wells SA Jr, Asa SL, Dralle H, Elisei R, Evans DB, Gagel RF, Lee N, Machens A, Moley JF, Pacini F, Raue F (2015) Revised American Thyroid Association guidelines for the management of medullary thyroid carcinoma: the American Thyroid Association Guidelines Task Force on medullary thyroid carcinoma. Thyroid 25(6):567–610
155. Farndon JR, Leight GS, Dilley WG et al (1986) Familial medullary thyroid carcinoma without associated endocrinopathies: a distinct clinical entity. Br J Surg 73(4):278–281
156. Nunziata V, Giannattasio R, Di Giovanni G, D'Armiento MR, Mancini M (1989) Hereditary localized pruritus in affected members of a kindred with multiple endocrine neoplasia type 2A (Sipple's syndrome). Clin Endocrinol 30(1):57–63
157. Donovan DT, Levy ML, Furst EJ et al (1989) Familial cutaneous lichen amyloidosis in association with multiple endocrine neoplasia type 2A: a new variant. Henry Ford Hosp Med J 37(3–4):147–150
158. Verdy M, Weber AM, Roy CC, Morin CL, Cadotte M, Brochu P (1982) Hirschsprung's disease in a family with multiple endocrine neoplasia type 2. J Pediatr Gastroenterol Nutr 1(4):603–607
159. Kakudo K, Carney JA, Sizemore GW (1985) Medullary carcinoma of thyroid. Biologic behavior of the sporadic and familial neoplasm. Cancer 55(12):2818–2821
160. Pacini F, Fontanelli M, Fugazzola L et al (1994) Routine measurement of serum calcitonin in nodular thyroid diseases allows the preoperative diagnosis of unsuspected sporadic medullary thyroid carcinoma. J Clin Endocrinol Metab 78(4):826–829
161. Guyetant S, Josselin N, Savagner F, Rohmer V, Michalak S, Saint-Andre JP (2003) C-cell hyperplasia and medullary thyroid carcinoma: clinicopathological and genetic correlations in 66 consecutive patients. Mod Pathol 16(8):756–763

162. Machens A, Niccoli-Sire P, Hoegel J et al (2003) Early malignant progression of hereditary medullary thyroid cancer. N Engl J Med 349(16):1517–1525
163. Cohen MS, Moley JF (2003) Surgical treatment of medullary thyroid carcinoma. J Intern Med 253(6):616–626
164. Szinnai G, Meier C, Komminoth P, Zumsteg UW (2003) Review of multiple endocrine neoplasia type 2A in children: therapeutic results of early thyroidectomy and prognostic value of codon analysis. Pediatrics 111(2):E132–E139
165. Robbins J, Merino MJ, Boice JD Jr et al (1991) Thyroid cancer: a lethal endocrine neoplasm. Ann Intern Med 115(2):133–147
166. Kebebew E, Ituarte PH, Siperstein AE, Duh QY, Clark OH (2000) Medullary thyroid carcinoma: clinical characteristics, treatment, prognostic factors, and a comparison of staging systems. Cancer 88(5):1139–1148
167. Sippel RS, Kunnimalaiyaan M, Chen H (2008) Current management of medullary thyroid cancer. Oncologist 13(5):539–547
168. Inabnet WB, Caragliano P, Pertsemlidis D (2000) Pheochromocytoma: inherited associations, bilaterality, and cortex preservation. Surgery 128(6):1007–1011; discussion 11–2
169. Rodriguez JM, Balsalobre M, Ponce JL et al (2008) Pheochromocytoma in MEN 2A syndrome. Study of 54 patients. World J Surg 32(11):2520–2526
170. Frank-Raue K, Rybicki LA, Erlic Z et al (2011) Risk profiles and penetrance estimations in multiple endocrine neoplasia type 2A caused by germline RET mutations located in exon 10. Hum Mutat 32(1):51–58
171. Pomares FJ, Canas R, Rodriguez JM, Hernandez AM, Parrilla P, Tebar FJ (1998) Differences between sporadic and multiple endocrine neoplasia type 2A phaeochromocytoma. Clin Endocrinol 48(2):195–200
172. Pacak K, Ilias I, Adams KT, Eisenhofer G (2005) Biochemical diagnosis, localization and management of pheochromocytoma: focus on multiple endocrine neoplasia type 2 in relation to other hereditary syndromes and sporadic forms of the tumour. J Intern Med 257(1):60–68
173. Pacak K, Eisenhofer G, Ilias I (2009) Diagnosis of pheochromocytoma with special emphasis on MEN2 syndrome. Hormones (Athens) 8(2):111–116
174. Modigliani E, Vasen HM, Raue K et al (1995) Pheochromocytoma in multiple endocrine neoplasia type 2: European study. The Euromen Study Group. J Intern Med 238(4):363–367
175. Schuffenecker I, Virally-Monod M, Brohet R et al (1998) Risk and penetrance of primary hyperparathyroidism in multiple endocrine neoplasia type 2A families with mutations at codon 634 of the RET proto-oncogene. Groupe D'etude des Tumeurs a Calcitonine. J Clin Endocrinol Metab 83(2):487–491
176. Machens A, Lorenz K, Dralle H (2013) Peak incidence of pheochromocytoma and primary hyperparathyroidism in multiple endocrine neoplasia 2: need for age-adjusted biochemical screening. J Clin Endocrinol Metab 98(2):E336–E345
177. Gagel RF, Levy ML, Donovan DT, Alford BR, Wheeler T, Tschen JA (1989) Multiple endocrine neoplasia type 2a associated with cutaneous lichen amyloidosis. Ann Intern Med 111(10):802–806
178. Ceccherini I, Romei C, Barone V et al (1994) Identification of the Cys634-->Tyr mutation of the RET proto-oncogene in a pedigree with multiple endocrine neoplasia type 2A and localized cutaneous lichen amyloidosis. J Endocrinol Investig 17(3):201–204
179. Machens A, Dralle H (2006) Multiple endocrine neoplasia type 2 and the RET protooncogene: from bedside to bench to bedside. Mol Cell Endocrinol 247(1–2):34–40
180. Machens A, Gimm O, Hinze R, Hoppner W, Boehm BO, Dralle H (2001) Genotype-phenotype correlations in hereditary medullary thyroid carcinoma: oncological features and biochemical properties. J Clin Endocrinol Metab 86(3):1104–1109
181. Angrist M, Kauffman E, Slaugenhaupt SA et al (1993) A gene for Hirschsprung disease (megacolon) in the pericentromeric region of human chromosome 10. Nat Genet 4(4):351–356
182. Romeo G, Ronchetto P, Luo Y et al (1994) Point mutations affecting the tyrosine kinase domain of the RET proto-oncogene in Hirschsprung's disease. Nature 367(6461):377–378

183. Edery P, Lyonnet S, Mulligan LM et al (1994) Mutations of the RET proto-oncogene in Hirschsprung's disease. Nature 367(6461):378–380
184. Tallini G, Santoro M, Helie M et al (1998) RET/PTC oncogene activation defines a subset of papillary thyroid carcinomas lacking evidence of progression to poorly differentiated or undifferentiated tumor phenotypes. Clin Cancer Res 4(2):287–294
185. Santoro M, Papotti M, Chiappetta G et al (2002) RET activation and clinicopathologic features in poorly differentiated thyroid tumors. J Clin Endocrinol Metab 87(1):370–379
186. Brauckhoff M, Gimm O, Hinze R, Ukkat J, Brauckhoff K, Dralle H (2002) Papillary thyroid carcinoma in patients with RET proto-oncogene germline mutation. Thyroid 12(7):557–561
187. Asai N, Jijiwa M, Enomoto A, Kawai K, Maeda K, Ichiahara M, Murakumo Y, Takahashi M (2006) RET receptor signaling: dysfunction in thyroid cancer and Hirschsprung's disease. Pathol Int 56:164–172
188. Williams ED, Pollock DJ (1966) Multiple mucosal neuromata with endocrine tumours: a syndrome allied to von Recklinghausen's disease. J Pathol Bacteriol 91(1):71–80
189. Shekitka KM, Sobin LH (1994) Ganglioneuromas of the gastrointestinal tract. Relation to Von Recklinghausen disease and other multiple tumor syndromes. Am J Surg Pathol 18(3):250–257
190. Skinner MA, DeBenedetti MK, Moley JF, Norton JA, Wells SA Jr (1996) Medullary thyroid carcinoma in children with multiple endocrine neoplasia types 2A and 2B. J Pediatr Surg 31(1):177–181; discussion 81–2
191. Shapiro B, Fig LM (1989) Management of pheochromocytoma. Endocrinol Metab Clin N Am 18(2):443–481
192. Carney JA, Sizemore GW, Sheps SG (1976) Adrenal medullary disease in multiple endocrine neoplasia, type 2: pheochromocytoma and its precursors. Am J Clin Pathol 66(2):279–290
193. Wray CJ, Rich TA, Waguespack SG, Lee JE, Perrier ND, Evans DB (2008) Failure to recognize multiple endocrine neoplasia 2B: more common than we think? Ann Surg Oncol 15(1):293–301
194. Brauckhoff M, Machens A, Hess S et al (2008) Premonitory symptoms preceding metastatic medullary thyroid cancer in MEN 2B: an exploratory analysis. Surgery 144(6):1044–1050; discussion 50–3
195. Kasprzak L, Nolet S, Gaboury L et al (2001) Familial medullary thyroid carcinoma and prominent corneal nerves associated with the germline V804M and V778I mutations on the same allele of RET. J Med Genet 38(11):784–787
196. Lee R, Hyer J, Chowdhury H, Teimory M (2012) Ocular signs of multiple endocrine neoplasia type 2B (MEN2B). J Clin Endocrinol Metab 97(3):725–726
197. Eter N, Klingmuller D, Hoppner W, Spitznas M (2001) Typical ocular findings in a patient with multiple endocrine neoplasia type 2b syndrome. Graefes Arch Clin Exp Ophthalmol 239(5):391–394
198. Jacobs JM, Hawes MJ (2001) From eyelid bumps to thyroid lumps: report of a MEN type IIb family and review of the literature. Ophthalmic Plast Reconstr Surg 17(3):195–201
199. Parker DG, Robinson BG, O'Donnell BA (2004) External ophthalmic findings in multiple endocrine neoplasia type 2B. Clin Exp Ophthalmol 32(4):420–423
200. Shields JA, Shields CL, Perez N (2002) Choroidal metastasis from medullary thyroid carcinoma in multiple endocrine neoplasia. Am J Ophthalmol 134(4):607–609
201. d'Amore ES, Manivel JC, Pettinato G, Niehans GA, Snover DC (1991) Intestinal ganglioneuromatosis: mucosal and transmural types. A clinicopathologic and immunohistochemical study of six cases. Hum Pathol 22(3):276–286
202. Lips CJ (1998) Clinical management of the multiple endocrine neoplasia syndromes: results of a computerized opinion poll at the sixth international workshop on multiple endocrine neoplasia and von Hippel-Lindau disease. J Intern Med 243(6):589–594
203. Cohen R, Campos JM, Salaun C et al (2000) Preoperative calcitonin levels are predictive of tumor size and postoperative calcitonin normalization in medullary thyroid carcinoma. Groupe d'Etudes des Tumeurs a Calcitonine (GETC). J Clin Endocrinol Metab 85(2):919–922

204. Ismailov SI, Piulatova NR (2004) Postoperative calcitonin study in medullary thyroid carcinoma. Endocr Relat Cancer 11(2):357–363
205. Kloos RT, Eng C, Evans DB et al (2009) Medullary thyroid cancer: management guidelines of the American Thyroid Association. Thyroid 19(6):565–612
206. Costante G, Meringolo D, Durante C et al (2007) Predictive value of serum calcitonin levels for preoperative diagnosis of medullary thyroid carcinoma in a cohort of 5817 consecutive patients with thyroid nodules. J Clin Endocrinol Metab 92(2):450–455
207. Pomares FJ, Rodriguez JM, Nicolas F et al (2002) Presurgical assessment of the tumor burden of familial medullary thyroid carcinoma by calcitonin testing. J Am Coll Surg 195(5):630–634
208. Neumann HP, Bausch B, McWhinney SR et al (2002) Germ-line mutations in nonsyndromic pheochromocytoma. N Engl J Med 346(19):1459–1466
209. Gimenez-Roqueplo AP, Lehnert H, Mannelli M et al (2006) Phaeochromocytoma, new genes and screening strategies. Clin Endocrinol 65(6):699–705
210. Erlic Z, Rybicki L, Peczkowska M et al (2009) Clinical predictors and algorithm for the genetic diagnosis of pheochromocytoma patients. Clin Cancer Res 15(20):6378–6385
211. Ilias I, Pacak K (2009) Diagnosis, localization and treatment of pheochromocytoma in MEN 2 syndrome. Endocr Regul 43(2):89–93
212. Amodru V, Guerin C, Delcourt S, Romanet P, Loundou A, Viana B, Brue T, Castinetti F, Sebag F, Pacak K, Taïeb D (2018) Quantitative 18 F-DOPA PET/CT in pheochromocytoma: the relationship between tumor secretion and its biochemical phenotype. Eur J Nucl Med Mol Imaging 45(2):278–282
213. Brenner ME, Jacene HA (2008) Recurrent or residual hyperparathyroidism and thyroid cancer effectively evaluated with scintigraphy. Otolaryngol Clin N Am 41(6):1117–1133, viii–ix
214. Yen TW, Shapiro SE, Gagel RF, Sherman SI, Lee JE, Evans DB (2003) Medullary thyroid carcinoma: results of a standardized surgical approach in a contemporary series of 80 consecutive patients. Surgery 134(6):890–899; discussion 99–901
215. Buhr HJ, Kallinowski F, Raue F, Frank-Raue K, Herfarth C (1993) Microsurgical neck dissection for occultly metastasizing medullary thyroid carcinoma. Three-year results. Cancer 72(12):3685–3693
216. Ukkat J, Gimm O, Brauckhoff M, Bilkenroth U, Dralle H (2004) Single center experience in primary surgery for medullary thyroid carcinoma. World J Surg 28(12):1271–1274
217. Gimm O, Ukkat J, Niederle BE et al (2004) Timing and extent of surgery in patients with familial medullary thyroid carcinoma/multiple endocrine neoplasia 2A-related RET mutations not affecting codon 634. World J Surg 28(12):1312–1316
218. Moley JF, Debenedetti MK, Dilley WG, Tisell LE, Wells SA (1998) Surgical management of patients with persistent or recurrent medullary thyroid cancer. J Intern Med 243(6):521–526
219. Brauckhoff M, Lorenz K, Ukkat J, Brauckhoff K, Gimm O, Dralle H (2004) Medullary thyroid carcinoma. Scand J Surg 93(4):249–260
220. Scollo C, Baudin E, Travagli JP et al (2003) Rationale for central and bilateral lymph node dissection in sporadic and hereditary medullary thyroid cancer. J Clin Endocrinol Metab 88(5):2070–2075
221. Niccoli-Sire P, Murat A, Baudin E et al (1999) Early or prophylactic thyroidectomy in MEN 2/FMTC gene carriers: results in 71 thyroidectomized patients. The French Calcitonin Tumours Study Group (GETC). Eur J Endocrinol 141(5):468–474
222. Machens A, Hauptmann S, Dralle H (2008) Prediction of lateral lymph node metastases in medullary thyroid cancer. Br J Surg 95(5):586–591
223. Dralle H, Machens A (2013) Surgical management of the lateral neck compartment for metastatic thyroid cancer. Curr Opin Oncol 25(1):20–26
224. Fleming JB, Lee JE, Bouvet M et al (1999) Surgical strategy for the treatment of medullary thyroid carcinoma. Ann Surg 230(5):697–707
225. Massoll N, Mazzaferri EL (2004) Diagnosis and management of medullary thyroid carcinoma. Clin Lab Med 24(1):49–83

226. Gottlieb JA, Hill CS Jr (1974) Chemotherapy of thyroid cancer with adriamycin. Experience with 30 patients. N Engl J Med 290(4):193–197
227. Martinez SR, Beal SH, Chen A, Chen SL, Schneider PD (2010) Adjuvant external beam radiation for medullary thyroid carcinoma. J Surg Oncol 102(2):175–178
228. Gild ML, Bullock M, Robinson BG, Clifton-Bligh R (2011) Multikinase inhibitors: a new option for the treatment of thyroid cancer. Nat Rev Endocrinol 7(10):617–624
229. Wells SA Jr, Robinson BG, Gagel RF et al (2012) Vandetanib in patients with locally advanced or metastatic medullary thyroid cancer: a randomized, double-blind phase III trial. J Clin Oncol 30(2):134–141
230. Schoffski PER, Müller S, Brose MS, Shah MH, Licitra LF, Jarzab B, Medvedev V, Kreissl M, Niederle B, Cohen EEW, Wirth LJ, Ali HY, Hessel C, Yaron Y, Ball DW, Nelkin B, Sherman SI, Schlumberger M (2012) An international, double-blind, randomized, placebo-controlled phase III trial (EXAM) of cabozantinib (XL184) in medullary thyroid carcinoma (MTC) patients (pts) with documented RECIST progression at baseline [abstract]. J Clin Oncol 30:5508
231. Smit J (2013) Treatment of advanced medullary thyroid cancer. Thyroid Res 6(Suppl 1):S7
232. Bargellini T, Cantelli G, Bruscino A, et al (2011) [Left laparoscopic adrenalectomy for pheochromocytoma in MEN 2B: case report]. G Chir 32(3):132–134
233. Fassbender WJ, Krohn-Grimberghe B, Gortz B et al (2000) Multiple endocrine neoplasia (MEN)—an overview and case report—patient with sporadic bilateral pheochromocytoma, hyperparathyroidism and marfanoid habitus. Anticancer Res 20(6C):4877–4887
234. Nguyen L, Niccoli-Sire P, Caron P et al (2001) Pheochromocytoma in multiple endocrine neoplasia type 2: a prospective study. Eur J Endocrinol 144(1):37–44
235. Eisenhofer G, Rivers G, Rosas AL, Quezado Z, Manger WM, Pacak K (2007) Adverse drug reactions in patients with phaeochromocytoma: incidence, prevention and management. Drug Saf 30(11):1031–1062
236. Bilezikian JP, Khan AA, Potts JT Jr (2009) Guidelines for the management of asymptomatic primary hyperparathyroidism: summary statement from the third international workshop. J Clin Endocrinol Metab 94(2):335–339
237. Twigt BA, Scholten A, Valk GD, Rinkes IH, Vriens MR (2013) Differences between sporadic and MEN related primary hyperparathyroidism; clinical expression, preoperative workup, operative strategy and follow-up. Orphanet J Rare Dis 8:50
238. Hansford JR, Mulligan LM (2000) Multiple endocrine neoplasia type 2 and RET: from neoplasia to neurogenesis. J Med Genet 37(11):817–827
239. Punales MK, Graf H, Gross JL, Maia AL (2003) RET codon 634 mutations in multiple endocrine neoplasia type 2: variable clinical features and clinical outcome. J Clin Endocrinol Metab 88(6):2644–2649
240. Gimm O, Neuberg DS, Marsh DJ et al (1999) Over-representation of a germline RET sequence variant in patients with sporadic medullary thyroid carcinoma and somatic RET codon 918 mutation. Oncogene 18(6):1369–1373
241. Romeo G, Ceccherini I, Celli J et al (1998) Association of multiple endocrine neoplasia type 2 and Hirschsprung disease. J Intern Med 243(6):515–520
242. Aiello A, Cioni K, Gobbo M et al (2005) The familial medullary thyroid carcinoma-associated RET E768D mutation in a multiple endocrine neoplasia type 2A case. Surgery 137(5):574–576
243. Jimenez C, Habra MA, Huang SC et al (2004) Pheochromocytoma and medullary thyroid carcinoma: a new genotype-phenotype correlation of the RET protooncogene 891 germline mutation. J Clin Endocrinol Metab 89(8):4142–4145
244. Gibelin H, Bezieau S, Misso C, Bouin-Pineau MH, Marechaud R, Kraimps JL (2004) Germline RET V804M mutation associated with multiple endocrine neoplasia type 2A. Br J Surg 91(11):1458–1459
245. Feldman GL, Edmonds MW, Ainsworth PJ et al (2000) Variable expressivity of familial medullary thyroid carcinoma (FMTC) due to a RET V804M (GTG-->ATG) mutation. Surgery 128(1):93–98

246. Frohnauer MK, Decker RA (2000) Update on the MEN 2A c804 RET mutation: is prophylactic thyroidectomy indicated? Surgery 128(6):1052–1057; discussion 57–8
247. Rothberg AE, Raymond VM, Gruber SB, Sisson J (2009) Familial medullary thyroid carcinoma associated with cutaneous lichen amyloidosis. Thyroid 19(6):651–655
248. Kahraman T, de Groot JW, Rouwe C et al (2003) Acceptable age for prophylactic surgery in children with multiple endocrine neoplasia type 2a. Eur J Surg Oncol 29(4):331–335
249. Moline J, Eng C (2011) Multiple endocrine neoplasia type 2: an overview. Genet Med 13(9):755–764

Thyroid Cancer

22

Per Hellman, Olov Norlén, Peter Stålberg, and Kosmas Daskalakis

22.1 Introduction

The most common endocrine malignancy is thyroid cancer (95% of all endocrine malignancies), and accounts for approximately 2% of all cancers diagnosed world-wide [1]. The incidence is increasing world-wide, and although the reasons thereof are debated, the increased detection rate through ultrasound is mostly appreciated [2]. While many have raised the reason for increased diagnosis due to screening, and the use of ultrasound, there may be a slight increase in cancer-specific mortality [3]. In the USA, the incidence has increased by on average 3.6% per year between 1974 and 2013 and is now 14.42/100,000 person-years [3]. In China, the age-standardized incidence rate increased from 2.75/100,000 in 2000 to 19.42/100,000 in 2012, while the mortality rate was constant at about 0.25/100,000 [4]. The prognosis is generally very good for thyroid carcinoma, and the risk for mortality after diagnosis has dropped considerably, but due to the increased incidence, there is still a high number of deaths per year in thyroid cancer. In the USA around 1800–2000 people will die yearly due to thyroid cancer [5].

Thyroid cancer is two- to threefold more common in females than males, although the latter gender dies of cancer more often than women (45,310 and 14,910 new thyroid cancer cases and 810 and 1040 deaths from thyroid cancer in women and men, respectively, estimated in 2013 in the USA) [5]. It is now the fifth-most common cancer (6% of all female cancers) among women in the USA [5].

The frequency of thyroid cancer is highest in younger age groups, and the age onset is bell-shaped with the highest incidence between 20 and 50 years of age [6].

P. Hellman (✉) · O. Norlén · P. Stålberg
Department of Surgical Sciences, Uppsala University, Uppsala, Sweden
e-mail: per.hellman@uu.se; olov.norlen@surgsci.uu.se; peter.stalberg@uu.se

K. Daskalakis
Faculty of Medicine and Health, Department of Surgery, Örebro University, Örebro, Sweden
e-mail: kosmas.daskalakis@oru.se

S. Yalcin, K. Öberg (eds.), *Neuroendocrine Tumours*,
https://doi.org/10.1007/978-3-031-56968-5_22

During recent years there has been a rise in the incidence in the somewhat older age groups.

Thyroid cancer derived from follicular cells is the most common papillary (PTC) and follicular thyroid cancer (FTC). Hürtle cell or oncocytic cancer (HCC) is considered a variant with a somewhat worse prognosis, and anaplastic thyroid cancer (ATC) has a dismal prognosis. Medullary thyroid cancer (MTC) arises from parafollicular C-cells which produce calcitonin and account for 5% of thyroid cancers. PTC and FTC are commonly referred together as differentiated thyroid cancer (DTC) which accounts for 94% of thyroid cancers. Less than 1–3% of thyroid cancers are ATC [7].

22.2 Etiology

22.2.1 External Radiation

The only well-established risk factor for differentiated thyroid cancer, specifically PTC, is external head and neck radiation during infancy, childhood period, and young adulthood [8]. The risk increases linearly after exposure to doses above 0.05–0.1 Gy, and the risk is highest in childhood [9]. Papillary thyroid cancer is the most associated cancer to radiation, after a lag time of 5–10 years. Genetic analyses have shown an increased rate of *RET*/PTC rearrangements (see below), and a high number of driver mutations (96.9%). In the latter study of a population exposed after the Chernobyl accident, the mean radiation dose for causing point mutations was 0.2 Gy, and higher doses for gene fusions, which were also noted in 70.8% of cases [10]. The younger the patient was at the time of exposure, the higher the risk of developing cancer. Iodine deficiency increases the risk of radiation-induced thyroid cancer [11]. From the 1920s to 1960s, external low-dose radiation therapy had been used for the treatment of a variety of benign diseases such as acne, tonsillitis, enlarged thymus, and fungal disease of the scalp [12]. More high-dose radiation (>20 Gy) was given as treatment for Hodgkin's disease, non-Hodgkin's lymphoma, Wilms' tumor, and neuroblastoma is also associated with development of thyroid cancer [12].

The average time duration between irradiation and thyroid tumor is 10–20 years; however, periods from 5 to 50 years have been reported [13]. In some regions of Japan, the incidence of thyroid cancer in a screened population is as high as 0.1%, tenfold higher than expected on US incidence rates. Within the first decade after the Chernobyl accident, some regions of Belarus showed a 100-fold increase in thyroid cancer in individuals, below the age of 15 at the time of exposure [14]. The risk for development of thyroid cancer after radiation is significant within 10 years of exposure (2.76), but remained elevated up to at least 50 years, based on studies from Japan [15].

There is no evidence that the diagnostic use of ^{131}I increased the risk of thyroid cancer. The therapeutic use of ^{131}I for ablation of thyroid tissue to treat hyperthyroidism seems to be associated with a very modest increased risk of thyroid cancer [16].

22.2.2 Dietary Factors

Thyroid cancer incidence is different in different geographic areas. Iodine deficiency has been considered as a risk factor for thyroid cancer, and iodine-rich diet such as shellfish, but also other types of fish, has been found to be protective [17, 18]. Consumption of the so-called goitrogenic food (cruciferous vegetables) has been noted with a minor increased risk, but also high consumption of meat, mostly chicken and pork [17, 18].

22.2.3 Autoimmune Disease and Thyroid Cancer

There seems to be an increased risk for thyroid cancer in the course of Grave's disease, although the criticism of the reason for the higher incidence is due to the finding of microcarcinomas after surgery [19]. Once established in a hyperthyroid patients, thyroid cancer is more aggressive in Grave's disease [20]. Stimulation of the TSH receptor, presumably through the thyroid-stimulating antibodies has been suggested as a causative factor. A recent review of 36 published studies also found an association between Hashimoto's disease and papillary thyroid cancer (not FTC, MTC, or ATC) [21]. There is no increased incidence of thyroid cancer among patients with primary hypothyroidism.

22.2.4 Familial Thyroid Cancer

Familial thyroid cancer is mostly associated with medullary thyroid cancer (MTC), which occurs in multiple endocrine neoplasia type 2A and 2B (MEN2A, MEN2B), as well as familial mMTC. All these syndromes exhibit a mutation in the RET protooncogene, and if this is noted early prophylactic thyroidectomy eliminates the risk of MTC [22]. Follicular cell-derived thyroid cancer may develop in several syndromes, although with low penetrance; Familial adenomatous polyposis (FAP), Carney Complex (CC), Cowden's syndrome (CS), McCune-Albright's syndrome, Pendreds syndrome, and Werner's syndrome [23]. Epidemiologic studies have demonstrated a four- to tenfold increased risk of DTC in first-degree relatives of the patients [24].

22.3 Pathology

There are four major types of thyroid carcinomas according to morphology and biological behavior: papillary (PTC), follicular (FTC), medullary (MTC), and anaplastic carcinomas (ATC). Highly differentiated papillary and follicular carcinomas may together be denoted differentiated thyroid carcinomas (DTC). The WHO (World Health Organization) classification of thyroid carcinomas is shown in Table 22.1 [25].

Table 22.1 Tumors of the thyroid according to the WHO classification, distribution, survival, and common genetic disturbances [22, 25]

Tumors	Fq %	10-year survival (%)	Genetic derangement [22]
Papillary carcinoma	84	93	
Classic papillary			*BRAF, RTK, RET/PTC*
Follicular variant—without invasion			*RAS*
Follicular variant—with invasion			*RAS, PAX8-PPARγ*
Tall cell variant			*BRAF*
Non-tall cell infiltrative			*BRAF, RAS*
Papillary microcarcinomas			
Follicular carcinoma	2	85	
Oncocytic variant (Hürtle cell)	2	76	
Poorly differentiated carcinoma	6	34	*TP53, BRAF, RAS, CTNNB1*
Undifferentiated (anaplastic) carcinoma	1	0	*TP53, BRAF, RAS*
Medullary thyroid carcinoma	4	75	
Other	1		

22.3.1 Differentiated Thyroid Carcinomas (DTC)

A total of 88% of all thyroid carcinomas are DTC. Papillary tumors arise from the thyroglobulin (Tg)-producing follicular cells, and 85% of DTC are PTC in developed countries where sufficient iodine is present in the diet [25].

PTC is the most well-differentiated type and accounts for 84% of all thyroid cancers. Microscopically they consist of several characteristic papillae, and also often evident are nuclear changes, especially the ground glass nuclei. They may be multifocal and usually are associated with a high rate of lymph node metastases [25].

They may also invade the thyroid capsule and the surrounding structures, such as the esophagus, the trachea, or the internal jugular vein. Psammoma bodies, calcified scarred remnants of tumor papillae, are commonly seen in about 50% of PTC and pathognomonic for PTC [25]. PTC less than 1 cm are often referred to as micro-carcinomas.

Genetically, PTC has a well-conserved genome, with a few copy number variations and few mutations. Among these the mitogen-activated protein kinase (MAPK) pathway may be affected, usually through mutations in *BRAF* V600E (60%). Mutations in *RAS* genes (15%) and derangements that involves *BRAF* or receptor kinases may also be present [22]. Such PTCs often bear lymph node metastases and may display various histopathologic features. The tall cell variant is associated with mutations in *BRAF* and may have a poor response to radioiodine therapy. The reason is the oncogene effect by the V600E variant, activating the downstream MAPK pathway which suppresses the expression of genes involved in handling iodine [26]. Detection of *BRAF* mutation on FNA specimens before surgery is recommended as a useful diagnostic marker and prognostic indicator for PTC and thus influences the surgeon's decision on the management of PTC [27]. Tumors with a more invasive feature, and perhaps a lower rate of lymph node metastases are associated with the follicular variant of PTC and may have *RAS* mutations, Activating *RET* mutations may be the result of ionizing radiation, but also chromosomal rearrangements, such as *RET-PTC, ETV6-NTRK3,* and *AKAP9-BRAF* [28–30]. *RET/PTC* genetic alterations are the most common mutation found in the Chernobyl radiation-induced thyroid carcinomas [31]. The prevalence of genetic alterations in patients with various thyroid carcinomas is outlined in Table 22.2 [30].

FTC is 12% of DTC. The true FTC are rarer than previously anticipated, and consist of 2(−5)% of all thyroid cancers, and may besides mutations in RAS mutually exclusive display the *PAX8-PPARγ* fusion gene. Prior to the introduction of iodinated salt, follicular carcinoma was much more frequently diagnosed. Follicular tumors display, to the contrary follicular adenomas, microscopic vascular, and capsular invasion, which distinguishes benign from malignant follicular neoplasm. Therefore, cytology alone cannot be used to diagnose follicular carcinoma.

HCC or oncocytic carcinoma is a histological variant of FTC often expressing a more aggressive behavior and accounts for 2% of DTCs.

Many tumors have both papillary and follicular elements histologically, and they are called follicular variants of papillary carcinoma and should be classified as papillary carcinoma because the clinical behavior of these tumors is not different from pure PTC. DTCs most often secrete thyroglobulin, and it can be used as a tumor marker.

Poorly differentiated thyroid carcinoma was defined in the 1980s [32], and have an aggressive histologic behavior with necrosis, increased mitotic rate, and vascular invasion. They account for 4–7% of all thyroid cancers [30]. *Also, TP53* mutations are present in 20–30% of cases [30] (Table 22.2). Poorly differentiated thyroid cancers are more aggressive than DTC and less aggressive than ATC. Recently, Nikoforov et al. mounted the term *noninvasive follicular* ***thyroid*** *neoplasm with papillary-like nuclear features* (NIFTP), showing that this tumor is indeed very indolent and has likely been overtreated earlier and classified as a papillary

Table 22.2 Prevalence of genetic alterations in patients with various thyroid carcinomas [30]

Altered gene	Poorly differentiated thyroid carcinoma (%)	Papillary thyroid carcinoma (%)	Follicular thyroid carcinoma (%)	Anaplastic thyroid carcinoma (%)
RET/PTC	0	20	0	0
TP53	20–30	0	0	65–70
BRAF	15	45	0	20–25
RAS	30–35	10–15	4	50–55
Beta-catenin	20–25	0	0	65
PAX8-PPARγ	0	0	35	0

carcinoma [33]. The ramifications on decrease of true malignancy when accounting for NIFTP is under scrutiny. A marked decrease in the risk of malignancy for the Bethesda 5 Category suspicious for malignancy has been shown, although further studies are needed [34].

22.3.2 Medullary Thyroid Carcinoma (MTC)

MTCs are derived from parafollicular cells or calcitonin-secreting C cells. RET proto-oncogene mutations are characteristic, with germline activating *RET* mutations as seen in FMTC and MEN 2A predisposing factors. Calcitonin and carcinoembryonic antigen (CEA) can be used as tumor markers [35].

22.3.3 Anaplastic Thyroid Cancer (ATC)

ATC is the most aggressive form of thyroid carcinomas and typically the cause of death within 6 months. One-year survival is about 20%. This type is about 1% of thyroid malignancies. ATC can occur de novo or has arisen from more differentiated cancer that went undiagnosed for many years. In some cases, there is a spectrum from papillary to anaplastic cancer. ATC is distinguished from poorly differentiated (grade 3) thyroid carcinoma in part by loss of TTF-1 expression and abnormalities in *p53* signaling pathway [29, 30]. *BRAF* and *RAS* mutations are also noted in ATC (Table 22.2).

22.3.4 Other Cancers of the Thyroid Gland

Thyroid lymphoma (5%), thyroid sarcoma (<1%), and squamous carcinoma of the thyroid (<1%) are the other very rare cancers of the thyroid gland. Breast, lung, and kidney cancers are the most frequent cancers that metastasize to the thyroid.

22.4 Diagnosis

The majority of patients with thyroid cancer present with a clinically or ultrasonographically (USG) detectable solitary nodule. While the risk of the solitary being malignant varies between 10% and 30% in different studies, the risk in multinodular disease is dramatically lower. History, physical examination, USG, and FNA are the four most important methods that help in the diagnostic work-up. History and patient characteristics speaking in favor of malignancy are history of dyspnea, dysphagia, persistent dysphonia, male sex, age <14 years or >70 years, personal thyroid cancer history with lobectomy, radiation exposure in childhood or adolescent period, first-degree relative with thyroid cancer or MEN2, personal history of familial adenomatous polyposis, Carney complex, Cowden syndrome, FDG avid on PET scan. Upon examination firm and hard fixed nodule/s or rapidly growing nodules and cervical lymph node/nodes are important findings for malignancy.

Neck and thyroid USG and fine needle aspiration (FNA) are very important in the differential diagnosis of thyroid nodules: sonographic features and thresholds for FNA, according to the American Thyroid Association (ATA) and National Cancer Center Network (NCCN) guidelines, are outlined in Table 22.3 [36].

The Bethesda system is widely used, using a six-category classification system to report thyroid FNA biopsy (FNAB) results (Table 22.4) [37], and which has been validated in a meta-analysis of 8 published studies including 25,445 thyroid FNABs [38].

Thus, the Bethesda level itself cannot alone be decisive in whether to perform surgery or not, and other factors, such as USG findings (Tables 22.3 and 22.4), personal history, and nodule size, should be considered. It is usually recommended to repeat FNAB when the diagnosis is indeterminate [38]. In this group, molecular markers (BRAF, RET/PTC, RAS, PAX8/PPAR mutations) (Table 22.2) may help to find out in which patients surgery is necessary [39]. In the diagnosis of a follicular lesion with undetermined significance (other used terms are "atypia of undetermined significance," "rule out neoplasm," "atypical follicular lesion," "follicular cell-rich aspirate," and "cellular follicular lesion") the estimated risk of malignancy is 5–10%. Here FNA can be repeated or surgery can be considered according to the clinical and USG findings [36]. Molecular diagnostics may be useful to allow reclassification of follicular lesions, such as follicular neoplasm or follicular lesions with undetermined significance [40]. Recently, promising results with DNA- and

Table 22.3 Thyroid carcinoma: nodule evaluation according to the sonographic features and thresholds for fine needle aspiration according to NCCN [Ny REF NCCN Clinical Practice Guidelines in Oncology. Thyroid carcinoma Version 1. 2017. NCCN.org]

Sonographic features	Threshold for FNA
Solid nodule	
With suspicious sonographic features (hypoechoic, increased central vascularity, infiltrative margins, microcalcifications, taller than wide in transverse plane)	≥1.0 cm
Without suspicious sonographic features	≥1.5 cm
Mixed cystic-solid nodule	
With suspicious sonographic features (hypoechoic, increased central vascularity, infiltrative margins, microcalcifications, taller than wide in transverse plane)	≥1.5 to 2.0 cm
Without suspicious sonographic features	≥2.0 cm
Spongiform nodule (aggregation of multiple microcystic components in more than 50% of the volume of the nodule)	≥2.0 cm
Purely cystic nodule	Not indicated except as therapeutic modality
Abnormal cervical lymph nodes	FNA node ± FNA-associated thyroid nodule(s)

NCCN thyroid cancer guideline, v.1.2017

Table 22.4 The Bethesda system for classification of thyroid FNAB [37]

1. Nondiagnostic/unsatisfactory: 13% of all FNABs; of those 16.8% were cancer at final pathology
2. Benign/noncancerous: 59% of all FNABs; of those only 3.7% were cancer at final pathology
3. Indeterminate: 9.6% of all FNABs; of those 15.9% were cancer at final pathology
4. Suspicious for follicular cancer: 10.1% of all FNABs; of those 26.1% were cancer at final pathology
5. Suspicious for cancer: 2.6% of all FNABs; of those 75.2% were cancer at final pathology
6. Positive for cancer: 5.4% of all FNABs; of those 98.6% were cancer at final pathology

RNA-based next-generation sequencing assays that analyzes 112 genes for a variety of genetic alterations, including point mutations, insertions/deletions, gene fusions, copy number alterations, and abnormal gene expression, using a genomic classifier (GC) to separate malignant lesions from benign lesions have been presented. The new version 3 of this test correctly classified most papillary, follicular, and Hurthle cell lesions, medullary thyroid carcinomas, and parathyroid lesions. In the FNA validation set, the GC sensitivity was 98.0%, the specificity was 81.8%, and the accuracy was 90.9% [41]. Unfortunately, version 2 of the formerly mentioned test and genomic classifier was uninformative in B-III nodules (area under the curve 0.57) [42].

Thyroid ultrasound has become very useful in diagnosis of thyroid nodules, is cost-effective and non-invasive, and is now a routine procedure. It is widely debated its role in comparison to cytology [43]. Structuring the investigation by using TIRADS (Thyroid Imaging Reporting and Data System) has even more clarified the usefulness [44]. Here, a structured report with clear definitions discriminating between benign, low-intermediate- and high-risk nodules as well as indications for FNA.

EU-TIRADS

Category		US features	Malignancy risk, %
EU-TIRADS 1	Normal	No nodules	None
EU-TIRADS 2	Benign	Pure cyst, entirely spongiform	0
EU-TIRADS 3	Low risk	Ovoid, smooth isoechoic/hyperechoic. No features of high suspicion	2–4
EU-TIRADS 4	Intermediate risk	Ovoid, smooth, mildly hypoechoic. No features of high suspicion	6–17
EU-TIRADS 5	High risk	At least one of the following features of high suspicion: – Irregular shape – Irregular margins – Microcalcifications – Marked hypoechogenicity (and solid)	26–87

TIRADS 5-lesions should undergo FNA, EU-TIRADS 4-lesions if >15 mm, EU-TIRADS 3-lesions if >20 mm, while EU-TIRADS 2-lesions do not need to be punctured for cytology. Thus, not all nodules need to be investigated by cytology [44].

Another diagnostic method is the radionuclide scan: In the last years, it is not used in the initial evaluation of thyroid nodules, except in the case of suppressed TSH levels. In this situation, a radionuclide scan is done to assess for a functioning (hot) adenoma. Malignant lesions usually are documented as hypofunctioning or cold lesions, but the sensitivity of radionuclide scan for determination of malignancy is only 12–15%.

Serum calcitonin measurement may be helpful for the diagnosis of MTC, but the yield is low when used for the initial evaluation of thyroid nodules [45].

22.5 Staging and Prognosis

There are many prognostic factors for DTC. Age, sex, histologic type, tumor size, tumor grade, multicentricity, extrathyroidal extension, type of surgery, ploidy, lymph node metastases, vascular invasion, and ^{131}I radioiodine ablation therapy (RAI) are important prognostic factors [25, 46]. Also, there are multiple prognostic scoring systems for DTC. These are AGES, AMES, DAMES (ploidy + AMES), MACIS, and the AJCC-TNM staging system 2018 eighth edition (Tables 22.5, 22.6, and 22.7) [47–49]. Age, size, and extent of the tumor are present in all prognostic scoring systems. There are some major changes in the newest eighth edition of the AJCC-TNM classification including the definition of T-stages and staging. For example, the age cut is 55 years instead of 45 years, anaplastic cancer is now staged as DTC and T3 is divided into T3a and T3b (Tables 22.5, 22.6, and 22.7). Comparison of prognoses according to the type of cancer and stage for the seventh and eighth editions are outlined in Table 22.8. Death related to DTC is very rare and associated with distant metastases, mostly pulmonary [50, 51]. Both PTC and FTC may lead to death, with an associated tendency towards higher T/N-values.

22.5.1 Age and Sex

Age is the most important prognostic factor for thyroid cancer mortality [46]. Thyroid carcinoma is more lethal in patients older than 40 years. The mortality rate increases dramatically after the age of 60. Recurrence frequencies are highest (40%) in patients younger than 20 years or older than 60 years. Male sex is a bad prognostic sign for PTCs, especially those larger than 1 cm [52]. The overall 5-year survival rate for all thyroid cancer is 85% for females and 74% for males.

22.5.2 Tumor Characteristics

The most important prognostic tumor characteristics are tumor histology, tumor size, vascular invasion, necrosis, *BRAF* mutation, local invasion, and metastases.

Table 22.5 American Joint Committee on Cancer (AJCC) eighth edition: thyroid cancer TNM staging [47]

Definition of primary tumor (T)	
T category	**T criteria**
TX	Primary tumor cannot be assessed
T0	No evidence of primary tumor
T1	Tumor ≤2 cm in greatest dimension limited to the thyroid
T1a	Tumor ≤1 cm in greatest dimension limited to the thyroid
T1b	Tumor >1 cm but ≤2 cm in greatest dimension limited to the thyroid
T2	Tumor >2 cm but ≤4 cm in greatest dimension limited to the thyroid
T3a	Tumor >4 cm limited to the thyroid or gross extrathyroidal extension invading only strap muscles
T3aa	Tumor >4 cm limited to the thyroid
T3ba	Gross extrathyroidal extension invading only strap muscles (sternohyoid, sternothyroid, thyrohyoid, or omohyoid muscles) from a tumor of any size
T4	Includes gross extrathyroidal extension into major neck structures
T4a	Gross extrathyroidal extension invading subcutaneous soft tissues, larynx, trachea, esophagus, or recurrent laryngeal nerve from a tumor of any size
T4b	Gross extrathyroidal extension invading prevertebral fascia or encasing carotid artery or mediastinal vessels from a tumor of any size
Definition of regional lymph node (N)	
N category	**N criteria**
NX	Regional lymph nodes cannot be assessed
N0	No evidence of regional lymph nodes metastasis
N0aa	One or more cytologic or histologically confirmed benign lymph node
N0ba	No radiologic or clinical evidence of locoregional lymph node metastasis
N1a	Metastasis to regional nodes
N1aa	Metastasis to level VI or VII (pretracheal, paratracheal, or prelaryngeal/Delphian, or upper mediastinal) lymph nodes; this can be unilateral or bilateral disease
N1ba	Metastasis to unilateral, bilateral, or contralateral lateral neck lymph nodes (levels I, II, III, IV, or V) or retropharyngeal lymph nodes
Definition of distant metastasis (M)	
M category	**M criteria**
M0	No distant metastasis
M1	Distant metastasis

PTC has the most favorable prognosis. Tall or columnar cells, diffuse sclerosing variants, and anaplastic tumor transformation have worse prognoses. The follicular variant of PTC has the same prognosis as pure PTC.

Many FTCs are minimally invasive tumors, exhibiting only slight tumor capsule penetration without vascular invasion. They are less likely to produce distant metastases and prognosis are good. Widely invasive FTCs are much less common and has a remarkably worse prognosis.

Table 22.6 Pathologic TNM staging system for differentiated thyroid cancer (AJCC)

Differentiated thyroid cancer				
When age at diagnosis is…	And T is…	And N is…	And M is…	Then the stage group is…
<55 years	Any T	Any N	M0	I
	Any T	Any N	M1	II
≥55 years	T1	N0/NX	M0	I
	T1	N1	M0	II
	T2	N0/NX	M0	I
	T2	N1	M0	II
	T3a/T3b	Any N	M0	II
	T4a	Any N	M0	III
	T4b	Any N	M0	IVA
	Any T	Any N	M1	IVB

Table 22.7 Pathologic TNM staging system for anaplastic thyroid cancer (AJCC)

Anaplastic thyroid cancer			
T is…	And N is…	And M is…	Then the stage group is…
T1-T3a	N0/NX	M0	IVA
T1-T3a	N1	M0	IVB
T3b	Any N	M0	IVB
T4	Any N	M0	IVB
Any T	Any N	M1	IVC

HCC is usually regarded as an aggressive variant of FTC, develops at an older age commonly displays vascular invasion, and also has a worse prognosis. HCC also more frequently metastasizes than FTC [53].

PTCs smaller than 1 cm are termed microcarcinoma or incidentaloma [25]. The risk of recurrence ranges from 1% to 2% in unifocal papillary microcarcinoma, and 4–6% in multifocal papillary microcarcinoma [54]. Their cancer-specific mortality rates are near zero. DTC tumors, with a size less than 1.5 cm and confined to the thyroid, almost never cause distant metastases [55]. Thirty-year recurrence rates are one-third of >1.5 cm tumors; 30-year cancer-specific mortality is 0.4% compared to 7% for ≥1.5 cm tumors [49].

Poorly differentiated thyroid cancers are more aggressive than DTC but less aggressive than ATC [30, 32], and are typically diagnosed in the sixth and seventh decade. Extrathyroidal extension and extensive local invasion are typically present at the diagnosis. Regional lymph node metastases (50–83%) and distant metastases (36–85%), most commonly to the lungs and bones, are frequently seen. Five-, 10-, and 15-year survival rates are 50%, 34%, and 0%, respectively [30, 56].

MTC is the intermediate differentiated thyroid carcinoma (Table 22.1). Overall, the 5-year survival is 80–86% and the 10-year survival is 75% (Table 22.8). In patients with sporadic MTC, a somatic RET oncogene mutation confers an adverse prognosis [57].

Table 22.8 Comparison of the American Joint Committee on Cancer Seventh and Eighth Edition Staging System

Stage	Seventh edition: Description	Seventh edition: 10-year DSS, %	Eighth edition: Description	Eighth edition: Expected 10-year DSS, %
Younger patients				
I	Age <45 years; all patients without distant metastases regardless of tumor size, lymph node status, or extrathyroidal extension	97–100	Age <55 years; all patients without distant metastases regardless of tumor size, lymph node status, or extrathyroidal extension	98–100
II	Age <45 years; distant metastases	95–99	Age <55 years; distant metastases	85–95
Older patients				
I	Age ≥45 years; tumor ≤2 cm; confined to thyroid	97–100	Age ≥55 years; tumor ≤4 cm; confined to thyroid	98–100
II	Age ≥45 years; tumor 2–4 cm; confined to thyroid	97–100	Age ≥55 years; tumor >4 cm; or tumor of any size with central or lateral neck lymph nodes or gross extrathyroidal extension into strap muscles	85–95
III	Age ≥45 years; tumor >4 cm; or minimal extrathyroidal extension or central neck lymph node metastasis	88–95	Age ≥55 years; tumor of any size with gross extrathyroidal extension into subcutaneous tissue, larynx, trachea, esophagus, recurrent laryngeal nerve	60–70
IV	Age ≥45 years; gross extrathyroidal extension, or lateral neck lymph node metastasis, or distant metastasis	50–75	Age ≥55 years; tumor of any size or lymph node status with gross extrathyroidal extension into prevertebral fascia, encasing major vessels; or distant metastasis	

ATC has the worst prognosis, with a median survival of 4–5 months after diagnosis. Favorable prognostic features seem to be unilateral tumors, tumor size less than 5 cm, no invasion of adjacent tissue, and absence of nodal involvement or distant metastases, but also fast handling from diagnosis to first treatment. Older age (>74 years of age) and high white blood cell count are bad prognostic factors [25, 58].

22.5.3 Regional Lymph Node Metastases

The prognostic impact of lymph node metastases is according to the 8th edition of the AJCC TNM classification of no significance, which supports previous general acceptance [6, 25]. However, recent findings of an increased risk for N1B have been presented, challenging the new classification [59, 60]. Lymph node metastases are frequent in PTC, especially multifocal PTC. The lymph node metastases rate is 35% in adults and 80% in children with PTC. The lymph node metastases ratio is much lower in FTC (15%), more prone to hematogenous spread.

22.5.4 Distant Metastases

Distant metastases, especially pulmonary which cause respiratory failure, are the main cause of death from DTC [50, 61]. In general, however, death from DTC is a very rare event. Ten percent of patients with PTC and 25% of patients with FTC develop distant metastases. The lungs, bones, soft tissues, and central nervous system are the most frequent metastatic sites. The main predictors of outcome for patients with distant metastases are the patient's age, site of metastases, and ^{131}I RAI uptake of the metastatic site. Younger patients have better and those being refractory to ^{131}I RAI treatment worse prognosis.

22.6 Management of Differentiated Thyroid Carcinoma

There are four major components in the management of DTC:

- Active Surveillance.
- Surgery.
- Postoperative ^{131}I RAI ablation therapy.
- TSH suppression with thyroid hormone therapy.

External beam radiotherapy (EBRT) can be used in the adjuvant treatment of selected patients with locally advanced, recurrent, and/or metastatic disease e.g., to the bones.

22.6.1 Active Surveillance

The recent development and spread of USA and US-guided FNA has facilitated the detection of small PTCs. In the large Japanese series of Ito et al., patients with PTCs measuring 1 cm or less not associated with unfavorable features, could be candidates for observation [62]. However, patient age was significantly related to progression under observation, as older patients with subclinical low-risk microPTCs were the best candidates for active surveillance [63]. Importantly, even if there were subsequent signs of progression, such as tumor enlargement in 15.9% and novel nodal metastasis in 3.4% of the patients on 10-year follow-up, it was not too late to perform surgical treatment [63]. Tuttle et al. published in 2017 the Memorial Sloan Kettering Cancer Center series on tumors ≤15 mm in size subjected to active surveillance [55]. The change in tumor volume kinetics during active surveillance in this US cohort with PTCs was as low as 3.8% on a relatively short-term follow-up of a median of 25 months. Younger age was linked with increased likelihood of tumor growth. Importantly, there were no patients who developed lymph nodes or distant metastases while on an active surveillance, and additionally there was no disease-specific mortality [55]. The change in tumor volume kinetics during active surveillance in a US cohort with PTCs measuring up to 1.5 cm were as low as 3.8% on a relatively short term follow-up of a median of 25 months [55]. However, these findings could not be replicated in the Korean experience where the growth rates during active surveillance of microPTCs were as high as 14% on short term follow-up of a median of 31 months and pathology findings, e.g., tall cell carcinoma in patients subsequently operated upon were concerning [64].

Generally, an active surveillance management approach may be considered in adult patients with very low-risk small tumors (e.g., microPTCs) without clinically evident metastases, extrathyroidal extension, or local invasion of the trachea and the RLN and also no convincing cytology of aggressive disease [36]. To date, biomarkers that may be utilized in such an approach are largely missing.

22.6.2 Surgical Management of DTC

Surgery is an important element in the multifaceted treatment approach to DTC, but the extent of it has long been a matter of debate. In 1977, a report of 576 DTC patients in the US Air Force Central Tumor Registry found that total thyroidectomy was associated with lower rates of recurrence and higher survival [65]. Clinicians would use this evidence to support an approach of total thyroidectomy for all cases of DTC. In contrast, other groups found that, in lower risk patients, outcomes were similar following thyroid lobectomy only [66, 67]. The recommendation of total thyroidectomy was later established following an analysis of population-level data from the National Cancer Database (NCDB) by Bilimoria et al. of more than 50,000 patients who either underwent total thyroidectomy or lobectomy for PTC, with the former being associated with longer overall survival for PTCs $\geq$1 cm [68]. However, an analysis of 22,724 PTC patients from the Surveillance, Epidemiology, and End Results (SEER) database showed no survival benefit for total thyroidectomy, raising concerns about the Bilimoria study's multivariable analysis [69]. Finally, patients with DTC smaller than 4 cm without extrathyroidal extension and without clinical evidence of lymph node metastases could be safely managed by thyroid lobectomy alone in terms of overall survival, local, and regional recurrence [70]. These studies had a great impact and led to the change of the 2015 American Thyroid Association guidelines [36], due to the lack of survival benefit with more extensive surgery and the apparent associated risks of hypoparathyroidism and recurrent laryngeal nerve injury, also confirmed in more recent studies [71–73]. Nevertheless, total thyroidectomy is still mandated in cases of multifocal bilateral disease, undiagnosed nodularity in the contralateral lobe, nodal metastases, extrathyroidal extension, and any high-grade disease that requires radioiodine treatment, such as very large tumors and aggressive pathology. Additionally, total thyroidectomy is the mainstay approach in patients with an underlying genetic predisposition to oncogenic changes throughout the thyroid gland, such as patients who previously received low-dose radiation to the neck, dental workers, Chernobyl population in the 1980s, Philippinos, patients with a strong family history of DTC as well as patients with syndromes associated to DTC, such as Familial Polyposis, Cowden or Pendred's syndrome.

For patients with cytologically characterized follicular lesion of unknown significance (FLUS) or suspicious follicular neoplasm (Bethesda group III and IV respectively), a diagnostic unilateral lobectomy and isthmectomy are the initial procedures of choice, as the value of currently commercially available, novel molecular tests (Thyroseq, Afirma Gene Expression Classifier, and ThyGenX) in the clinical setting remains to be proven. If a malignant follicular lesion is confirmed on final pathology, then a completion thyroidectomy may be warranted to allow for treatment with radioiodine therapy in patients with large tumors and/or aggressive histopathological findings (e.g., widely invasive FTC) similar to the papillary counterpart. Nodal metastases, however, represent an uncommon finding in follicular carcinoma, but when present may indicate a dismal prognosis.

In patients with papillary thyroid cancer, 35% have clinically apparent central lymph nodes involved on physical examination and/or imaging (US or CT scan) at the time of initial presentation or grossly abnormal appearance at surgery, even in low-risk patients [74, 75]. Therapeutic central lymph node dissection is considered to be common practice for these patients. However, it is controversial to perform routine prophylactic central lymph node dissection during total thyroidectomy. Central lymph node dissection is a comprehensive compartment-oriented removal of prelaryngeal (delphian) and pretracheal lymph nodes and at least one paratracheal nodal basin or both. Lymphoareolar tissue anterior and posterior to the RLN is removed on one or both sides. Interestingly, 23–81% of the patients receiving a prophylactic central lymph node dissection indeed have micro-metastases in the final pathology report [76–78]. However, these appear to be clinically irrelevant as rates of nodal recurrence after central node dissection were found 4% in pathologically node-negative patients and 6% in patients with micro-metastases receiving prophylactic central node dissection, whereas as high as 21% in patients with clinical apparent nodal disease receiving therapeutic central lymph node dissection [74, 75, 79, 80]. No difference in recurrence or long-term complication rates, with the exception of permanent hypoparathyroidism, has been found between patients undergoing total thyroidectomy with or without prophylactic central lymph node dissection [81, 82]. However, given the low rates of both newly identified structural disease and morbidity after surgery for clinically node-negative PTC, prohibitively large sample sizes would be required for sufficient statistical power to demonstrate significant differences in outcomes in a prospective randomized controlled trial of prophylactic central lymph node dissection in these patients; thus, such a task is not readily feasible [83].

Lymph nodes in the lateral neck may also be involved in thyroid cancer. Although unilateral and bilateral therapeutic lateral cervical lymph node dissection with curative intent is widely recognized, prophylactic lateral neck dissection is not advisable. However, in Japan, because of legal restrictions, most patients will not undergo radioactive iodine ablation, thus patients with high-risk DTC such as those with large tumors or clinical central lymph node metastases may undergo a prophylactic lateral neck dissection, although there is no evidence that such an approach would increase cause-specific survival [84]. For those patients in whom nodal disease is clinically evident, surgical resection may reduce the risk of recurrence and possibly mortality. Planned compartmental dissection should be titrated and be more selective depending on the surgeon's judgment of procedural safety, however, node "picking" is considered unacceptable. For more advanced cases with bulky lateral disease, a comprehensive clearance of the target basins has been recommended, following the planes of coalescence of different fascial layers, which are avascular and allow to remove the target nodes en bloc with their investing fascial layers, known as fascial neck dissection [85, 86].

22.6.2.1 Postoperative RAI Ablation Therapy

Radioiodine (RAI) therapy with iodine-131 isotope (^{131}I) is a well-established adjuvant therapy, which is performed after surgery for DTC patients. The principle of the therapy is that ^{131}I is preferentially taken up and trapped by thyroid follicular cells, with just the same mechanism as its chemical analog nonradioactive (cold) iodine. Contrary to cold iodine, ^{131}I emits beta radiation as well as high-energetic gamma radiation. Beta radiation from ^{131}I is responsible for its therapeutic effect, while imaging can be done with the use of its gamma radiation. Therefore, postoperative radioiodine allows the identification of residual regional and/or distant metastatic disease as well as exerts therapeutic effect to destroy tumor foci by internal radiation exposure.

The major aims of postoperative radioiodine therapy are:

1. To destroy any postoperative microscopic residual tumor foci, with internal radiation exposure by beta particles. The destroy process of residual regional tissue is preferably called "ablation."
2. To ablate residual normal thyroid tissue and therefore to increase the specificity of subsequent ^{131}I scintigraphy in the follow-up to detect any recurrence or metastasis.
3. To provide the use of serum Tg as a tumor marker for thyroid cancer in the follow-up of patients. After ablation of residual tissue postoperatively, any increase in Tg level would represent the presence of recurrent or metastatic disease.
4. To assess the postoperative staging of the patient. Whole-body scintigraphic imaging after administration of high dose of ^{131}I for postoperative ablation makes it possible for unexpected metastases to be detected easily. Therefore, the patients would be upstaged and additional ^{131}I or other treatment options could be planned sequentially.

Over the long term, for tumors larger than 1.5 cm, total thyroidectomy followed by RAI plus thyroid hormone suppression therapy confers a distinct outcome advantage, with a reduction in tumor recurrence and mortality sufficiently to offset some of the bad prognostic signs (age >40 years at the time of diagnosis, multicentric large or locally invasive tumors, or those with regional metastases) [49, 87].

However, no survival benefit has been demonstrated for low and even intermediate-risk tumors. Additionally, the risk of persistent disease postoperatively in patients, who are correctly identified at low risk, is only 2–3%, raising the question of how we can avoid useless adjuvant radioiodine in the 97–98% of patients with no residual disease [49, 88–92]. Indeed, when criteria of excellent response are met before ablation, this may be unnecessary, e.g., in patients with undetectable serum thyroglobulin prior to radioiodine administration [88, 91]. Additionally, the high prevalence of adjuvant RAI utilization for early stage PTC is causing a financial burden on the health system with no evidence of survival benefit [93]. Therefore, radioiodine remnant ablation is not routinely recommended after thyroidectomy for low-risk DTC patients. Low dose RAI of 30 mCi is generally favored over higher administered activities, with an excellent response, high long-term-remission rates, and lower rates of adverse effects in the HiLo study [94, 95]. Nevertheless, prospective randomized controlled trials on the use of radioiodine in low-risk DTC are feasible, with the paradigm of the aforementioned ESTIMABL and HiLo studies [91, 94].

Basically, the efficacy of ^{131}I therapy depends on several factors such as patient preparation, tumor characteristics, extent and sites of disease, and the therapeutic dose of ^{131}I. Iodine uptake by thyroid follicular cells, whether it is radioactive or not, is closely and directly related to the serum TSH level, while it is inversely related to the level of iodine pool within the body. Therefore, the patient should express high TSH values (at least 30 mU/L) at the time of RAI treatment. This can be achieved either the classical way by being off thyroxine (T4) at least for 3–4 weeks, or by 2 consecutive days before RAI treatment giving subcutaneous injection with recombinant TSH. The latter procedure omits the need for withdrawal of thyroxine.

Recombinant TSH is mostly preferred for patients who have major risks for prolonged hypothyroidism in order to avoid serious complications and also for the patients in whom endogenous TSH level cannot be increased due to hypopituitarism or due to the presence of functioning bulky metastases. A combination of radioiodine WBS and serum Tg after rhTSH stimulation detected thyroid tissue or cancer in more than 90% of patients with persistent disease or remnant tissue limited to the thyroid bed and 100% of patients with metastatic disease. Thus, rh TSH administration is a safe and effective means of RAI uptake and serum Tg levels in patients undergoing evaluation for thyroid cancer persistence and recurrence [96]. Recombinant TSH is administered intramuscularly on 2 consecutive days, followed by radioiodine administration on the third day and imaging on the fifth day. A major drawback of rhTSH is its relatively high cost and less availability, especially in developing countries which hamper its wide use.

During 2 weeks before ^{131}I administration, the patient may be put on a low-iodine diet, in order to decrease the level of iodine pool, which has the potential to competitively inhibit ^{131}I uptake and decrease the treatment efficiency. Radiocontrast media and some other agents such as hair dyes, which are very rich in iodine, are strictly forbidden to avoid competitive inhibition with ^{131}I. Since ^{131}I is orally administered, the patient should be in a fasting state at least for 4 h and continue to fast for a few hours to establish a good gastric absorption, following the oral administration of the therapeutic dose. Then, the patient is encouraged to be well hydrated, especially on the first day of the therapy, in order to both decrease radiation exposure from the unbound ^{131}I by increasing excretion and lower the glandular tissue exposure which may cause some side effects such as sialadenitis. To overcome such side effects, saliva stimulants like lemon juice or sour candies as well as antacids to protect the gastric mucosa are recommended.

^{131}I is known as a quite safe treatment option, with relatively low major side effects or complications. The rare long-term side effects include xerostomia, lacrimal gland obstruction, pulmonary fibrosis if pulmonary metastases are present and treated with higher doses, and secondary malignancies, like leukemia and salivary gland, breast, and colon cancer. Importantly, the overall risk of second primary malignancies is increased for thyroid cancer survivors by 19–27% and varies by radioisotope therapy, latency, and age at diagnosis [97–99]. The only contraindication of ^{131}I therapy is pregnancy and most centers recommend their female patients not to get pregnant for at least 6 months, to avoid possible teratogenic effects on fetus growth. Similarly, male patients are strongly encouraged to use birth control methods for at least for 4–6 months, following treatment, to avoid potential teratogenic effects.

22.6.2.2 TSH Suppression with Thyroid Hormone Therapy

Patients have to receive thyroid hormone therapy after surgery and ^{131}I RAI ablation therapy for two reasons: (a) for the correction of iatrogenic hypothyroidism and (b) because TSH is a trophic hormone that can stimulate the growth of cells derived from follicular epithelium. For low-risk patients and patients with excellent response to initial therapy, thyroid hormone should be given to suppress the TSH level to 0.1–0.5 mU/L. For high-risk patients and patients with known residual disease, the recommended TSH level is below 0.1 mU/L. The risk and benefit of TSH suppression therapy must be balanced for each individual patient. Osteopenia, possible cardiac hypertrophy, and atrial fibrillation are some of the side effects of TSH suppression therapy. For patients whose TSH levels are chronically suppressed, particularly postmenopausal women, an adequate daily intake of calcium 1200 mg/day and vitamin D 1000 units/day is recommended. Excessive TSH suppression (into the undetectable level or thyrotoxic level) is not required to prevent disease progression in all DTC patients.

22.6.2.3 Adjuvant External Beam Radiation Therapy (EBRT)

There is no prospective randomized trial, but EBRT has a role in the treatment of locally invasive DTC [25, 100]. The development of additional treatments during recent years now offers several treatments for the more complicated patient groups, but where EBRT still has an important role [101, 102].

Doses in the range of 40–50 Gy EBRT may be included in the treatment of DTC patients who are older than 45 years, display gross extrathyroidal extension, microscopic residual disease, and incomplete resection near the aerodigestive tract (R1 resection), and for those patients with gross residual disease, in whom further surgery or RAI would likely be ineffective, in order to increase local-regional control.

Patients younger than 45 years generally are not treated with EBRT because of their better prognosis and the possible late side effects, especially secondary malignancies. Additionally, for multiple DTC recurrences in the thyroid bed with local invasion into the tracheo-esophageal groove or adjacent structures and positive resection margins, EBRT may be considered after adjuvant radioiodine treatment.

22.6.3 Assessment and Management After Initial Treatment

After initial surgery and ^{131}I RAI ablation therapy in a subset of patients with DTC, the patients are then subjected to follow-up with clinical and radiologic data. Serum Tg, neck USG, whole-body ^{131}I RAI scan, and other modalities, such as FDG-PET detect recurrent or residual disease in most patients.

22.6.3.1 Follow-Up

The follow-up of patients after thyroid surgery and eventually added radioiodine ablation includes clinical examination, biochemical evaluation and imaging procedures. Many consensus guidelines recommend radioiodine scintigraphy 6–12 months after initial radioiodine ablation where radioiodine scintigraphy at the sixth month has been reserved only for patients with poor prognostic factors or some suspicious clinical, laboratory, or ultrasonographic findings [36]. The predictive value for 10-year disease-free survival is reported to be approximately 90% if the first follow-up scintigraphy is normal. Neck ultrasonography is indeed the imaging method of choice for long-term follow-up to detect recurrent disease and more importantly lymph node metastases. Neck ultrasonography in the 3-to-12-month monitoring of the patients with extrathyroidal invasion and/or regional lymph node metastases is recommended on a routine basis in consensus guidelines [36]. Generally, whenever a suspicious finding is encountered, fine needle aspiration biopsy is strongly advocated to confirm diagnosis. During follow-up, serum Tg and anti-Tg antibody levels should also be monitored. Any increase in serum Tg levels should be accepted as suspicious for recurrence or metastasis and should lead to other modalities. Tg measured 3–4 months after total thyroidectomy is important in the risk restratification of DTC patients and is combination with neck US a sensitive tool for detection of recurrences and in the decision to perform remnant radioiodine ablation [103–105].

Serum Tg determination on I-T4 suppression treatment can be used for follow-up of DTC even in the absence of RAI administration. An increasing trend of Tg over time may subsequently lead to imaging and RAI administration. Delayed treatment of persistent disease will provide similar outcome. On the other hand, in patients with postoperative undetectable or low serum Tg and without any suspicious findings on neck US, the risk of persistent disease is very low.

Importantly, upon recent reclassification according to the eighth AJCC TNM staging edition, approximately one-third of patients are now down-staged. In a Korean study by Kim et al. the proportions of stage I and II tumors increased from 61.9% to 81.1% and from 1.7% to 16.0%, respectively, whereas those of stage III and IVB (formerly IVC in the seventh edition) decreased from 27.6% to 2.3% and

0.8% to 0.5%, respectively, resulting in a higher prognostic value of the eighth edition in terms of cancer-specific survival [106].

A dynamic risk stratification for the follow-up of patients with DTC, estimating changes over time based on response to therapy and the course of the disease is necessary to effectively tailor ongoing follow-up recommendations [107]. However, the marked rise in the use of imaging tests after primary treatment of DTC has been associated with an increased treatment for recurrence. This association has shown no clear improvement in disease-specific survival, emphasizing the importance of curbing unnecessary imaging and tailoring imaging after primary treatment to patient risk [108]. Specifically, low-risk DTC is associated with low recurrence rates and mortality compared to other groups, and for the younger patients without distant metastases at diagnosis, there is no proven survival benefit from lifelong follow-up following primary treatment and first follow-up [109]. In these patients routine screening US is substantially more likely to identify false-positive results than clinically significant structural disease recurrence [110]. Extending postoperative surveillance to 3-year intervals after 5 years of annual surveillance in patients with low-risk PTC with excellent response to therapy was more cost-effective than annual surveillance [111].

22.6.3.2 Imaging Techniques

Radioiodine Scintigraphy

Radioiodine scintigraphy can be performed by oral administration of either 2–5 mCi of ^{131}I or ^{123}I, the latter having some dosimetric and imaging advantages over ^{131}I, given that it only emits gamma radiation, despite its high cost and low availability as a disadvantage. In addition, another disadvantage of ^{131}I is its potential for "stunning," defined as the phenomenon that the diagnostic dose of ^{131}I administered before the treatment decreases the therapeutic dose uptake of thyroid cancer cells, possibly as a result of the indeed small but still significant cell-killing effect also of a lower radiation dose [112]. However, there are some recent studies that conclude that when a low-activity diagnostic dose is used and therapeutic dose is given within the following 3 days, stunning does not occur, even if there is still controversy [113]. The patient needs to be off T4 medication for a period of 3–4 weeks for serum TSH level to be at least 30 mU/L. Alternatively, recombinant human TSH can be administered, without the need of ceasing T4 medication, especially for patients who cannot tolerate hypothyroidism. Whole-body imaging and spot views from various body parts are acquired 4–24 and 48 h after ^{123}I and ^{131}I administration, respectively (Fig. 22.1). TSH-stimulated low-dose ^{131}I whole-body scanning with serum thyroglobulin either by standard LT4 withdrawal or rhTSH stimulation is the preferred test for monitoring patients without palpable disease or elevated serum thyroglobulin on LT4 therapy. This approach has the advantage of finding disease that may be amenable to ^{131}I therapy, although low-dose ^{131}I scans are less sensitive than are scans with other imaging agents, e.g., ^{123}I which has better imaging characteristics than ^{131}I and has been shown to be equivalent or superior to low-dose ^{131}I [114]. A combination of RAI WBS and serum Tg after recombinant human TSH

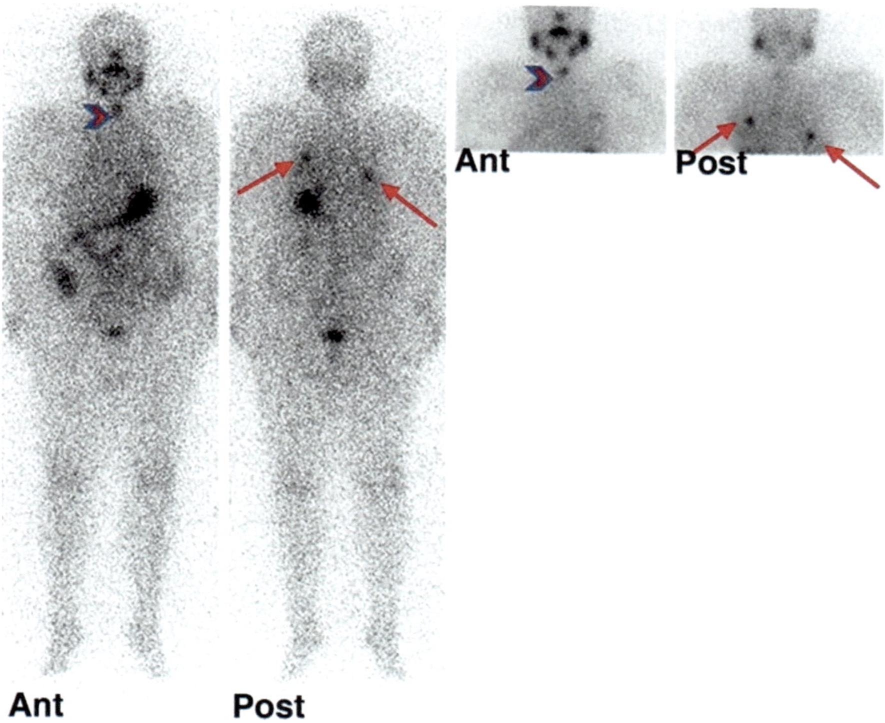

Fig. 22.1 Diagnostic I^{131} scintigraphy anterior and posterior whole-body and spot planar images of a 64-year-old female patient with papillary thyroid carcinoma (TSH, 98 uIU/mL; Tg, 278 ng/mL; anti-Tg Ab <20 IU/mL) shows radioiodine uptake consistent with residual disease in the neck region (*arrowhead*) as well as bilateral lung metastases (*arrows*). *ant* anterior, *post* posterior

stimulation detected thyroid tissue or cancer in 93% of patients with disease or remnant tissue limited to the thyroid bed and 100% of patients with metastatic disease [96].

Neck USG

It is a useful method to detect them as small as 3 mm lesions. Neck USG visualizes central and lateral lymph nodes. It can, especially when using TIRADS distinguish benign lesions from malign lesions; and may be used for the selection of which lesions to perform FNA upon. USG combined with rhTSH-stimulated Tg test has the highest diagnostic accuracy in detecting persistent disease in the follow-up of DTC. A detectable level of serum Tg on L-T [4], its conversion from undetectable to detectable after rhTSH, and/or a suspicious finding at ultrasound will allow the identification of patients requiring therapeutic procedures without the need for diagnostic RAI-WBS [115]. Additionally, US may identify lymph node metastases even in patients with low or undetectable serum Tg levels [116].

CT and MR Imaging Techniques

Other imaging techniques are CT scan or MRI (magnetic resonance imaging) of the neck, CT scan of the chest, chest X-ray, and FDG-PET imaging [117]. Chest X-ray may show macronodular lung metastases. Chest CT scan shows micronodular lung metastases. CT scan and MRI are not more sensitive than neck USG, but less operator dependent and may visualize local invasion into surrounding tissues. Indeed, some authors question the use of PET/CT as its added-on value is low [118].

Positron Emission Tomography with F-18: Fluorodeoxyglucose (FDG-PET)

FDG-PET serves as a molecular in vivo imaging modality to show glycolytic activity, which is the preferred metabolic pathway for most of the tumors. Current hybrid imaging systems combine PET with CT to provide the advantages of both functional and morphological imaging. In differentiated thyroid cancer, FDG-PET/CT is reserved only for patients with high serum Tg levels along with no uptake on radioiodine imaging during follow-up [119]. There is a "flip-flop mechanism" that FDG uptake in differentiated thyroid cancer cells increases as the tumor grade increases and on contrary radioiodine uptake increases as the grade decreases. Therefore, FDG acts as a marker of dedifferentiation and its degree of uptake correlates with poor prognosis. Indeed, the possibility of detecting metastases is higher if the tumor confers a V600E BRAF mutation [120]. The possibility of detecting metastases on FDG-PET/CT also increases as serum Tg increases; thus, it is generally recommended at a setting of serum Tg >10 ng/L along with negative radioiodine scintigraphy (Fig. 22.2a, b). A positive FDG-PET/CT result can lead to surgery, especially when there are isolated lymph nodes or soft tissue metastases around the neck region, also allowing the use of PET probe-guided surgery, just like gamma probe-guided approaches. It also leads to other therapeutic modalities such as external radiation therapy for unexpected bone metastases which show no radioiodine uptake and some other systemic therapy options in advanced cases [121]. The patient should be fasting for at least 4 h and the serum glucose level should not be over 200 mg/dL on the day of FDG i.v. injection. Thyroid hormone withdrawal is encouraged by most of the literature data, given that the hypothyroid state increases glycolytic activity and increases the diagnostic efficacy of FDG-PET/CT imaging.

22.6.3.3 Monitoring Serum Thyroglobulin (Tg)

Thyroglobulin is a protein synthesized only by thyroid follicular cells (benign or malignant). After total thyroidectomy and ablation therapy, Tg should be undetectable. Therefore, it is a good marker to assess the presence of recurrent, residual, or metastatic disease. The nadir should be reached within 3 months post-treatment, but it may take as long as 1–2 years. Tg and TSH must be measured together because Tg production is dependent on TSH secretion. The sensitivity of Tg is only 50% under TSH suppression therapy, but if measurable during thyroxin therapy suggestive of recurrence. After thyroid hormone withdrawal and TSH elevation, the sensitivity to detect cancer is increased to 85–95%. Anti-Tg antibodies are present in nearly 20% of patients with thyroid carcinoma, compared to 10% in the general population. The presence of antibodies after total thyroidectomy and RAI ablation

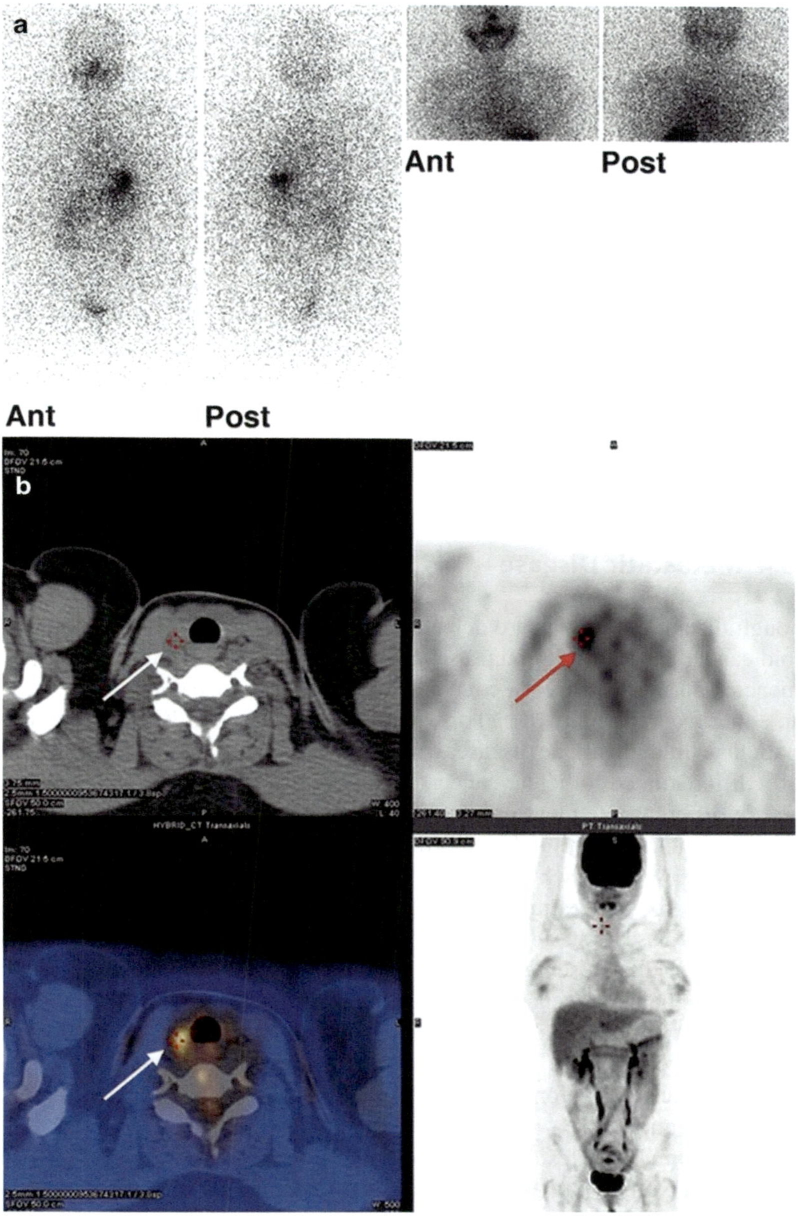

Fig. 22.2 (**a**) Follow-up diagnostic I^{131} scintigraphy of a 38-year-old female patient with the diagnosis of diffuse sclerosing type of thyroid cancer does not show any uptake consistent with recurrent or metastatic disease. (**b**) The same patient underwent FDG-PET/CT imaging since Tg is 46.7 ng/mL (anti-Tg Ab <20 IU/mL, TSH >100 uIU/mL) with a negative radioiodine scintigraphy, which displays focal FDG hypermetabolism of a middle-jugular lymph node (*arrow*). The biopsy was consistent with thyroid cancer metastasis and the patient was referred to surgery

therapy may prohibit the use of Tg measurements as a tumor marker in such patients, due to interference with analytical methods [122, 123]. Thus, a false negative Tg value may be due to the presence of anti-TG antibodies. Immunometric assays are more prone to detect these antibodies than radioimmunometric methods [123], The anti-Tg antibodies may disappear, although sometimes after many years. Optimal follow-up exhibits negative neck USG, stimulated Tg level <2 ng/mL with negative anti-Tg antibodies and negative RAI imaging after RAI ablation therapy. Tumor recurrence amenable to early therapy may be found when rhTSH-stimulated serum Tg rises above 2 ng/mL without performing a diagnostic whole body scan, which merely provides data concerning the completeness of thyroid ablation, but not persistent tumor. An elevated rhTSH-stimulated Tg greater than 2 ng/mL warrants further study [124]. As previously mentioned, the rhTSH-stimulated Tg test combined with neck ultrasonography has the highest diagnostic accuracy in detecting persistent disease in the follow-up of DTC [115]. However, the optimum cut-off value for postop serum Tg to guide decision-making regarding RAI administration is not known.

22.6.4 Metastatic Disease

Although distant metastases are detected in only less than 1% of all differentiated thyroid cancer patients at initial presentation, they can be encountered with various frequencies during the disease course. Nearly 15–20% of patients with DTC will recur, either locoregionally (80%) or with distant metastases (20%). Five percent of the patients will die with the disease, with types associated with poor differentiation (poorly differentiated follicular cancer, anaplastic cancer, Hürthle cell cancer) [51]. There are different treatment options for metastatic DTC. These are surgery, RAI therapy, systemic therapy, and supportive therapy. Only about 50–80% of primary tumors and their metastases take up ^{131}I RAI.

The most common treatment option for lymph node metastases is surgical excision and neck dissection, whenever possible, followed by radioiodine therapy for microscopic residual disease. Surgery decreases tumor burden significantly and thus increases the effectiveness of radioiodine therapy.

The dose of ^{131}I in nodal metastases is generally 150 mCi. In addition to this fixed-dose approach, there are some dosimetric methods, in which basically the pharmacokinetics of ^{131}I for each individual patient is estimated to define a more precise therapeutic dose.

The most common sites of metastases are the lungs (60%), bones (35%), bone and lung (15%), other soft issues, and rarely the brain (10%). As the rate of poorly differentiated tumors rises with age, it is more common with metastases at higher ages. Lung metastases were most frequent in patients with HCC and were least common in patients with PTC. Pulmonary metastases may be micronodular (Fig. 22.3a, b) or macronodular (Fig. 22.4a, b). The micronodular type usually has a diffuse miliary pattern and shows diffuse RAI accumulation, and therefore may be treatable by RAI. Especially in children, this may be successful and even curative. Patients with age less than 40 and RAI uptake in lung metastases generally have better prognosis (5-year survival 60% for ^{131}I RAI-positive metastases and 30% for ^{131}I RAI-negative metastases). ^{131}I RAI dose in the range of 150–175 mCi is used to treat pulmonary metastases; higher doses may cause pulmonary fibrosis. However, macronodular metastases are more frequent and RAI uptake is usually not present.

Bone metastases are more frequently seen in follicular thyroid cancer compared to the papillary type, where the preferred ^{131}I dose should be about 250 mCi or at least 200 mCi as a fixed-dose approach. Bone lesions mostly show high ^{131}I uptake; however, complete resolution is achieved in only about 10% of the patients. Surgical therapy especially to avoid vertebral collapse along with external radiation therapy is usually accompanied by radioiodine therapy in this setting.

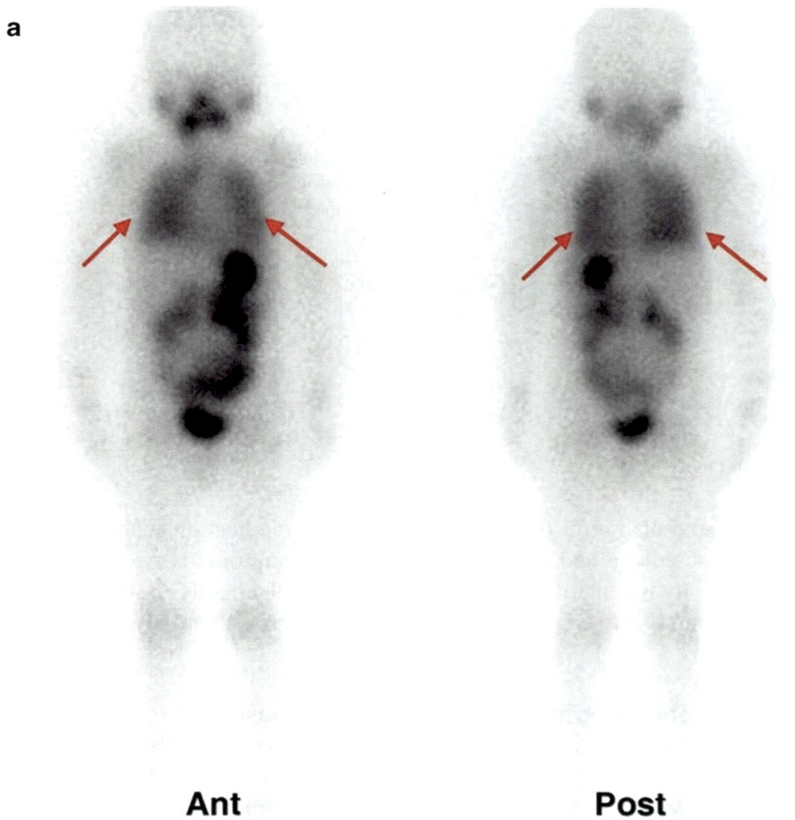

Fig. 22.3 (**a**) Diffuse lung uptake consistent with micronodular lung metastases (*arrows*) on post-therapy whole-body imaging following 200 mCi I^{131} therapy dose to a 5-year-old girl with the diagnosis of papillary thyroid carcinoma (TSH >100 uIU/mL; Tg, 695 ng/mL; anti-Tg Ab <20 IU/mL). (**b**) SPECT/CT I^{131} images of the same patient display diffuse lung uptake especially in the posterobasal parts of both lungs, consistent with micronodular lung metastases

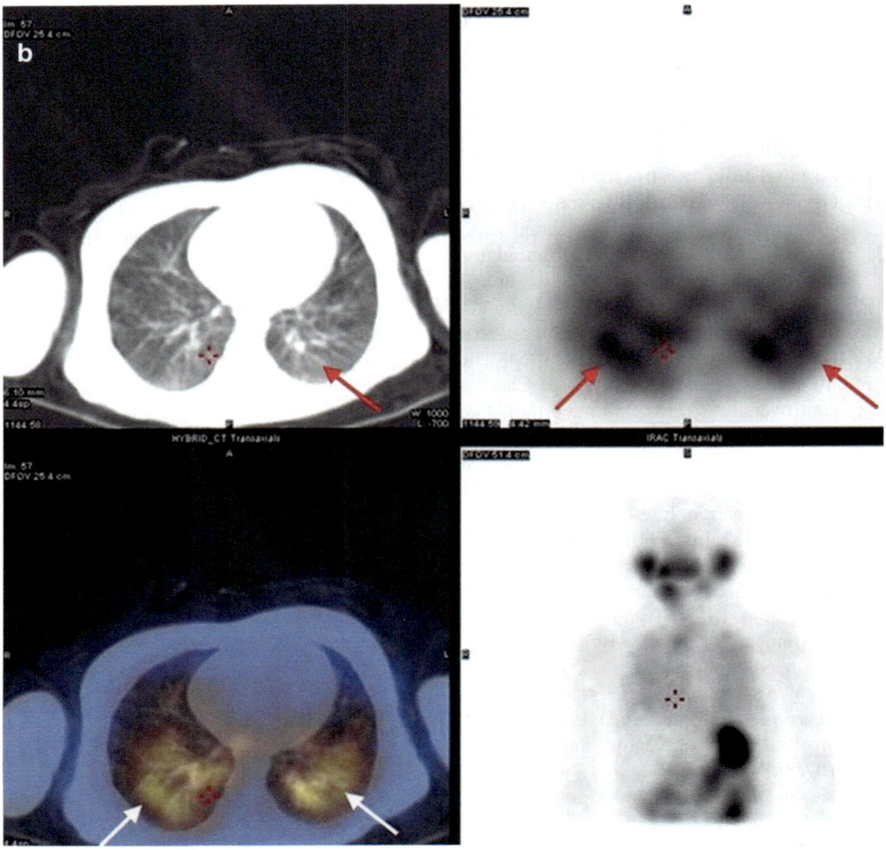

Fig. 22.3 (continued)

Before the administration of high dose of ^{131}I, premedication with glucocorticoids to decrease edema and to avoid compression symptoms is strongly recommended for the treatment of brain metastases as well as soft tissue metastatic recurrences around the midline neck region, which potentially may block respiration.

22.6.4.1 Systemic Treatment of Metastatic Disease

Metastatic DTC can be stable and silent for many years. Because of this, only patients with symptomatic or progressive disease should be treated with systemic treatment. RAI therapy is the first option for patients with RAI uptake-positive distant metastatic disease except for local therapies such as surgery and EBRT. However, tumor dedifferentiation and loss of iodine avidity may occur in the disease course. The long-term management of RAI-refractory (^{131}I refractory) DTC may be divided into four basic decision-making groups: patients who should undergo monitoring, patients who should undergo directed therapies, patients who should undergo systemic therapies, and patients who should be offered entry into clinical trials [125].

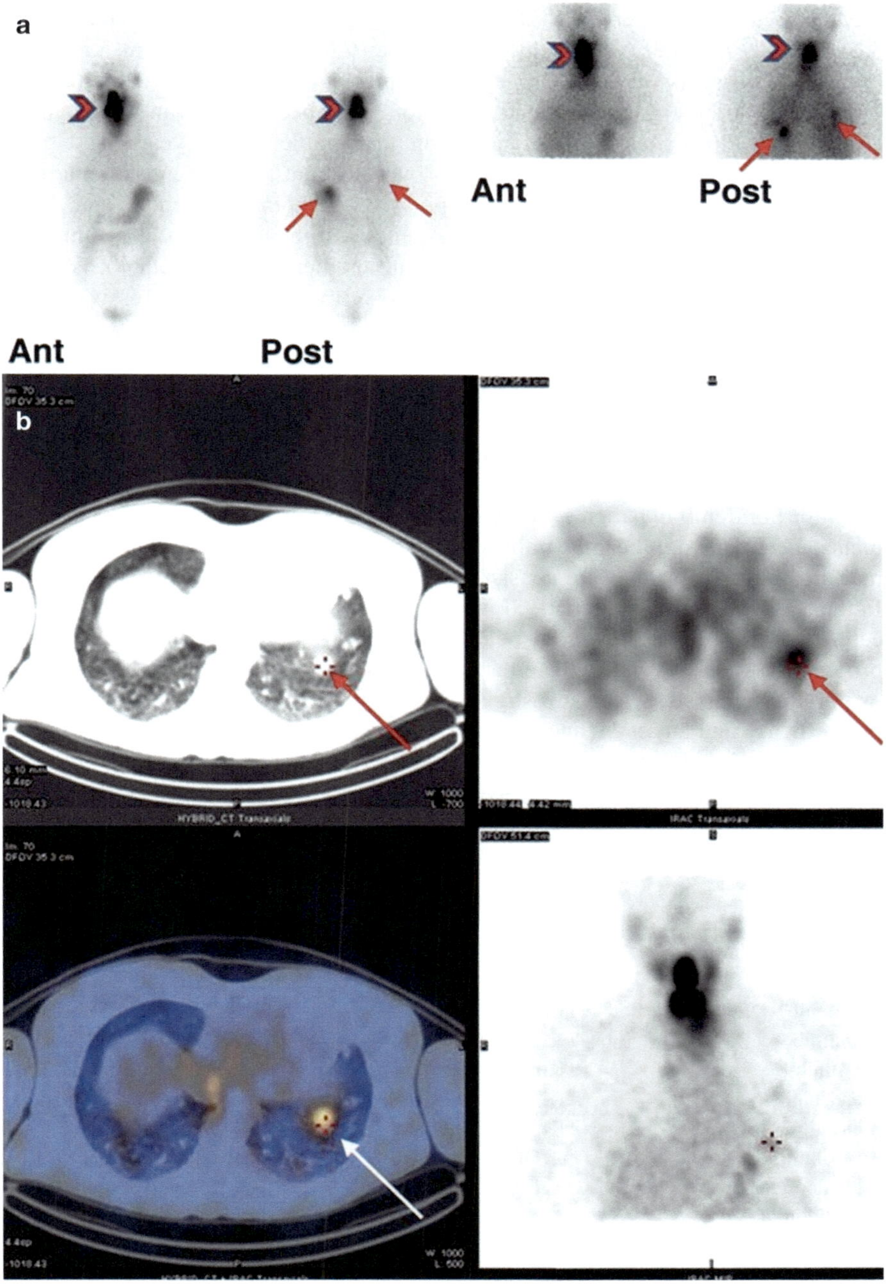

Fig. 22.4 (**a**) Post-therapy scintigraphy which was performed 4 days after the administration of 200 mCi of I^{131} in a 40-year-old woman with papillary thyroid cancer along with low differentiated thyroid cancer (TSH, 31 uIU/mL; Tg, 4508 ng/mL; anti-Tg Ab <20 IU/mL) displays prominent radioiodine uptake around the neck region consistent with recurrent disease (*arrowhead*) as well as faint radioiodine uptake suggesting macronodular lung metastases (*arrows*). (**b**) Macronodular lung metastases are better delineated on SPECT/CT transaxial images (*arrows*)

A key molecular element in the biology of DTC is the tyrosine kinase *RAS/RAF/MEK MAPK/ERK* pathway [22]. The *PI3K/Akt* pathway is also involved in the pathogenesis of DTC. Targeted therapies to these pathways, multikinase inhibitors, and other antiangiogenic inhibitors have been studied in various trials (Table 22.9). Great advancements have been made in the last few years in the treatment of RAI-refractory DTC. At present, two different tyrosine kinase inhibitors (TKIs), lenvatinib and sorafenib, approved by both US Food and Drug Administration and European Medicine Agency, can be used for the treatment of RAI-refractory DTCs [129, 132] In addition, another TKI, vandetanib, is under Phase III investigation in patients with RAI-refractory and progressive DTCs (VERIFY study) [130].

VEGF autocrine action in DTC plays a crucial role in tumor cell survival and represents a useful therapeutic target for thyroid tumors [135]. Interestingly, the level of VEGF expression in BRAF V600E(+) PTC was closely correlated with tumor size, extrathyroidal invasion, and stage and linked with poorer clinical outcomes and recurrences [136]. As shown in the DECISION trial, the use of the VEGF inhibitor Sorafenib in patients with progressive RAI-refractory locally advanced or metastatic DTC, significantly improved progression-free survival compared with placebo. Adverse events were consistent with the safety profile of sorafenib [129]. In the SELECT trial, another VEGF inhibitor, Lenvatinib, was compared with placebo and the use of it was also associated with significant improvements in progression-free survival with remarkable response rates as high as 65%. In an exploratory analysis, which investigated potential predictive biomarkers of lenvatinib efficacy and target engagement, the PFS benefit was maintained regardless of baseline CAF or BRAF/RAS status. Baseline Ang2 was predictive of PFS in a

Table 22.9 Targeted agents for the treatment of advanced thyroid cancer

Compound	Class	Thyroid cancers
Axitinib	TKI[a]	DTC, MTC, ATC [126]
Motesanib diphosphate	TKI	DTC, MTC [127]
Pazopanib	TKI	DTC [128]
Sorafenib[b] (DECISION)	TKI, VEGF inhibitor	DTC [129]
Sunitinib	TKI	DTC, MTC, ATC
Gefitinib	TKI	Advanced thyroid cancer
Vandetanib (VERIFY)	TKI	DTC, MTC, ATC [130, 131]
Lenvatinib[b] (SELECT)	TKI, VEGF inhibitor	DTC [132]
Everolimus	m-TOR inhibitor	Advanced thyroid cancer
Thalidomide	Angiogenesis inhibitor	DTC, MTC
Lenalidomide	Angiogenesis inhibitor	DTC
Cabozantinib	TKI	DTC, MTC [133]
Dabrafenib	BRAF inhibitor	DTC [134]
Trematinib	MEK inhibitor	DTC

[a] *TKI* tyrosine kinase inhibitor, *DTC* differentiated thyroid cancer, *MTC* medullary thyroid cancer, *ATC* anaplastic thyroid cancer
[b] US Food and Drug Administration and European Medicine Agency approved

subgroup of lenvatinib-treated patients, indicating that Ang2 may be predictive of lenvatinib sensitivity. Improved outcomes were associated with upregulated FGF23 suggesting that lenvatinib-induced FGF receptor inhibition contributes to lenvatinib efficacy [137].

Combined analyses of genomic variants, gene expression, and methylation have demonstrated that different driver groups lead to different pathologies with distinct signaling and differentiation characteristics. Similarly, distinct molecular subgroups of BRAF-mutant tumors have been identified and potential involvement of oncomiRs in less-differentiated tumors has been recognized [138]. Across solid tumors, PTC had the highest rate of recurrent oncogenic kinase fusions, indicating a prominent role for kinase fusions in PTC tumorigenesis [139]. A similar study by Yoo et al. in FTC has demonstrated a high rate of potentially actionable, drugable oncogenic driver mutations, including the N/H/K RAS mutations and the expected fusions of PAX-PPARG, but also ALK, NTRK, and RET fusions [140].

As far as immunotherapy is concerned, PD-1+ Tim-3+ CD8+ T Lymphocytes display varied degrees of functional exhaustion in patients with metastatic DTC. Identification of PD-L1 expression may have direct therapeutic relevance as therapies that release the effects of PD-1 and Tim-3 and reduce the suppressive effects of Tregs may encourage tumor elimination in patients with metastatic RAI-refractory DTC [141, 142].

The results of ongoing trials on Dabrafenib (BRAF inhibitor) and Trematinib (MEK inhibitor) in RAI refractory PTC are eagerly anticipated. Additionally, combined VEGFR multikinase inhibitors and immunotherapy may be applicable, but further studies on such combinations are necessary.

Other targeted agents, such as sunitinib, pazopanib, vemurafenib, gefitinib, axitinib, everolimus, motesanib, and cabozantinib are also under clinical investigation. Importantly, a major limitation of using TKIs is the significant toxicity from off-target effects encountered in many patients, limiting their use and leading to either drug discontinuation or dose reduction.

The combinatorial effect of TKIs plus the standard radiotherapy or combination of different specific inhibitors may decrease the likelihood of a tumor developing therapy resistance. The ASTRA phase III trial studied the effect of Selumetinib, a specific MEK inhibitor, in high-risk patients with DTC plus adjuvant radiotherapy but showed no improvement in complete remission outcomes [143]. Sorafenib combined with temsirolimus, an inhibitor of the mTOR pathway, in RAI-refractory DTC, had promising results [144]. Finally, several small BRAF kinase inhibitors have been developed targeting protein degradation. These new molecules target the ubiquitin-proteasome system, degrading selectively the $BRAF^{V600E}$ [145]. Redifferentiation therapy is another treatment option for these patients [146].

22.6.4.2 Surgery, EBRT, and Supportive Therapy

Surgery is a useful treatment option for loco-regional recurrences, localized painful bone lesions, spinal cord-compressing lesions, selected brain metastases, and localized soft tissue metastases. Bone metastases are more frequent in widely invasive FTC than in PTC. Bone lesions are generally osteolytic. ^{131}I RAI therapy, EBRT, intravenous bisphosphonates therapy, and denosumab are effective treatment options for bone metastases. EBRT is a useful treatment in patients with unresectable, grossly invasive, or metastatic disease to the neck.

22.6.4.3 Redifferentiation Therapy in RAI-Refractory DTC

Although DTC is a well-treated and even curable malignancy for most patients, approximately 10–15% of them present with recurrence during the disease course, and about 30% of thyroid cancer patients with recurrence and/or metastases show dedifferentiation of tumor cells with regard to morphology and function [147]. As tumor cell dedifferentiation proceeds, sodium/iodide symporter system expression decreases and the tumor cell loses its ability to take up radioiodine, which eventually results in a radioiodine therapy-resistant thyroid cancer.

Redifferentiating pharmaceuticals can potentially reactivate the radioiodine uptake of tumor cells and thus make radioiodine therapy possible [146, 148]. Retinoic acid derivatives, which are chemically similar to vitamin A, are the first agents used in redifferentiation therapy. Therapy includes oral administration of 1–1.5 mg/kg/day of isotretinoin or 13-cis-retinoic acid for 5–8 weeks. Some studies in the literature using similar therapy protocols reported that retinoids could cause a slight increase in the radioiodine uptake; however, the increased rate of radioiodine uptake was not always correlated with therapy efficacy. Incorporation of oral isotretinoin to induce redifferentiation and increased efficiency of radioiodine therapy has been investigated, the overall therapy response rate at 6-month follow-up was 21.3% [149]. An antidiabetic pharmaceutical thiazolidinedione which acts as a peroxisome-proliferator-activated receptor agonist was also reported to have both redifferentiating and antiproliferative effects and thus can potentially be used as a redifferentiating agent. In an open phase II study on 20 patients with radioiodine-refractory thyroid cancer, 5 patients had an overall partial response with regard to the decrease in Tg levels and increase in radioiodine uptake on scintigraphy, even though no partial or complete response regarding the RECIST criteria was reported [150]. Digitalis-like compounds may also be an alternative, and findings of increased iodine uptake in vitro have been presented [148].

Of note, the MAPK pathway activation may result in RAI refractoriness, while TKI therapy could lead to re-differentiation of RAI-refractory DTC [151]. The activation of the receptor tyrosine kinase erbB-3 (HER3) mitigates the MAPK activation achieved by BRAF inhibitors in $BRAF^{V600E}$ mutant thyroid cancers. Combined inhibition of BRAF and HER3 using Vemurafenib and CDX-3379, could restore RAI avidity by potently inhibiting MAPK activation in BRAF-mutant patients in this setting [152].

22.7 Anaplastic Thyroid Carcinoma (ATC)

ATC is a rare but highly lethal form of thyroid cancer. It is both a locally and systemically aggressive undifferentiated tumor derived from follicular cells. Geographically, the prevalence of ATC ranges from 1.3% to 9.8%, and patients have a median survival of 5 months and a 20% 1-year survival rate. More than 90% of patients with this disease are over the age of 50 years, and a male/female ratio is 2:3. The incidence of ATC has been decreasing in the last years.

The patient uniformly presents with a rapidly progressive palpable mass, frequently in a preexisting goiter. The median tumor size is 8–9 cm, with a range of 3–30 cm [25]. In 50% of cases, this disease arises from preexisting DTC [153]. Tg immunoreactivity is absent in the pathology specimens. Compared to poorly DTCs, ATCs had a greater mutation burden, including a higher frequency of mutations in TP53 (65–70%), TERT promoter, PI3K/AKT/mTOR pathway effectors, SWI/SNF subunits, and histone methyltransferases. Mutations of EIF1AX, a component of the translational preinitiation complex, are markedly enriched in ATCs and had a striking pattern of co-occurrence with RAS mutations [22]. *Beta-catenin* gene alterations are present in 65% of the cases [30]. In one study, *PI3K* mutations were found in 14% of the cases, but the *PI3K* gain of copy number was found in 39% [154]. Vandetinib, a multikinase inhibitor, has been demonstrated to inhibit growth of anaplastic thyroid cancer tissue [131].

TERT promoter mutations are clonal and highly prevalent in ATC. Application of the TCGA-derived BRAF-RAS score (a measure of MAPK transcriptional output) revealed a preserved relationship with BRAF/RAS mutation in poorly DTCs, whereas ATCs were BRAF-like irrespective of driver mutation. Thus, poorly DTCs and ATCs arise from well-differentiated tumors through the accumulation of key additional genetic abnormalities, many of which have prognostic and possible therapeutic relevance. The widespread genomic disruptions in ATC compared with poorly DTC underscore their greater virulence and higher mortality [155].

22.7.1 Treatment of ATC

22.7.1.1 Surgery

Unfortunately, not much progress has been made over the last 5 years in the treatment of ATC and tri-modality therapy (surgery, radiation, and cytotoxic chemotherapy) remains the mainstay of therapy. The initial approach to patients with stage IVA or IVB disease depends on whether the tumor is resectable or unresectable at the time of diagnosis. Patients with locoregional disease should be offered a resection if gross tumor resection can be achieved with minimal morbidity. Gross tumor resection, not debulking, is the goal of surgery. Most studies suggest that complete resection (R0/R1) is associated with prolonged disease-free survival and/or overall survival with or without combination chemotherapy and radiotherapy [156]. Patients with unresectable stage IVB disease may also respond to aggressive multimodal therapy. In patients with systemic disease, resection of locoregional disease for palliation may be considered if there is impending airway obstruction. Patients with distant metastases (stage IVC) only rarely have responded to traditional therapies, and if an aggressive approach is desired by the patient, a clinical trial should be considered. Hospice or palliative care is also an important component of managing patients with stage IVC disease.

22.7.1.2 Chemotherapy, Radiotherapy, and Targeted Therapies

RAI therapy has no role in this tumor. Except for surgery, chemoradiotherapy with paclitaxel/carboplatin combination, paclitaxel, docetaxel, cisplatin (C), and doxorubicin (D) weekly or 3-weekly can be used in local-regional disease control [156]. Clinical trials with chemotherapy and targeted agents (combretastatin, fosbretabulin, and crinobulin), which are vascular disrupting agents; CS-71-07 and oral *PPAR gamma* agonist; TKIs such as sorafenib, sunitinib, pazopanib, and imatinib; bevacizumab and biologic response modifiers aimed at restoring the dedifferentiated functions of thyroid tissue in combination with chemotherapy are under clinical investigation. Interestingly, patients with ATC amenable to aggressive tri-modal therapy demonstrate improved survival. Recently, dabrafenib plus trametinib demonstrated improved long-term survival and manageable toxicity in BRAF V600E-mutant ATC representing a meaningful treatment option for this rare, aggressive cancer [157, 158].

Immunotherapy is recently being explored in ATC as well. The addition of pembrolizumab as salvage to ongoing TKI demonstrated partial response in 42% of ATC patients and stable disease in another 33% in a study by Iyer et al. [159]. In the phase 2 ATLEP study, combination of pembrolizumab and lenvatinib resulted in an objective response rate as high as 35.7% of ATC patients. Pembrolizumab is currently FDA-approved for use in patients with thyroid cancer of any histology with high microsatellite instability (MSI-high) and/or high mutation burden [160]. Generally, the short time to treatment failure, due primarily to distant metastatic disease, highlights the potential opportunity for improved outcomes with earlier initiation of systemic therapy including adjuvant or neoadjuvant therapy [161]. Generally, even if early intensive multimodality therapy seems to improve the survival outcomes of patients with ATC, salvage therapies are of uncertain benefit. Additional innovative, rationally designed therapeutic strategies are under active development both for patients with ATC, with multiple ongoing phase II and phase III randomized clinical trials.

References

1. Sipos JA, Mazzaferri EL (2010) Thyroid cancer epidemiology and prognostic variables. Clin Oncol (R Coll Radiol) 22:395–404
2. Davies L, Welch HG (2014) Current thyroid cancer trends in the United States. JAMA Otolaryngol Head Neck Surg 140:317–322
3. Lim H, Devesa SS, Sosa JA, Check D, Kitahara CM (2017) Trends in thyroid cancer incidence and mortality in the United States, 1974–2013. JAMA 317:1338–1348
4. Du L et al (2018) Thyroid cancer: trends in incidence, mortality and clinical-pathological patterns in Zhejiang Province, Southeast China. BMC Cancer 18:291
5. Siegel R, Naishadham D, Jemal A (2013) Cancer statistics, 2013. CA Cancer J Clin 63:11–30
6. Shah JP (2015) Thyroid carcinoma: epidemiology, histology, and diagnosis. Clin Adv Hematol Oncol 13:3–6
7. Haddad RI et al (2015) Anaplastic thyroid carcinoma, version 2.2015. J Natl Compr Cancer Netw 13:1140–1150
8. Iglesias ML et al (2017) Radiation exposure and thyroid cancer: a review. Arch Endocrinol Metab 61:180–187

9. Lubin JH et al (2017) Thyroid cancer following childhood low-dose radiation exposure: a pooled analysis of nine cohorts. J Clin Endocrinol Metab 102:2575–2583
10. Efanov AA et al (2018) Investigation of the relationship between radiation dose and gene mutations and fusions in post-chernobyl thyroid cancer. J Natl Cancer Inst 110(4):371–378
11. Cardis E et al (2005) Risk of thyroid cancer after exposure to 131I in childhood. J Natl Cancer Inst 97:724–732
12. Ron E et al (1995) Thyroid cancer after exposure to external radiation: a pooled analysis of seven studies. Radiat Res 141:259–277
13. Schneider AB, Sarne DH (2005) Long-term risks for thyroid cancer and other neoplasms after exposure to radiation. Nat Clin Pract Endocrinol Metab 1:82–91
14. Ron E (2007) Thyroid cancer incidence among people living in areas contaminated by radiation from the Chernobyl accident. Health Phys 93:502–511
15. Veiga LH et al (2016) Thyroid cancer after childhood exposure to external radiation: an updated pooled analysis of 12 studies. Radiat Res 185:473–484
16. Dickman PW, Holm LE, Lundell G, Boice JD Jr, Hall P (2003) Thyroid cancer risk after thyroid examination with 131I: a population-based cohort study in Sweden. Int J Cancer 106:580–587
17. Choi WJ, Kim J (2014) Dietary factors and the risk of thyroid cancer: a review. Clin Nutr Res 3:75–88
18. Liu ZT, Lin AH (2014) Dietary factors and thyroid cancer risk: a meta-analysis of observational studies. Nutr Cancer 66:1165–1178
19. Boutzios G et al (2014) Higher incidence of tall cell variant of papillary thyroid carcinoma in Graves' Disease. Thyroid 24:347–354
20. Medas F et al (2018) Does hyperthyroidism worsen prognosis of thyroid carcinoma? A retrospective analysis on 2820 consecutive thyroidectomies. J Otolaryngol Head Neck Surg 47:6
21. Resende de Paiva C, Gronhoj C, Feldt-Rasmussen U, von Buchwald C (2017) Association between Hashimoto's thyroiditis and thyroid cancer in 64,628 patients. Front Oncol 7:53
22. Fagin JA, Wells SA Jr (2016) Biologic and clinical perspectives on thyroid cancer. N Engl J Med 375:1054–1067
23. Guilmette J, Nose V (2018) Hereditary and familial thyroid tumours. Histopathology 72:70–81
24. Nose V (2008) Familial non-medullary thyroid carcinoma: an update. Endocr Pathol 19:226–240
25. Carling T, Udelsman R (2014) Thyroid cancer. Annu Rev Med 65:125–137
26. Chakravarty D et al (2011) Small-molecule MAPK inhibitors restore radioiodine incorporation in mouse thyroid cancers with conditional BRAF activation. J Clin Invest 121:4700–4711
27. Decaussin-Petrucci M et al (2017) Molecular testing of BRAF, RAS and TERT on thyroid FNAs with indeterminate cytology improves diagnostic accuracy. Cytopathology 28:482–487
28. Bounacer A et al (1997) High prevalence of activating ret proto-oncogene rearrangements, in thyroid tumors from patients who had received external radiation. Oncogene 15:1263–1273
29. Acquaviva G et al (2018) Molecular pathology of thyroid tumours of follicular cells: a review of genetic alterations and their clinicopathological relevance. Histopathology 72:6–31
30. Hannallah J, Rose J, Guerrero MA (2013) Comprehensive literature review: recent advances in diagnosing and managing patients with poorly differentiated thyroid carcinoma. Int J Endocrinol 2013:317487
31. Jhiang SM (2000) The RET proto-oncogene in human cancers. Oncogene 19:5590–5597
32. Sakamoto A, Kasai N, Sugano H (1983) Poorly differentiated carcinoma of the thyroid. A clinicopathologic entity for a high-risk group of papillary and follicular carcinomas. Cancer 52:1849–1855
33. Nikiforov YE et al (2016) Nomenclature revision for encapsulated follicular variant of papillary thyroid carcinoma: a paradigm shift to reduce overtreatment of indolent tumors. JAMA Oncol 2:1023–1029
34. Baloch ZW et al (2016) Noninvasive follicular thyroid neoplasm with papillary-like nuclear features (NIFTP): a changing paradigm in thyroid surgical pathology and implications for thyroid cytopathology. Cancer Cytopathol 124:616–620

35. Rajabi S, Hedayati M (2017) Medullary thyroid cancer: clinical characteristics and new insights into therapeutic strategies targeting tyrosine kinases. Mol Diagn Ther 21:607–620
36. Haugen BR et al (2016) 2015 American Thyroid Association management guidelines for adult patients with thyroid nodules and differentiated thyroid cancer: The American Thyroid Association Guidelines Task Force on thyroid nodules and differentiated thyroid cancer. Thyroid 26:1–133
37. Cibas ES, Ali SZ, NCI Thyroid FNA State of the Science Conference (2009) The Bethesda System for reporting thyroid cytopathology. Am J Clin Pathol 132:658–665
38. Bongiovanni M, Spitale A, Faquin WC, Mazzucchelli L, Baloch ZW (2012) The Bethesda System for reporting thyroid cytopathology: a meta-analysis. Acta Cytol 56:333–339
39. Nikiforov YE et al (2011) Impact of mutational testing on the diagnosis and management of patients with cytologically indeterminate thyroid nodules: a prospective analysis of 1056 FNA samples. J Clin Endocrinol Metab 96:3390–3397
40. Ohori NP et al (2010) Contribution of molecular testing to thyroid fine-needle aspiration cytology of "follicular lesion of undetermined significance/atypia of undetermined significance". Cancer Cytopathol 118:17–23
41. Nikiforova MN et al (2018) Analytical performance of the ThyroSeq v3 genomic classifier for cancer diagnosis in thyroid nodules. Cancer 124(8):1682–1690
42. Valderrabano P et al (2017) Evaluation of ThyroSeq v2 performance in thyroid nodules with indeterminate cytology. Endocr Relat Cancer 24:127–136
43. Remonti LR, Kramer CK, Leitao CB, Pinto LC, Gross JL (2015) Thyroid ultrasound features and risk of carcinoma: a systematic review and meta-analysis of observational studies. Thyroid 25:538–550
44. Russ G et al (2017) European Thyroid Association Guidelines for ultrasound malignancy risk stratification of thyroid nodules in adults: the EU-TIRADS. Eur Thyroid J 6:225–237
45. Henry JF et al (1996) [Early diagnosis of sporadic medullary cancers of the thyroid: value of systematic assay of calcitonin]. Presse Med 25:1583–1588
46. Glikson E, Alon E, Bedrin L, Talmi YP (2017) Prognostic factors in differentiated thyroid cancer revisited. Isr Med Assoc J 19:114–118
47. Perrier ND, Brierley JD, Tuttle RM (2018) Differentiated and anaplastic thyroid carcinoma: major changes in the American Joint Committee on Cancer eighth edition cancer staging manual. CA Cancer J Clin 68:55–63
48. Edge SB, Compton CC (2010) The American Joint Committee on Cancer: the 7th edition of the AJCC cancer staging manual and the future of TNM. Ann Surg Oncol 17:1471–1474
49. Mazzaferri EL, Jhiang SM (1994) Long-term impact of initial surgical and medical therapy on papillary and follicular thyroid cancer. Am J Med 97:418–428
50. Leite AKN et al (2017) Deaths related to differentiated thyroid cancer: a rare but real event. Arch Endocrinol Metab 61:222–227
51. Wu HS et al (2000) Death from thyroid cancer of follicular cell origin. J Am Coll Surg 191:600–606
52. Liu C et al (2017) Reevaluating the prognostic significance of male gender for papillary thyroid carcinoma and microcarcinoma: a SEER database analysis. Sci Rep 7:11412
53. Grani G, Lamartina L, Durante C, Filetti S, Cooper DS (2018) Follicular thyroid cancer and Hurthle cell carcinoma: challenges in diagnosis, treatment, and clinical management. Lancet Diabetes Endocrinol 6(6):500–514
54. Roti E, degli Uberti EC, Bondanelli M, Braverman LE (2008) Thyroid papillary microcarcinoma: a descriptive and meta-analysis study. Eur J Endocrinol 159:659–673
55. Tuttle RM et al (2017) Natural history and tumor volume kinetics of papillary thyroid cancers during active surveillance. JAMA Otolaryngol Head Neck Surg 143:1015–1020
56. Patel KN, Shaha AR (2006) Poorly differentiated and anaplastic thyroid cancer. Cancer Control 13:119–128
57. Elisei R et al (2008) Prognostic significance of somatic RET oncogene mutations in sporadic medullary thyroid cancer: a 10-year follow-up study. J Clin Endocrinol Metab 93:682–687

58. Hvilsom GB et al (2018) Anaplastic thyroid carcinoma in Denmark 1996–2012: a national prospective study of 219 patients. Cancer Epidemiol 53:65–71
59. Sapuppo G et al (2018) Lymph node location is a risk factor for papillary thyroid cancer-related death. J Endocrinol Investig 41(11):1349–1353
60. Kim HI et al (2018) Refining the eighth edition AJCC TNM classification and prognostic groups for papillary thyroid cancer with lateral nodal metastasis. Oral Oncol 78:80–86
61. Shaha AR, Loree TR, Shah JP (1995) Prognostic factors and risk group analysis in follicular carcinoma of the thyroid. Surgery 118:1131–1136; discussion 1136–1138
62. Ito Y et al (2010) An observational trial for papillary thyroid microcarcinoma in Japanese patients. World J Surg 34:28–35
63. Ito Y et al (2014) Patient age is significantly related to the progression of papillary microcarcinoma of the thyroid under observation. Thyroid 24:27–34
64. Kwon H et al (2017) Active surveillance for patients with papillary thyroid microcarcinoma: a single center's experience in Korea. J Clin Endocrinol Metab 102:1917–1925
65. Mazzaferri EL, Young RL, Oertel JE, Kemmerer WT, Page CP (1977) Papillary thyroid carcinoma: the impact of therapy in 576 patients. Medicine (Baltimore) 56:171–196
66. Hay ID, Grant CS, Taylor WF, McConahey WM (1987) Ipsilateral lobectomy versus bilateral lobar resection in papillary thyroid carcinoma: a retrospective analysis of surgical outcome using a novel prognostic scoring system. Surgery 102:1088–1095
67. Shah JP, Loree TR, Dharker D, Strong EW (1993) Lobectomy versus total thyroidectomy for differentiated carcinoma of the thyroid: a matched-pair analysis. Am J Surg 166:331–335
68. Bilimoria KY et al (2007) Utilization of total thyroidectomy for papillary thyroid cancer in the United States. Surgery 142:906–913; discussion 913.e901–902
69. Mendelsohn AH, Elashoff DA, Abemayor E, St John MA (2010) Surgery for papillary thyroid carcinoma: is lobectomy enough? Arch Otolaryngol Head Neck Surg 136:1055–1061
70. Nixon IJ et al (2012) Thyroid lobectomy for treatment of well differentiated intrathyroid malignancy. Surgery 151:571–579
71. Choi JB et al (2019) Oncologic outcomes in patients with 1-cm to 4-cm differentiated thyroid carcinoma according to extent of thyroidectomy. Head Neck 41:56–63
72. Liu J et al (2019) Total thyroidectomy versus lobectomy for intermediate-risk papillary thyroid carcinoma: a single-institution matched-pair analysis. Oral Oncol 90:17–22
73. Zambeli-Ljepovic A et al (2019) Extent of surgery for low-risk thyroid cancer in the elderly: equipoise in survival but not in short-term outcomes. Surgery 166:895–900
74. Gemsenjager E et al (2003) Lymph node surgery in papillary thyroid carcinoma. J Am Coll Surg 197:182–190
75. Bardet S et al (2008) Macroscopic lymph-node involvement and neck dissection predict lymph-node recurrence in papillary thyroid carcinoma. Eur J Endocrinol 158:551–560
76. Gimm O, Rath FW, Dralle H (1998) Pattern of lymph node metastases in papillary thyroid carcinoma. Br J Surg 85:252–254
77. Mirallie E et al (1999) Localization of cervical node metastasis of papillary thyroid carcinoma. World J Surg 23:970–973; discussion 973–974
78. Qubain SW, Nakano S, Baba M, Takao S, Aikou T (2002) Distribution of lymph node micrometastasis in pN0 well-differentiated thyroid carcinoma. Surgery 131:249–256
79. Cranshaw IM, Carnaille B (2008) Micrometastases in thyroid cancer. An important finding? Surg Oncol 17:253–258
80. Wada N et al (2008) Clinical outcomes in older or younger patients with papillary thyroid carcinoma: impact of lymphadenopathy and patient age. Eur J Surg Oncol 34:202–207
81. Viola D et al (2015) Prophylactic central compartment lymph node dissection in papillary thyroid carcinoma: clinical implications derived from the first prospective randomized controlled single institution study. J Clin Endocrinol Metab 100:1316–1324
82. Wang TS, Cheung K, Farrokhyar F, Roman SA, Sosa JA (2013) A meta-analysis of the effect of prophylactic central compartment neck dissection on locoregional recurrence rates in patients with papillary thyroid cancer. Ann Surg Oncol 20:3477–3483

83. Carling T et al (2012) American Thyroid Association design and feasibility of a prospective randomized controlled trial of prophylactic central lymph node dissection for papillary thyroid carcinoma. Thyroid 22:237–244
84. Ito Y, Miyauchi A (2007) Lateral and mediastinal lymph node dissection in differentiated thyroid carcinoma: indications, benefits, and risks. World J Surg 31:905–915
85. Bocca E, Pignataro O (1967) A conservation technique in radical neck dissection. Ann Otol Rhinol Laryngol 76:975–987
86. Ferlito A, Robbins KT, Silver CE, Hasegawa Y, Rinaldo A (2009) Classification of neck dissections: an evolving system. Auris Nasus Larynx 36:127–134
87. Jonklaas J et al (2006) Outcomes of patients with differentiated thyroid carcinoma following initial therapy. Thyroid 16:1229–1242
88. Avram AM, Fig LM, Frey KA, Gross MD, Wong KK (2013) Preablation 131-I scans with SPECT/CT in postoperative thyroid cancer patients: what is the impact on staging? J Clin Endocrinol Metab 98:1163–1171
89. Durante C et al (2012) Long-term surveillance of papillary thyroid cancer patients who do not undergo postoperative radioiodine remnant ablation: is there a role for serum thyroglobulin measurement? J Clin Endocrinol Metab 97:2748–2753
90. Hay ID, McConahey WM, Goellner JR (2002) Managing patients with papillary thyroid carcinoma: insights gained from the Mayo Clinic's experience of treating 2512 consecutive patients during 1940 through 2000. Trans Am Clin Climatol Assoc 113:241–260
91. Schlumberger M et al (2012) Strategies of radioiodine ablation in patients with low-risk thyroid cancer. N Engl J Med 366:1663–1673
92. Schvartz C et al (2012) Impact on overall survival of radioactive iodine in low-risk differentiated thyroid cancer patients. J Clin Endocrinol Metab 97:1526–1535
93. Al-Qurayshi Z, Bu Ali D, Srivastav S, Kandil E (2017) Financial implication of radioactive iodine therapy for early-stage papillary thyroid cancer. Oncology 93:122–126
94. Mallick U et al (2012) Ablation with low-dose radioiodine and thyrotropin alfa in thyroid cancer. N Engl J Med 366:1674–1685
95. Mujammami M, Hier MP, Payne RJ, Rochon L, Tamilia M (2016) Long-term outcomes of patients with papillary thyroid cancer undergoing remnant ablation with 30 milliCuries radioiodine. Thyroid 26:951–958
96. Haugen BR et al (1999) A comparison of recombinant human thyrotropin and thyroid hormone withdrawal for the detection of thyroid remnant or cancer. J Clin Endocrinol Metab 84:3877–3885
97. Brown AP et al (2008) The risk of second primary malignancies up to three decades after the treatment of differentiated thyroid cancer. J Clin Endocrinol Metab 93:504–515
98. Rubino C et al (2003) Second primary malignancies in thyroid cancer patients. Br J Cancer 89:1638–1644
99. Sawka AM et al (2009) Second primary malignancy risk after radioactive iodine treatment for thyroid cancer: a systematic review and meta-analysis. Thyroid 19:451–457
100. Brierley J, Tsang R, Panzarella T, Bana N (2005) Prognostic factors and the effect of treatment with radioactive iodine and external beam radiation on patients with differentiated thyroid cancer seen at a single institution over 40 years. Clin Endocrinol 63:418–427
101. Tam S et al (2017) Adjuvant external beam radiotherapy in locally advanced differentiated thyroid cancer. JAMA Otolaryngol Head Neck Surg 143:1244–1251
102. Tumino D, Frasca F, Newbold K (2017) Updates on the management of advanced, metastatic, and radioiodine refractory differentiated thyroid cancer. Front Endocrinol (Lausanne) 8:312
103. Matrone A et al (2017) Postoperative thyroglobulin and neck ultrasound in the risk restratification and decision to perform 131I ablation. J Clin Endocrinol Metab 102:893–902
104. Bandeira L et al (2017) Thyroglobulin levels before radioactive iodine therapy and dynamic risk stratification after 1 year in patients with differentiated thyroid cancer. Arch Endocrinol Metab 61:590–599
105. Zhang L, Zou G (2019) Role of thyroid ultrasound combined with thyroglobulin in the diagnosis of postoperative recurrence of thyroid cancer. Minerva Endocrinol 44(2):192–198

106. Kim TH et al (2017) Prognostic value of the eighth edition AJCC TNM classification for differentiated thyroid carcinoma. Oral Oncol 71:81–86
107. Tuttle RM et al (2010) Estimating risk of recurrence in differentiated thyroid cancer after total thyroidectomy and radioactive iodine remnant ablation: using response to therapy variables to modify the initial risk estimates predicted by the new American Thyroid Association staging system. Thyroid 20:1341–1349
108. Banerjee M, Wiebel JL, Guo C, Gay B, Haymart MR (2016) Use of imaging tests after primary treatment of thyroid cancer in the United States: population based retrospective cohort study evaluating death and recurrence. BMJ 354:i3839
109. Garas G et al (2013) Is there survival benefit from life-long follow-up after treatment for differentiated thyroid cancer? Int J Surg 11:116–121
110. Yang SP, Bach AM, Tuttle RM, Fish SA (2015) Serial neck ultrasound is more likely to identify false-positive abnormalities than clinically significant disease in low-risk papillary thyroid cancer patients. Endocr Pract 21:1372–1379
111. Wu JX, Beni CE, Zanocco KA, Sturgeon C, Yeh MW (2015) Cost-effectiveness of long-term every three-year versus annual postoperative surveillance for low-risk papillary thyroid cancer. Thyroid 25:797–803
112. Walrand S, Hesse M, Jamar F (2015) Statistical and radiobiological analysis of the so-called thyroid stunning. EJNMMI Res 5:67
113. Norden MM et al (2007) Down-regulation of the sodium/iodide symporter explains 131I-induced thyroid stunning. Cancer Res 67:7512–7517
114. Haugen BR, Lin EC (2001) Isotope imaging for metastatic thyroid cancer. Endocrinol Metab Clin N Am 30:469–492
115. Pacini F et al (2003) Recombinant human thyrotropin-stimulated serum thyroglobulin combined with neck ultrasonography has the highest sensitivity in monitoring differentiated thyroid carcinoma. J Clin Endocrinol Metab 88:3668–3673
116. Torlontano M et al (2003) Serum thyroglobulin and 131I whole body scan after recombinant human TSH stimulation in the follow-up of low-risk patients with differentiated thyroid cancer. Eur J Endocrinol 148:19–24
117. Hempel JM et al (2016) Impact of combined FDG-PET/CT and MRI on the detection of local recurrence and nodal metastases in thyroid cancer. Cancer Imaging 16:37
118. Schutz F, Lautenschlager C, Lorenz K, Haerting J (2018) Positron emission tomography (PET) and PET/CT in thyroid cancer: a systematic review and meta-analysis. Eur Thyroid J 7:13–20
119. Lee JW, Lee SM, Lee DH, Kim YJ (2013) Clinical utility of 18F-FDG PET/CT concurrent with 131I therapy in intermediate-to-high-risk patients with differentiated thyroid cancer: dual-center experience with 286 patients. J Nucl Med 54:1230–1236
120. Santhanam P, Khthir R, Solnes LB, Ladenson PW (2018) The relationship of BRAF(V600e) mutation status to Fdg Pet/Ct avidity in thyroid cancer: a review and meta-analysis. Endocr Pract 24:21–26
121. Farina E et al (2017) (18)F-FDG Pet-guided external beam radiotherapy in iodine-refractory differentiated thyroid cancer: a pilot study. J Thyroid Res 2017:9807543
122. Algeciras-Schimnich A (2018) Thyroglobulin measurement in the management of patients with differentiated thyroid cancer. Crit Rev Clin Lab Sci 55:205–218
123. Spencer CA, Lopresti JS (2008) Measuring thyroglobulin and thyroglobulin autoantibody in patients with differentiated thyroid cancer. Nat Clin Pract Endocrinol Metab 4:223–233
124. Mazzaferri EL, Kloos RT (2002) Is diagnostic iodine-131 scanning with recombinant human TSH useful in the follow-up of differentiated thyroid cancer after thyroid ablation? J Clin Endocrinol Metab 87:1490–1498
125. Haugen BR (2017) 2015 American Thyroid Association Management guidelines for adult patients with thyroid nodules and differentiated thyroid cancer: what is new and what has changed? Cancer 123:372–381
126. Capdevila J et al (2017) Axitinib treatment in advanced RAI-resistant differentiated thyroid cancer (DTC) and refractory medullary thyroid cancer (MTC). Eur J Endocrinol 177:309–317

127. Sherman SI et al (2008) Motesanib diphosphate in progressive differentiated thyroid cancer. N Engl J Med 359:31–42
128. Bible KC et al (2010) Efficacy of pazopanib in progressive, radioiodine-refractory, metastatic differentiated thyroid cancers: results of a phase 2 consortium study. Lancet Oncol 11:962–972
129. Brose MS et al (2014) Sorafenib in radioactive iodine-refractory, locally advanced or metastatic differentiated thyroid cancer: a randomised, double-blind, phase 3 trial. Lancet 384:319–328
130. Leboulleux S et al (2012) Vandetanib in locally advanced or metastatic differentiated thyroid cancer: a randomised, double-blind, phase 2 trial. Lancet Oncol 13:897–905
131. Ferrari SM et al (2018) Vandetanib has antineoplastic activity in anaplastic thyroid cancer, in vitro and in vivo. Oncol Rep 39:2306–2314
132. Schlumberger M et al (2015) Lenvatinib versus placebo in radioiodine-refractory thyroid cancer. N Engl J Med 372:621–630
133. Markowitz JN, Fancher KM (2018) Cabozantinib: a multitargeted oral tyrosine kinase inhibitor. Pharmacotherapy 38:357–369
134. Falchook GS et al (2012) Dabrafenib in patients with melanoma, untreated brain metastases, and other solid tumours: a phase 1 dose-escalation trial. Lancet 379:1893–1901
135. Vieira JM et al (2005) Expression of vascular endothelial growth factor (VEGF) and its receptors in thyroid carcinomas of follicular origin: a potential autocrine loop. Eur J Endocrinol 153:701–709
136. Jo YS et al (2006) Influence of the BRAF V600E mutation on expression of vascular endothelial growth factor in papillary thyroid cancer. J Clin Endocrinol Metab 91:3667–3670
137. Tahara M et al (2017) Exploratory analysis of biomarkers associated with clinical outcomes from the study of lenvatinib in differentiated cancer of the thyroid. Eur J Cancer 75:213–221
138. Cancer Genome Atlas Research Network (2014) Integrated genomic characterization of papillary thyroid carcinoma. Cell 159:676–690
139. Stransky N, Cerami E, Schalm S, Kim JL, Lengauer C (2014) The landscape of kinase fusions in cancer. Nat Commun 5:4846
140. Yoo SK et al (2016) Comprehensive analysis of the transcriptional and mutational landscape of follicular and papillary thyroid cancers. PLoS Genet 12:e1006239
141. Severson JJ et al (2015) PD-1+Tim-3+ CD8+ T lymphocytes display varied degrees of functional exhaustion in patients with regionally metastatic differentiated thyroid cancer. Cancer Immunol Res 3:620–630
142. Ahn S et al (2017) Comprehensive screening for PD-L1 expression in thyroid cancer. Endocr Relat Cancer 24:97–106
143. Ho AL et al (2022) Selumetinib plus adjuvant radioactive iodine in patients with high-risk differentiated thyroid cancer: a phase III, randomized, placebo-controlled trial (ASTRA). J Clin Oncol 40(17):1870–1878
144. Sherman EJ et al (2017) Phase 2 study evaluating the combination of sorafenib and temsirolimus in the treatment of radioactive iodine-refractory thyroid cancer. Cancer 123:4114–4121
145. Hyman DM et al (2015) Vemurafenib in multiple nonmelanoma cancers with BRAF V600 mutations. N Engl J Med 373:726–736
146. Verburg FA, Luster M (2017) Thyroid cancer: redifferentiation—a 'new' option for (131) I-negative DTC. Nat Rev Endocrinol 13:9–10
147. Kim EY et al (2009) Coexistence of chronic lymphocytic thyroiditis is associated with lower recurrence rates in patients with papillary thyroid carcinoma. Clin Endocrinol 71:581–586
148. Tesselaar MH et al (2018) Digitalis-like compounds restore hNIS expression and iodide uptake capacity in anaplastic thyroid cancer. J Nucl Med 59(5):780–786
149. Oh SW et al (2011) Combined therapy with 131I and retinoic acid in Korean patients with radioiodine-refractory papillary thyroid cancer. Eur J Nucl Med Mol Imaging 38:1798–1805
150. Kebebew E et al (2009) Results of rosiglitazone therapy in patients with thyroglobulin-positive and radioiodine-negative advanced differentiated thyroid cancer. Thyroid 19:953–956

151. Buffet C et al (2020) Redifferentiation of radioiodine-refractory thyroid cancers. Endocr Relat Cancer 27:R113–R132
152. Tchekmedyian V et al (2022) Enhancing radioiodine incorporation in BRAF-mutant, radioiodine-refractory thyroid cancers with vemurafenib and the anti-ErbB3 monoclonal antibody CDX-3379: results of a pilot clinical trial. Thyroid 32:273–282
153. Are C, Shaha AR (2006) Anaplastic thyroid carcinoma: biology, pathogenesis, prognostic factors, and treatment approaches. Ann Surg Oncol 13:453–464
154. Santarpia L, El-Naggar AK, Cote GJ, Myers JN, Sherman SI (2008) Phosphatidylinositol 3-kinase/akt and ras/raf-mitogen-activated protein kinase pathway mutations in anaplastic thyroid cancer. J Clin Endocrinol Metab 93:278–284
155. Landa I et al (2016) Genomic and transcriptomic hallmarks of poorly differentiated and anaplastic thyroid cancers. J Clin Invest 126:1052–1066
156. Tiedje V et al (2018) Anaplastic thyroid carcinoma: review of treatment protocols. Endocr Relat Cancer 25:R153–R161
157. Subbiah V et al (2018) Dabrafenib and trametinib treatment in patients with locally advanced or metastatic BRAF V600-mutant anaplastic thyroid cancer. J Clin Oncol 36:7–13
158. Subbiah V et al (2022) Dabrafenib plus trametinib in patients with BRAF V600E-mutant anaplastic thyroid cancer: updated analysis from the phase II ROAR basket study. Ann Oncol 33:406–415
159. Iyer PC et al (2018) Salvage pembrolizumab added to kinase inhibitor therapy for the treatment of anaplastic thyroid carcinoma. J Immunother Cancer 6:68
160. Marcus L, Lemery SJ, Keegan P, Pazdur R (2019) FDA approval summary: pembrolizumab for the treatment of microsatellite instability-high solid tumors. Clin Cancer Res 25:3753–3758
161. Rao SN et al (2017) Patterns of treatment failure in anaplastic thyroid carcinoma. Thyroid 27:672–681

Medullary Thyroid Cancer

23

Şahin Laçin and Suayib Yalcin

23.1 Introduction

Medullary thyroid cancers (MTC) account for 1–2% of all thyroid cancers, making it the third most common thyroid malignancy after papillary and follicular thyroid carcinoma. MTC's incidence is 0.28 per 100,000 in the USA and 0.11 per 100,000 in Europe [1, 2]. The characteristic feature of this tumor is the production of calcitonin. Calcitonin is a hormone that is produced in humans by the parafollicular cells (commonly known as C-cells) of the thyroid gland. MTC is a neuroendocrine tumor that originates from the C cells or parafollicular cells of the thyroid gland. Parafollicular C cells originate from the neuroectoderm and are concentrated in the specific area of the thyroid gland [3–5]. MTC most often develops sporadically, however, about 25% of MTC are hereditary as part of the multiple endocrine neoplasia type 2 (MEN2) syndrome. Hereditary multiple endocrine neoplasia type 2 (MEN2) syndrome is divided into two different subgroups, MEN 2A and MEN 2B. MEN 2A is the most common subtype of all MEN2 syndromes, constitutes 95% of all cases, and is further subdivided into 4 groups. The first, classical MEN2A, which includes MTC with pheochromocytoma or hyperparathyroidism or both; the second, MEN2A with Hirschsprung's disease; third, MEN2A with cutaneous lichen amyloidosis; fourth, the familial MTC (FMTC). The FMTC, which is characterized by the presence of only MTC without hyperparathyroidism or pheochromocytoma, was used to be classified as a separate entity of hereditary thyroid medullary cancer in the past, but it is now determined as a variant of MEN2A [6, 7]. MEN2B syndrome is a much less frequent form that constitutes 5% of all MEN2 cases and includes pheochromocytoma, ganglioneuromatosis, and Marfanoid habitus.

Ş. Laçin
Department of Medical Oncology, Yeditepe University Faculty of Medicine, Istanbul, Turkey

S. Yalcin (✉)
Department of Medical Oncology, Hacettepe University Cancer Institute, Ankara, Turkey
e-mail: syalcin@hacettepe.edu.tr

S. Yalcin, K. Öberg (eds.), *Neuroendocrine Tumours*,
https://doi.org/10.1007/978-3-031-56968-5_23

However, MEN2B is the most aggressive subtype of MEN2 syndrome. The sporadic MTC is most commonly presenting as a solitary thyroid nodule, however, hereditary MTC typically emerges bilateral and multicentric. Rearranged during transfection (RET) pro-oncogene germline mutation is responsible for nearly all cases of hereditary or familial MTC, but studies of unselected patients with MTC have reported germline RET mutations in approximately 60–70% in patients with sporadic medullary thyroid cancer [8, 9]. The parafollicular C-cells of the thyroid gland secrete several hormones besides calcitonin, these substances include serotonin, vasoactive intestinal peptide (VIP), adrenocorticotropic hormone (ACTH), B-melanocyte stimulating hormone, carcinoembryonic antigen (CEA), chromogranin, histaminase, neurotensin, and somatostatin. Systemic symptoms may occur due to hormonal secretion by the tumor, such as cause diarrhea or facial flushing in patients with advanced disease [10–12].

23.2 Genetic Characteristics of MTC

While 25% of the disease develops in the form of autosomal dominant inheritance, the remaining vast majority of the disease occurs sporadically. The main genetic abnormality in the development of the MTC is the RET proto-oncogene discovered in 1985. It is located on chromosome 10q11.2 and encodes a single-pass transmembrane receptor of the tyrosine kinase family [13, 14]. Most mutation carriers can be detected by currently available genetic tests, and these tests are considered the standard of care for all first-degree relatives of patients with newly diagnosed hereditary MTC [15]. Different mutations of the RET proto-oncogene may be responsible for hereditary MTC and approximately 50% of sporadic MTC tumors have somatic RET mutations, among these mutations, 85% emerge particularly at codon 918 which is associated with a poor prognosis [16]. Some recent studies have shown some sporadic MTCs without somatic RET mutations, instead, they have different somatic mutations like HRAS, KRAS, or rarely NRAS [17, 18]. The patients with sporadic MTC who have the somatic RET codon M918T mutation have a more aggressive clinical course and a poorer prognosis compared to the patients without. In a recent study, the relationship between the prevalence of somatic RET codon M918T mutations and tumor size has been reported, and the frequency of the mutation was found to higher with the increased tumor size [16, 19]. After the discovery of the RET oncogene, numerous mutations, duplications, insertions, or deletions related RET have been identified in patients with hereditary MTC. MEN type 2, in contrast to the previously described as the hereditary disease by Steiner and colleagues in 1968 as the occurrence of MTC, pheochromocytoma (PHEO), hyperparathyroidism (HPTH), and Cushing's syndrome at the same time [20]. The syndrome that was described by the investigators with multiple endocrine disorders is now known as MEN2A. Similarly, the MEN2B syndrome described by investigators as a syndrome of bilateral pheochromocytoma, medullary thyroid carcinoma, and multiple neuromas, consists of 5% of hereditary MTCs [21–23]. The third hereditary MTC was known as familial MTC (FMTC) which is characterized by RET codon G533C mutation in exon 8. Although FMTC was known as hereditary MTC without hyperparathyroidism or pheochromocytoma, in the past, defining and separating FMTC from MEN2A was challenging. Since families with RET codon G533C mutant MTC emerged pheochromocytoma during their follow-up, therefore, currently, the recommendation is that FMTC should not be an independent or distinct syndrome; rather it should be considered as a variant of MEN2A [24–27]. In patients with hereditary MTC, the most commonly mutated RET cysteine codons are exons 10, 11, 13, 14, 15, and 16 [28]. The most common RET germline mutations in MEN2A occur in codons 609, 611, 618, or 620 of exon 10 or codon 634 of exon 11 [29]. On the other hand, the most common RET germline mutations in MEN2B occur in codon M918T of exon 16 and less than 5% of patients have RET germline mutations in codon A883F of exon 15 [7, 30, 31]. The genetic and clinical features of MTC are listed in Table 23.1.

Table 23.1 Genetic and clinical features of medullary thyroid carcinoma subtypes

Subtype		Frequency (%)	Clinical presentation	Associated endocrinopathies and clinical findings	Genetic predisposition
Sporadic MTC		75	Unifocal thyroid nodule, occurs between the fourth and sixth decades of life		RET codon M918T mutation, HRAS, KRAS, NRAS
Hereditary MTC	MEN-2A	20–23	Multifocal, bilateral thyroid nodule, occurs at third decade of life	Pheochromocytoma Primary parathyroid hyperplasia Cutaneous lichen planus amyloidosis Hirschsprung disease	RET mutations in codons 609, 611, 618, and 620 of exon 10, in codons 630 and 634 of exon 11, and exons 8, 13, 14, 15, and 16
	MEN-2B	2–5	Multifocal, bilateral thyroid nodule, occurs at the 1th decade of life	Pheochromocytoma Multiple mucosal ganglioneuromas Marfanoid body habitus	RET codon M918T mutation of exon 16, codon A883F mutation of exon 15

23.3 Clinical Manifestations

The sporadic MTC has a slight female predominance, while familial cases have no gender predilection or dominance due to their autosomal dominant inheritance pattern. Although the age at which inherited MTC occurs varies according to the underlying RET mutation subtype, it usually occurs in second and third decades, whereas somatic MTCs usually occur in the fourth and fifth decades [32]. Majority of sporadic MTC patients present with a solitary thyroid nodule, in contrast, hereditary MTC patients present with bilateral, multicentric nodules [33, 34]. The MTC is usually a slow-growing and indolent neuroendocrine tumor with good prognosis, a 10-year disease-specific survival is about 75%, however, survival rates depend on the tumor stage at diagnosis [35]. After the patient is diagnosed with MTC, the clinician needs to evaluate the extent of the disease, and classify the MTC as sporadic or hereditary by DNA testing, and by screening for associated endocrinopathies if it is hereditary. The parafollicular C cells of thyroid gland are predominantly located in the upper portion of each thyroid lobe; therefore, these areas are the most common locations where MTC emerge. Patients diagnosed with only palpable cervical lymphadenopathy refer to locally advanced disease. Icterus and rarely bone tenderness may occur in patients with systemic metastases. The identification of patients with MTC in early stage has changed the presentation from clinical tumors to preclinical disease, resulting in the highest cure rate for affected patients and a much better prognosis. Cutaneous lichen amyloidosis can manifest itself as multiple itchy, hyperpigmented, lichenoid papules in the scapular region of the back, especially in MEN 2A patients. Pheochromocytoma should be considered in patients with labile hypertension. MEN 2B patients may have a marfanoid habitus with mucosal neuromas. MTC is a neuroendocrine disease and systemic symptoms occur due to hormonal secretion by the tumor cells. Due to different hormone secretion, it can proceed with different clinical findings like diarrhea, facial flushing, and ectopic Cushing's syndrome.

23.4 Diagnosis and Staging

Locoregional lymph node involvement is the most common finding of early spreading of MTC, it occurs before the primary tumor is diagnosed. The central, lateral cervical, and mediastinal lymph nodes of the neck that are invaded by MTC can be found in around 10% of patients with a micro-MTC and in 90% of patients with clinically determined MTC, respectively. On the other hand, metastatic disease is observed in 7–23% of MTC cases [15]. The fine-needle aspiration (FNA) biopsy is generally the first procedure in a patient with a solitary thyroid nodule for diagnosis. Solely the sensitivity of FNA is low but it can be increased with additional immunohistochemical staining to 50–80% [36, 37]. The diagnosis of MTC is not possible for all cases by FNA, and in some cases, the diagnosis can be made after thyroid lobectomy for a suspicious or indeterminate FNA biopsy. Surgical specimens from patients with MTC demonstrate specific characteristics of MTC. Around 50–80%

of MTC patients have amyloid in tumor-stromal tissues, and this is one of the characteristic features of the disease. The tumor-stromal amyloid deposits are staining positive with Congo red, and brightening green birefringence under polarized light [38]. Currently, immunohistochemical staining with antibodies to calcitonin and thyroglobulin is standard for diagnosis, and classically MTC is thyroglobulin-negative and calcitonin-positive tumor. As neuroendocrine tumors, MTCs are immunostained with antibodies to chromogranin, synaptophysin, and neuron-specific enolase. Additionally, they may positively stain with somatostatin, bombesin, serotonin, and carcinoembryonic antigen (CEA) as well [39].

Numerous situations are included in the differential diagnosis of patients presenting with a mass in the neck, and comprehensive evaluation is required. The patient with neck mass detected is generally grouped into three subheadings according to mass characteristics such as the time of mass emerge, mass mobility, and present or absent of pain. In terms of these characteristics, the mass may be due to inflammatory, and neoplastic involvement or congenital. Congenital neck mass may due to branchial cleft or thyroglossal duct cyst, vascular anomalies, laryngocele, ranula, teratoma, dermoid cyst, and thymic cyst [40–43]. Inflammatory neck mass may be due to infectious inflammatory disorders like reactive viral lymphadenopathy, bacterial, and parasitic lymphadenopathies, also, noninfectious inflammatory disorders may cause neck mass [44]. Neoplastic disorders may be due to metastatic head and neck carcinoma, thyroid masses, salivary gland neoplasm, paragangliomas, schwannoma, lymphoma, and lipoma [45].

Calcitonin is a 32-amino acid monomeric peptide and precursor derived from preprocalcitonin which is the cleavage and posttranslational processing of procalcitonin. It is secreted as the primary product of MTC [46]. The method of measurement of calcitonin is very important, and need to be specific for avoiding cross-reactivity with procalcitonin or other calcitonin-related peptides. The prevention of cross-reactivity is important because various conditions like sepsis and general inflammation may cause serious elevation and secretion of procalcitonin in tissues that do not normally transcribe the calcitonin gene [47]. In this context, immunochemiluminometric two-site assays (ICMAs) are the most sensitive and specific way to test for intact, monomeric calcitonin [48, 49]. Basal serum calcitonin level according to sex is higher in men than in women which is due to a larger C cell mass in men compared to women [50, 51]. The tumor mass size and differentiation are associated with serum calcitonin levels; however, the level is almost always high in patients with palpable thyroid masses [52]. When ideally measured, the presence of MTC diagnosis is approximately 100% if baseline serum calcitonin levels are higher than 100 pg/mL or calcitonin levels with pentagastrin stimulation are higher than 1000 pg/mL [53, 54]. Pentagastrin stimulation test is very valuable to differ MTC from other conditions that are not related to MTC. Because the serum calcitonin levels in patients with non-MTC malignancies or conditions are not expected to significantly increase in response to calcium or pentagastrin stimulation. These conditions that may cause increased calcitonin levels include early childhood, pregnancy, chronic renal failure, autoimmune thyroiditis, proton pump inhibitors usage, smoking, small-cell or large-cell lung cancers, prostate cancer, mastocytosis, and enteric and pulmonary neuroendocrine tumors [55–58]. Undetectable serum calcitonin levels are expected after curative surgical resection, therefore elevated plasma calcitonin levels following surgery are indicative of persistent or recurrent disease [59]. The ultrasound for the preoperative detection of neck metastases are superior to computed tomography in terms of sensitivity, specificity, and diagnostic accuracy [60]. However, in patients with suspected skeletal metastases, magnetic resonance imaging (MRI) is superior to other imaging modalities [61]. Despite around 78% sensitivity in patients with high calcitonin levels (higher than 1000 pg/mL), 18-fluoro-2-deoxyglucose positron emission tomography (FDG-PET) or 6-Fluoro-(^{18}F)-L-3,4-dihydroxyphenylalanine (FDOPA) receptor imaging are not recommended to use in routine initial screening for metastatic disease [62–64].

The parafollicular cells that medullary thyroid cancer cells arise have the capability of secreting carcinoembryonic antigen (CEA) as a serum protein [65]. In contrast to calcitonin, CEA is integrated into the cell membrane, therefore, as a membrane-bound protein, CEA is less susceptible to stimulation [66]. The high level of serum CEA has been associated with tumor aggressiveness, tumor recurrence, tumor cell mass, and poor prognosis in numerous trials [67]. The majority of preoperative serum markers have a prognostic role, and in previous studies, the correlation between preoperative serum CEA level and regional lymph node involvement or overall stage of the disease has been reported. In one of these studies, serum CEA level that is higher than 30.0 ng/mL has been related to a higher possibility of the central neck and ipsilateral lateral neck lymph node metastases. Similarly, the level higher than 100.0 ng/mL has been related to a higher possibility of contralateral lateral neck lymph node metastases and distant metastases [68]. A similar relation between tumor mass and serum CEA level has been observed in different stages of metastatic disease, in this study the 25-fold difference of serum CEA levels between stage III and stage IVC, and fivefold difference between stage IVA and stage IVC, and the threefold difference between stage IVB and stage IVC has been reported [69]. In addition, it has been shown that patients with a serum CEA doubling time shorter than 24 months may not respond adequately to TKI treatments [70]. In patients with medullary thyroid cancer, because of the relation between serum CEA level and the presence of larger tumors, regional lymph node metastases, and systemic metastases, preoperative or before systemic treatment, serum CEA level measurement is very useful for planning the extent of surgery or deciding systemic treatment type.

23.5 Treatment

Regardless of the MTC subtypes, either sporadic or familial, surgery is the only definitive treatment for primary or recurrent MTC [71]. However, in the presence of metastatic disease, the goal of surgery is to provide palliative benefit. External beam radiation therapy (EBRT) is the treatment modality that can play a role in patients at high risk for local recurrence, however, this role is known as minimally effective in the control of MTC. Therefore, high-risk MTC patients are still being evaluated postoperatively for consideration of EBRT [72]. Patients with progressive or symptomatic metastatic MTC who are not candidates for surgery, local management, or radiotherapy should be referred to a medical oncologist to be treated with systemic therapy. The cytotoxic agents such as dacarbazine, doxorubicin, cyclophosphamide, streptozocin, vincristine, 5-fluorouracil, capecitabine, and temozolamide are the most commonly used systemic agents with limited benefit and considerable toxicity [73–75]. As a new treatment option, tyrosine kinase inhibitors changed the standard approach to treating these patients, further limited the role of cytotoxic agents.

23.5.1 Surgery

Surgery constitutes the only curative therapeutic strategy, and prophylactic thyroidectomy is absolutely necessary and makes the cure of MTC possible in MEN2 patients. By contrast, unilateral lobectomy is enough in a patient with sporadic MTC, because these patients generally have a single, unifocal tumor that is limited to the thyroid gland. The successful surgical procedure is defined with tumor-free surgical margins and undetectable postoperative plasma calcitonin levels. Since diagnosis is often made late in patients with sporadic MTC, unfortunately in most patients the tumor has already metastasized beyond the thyroid, so patients are often too late for curative therapy. The timing of prophylactic thyroidectomy in hereditary MTC patients is based on a model that uses genotype–phenotype correlations that to stratify mutations into three risk groups, such as moderate, high, and highest risk [76]. Additionally, in hereditary MTC patients, surgery may be delayed until the patient has an abnormal basal calcitonin level or C-cell stimulation test result. MTCs are a distinct disease that differs in their numerous features from follicular cell-derived papillary, follicular, poorly differentiated or undifferentiated thyroid cancers. These features are not only in terms of embryological origin, morphology, and predisposition factors but also functionally and tumor biology. For instance, despite high effective role in well-differentiated thyroid cancers, radioiodine therapy remains ineffective in MTC due to insufficient of the sodium-iodine symporter that is necessary to concentrate iodine in medullary cells. Therefore, surgery is the only curative treatment modality that constitutes the mainstay in disease management. The ideal type of surgery for MTC is total thyroidectomy with central node dissection and to dissect unilateral or bilateral neck lymph nodes for those with evidence of or at high risk of nodal involvement is necessary [77]. In order to staging disease and the prevention of later midline complications related to local metastatic disease, central lymph node dissection is necessary. In the condition that has a lack of evidence of local lymph node metastases during the primary surgical procedure, further neck dissection may be unnecessary. There is a correlation that has been reported between serum calcitonin levels and the extent of disease. In one study, no lymph node metastasis was found in patients with calcitonin levels less than 53 pg/mL [78]. In another study, the level of calcitonin that reflects patients without lymph node metastasis was found less than 20 pg/mL [77]. Surgical approaches should be done carefully in patients with MEN2 who may have pheochromocytoma at the time of diagnosis, and all necessary measures must be met in order to prevent pheochromocytoma complications.

23.5.2 Radiotherapy

MTC is not a frequent cancer, randomized studies are more difficult to design and conduct effectively in such disease, therefore, efficacy of EBRT for MTC has not been able to establish prospectively. On the other hand, the data from non-randomized studies have a higher risk of bias which needs comprehensive assessment. In this context, available reliable data regarding radiation treatment in MTC is limited and recommendations for patient management need to be discussed very carefully. In the past, MTC has been defined as a radiotherapy-resistant disease, so the role of EBRT in MTC management is controversial. However, radiotherapy techniques have changed markedly over the decades, and now tumor doses are higher and normal tissue doses lower than 20–30 years ago. The techniques that were used in the past had low effectiveness and high toxicity, therefore, may not be reliable to compare with radiotherapy practices today. For instance, in a much-quoted study conducted in the past, MTC patients who were treated with radiotherapy had worse survival than those not treated [79]. Risk stratification is one of the most important factors for treating patients. The several characteristics of the patients with MTC have been defined as high-risk features, which include T4 disease, node-positive disease, extrathyroidal extension (ETE), extranodal extension (ENE), and positive surgical margins. Patients with these features may benefit from radiation treatment. For example, the general risk of lung metastasis of a patient with MTC is around 3%, but if patient has extrathyroidal extension and 1–10 nodes involved risk is 13%, and is 28% with tumors larger than 4 cm and 11–20 or more than 20 nodes involved [80]. Intensity-modulated radiation therapy (IMRT) is one of the most common current techniques of radiation treatment, and it is possible to perform more doses without serious complications than old techniques. In two studies, higher radiation doses greater than 60 Gy that were performed with IMRT compared to earlier techniques have been reported more effective [81, 82]. As it has been reported in head and neck cancers, delaying radiotherapy increased locoregional relapse rate in patients with MTC as well. Therefore, if decided to perform, radiation therapy is recommended starting within 6 weeks of surgery [83]. EBRT with new techniques, particularly in high-risk patients reduces the risk of locoregional relapse and improves locoregional relapse-free survival without a consistent effect on overall survival [84].

23.5.3 Chemotherapy

There is clearly no role of cytotoxic chemotherapy in the adjuvant treatment of MTC. In patients with metastatic MTC, chemotherapy may provide significant benefits. Single-agent or combination cytotoxic chemotherapy response rates vary between 15% and 20%, and unfortunately, this response duration is usually short [85, 86]. The most common agents that have been used in the treatment of metastatic MTC are dacarbazine, doxorubicin, vincristine, fluorouracil, cyclophosphamide, streptozotocin, bleomycin, cisplatin, capecitabine, and temozolomide. Most of the data regarding the use of cytotoxic chemotherapy in MTC patients have been reported from old studies that started from 1974 to the tyrosine kinase era [75, 86–93]. Doxorubicin was the first agent that reported measurable tumor response in the treatment of MTC patients [87]. After that, cisplatin has been used as a cytotoxic agent for treatment of MTC. These two drugs were compared head to head in the first phase II trial conducted in MTC patients; the study concluded with a 15% response rate for doxorubicin and 21% for cisplatin treatment [88]. The combination of doxorubicin and cisplatin was compared with single-agent doxorubicin and experienced as an option with increased toxicity for patients with metastatic MTC [75]. Similarly, numerous cytotoxic agents were added to the doxorubicin and cisplatin combination, and their different combinations were compared with different agents. One of these combinations is dacarbazine and 5-fluorouracil combination, which has been reported as similar effective to doxorubicin and cisplatin but less toxic [86]. Oral cytotoxic agents capecitabine and temozolomide have been used, and promising response rates have been demonstrated [93, 94]. However, the use of these drugs has been reported as case reports or series, and there are no studies that have been conducted with a large number of cases. However, although anecdotal CAPTEM ± bevacizumab can be used with potential clinical benefit either in first line or as a salvage with acceptable toxicity. To summarize, there is no predictive biomarkers or factors regarding response to chemotherapy in MTC patients, the role of RET mutation in cytotoxic chemotherapy and its effect on the response of treatment not reveal yet. However, cytotoxic chemotherapy has still role in treatment of patients who have progressed during tyrosine kinase inhibitors, and their role and effectiveness should be evaluated with the prospective studies for the treatment of metastatic MTC patients.

23.5.4 Tyrosine Kinase Inhibitors

Regardless of the subtype of MTC, activating mutations of the RET gene in MTC patients is the main driver mutation that encodes tyrosine kinase receptor. Besides different somatic mutations like HRAS, KRAS, or rarely NRAS have also been reported. These RAS mutations have been found in around 70% of MTC tumors without RET mutation and rarely in MTC that harbors a RET mutation [17, 95]. Numerous other factors playing a role in MTC are tyrosine kinase receptor (TKR), vascular endothelial growth factor (VEGF), epidermal growth factor (EGF), fibroblast growth factor (FGF), and platelet-derived growth factor (PDGF). These factors are necessary for tumor proliferation, angiogenesis, invasion, and metastasis in patients with MTC. The main targets of agents used in MTC patients are the RET kinases and VEGF receptor kinase activity. The specific feature of the subtype RET mutation may also have effect on the choice of therapy or outcome. Efforts continue to find inhibitors that inhibit more selectively RET kinase and less VEGF receptor kinase activity, and Selpercatinib was discovered as an option that first met these features [96]. Therefore, molecular-targeted therapies for MTC have been divided into two groups, mutation-selective kinase inhibitors and multi-targeted kinase inhibitors. All tyrosine kinase inhibitors for MTC and their studies are listed in Table 23.2, and the most effective agents and their comparisons are listed in Table 23.3.

Table 23.2 Kinase inhibitors for the treatment of MTC and their studies

Phase of study	Line of systemic treatment	Drug	Mechanism of action	First end-point	References
Phase 3	1.line and beyond	Vandetanib	RET VEGFR EGFR cKIT	PFS 30.5 Months vs. 19.3 months	[97]
	1.line and beyond	Cabozantinib	AXL, VEGFR 1–3, c-MET, RET, ROS1, TIE-2, TRKB, TYRO3, FLT-3, KIT, and MER	PFS 11.2 months vs. 4.0 months	[98]
Phase 2	2.and beyond (except previous vandetanib, or motesanib)	Sorafenib	RAF, VEGFR 2, and 3, PDGFR-beta, cKIT, FLT-3, and RET	PFS 18 months	[99]
	2.line	Sunitinib	PDGFRα and PDGFRβ, VEGFR 1, 2 and 3, FLT3, RET	PFS 16.5 months	[100]
	2.and beyond	Pazopanib	VEGFR 1–3, PDGFR-α and -β; and c-Kit	PFS 9.4 months	[101]
	1.line and beyond	Lenvatinib	VEGFR 1–3, FGFR 1–4, PDGFRα, RET, and KIT	PFS 9 months	[102]
	2.line and beyond (except previous motesanib, RET, or VEGFR inhibitors)	Motesanib	VEGFR, PDGFR cKIT, RET	PFS 11 months	[103]
	2.line	Axitinib	VEGFR-1, VEGFR-2, and VEGFR-3	PFS 16.1 months	[104]
	1.line	Imatinib	RET, cKIT, PDGFR	PFS 6 months	[105]
Phase 1–2	1.line and beyond	Selpercatinib	ATP-competitive, selective RET inhibition	PFS 27.4 months	[106]

Table 23.3 The most effective agents and their comparison between each other

Compared parameter	Vandetanib	Cabozantinib	Selpercatinib
Phase of trial	Phase III	Phase III	Phase I-II
Patient population	MTC	MTC	MTC
Treatment line	1.line and beyond	1.line and beyond	2.line and beyond
Previous treatment rate	39%	38.8%	100%
Objective response rate	45%	28%	69%
The median PFS, months	30.5 months	11.2 months	27.4 months

23.5.4.1 Vandetanib

Vandetanib is a low molecular weight oral multi-kinase inhibitor. It inhibits tyrosine kinases including RET, EGFR, VEGFR, and other kinase receptors. However, vandetanib selectively inhibits the tyrosine kinase activity of RET, EGFR, and VEGF receptor 2 (VEGFR 2), particularly preventing endothelial cell proliferation and migration stimulated by VEGF and decreasing tumor capillary permeability [107]. The efficacy and tolerability of vandetanib were first evaluated in hereditary metastatic or unresectable medullary thyroid cancer patients. The study has resulted in considerable objective partial responses and disease control, and the drug-related adverse events that have been reported during the study were tolerable [70]. The rate of confirmed partial response and stable disease was 20% and 53%, respectively. Diarrhea, rash, fatigue, and nausea were the most common adverse events that occurred in more than half of the patients during the study. Following the promising results obtained with vandetanib in patients with hereditary MTC, the drug was planned to be used in also sporadic metastatic patients, and a phase III study was conducted. In this study, over 300 patients with advanced unresectable or metastatic hereditary or sporadic MTC were randomly allocated in a 2:1 ratio to take vandetanib 300 mg daily or placebo. Wells et al. reported a significant improvement in progression-free survival (PFS), objective response rate (ORR), disease control rate (DCR), and biochemical response in the vandetanib group compared to the placebo group. The objective response rate for the vandetanib and placebo groups was 45% and 13%, respectively, difference was significantly higher in the vandetanib group. Although the median progression-free survival had not yet been reached for the vandetanib group with a median follow-up of 24 months, progression-free survival has been reported significantly prolonged for patients randomly allocated to vandetanib versus placebo. The median PFS was 19.3 months for the placebo group, predicted PFS found with the Weibull prediction model was 30.5 months. The biochemical response rate was 69% for calcitonin and 52% for CEA level, both of them were significantly higher in vandetanib group compared to placebo [97]. In subgroup analysis, it has been determined that the patients who had a shorter doubling time of CEA than 24 months and M918T mutation more benefited from vandetanib treatment. Recently, the results of a post-hoc analysis of phase III vandetanib trial have been released at American Society of Clinical Oncology (ASCO) 2020 meeting. In this study, despite the efficacy and safety of vandetanib have been evaluated in four disease severity subgroups of patients with MTC, analysis has focused on particularly patients with symptomatic and aggressive disease. Among these subgroups, the group that the most benefited from vandetanib was patients with both symptoms and progression.

23.5.4.2 Cabozantinib

Cabozantinib is a potent inhibitor of receptor tyrosine kinases (RTKs) which include AXL, VEGFR-1, -2, and -3, c-MET, RET, ROS1, TIE-2, TRKB, TYRO3, FLT-3, KIT, and MER; also, cabozantinib induces apoptosis of cancer cells and suppresses tumor growth, metastasis, and angiogenesis [108]. The preclinical studies have demonstrated significant antiangiogenic and antitumor activity of cabozantinib in diverse types of tumor models which included medullary thyroid cancer (MTC) with an activating RET mutation [109]. After preclinical trial results, a phase I trial has been conducted to find the best dose of cabozantinib with the fewest side effects in metastatic medullary thyroid cancer. In this study, 35 patients with MTC with measurable disease were evaluated 10 of them had a partial response and 15 of them had stable disease that lasted more than 6 months, overall response rate was around 72%. The MTC patients without RET mutation were also included in the study, and responses were seen in patients regardless of the RET mutation status of their tumors. Therefore, cabozantinib is considered to be active also in patients without RET-activating mutations [110]. After these promising findings of cabozantinib efficacy, a double-blind, phase III trial comparing cabozantinib with a placebo study was initiated in patients with clinically documented disease progression, and cross over was not allowed in case of progression in the placebo group. The patient population included in the study differed from the previous study with vandetanib. RET mutation was positive in 46.1% of the patients, 14.2% had no mutation, and 39.7% were unknown. The majority of patients had sporadic MTC disease. RET M918T mutation, which is one of the determining factors in treatment efficiency, was present in 34.2% of the patients. Around 40% of the patients had received systemic treatment, and 20% of the patients received any TKI treatment. The proportion of patients who received two or more treatments, which means treatment-resistant disease, was 23.7%. The median PFS was significantly longer in cabozantinib-treated patients versus placebo, it was 11.2 and 4 months, respectively (P <0.001). As primary endpoint of the study, the median PFS was significantly longer in cabozantinib-treated patients versus placebo, it was 11.2 and 4 months, respectively (P <0.001). However, in an updated analysis of the study with a minimum 42 months follow-up, despite the 5-month difference, difference between the overall survival of two groups was not significant, which was 26.6 versus 21.1 months. In contrast, in patients with RET M918T-positive disease who have been reported in other TKI previous studies as well, the difference was significant, median OS was 44.3 months for cabozantinib versus 18.9 months for placebo (P = 0.03). So, this exploratory analysis demonstrated that patients with RET M918T-positive tumors may have a greater treatment benefit with cabozantinib, this factor should be taken into account when patients stratification in future studies [98]. The side effects that occurred during treatment in more than 25% of patients were diarrhea, stomatitis, palmar-plantar erythron dysesthesia syndrome, hypertension, and abdominal pain. Fistula formation and osteonecrosis of the jaw were observed, which were reported to be uncommon but serious side effects. Additionally, 16% of patients who were receiving cabozantinib discontinued treatment and around 80% of them required dose reduction because of an adverse event.

23.5.4.3 Other Non-selective Tyrosine Kinase Inhibitors

As a multikinase inhibitor, Sorafenib inhibits intracellular Raf kinases (CRAF, BRAF, and mutant BRAF), and cell surface kinase receptors (VEGFR-1, VEGFR-2, VEGFR-3, PDGFR-beta, cKIT, FLT-3, and RET) to prevent tumor growth and angiogenesis [111]. Sorafenib efficacy has been evaluated in a pilot study in small number of patients with MTC. Symptomatic response was reported in all patients, but the objective response was confirmed in two of them. Due to effective vandetanib and cabozantinib treatment in patients with MTC, the role of sorafenib is not sufficiently evaluated in metastatic MTC. There are only two phase II studies and a few retrospective case reports that tried to figure out its role in this disease [99, 112, 113]. Final sorafenib efficacy evaluation has been reported in Hungary that vandetanib and cabozantinib were not available until 2016, Among 10 patients, the partial response has been reported in 5 (40%) patients and 5 patients have confirmed with stable disease beyond 12 months (50%) and 1 patient has been progressive disease (10%). The median PFS was 19.1 months [114]. The PFS, disease control rate, and clinical benefit obtained with sorafenib treatment were found to be comparable to vandetanib or cabozantinib, therefore it may be considered for use in selected patients with advanced MTC who could not participate in clinical trials.

Sunitinib is a multi-kinase inhibitor such as platelet-derived growth factors (PDGFRα and PDGFRβ), VEGF receptors 1, 2 and 3, FLT3, RET, etc. [115]. Nevertheless, sunitinib has not been evaluated specifically in patients with metastatic MTC. The data regarding sunitinib efficacy in these patients come from subgroup analysis of studies that included MTC patients besides other types of cancer [100]. Therefore, it is not possible to define the exact efficacy of sunitinib for this rare disease.

Pazopanib is an oral small-molecule multi-kinase inhibitor, it is inhibiting VEGF receptors-1, -2, and -3; PDGF receptors-α and -β; and c-Kit [116]. In a preclinical trial, the proliferation of MTC cell lines has significantly reduced in response to pazopanib treatment in each line, and this result suggested to the investigators that pazopanib might have therapeutic promise in MTC. Then phase II study was conducted with 35 MTC patients, 5 patients achieved partial response (14.3%), and median PFS and overall survival were 9.4 and 19.9 months, respectively. The most common adverse effects were hypertension (33%), fatigue (14%), diarrhea (9%), and abnormal liver tests (6%); 3 (8.6%) patients have discontinued therapy due to adverse events [101]. Pazopanib has demonstrated promising clinical activity in metastatic MTC with overall manageable toxicities; these results are a rationale for pazopanib further study in patients with MTC.

Axitinib is an oral, potent, and selective inhibitor of VEGF receptors-1, 2, and 3 kinases activity [117]. Axitinib has been used for the treatment of thyroid cancer in the mixed patient population. In a study, Capdevila et al. used axitinib in advanced

RAI-resistant differentiated thyroid cancer (DTC) and refractory MTC patients. A total of 47 patients were included in this study, 13 patients had MTC diagnosis, among these 13 patients, the partial response rate was 23.1%, and stable disease was 38.5% under axitinib treatment. Consequently, in this study, axitinib showed promising efficacy and safety profiles in first-line treatment in MTC histology [104, 118]. Axitinib was well tolerated and had a good safety profile in the study as expected from previous clinical trials. The most common adverse events of axitinib seen in the study were diarrhea, hypertension, fatigue, dysphonia, nausea, decreased appetite, and the hand-foot syndrome and they were defined from mild to moderate in severity.

Lenvatinib is an oral, multi-targeted tyrosine kinase inhibitor that inhibits VEGF receptors 1–3, fibroblast growth factor receptors (FGFR)1–4, PDGFRα, RET, and KIT [102, 119]. In preclinical and phase I trials, lenvatinib has demonstrated promising antitumor efficacy in a variety of solid tumor types that included MTC as well [120–122]. These results supported the initiation of a phase 2 trial of lenvatinib in patients with advanced, unresectable progressive MTC. In the study, a total of 59 patients with unresectable progressive MTC were included. The patients who were treated with lenvatinib achieved a 36% partial response rate and 44% stable disease, thereby reporting a total disease control rate reached 80%. The median PFS was reported 9.0 months. The most common adverse events reported were diarrhea, hypertension, decreased appetite, fatigue, dysphagia, and increased alanine aminotransferase levels [102].

Motesanib and imatinib have been used to treat metastatic MTC patients, however, response and disease control rates were far below expected [103, 105]. In conclusion, the results of studies that have used these multiple kinase inhibitors were overall disappointing.

23.5.4.4 Selective Tyrosine Kinase Inhibitor

Vandetanib and cabozantinib are multi-targeted kinase inhibitors that have been approved for MTC treatment; however, these inhibitors simultaneously target many other kinases in addition to RET. Although very good percentage of patients' respond to these agents, the responses and tolerability are being challenged by toxic effects [123]. Drugs-related adverse events are primarily associated with the less potent inhibition of RET kinase than non-RET kinases inhibition, particularly to VEGF receptor 2. Therefore, selective RET inhibition can increase tolerability by overcoming these adverse events.

Selpercatinib (LOXO-292) is a novel, ATP-competitive, highly selective, small-molecule RET kinase inhibitor, it has been shown to have nanomolar potency against diverse RET alterations, including the acquired gatekeeper resistance mutation [124]. The safety and efficacy of selpercatinib have been evaluated in phase 1–2 clinical trials that included adolescent and adult patients with different types of thyroid cancers. This open-label LIBRETTO-001trial comprised 3 different groups of patients, the first group was included 55 patients with metastatic MTC who previously treated with vandetanib, cabozantinib, or both, the second group included 88 metastatic MTC who treatment-naive, the third group included the patients with non-MTC who previously treated. Among 143 patients with advanced or metastatic RET-mutant MTC, previously treated or not treated with cabozantinib, vandetanib or both, the objective response rate (ORR) was 69% and 73%, respectively. As more striking result, the complete response rate of the previously treated or not treated group was 9% and 11%, respectively. Despite the median PFS not been reached yet, 12-month PFS rates of the previously treated or not treated group were 82% and 92%, respectively [106]. These promising results prompted selpercatinib to be evaluated with the phase III randomized trial, in which it will be compared with the physician's choice of cabozantinib or vandetanib. Hypertension, increased liver function enzymes, hyponatremia, and diarrhea were the most common adverse events that have been reported grade 3 or higher during the study.

23.6 Conclusion

Medullary thyroid cancer (MTC) is a rare neuroendocrine tumor that emerges from thyroid parafollicular cells that do not concentrate iodine. Currently, MTC accounts for 1–2% of all thyroid cancers and mostly develops sporadically, however, about 25% of MTC are hereditary as part of the multiple endocrine neoplasia type 2 (MEN2) syndrome. REarranged during Transfection (RET) pro-oncogene germline mutation is responsible for nearly all cases of hereditary or familial MTC, however in unselected patients with MTC germline RET mutations are reported in approximately 60–70% in patients with sporadic medullary thyroid cancer. It is very important to determine hereditary MTC patients through genetic counseling and analysis because diagnosing them early would make it possible to apply curative treatments and save their life. The curative and the most effective treatment of MTC is surgery, however, the main treatment of advanced unresectable or metastatic MTC is tyrosine kinase inhibitors. The development in genetic analysis has led to a much more understanding of the molecular biology of disease and the discovery of diverse, novel, and more selective targeted inhibitors against mutations in MTC patients, and have changed the treatment paradigm of metastatic disease. Promising results have been obtained in the treatment of metastatic disease with mutation-targeted drugs, with the developments in this area, fewer side effects and higher responses can be obtained.

References

1. Noone A, Howlader N, Krapcho M, Miller D, Brest A, Yu M et al (2018) Surveillance, epidemiology, and end results (SEER) program cancer statistics review, 1975–2015. National Cancer Institute, Bethesda
2. Filetti S, Durante C, Hartl D, Leboulleux S, Locati L, Newbold K et al (2019) Thyroid cancer: ESMO clinical practice guidelines for diagnosis, treatment and follow-up. Ann Oncol 30(12):1856–1883
3. Siegel RL, Miller KD, Jemal A (2019) Cancer statistics, 2019. CA Cancer J Clin 69(1):7–34
4. Wells SA Jr, Asa SL, Dralle H, Elisei R, Evans DB, Gagel RF et al (2015) Revised American Thyroid Association guidelines for the management of medullary thyroid carcinoma. Thyroid 25(6):567–610

5. Davies L, Welch HG (2006) Increasing incidence of thyroid cancer in the United States, 1973-2002. JAMA 295(18):2164–2167
6. Romei C, Elisei R, Pinchera A, Ceccherini I, Molinaro E, Mancusi F et al (1996) Somatic mutations of the ret protooncogene in sporadic medullary thyroid carcinoma are not restricted to exon 16 and are associated with tumor recurrence. J Clin Endocrinol Metab 81(4):1619–1622
7. Hofstra RM, Landsvater RM, Ceccherini I, Stulp RP, Stelwagen T, Luo Y et al (1994) A mutation in the RET proto-oncogene associated with multiple endocrine neoplasia type 2B and sporadic medullary thyroid carcinoma. Nature 367(6461):375–376
8. Eng C, Mulligan LM, Smith DP, Healey CS, Frilling A, Raue F et al (1995) Low frequency of germline mutations in the RET proto-oncogene in patients with apparently sporadic medullary thyroid carcinoma. Clin Endocrinol 43(1):123–127
9. Elisei R, Romei C, Cosci B, Agate L, Bottici V, Molinaro E et al (2007) RET genetic screening in patients with medullary thyroid cancer and their relatives: experience with 807 individuals at one center. J Clin Endocrinol Metab 92(12):4725–4729
10. Abe K, Adachi I, Miyakawa S, Tanaka M, Yamaguchi K, Tanaka N et al (1977) Production of calcitonin, adrenocorticotropic hormone, and beta-melanocyte-stimulating hormone in tumors derived from amine precursor uptake and decarboxylation cells. Cancer Res 37(11):4190–4194
11. Baylin SB, Beaven MA, Engelman K, Sjoerdsma A (1970) Elevated histaminase activity in medullary carcinoma of the thyroid gland. N Engl J Med 283(23):1239–1244
12. Ishikawa N, Hamada S (1976) Association of medullary carcinoma of the thyroid with carcinoembryonic antigen. Br J Cancer 34(2):111–115
13. Takahashi M, Ritz J, Cooper GM (1985) Activation of a novel human transforming gene, ret, by DNA rearrangement. Cell 42(2):581–588
14. Ishizaka Y, Itoh F, Tahira T, Ikeda I, Sugimura T, Tucker J et al (1989) Human ret proto-oncogene mapped to chromosome 10q11.2. Oncogene 4(12):1519–1521
15. F. American Thyroid Association Guidelines Task, Kloos RT, Eng C, Evans DB, Francis GL, Gagel RF et al (2009) Medullary thyroid cancer: management guidelines of the American Thyroid Association. Thyroid 19(6):565–612
16. Elisei R, Cosci B, Romei C, Bottici V, Renzini G, Molinaro E et al (2008) Prognostic significance of somatic RET oncogene mutations in sporadic medullary thyroid cancer: a 10-year follow-up study. J Clin Endocrinol Metab 93(3):682–687
17. Moura MM, Cavaco BM, Pinto AE, Leite V (2011) High prevalence of RAS mutations in RET-negative sporadic medullary thyroid carcinomas. J Clin Endocrinol Metab 96(5):E863–E868
18. Ciampi R, Mian C, Fugazzola L, Cosci B, Romei C, Barollo S et al (2013) Evidence of a low prevalence of RAS mutations in a large medullary thyroid cancer series. Thyroid 23(1):50–57
19. Romei C, Ugolini C, Cosci B, Torregrossa L, Vivaldi A, Ciampi R et al (2012) Low prevalence of the somatic M918T RET mutation in micro-medullary thyroid cancer. Thyroid 22(5):476–481
20. Steiner AL, Goodman AD, Powers SR (1968) Study of a kindred with pheochromocytoma, medullary thyroid carcinoma, hyperparathyroidism and Cushing's disease: multiple endocrine neoplasia, type 2. Medicine (Baltimore) 47(5):371–409
21. Schimke RN, Hartmann WH, Prout TE, Rimoin DL (1968) Syndrome of bilateral pheochromocytoma, medullary thyroid carcinoma and multiple neuromas. A possible regulatory defect in the differentiation of chromaffin tissue. N Engl J Med 279(1):1–7
22. Gorlin RJ, Sedano HO, Vickers RA, Cervenka J (1968) Multiple mucosal neuromas, pheochromocytoma and medullary carcinoma of the thyroid—a syndrome. Cancer 22(2):293–299. passim
23. Williams ED, Pollock DJ (1966) Multiple mucosal neuromata with endocrine tumours: a syndrome allied to von Recklinghausen's disease. J Pathol Bacteriol 91(1):71–80
24. Oliveira MN, Hemerly JP, Bastos AU, Tamanaha R, Latini FR, Camacho CP et al (2011) The RET p.G533C mutation confers predisposition to multiple endocrine neoplasia type 2A in a

Brazilian kindred and is able to induce a malignant phenotype in vitro and in vivo. Thyroid 21(9):975–985
25. Peppa M, Boutati E, Kamakari S, Pikounis V, Peros G, Panayiotides IG et al (2008) Multiple endocrine neoplasia type 2A in two families with the familial medullary thyroid carcinoma associated G533C mutation of the RET proto-oncogene. Eur J Endocrinol 159(6):767–771
26. Bethanis S, Koutsodontis G, Palouka T, Avgoustis C, Yannoukakos D, Bei T et al (2007) A newly detected mutation of the RET protooncogene in exon 8 as a cause of multiple endocrine neoplasia type 2A. Hormones (Athens) 6(2):152–156
27. Castro MR, Thomas BC, Richards ML, Zhang J, Morris JC (2013) Multiple endocrine neoplasia type 2A due to an exon 8 (G533C) mutation in a large North American kindred. Thyroid 23(12):1547–1552
28. Conzo G, Circelli L, Pasquali D, Sinisi A, Sabatino L, Accardo G et al (2012) Lessons to be learned from the clinical management of a MEN 2A patient bearing a novel 634/640/700 mutation of the RET proto-oncogene. Clin Endocrinol 77(6):934–936
29. Raue F, Frank-Raue K (2012) Genotype-phenotype correlation in multiple endocrine neoplasia type 2. Clinics (Sao Paulo) 67(Suppl 1):69–75
30. Carlson KM, Dou S, Chi D, Scavarda N, Toshima K, Jackson CE et al (1994) Single missense mutation in the tyrosine kinase catalytic domain of the RET protooncogene is associated with multiple endocrine neoplasia type 2B. Proc Natl Acad Sci U S A 91(4):1579–1583
31. Gimm O, Marsh DJ, Andrew SD, Frilling A, Dahia PL, Mulligan LM et al (1997) Germline dinucleotide mutation in codon 883 of the RET proto-oncogene in multiple endocrine neoplasia type 2B without codon 918 mutation. J Clin Endocrinol Metab 82(11):3902–3904
32. Rich TA, Feng L, Busaidy N, Cote GJ, Gagel RF, Hu M et al (2014) Prevalence by age and predictors of medullary thyroid cancer in patients with lower risk germline RET proto-oncogene mutations. Thyroid 24(7):1096–1106
33. Saad MF, Ordonez NG, Rashid RK, Guido JJ, Hill CS Jr, Hickey RC et al (1984) Medullary carcinoma of the thyroid. A study of the clinical features and prognostic factors in 161 patients. Medicine (Baltimore) 63(6):319–342
34. Kebebew E, Ituarte PH, Siperstein AE, Duh QY, Clark OH (2000) Medullary thyroid carcinoma: clinical characteristics, treatment, prognostic factors, and a comparison of staging systems. Cancer 88(5):1139–1148
35. Barbet J, Campion L, Kraeber-Bodere F, Chatal JF, G.T.E.S. Group (2005) Prognostic impact of serum calcitonin and carcinoembryonic antigen doubling-times in patients with medullary thyroid carcinoma. J Clin Endocrinol Metab 90(11):6077–6084
36. Trimboli P, Treglia G, Guidobaldi L, Romanelli F, Nigri G, Valabrega S et al (2015) Detection rate of FNA cytology in medullary thyroid carcinoma: a meta-analysis. Clin Endocrinol 82(2):280–285
37. Bhanot P, Yang J, Schnadig VJ, Logrono R (2007) Role of FNA cytology and immunochemistry in the diagnosis and management of medullary thyroid carcinoma: report of six cases and review of the literature. Diagn Cytopathol 35(5):285–292
38. Khurana R, Agarwal A, Bajpai VK, Verma N, Sharma AK, Gupta RP et al (2004) Unraveling the amyloid associated with human medullary thyroid carcinoma. Endocrinology 145(12):5465–5470
39. Mendelsohn G, Wells SA Jr, Baylin SB (1984) Relationship of tissue carcinoembryonic antigen and calcitonin to tumor virulence in medullary thyroid carcinoma. An immunohistochemical study in early, localized, and virulent disseminated stages of disease. Cancer 54(4):657–662
40. Ibrahim M, Hammoud K, Maheshwari M, Pandya A (2011) Congenital cystic lesions of the head and neck. Neuroimaging Clin 21(3):621–639
41. Abuabara A, Baratto Filho F, Fuzza RF (2010) Thyroglossal duct cyst. RSBO Revista Sul-Brasileira de Odontologia 7(2):244–246
42. Cătălina R, Alina O, Mioriţa T (2015) Compressing dermoid cyst of the neck. Ther Pharmacol Clin Toxicol 19(4)

43. April MM, Ward RF, Garelick JM (1998) Diagnosis, management, and follow-up of congenital head and neck teratomas. Laryngoscope 108(9):1398–1401
44. Leung AK, Davies HD (2009) Cervical lymphadenitis: etiology, diagnosis, and management. Curr Infect Dis Rep 11(3):183–189
45. Schwetschenau E, Kelley DJ (2002) The adult neck mass. Am Fam Physician 66(5):831
46. Steenbergh P, Höppener J, Zandberg J, Visser A, Lips C, Jansz H (1986) Structure and expression of the human calcitonin/CGRP genes. FEBS Lett 209(1):97–103
47. Whang KT, Steinwald PM, White JC, Nylen ES, Snider RH, Simon GL et al (1998) Serum calcitonin precursors in sepsis and systemic inflammation. J Clin Endocrinol Metabol 83(9):3296–3301
48. Kratzsch J, Petzold A, Raue F, Reinhardt W, Brocker-Preuss M, Gorges R et al (2011) Basal and stimulated calcitonin and procalcitonin by various assays in patients with and without medullary thyroid cancer. Clin Chem 57(3):467–474
49. Becker KL, Nylen ES, White JC, Muller B, Snider RH Jr (2004) Clinical review 167: procalcitonin and the calcitonin gene family of peptides in inflammation, infection, and sepsis: a journey from calcitonin back to its precursors. J Clin Endocrinol Metab 89(4):1512–1525
50. Guyetant S, Rousselet MC, Durigon M, Chappard D, Franc B, Guerin O et al (1997) Sex-related C cell hyperplasia in the normal human thyroid: a quantitative autopsy study. J Clin Endocrinol Metab 82(1):42–47
51. Basuyau JP, Mallet E, Leroy M, Brunelle P (2004) Reference intervals for serum calcitonin in men, women, and children. Clin Chem 50(10):1828–1830
52. Machens A, Dralle H (2010) Peak calcitonin cut-off levels for the diagnosis of occult medullary thyroid cancer: evidence of confounding by gender. Clin Endocrinol 73(2):274
53. Scheuba C, Kaserer K, Moritz A, Drosten R, Vierhapper H, Bieglmayer C et al (2009) Sporadic hypercalcitoninemia: clinical and therapeutic consequences. Endocr Relat Cancer 16(1):243–253
54. Costante G, Meringolo D, Durante C, Bianchi D, Nocera M, Tumino S et al (2007) Predictive value of serum calcitonin levels for preoperative diagnosis of medullary thyroid carcinoma in a cohort of 5817 consecutive patients with thyroid nodules. J Clin Endocrinol Metab 92(2):450–455
55. Whang KT, Steinwald PM, White JC, Nylen ES, Snider RH, Simon GL et al (1998) Serum calcitonin precursors in sepsis and systemic inflammation. J Clin Endocrinol Metab 83(9):3296–3301
56. Schuetz M, Duan H, Wahl K, Pirich C, Antoni A, Kommata S et al (2006) T lymphocyte cytokine production patterns in Hashimoto patients with elevated calcitonin levels and their relationship to tumor initiation. Anticancer Res 26(6B):4591–4596
57. Machens A, Haedecke J, Holzhausen HJ, Thomusch O, Schneyer U, Dralle H (2000) Differential diagnosis of calcitonin-secreting neuroendocrine carcinoma of the foregut by pentagastrin stimulation. Langenbecks Arch Surg 385(6):398–401
58. Toledo SP, Lourenco DM Jr, Santos MA, Tavares MR, Toledo RA, Correia-Deur JE (2009) Hypercalcitoninemia is not pathognomonic of medullary thyroid carcinoma. Clinics (Sao Paulo) 64(7):699–706
59. Cohen EG, Shaha AR, Rinaldo A, Devaney KO, Ferlito A (2004) Medullary thyroid carcinoma. Acta Otolaryngol 124(5):544–557
60. Lee KB, Jang IM, Roh H, Ahn MY, Woo HY (2008) Transient urinary retention in acute right lateral medullary infarction. Neurologist 14(5):312–315
61. Mirallie E, Vuillez JP, Bardet S, Frampas E, Dupas B, Ferrer L et al (2005) High frequency of bone/bone marrow involvement in advanced medullary thyroid cancer. J Clin Endocrinol Metab 90(2):779–788
62. Oudoux A, Salaun PY, Bournaud C, Campion L, Ansquer C, Rousseau C et al (2007) Sensitivity and prognostic value of positron emission tomography with F-18-fluorodeoxyglucose and sensitivity of immunoscintigraphy in patients with medullary thyroid carcinoma treated with anticarcinoembryonic antigen-targeted radioimmunotherapy. J Clin Endocrinol Metab 92(12):4590–4597

63. Giraudet AL, Vanel D, Leboulleux S, Auperin A, Dromain C, Chami L et al (2007) Imaging medullary thyroid carcinoma with persistent elevated calcitonin levels. J Clin Endocrinol Metab 92(11):4185–4190
64. Ong SC, Schoder H, Patel SG, Tabangay-Lim IM, Doddamane I, Gonen M et al (2007) Diagnostic accuracy of 18F-FDG PET in restaging patients with medullary thyroid carcinoma and elevated calcitonin levels. J Nucl Med 48(4):501–507
65. Osamura RY, Yasuda O, Kawakami T, Itoh Y, Inada K, Kakudo K (1997) Immunoelectron microscopic demonstration of regulated pathway for calcitonin and constitutive pathway for carcinoembryonic antigen in the same cells of human medullary carcinomas of thyroid glands. Mod Pathol 10(1):7–11
66. Wells SA Jr, Haagensen DE Jr, Linehan WM, Farrell RE, Dilley WG (1978) The detection of elevated plasma levels of carcinoembryonic antigen in patients with suspected or established medullary thyroid carcinoma. Cancer 42(3 Suppl):1498–1503
67. Rougier P, Calmettes C, Laplanche A, Travagli JP, Lefevre M, Parmentier C et al (1983) The values of calcitonin and carcinoembryonic antigen in the treatment and management of nonfamilial medullary thyroid carcinoma. Cancer 51(5):855–862
68. Machens A, Ukkat J, Hauptmann S, Dralle H (2007) Abnormal carcinoembryonic antigen levels and medullary thyroid cancer progression: a multivariate analysis. Arch Surg 142(3):289–293; discussion 294
69. Turkdogan S, Forest VI, Hier MP, Tamilia M, Florea A, Payne RJ (2018) Carcinoembryonic antigen levels correlated with advanced disease in medullary thyroid cancer. J Otolaryngol Head Neck Surg 47(1):55
70. Wells SA Jr, Gosnell JE, Gagel RF, Moley J, Pfister D, Sosa JA et al (2010) Vandetanib for the treatment of patients with locally advanced or metastatic hereditary medullary thyroid cancer. J Clin Oncol 28(5):767–772
71. Machens A, Dralle H (2015) Surgical treatment of medullary thyroid cancer. Recent Results Cancer Res 204:187–205
72. Brierley J, Tsang R, Simpson WJ, Gospodarowicz M, Sutcliffe S, Panzarella T (1996) Medullary thyroid cancer: analyses of survival and prognostic factors and the role of radiation therapy in local control. Thyroid 6(4):305–310
73. Wu LT, Averbuch SD, Ball DW, de Bustros A, Baylin SB, McGuire WP III (1994) Treatment of advanced medullary thyroid carcinoma with a combination of cyclophosphamide, vincristine, and dacarbazine. Cancer 73(2):432–436
74. Nocera M, Baudin E, Pellegriti G, Cailleux AF, Mechelany-Corone C, Schlumberger M (2000) Treatment of advanced medullary thyroid cancer with an alternating combination of doxorubicin-streptozocin and 5 FU-dacarbazine. Groupe d'Etude des Tumeurs a Calcitonine (GETC). Br J Cancer 83(6):715–718
75. Shimaoka K, Schoenfeld DA, DeWys WD, Creech RH, DeConti R (1985) A randomized trial of doxorubicin versus doxorubicin plus cisplatin in patients with advanced thyroid carcinoma. Cancer 56(9):2155–2160
76. Kloos RT, Eng C, Evans DB, Francis GL, Gagel RF, Gharib H et al (2009) Medullary thyroid cancer: management guidelines of the American Thyroid Association. Thyroid 19(6):565–612
77. Machens A, Dralle H (2010) Biomarker-based risk stratification for previously untreated medullary thyroid cancer. J Clin Endocrinol Metab 95(6):2655–2663
78. Yip DT, Hassan M, Pazaitou-Panayiotou K, Ruan DT, Gawande AA, Gaz RD et al (2011) Preoperative basal calcitonin and tumor stage correlate with postoperative calcitonin normalization in patients undergoing initial surgical management of medullary thyroid carcinoma. Surgery 150(6):1168–1177
79. Samaan NA, Schultz PN, Hickey RC (1988) Medullary thyroid carcinoma: prognosis of familial versus sporadic disease and the role of radiotherapy. J Clin Endocrinol Metab 67(4):801–805
80. Jimenez-Fonseca P, Carmona-Bayonas A, Font C, Plasencia-Martinez J, Calvo-Temprano D, Otero R et al (2018) The prognostic impact of additional intrathoracic findings in patients with cancer-related pulmonary embolism. Clin Transl Oncol 20(2):230–242

81. Esik O, Tusnady G, Tron L, Boer A, Szentirmay Z, Szabolcs I et al (2002) Markov model-based estimation of individual survival probability for medullary thyroid cancer patients. Pathol Oncol Res 8(2):93–104
82. Fife KM, Bower M, Harmer CL (1996) Medullary thyroid cancer: the role of radiotherapy in local control. Eur J Surg Oncol 22(6):588–591
83. Stankovic V, Borojevic N, Dzodic R, Golubicic I (2003) [Medullary carcinoma of the thyroid gland: effect of postoperative transcutaneous radiotherapy on local control and results of treatment]. Acta Chir Iugosl 50(3):125–130
84. Rowell NP (2019) The role of external beam radiotherapy in the management of medullary carcinoma of the thyroid: a systematic review. Radiother Oncol 136:113–120
85. Orlandi F, Caraci P, Berruti A, Puligheddu B, Pivano G, Dogliotti L et al (1994) Chemotherapy with dacarbazine and 5-fluorouracil in advanced medullary thyroid cancer. Ann Oncol 5(8):763–765
86. Petursson SR (1988) Metastatic medullary thyroid carcinoma. Complete response to combination chemotherapy with dacarbazine and 5-fluorouracil. Cancer 62(9):1899–1903
87. Gottlieb JA, Hill CS Jr (1974) Chemotherapy of thyroid cancer with adriamycin. Experience with 30 patients. N Engl J Med 290(4):193–197
88. Droz JP, Rougier P, Goddefroy V, Schlumberger M, Gardet P, Parmentier C (1984) [Chemotherapy for medullary cancer of the thyroid. Phase II trials with adriamycin and cis-platinum administered as monochemotherapy]. Bull Cancer 71(3):195–199
89. De Besi P, Busnardo B, Toso S, Girelli ME, Nacamulli D, Simioni N et al (1991) Combined chemotherapy with bleomycin, adriamycin, and platinum in advanced thyroid cancer. J Endocrinol Investig 14(6):475–480
90. Deutschbein T, Matuszczyk A, Moeller LC, Unger N, Yuece A, Lahner H et al (2011) Treatment of advanced medullary thyroid carcinoma with a combination of cyclophosphamide, vincristine, and dacarbazine: a single-center experience. Exp Clin Endocrinol Diabetes 119(9):540–543
91. Schlumberger M, Abdelmoumene N, Delisle MJ, Couette JE (1995) Treatment of advanced medullary thyroid cancer with an alternating combination of 5 FU-streptozocin and 5 FU-dacarbazine. The Groupe d'Etude des Tumeurs a Calcitonine (GETC). Br J Cancer 71(2):363–365
92. Gilliam LK, Kohn AD, Lalani T, Swanson PE, Vasko V, Patel A et al (2006) Capecitabine therapy for refractory metastatic thyroid carcinoma: a case series. Thyroid 16(8):801–810
93. Lacin S, Esin E, Karakas Y, Yalcin S (2015) Metastatic medullary thyroid cancer: a dramatic response to a systemic chemotherapy (temozolomide and capecitabine) regimen. Onco Targets Ther 8:1039–1042
94. Paiva CE, Michelin OC (2008) Use of capecitabine in refractory metastatic medullary thyroid carcinoma. Thyroid 18(5):587
95. Boichard A, Croux L, Al Ghuzlan A, Broutin S, Dupuy C, Leboulleux S et al (2012) Somatic RAS mutations occur in a large proportion of sporadic RET-negative medullary thyroid carcinomas and extend to a previously unidentified exon. J Clin Endocrinol Metab 97(10):E2031–E2035
96. Drilon A, Oxnard G, Wirth L, Besse B, Gautschi O, Tan S et al (2019) PL02.08 registrational results of LIBRETTO-001: a phase 1/2 trial of LOXO-292 in patients with RET fusion-positive lung cancers. J Thorac Oncol 14(10):S6–S7
97. Wells SA Jr, Robinson BG, Gagel RF, Dralle H, Fagin JA, Santoro M et al (2012) Vandetanib in patients with locally advanced or metastatic medullary thyroid cancer: a randomized, double-blind phase III trial. J Clin Oncol 30(2):134–141
98. Schlumberger M, Elisei R, Muller S, Schoffski P, Brose M, Shah M et al (2017) Overall survival analysis of EXAM, a phase III trial of cabozantinib in patients with radiographically progressive medullary thyroid carcinoma. Ann Oncol 28(11):2813–2819
99. Lam ET, Ringel MD, Kloos RT, Prior TW, Knopp MV, Liang J et al (2010) Phase II clinical trial of sorafenib in metastatic medullary thyroid cancer. J Clin Oncol 28(14):2323–2330

100. Carr LL, Mankoff DA, Goulart BH, Eaton KD, Capell PT, Kell EM et al (2010) Phase II study of daily sunitinib in FDG-PET-positive, iodine-refractory differentiated thyroid cancer and metastatic medullary carcinoma of the thyroid with functional imaging correlation. Clin Cancer Res 16(21):5260–5268
101. Bible KC, Suman VJ, Molina JR, Smallridge RC, Maples WJ, Menefee ME et al (2014) A multicenter phase 2 trial of pazopanib in metastatic and progressive medullary thyroid carcinoma: MC057H. J Clin Endocrinol Metab 99(5):1687–1693
102. Schlumberger M, Jarzab B, Cabanillas ME, Robinson B, Pacini F, Ball DW et al (2016) A phase II trial of the multitargeted tyrosine kinase inhibitor lenvatinib (E7080) in advanced medullary thyroid cancer. Clin Cancer Res 22(1):44–53
103. Schlumberger MJ, Elisei R, Bastholt L, Wirth LJ, Martins RG, Locati LD et al (2009) Phase II study of safety and efficacy of motesanib in patients with progressive or symptomatic, advanced or metastatic medullary thyroid cancer. J Clin Oncol 27(23):3794–3801
104. Cohen EE, Rosen LS, Vokes EE, Kies MS, Forastiere AA, Worden FP et al (2008) Axitinib is an active treatment for all histologic subtypes of advanced thyroid cancer: results from a phase II study. J Clin Oncol 26(29):4708–4713
105. de Groot JW, Zonnenberg BA, van Ufford-Mannesse PQ, de Vries MM, Links TP, Lips CJ et al (2007) A phase II trial of imatinib therapy for metastatic medullary thyroid carcinoma. J Clin Endocrinol Metab 92(9):3466–3469
106. Wirth LJ, Sherman E, Robinson B, Solomon B, Kang H, Lorch J et al (2020) Efficacy of Selpercatinib in RET-altered thyroid cancers. N Engl J Med 383(9):825–835
107. Carlomagno F, Vitagliano D, Guida T, Ciardiello F, Tortora G, Vecchio G et al (2002) ZD6474, an orally available inhibitor of KDR tyrosine kinase activity, efficiently blocks oncogenic RET kinases. Cancer Res 62(24):7284–7290
108. Yakes FM, Chen J, Tan J, Yamaguchi K, Shi Y, Yu P et al (2011) Cabozantinib (XL184), a novel MET and VEGFR2 inhibitor, simultaneously suppresses metastasis, angiogenesis, and tumor growth. Mol Cancer Ther 10(12):2298–2308
109. Sennino B, Naylor RM, Tabruyn SP, You WK, Aftab DT, McDonald DM (2009) Abstract A13: reduction of tumor invasiveness and metastasis and prolongation of survival of RIP-Tag2 mice after inhibition of VEGFR plus c-met by XL184. AACR 8:A13
110. Kurzrock R, Sherman SI, Ball DW, Forastiere AA, Cohen RB, Mehra R et al (2011) Activity of XL184 (Cabozantinib), an oral tyrosine kinase inhibitor, in patients with medullary thyroid cancer. J Clin Oncol 29(19):2660–2666
111. Wilhelm SM, Carter C, Tang L, Wilkie D, McNabola A, Rong H et al (2004) BAY 43-9006 exhibits broad spectrum oral antitumor activity and targets the RAF/MEK/ERK pathway and receptor tyrosine kinases involved in tumor progression and angiogenesis. Cancer Res 64(19):7099–7109
112. Frank-Raue K, Ganten M, Kreissl MC, Raue F (2011) Rapid response to sorafenib in metastatic medullary thyroid carcinoma. Exp Clin Endocrinol Diabetes 119(3):151–155
113. Benekli M, Yalcin S, Ozkan M, Elkiran ET, Sevinc A, Cabuk D et al (2015) Efficacy of sorafenib in advanced differentiated and medullary thyroid cancer: experience in a Turkish population. Onco Targets Ther 8:1–5
114. Kocsis J, Szekanecz E, Bassam A, Uhlyarik A, Papai Z, Rubovszky G et al (2019) First line sorafenib treatment for metastatic medullary thyroid cancer: efficacy and safety analysis. Exp Clin Endocrinol Diabetes 127(4):240–246
115. Mendel DB, Laird AD, Xin X, Louie SG, Christensen JG, Li G et al (2003) In vivo antitumor activity of SU11248, a novel tyrosine kinase inhibitor targeting vascular endothelial growth factor and platelet-derived growth factor receptors: determination of a pharmacokinetic/pharmacodynamic relationship. Clin Cancer Res 9(1):327–337
116. Kumar R, Knick VB, Rudolph SK, Johnson JH, Crosby RM, Crouthamel MC et al (2007) Pharmacokinetic-pharmacodynamic correlation from mouse to human with pazopanib, a multikinase angiogenesis inhibitor with potent antitumor and antiangiogenic activity. Mol Cancer Ther 6(7):2012–2021

117. Hu-Lowe DD, Zou HY, Grazzini ML, Hallin ME, Wickman GR, Amundson K et al (2008) Nonclinical antiangiogenesis and antitumor activities of axitinib (AG-013736), an oral, potent, and selective inhibitor of vascular endothelial growth factor receptor tyrosine kinases 1, 2, 3. Clin Cancer Res 14(22):7272–7283
118. Capdevila J, Trigo JM, Aller J, Manzano JL, Adrian SG, Llopis CZ et al (2017) Axitinib treatment in advanced RAI-resistant differentiated thyroid cancer (DTC) and refractory medullary thyroid cancer (MTC). Eur J Endocrinol 177(4):309–317
119. Matsui J, Yamamoto Y, Funahashi Y, Tsuruoka A, Watanabe T, Wakabayashi T et al (2008) E7080, a novel inhibitor that targets multiple kinases, has potent antitumor activities against stem cell factor producing human small cell lung cancer H146, based on angiogenesis inhibition. Int J Cancer 122(3):664–671
120. Tohyama O, Matsui J, Kodama K, Hata-Sugi N, Kimura T, Okamoto K et al (2014) Antitumor activity of lenvatinib (e7080): an angiogenesis inhibitor that targets multiple receptor tyrosine kinases in preclinical human thyroid cancer models. J Thyroid Res 2014:638747
121. Boss DS, Glen H, Beijnen JH, Keesen M, Morrison R, Tait B et al (2012) A phase I study of E7080, a multitargeted tyrosine kinase inhibitor, in patients with advanced solid tumours. Br J Cancer 106(10):1598–1604
122. Matsui J, Minoshima Y, Tsuruoka A, Funahashi Y (2010) Multi-targeted kinase inhibitor E7080 showed anti-tumor activity against medullary thyroid carcinoma and squamous thyroid carcinoma cell line based on RET and VEGFR2 tyrosine kinase inhibition. AACR 70:3614
123. Brose MS, Bible KC, Chow LQM, Gilbert J, Grande C, Worden F et al (2018) Management of treatment-related toxicities in advanced medullary thyroid cancer. Cancer Treat Rev 66:64–73
124. Subbiah V, Velcheti V, Tuch BB, Ebata K, Busaidy NL, Cabanillas ME et al (2018) Selective RET kinase inhibition for patients with RET-altered cancers. Ann Oncol 29(8):1869–1876

Adrenocortical Carcinoma

24

Bülent Orhan, Ömer Dızdar, Suayib Yalcin, and Özcan Yıldız

24.1 Introduction

Adrenocortical adenomas (ACA) and adrenocortical carcinomas (ACC) are diagnosed more often with the improvement in imaging techniques. The detection rate of incidental adrenal lesions in computed tomography (CT) or magnetic resonance imaging (MRI) can be 5% with an estimated incidence of 7.3% from autopsy series [1]. If the lesion has apparently benign imaging features, no follow-up is necessary. Although the majority of those lesions are benign adrenocortical adenomas, some lesions are malignant, dubbed as adrenocortical carcinoma (ACC). ACC is a rare and highly aggressive tumor and is usually resistant to most of the conventional chemotherapeutics, although new drugs with different mechanism of action such as immune check point inhibitors are being tested in clinical trials [2]. Often, the disease is diagnosed late, and in advanced stage, 5-year survival is <15% with a high recurrence rate even after radical surgery. Significant progress has been made in exploring the pathogenesis of ACC over the past 20 years through genomic and molecular analysis facilitating to develop targeted drugs [3]. Surgery is the treatment of choice for localized ACC with the aim to achieve complete resection with clear margins. Unfortunately, current treatment options other than surgery have limited efficacy in the neoadjuvant, adjuvant, and advanced setting. Given the low

B. Orhan
Ceylan International Hospital, Bursa, Turkey

Ö. Dızdar
Hacettepe University Cancer Institute, Ankara, Turkey

S. Yalcin (✉)
Department of Medical Oncology, Hacettepe University Cancer Institute, Ankara, Turkey
e-mail: syalcin@hacettepe.edu.tr

Ö. Yıldız
Bağcılar Medipol Mega University Hospital, Istanbul, Turkey
e-mail: ozcan.yildiz@medipol.com.tr

S. Yalcin, K. Öberg (eds.), *Neuroendocrine Tumours*,
https://doi.org/10.1007/978-3-031-56968-5_24

incidence of the disease, the number of clinical trials in patients with ACC is limited and mostly retrospective; therefore, treatment recommendations are generally based on retrospective data or expert opinion. In order to understand molecular mechanisms underlying the disease and develop more effective treatment for ACC, clinical and translational studies with international collaboration are needed [1–3].

24.2 Epidemiology

Adrenocortical carcinomas (ACCs) are not common, and its incidence is yearly one to two per million population. The incidence is higher in children in some parts of the world where environmental and genetic factors can be causative factors [4–6]. There seems to be two peaks in age distribution: one is at the age of 5, and the other is in the forth and fifth decade of life [4]. Female-to-male ratio is 1.5 to 2.5:1 probably due to hormonal factors, and disease progression is more rapid in adults than that of children [1, 7, 8].

The median age at diagnosis is 55 years, median tumor size is 13 cm, and distant metastasis is found on presentation in 21.6% of patients. ACC may present with symptoms due to the mass effect of tumor or with hormone-secreting features in 40–70% of patients. Abdominal mass may cause abdominal discomfort, indigestion, or pain. Hormonal symptoms may vary and depend on the type of hormone produced such as cortisol, aldosterone, testesterone, prolactin, or estradiol.

24.3 Pathogenesis

The etiopathogenesis of ACC is rather complex, and there is no identified causative environmental agent described yet. ACC cases are mostly sporadic, with no identifible family history. However, some cases may be associated with hereditary cancer syndromes [9, 10] such as Li-Fraumeni syndrome (the sarcoma, breast, leukemia, and adrenal gland [SBLA] cancer syndrome) in which an autosomal dominant *TP53* tumor suppressor gene mutation on chromosome 17p is the causative factor. Other conditions associated with ACC are Beckwith-Wiedemann syndrome (Wilms' tumor, neuroblastoma, hepatoblastoma, and ACC), Carney complex, multiple endocrine neoplasia type 1 (MEN1; parathyroid, pituitary, and pancreatic neuroendocrine tumors and adrenal adenomas, as well as carcinomas), congenital adrenal hyperplasia, and familial adenomatous polyposis (FAP).

Although the molecular mechanisms of tumorigenesis in these syndromes are well defined, the pathogenesis of sporadic ACCs is poorly understood [11]. Similar to progression model of colorectal cancer, a multistep tumor progression model is proposed for this disease [9, 12, 13].

Located on chromosome 17p13, *TP53* gene is the most frequently mutated gene in human cancers, as in the case of sporadic ACCs as well due to the fact that there is a frequent finding of loss of heterozygosity at the 17p13 locus [14, 15]. A distinct germline *TP53* mutation (R337H) has been identified in a high percentage of children with adrenocortical tumors from southern Brazil [16, 17] and North America [18, 19], which may in part explain the higher frequency of ACC in this population. Amplification of the steroidogenic factor 1 (SF-1) gene in tumors also has been reported in this population [20].

In one study, next-generation sequencing was used to assess predisposing gene mutations in children and adolescents with cancer. Among 1120 patients, 8.5% (95 patients) had germline pathogenic or probably pathogenic mutations. Patients with adrenocortical cancers had the highest prevalence of mutations (27 of 39 patients, 69%), mostly in the TP53 gene, compared with other cancers [21]. It is imperative to know that it was not possible to judge the presence of an underlying predisposition syndrome in many patients by looking at the family history.

The chromosomal locus 11p, the area of abnormality in Beckwith-Wiedemann syndrome [22], LOH at the 11p15 locus, and the site of the insulin-like growth factor-2 (IGF-2) gene are other alterations implicated in the pathogenesis of ACCs [14, 23, 24]. Activating CTNNB1 somatic mutation is found in ACCs. Wnt/beta-catenin pathway activation was found as an independent predictor of disease free and overall survival [25]. Exome sequencing and SNP array analysis of 45 ACCs identified recurrent alterations in known driver genes (CTNNB1, TP53, CDKN2A, RB1, and MEN1) and in genes not previously reported in ACC (ZNRF3, DAXX, TERT, and MED12), which was validated in an independent cohort of 77 ACCs. ZNRF3, encoding a cell-surface E3 ubiquitin ligase, was identified in 21% of cases [15]. Being related to the beta-catenin pathway, ZNRF3 is considered to be possible tumor suppressor gene. Some other known mutations related to ACC such as CTNNB1, TP53, CDKN2A (cyclin-dependent kinase inhibitor 2A), RB1 (retinoblastoma 1), and MEN1 (multiple endocrine neoplasias) were diagnosed. Other driver genes including PRKAR1A, RPL22, TERF2, CCNE1, and NF1 are diagnosed by comprehensive Cancer Genome Atlas (TCGA) group for characterization of ACC. Aggressive clinical course was found to be related to the whole-genome doubling which expands telomerase reverse transcriptase (TERT) [26].

For the follow-up of the patients with ACC, an emerging method is to discover these kind of mutations in circulating cell-free tumor DNA [27].

24.4 Clinical Presentation and Diagnosis

Approximately 60–70% of adult patients with ACC present with clinical findings of hormone excess, mostly with Cushing's syndrome. Signs and symptoms of hyperandrogenism, pheochromocytoma, and hyperaldosteronism should also be assessed. Weight gain, virilization, feminization, weakness, or hyperaldosteronism may occur depending on the hormone secreted. Diagnosis is based on clinical, laboratory, and radiologic findings. Laboratory evaluation should include corticotropin (ACTH), serum cortisol, 24-h free cortisol in urine, total testosterone, dehydroepiandrosterone sulfate, and estradiol. Serum chemistries and complete blood count should also be obtained [28]. The European Network for the Study of Adrenal Tumors recommends plasma aldosterone and renin measurement if hypertension or hypokalemia is present and plasma metanephrine or urinary metanephrine and catecholamine measurement in all patients to exclude pheochromocytoma. In recent studies, excessive amounts of adrenal steroid precursors are detected in urine; these markers may aid in the diagnosis and also follow-up to detect the presence of tumor recurrence in patients with ACC [29]. Computed tomography (CT) is widely used in the diagnosis and differentiation of benign from malignant lesions. Increased size of the adrenal mass usually a sign of malignancy. An adrenal tumor diameter >5 cm identifies ACC with a sensitivity of 93% and a specificity of 64% [30]. Second, the radiologic appearance of the suspected mass helps to decide; benign adenomas usually have higher lipid content, and this results in a low attenuation on CT scans (i.e., 10%).

24.5 Pathology

The only definitive criterion for malignant adrenal tumors is the presence of local invasion or distant metastases. Fine-needle aspiration biopsy cannot discriminate between adrenal adenoma and ACC but may be useful in distinguishing adrenal metastases. On macroscopic examination, ACCs are often large, with a tan-yellow cut surface, and areas of hemorrhage and necrosis may be seen. The tumors are usually encapsulated or lobulated and can be solid or cystic [31]. On microscopic examination, the tumor usually displays sheets of atypical, eosinophilic cells with some resemblance to the cells of the normal adrenal cortex. Polygonal cells are arranged in sheets, nests, trabeculae, or ribbons and may contain anaplastic features. Other signs of malignancy are increased mitotic activity and vascular and capsular invasion. Immunohistochemistry may help to differentiate ACCs from adrenal adenomas. ACCs usually show immunostaining with Ki-67 (>10%) and overexpression of insulin-like growth factor 2. The presence of invasion and increased mitotic activity helps differentiate small cancers from adrenocortical adenomas [31–33].

Differential diagnostic scores have been developed for pathological diagnosis; currently, the Weiss and modified Weiss scores are the most widely accepted scoring systems and are based on histological findings. The updated Weiss score consists of five criteria including mitotic rate >5 mitoses/50 high-power fields, cytoplasm (clear cells comprising 25% or less of the tumor), abnormal mitoses, necrosis, and capsular invasion. Each criterion is scored 0 when absent, 2 for the first two criteria, and 1 for the last three when present; a total score ≥3 is highly suggestive of ACC [32].

There are several relatively rare variants of ACC. These histologic variants are oncocytic adrenal cortical carcinoma, myxoid adrenal cortical carcinoma, carcinosarcoma, adenosquamous adrenocortical carcinoma, and clear cell adrenal cortical carcinoma [31].

24.6 Staging

There are several staging systems for ACC. Macfarlene et al. proposed a staging system in 1958. This system was modified by Sullivan et al. in 1978 and Lee et al. in 1995. The eighth tumor, node, metastases (TNM) staging system from the combined American Joint Committee on Cancer (AJCC)/Union for International Cancer Control (UICC) was revised in 2017 for implementation in January 2018 (Table 24.1) [29]. The TNM classification definitions were the same as those initially proposed by the UICC/World Health Organization (WHO) in 2004 [34], which were in turn based upon the Sullivan modification of the original McFarlane staging system [22].

Table 24.1 Tumor-node-metastasis (TNM) classification of adrenal carcinoma

T category	T criteria
Tx	Primary tumor cannot be assessed
T0	No evidence of primary tumor
T1	Tumor ≤5 cm in greatest dimension, no extra-adrenal invasion
T2	Tumor >5 cm, no extra-adrenal invasion
T3	Tumor of any size with local invasion but not invading adjacent organs
T4	Tumor of any size that invades adjacent organs (kidney, diaphragm, pancreas, spleen, or liver) or large blood vessels (renal vein or vena cava)

Regionel lymph nodes (N)	
N category	
Nx	Regional lymph nodes cannot be assessed
N0	No regional lymph node metastasis
N1	Metastasis in regional lymph node(s)
Distant metastasis (M)	
M category	
M1	No distant metastasis
M2	Distant metastasis

Prognositic stage groups			
When T is	**And N is**	**And M is**	**The stage group is**
T1	N0	M0	I
T2	N0	M0	II
T1	N1	M0	III
T2	N1	M0	III
T3	Any N	M0	III
T4	Any N	M0	III
Any T	Any N	M1	IV

Used with permission of the American College of Surgeons, Chicago, Illinois. The original source for this information is the AJCC Cancer Staging Manual, Eighth Edition (2017) published by Springer International Publishing

Phan AT, Grogan RH, Rohren E, Perrier ND. Adrenal Cortical Carcinoma. In: AJCC Cancer Staging Manual, 8th, Amin MB (Ed), Springer, New York 2017. p. 911

In the eighth edition of the TNM staging system, stage IV disease now, in contrast to the previous 2004 AJCC/UICC classification (Table 24.1), is limited to patients with distant metastases, and those with local invasion or invasion of adjacent organs (T3 or T4) but without distant metastases are classified as having stage III disease. These changes are consistent with the modifications initially proposed by the ENSAT group and confirmed by others [35, 36].

Proper staging should include computed tomography of the abdomen and chest. Magnetic resonance imaging may help discriminate benign from malignant lesions. Extracapsular tumor invasion, extension into the vena cava, or metastases to other organs may be detected more accuratelly with MRI.

24.7 Treatment

24.7.1 Surgery

Complete surgical resection is the only potentially curative treatment for adrenocortical carcinoma (ACC) [37–40]. Although resection is technically possible for most patients with stage I–III disease, it is not curative for many, presumably because occult micrometastases are present at the time of initial presentation, even in patients with stage I disease [41].

Complete, en bloc, margin-negative resection should be the surgical goal [42]. Along with complete resection, lymph node dissection is recommended [42]. Resection of adjacent organs including the spleen, kidney, liver, or pancreas might be required if local invasion is present. Tumor infiltration into the inferior vena cava is not a contraindication to surgery, and resection can be performed by cardiopulmonary bypass.

The role of laparoscopy is controversial; a number of previous studies showed that laparoscopic surgery for ACC increased the risk of local recurrence, peritoneal dissemination, and metastases [43, 44], while others reported comparable results with open surgery particularly if the adrenal tumor is small [45]. Open surgery is currently the preferred approach by NCCN guidelines [46]. If resection is incomplete, repeated surgery should be considered because achieving clear margins is the most important goal.

Before proceeding to a surgical excision, all patients must undergo a complete hormonal assessment to determine the secretory activity of the tumor. Some patients may have some degree of hypothalamic–pituitary–adrenal (HPA) axis suppression and require glucocorticoid coverage to prevent postoperative adrenal insufficiency [39].

The benefit of the maximal debulking is not proven yet. For patients with advanced functioning tumors, debulking may help to control hormone hypersecretion and increases the efficacy of further therapies, and surgery may be an option to control the symptoms for those patients [40]. Overall, however, patients with unresectable disease have a poor prognosis, particularly with high-grade disease, often surviving only 3–9 months, and they are often better palliated with medical management [28]. Patient who undergo complete resection of local recurrences or distant metastases may also have improved survival [27].

The role of neoadjuvant systemic therapy prior to surgery for patients with locally advanced disease is not defined, and this is not considered a standard approach. The value of neoadjuvant cisplatin-based chemotherapy is being addressed in a clinical trial from the Children's Oncology Group that is enrolling individuals up to age 21 years with ACC [47]. In adults, one retrospective study suggested that patients with locoregionally advanced tumors might benefit from cisplatin-based neoadjuvant chemotherapy [48]. However, definitive evidence is still lacking, and therapeutic decisions should be individualized.

24.7.2 Adjuvant Treatment

Since adrenocortical carcinoma is a rare tumor, data on adjuvant therapy are limited. Most patients (up to 80%) have recurrences after resection, and this is the rationale behind adjuvant therapy.

The only treatment with benefit in terms of disease-free survival and overall survival is mitotane. Mitotane (o,p′-DDD, a congener of the pesticide dichlorodiphenyltrichloroethane [DDT or rothane]) is an adrenocorticolytic drug that has efficacy in patients with ACC [22–24]. Mitotane leads to the necrosis of zona fasiculata, and reticularis of the adrenal cortex inhibits adrenocortical hormone production.

The European Society of Endocrinology clinical guidelines on ACC suggest adjuvant mitotane use (alone, without chemotherapy) for patients at the highest risk of recurrence, e.g., those who have histologically high-grade disease (Ki67 staining of >10% of tumor cells, >20 mitotic figures per 50 HPF regardless of tumor size [21]), intraoperative tumor spillage or fracture, and some large tumors that are low grade but have vascular or capsular invasion.

While a number of uncontrolled reports suggest that adjuvant mitotane may delay or prevent recurrence after complete primary resection for nonmetastatic disease [27, 37], others have failed to show any benefit in terms of disease free or overall survival [1, 5, 37].

Benefit of adjuvant mitotane was supported by some studies [49, 50] One of the largest series of adjuvant mitotane treatment after surgery is a retrospective analysis of 177 patients who had undergone macroscopically complete radical surgery at 8 Italian and 47 German centers between 1985 and 2005 [26]. In the Italian cohort, 47 patients received adjuvant mitotane, whereas 55 patients did not (Italian control group). None of the 75 patients in the German cohort, who were more likely to have stage I or II disease, received adjuvant mitotane (German control group). With a median follow-up between 43 and 68 months and the median treatment duration of 29 months in the 3 groups, the following results were seen: mitotane treatment was associated with a significantly longer recurrence-free survival as compared with either control group (median recurrence-free survival 42 versus 10 and 25 months in the Italian and German control groups, respectively). There were also fewer deaths from ACC in the mitotane group than in either control group (25% vs. 55%

and 41%, respectively). Median overall survival durations were 110 months in the mitotane group, 52 months in the Italian control group, and 67 months in the German control group.

In a retrospective study of 100 patients treated with adjuvant mitotane and 52 who did not receive mitotane, adjuvant therapy lowered the risk of recurrence but did not improve overall survival [50]. However, a survival benefit was seen in a subset of mitotane-treated patients with stage III ACC or an elevated Ki67 index.

These data support the view that adjuvant mitotane therapy, even at relatively low doses, improves recurrence-free and overall survival after macroscopically complete radical resection for stage I, II, or III ACC. Adjuvant mitotane should be used as soon as possible after surgery (within 3 months) for patients at the highest risk of recurrence (i.e., in patients with intraoperative tumor spillage, tumors with high ki67 index, tumor size >8 cm, or invasion of tumor capsule or blood vessels) [21, 51]. The role of adjuvant mitotane therapy for patients with low-grade ACC who have an open resection and no tumor fracture or spillage at the time of surgery is unclear.

National Comprehensive Cancer Network (NCCN) guidelines suggest that mitotane be "considered" for all patients with resected low- or high-grade localized ACC regardless of stage or tumor size (category 3 recommendation, with major disagreement that the intervention is appropriate).

If available, serum mitotane level should be monitored and maintained between 14 and 20 μg/mL during therapy to achieve therapeutic levels and avoid toxicity. It is not known if cytotoxic chemotherapy alone or in combination with mitotane is more effective than adjuvant mitotane alone. The use of Ki67 labeling index to select patients for adjuvant chemotherapy in addition to mitotane has been suggested [52].

The efficacy of cisplatin and etoposide was explored in the adjuvant setting in a small series of 5 individuals aged 1.2–21 years, and all remained in remission 29–109 months later [53]. The combination of mitotane plus streptozotocin as adjuvant therapy was evaluated in a nonrandomized phase II trial. The trial included 17 patients who had undergone complete tumor resection. In patients who received adjuvant mitotane-streptozotocin therapy, disease-free survival was significantly better compared with a separate cohort of 11 patients who did not receive any adjuvant therapy after complete resection (49 vs. 12 months) [54]. However, in the absence of a comparator group receiving mitotane alone, it cannot be concluded that combined therapy is superior.

The role of adjuvant radiotherapy (RT) for patients with adrenocortical carcinoma (ACC) has been controversial. Radiotherapy is not routinelly used in the treatment of ACC as it was considered radioresistant. Recently, conformal radiotherapy techniques resulted in better efficacy, less toxicity, and better dose delivery to the target volume. The benefit of adjuvant RT is limited to improved local control; no clear survival benefit has been shown except in one study. A recent meta-analysis (8 case series [48 patients] and 4 cohort studies [136 patients]) showed that adjuvant RT dramatically reduced local recurrence of ACC after surgery.

In conclusion, radiotherapy in high-risk patients seems to reduce local recurrence, and adjuvant radiotherapy should be recommended to all patients with incompletely resected ACC, stage III disease (regardless of resection status), those who have tumor spillage at the time of resection, and patients with indeterminate or microscoically involved margins. Radiotherapy ideally should also be started for all patients with high-grade ACC (>20 mitotic figures per 50 HPF) [55] within 3 months of surgery.

24.8 Recurrent or Advanced Adrenocortical Cancer

Complete removal is the main target in the treatment of ACC. Locally recurrent disease should be resected with the aim of achieving negative surgical margins [26, 27, 56]. The best candidates for aggressive surgery are those who have potentially resectable disease with a disease-free interval of at least 1 year after initial treatment. Surgery may also be considered in patients who present with synchronous limited, potentially resectable hepatic or pulmonary metastases or in patients with oligometastatic disease [57].

Resection of locally recurrent disease may also be indicated for patients in whom surgery will be able to remove a majority of tumor burden or decrease severe hypercortisolism that is otherwise difficult to control; however, recovery from surgery may be slow, delaying administration of systemic therapy [46].

For palliation of symptoms from locally advanced or distant metastatic disease (e.g., a bone metastasis), we use palliative radiation therapy (RT).

Percutaneous image-guided radiofrequency ablation (RFA) is a minimally invasive and reasonable method for unresectable localised disease. Studies have shown that RFA can produce local control of primary ACC particularly for tumors less than 50 mm in size if they are anatomically suitable. RFA may provide short-term local control of an unresectable primary tumor, particularly for those <5 cm in diameter [58, 59]. The long-term impact on survival is unknown. RFA has also been used to treat small liver metastases [58, 59].

For unresectable disease which is not suitable for local therapy techniques such as radiotherapy or RFA, mitotane is the treatment of choice. The main benefit of mitotane for patients with unresectable advanced disease is usually reduction in symptoms of hypercortisolism (weakness, myopathy, diabetes, immunosuppression, and insomnia). Mitotane may decrease hormone secretion and also tumor volume at the same time. Excess hormone production is reported to be decreased in up to 75% of patients, and tumor size is reduced in as many as one-third of cases [23, 60]. mMitotane therapy alone is usually not sufficient to significantly decrease cortisol levels to normal levels or have long-lasting effects on tumor growth.

We reserve mitotane monotherapy for the few patients who have a minimal disease burden (low number of tumor-involved organs) or patients with low-grade (i.e., low mitotic rate) disease and have recurred relatively late (2–3 years) after surgery. These are the patients who are likely to have a prolonged survival [10].

Determinants of mitotane efficacy are unknown; CYP2W1, which is highly expressed in ACC, may represent a new predictive marker of response to mitotane treatment [53]. For patients with active disease and visible lesions, mitotane is typically continued lifelong or until disease progression. Treatment benefits are generally short lived [61], and survival is not consistently prolonged. In several studies of primary mitotane therapy, response rates are between 13% and 33%, and the median survival was only 6.5 months [23, 60], no different from that expected in untreated patients [62]. The main benefit of mitotane in advanced disease is reduction of excess hormone production rather than prolonging survival.

Response rates are higher when mitotane is administered in combination with cytotoxic chemotherapy and should be preferred if there is extensive (multiple tumor-involved organs), rapidly progressive, and high-grade disease.

Side effects of mitotane include anorexia, nausea, vomiting, and diarrhea. These side effects can limit mitotane use as long-term treatment. As mitotane has considerabe side effects, monitoring blood levels is essential for effective treatment. Mitotane treatment starts 1 g twice dail orally, and the dose is escalated up to 10 g/day. Target serum mitotane level is between 14 and 20 mg/L for obtaining optimal response and decreased toxic side effects.

Mitotane induces atrophy and/or inhibition of the normal adrenal glands; therefore, cortisol replacement therapy is necessary; the zona glomerulosa is more resistant to the adrenolytic effect of mitotane, and aldosterone deficiency may occur after several months of therapy. Monitoring of blood sodium, potassium, creatinine, and 24-h urinary-free cortisol levels is mandatory to assess adrenal insufficiency. Higher doses than the routine maintenance can be needed to avoid adrenal insufficiency. If signs or symptoms of mineralocorticoid deficiency (i.e., postural hypotension, hyperkalemia, etc.) develop, fludrocortisone should be added. Patients should also be monitored for hypogonadism and hypothyroidism. The most common side effects are fatigue, nausea, vomiting, and anorexia, but skin rash, diarrhea, lethargy, sedation, confusion, dizziness, ataxia, gynecomastia, arthralgias, leukopenia, prolonged bleeding time, and hematuria. Mitotane has significant drug interactions and can reduce efficacy of some calcium channel antagonists, opioids, benzodiazepines, macrolide-type antibiotics, and many other drugs.

As ACC is a rare disease, few non-mitotane-containing chemotherapy regimens have been tested in ACC. Single agents such as cisplatin or doxorubicin are associated with response rates that are generally less than 30% and of short duration [63]. Chemotherapy plus mitotane produces better responses than mitotane alone. Mitotane in combination with etoposide, doxorubicin, and cisplatin (EDP) is the preferred front-line therapy.

One of the largest trial of advanced ACC to date is the First International Randomized trial in Locally Advanced and Metastatic Adrenocortical Carcinoma Treatment (FIRM-ACT), which randomly assigned 304 patients with advanced ACC not suitable for radical surgery to mitotane plus either EDP or streptozotocin [64]. Rates of objective tumor response (23% vs. 9%) and median progression-free survival (5 vs. 2.1 months) were both significantly better in the EDP-mitotane (EDP-M) group, although these benefits did not translate into a significantly prolonged survival (median 14.8 vs.12 months), possibly because of high cross-over rate. Nevertheless, the preferred treatment of choice is EDP-M because of better rates of objective tumor response and longer progression-free survival. Serious adverse events were similar in both treatment arms.

Multidrug resistance (MDR) protein is found in high concentrations in ACC. Mitotane increases the cytotoxic activity of other chemotherapeutic drugs on human adrenal carcinoma cells, most probably by acting as an antagonist of the MDR protein [65]. These data provide a rationale for combination therapy.

ACC patients which could be defined as less aggressive disease (slow tumor growth, long disease-free interval after initial surgery) might receive mitotane monotherapy in the first line followed by combination chemotherapy upon progression. Second, this patient group might also be good candidates for upfront experimental therapies as efficacy of several drugs is diminished once mitotane is used due to increased drug metabolism.

Patients receiving mitotane alone or with chemotherapy should be assessed regularly at 2-month intervals for tumor progression. Patients who have tumor regression might be considered for surgical resection. Patients with progressive disease can be considered for further lines of chemotherapy or enrolled in a clinical trial. There are currently no established second- or third-line chemotherapy regimens for systemic disease. However, there are phase II trials of gemcitabine plus capecitabine showing response rates as high as 46%. This combination might represent a promising second-line regimen.

24.8.1 Investigational Approaches

Using checkpoint inhibitor therapy is a growing interest in the treatment of ACC because increased PD-L1 (programmed cell death ligand) expression is seen in some ACCs. PDL1 expression is also increased in associated tumor-infiltrating lymphocytes [66]. Pembrolizumab has been used in phase II studies in both adult and pediatric population. Response rates of pembrolizumab ranged between 14% and 50% in those studies, with a good safety profile [66]. Majority had received prior systemic therapy (either mitotane- or platinum-based chemotherapy). Median follow-up time of patients treated with pembrolizumab was nearly 18 months. Median progression-free and overall survival were 2 and 24 months, respectively. The objective response rate was 23%. Rates of grade ≥3 toxicity were low (13%) [66, 67].

In a phase I–II open label trial of pembrolizumab (KEYNOTE-051) in pediatric patients with various solid tumors (n = 154), 4 patients had ACC and 2 of those 4 patients achieved a partial response [68].

Another checkpoint inhibitor avelumab was studied in a phase 1b JAVELIN tiral The study enrolled 50 patients who were previously treated with more than 2 lines of therapy. The patients recieved avelumab for a median of 16.5 months. The objective response rate (ORR) was 6.0% (3/50 patients) (95% CI, 1.3–16.5%). Twenty-one patients (42.0%) had stable disease (disease control rate 48.0%). Median progression-free survival was 2.6 months, median overall survival (OS) was 10.6 months, and the 1-year OS rate was 43.4% [69].

In a single-arm, multicenter, phase 2 clinical trial to determine the efficacy of checkpoint inhibitors in ACC, 10 adult patients with metastatic ACC previously treated with platinum-based chemotherapy and/or mitotane as well as patients who declined front-line chemotherapy recieved nivolumab (240 mg) IV every 2 weeks. After median follow-up of 4.5 months (range, 0.1–25.6 months), the median PFS was 1.8 months. Two patients had stable disease for a duration of 48 and 11 weeks, respectively. One patient had an unconfirmed partial response but discontinued the study due to an AE. Most AEs were grade 1/2 [70].

In a phase I study, combination of lenvatinib and pembrolizumab as salvage therapy was investigated in patients with heavily pretreated ACC. In the combination group, objective responses were seen in a subset of patients without significant toxicity. This combination should be further investigated in phase II clinical trial with robust correlative studies to identify predictors for response [71].

Approximately 80% of ACCs overexpress insulin-like growth factor type 2 (IGF-2). IGF-2 is known to signal predominantly through the IGF-1 receptor (IGF1R). Preclinical and early-phase studies of monoclonal antibodies or small molecules inhibiting IGF1R were initially promising [72–75]. A subsequent phase I–II trial of the anti-IGF1R antibody cixutumumab demonstrated only limited overall efficacy [76]. Linsitinib, an oral small molecule of both the IGF1R and insulin receptor, did not demonstrate an improvement in disease free or overall survival in patients with advanced ACC in a placebo-controlled phase III trial [77]. However, disease stabilization and partial responses in a subset of patients were observed with these drugs as single agents [76–78] and in combination with other drugs (such as temsirolimus) [79]. Further studies may determine molecular markers that can predict which patients may benefit from this approach.

Vascular endothelial growth factor (VEGF) is upregulated in ACC tumor tissue, and some studies have found that circulating VEGF levels are significantly greater in patients with ACC as compared with those with adrenal adenomas. While case reports suggested activity of antiangiogenic agents thalidomide [80, 81], sorafenib, and sunitinib [80–83], subsequent phase II trials have demonstrated limited efficacy of VEGF inhibitors both as single agents (e.g., axitinib [84], sunitinib [85]), or in combination with chemotherapy (e.g., bevacizumab plus capecitabine [86]; sorafenib plus weekly paclitaxel [87]).

The finding that over 80% of ACCs express the epidermal growth factor receptor (EGFR) [88, 89] provides a rationale for the study of agents that target the EGFR. Unfortunately, salvage therapy with the small-molecule EGFR inhibitor erlotinib in combination with gemcitabine was of little benefit in a trial of ten patients with advanced ACC who had failed at least two other systemic chemotherapy regimens [90]. Only one patient experienced a minor response, while eight patients experienced disease progression.

Radionuclide therapy—ACC can also be targeted with therapeutic radionuclides. In a study testing, in the efficacy of iodine-131-metomidate in 11 patients with refractory/advanced ACC, there was only a single partial response; however, long-term disease stabilization was achieved in 5 patients [91].

24.9 Conclusion

In recent years, major progress has been made in understanding the pathogenesis and treatment of ACC. Molecular profiling studies in patients with ACC showed that ACC is a very heterogeneous disease. Exon-sequencing studies identified some alterations in known driver genes and in genes which are not previously reported in ACC. Chemotherapy is not highly effective and further trials are needed. Mitotane treatment in adjuvant setting and in metastatic disease show promising results. More recently, immune checkpoint inhibitors such as pembrolizumab and nivolumab have attracted attention in the metastatic setting. Nevertheless, overall prognosis is still poor. International collaboration is needed to design translational research and prospective clinical trials. New insights into the pathogenesis of ACC and identification of potential "driver" pathways will highlight the opportunity for more personalized treatment strategies in the future.

References

1. Vassilopoulou-Sellin R, Schultz PN (2001) Adrenocortical carcinoma. Clinical outcome at the end of the 20th century. Cancer 92:1113
2. Pittaway JFH, Guasti L (2019) Pathobiology and genetics of adrenocortical carcinoma. J Mol Endocrinol 62(2):R105–R119. https://doi.org/10.1530/JME-18-0122
3. Armignacco R, Cantini G, Canu L, Poli G, Ercolino T, Mannelli M, Luconi M (2018) Adrenocortical carcinoma: the dawn of a new era of genomic and molecular biology analysis. J Endoccrinol Invest 41(5):499–507. https://doi.org/10.1007/s40618-017-0775-y. Epub 2017 Oct 28
4. Else T, Kim AC, Sabolch A et al (2014) Adrenocortical carcinoma. Endocr Rev 35:282
5. Icard P, Goudet P, Charpenay C et al (2001) Adrenocortical carcinomas: surgical trends and results of a 253-patient series from the French Association of Endocrine Surgeons study group. World J Surg 25:891
6. Michalkiewicz E, Sandrini R, Figueiredo B et al (2004) Clinical and outcome characteristics of children with adrenocortical tumors: a report from the International Pediatric Adrenocortical Tumor Registry. J Clin Oncol 22:838
7. Lucon AM, Pereira MA, Mendonça BB et al (2002) Adrenocortical tumors: results of treatment and study of Weiss's score as a prognostic factor. Rev Hosp Clin Fac Med Sao Paulo 57:251
8. Bilimoria KY, Shen WT, Elaraj D et al (2008) Adrenocortical carcinoma in the United States: treatment utilization and prognostic factors. Cancer 113:3130
9. Morimoto R, Satoh F, Murakami O et al (2008) Immunohistochemistry of a proliferation marker Ki67/MIB1 in adrenocortical carcinomas: Ki67/MIB1 labeling index is a predictor for recurrence of adrenocortical carcinomas. Endocr J 55:49
10. Assié G, Antoni G, Tissier F et al (2007) Prognostic parameters of metastatic adrenocortical carcinoma. J Clin Endocrinol Metab 92:148
11. Beuschlein F, Weigel J, Saeger W et al (2015) Major prognostic role of Ki67 in localized adrenocortical carcinoma after complete resection. J Clin Endocrinol Metab 100:841

12. de Reyniès A, Assié G, Rickman DS et al (2009) Gene expression profiling reveals a new classification of adrenocortical tumors and identifies molecular predictors of malignancy and survival. J Clin Oncol 27:1108
13. Giordano TJ, Kuick R, Else T et al (2009) Molecular classification and prognostication of adrenocortical tumors by transcriptome profiling. Clin Cancer Res 15:668
14. Fragoso MC, Almeida MQ, Mazzuco TL et al (2012) Combined expression of BUB1B, DLGAP5, and PINK1 as predictors of poor outcome in adrenocortical tumors: validation in a Brazilian cohort of adult and pediatric patients. Eur J Endocrinol 166:61
15. Assié G, Letouzé E, Fassnacht M et al (2014) Integrated genomic characterization of adrenocortical carcinoma. Nat Genet 46:607
16. Ross JS, Wang K, Rand JV et al (2014) Next-generation sequencing of adrenocortical carcinoma reveals new routes to targeted therapies. J Clin Pathol 67:968
17. Zheng S, Cherniack AD, Dewal N et al (2016) Comprehensive pan-genomic characterization of adrenocortical carcinoma. Cancer Cell 29:723
18. Heaton JH, Wood MA, Kim AC et al (2012) Progression to adrenocortical tumorigenesis in mice and humans through insulin-like growth factor 2 and β-catenin. Am J Pathol 181:1017
19. Mohan DR, Lerario AM, Else T et al (2019) Targeted assessment of G0S2 methylation identifies a rapidly recurrent, routinely fatal molecular subtype of adrenocortical carcinoma. Clin Cancer Res 25:3276
20. Libè R, Fratticci A, Bertherat J (2007) Adrenocortical cancer: pathophysiology and clinical management. Endocr Relat Cancer 14:13
21. Giordano TJ (2011) The argument for mitotic rate-based grading for the prognostication of adrenocortical carcinoma. Am J Surg Pathol 35:471
22. Henley DJ, van Heerden JA, Grant CS et al (1983) Adrenal cortical carcinoma—a continuing challenge. Surgery 94:926
23. Hutter AM Jr, Kayhoe DE (1966) Adrenal cortical carcinoma. Clinical features of 138 patients. Am J Med 41:572
24. Nader S, Hickey RC, Sellin RV, Samaan NA (1983) Adrenal cortical carcinoma. A study of 77 cases. Cancer 52:707
25. Khorram-Manesh A, Ahlman H, Jansson S et al (1998) Adrenocortical carcinoma: surgery and mitotane for treatment and steroid profiles for follow-up. World J Surg 22:605
26. Terzolo M, Angeli A, Fassnacht M et al (2007) Adjuvant mitotane treatment for adrenocortical carcinoma. N Engl J Med 356:2372
27. Kendrick ML, Lloyd R, Erickson L et al (2001) Adrenocortical carcinoma: surgical progress or status quo? Arch Surg 136:543
28. Strong VE, Kennedy T, Al-Ahmadie H et al (2008) Prognostic indicators of malignancy in adrenal pheochromocytomas: clinical, histopathologic, and cell cycle/apoptosis gene expression analysis. Surgery 143:759–768
29. Arlt W, Biehl M, Taylor AE et al (2011) Urine steroid metabolomics as a biomarker tool for detecting malignancy in adrenal tumors. J Clin Endocrinol Metab 96(12):3775–3784
30. Dackiw AP, Lee JE, Gagel RF, Evans DB (2001) Adrenal cortical carcinoma. World J Surg 25(7):914–926
31. Cote R, Suster S, Weiss L, Weidner N (eds) (2002) Modern surgical pathology (2 volume set). W B Saunders, London
32. Aubert S, Wacrenier A, Leroy X et al (2002) Weiss system revisited: a clinicopathologic and immunohistochemical study of 49 adrenocortical tumors. Am J Surg Pathol 26(12):1612–1619
33. Weiss LM (1984) Comparative histologic study of 43 metastasizing and non-metastasizing adrenocortical tumors. Am J Surg Pathol 8(3):163–169
34. Deandreis D, Leboulleux S, Caramella C et al (2011) FDG PET in the management of patients with adrenal masses and adrenocortical carcinoma. Horm Cancer 2:354
35. De León DD, Lange BJ, Walterhouse D, Moshang T (2002) Long-term (15 years) outcome in an infant with metastatic adrenocortical carcinoma. J Clin Endocrinol Metab 87:4452
36. Robinson BG, Hales IB, Henniker AJ et al (1987) The effect of o,p′-DDD on adrenal steroid replacement therapy requirements. Clin Endocrinol 27:437

37. Schteingart DE, Doherty GM, Gauger PG et al (2005) Management of patients with adrenal cancer: recommendations of an international consensus conference. Endocr Relat Cancer 12:667
38. Stojadinovic A, Ghossein RA, Hoos A et al (2002) Adrenocortical carcinoma: clinical, morphologic, and molecular characterization. J Clin Oncol 20:941
39. Fassnacht M, Dekkers O, Else T et al (2018) European Society of Endocrinology Clinical Practice Guidelines on the management of adrenocortical carcinoma in adults, in collaboration with the European Network for the Study of Adrenal Tumors. Eur J Endocrinol 179(4):G1–G46
40. Allolio B, Hahner S, Weismann D, Fassnacht M (2004) Management of adrenocortical carcinoma. Clin Endocrinol (Oxf) 60:273
41. Reibetanz J, Rinn B, Kunz AS et al (2019) Patterns of lymph node recurrence in adrenocortical carcinoma: possible implications for primary surgical treatment. Ann Surg Oncol 26:531
42. Shen WT, Sturgeon C, Duh QY (2005) From incidentaloma to adrenocortical carcinoma: the surgical management of adrenal tumors. J Surg Oncol 89(3):186–192
43. Schlamp A, Hallfeldt K, Mueller-Lisse U, Pfluger T, Reincke M (2007) Recurrent adrenocortical carcinoma after laparoscopic resection. Nat Clin Pract Endocrinol Metab 3(2):191–195; quiz 1 p following 5
44. Ushiyama T, Suzuki K, Kageyama S, Fujita K, Oki Y, Yoshimi T (1997) A case of Cushing's syndrome due to adrenocortical carcinoma with recurrence 19 months after laparoscopic adrenalectomy. J Urol 157(6):2239
45. Brix D, Allolio B, Fenske W et al (2010) Laparoscopic versus open adrenalectomy for adrenocortical carcinoma: surgical and oncologic outcome in 152 patients. Eur Urol 58(4):609–615
46. Sgourakis G, Lanitis S, Kouloura A et al (2015) Laparoscopic versus open adrenalectomy for stage I/II adrenocortical carcinoma: meta-analysis of outcomes. J Investig Surg 28:145
47. Information on Children's Oncology Group NCT00304070 protocol. http://clinicaltrials.gov/ct2/show/NCT00304070?term=adrenocortical+cancer&type=Intr&age=0&rank=1. Accessed 23 Jul 2012
48. Bednarski BK, Habra MA, Phan A et al (2014) Borderline resectable adrenal cortical carcinoma: a potential role for preoperative chemotherapy. World J Surg 38:1318
49. Else T, Williams AR, Sabolch A et al (2014) Adjuvant therapies and patient and tumor characteristics associated with survival of adult patients with adrenocortical carcinoma. J Clin Endocrinol Metab 99:455
50. Calabrese A, Basile V, Puglisi S et al (2019) Adjuvant mitotane therapy is beneficial in non-metastatic adrenocortical carcinoma at high risk of recurrence. Eur J Endocrinol 180:387
51. Miller BS, Gauger PG, Hammer GD et al (2010) Proposal for modification of the ENSAT staging system for adrenocortical carcinoma using tumor grade. Langenbecks Arch Surg 395:955
52. Fassnacht M, Libé R, Kroiss M, Allolio B (2011) Adrenocortical carcinoma: a clinician's update. Nat Rev Endocrinol 7:323
53. Hovi L, Wikström S, Vettenranta K et al (2003) Adrenocortical carcinoma in children: a role for etoposide and cisplatin adjuvant therapy? Preliminary report. Med Pediatr Oncol 40:324
54. Khan TS, Imam H, Juhlin C et al (2000) Streptozocin and o,p′DDD in the treatment of adrenocortical cancer patients: long-term survival in its adjuvant use. Ann Oncol 11:1281
55. Viani GA, Viana BS (2019) Adjuvant radiotherapy after surgical resection for adrenocortical carcinoma: a systematic review of observational studies and meta-analysis. J Cancer Res Ther 15:S20
56. Schulick RD, Brennan MF (1999) Long-term survival after complete resection and repeat resection in patients with adrenocortical carcinoma. Ann Surg Oncol 6:719
57. Dy BM, Strajina V, Cayo AK et al (2015) Surgical resection of synchronously metastatic adrenocortical cancer. Ann Surg Oncol 22:146
58. Wood BJ, Abraham J, Hvizda JL et al (2003) Radiofrequency ablation of adrenal tumors and adrenocortical carcinoma metastases. Cancer 97:554
59. Mayo-Smith WW, Dupuy DE (2004) Adrenal neoplasms: CT-guided radiofrequency ablation—preliminary results. Radiology 231:225

60. Lubitz JA, Freeman L, Okun R (1973) Mitotane use in inoperable adrenal cortical carcinoma. JAMA 223:1109
61. Luton JP, Cerdas S, Billaud L et al (1990) Clinical features of adrenocortical carcinoma, prognostic factors, and the effect of mitotane therapy. N Engl J Med 322:1195
62. Bodie B, Novick AC, Pontes JE et al (1989) The Cleveland Clinic experience with adrenal cortical carcinoma. J Urol 141:257
63. Haq MM, Legha SS, Samaan NA et al (1980) Cytotoxic chemotherapy in adrenal cortical carcinoma. Cancer Treat Rep 64:909
64. Fassnacht M, Terzolo M, Allolio B et al (2012) Combination chemotherapy in advanced adrenocortical carcinoma. N Engl J Med 366:2189
65. Flynn SD, Murren JR, Kirby WM et al (1992) P-glycoprotein expression and multidrug resistance in adrenocortical carcinoma. Surgery 112:981
66. Raj N, Zheng Y, Kelly V et al (2020) PD-1 blockade in advanced adrenocortical carcinoma. J Clin Oncol 38:71
67. Habra MA, Stephen B, Campbell M et al (2019) Phase II clinical trial of pembrolizumab efficacy and safety in advanced adrenocortical carcinoma. J Immunother Cancer 7:253
68. Geoerger B, Kang HJ, Yalon-Oren M et al (2020) Pembrolizumab in paediatric patients with advanced melanoma or a PD-L1-positive, advanced, relapsed, or refractory solid tumour or lymphoma (KEYNOTE-051): interim analysis of an open-label, single-arm, phase 1-2 trial. Lancet Oncol 21:121
69. Christophe Le T, Christopher H, Corrine Z et al (2018) Avelumab in patients with previously treated metastatic adrenocortical carcinoma: phase 1b results from the JAVELIN solid tumor trial. J Immunother Cancer 6(1):111
70. Benedito AC, Bhavana K, Rubens BC et al (2019) Nivolumab in metastatic adrenocortical carcinoma: results of a phase 2 trial. J Clin Endocrinol Metab 104(12):6193–6200
71. Sara B, Kevin CM, Lina A et al (2020) Combined lenvatinib and pembrolizumab as salvage therapy in advanced adrenal cortical carcinoma. J Immunother Cancer 8(2):e001009
72. Barlaskar FM, Spalding AC, Heaton JH et al (2009) Preclinical targeting of the type I insulin-like growth factor receptor in adrenocortical carcinoma. J Clin Endocrinol Metab 94:204
73. Haluska P, Worden F, Olmos D et al (2010) Safety, tolerability, and pharmacokinetics of the anti-IGF-1R monoclonal antibody figitumumab in patients with refractory adrenocortical carcinoma. Cancer Chemother Pharmacol 65:765
74. Puzanov I, Lindsay CR, Goff L et al (2015) A phase I study of continuous oral dosing of OSI-906, a dual inhibitor of insulin-like growth factor-1 and insulin receptors, in patients with advanced solid tumors. Clin Cancer Res 21:701
75. Carden CP, Frentzas S, Langham M et al (2009) Preliminary activity in adrenocortical tumor (ACC) in phase I dose escalation study of intermittent oral dosing of OSI-906, a small-molecule insulin-like growth factor-1 receptor (IGF-1R) tyrosine kinase inhibitor in patients with advanced solid tumors (abstract 3544). J Clin Oncol 27:15s. Abstract. http://www.asco.org/ASCOv2/Meetings/Abstracts?&vmview=abst_detail_view&confID=65&abstractID=31413. Accessed 11 Jun 2012
76. Lerario AM, Worden FP, Ramm CA et al (2014) The combination of insulin-like growth factor receptor 1 (IGF1R) antibody cixutumumab and mitotane as a first-line therapy for patients with recurrent/metastatic adrenocortical carcinoma: a multi-institutional NCI-sponsored trial. Horm Cancer 5:232
77. Fassnacht M, Berruti A, Baudin E et al (2015) Linsitinib (OSI-906) versus placebo for patients with locally advanced or metastatic adrenocortical carcinoma: a double-blind, randomised, phase 3 study. Lancet Oncol 16:426
78. https://clinicaltrials.gov/ct2/show/NCT00778817?term=cixutumumab+and+adrenocortical+carcinoma&rank=2. Accessed 19 Feb 2015
79. Naing A, Lorusso P, Fu S et al (2013) Insulin growth factor receptor (IGF-1R) antibody cixutumumab combined with the mTOR inhibitor temsirolimus in patients with metastatic adrenocortical carcinoma. Br J Cancer 108:826

80. Chacón R, Tossen G, Loria FS, Chacón M (2005) CASE 2. Response in a patient with metastatic adrenal cortical carcinoma with thalidomide. J Clin Oncol 23:1579
81. Boudou-Rouquette P, Alexandre J, Soubrane O et al (2009) Antitumoral effect of the bisphosphonate zoledronic acid against visceral metastases in an adrenocortical cancer patient. Ann Oncol 20:1747
82. Butler C, Butler WM, Rizvi AA (2010) Sustained remission with the kinase inhibitor sorafenib in stage IV metastatic adrenocortical carcinoma. Endocr Pract 16:441
83. Lee JO, Lee KW, Kim CJ et al (2009) Metastatic adrenocortical carcinoma treated with sunitinib: a case report. Jpn J Clin Oncol 39:183
84. O'Sullivan C, Edgerly M, Velarde M et al (2014) The VEGF inhibitor axitinib has limited effectiveness as a therapy for adrenocortical cancer. J Clin Endocrinol Metab 99:1291
85. Kroiss M, Quinkler M, Johanssen S et al (2012) Sunitinib in refractory adrenocortical carcinoma: a phase II, single-arm, open-label trial. J Clin Endocrinol Metab 97:3495
86. Wortmann S, Quinkler M, Ritter C et al (2010) Bevacizumab plus capecitabine as a salvage therapy in advanced adrenocortical carcinoma. Eur J Endocrinol 162:349
87. Berruti A, Sperone P, Ferrero A et al (2012) Phase II study of weekly paclitaxel and sorafenib as second/third-line therapy in patients with adrenocortical carcinoma. Eur J Endocrinol 166:451
88. Edgren M, Eriksson B, Wilander E et al (1997) Biological characteristics of adrenocortical carcinoma: a study of p53, IGF, EGF-r, Ki-67 and PCNA in 17 adrenocortical carcinomas. Anticancer Res 17:1303
89. Kamio T, Shigematsu K, Sou H et al (1990) Immunohistochemical expression of epidermal growth factor receptors in human adrenocortical carcinoma. Hum Pathol 21:277
90. Quinkler M, Hahner S, Wortmann S et al (2008) Treatment of advanced adrenocortical carcinoma with erlotinib plus gemcitabine. J Clin Endocrinol Metab 93:2057
91. Hahner S, Kreissl MC, Fassnacht M et al (2012) [131I]iodometomidate for targeted radionuclide therapy of advanced adrenocortical carcinoma. J Clin Endocrinol Metab 97:914

Pheochromocytoma and Paraganglioma 25

Eleonora Patricia Corssmit
and Leonie Theresia van Hulsteijn

25.1 The Paraganglion System

Paragangliomas (PGLs) are rare vascular, neuroendocrine tumors of paraganglia, cell clusters originating from the neural crest that have co-migrated with the autonomic nervous system [1]. PGLs derive from either sympathetic tissue in adrenal and extraadrenal locations (PPGLs) or parasympathetic tissue of the head and neck (HNPGL, formerly called glomus tumors) [1]. Approximately 70–80% of PGLs arise from the adrenal medulla and are also referred to as pheochromocytoma (PCC) [1, 2]. PGLs can be found from the skull base to the sacrum, with a predilection for the middle ear (tympanic PGL), the dome of the internal jugular vein (jugular PGL), the bifurcation of the common carotid arteries (carotid body PGL), along the vagus nerve (vagal PGL), in the mediastinum (from the aortopulmonary body or the thoracic sympathetic chain), in the adrenal medulla, and in the abdominal and pelvic paraaortic regions, including the organ of Zuckerkandl.

25.2 Pathology

PGLs are usually well demarcated and often encapsulated. PGLs are characterized by their architecture, the tumor cells being arranged in distinctive cell balls, or Zellballen. These cell balls are separated by a fibrovascular stroma. The Zellballen are composed of clusters of chief cells that are surrounded by supportive

E. P. Corssmit (✉)
Department of Endocrinology, Leiden University Medical Center, Leiden, The Netherlands
e-mail: E.P.M.van_der_Kleij-Corssmit@lumc.nl

L. T. van Hulsteijn
Department of Endocrinology, Groningen University Medical Center, Groningen, The Netherlands
e-mail: l.t.van.hulsteijn@umcg.nl

S. Yalcin, K. Öberg (eds.), *Neuroendocrine Tumours*,
https://doi.org/10.1007/978-3-031-56968-5_25

sustentacular cells at the periphery. The chief cells, which are neuroendocrine cells, express neuron-specific enolase, serotonin, and chromogranin, and the sustentacular cells express S-100 protein [3]. Membrane-bound electron-dense neurosecretory granules may be seen on electron microscopy [4, 5]. These neurosecretory granules vary in size, configuration, and electron density of their cores [5]. PGLs originate from chief cells. The sustentacular cells are spindled and devoid of granules. The histologic features of malignant PGLs are basically identical to those of benign tumors, but may exhibit the following features: central necrosis of Zellballen, vascular and lymphatic invasion, and the presence of mitotic spindles [6]. Because there are no accepted pathological or immunohistochemical markers that distinguish malignant from benign tumors, malignancy is only diagnosed when metastasis to non-neuroendocrine tissue is demonstrated [7]. The TNM staging for PPGLs has adopted a cutoff of 5 cm and extra-adrenal localization as important determinants of malignancy risk [8]. In addition,the presence of an *SDHB* mutation [9], a PASS score (pheochromocytoma of the Adrenal Gland Scale Score) >6 [10] and a Ki-67 index >3% [11] have been associated with an increased risk of malignancy.

25.3 Clinical Presentation

The exact prevalence of PGLs is unknown but has been estimated to lie between 1:6500 and 1:2500 in the United States [12]. Their prevalence is higher in autopsy series (1:2000), suggesting that many tumors remain undiagnosed [13]. The annual incidence has been reported to be two to ten cases per million [14]. The tumors may occur in all ages but have the highest incidence between 40 and 50 years, with an approximately equal sex distribution [15, 16]. From all PGLs, PCCs have the highest relative incidence. In 340 unselected PGL patients, about 73% of the patients had PCC, 9% had sPGL, and 20% had HNPGL [16].

HNPGLs usually grow slowly; the majority has a tumor doubling time of more than 10 years [17]. Because of this slow growth rate, HNPGLs may remain clinically silent for years. Although these tumors are usually benign and only a minority produces catecholamines [18], their location in the close proximity of nerves and vascular structures often results in considerable morbidity due to compression or infiltration of the adjacent structures, causing symptoms like hearing loss, tinnitus, dysphagia, and cranial nerve palsy. Carotid body tumors are the most common HNPGL, usually presenting as a painless cervical mass [19]. Large compressive tumors may result in cranial nerve paralysis. Vagal body tumors present as painless neck masses, located behind the angle of the mandible, occasionally accompanied by dysphagia and hoarseness [20]. Tympanic and jugular foramen tumors most commonly present as a vascular middle ear mass causing pulsatile tinnitus and hearing loss. Difficulties in speech, swallowing, and airway function may be the result of dysfunction of cranial nerves traversing the jugular foramen [21].

The majority of PPGLs produce catecholamines, causing symptoms of catecholamine excess. The clinical presentation is highly variable due to different profiles of catecholamines secreted, secretion of different other vasoactive peptides (e.g., neuropeptide Y, adrenomedullin, and atrial natriuretic peptide), presentation of symptoms related to tumor mass or other organ involvement in syndromic forms, and desensitization of adrenoreceptors (most likely due to long-term exposure to high circulating catecholamine levels) [22]. Hypertension, continuous or paroxysmal, is the most common feature of PCCs and sPGLs. Hypertensive crises are frequently associated with the classic triad of severe headache, palpitations, and diaphoresis. Paroxysms can last minutes to hours, vary in interval, and occur spontaneously or be triggered by direct stimulation of the tumor (e.g., bladder localization), physical activity, diagnostic procedures, or certain drugs (e.g., metoclopramide) [23]. Other symptoms may include anxiety, nausea, vomiting, dyspnea, and weakness [24, 25]. In addition, hyperglycemia, resulting from metabolic actions of catecholamines, may be the presenting symptom, which could lead to delayed diagnosis [26]. Morbidity and mortality in PPGL patients are predominantly the result of cardiovascular complications (e.g., sudden death, myocardial infarction, heart failure, and cerebrovascular accidents). In addition, malignant PGLs may also present with systemic symptoms such as weight loss or clinical manifestations related to metastatic spread such as pain in bones.

25.4 Pathophysiology

Genomic alterations largely drive the pathophysiology of PGL. At least 35% of PGLs are part of a hereditary disease [27–29]. In contrast to sporadic PGLs, familial PGLs are more often bilateral, extra-adrenal, multifocal, and occurring during childhood. Hereditary PGL is caused by mutations in an increasing number of tumor susceptibility genes, in particular succinate dehydrogenase subunits A, B, C, and D and assembly factor 2, Von Hippel-Lindau, *RET* (causing multiple endocrine neoplasia type 2), neurofibromatosis type 1, MAX, *TMEM127*, and more recently discovered fumarate hydratase and malate dehydrogenase 2. In addition to these germline mutations, in 30–40% of PPGLs, tumorigenesis is driven by somatic mutations, mainly in HRAS, neurofibromatosis type 1, EPAS1/HIF2A, RET, *V*on Hippel-Lindau and CSDE1, or by fusions of mastermindlike transcriptional coactivator 3 [30, 31].

PGLs can be classified into different clusters based on transcriptional profiling studies [27, 32]. Tumors in cluster one include those associated with succinate dehydrogenase, Von Hippel-Lindau, fumarate hydratase, malate dehydrogenase and EPAS1/HIF2A and are characterized by increased expression of genes involved in (pseudo)hypoxia, cell proliferation, angiogenesis, electron transport chain and the Krebs cycle and abnormal function of oxidoreductases. Tumors in Cluster II include those associated with RET, neurofibromatosis type 1, TMEM127, and MAX and show an increased expression of genes involved in kinase signaling, protein synthesis, endocytosis, and maintenance of a differentiated chomaffin cell catecholamine biosynthetic and secretory phenotype. Cluster III involves alterations in the Wnt signaling pathway of tumourigenesis and is driven by MAML3 and CSDE1.

There are clear genotype–phenotype correlations (Table 25.1). For example, succinate dehydrogenase subunit B mutations are associated with increased risk of malignancy [33, 34]. Succinate dehydrogenase serves as complex II of the

Table 25.1 Genotype–phenotype correlations in the most frequently occurring hereditary forms of PGL

Syndrome	Gene	HNPGL	sPGL	PCC	Multiple PGL	Bilateral PCC	Malignancy risk	Parent of origin preference
MEN2	*RET*	Extremely rare	–	++	–	++	+/–	–
VHL	*VHL*	Rare	+	++	+	++	+	–
NF1	*NF1*	–	–	+	–	–	+	–
PGL1	*SDHD*	+++	++	+	+++	+	+	Paternal
PGL2	*SDHAF2*	+++	–		++	–	Not known	Paternal
PGL3	*SDHC*	++	+	+/–	+	–	+/–	–
PGL4	*SDHB*	++	+++	++	++	+	++	–
PGL5	*SDHA*	+	+	–	–	–	Not known	–
–	*TMEM127*	+/–	+/–	+++	+/–	++	+	–
–	*MAX*	–	–	++	–	++	+	Paternal
–	*KIF1β*	–	–	+	–	+	Not known	–
–	*FH*	–	+/–	+/–	–	–	Not known	–

+: present; –: absent
HNPGL = head and neck paraganglioma, sPGL = sympathetic paraganglioma, PCC = pheochromocytoma, PGL = paraganglioma
MEN2 = multiple endocrine neoplasia type 2, VHL = von Hippel Lindau disease, NF1 = neurofibromatosis type 1, PGL1–5 = familial paraganglioma syndrome type 1–5

mitochondrial electron transport chain and is also part of the tricarboxylic acid cycle where it converts succinate to fumarate. Succinate dehydrogenase deficiency results in the accumulation of the oncometabolite succinate, which triggers stabilization of hypoxia-inducible transcription factors that support tumor progression via different signaling pathways. Also, succinate causes global histone and DNA hypermethylation through inactivation of histone demethylases [35]. Epigenetic changes account for several of the characteristics of this subset of tumors, including cell migration/metastatic capacity and catecholamine secretory profile.

A small fraction of PPGLs is associated with other syndromes, including Carney triad, Carney–Stratakis syndrome, and multiple endocrine neoplasia type 1 (MEN1) [36, 37]. In addition, other tumors have been documented in SDH mutations, like gastrointestinal stromal tumors [38], renal cell carcinomas [39], growth hormone producing pituitary adenomas [40], and pancreas NET [41]. Apart from RET, which is a proto-oncogene, all the other susceptibility genes for PPGL are tumor suppressor genes. All familial PGL syndromes have an autosomal dominant mode of inheritance; interestingly, SDHD, SDHAF2, and MAX are characterized by paternal transmission only of the disease [41–43]. This observation strongly suggests that these genes are subject to genetic imprinting, although the exact molecular mechanism remains unknown [44, 45].

25.5 Diagnosis

25.5.1 Biochemistry

Biochemical diagnosis of PPGL relies on the measurement of catecholamine metabolites in plasma or 24-h urine. Within adrenal chromaffin cells, adrenaline and noradrenaline are metabolized into the *O*-methylated metabolites metanephrine and normetanephrine (Fig. 25.1). Plasma-free and 24-h urinary fractionated

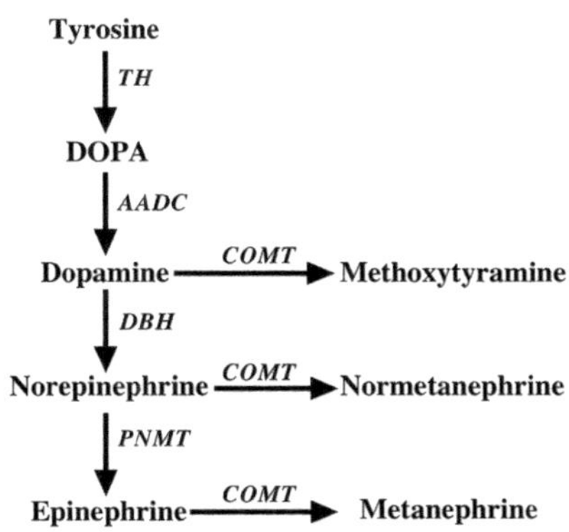

Fig. 25.1 Pathways of catecholamine synthesis and O-methylation. *TH* tyrosine hydroxylase, *DOPA* 3,4-dihydroxyphenylalanine, *AADC* aromatic amino acid decarboxylase, *COMT* catechol-*O*-methyltransferase, *DBH* dopamine β-hydroxylase, *PNMT* phenylethanolamine-*N*-methyltransferase

metanephrines offer high sensitivities between 96% and 99% and a specificity between 69% and 93% [46, 47]. To avoid false-positive results, blood sampling should ideally be done after supine rest in a quiet room for at least 20–30 min, following abstinence of caffeine, smoking, and interfering medications. Also, some medications can interfere analytically, pharmacodynamically, and pharmacokinetically, resulting in usually false-positive test results. Tandem mass spectroscopy is generally less susceptible to analytical interference than light chromatography with electrochemical detection assays. Pharmacodynamic and pharmacokinetic interference involves the effects of drugs on secretion, metabolism, and excretion of catecholamines or metabolites. Many drugs are known to increase catecholamine and metabolite concentrations [48]. Examples are sympathomimetic agents such as ephedrine, amphetamine, cocaine, caffeine, and nicotine, agents that inhibit reuptake of noradrenaline such as serotonin/noradrenaline reuptake inhibitors and tricyclic antidepressants, and agents that inhibit catecholamine metabolisation such as mono-amino oxidase inhibitors and vasodilators such as calcium channel blockers and alpha- and beta-adrenergic receptor blockers. False-positive results can also occur with Levodopa. In case of inconclusive tests despite ruling out sources of false-positive results, a clonidine suppression test can be performed, being abnormal in PPGL as indicated by elevated plasma normetanephrine at 3 h after clonidine administration and a less than 40% decrease in levels compared with baseline [47]. If these criteria are not met, sympathetic activation rather than PPGL is the cause of elevation. Both sensitivity and specificity of the test are high.

Chromogranin A (CgA) is secreted from neurosecretory vesicles, along with catecholamines [49]. Plasma CgA level is often elevated in functioning and nonfunctioning PGLs [50]. The levels correlate with tumor mass, making CgA a useful tumor marker [51]. Sensitivity for identifying PGLs is 83–89%, and false-positive results, however, occur often due to liver or kidney failure or use of proton pump inhibitors [52]. Plasma CgA levels are particularly elevated in patients with malignant PGL [53].

25.5.2 Anatomical and Functional Imaging

Once a biochemical diagnosis of PPGL has been established, the source of catecholamine excess is subsequently localized by anatomical and functional imaging studies. Anatomical imaging such as computed tomography (CT) or magnetic resonance imaging (MRI) has an excellent sensitivity (77–98% and 90–100%, resp.) but lack specificity (29–92% and 50–100%, respectively) for detecting PPGL [54, 55]. On CT, PCCs usually present as homogenous tumors with soft tissue density of more than 10 Hounsfield Units (HU) and uniform enhancement with contrast; however, larger PCCs may undergo hemorrhage and necrosis resulting in areas of low density [56]. On MRI, PCCs present as a mass absent of fat on chemical shift, with a high signal on T2 sequences as a result of their hypervascularity [57]. MR imaging with pre- and post-contrast enhanced 3D time of flight (TOF) MR angiography sequence represents the most important imaging technique for evaluation and characterization of HNPGLs [58]. MR imaging of HNPGL provides more diagnostic information than does CT scanning because of the better soft tissue contrasts as compared to CT [59]. MRI enables multiplanar imaging of tumor extension and vessel encasement. Ultrasound has a limited diagnostic yield but can be of use in imaging HNPGL [60]. Tumors detected by anatomical imaging can subsequently be identified as PGL by functional imaging agents that specifically target the catecholamine synthesis, storage, and secretion pathway of chromaffin tumor cells. 123I-metaiodobenzylguanidine (MIBG) scintigraphy is the most widely used nuclear technique for this purpose, despite its limited sensitivity of only around 80% [54, 60–62]. The use of positron emission tomography (PET) is recommended, and the choice of radiopharmaceutical (labeled fluorodeoxyglucose/DOPA or somatostatin analogs (Ga-DOTATATE)) depends on, among others, location and germline mutation [63, 64].

Functional imaging is also recommended in patients with an increased risk for multiple or metastatic PPGLs due to an underlying hereditary diseases, large tumor size (>4 cm), extra-adrenal location, and recurrence. For the detection and monitoring of metastatic PPGL, PET using Ga-DOTATATE is preferred [65].

25.6 Treatment

The treatment of choice for PPGLs is surgical resection, preferably laparoscopically [66], but in cases of large tumors with a high risk of malignancy, conventional laparotomy should be considered. In order to avoid surgical complications (hypertensive crisis, arrhythmias), all patients with preoperative catecholamine excess should be adequately pretreated with α-blockade (phenoxybenzamin, doxazosin), if necessary followed by β-blockade (propanolol, atenolol) and volume expansion as these patients are in a constant status of volume depletion. This has been shown to reduce operative mortality to below 1% [67]. To evaluate postoperative cure, plasma or urinary metanephrines should be checked 2–6 weeks after recovery of surgery. In the long term, new events can occur. Therefore, a minimum follow-up of 10 years by yearly clinical and biochemical investigations is recommended. In addition, in high-risk patients, i.e., young patients and those with a hereditary disease, a large tumor and/or an extra-adrenal PPGL, lifelong annual follow-up should be offered [68].

Treatment for HNPGL must be considered in relation to tumor growth velocity, biological activity of the tumor, patient age and medical condition, tumor size and site, and potential for treatment-related morbidity [17]. Because most tumors grow slowly, a wait-and-scan policy is often advised [17]. However, although HNPGLs are indolent tumors, tumor growth may lead to serious morbidity and cranial nerve impairment due to their location in close proximity to important neurovascular structures. The main treatment modalities for HNPGL are surgery and radiotherapy. A multidisciplinary team approach is recommended for the choice of treatment of most HNPGL except for the very small and easy to resect tumors. With surgery, it is possible to remove the tumor without recurrence. Preoperatively, HNPGL should be tested for catecholamine excretion, and pharmacological preparation should be started in positive cases [69]. The rate of surgical complications rises with the size of the tumor [70]. The most common complications are cranial nerve damage and vascular complications [71–74]. External beam radiotherapy and radiosurgery are alternative treatment modalities for HNPGL patients, resulting in local tumor control and sometimes regression by producing fibrosis and vascular sclerosis. These may be options in patients with large growing tumors, in which resection may result in considerable morbidity, or after incomplete resection of tumor with intracranial or skull base invasion [75].

25.7 Malignant Paragangliomas

Because there is no definite histological substrate for malignant PGL [76, 77], malignancy is defined by the presence of metastases: tumor spread in sites where chromaffin tissue is normally absent [7, 8]. Depending on the genetic background, up to 50% of sPGLs are malignant [78, 79], whereas HNPGLs are usually benign [80]. Malignant HNPGLs are confirmed by the presence of local metastases in cervical lymph nodes or systemic metastases, usually to bones, lung, and liver [80]. The primary management of patients with malignant HNPGLs should be directed toward complete surgical resection of the primary tumor and regional lymph nodes. Postoperative radiation may be beneficial in slowing down the progression of residual disease. In half of the patients who develop malignant PPGLs, metastases are discovered synchronously at the initial diagnosis. Treatment for malignant PPGLs include surgical debulking, pharmacological control of catecholamine-induced symptoms, external radiation, and systemic antineoplastic therapy. There is no effective treatment for malignant PPGLs. Although the usefulness of debulking of tumor has not been established, it may reduce catecholamine-related problems and improve response to further treatment. Currently, the practiced standard of therapy includes radionuclide therapy (^{131}I-MIBG, ^{177}Lu-DOTATATE), chemotherapy (CVD scheme or temozolomide monotherapy), tyrosine kinase inhibitors (sunitinib), and immunotherapy [81]. Conventional radiotherapy may provide effective palliation in patients with painful bone metastases; arterial embolization, chemoembolization, or radiofrequency ablation may be useful in case of liver metastases [82, 83]. Catecholamine-induced signs and symptoms can be treated with catecholamine synthesis inhibitors (alpha-methyl-para-tyrosine) or α-receptor blocking medication. Depending on the cluster, new effective molecular-targeted therapies are developed, like antiangiogenic therapy, HIF inhibitors, PARP (polyADP-ribose polymerase) inhibition and immunotherapy for Cluster I, and mTOR (mammalian target of rapamycin) inhibitors for Cluster II. Currently, there are no Cluster III Wnt signaling-targeted therapies for PPGL patients [84]. Malignant PGLs occur most frequently in patients with *SDHB* gene mutations [79, 80]. The natural course of metastasized disease is highly variable, with 5-year survival rates ranging from 40% to 85% [85], rapid progression of disease being associated with male sex, older age at diagnosis, synchronous metastases, larger tumor size, elevated dopamine, and not undergoing resection of the primary tumor. In addition, extra-adrenal tumors have been associated with a higher risk for metastatic spread, whereas malignant skull base and neck PGL showed more indolent courses of disease with longer survival (overall 5-year survival rate 85.4%) [86]. For the individual patient, overall survival, progression-free survival, and clinical outcome are difficult to predict.

25.8 Genetic Testing

To date, more than 20 susceptibility PGL genes have been identified, and at least 35% of cases are classified as genetically determined. Owing to the large number of susceptibility genes implicated in the diagnosis of inherited PGLs, next-generation sequencing technology is ideally suited for carrying out genetic screening of these individuals [87]. Genetic testing can be of great importance for patients and their relatives because it gives the opportunity for early diagnosis through periodical imaging studies in family members of the affected individual [88]. Early detection of a familial PGL allows early detection of potentially malignant PGLs, especially in SDHB mutation carriers, and early surgical treatment, reducing the complication rate of this operation [89, 90]. Genetic testing algorithms can be made to reduce time and costs. The clinical and biochemical phenotype and SDHB and SDHA immunohistochemistry of the tumor tissue [91, 92] may be valuable tools to guide the order of genetic testing [34]. Mutation-positive carriers need regular clinical follow-up [93], except for the children of female mutation carriers of SDHD, SDHAF2, and MAX because of maternal imprinting. Annual biochemical testing, e.g., plasma-free metanephrines and/or urine fractionated metanephrines, and every 1–2 years radiological imaging of neck and/or thorax/abdomen/pelvis, depending on the mutation, with additional functional imaging in selected cases can be recommended as a surveillance program [68]. Recently, a consensus algorithm was established for the initial screening and follow-up of SDHx mutation carriers by an international panel of 29 experts from 12 countries using the Delphi method [93].

References

1. De Lellis RA, Lloyd RV, Heitz PU, Eng C (2004) World Health Organization classification of tumours. Pathology and genetics of tumours of endocrine organs. IARC Press, Lyon
2. Pacak K, Keiser H, Eisenhofer G (2005) Pheochromocytoma. In: DeGroot LS, Jameson JL (eds) Textbook of endocrinology, 5th edn. Elsevier Saunders, Philadelphia, pp 2501–2534
3. Kliewer KE, Wen DR, Cancilla PA, Cochran AJ (1989) Paragangliomas: assessment of prognosis by histologic, immunohistochemical, and ultrastructural techniques. Hum Pathol 20:29–39
4. Sennaroglu L, Sungur A (2002) Histopathology of paragangliomas. Otol Neurotol 23:104–105
5. Warren WH, Lee I, Gould VE, Memoli VA, Jao W (1985) Paragangliomas of the head and neck: ultrastructural and immunohistochemical analysis. Ultrastruct Pathol 8:333–343
6. Lack EE, Cubilla AL, Woodruff JM (1979) Paragangliomas of the head and neck region. A pathologic study of tumors from 71 patients. Hum Pathol 10:191–218
7. Scholz T, Schulz C, Klose S, Lehnert H (2007) Diagnostic management of benign and malignant pheochromocytoma. Exp Clin Endocrinol Diabetes 115:155–159

8. Jimenez C, Libutti SK, Landry CS et al (2017) The first TNM staging system for patients with pheochromocytomas and paragangliomas. In: Amin MB (ed) AJCC cancer staging manual, 8th edn. Springer, New York, pp 919–927
9. Amar L, Baudin E, Burnichon N et al (2007) Succinate dehydrogenase B gene mutations predict survival in patients with malignant pheochromocytomas or paragangliomas. J Clin Endocrinol Metab 92:3822–3828
10. Strong VE, Kennedy T, Al-Ahmadie H et al (2008) Prognostic indicators of malignancy in adrenal pheochromocytomas: clinical, histopathologic, and cell cycle/apoptosis gene expression analysis. Surgery 143:759–768
11. Liu TH, Chen YJ, Wu SF et al (2004) [Distinction between benign and malignant pheochromocytomas]. Zhonghua Bing Li Xue Za Zhi 33:198–202
12. Chen H, Sippel RS, O'Dorisio MS, Vinik AI, Lloyd RV, Pacak K (2010) The North American Neuroendocrine Tumor Society consensus guideline for the diagnosis and management of neuroendocrine tumors: pheochromocytoma, paraganglioma, and medullary thyroid cancer. Pancreas 39:775–783
13. McNeil AR, Blok BH, Koelmeyer TD, Burke MP, Hilton JM (2000) Phaeochromocytomas discovered during coronial autopsies in Sydney, Melbourne and Auckland. Aust N Z J Med 30:648–652
14. Beard CM, Sheps SG, Kurland LT, Carney JA, Lie JT (1983) Occurrence of pheochromocytoma in Rochester, Minnesota, 1950 through 1979. Mayo Clin Proc 58:802–804
15. Cascon A, Pita G, Burnichon N et al (2009) Genetics of pheochromocytoma and paraganglioma in Spanish patients. J Clin Endocrinol Metab 94:1701–1705
16. Mannelli M, Castellano M, Schiavi F et al (2009) Clinically guided genetic screening in a large cohort of Italian patients with pheochromocytomas and/or functional or nonfunctional paragangliomas. J Clin Endocrinol Metab 94:1541–1547
17. Jansen JC, van den Berg R, Kuiper A, van der Mey AG, Zwinderman AH, Cornelisse CJ (2000) Estimation of growth rate in patients with head and neck paragangliomas influences the treatment proposal. Cancer 88:2811–2816
18. van Duinen N, Steenvoorden D, Kema IP et al (2010) Increased urinary excretion of 3-methoxytyramine in patients with head and neck paragangliomas. J Clin Endocrinol Metab 95:209–214
19. Gardner P, Dalsing M, Weisberger E, Sawchuk A, Miyamoto R (1996) Carotid body tumors, inheritance, and a high incidence of associated cervical paragangliomas. Am J Surg 172:196–199
20. Netterville JL, Jackson CG, Miller FR, Wanamaker JR, Glasscock ME (1998) Vagal paraganglioma: a review of 46 patients treated during a 20-year period. Arch Otolaryngol Head Neck Surg 124:1133–1140
21. Jackson CG (2001) Glomus tympanicum and glomus jugulare tumors. Otolaryngol Clin N Am 34:941–970, vii
22. Bravo EL (1994) Evolving concepts in the pathophysiology, diagnosis, and treatment of pheochromocytoma. Endocr Rev 15:356–368
23. Lenders JW, Eisenhofer G, Mannelli M, Pacak K (2005) Phaeochromocytoma. Lancet 366:665–675
24. Kebebew E, Duh QY (1998) Benign and malignant pheochromocytoma: diagnosis, treatment, and follow-up. Surg Oncol Clin N Am 7:765–789
25. Werbel SS, Ober KP (1995) Pheochromocytoma. Update on diagnosis, localization, and management. Med Clin North Am 79:131–153
26. La Batide-Alanore A, Chatellier G, Plouin PF (2003) Diabetes as a marker of pheochromocytoma in hypertensive patients. J Hypertens 21:1703–1707
27. Jhawar S, Arakawa Y, Kumar S et al (2022) New insights on the genetics of pheochromocytoma and paraganglioma and its clinical implications. Cancers (Basel) 14:594
28. Fishbein L, Leshchiner I, Walter V et al (2017) Comprehensive molecular characterization of pheochromocytoma and paraganglioma. Cancer Cell 31:181–193

29. Favier J, Amar L, Gimenez-Roqueplo A (2015) Paraganglioma and phaeochromocytoma: from genetics to personalized medicine. Nat Rev Endocrinol 11:101–111
30. Dahia PL (2014) Pheochromocytoma and paraganglioma pathogenesis.: learning from genetic heterogeneity. Nat Rev Cancer 14:108–119
31. Curras-Freixes M, Inglada-Perez L, Mancikova V et al (2015) Recommendations for somatic and germline testing of single pheochromocytoma and paraganglioma based on findings from a series of 329 patients. J Med Genet 52:647–656
32. Crona J, Taieb D, Pacak K (2017) New perspectives on pheochromocytoma and paraganglioma: toward a molecular classification. Endocr Rev 38:489–515
33. van Hulsteijn LT, Dekkers OM, Hes FJ, Smit JW, Corssmit EP (2012) Risk of malignant paraganglioma in SDHB-mutation and SDHD-mutation carriers: a systematic review and meta-analysis. J Med Genet 49:768–776
34. Welander J, Soderkvist P, Gimm O (2011) Genetics and clinical characteristics of hereditary pheochromocytomas and paragangliomas. Endocr Relat Cancer 18:R253–R276
35. Letouze E, Martinelli C, Loriot C et al (2013) SDH mutations establish a hypermethylator phenotype in paraganglioma. Cancer Cell 23:739–752
36. Carney JA, Stratakis CA (2002) Familial paraganglioma and gastric stromal sarcoma: a new syndrome distinct from the Carney triad. Am J Med Genet 108:132–139
37. Schussheim DH, Skarulis MC, Agarwal SK et al (2001) Multiple endocrine neoplasia type 1: new clinical and basic findings. Trends Endocrinol Metab 12:173–178
38. McWhinney SR, Pasini B, Stratakis CA (2007) Familial gastrointestinal stromal tumors and germ-line mutations. N Engl J Med 357:1054–1056
39. Vanharanta S, Buchta M, McWhinney SR et al (2004) Early-onset renal cell carcinoma as a novel extraparaganglial component of SDHB-associated heritable paraganglioma. Am J Hum Genet 74:153–159
40. Xekouki P, Pacak K, Almeida M et al (2012) Succinate dehydrogenase (SDH) D subunit (SDHD) inactivation in a growth-hormone-producing pituitary tumor: a new association for SDH? J Clin Endocrinol Metab 97:E357–E366
41. Niemeijer ND, Papathomas TG, Korpershoek E et al (2015) Succinate dehydrogenase (SDH)-deficient pancreatic neuroendocrine tumor expands the SDH-related tumor spectrum. J Clin Endocrinol Metab 100(10):E1386–E1393
42. Baysal BE, Farr JE, Rubinstein WS et al (1997) Fine mapping of an imprinted gene for familial nonchromaffin paragangliomas, on chromosome 11q23. Am J Hum Genet 60:121–132
43. Heutink P, van der Mey AG, Sandkuijl LA et al (1992) A gene subject to genomic imprinting and responsible for hereditary paragangliomas maps to chromosome 11q23-qter. Hum Mol Genet 1:7–10
44. van der Mey AG, Maaswinkel-Mooy PD, Cornelisse CJ, Schmidt PH, van de Kamp JJ (1989) Genomic imprinting in hereditary glomus tumours: evidence for new genetic theory. Lancet 2:1291–1294
45. Hensen EF, Jordanova ES, van Minderhout IJ et al (2004) Somatic loss of maternal chromosome 11 causes parent-of-origin-dependent inheritance in SDHD-linked paraganglioma and phaeochromocytoma families. Oncogene 23:4076–4083
46. Lenders JW, Pacak K, Walther MM et al (2002) Biochemical diagnosis of pheochromocytoma: which test is best? JAMA 287:1427–1434
47. Eisenhofer G, Goldstein DS, Walther MM et al (2003) Biochemical diagnosis of pheochromocytoma: how to distinguish true-from false-positive test results. J Clin Endocrinol Metab 88:2656–2666
48. Neary NM, King KS, Pacak K (2011) Drugs and pheochromocytoma—don't be fooled by every elevated metanephrine. N Engl J Med 364:2268–2270
49. Montesinos MS, Machado JD, Camacho M et al (2008) The crucial role of chromogranins in storage and exocytosis revealed using chromaffin cells from chromogranin A null mouse. J Neurosci 28:3350–3358

50. Guignat L, Bidart JM, Nocera M, Comoy E, Schlumberger M, Baudin E (2001) Chromogranin A and the alpha-subunit of glycoprotein hormones in medullary thyroid carcinoma and phaeochromocytoma. Br J Cancer 84:808–812
51. d'Herbomez M, Gouze V, Huglo D et al (2001) Chromogranin A assay and (131)I-MIBG scintigraphy for diagnosis and follow-up of pheochromocytoma. J Nucl Med 42:993–997
52. Algeciras-Schimnich A, Preissner CM, Young WF Jr, Singh RJ, Grebe SK (2008) Plasma chromogranin A or urine fractionated metanephrines follow-up testing improves the diagnostic accuracy of plasma fractionated metanephrines for pheochromocytoma. J Clin Endocrinol Metab 93:91–95
53. Rao F, Keiser HR, O'Connor DT (2000) Malignant pheochromocytoma. Chromaffin granule transmitters and response to treatment. Hypertension 36:1045–1052
54. Ilias I, Pacak K (2004) Current approaches and recommended algorithm for the diagnostic localization of pheochromocytoma. J Clin Endocrinol Metab 89:479–491
55. Maurea S, Cuocolo A, Reynolds JC, Neumann RD, Salvatore M (1996) Diagnostic imaging in patients with paragangliomas. Computed tomography, magnetic resonance and MIBG scintigraphy comparison. Q J Nucl Med 40:365–371
56. Sohaib SAA, Bomanji J, Evanson J, Reznek RH (2001) Imaging of the endocrine system. In: Grainger R, Allison D, Adam A, Dixon A (eds) Diagnostic radiology: a textbook of medical imaging, 4th edn. Churchill Livingston, London, pp 1367–1399
57. Fink IJ, Reinig JW, Dwyer AJ, Doppman JL, Linehan WM, Keiser HR (1985) MR imaging of pheochromocytomas. J Comput Assist Tomogr 9:454–458
58. van den Berg R, Verbist BM, Mertens BJ, van der Mey AG, van Buchem MA (2004) Head and neck paragangliomas: improved tumor detection using contrast-enhanced 3D time-of-flight MR angiography as compared with fat-suppressed MR imaging techniques. AJNR Am J Neuroradiol 25:863–870
59. Olsen WL, Dillon WP, Kelly WM, Norman D, Brant-Zawadzki M, Newton TH (1987) MR imaging of paragangliomas. AJR Am J Roentgenol 148:201–204
60. Shulkin BL, Ilias I, Sisson JC, Pacak K (2006) Current trends in functional imaging of pheochromocytomas and paragangliomas. Ann N Y Acad Sci 1073:374–382
61. Nielsen JT, Nielsen BV, Rehling M (1996) Location of adrenal medullary pheochromocytoma by I-123 metaiodobenzylguanidine SPECT. Clin Nucl Med 21:695–699
62. van der Harst E, de Herder WW, Bruining HA et al (2001) [(123)I]metaiodobenzylguanidine and [(111)In]octreotide uptake in benign and malignant pheochromocytomas. J Clin Endocrinol Metab 86:685–693
63. Archier A, Varoquaux A, Garrique P et al (2016) Prospective comparison of (68) Ga-DOTATATE and (18)F-FDOPA PET/CT in patients with various pheochromocytomas and paragangliomas with emphasis on sporadic cases. Eur J Nucl Med Mol Imaging 43(7):1248–1257
64. Taieb D, Hicks RJ, Hindie E, Guillet BA, Avram A, Ghedini P et al (2019) European Association of Nuclear Medicine Practice Guideline/Society of Nuclear Medicine and Molecular Imaging Procedure Standard 2019 for radionuclide imaging of phaeochromocytoma and paraganglioma. Eur J Nucl Med Mol Imaging 46:2112–2137. [PubMed: 31254038]
65. Janssen I, Blanchet EM, Adams K et al (2015) Superiority of [68]-DOTATATE PET/CT to other functional imaging modalities in the localization of SDHB-associated metastatic pheochromocytoma and paraganglioma. Clin Cancer Res 21:3888–3895
66. Janetschek G, Finkenstedt G, Gasser R et al (1998) Laparoscopic surgery for pheochromocytoma: adrenalectomy, partial resection, excision of paragangliomas. J Urol 160:330–334
67. Niemann U, Hiller W, Behrend M (2002) 25 years experience of the surgical treatment of phaeochromocytoma. Eur J Surg 168:716–719
68. Plouin PF, Amar L, Dekkers OM et al (2016) European Society of Endocrinology Clinical Practice Guideline for long-term follow-up of patients operated on for a phaeochromocytoma or a paraganglioma. Eur J Endocrinol 174:G1–G10
69. van Duinen N, Corssmit EPM, de Jong WHA et al (2013) Plasma levels of free metanephrines and 3-methoxytyramine indicate a higher number of biochemically active HNPGL than 24-h urinary excretion rates of catecholamines and metabolites. Eur J Endocrinol 169:377–382

70. Lim JY, Kim J, Kim SH et al (2010) Surgical treatment of carotid body paragangliomas: outcomes and complications according to the shamblin classification. Clin Exp Otorhinolaryngol 3:91–95
71. Hamming JF, Schepers A (2021) Assessing the complexity of a carotid body tumor resection. Eur J Surg Oncol 47:1811–1812
72. Suarez C, Rodrigo JP, Bodeker CC et al (2013) Jugular and vagal paragangliomas: systematic study of management with surgery and radiotherapy. Head Neck 35:1195–1204
73. Luna-Ortiz K, Rascon-Ortiz M, Villavicencio-Valencia V et al (2005) Carotid body tumors: review of a 20-year experience. Oral Oncol 41:56–61
74. Wang SJ, Wang MB, Barauskas TM et al (2000) Surgical management of carotid body tumors. Otolaryngol Head Neck Surg 123:202–206
75. Hawthorne MR, Makek MS, Harris JP et al (1988) The histopathological and clinical features of irradiated and nonirradiated temporal paragangliomas. Laryngoscope 98: 325–331
76. Boedeker CC, Ridder GJ, Schipper J (2005) Paragangliomas of the head and neck: diagnosis and treatment. Fam Cancer 4:55–59
77. Persky MS, Setton A, Niimi Y, Hartman J, Frank D, Berenstein A (2002) Combined endovascular and surgical treatment of head and neck paragangliomas—a team approach. Head Neck 24:423–431
78. Chrisoulidou A, Kaltsas G, Ilias I, Grossman AB (2007) The diagnosis and management of malignant phaeochromocytoma and paraganglioma. Endocr Relat Cancer 14:569–585
79. Niemeijer ND, Rijken JA, Eijkelenkamp K et al (2017) The phenotype of SDHB germline mutation carriers: a nationwide study. Eur J Endocrinol 177920:115–125
80. Boedeker CC, Neumann HP, Maier W, Bausch B, Schipper J, Ridder GJ (2007) Malignant head and neck paragangliomas in SDHB mutation carriers. Otolaryngol Head Neck Surg 137:126–129
81. Nölting S, Grossman A, Pacak K (2019) Metastatic phaeochromocytoma: spinning towards more promising treatment options. Exp Clin Endocrinol Diabetes 127:117–128
82. Maithel SK, Fong Y (2009) Hepatic ablation for neuroendocrine tumor metastases. J Surg Oncol 100:635–638
83. Takahashi K, Ashizawa N, Minami T et al (1999) Malignant pheochromocytoma with multiple hepatic metastases treated by chemotherapy and transcatheter arterial embolization. Intern Med 38:349–354
84. Ilanchezhian M, Jha A, Pacak K, Del Rivero J (2020) Emerging treatments for advanced/metastatic pheochromocytoma and paraganglioma. Curr Treat Options Oncologia 21:85
85. Yound WF Jr, Iniguez-Ariza NM et al (2017) Malignant pheochromocytoma and paraganglioma: 272 patients over 55 years. J Clin Endocrinol Metab 102:3296–3305
86. Korevaar TI, Grossman AB (2011) Pheochromocytomas and paragangliomas: assessment of malignant potential. Endocrine 40:354–365
87. NGS in PPGL (NGSnPPGL) Study Group, Toledo RA, Burnichon N, Cascon A et al (2017) Consensus statement on next generation-sequencing-based diagnostic testing of hereditary phaeochromocytomas and paragangliomas. Nat Rev Endocrinol 13(4):233–247
88. van Gils AP, van der Mey AG, Hoogma RP et al (1992) MRI screening of kindred at risk of developing paragangliomas: support for genomic imprinting in hereditary glomus tumours. Br J Cancer 65:903–907
89. Hermsen MA, Sevilla MA, Llorente JL et al (2010) Relevance of germline mutation screening in both familial and sporadic head and neck paraganglioma for early diagnosis and clinical management. Cell Oncol 32:275–283
90. van Duinen N, Steenvoorden D, Bonsing BA et al (2010) Pheochromocytomas detected by biochemical screening in predisposed subjects are associated with lower prevalence of clinical and biochemical manifestations and smaller tumors than pheochromocytomas detected by signs and symptoms. Eur J Endocrinol 163:121–127
91. Gill AJ, Benn DE, Chou A et al (2010) Immunohistochemistry for SDHB triages genetic testing of SDHB, SDHC, and SDHD in paraganglioma-pheochromocytoma syndromes. Hum Pathol 41:805–814

92. van Nederveen FH, Gaal J, Favier J et al (2009) An immunohistochemical procedure to detect patients with paraganglioma and phaeochromocytoma with germline SDHB, SDHC, or SDHD gene mutations: a retrospective and prospective analysis. Lancet Oncol 10:764–771
93. Amar L, Pacak K, Steichen O et al (2021) International consensus on initial screening and follow-up of asymptomatic SDHx mutation carriers. Nat Rev Endocrinol 17:435–444

Surgical Approach in the Treatment of Neuroendocrine Neoplasms

26

P. Stålberg, P. Hellman, B. Klimácek, and O. Norlén

26.1 Classification

GEP-NENs are classified according to the WHO Classification of Digestive System Tumours 2019, IUCC's TNM classification of Malignant Tumours or ENETS TNM classification [1]. Moreover, GEP-NENs are by the WHO 2019 classifications graded as well-differentiated neuroendocrine neoplasms (NEN) grade 1, 2, 3 or poorly differentiated neuroendcrine carcinomas (NEC) [1]. Grade 1 neoplasms with a Ki-67 index ≤3%, or mitotic counts (MC) <2/10 high power fields (HPF); grade 2 neoplasms with Ki-67 index of 3–20%, or 2–20 MC/10 HPF; and grade 3 neoplasms with Ki-67 index >20%, or > 20 MC/10 HPF).

Distant metastases should be expected also in grade 1 NET with the lowest Ki67 index, but the progression is often less aggressive with the lower grade.

26.2 Diagnosis

Ultrasound (US)-guided fine-needle aspiration biopsy (FNAB) has been commonly used for cytologic diagnosis of primary and metastatic NENs. Formalin-fixed paraffin-embedded US guided semifine (1.2 mm) needle tissue biopsies, or surgical tumor specimens, are now routinely used for final diagnosis to allow appropriate diagnostic immunohistochemical staining, and evaluation of proliferation by Ki67 index, which has become the important parameter for grading [2]. Positive staining for either of the general neuroendocrine markers chromogranin A (CgA) or synaptophysin confirms the NEN diagnosis [3]. Other IHC markers such as thyroid

P. Stålberg (✉) · P. Hellman · B. Klimácek · O. Norlén
Department of Surgical Sciences, University Hospital, Uppsala, Sweden
e-mail: peter.stalberg@surgsci.uu.se; per.hellman@surgsci.uu.se; Branislav.klimacek@surgsci.uu.se; olov.norlen@surgsci.uu.se

S. Yalcin, K. Öberg (eds.), *Neuroendocrine Tumours*,
https://doi.org/10.1007/978-3-031-56968-5_26

transcription factor-1 (TTF-1), serotonin, CDX2, islet1, and vesicular monoamine transporter type 2 (VMAT2) may indicate the primary tumor site.

For poorly differentiated lesions chromogranin A staining may be variable and involve only subsets of cells, and synaptophysin reactivity more intense [3].

26.3 Biochemical Markers

Plasma chromogranin A (CgA) levels are sensitive and early markers for NENs with relation to tumor load and has been used to monitor effects of treatment [3–5]. However, CgA levels are unspecific as they are raised with all types of NENs and some non-endocrine malignancies (as prostate carcinoma). CgA values are also raised due to endocrine cell hyperplasia in chronic atrophic gastritis (CAG) (high levels), and in patients with renal, liver, or heart failure, stress, inflammatory bowel disease, and as result of chronic proton-pump inhibitor (PPI) therapy (moderately raised values). Chromogranin A decrease of $\geq$80% has predicted resolution of symptoms and disease stabilization, however, as it has been shown to be inadequate to fully predict tumor progression, it should be combined with radiology in tumor follow-up [6, 7]. Depending on the primary tumor and symptoms of the patient, measurement of specific markers, such as gastrin, insulin, c-peptide, pro-insulin, glucagon, VIP, somatostatin, ACTH, or calcitonin, should be performed. In small intestinal NENs (Si-NENs), raised levels of the serotonin metabolite 5-hydroxyindoleacetic acid (5HIAA) are often elevated and should be measured, preferably in blood [8], although urinary tests are also available [3]. False-positive elevation of 5-HIAA may be caused by tryptophan/serotonin-rich foods (bananas, avocados, plums, eggplant, chocolate, figs, tomatoes, pineapples, pecan nuts, walnuts, nicotin, and wine), which should be avoided prior to urine collection for the 5-HIAA measurements [3, 4].

26.4 Localisation and Radiology

Endoscopy is used to detect NENs in the oesophagus, stomach, duodenum, pancreas, and rectum. It may be complemented by **endoscopic ultrasonography (EUS)** to allow determination of submucosal invasion and presence of regional metastases for staging. EUS-guided biopsy can also be performed for diagnosis or approximation of Ki-67.

Percutaneous US with dynamic i.v. contrast enhancement has been sensitive for detection of liver metastases and commonly used to guide semi-fine or fine-needle biopsy for tissue sample [3].

Computed tomography (CT) with i.v. contrast enhancement is the most common method to detect NENs. Primary Si-NENs neoplasms are often too small to be visualized, though associated mesenteric metastases often show typical features. The presence of a circumscribed mesenteric mass with radiating densities due to fibrotic strands is highly suspicious of a Si-NENs mesenteric metastasis [3]. For optimal detection of liver metastases, 3-phase CT scans for arterial and venous portal phase studies are needed. Pancreatic NEN are generally hyperattenuating in contrast phases.

Magnetic resonance imaging (MRI) may be more sensitive than CT for detection of small liver metastases, with use of contrast, arterial phase and T-2 weighted images [3]. MRI during follow-up may reduce radiation exposure.

26.5 Functional Imaging

Somatostatin receptor scintigraphy (SRS), OctreoScan (with ^{111}indium pentreotide) has been the routine during primary investigations and follow-up of patients with NENs [9]; however, it has in most centers largely been replaced by positron emission tomography (PET). PET-imaging has been developed with specific radiotracers for NEN, including ^{11}C-5-hydroxytryptophan [^{11}C-5-HTP], ^{18}F-L-dihydroxy-phenyl-alanine [^{18}F-DOPA], and ^{64}Cu/^{68}Ga coupled to a somatostatin receptor analog (i.e. DOTATOC/DOTANOC) and combined with a fully diagnostic CT or MRI if needed and available [3, 4, 9]. These PET studies provide higher resolution and improved sensitivity compared to conventional SRS and has proved of considerable value in patients with NENs and negative or inconclusive results on SRS [3, 4, 10]. ^{68}Ga-DOTATOC/DOTANOC-PET/CT has shown the highest sensitivity and commonly been able to detect additional metastases, especially within the skeletal system (in >30%) [11], and established localization of unknown primary NENs in up to 39% of cases [4, 12]. In a recent study, ^{68}Ga-DOTATOC-PET/CT revealed additional hepatic or extra-hepatic metastases in ~50% of patient planned for liver resection or liver transplantation, which strongly impacted treatment decisions based on CT and/or MRI investigations, that had failed to reveal these additional metastases [13]. ^{18}F-DOPA-PET has also been efficient for visualization of Si-NENs [3]. ^{18}F-fluorodeoxyglucose (FDG)-PET imaging may be used to detect intermediate and high-grade NEN or poorly differentiated neuroendocrine carcinoma (NEC) (sensitivity of 92% with Ki-67 > 15%), but will often not visualize low-grade, well-differentiated lesions [14].

26.6 Specifics for NENs with Different Location

26.6.1 Esophageal NENs

Esophageal NENs are rare (<1% of all NENs) and reported to occur with male predominance at around 60 years of age [3, 15]. Symptoms are usually similar to adenocarcinoma with dysphagia and retro-sternal pain. Most tumors have been located in the lower third of the esophagus or in the gastro-esophageal junction. Most have been poorly differentiated small cell NEC, often with components of adenocarcinoma and with lymph node spread reported in 50% of patients. The tumors should only be operated if radical resection is possible, and preoperative chemo-radiation has been suggested to improve outcome. Survival depends on disease stage and has been overall poor [3, 15].

26.6.2 Gastric NENs

The WHO guidelines depict three groups of enterochromaffine cell-like (ECL)-cell derived gastric NENs, types 1, 2, and 3 [3]. The majority of gastric NENs, type 1 (70–80%), occurs in patients with hypergastrinemia due to chronic atrophic gastritis (CAG). Type 2 patients (5–8%) also have hypergastinemia, but due to a Zollinger Ellison syndrome (ZES) as part of a familial multiple endocrine neoplasia type 1 syndrome (MEN1). Type 3 gastric NENs (15–20%) occur as sporadic, solitary lesions in patients without hypergastrinemia. These type 3 neoplasms are often larger, more aggressive, and prone to metastazise.

26.6.3 Type 1 Gastric NENs

The type 1 NENs occur with female predominance (3:1 vs males) at a mean age of around 65 years [3, 4]. The tumors arise in patients with chronic atrophic gastritis (CAG) with hypo- or achlorhydria due to destruction of acid secreting parietal cells. CAG may be autoimmune or nonimmune. Hypergastrinemia occurs because gastrin-secreting G-cells of the antrum are not inhibited in absence of gastric acid. The excessive gastrin secretion will in combination with other predisposing factors, such as diet or possibly bacteria, further stimulate the ECL-cell hyperplasia and development of the ECL cell tumors. Hypergastrinemia alone does not appear to cause gastric NENs, as tumors occur in a minority of CAG patients, and not due to chronic PPI treatment or vagotomy [3, 15–17]. More than half of the patients have vitamin B12 malabsorption and pernicious anaemia, and in this population, the NENs have often been accidentally revealed by endoscopy, as the patients have generally been without symptoms. Although CAG is common in elderly individuals, only few patients (1%) with long duration of markedly raised serum gastrin values develop gastric NENs. The NENs will typically occur as multiple (60%), small polyps in the gastric body and fundus, or in the transitional zone to the antrum, developing in a surrounding atrophic mucosa where ECL cell hyperplasia and dysplasia can be detected. Individual tumors can present as broad-based, round polypoid lesions, some can be flat and broad, or appear as discolored spots or slight mucosal protrusions. The number and size vary from uncountable pinpoint size to few prominent lesions measuring up to 1–1.5 cm, and uncommonly up to 2 cm or more [3, 16]. Some are solitary and may be difficult to distinguish from adenopolyps, which also occur in CAG patients. Only rare larger lesions may be ulcerated or bleeding. The small type 1 gastric NENs are benign with low proliferation (grade 1), and low risk of invasion beyond the submucosa. Larger lesions (>1 cm) are also predominantly benign, but may occasionally invade the muscularis propria (<10%) or have higher grade. The incidence of regional lymph node metastases is low

(<2–5%), distant liver metastases are exceptional (<2%), and disease related death is rare, though earlier reports with greater proportion of larger lesions described more frequent metastases [3, 16, 17].

26.6.4 Type 2 Gastric NENs

ECL cell hyperplasia can be detected in 80% of MEN1 patients with ZES, and 5–30% of MEN1-ZES patients develop the type 2 gastric NENs [3, 15, 17]. The patients have high gastric acid secretion and present with typical increased mucosa thickness in contrast to the distinct atrophy of type 1 lesions. Patients with sporadic ZES may also often exhibit ECL cell hyperplasia, but rarely (<1%) develop gastric NENs. Type 2 gastric NENs occur in the gastric body and fundus and occasionally in the antrum [11, 20, 22]. They are also often multiple and usually small (<1–2 cm), but generally larger than type 1 tumours, and occasionally markedly larger in size, of up to 4–5 cm or more. The biopsies from the surrounding gastric mucosa show hypertrophy rather than atrophy. The tumor grade may be 1 or 2, and the malignant potential is intermediate between CAG associated and sporadic gastric NENs. Lymph node metastases occur in ~30% of patients and liver metastases in 10–20% [3, 17]. More aggressive tumors with liver metastases and higher grade have been more frequent with long-standing ZES. Poorly differentiated gastric NECs with local invasion, angioinvasion, and high proliferation rate have occasionally been associated with MEN1.

26.6.5 Type 3 Sporadic Gastric NENs

The type 3 sporadic gastric NENs occur in patients with normal serum gastrin. The tumors are most common in males, with a mean age around 50 years [3, 15–17]. Determination of serum calcium and the family history helps exclude MEN1. A majority of patients have symptoms as with gastric adenocarcinoma with pain, weight loss and gastrointestinal bleeding.

The majority of type 3 NENs occur in the gastric body and fundus as solitary, often large tumors, usually >2 cm (Fig. 26.1), occasional tumors occur in the antral or prepyloric region [3, 15, 17]. The tumors develop in non-atrophic gastric mucosa, without ECL-cell proliferation, most tumours originate in ECL cells. Uncommon forms generally occurring in the antrum may originate from G (gastrin) cells or constitute a mixture of EC (serotonin) cells and other cell types and then be associated with worse prognosis. Most G cell tumors have sparse staining for gastrin. Tumors with intense gastrin reactivity are rare in the stomach, but can occur in the prepyloric mucosa and represent an exceptional cause of hypergastriemia and ZES.

Two thirds of type 3 neoplasms have infiltrated the muscularis layer and 50% have invaded all layers of the gastric wall. Regional lymph node metastases may be present in 20–50%, also with small tumours, and liver metastases eventually develop in two-thirds of the patients [3, 15]. The sporadic gastric NENs can have atypical

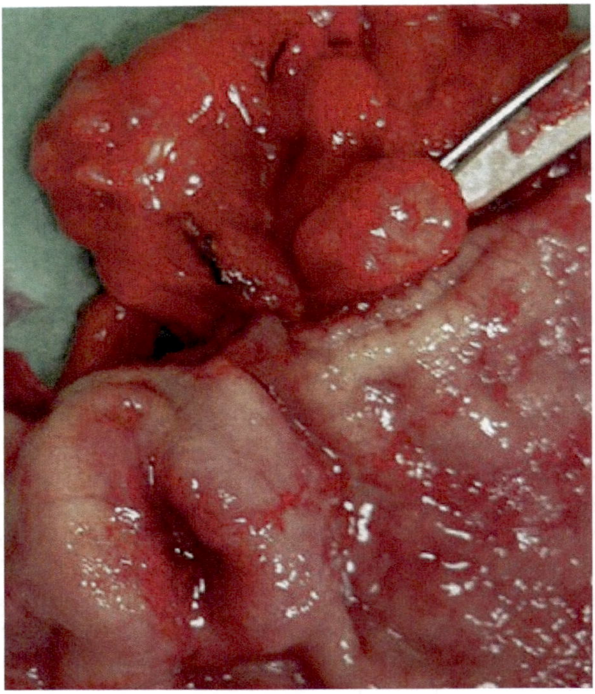

Fig. 26.1 Sporadic, solitary gastric NEN with lymph node metastasis removed by gastric resection. (From Åkerstrom G, et al. (2009) Gastrointestinal carcinoids. In Endocrine Surgery, fourth edn, pp. 147–176. Ed T Lennard. London: Saunders Elsevier)

histology, with pleomorphism, high mitosis rate, and high Ki67 index. The atypical tumours are larger, with mean size around 5 cm, more frequently invasive and have unfavorable survival [3].

26.6.6 Atypical Carcinoid Syndrome

The ECL cells have the ability to secrete histamine and disseminated lesions of type 3 gastric NENs may in 5–10% be associated with an "atypical carcinoid syndrome". The syndrome can occur also in exceptional patients with disseminated type 1 and 2 neoplasms [3]. The syndrome has a patchy "geographic" flush, urticarial rash, cutaneous edema, mucous membrane swelling, bronchospasm, salivary gland swelling, and lacrimation. Since the syndrome is caused by histamine release from tumour cells, urinary estimates of the histamine metabolite methylmidazol-acetic acid (MelmAA) serve as tumor marker. Most gastric NENs lack the enzyme L-amino acid decarboxylase, and few patients have elevated serotonin levels. Owing to this decarboxylation defect, the patients will have only minimal elevation of urinary 5-HIAA values [3].

26.7 Diagnosis

Diagnosis of CAG-related type 1 NENs is based on demonstration of high serum gastrin levels, lack of gastric acid secretion with high pH in gastric aspirate (pH > 3 in the gastric aspirate excludes ZES), and confirmation of mucosal atrophy together with ECL cell hyperplasia in endoscopic biopsies from the antrum (2 biopsies) and fundus (4 biopsies) [3]. Basal and pentagastrin stimulated gastric acid secretion studies is recommended. Endoscopy is used to evaluate multiplicity and size of the gastric NENs. Tumor biopsies should be stained with endocrine tumor markers (chromogranin A, synaptophycin, and VMAT2) and proliferation markers (Ki67 index) [3]. Multiple NENs in the gastric fundus in an elderly are most likely to represent CAG-associated NENs.

Diagnosis of MEN1-associated type 2 gastric NENs and ZES is based on demonstration of low gastric pH, raised basal acid output in gastric acid secretion studies, generally together with markedly raised gastrin levels [3]. Serum gastrin >1000 pg/m is diagnostic of ZES if gastric pH <2. The important differential diagnosis is CAG, where patients have high gastrin, without gastric acid (with high gastric pH, and pH > 3 excludes ZES). Biochemical screening for other MEN1 endocrinopathies includes measurements of serum calcium and parathyroid hormone, pituitary hormones (prolactin and insulin-like growth factor 1, IGF-1), and pancreatic hormones and CgA [3]. MEN1 genetic testing is done if the familial disease is not previously recognized.

Diagnosis of the type 3 gastric NENs is essentially settled by verifying absence of hypergastrinemia.

Radiology is generally not needed in type 1 gastric NENs without signs of spread. CT with contrast enhancement (3-phase) and functional studies (often ^{68}Ga-DOTATOC-PET/CT) are used to determine metastatic spread in type 2 and 3 NENs [3]. For type 3 lesions with higher proliferation FDG-PET may also be of value. EUS may be added to the endoscopic examination in type 1 and 2 lesions larger than 1 cm and some type 3 lesions to provide information about invasion and the depth and may reveal regional lymph node metastases (and possibly pancreatico-duodenal lesions in MEN1 patients).

26.8 Surgical Treatment

Type 1 gastric NENs < 1 cm are generally indolent and can be followed with yearly endoscopic surveillance [3, 4, 16, 17]. Neoplasms >1 cm, or multiple lesions without invasion can be treated with endoscopic mucosal resection or endoscopic submucosal resection [4, 18]. Few large invasive neoplasms require local surgical excision, and only rare larger, multifocal lesions need gastric resection [3, 16, 19]. Antrectomy combined with tumor excision may be considered in type 1 cases with invasion and repeated recurrence, but the effect on remaining clinically significant lesions may be limited [3, 16]. Treatment with somatostatin analogues has been associated with time-limited regression of type 1 lesions, but disease progression has been noted at follow-up 5 years after termination of therapy [4, 20–22].

Surgical treatment in type 2 gastric NENs is focused on removing the source of hypergastrinaemia, generally by excision of duodenal gastrinomas via duodenotomy, together with clearance of lymph node metastases (see below) [16, 17, 19]. The type 2 gastric NENs per se require endoscopic or surgical excision that should be radical. Gastric resection or gastrectomy combined with regional lymph node clearance is recommended for larger, and multifocal neoplasms, or those with deep gastric wall invasion or angioinvasion [16, 17]. If hypergastrinemia has not been reversed by surgery for gastrinoma, somatostatin analog treatment may be used to reduce tumor growth, especially in cases with multiple gastric NENs, though proton-pump inhibitors is most often the suggested therapy [20, 23, 24].

The type 3 sporadic gastric carcinoids should be radically treated with gastric resection and regional lymph node clearance. Tumors larger than 2 cm, and those with atypical histology or gastric wall invasion, are most appropriately treated with gastrectomy and nodal dissection [3, 4, 16, 17]. Endoscopic resection is only occasionally performed for small non-metastasized tumors [3, 4]. The overall 5-year survival for patients with type 3 lesions has been ~50%, but only 10% in cases with distant metastases [3, 4].

26.8.1 Gastrinoma

Tumors with sparse staining for gastrin may occur in association with CAG. Tumors with intense staining for gastrin are rare in the stomach and have been located in the prepyloric mucosa close to the duodenum. Few gastric NENs have caused hypergastrinaemia and peptic ulcer disease, but they still represent an exceptional but possible origin of gastrin excess and ZES [3]. Rare tumors may present with ectopic Cushing's syndrome due to ACTH secretion [3].

26.9 Duodenal NENs

NENs of the duodenum are rare and comprise less than 2% of all GEP-NENs [3, 25, 26]. Duodenal adenomas or adenocarcinomas are more frequent. Duodenal NENs comprise gastrinomas (48%) (not described here, see Chap. 13), somatostatinomas (44%), nonfunctioning tumors, staining for serotonin (28%), or calcitonin (9%), and rare gangliocytic paragangliomas or carcinomas [3, 25, 26]. The duodenal NENs generally present in the sixth decade of life. The majority (>90%) occurs in the first and second part of the duodenum, 20% in the periampullary region. The tumors are characteristically small (<1.5 cm), most are T1, but lymph node metastases have been reported to occur in around 50% and liver metastases in <10%.

26.9.1 Somatostatin-Rich NENs

NENs with somatostatin reactivity occur in the ampullary or periampullary region, almost exclusively in the ampulla of Vater, may cause obstructive jaundice, pancreatitis, or bleeding [3, 25, 27]. A clinical somatostatinoma syndrome is very rare. The tumors appear as 1–2 cm homogeneous ampulla nodules, which only occasionally are polypoid, larger, or ulcerated. Regional lymph node or liver metastases are present in nearly 50% of patients. Unlike conventional NENs, the tumors have a glandular growth pattern and may characteristically contain special laminated psammoma bodies. The lesions may be associated with von Recklinghausen's neurofibromatosis (neurofibromatosis type 1, NF1) and occasionally with pheochromocytoma [3, 25, 27]. The ampullary somatostatin-rich NENs may be locally excised, together with clearance of regional lymph glands, but since there is no established correlation between tumor size and metastases, pancreatico-duodenectomy has been recommended in younger patients [3, 25].

26.9.2 Gangliocytic Paragangliomas

Gangliocytic paragangliomas are rare tumors, occurring almost exclusively in the second portion of the duodenum, and are sometimes associated with NF1 [3, 25]. The tumors consist of a mixture of paraganglioma, ganglioneuroma, and NEN tissue, with reactivity for somatostatin and pancreatic polypeptide (PP). The tumors may be recognized incidentally or because of bleeding. They may be large but are generally benign and often have an excellent prognosis following surgical excision [3, 25].

26.9.3 Other Duodenal NENs

More unusual NENs have reactivity for other hormones, such as calcitonin, PP, and serotonin [3, 25, 28, 29]. Most of these tumors occur as small polyps (<2 cm) in the proximal duodenum. Multiple tumors should raise suspicion of an associated MEN 1 syndrome. The majority are low-grade malignant and often suitable for endocopic mucosal resection or local surgical excision, only rare large tumors require pancreatico-duodenectomy [3, 25, 28, 29].

A distinct group of duodenal NENs without release or staining for hormones is also recognised. These tumors have a somewhat different biology and have less often metastasized than the gastrinomas and somatostatinomas [3, 25, 28–30]. Some are asymptomatic and incidentally found at endoscopy, others present with nonspecific abdominal symptoms, gastrointestinal bleeding, and sometimes with vomiting or weight loss. Most tumors are located in the first portion of the duodenum, occasionally in the second part and rarely in the third portion (horizontal duodenum). The majority stains for chromogranin A, and some for synaptophysin and/or NSE [3, 28–30]. Up to one-third of the patients have had other primary malignancies as well, including adenocarcinomas of the gastrointestinal tract, prostate, or other organs [3, 25, 28–30]. More than half of the tumors are smaller than 2 cm and generally have a good prognosis after resection. Lesions smaller than 1 cm can be endoscopically excised, but re-examination with follow-up endoscopy is required to ensure complete removal. Size >2 cm, invasion beyond the submucosa, or presence of mitotic figures, are independent risk factors for metastases (Grade 2 tumors). Tumors with these risk factors are likely to recur also after apparently curative surgery, even if no lymph node metastases have been detected, whereas lesions smaller than 2 cm rarely metastasize [3, 28–30]. Rare duodenal neoplasms may cause an ectopic Cushing's syndrome due to ACTH secretion [25].

The treatment suggested for larger tumors is segmental duodenal resection or pancreatico-duodenectomy in order to decrease the risk of recurrence [3, 28–30]. Periampullary tumors behave in malignant fashion and need more radical surgery. Patients with metastasizing duodenal NENs may survive for decades, substantiating that NENs are less aggressive than adenocarcinomas.

26.9.4 Poorly Differentiated Duodenal Neuroendocrine Carcinomas (NEC)

NEC (large or small cell) in the duodenum are exceptionally rare, occurring most often in the ampulla of Vater, and the patients present with obstructive jaundice, and most often with a rapidly fatal course [3, 28–30].

26.9.5 Pancreatic NENs

(Pancreatic islet cell neoplasms are reported in Chap. X). Exceptional PNEN stain intensely for serotonin (and may also contain other biogenic amines) [3, 29]. They appear histologically as classical GEP-NENs, but few have been associated with the carcinoid syndrome. The tumors are managed surgically according to guidelines similar to those for nonfunctioning malignant pancreatic NENs. Hepatic metastases and a carcinoid syndrome may be treated with somatostatin analogs and interferon, or with chemotherapy in the presence of higher proliferation rate [3, 29].

26.10 Jejuno-Ileal Small Intestinal Neuroendocrine Neoplasms (Si-NENs)

The jejuno-ileal, small intestinal neurodoctrine neoplasms (Si-NENs), also named "classical" midgut carcinoids, originate from intestinal enterochromaffin (EC) cells in intestinal crypts, and can be recognized by typical tumor cell serotonin immunoreactivity. Carcinoids may be detected in up to 1/150 of routine autopsies, indicating that the tumors may remain silent throughout life [31, 32]. The Si-NENs are the most common cause of the carcinoid syndrome and have therefore often prevailed at referral centers, with possibility to offer combined medical and surgical treatment [3, 15]. The Si-NENs account for >75% of small-bowel neoplasms and have been diagnosed with slight male predominance at a mean age of 65 years.

The primary Si-NENs occur most often in the distal ileum, within 60–80 cm of the ileocecal valve, less often in the proximal ileum or the jejunum. Occasional tumors in the cecum with serotonin immunoreactivity are classified as Si-NENs [3, 15, 33, 34]. The primary tumor is typically a small, flat, and fibrotic submucosal lesion; occasional tumors may be polypoid and fungating [3, 35]. The tumors may be difficult to detect at surgery, often appearing only as a localized fibrosis or thickening of the intestinal wall (Fig. 26.2a), but may even with minimal fibrosis cause intestinal obstruction (Fig. 26.2b) [3, 35, 36]. More than 30% of patients subjected to surgery have multiple, submucosal tumor nodules in the small intestinal wall close to the primary tumor [3, 35, 36], and rare cases have had additional tumors in the proximal intestine, possibly representing additional primary tumors [3, 35, 37]. When growing close to the intestinal wall the metastases may be easily mistaken to represent primary tumors, and some primaries have extended directly into node metastases [3, 35, 37]. The mesenteric metastases have often grown larger than the primary tumor and evoked a desmoplastic reaction with pronounced mesenteric fibrosis (Fig. 26.3). The fibrosis may be because of local effects of serotonin, growth factors, and other substances released from the Si-NEN metastases [3, 37–39].

Larger metastases and more extensive fibrosis have often caused mesentery contraction and tethered the mesenteric root to the retroperitoneum, with fibrous binding to the horizontal duodenum [3, 35, 37]. The mesenteric tumors may extend high in the mesenteric root and may sometimes grow into the duodenal wall, into the pancreas, or spread to the hepatoduodenal ligament or to the retroperitoneum/and para-aortal space [3, 35, 37, 40]. The fibrotic adhesions will kink and entrap the intestines and cause partial or complete small bowel obstruction and at advanced stage occasionally duodenal obstruction [3, 35, 37, 40]. With extended mesenteric tumor growth and fibrosis, mesenteric vessels may be encased, and intestinal

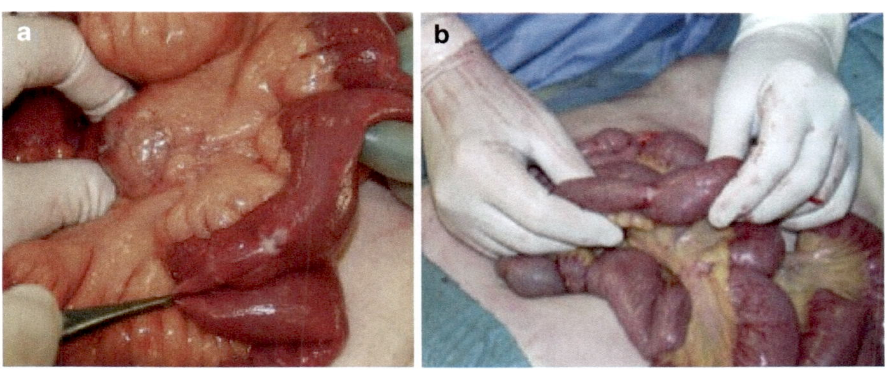

Fig. 26.2 (**a**) Si-NEN primary tumor visible as a localized fibrotic thickening of the intestinal wall; (**b**) Si-NEN primary tumor with minimal fibrosis causing partial intestinal obstruction

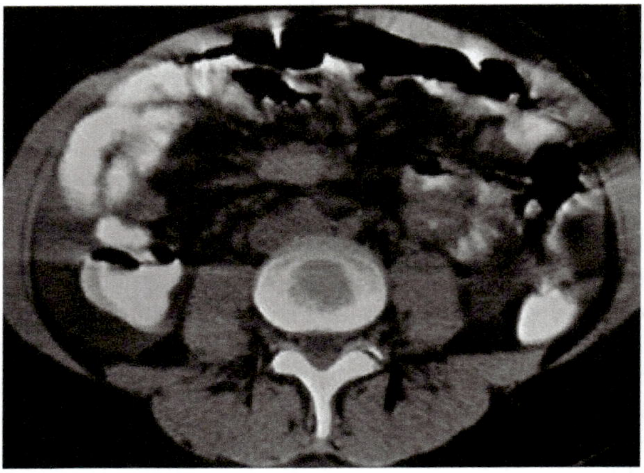

Fig. 26.3 CT image of a mesenteric metastasis from a Si-NEN surrounded by fibrosis (appearing like a "hurricane centre"). (From Åkerström G, et al. (2001) Midgut and hindgut carcinoid tumors. In: Doherty GM, Skogseid B (eds) Surgical endocrinology, first edn. Philadelphia: Lippincott Williams & Wilkins; pp. 448–52)

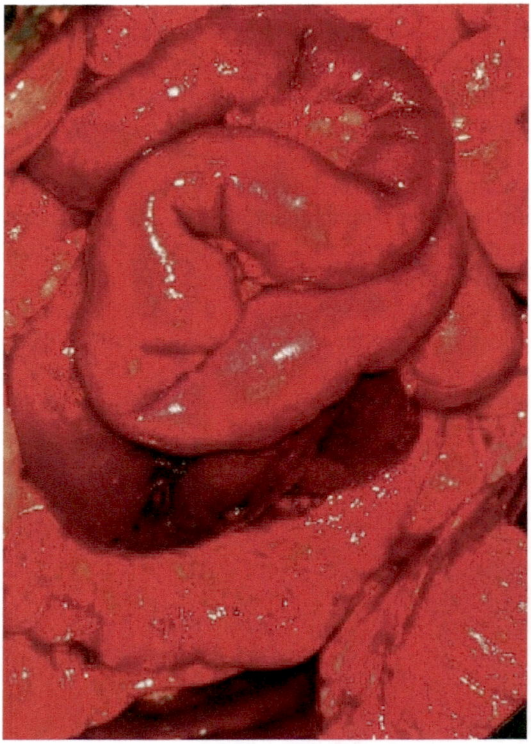

Fig. 26.4 Limited intestinal segment with venous ischemia due to Si-NEN mesenteric tumor. (From Åkerström G, et al. (2001) Midgut and hindgut carcinoid tumors. In: Doherty GM, Skogseid B (eds) Surgical endocrinology, first edn. Philadelphia: Lippincott Williams & Wilkins, 2001; pp. 448–52)

segments of variable length will appear blue-reddish due to incipient venous ischemia (Fig. 26.4). The patient may experience diarrhea, or functional obstruction, and occasionally abdominal angina [3, 35, 37, 40, 41]. A specific angiopathy, named vascular elastosis, with elastic tissue proliferation in the adventitia and marked thickening of mesenteric vessel walls has been reported with advanced Si-NENs [3, 42], though in our experience tumor compression and fibrosis has been the obvious cause of intestinal ischemia [3, 35, 36].

Cases with higher mesenteric root tumors and central mesenteric vein or artery occlusion may have longer involved intestinal segments with blue pale cyanosis or occasionally absent arterial circulation (Fig. 26.5). If the tumor and fibrosis has remained for longer time, bowel adhesions and kinking have often created a conglomerate of intestinal loops fixed to the abdominal walls, which sometimes need to be removed en bloc [3, 35, 37]. The incidence of mesenteric metastases at time of diagnosis has been at least 35% in reports based on imaging studies [43]. In operative series, the incidence of gross and microscopic mesenteric metastases has been as high as 70–90%, and have occurred in high frequency also with small primary Si-NENs, and microscopic spread has been almost invariably present (in contrast to GI-NENs at other sites) [3, 35, 37].

In a large series of Si-NEN patients, 93% of operated patients had mesenteric metastases at operation [33]. Distant metastases in retroperitoneal/ paraaortal location or more occasionally in the hepaticoduodenal ligament were identified in 18% of patients. Liver metastases were present at diagnosis or discovered at operation in 61% of patients and occurred during follow-up in an additional 99 patients (16%) [33]. The majority of patients had bilateral and multiple liver metastases; around 14% had fewer than 5 metastases in one liver lobe, occasional metastases were dominant with conspicuous growth [33]. Around 10% of patients presented with liver metastases without identified mesenteric lesions. Peritoneal carcinomatosis was revealed in 20% of operated patients, ovarian metastases in 4%, and pancreatic or splenic metastases each occurred in 0.5% [33]. Extra-abdominal spread to lymph nodes occurred at diagnosis in 4.0%, to other sites in 6.1% including bone, breast, and skin [33]. Many patients had multiple sites of extra-abdominal spread, most often to mediastinal and peripheral lymph nodes (including neck lymph glands, which occasionally was the first presentation) and bone [33]. During follow-up of this series, another 12% developed extra-abdominal spread [33]. In other series, especially bone metastases have been associated with poor prognosis [34, 44].

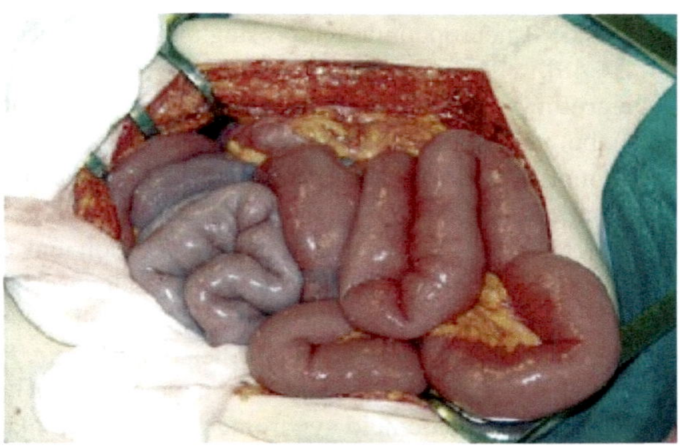

Fig. 26.5 Longer ischemic intestinal segment with compromized mesenteric vein and artery circulation, due to a high Si-NEN mesenteric tumor

26.10.1 Clinical Symptoms

Many patients with Si-NENs have experienced long periods of unspecific episodic abdominal pain, and diarrhea, often misinterpreted as irritable bowel syndrome or food allergy before the disease has been clinically diagnosed [4, 35, 37, 45]. Others have had unrecognized features of the carcinoid syndrome with discrete flush misinterpreted as menopausal complaints, or palpitations and intolerance for specific food or alcohol [4, 35, 36, 46]. Intestinal bleeding has generally been rare with Si-NENs due to the submucosal location of the primary tumor and has been more likely to occur with the more rare larger, polypoid, fungating primary tumors [3, 35, 37]. Bleeding may also occur when mesenteric metastases have grown into the horizontal duodenum, or in the presence of intestinal venous stasis and incipient ischemia [3, 35, 37]. Intermittent pain attacks have been common and often increased in frequency until the patient has developed subacute or acute intestinal obstruction requiring surgery. In around 50% of patients, the Si-NEN diagnosis has becomes evident after needle biopsy of liver metastases [3, 35, 37].

26.11 Carcinoid Syndrome

The carcinoid syndrome, described in 1954 by Thorson, has been reported to occur in approximately 20% of patients with jejuno-ileal NENs, though the frequency may be higher at referral centers [3, 32–36, 47]. The syndrome includes flushing, diarrhea, right-sided heart valve disease, and bronchoconstriction. Serotonin (5-hydroxytryptamine), derived from the amino acid tryptophan, has been identified as the major cause of the syndrome [3, 4, 34, 37]. Serotonin is inactivated by monoamine oxidase in the liver and in the kidney converted to 5-HIAA, which is excreted in urine. Presence of the carcinoid syndrome generally implies that the patient has liver metastases, with secretion directly into the systemic circulation [3, 34, 37]. Occasionally, the syndrome may occur in patients with large retroperitoneal or ovarian lesions, where the secretion exceeds the capacity of the monoamine detoxification, or can bypass the liver and drain directly into the systemic circulation [3, 34, 37]. The syndrome is related to release also of other vasoactive factors tachykinins (substance P, neuropeptide K), prostaglandins, and occasionally norepinephrine [3, 34, 37, 48].

Secretory diarrhea is the most common feature of the syndrome (reported in 73%), but may initially be mild and unspecific. Diarrhea tends to be most prevalent in the morning and is often meal related. The diarrhea may have other causes in NEN patients, especially when previously operated upon, or having advanced disease [3, 35, 37]. A distal small intestinal resection may cause moderate diarrhea due to removal of the intestinal segment for bile salt absorption; treatment with bile acid binding agents (cholestyramin) may provide relief. Somatostatin analogs in high doses may cause malabsorption diarrhea, with foamy, floating diarrhea after meals, which can be treated with pancreatic enzymes (Creon). Patients with long-standing poorly controlled carcinoid syndrome may develop niacin deficiency and pellagra, a syndrome consisting of diarrhea, dementia, and dermatitis, which can be prevented by niacin supplementation. Other causes are a short bowel, or partial intestinal obstruction. In patients with large mesenteric tumors, intestinal venous stasis or ischemia may contribute significantly to stool frequency. Occlusion of main mesenteric vein branches may cause severe watery diarrhea and malnutrition because of severely edematous, fluid-leaking intestinal segments of variable length [3, 35, 37, 49, 50].

Cutaneous flushing (reported in 65%) affects the face, neck, and upper chest and is the most characteristic feature of the carcinoid syndrome [3, 35, 37, 46, 50]. Flushing may nevertheless easily be overlooked, especially in females at menopause. The flush may be provoked by stress, alcohol, certain food, aged cheese, or coffee. It is often of short duration, lasting for 1–5 min, but may occasionally be prolonged for hours or even days. Flushing may occasionally be severe, and with longstanding flush the patients may develop telangiectasies and persistent blue-cyanotic discoloration of the skin on the nose and chins.

Heart valve fibrosis, with plaque-like fibrotic endocardial thickening affecting the tricuspid and pulmonary valves, is a late consequence of a severe and longstanding carcinoid syndrome with high serotonin levels [3, 34, 37, 51–53]. This will lead to retraction and fixation of the heart valves and subsequently regurgitation and stenosis. Serotonin (and possibly tachykinins) may influence the heart and cause fibrosis and valvular thickening with retraction and thickening of heart valves leading to tricuspid regurgitation and pulmonary valve stenosis. Tricuspid valve abnormalities were in one series reported in 65% of patients with the carcinoid syndrome, and 19% had pulmonary valve stenosis [53]. In less than 10%, the fibrosis may involve also the left-sided heart valves, in case of a patent oval foramen, or when the pulmonary monoamine oxidase activity is exceeded, and then possibly contribute to bronchoconstriction.

The carcinoid heart disease may lead to progressive right-sided heart failure and severe lethargy and used to be the cause of death in 50% of patients with the carcinoid syndrome [3, 32, 40, 51–53]. Nowadays, after introduction of somatostatin analogs, patients more often die from progressive tumor disease. Affected patients may require heart surgery and prostheses replacement of fibrotic heart valves [51, 53]. The operation may lead to substantial improvement, but can especially in older persons be associated with complications [53]. The heart disease is efficiently diagnosed by echocardiography, which should invariably be performed prior to major abdominal surgery.

Bronchial constriction as part of the carcinoid syndrome caused by small intestinal NENs is relatively rare, but may occur during anesthesia.

26.11.1 Imaging

The primary Si- NENs generally escape detection by conventional **bowel contrast studies or CT images** because of limited size [43]. Typical arcading of entrapped intestines, with segments of partial obstruction, may be revealed with advanced disease, and occasionally the signs of chronic obstruction, with edematous thickened bowel wall. In the presence of large-bowel symptoms, entrapment of the sigmoid or transverse colon may be important to identify prior to surgery.

CT can rarely visualize a primary Si-NEN, but will often reveal mesenteric lymph node metastases, retroperitoneal extension of such masses, and liver metastases. The presence of a circumscribed mesenteric mass with radiating densities is highly suspicious for an Si-NEN mesenteric metastasis [43]. Contrast-enhanced **CT** is important prior to operation, by possibility to reveal relation between the mesenteric metastases and the main mesenteric vessels [3, 37]. In cases with intestinal ischemia, CT may show a characteristic image of dilated peripheral veins and edematous loops of intestine (Fig. 26.6). CT with contrast enhancement is often the primary method for visualization of liver metastases, but fail to identify the smallest lesions. **MRI** can sometimes be more efficient than CT for demonstration of liver metastases [43]. **Percutaneous US** with power Doppler enhancement and use of US contrast may increase sensitivity for detection of liver metastases and is mainly used to visualize liver metastases, and to guide fine or semi-fine-needle biopsy of liver or mesenteric metastases for histological diagnosis and grading.

26.11.1.1 Positron Emission Tomography (PET)

In nearly 90% of cases, Si-NENs possess somatostatin receptors types 2 and 5, for which the somatostatin analogs octreotide has high affinity [3, 15, 37]. Somatostatin receptor scintigraphy, SRS (OctreoScan®), detects small intestinal NENs with a sensitivity of 90% and has been commonly utilized to determine metastatic spread; however, it has now largely been replaced by positron emission tomography (PET) [43]. ^{68}Ga-PET or PET with the serotonin precursor 5-hydroxytryptophan, labeled with ^{11}C (5HTP-PET), may identify the Si-NENs with a very high sensitivity and has been increasingly used to diagnose stage and monitor effects of therapy [3, 13, 37, 43, 54]. ^{68}Ga-DOTATOC PET/CT reveals additional hepatic or extrahepatic metastases in more than 60% of patient planned for liver resection or liver

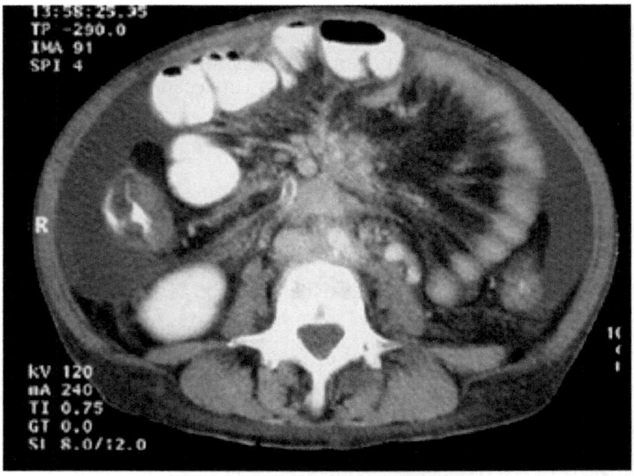

Fig. 26.6 CT image of Si-NEN case with intestinal ischemia showing mesenteric tumor surrounded by dilated peripheral mesenteric veins

transplantation, which may impact treatment decisions based on CT and/or MRI investigations that had failed to reveal these additional metastases [13]. In our institution, a baseline ^{68}Ga-DOTATOC-PET/CT is performed invariably in all Si-NENs. FDG-PET imaging may be used to detect intermediate and high-grade and poorly differentiated (NECs) (sensitivity of 92% with Ki-67 > 15%), but will not usually not visualize grade 1 or 2 lesions with lower proliferation [14, 43].

26.11.2 Diagnosis

Needle biopsy specimens from metastases are often used for diagnosis. The NEN cells stain immunocytochemically with neuroendocrine tumor markers, mainly chromogranin A, and synaptophysin, and reactivity with serotonin-specific antisera implies that a primary tumor should be searched for in the midgut [3, 15, 37]. Most jejuno-ileal NENs show a mixed insular and glandular growth pattern; occasional tumors have a pure insular and trabecular pattern and have been reported to have slightly less favorable prognosis [3, 15]. Proliferation rate determined with the Ki-67/MIB antibody is often very low <2% in classical Si-NENs. Occasional tumors have higher proliferation rate (grade 2) or may change to higher grade during the disease course [3, 15]. Rare lesions present as Si-NEC with poorly differentiated pattern and high proliferation rate with poor prognosis and sparse effects of surgery.

26.11.3 Surgery

Since Si-NENs patients may be subjected to acute laparotomy due to abdominal pain or intestinal obstruction with unknown diagnosis, it is important that surgeons in general learn that the Si-NENs are common small-bowel neoplasms and also learn to recognize the typical features of a small ileal tumor and conspicuously larger mesenteric metastases with surrounding fibrosis [3, 35, 37, 40, 41, 55, 56]. Since an intestinal by-pass may complicate more radical surgery, the locoregional tumor should if possible be removed by mesenteric wedge resection and limited intestinal resection, with clearance of lymph node metastases around the mesenteric artery and vein branches [3, 41]. The procedure is generally justified also in patients with distant metastases where R0 resection may be achieved and in patients with symptoms from a resectable mesenteric mass. In asymptomatic patients with unresectable metastatic disease, upfront surgery of the primary tumor is questionable, and standard oncologic treatment with surgery if symptoms develop seems to yield equal results in terms of survival [57]. If the primary tumor surgery has been inadequately performed, reoperation for removal of a remaining mesenteric tumor may be considered in all patients where R0 is deemed possible, as the patient may otherwise risk future abdominal complications [3, 35, 37, 40, 41, 56]. If grossly radical locoregional tumor removal has been accomplished, the Si-NENs patients often remain symptom free for long periods from treatment with somatostatin analogs. However, the Si-NENs are markedly tenacious and recurrence with liver metastases should be expected in the vast majority of patients (60–80%) if follow-up is long enough [3, 35, 37, 40, 41, 56]. Since the Si-NENs are slow-growing tumors, clinically overt recurrence may occur after long duration of up to 10–25 years [3, 37, 41, 56]. Recurrence may be diagnosed by serum chromogranin A, 5-HIAA measurements, or imaging.

Many Si-NENs patients present with liver metastases and sometimes also features of the carcinoid syndrome. Life expectancy used to be poor in patients with liver metastases and the carcinoid syndrome, now symptoms may be efficiently controlled with somatostatin analogs, which together with earlier detection of disease and other treatment modalities have markedly increased life expectancy and life quality [3, 37, 41, 56]. The carcinoid heart disease used to be a principal death cause in Si-NENs patients, together with abdominal complications, which played a significant role in 40% of patients [3, 56]. Possibly due to treatment with efficient biotherapy, the heart disease has become less common, and some patients now die with the disease rather than from the disease. Wide spread malignancy, liver failure, or bowel ischemia/obstruction are common causes of death after an extended disease course [3, 34, 56, 57].

Abdominal pain is unlikely to be caused merely by the carcinoid syndrome, and complications of the mesenteric tumor are important to recognize since considerable long-term palliation may be achieved by appropriate surgery [3, 55, 56]. Incipient venous ischemia may both cause diarrhea or functional obstruction. The authors advocate liberal surgical consultations when abdominal symptoms occur during periods of medical treatment [3, 56]. Too late surgical consultation may allow the disease to be increasingly difficult or impossible to manage surgically.

26.11.3.1 Surgical Technique for Removal of Mesenteric Metastases

The extension below or above the horizontal duodenum (as can be depicted with coronal CT) is crucial for preoperative evaluation, as this can determine if metastases are regional, or located high in the mesenteric root (Fig. 26.7). At operation, the advanced Si-NENs may appear inoperable, if high mesenteric metastases with surrounding fibrosis appear to encase the mesenteric root and the major intestinal vascular supply [3, 35, 37, 41, 56]. Incautious wedge resection in the fibrotic and contracted mesentery may risk to seriously compromise the intestinal circulation. It is recommended to begin with palpation of the small bowel from the Treitz ligament to the caecum, to identify the primary tumor, exclude presence of multiple intestinal tumors, and allow judgment of the length of the small intestine that needs to be removed. Ischemic changes and venous stasis can be found to comprise limited intestinal segments, and the locoregional tumor can then be safely removed by a common distal ileal resection. This may be combined with cecal resection or right hemicolectomy, with proximal vascular ligature, and extended wedge resection for improved clearance of regional metastases [34]. For tumors originating in the proximal intestine, segmental small intestinal resection is performed.

With advanced growth of bulky mesenteric tumors with higher location in the mesenteric root, above the horizontal duodenum, the management can be more complex (Fig. 26.8) [3, 37, 41, 56]. The majority of these metastases originate from

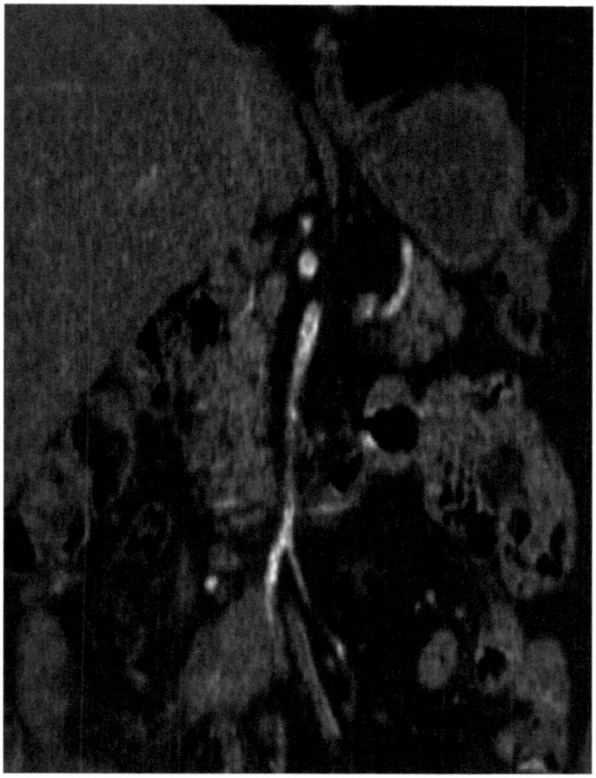

Fig. 26.7 The extension below or above the horizontal duodenum (depicted with coronal CT) is crucial for evaluation of operability of an Si-NEN mesenteric metastasis, as this can determine if metastases are regional, or located high in the mesenteric root

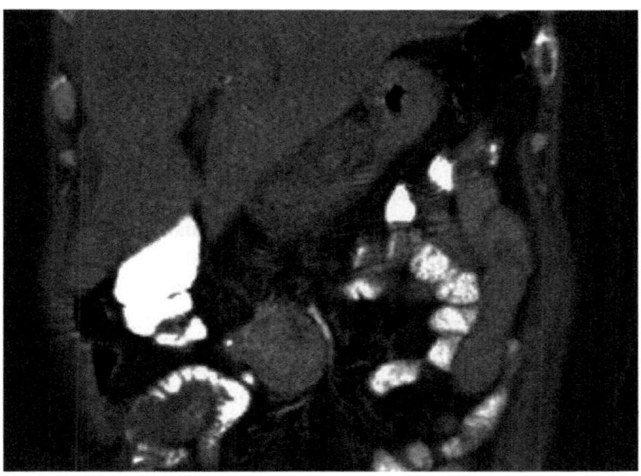

Fig. 26.8 CT image with contrast enhancement in a patient with Si-NEN, where a large and high mesenteric tumor has caused intestinal ischemia, with edema in the terminal ileum

distal intestinal tumors and tend to be deposited on to the right side of the main mesenteric vessels. A method has been proposed (Fig. 26.9), where the right colon and the mesenteric root are mobilized from adhesions to the retroperitoneum to the

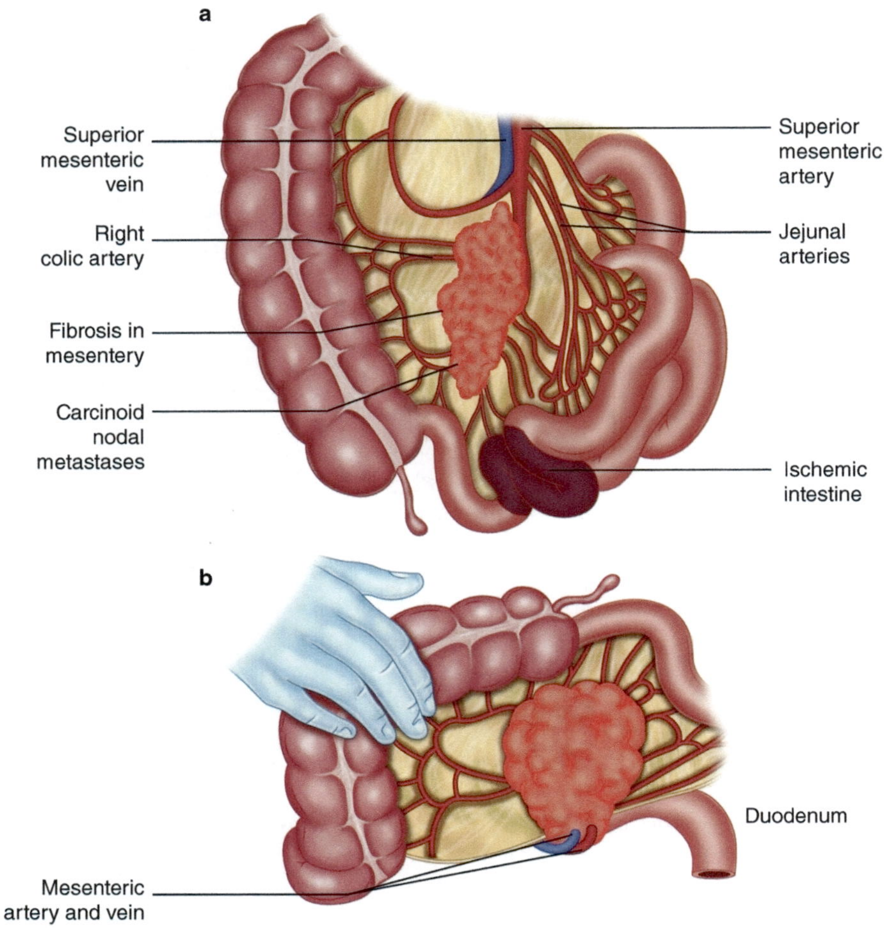

Fig. 26.9 Method for resection of the Si-NEN primary tumor and mesenteric metastases. (**a**) The mesenteric tumor may extensively involve the mesenteric root and appear impossible to remove; (**b**) mobilization of caecum, terminal ileum, and the mesenteric root by separation of retroperitoneal attachments, allows the tumor to be lifted, approached from a posterior angle, and separated from the duodenum and main mesenteric vessels; (**c**) tumor removed with preservation of collateral circulation along can maintain the intestinal length; the bowel can then be anastomosed and the mesenteric defect repaired. (Redrawn from Åkerström G, et al. Midgut and hindgut carcinoid tumors. In: Doherty GM, Skogseid B (eds) Surgical endocrinology, first edn. Philadelphia: Lippincott Williams & Wilkins, 2001; pp. 448–52)

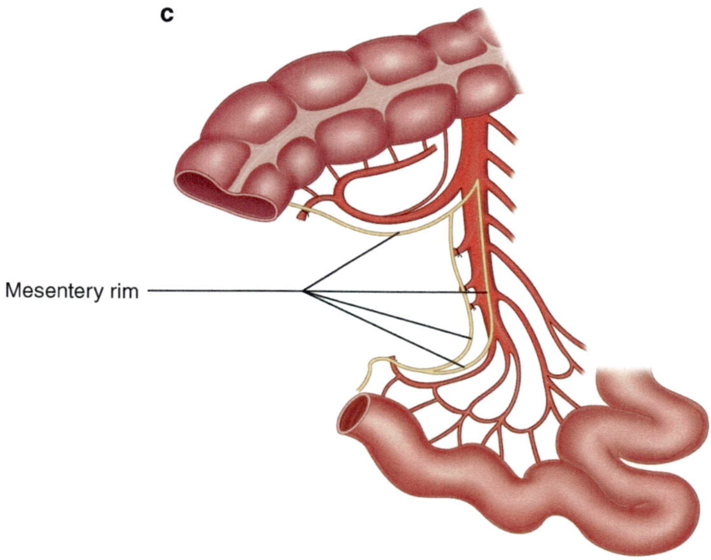

Fig. 26.9 (continued)

level of the horizontal duodenum and the pancreas [3, 37, 41]. Staple transection of the right colon then allows visualization of the mesenteric artery and vein from the right side, and possibility for vascular control above the mesenteric tumor during excision. With posterior view in the lifted mesenteric root, fibrotic bands can be transected and the tumor dissected from the serosa of the horizontal duodenum, occasionally, with duodenal wall excision or short duodenal resection in case of tumor invasion. It may then be possible to free-dissect the mesenteric tumor from the major vessels and carefully preserve the arcades of collateral circulation along the intestine and limit the required intestinal resection [3, 37, 41] (Fig. 26.10).

An own arbitrary staging of the mesenteric metastases has been suggested (Fig. 26.11) to describe the extension in the mesenteric root. Mesenteric tumors with very high extension, encircling major vessels with severe fibrosis, or with growth into the pancreas or the retroperitoneal/paraaortal spaces, have in our experience been irresectable. The median colic artery circulation should be carefully preserved [3, 37, 41]. Some of the cases with circumeferential involvement have originated from jejunal tumors.

Repeated surgery may sometimes be required in Si-NEN patients with chronic or intermittent abdominal main due to partial or complete intestinal obstruction, or segmental intestinal ischaemia [3, 37, 41]. These operations may be difficult due to fibrosis and carcinomatosis between loops of intestine. Re-operations, and indeed any surgery in patients with Si-NENs, should be done with caution, since mistakes may cause intestinal fistulation, or creation of a short-bowel syndrome [3, 37, 41].

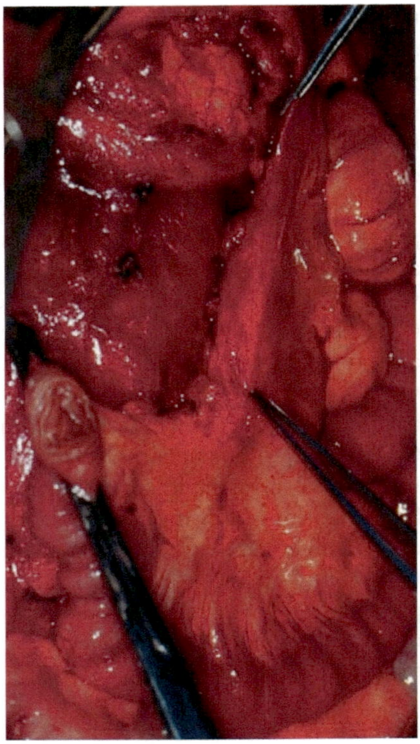

Fig. 26.10 Image from operation in Si-NEN patient with alleviation of intestinal ischemia after removal of a high mesenteric tumor, which was possible to free dissect from the mesenteric root, the pancreas and the duodenum. Maintenance of collateral circulation along the intestine allowed a limited resection of the ischemic part of the small bowel. (From Öhrvall U, et al. (2000) Method of dissection of mesenteric metastases in midgut carcinoid tumors. World J Surg 24:1402–8. Springer Science and Business Media)

26.11.4 Peritoneal Carcinomatosis

NEN peritoneal carcinomatosis (PC) has been most commonly encountered in the Si-NENs patients (reported to occur in 10–30%) and may have been incidentally detected at operation (or by histopathology), as a few mm large tumor nodules on peritoneal surfaces [33, 58, 59]. In some patients, CT may have revealed larger tumor nodules within the omentum or between the intestines, which occasionally have caused intestinal obstruction. Lateral deposits have rarely caused ureter block and hydronephrosis (the right ureter may also be blocked by a mesenteric lymph node metastasis with fibrosis). Larger deposits may also occur in the recto-uterine pouch (Douglasi pouch), on the uterus and on the rectum, and may then threaten to obstruct the rectum and both ureters. Occasional Si-NEN patients have been operated in Uppsala for pelvic NEN deposits with hystero-salpingooforectomy and anterior resection for pain relief and palliation. Ovarian deposits have been frequently noted in some series [34, 44].

A common Gilly's classification of PC is based on nodule size (>5 mm to >2 cm) and whether extent of involvement has been localized or diffused [59]. The ENETS has proposed an abdominal gravity PC scoring system (GPS), which incorporates the Gilly classification, together with the extent of lymph node and liver metastases

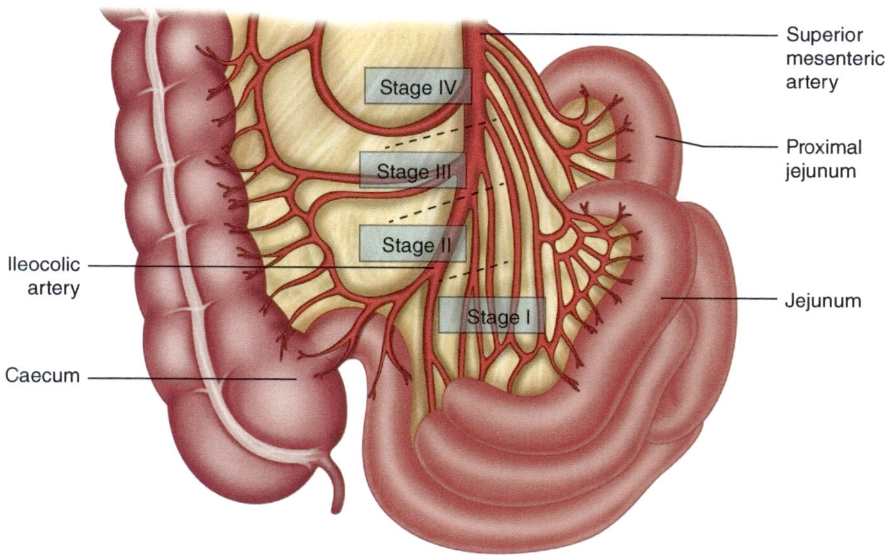

Fig. 26.11 Surgical/anatomical stages of Si-NEN mesenteric metastases. Stage I tumors located close to the intestine; Stage II tumors higher in the mesentery; Stage III tumors extending along, but without encircling the mesenteric trunk. Stage IV tumors growing around the mesenteric trunk, involving origins of proximal jejunal arteries, median colic artery, or extending to retroperitoneal/paraaortal spaces (have been inoperable). (From Öhrvall U, et al. Method of dissection of mesenteric metastases in mid-gut carcinoid tumors. World J Surg 2000; 24:1402–8. Springer Science and Business Media)

[59]. More often, the peritoneal carcinomatosis score (PCI) used for colorectal and appendicecal tumors may be used to date [59, 60]. Scoring may be done at the first laparotomy, by digital and visual exploration of subdiafragmatic spaces, the large and small omentum, and lateral abdominal spaces and can be combined with intraoperative US and palpation of the liver. PC was revealed as a strong prognostic factor, with markedly negative effect on in Si-NEN patients [33], and it is obviously important to have this spread diagnosed concomitant with the primary surgery. The ENETS guidelines have provided a low-grade recommendation that peritoneal cytoreductive surgery may be considered in Si-NENs patients, if they can be judged to be fit enough to undergo this somewhat extensive procedure [59]. Study evidence of long-term outcome of peritoneal cytoreductive surgery for NEN is still lacking, and there is a need to emphasize a risk for high morbidity, especially if treating peritoneal metastases and liver metastases at the same operation [58, 59]. A multistep procedure may be recommended if either operation is expected to be extensive [59]. The peritoneal cytoreductive surgery implies cautious dissection of all abdominal quadrants (right and left diaphragmatic peritoneum, small and great omentum, posterior face of stomach, mesenteric axes, and the pelvis) [59]. It has been recommended to remove both ovaries in females older than 55 years [59]. The PC resection

should be reported as completeness of cytoreduction (CCR) [59]. Perioperative hyperthermic intraperitoneal chemotherapy (HIPEC) has been performed for other malignancies, but remains experimental for Si-NENs, where most systemic chemotherapy has been inefficient [59].

26.11.5 Liver Metastases

Presence of liver metastases is crucial for the prognosis of NENs [4, 5, 61]. The most common origin of NEN liver metastases is the small intestine, and liver spread is also often seen with pancreatic and colonic NENs, less often with appendiceal, gastric, and rectal NENs [5, 61]. Metastases are found at diagnosis or develop during follow-up in about 40–90% of Si-NENs, pancreatic, and colonic NENs, in contrast to gastric, rectal, and appendiceal NENs, which in 85–90% remain as local tumors (and have often been incidentally discovered) [61]. Jejuno-ileal NENs have high probability of developing liver metastases despite low grade and Ki-67 index (<2%) [4, 33, 61–63].

Biopsy for grading with Ki-67 index should exclude NEC where liver surgery should not be considered due to poor survival. In patients with low to intermediate grade (G1 and G2), NENs surgical treatment of liver metastases should be considered in the absence of unresectable extra-hepatic disease, since this is the only potentially long-term cure [5, 61]. The benefit would be to achieve complete R0 resection, or efficient debulking leading to reduction of hormone levels and palliation of symptoms, and thereby reduce the risk to develop long-term complications such as the carcinoid heart disease. Long-term palliation of the carcinoid syndrome has been reported after removal of unilateral, large, or dominant liver metastases, and if 70–90% of the tumor burden has been removed. There has not been consensus on what amount of surgical debulking that would be needed to achieve symptomatic or survival benefit [64]. Liver surgery has proved to be safe and postresection 5-year survival has reached 85–94% at specialized centers, but early recurrence should be expected, with 5-year disease-free survival of <50% reported in most series [65–69]. A recent "thin slice" pathology examination could thus reveal that numerous small metastases often accompanied larger resected liver metastases, and only half of these additional metastases had been detected by preoperative imaging [70]. Liver resections combined with thermal ablation has been increasingly used in patients with multiple, bilateral metastases [66], but in a prospensity score matched study, a combination of liver surgery and thermal ablation (microwawe and radiofrequency ablation) could not demonstrate to have positive effects on survival [71].

Alternatives to surgical debulking of liver metastases are hepatic artery embolization/ chemoembolization, peptide receptor radionucleid therapy (PRRT) with ^{177}Lu-labelled DOTA-Tyr3-octreotate, the use of selective intrahepatic radiotherapy (SIRT), or medical treatment with long-acting somatostatin analogs [72–75]. Owing to high incidence of multifocal and bilateral liver metastases, radical liver resection is possible in less than 10- [20]%, and the majority of patients with advanced NENs are therefore mainly considered for other treatment modalities [72–75]. In cases with large colon or rectal NEN metastases, PRRT with Lu-labeled somatostatin analogs has occasionally provided successful preoperative treatment [74, 76].

26.11.5.1 Liver Surgery

A classification of NEN liver metastases based on morphological features has been proposed to facilitate patient selection; type I (simple), depicts single or multiple metastases confined to one lobe or adjacent segments; type II (complex), one major focus but with contralateral smaller satellites; type III disseminated spread with both lobes involved [65]. In cases with solitary, unilateral, or grossly dominant liver metastases, formal hepatic lobectomy or parenchyma-saving liver resections should be undertaken, and this may be combined with thermal ablation, wedge resections, or simple enucleations of superficially located, and even bilateral lesions [65, 71, 77].

Two-stage surgical resection may be performed to allow regeneration of the contralateral lobe to avoid liver insufficiency, and preoperative portal embolization may be used to induce regeneration of a hepatic lobe that is planned to remain after hepatic lobectomy for removal of metastatic tumor. The two-step surgery has allowed safe resection of bilateral tumors, though high recurrence has been evident [3, 64, 66, 69]. Up to 75% of the liver parenchyma may be resected if the remaining liver parenchyma is healthy.

Retrospective analyses have described series of patients who have undergone successful liver surgery with long survival, and with significant long-term symptom alleviation [78–81]. On the other hand, virtually every patient will recur with new metastases after liver resection or thermal ablation, if follow-up time is long enough. Five-year survival has been around 75–80% whether liver surgery was performed or not. Thus, although survival has not proved to be increased in G1 or G2 tumors after treatment of liver metastases with surgery or RFA, symptomatic improvement and palliation of the carcinoid syndrome and reduction of tumor markers are regularly seen [71, 82].

26.12 Thermal Ablation

RFA or microwave ablations are safe and efficient methods for moderately large NEN liver metastases (< 4 cm) [83, 84]. An ultrasound-guided insertion of the ablation needle and application of RF or microwave energy leads to ablation of an area surrounding the needle tip. This may be performed either percutaneously or intraoperatively (open or laparoscopically). Somewhat larger tumors may be coagulated by overlapping treatment, or by applying a Pringle's maneouvre to reduce the hepatic circulation during the procedure. While RFA can treat somewhat larger tumors than microwave, the latter is theoretically more efficient if the metastasis is situated close to larger vessels, due to less negative heat-sink effects, and microwave has like RFA been proven to provide symptom relief [85].

The use of RFA, microwave and surgery in combinations has allowed treatment of more or bilateral metastases. Although there has been no absolute maximum, we have advocated a highest number for this treatment of approximately 7 metastases, before choosing alternative methods (liver embolization, or PRRT, etc) [86–89]. The optimal method of assessing the number of metastases appears to be ^{68}Ga-DOTATOC/PET/CT in combination with MRI [13, 43]. However, also these investigations may underestimate the true number of metastases that can be detected intraoperatively by intraoperative ultrasound [70]. Therefore, the proper treatment for each patient may have to be decided during surgery. Since large vessels reduce the efficiency and bile ducts and bowel seem to be the most vulnerable structures, RFA and microwave should be avoided for tumors located in the hepatic hilum or very close to the surface of the liver. Also, patients who have undergone hepatico-jejunostomy or papillotomy are more prone to develop cholangitis or hepatic abscesses afterward and should be covered with proper antibiotic prophylaxis during the procedure and be carefully monitored afterwards.

26.13 Liver Transplantation

Liver transplantation should be considered experimental for most patients with liver metastases from Si-NENs. The new liver will often become the site for new metastases, emphasizing a possible need to combine with other treatment. Although a meta-analysis of patients with neuroendocrine tumors subjected to liver transplantation revealed a nearly 50% 1-year survival, and newer results indicate reduced operative risks and improved results after transplantation in NENs, with up to 77% 1-year tumor-free survival and 90% overall 5-year survival, and another theoretical study of non-transplanted patients with characteristics making them eligible for transplantation demonstrates a very favorable survival for such Si-NENs patients if only subjected to conventional oncologic therapy [90]. In fact these patients survival would overall exceed the expected survival if such patients were subjected to liver transplantation [90].

26.13.1 Prophylaxis Against Carcinoid Crisis

A carcinoid crisis with hyperthermia, shock, arrhythmia, excessive flush or bronchial obstruction is always a risk during treatment of patients with Si-NENs [91]. Initiation of somatostatin analogue treatment is recommended before surgery (patient's regular dose or daily 100 μg × 3 s.c.), and prophylaxis has to be given during operation, or any other intervention, preferably with octreotide (i.v. octreotide 500 μg in 500 mL saline, 50 μg/h), with possibility to increase the dose (to 100 μg/h) if symptoms should not resolve NENs [91]. Adrenergic drugs should be avoided if hypotension should occur during surgery. Patients with foregut NENs and an atypical carcinoid syndrome may be treated with octreotide, histamine blockade and cortisone, with recommendation to avoid histamine-releasing agents (morphine and tubocurarine).

26.13.2 Survival

Survival data from the Uppsala series of 603 Si-NEN patients admitted to various operations and treatments in Uppsala, between 1985–2010 were recently reported [33]. Median survival was related to stage and grade and was overall 8.4 years, with 67% 5-year survival. With adjustments for co-morbidity by multivariate analyses, survival advantage could be demonstrated in patients subjected to mesenteric tumor removal, with low mortality for the primary surgery (<1%) [33]. Previously recognized prognostic factors were carcinoid heart disease, old age at diagnosis, liver tumor load, and extra-abdominal metastases; new prognostic factors were remaining mesenteric metastases, distant abdominal metastases (paraaortal/retroperitoneal), and peritoneal carcinomatosis. A recent US series of 691 Si-NENs patients also showed strong relation to tumor stage and grade, and substantiated higher survival in patients with resectable compared to unresectable mesenteric tumors [92].

The ENETS Ki-67 grading appears increasingly important for long-term outcome and for results of surgery. The NEC are rare among Si-NENs (1%), but it has been emphasized that different metastases sites in the same patient may express different Ki67 levels [33, 93]. Upgrading may occur in Si-NEN metastases, and if carefully examined, there may be variable grading within metastases [93].

26.13.3 Appendiceal NENs

Appendiceal NENs constitute ~5% of GEP-NEN and has a recently estimated annual incidence of 0,5/100000, which is increasing. However, all NENs have rising incidence, and the share of appendiceal NENs is probably decreasing. It is found in approximately 1/300 appendectomies constitutes up to 80% of all types of appendix tumors [94, 95]. The majority of appendiceal NENs originate from serotonin-producing EC cells, but have a more benign course than other GI-NENs [96].

Appendiceal NENs are usually an incidental finding at surgery [94]. The majority are located in the tip of the appendix, and only few cases have had appendicitis due to an occluded appendix lumen [96]. The mean age for discovery of appendiceal NENs is between 38 and 41 years, somewhat younger than for other NENs. Also children are affected, in some series with higher incidence, which has led to the assumption that some appendiceal NENs undergo involution with age. The overall rate of metastasis has been 3.8%, with distant metastases in 0.7% [47].

Appendiceal NENs are usually small, <1 cm, and only few metastasize with a risk increasing with size. Therefore, small NENs in the tip of the appendix may be treated with simple appendectomy [97]. According to ENETS guidelines, tumors <1 cm, with a maximum invasion of 3 mm into the mesoappendix or subserosa and with clear surgical margins, have no risk of recurrence and appendectomy is sufficient. Lesions >2 cm, as well as cases with residual tumor at resection margins, or with lymph gland metastases, should be treated with right hemicolectomy and lymph node clearance. Tumors between1 and 2 cm in size are treated according to associated risk for metastases, where the pathology report is crucial. Tumors in the base of the appendix require hemicolectomy since they may represent colon-, rather than appendix-derived tumors.

The prognosis for appendiceal NENs is good, with a 5-year survival rate of 100% for the majority without metastases, 84% for patients with regional metastases, and 28% for the few patients with distant metastases (which presumably includes patients with adenocarcinoid appearance).

After surgery, regular CT scanning, or ^{68}Ga-DOTATOC-PET/CT, may reveal residual disease, since somatostatin receptors may be expressed. The only tumor marker is chromogranin A, which has low sensitivity. The carcinoid syndrome is absent, as well as hormone secretion, and there is no indication for urinary 5-HIAA measurements [98].

26.14 Colon NENs

Colon NENs are rare and constitute only about 7% of GEP-NENs and < 1% of colorectal neoplasms [99]. The incidence varies highly between different registers (0.06/100000 in Europe and 0.2/100000 in the United States). The 5-year survival rate for colon NENs has averaged around 40–50%, slightly better than the survival for colon adenocarcinoma [100]. The colon NENs are more common in elderly age groups compared with other NENs and have been most often located in the proximal colon. A fraction of colon NENs, originating in the cecum and right colon appear with serotonin immune-reactivity, and should be regarded and treated as Si-NENs, as they have similar behavior and comprise G1-G2 tumors. The carcinoid syndrome is exceedingly rare, and secretion of hormones measurable in serum or urine is absent apart from those treated as Si-NENs. Diagnostic procedures include s-CgA, p-5HIAA for those arising in the right colon and mandatory colonoscopy with biopsy. CT/MRI with somatostatin receptor analog-based PET (i.e., ^{64}Cu/^{68}Ga-DOTATATE). Tumors in the remaining part of the colon (the majority) are usually NECs, non-serotonin reactive, and have more aggressive behavior, but may still be slow growing, and the primary tumor may reach conspicuous size and lead to obstruction, bleeding or even a palpable mass as initial symptoms. With these tumors, metastases are common at diagnosis. The lower differentiation state is noted by higher Ki67 index and risk for presenting with spread disease at diagnosis [100]. Diagnosis may be difficult, but synaptophysin immuno-staining is usually positive, supporting the neuroendocrine origin. Left colon NENs may mimic rectal NENs (see below) with an accompanying L cell expression and other histopathological profiles.

Treatment of choice for loco-regional disease is surgery with bowel resection and lymph node clearance, similar to colon adenocarcinoma, because of the presence of very few G1-G2 tumors. Colon-NECs with distant metastases should be treated according to special protocols [1]. Owing to their generally slow growth rate, palliative tumor debulking, before or after down-staging treatment, may also be undertaken.

26.15 Rectal NENs

Rectal NENs have previously been regarded as uncommon, but the incidence is increasing, according to SEERS 0.86/100000/year. They constitute 25% of all GEP-NENs, but there is a similar difference between Europe and the United States as for colon NENs, with higher incidence in the United States [101]. The generally increased incidence compared with earlier reports may be due to improved awareness of the diagnosis and the increased use of new diagnostic methods including endosonography. The overall prognosis is favorable, with 5-year survival varying in different series between 45 and 88%.

26.15.1 Presentation and Diagnosis

Rectal NENs usually occur in the sixth decade, about 10 years earlier than non-NEN rectal tumors. The rectal NENs are generally small and polypoid, located between 4 and 20 cm above the dentate line (75% within 8 cm, reachable for palpation by a finger) [100, 102], and may be discovered after presenting symptoms, such as perianal pain or discomfort, or haematochezia that may lead to the endoscopic investigation. However, the small rectal NENs are generally not the cause of symptoms, and therefore more often an incidental finding. Diagnosis is made after histopathological evaluation of biopsies or after removal of the whole nodule. The most sensitive histological tumor markers are NSE (being positive in 87%) and prostate-specific acid phosphatase (positive in 80–100%), which can make differentiation from prostatic carcinoma difficult [103]. Other markers are glicentin and glucagon. Classical tumor markers like CA19–9, CA50, and alpha-fetoprotein are poorly expressed or absent, while carcino-embryonic antigen (CEA) has been demonstrated in up to 25% of cells. The CEA expression is possibly related to the occasional rectal NEN with histopathological signs of both adenocarcinoma and NEN.

Rectal NENs generally show focal and patchy multihormonal expression, in which glucagon, somatostatin, pancreatic polypeptide, substance P, and β-endorphins may be detected. A small and limited fraction of cells generally are positive for chromogranin A and synaptophysin, but negative for serotonin. Measurable release of these hormones in the circulation is anecdotal. These tumors have rarely metastasized at diagnosis.

Some patients have more aggressive disease with larger tumors, and more local symptoms, such as obstruction or bleeding. Even with these larger tumors, hormonal release or the carcinoid syndrome is extremely rare. Occasional large tumors can be fixed to perirectal tissues and may initially be difficult to distinguish from rectal adenocarcinoma. Metastases are common, and the larger the tumor, the higher is the risk for presentation of metastases. As with appendiceal NENs, tumors smaller than 1 cm rarely metastasize (<2%), while those >2 cm frequently do (60–80%). Patients with 1–2 cm large tumors have an intermediate risk for metastatic spread (10–15%). The main sites for tumor spread are regional lymph nodes and the liver, and less commonly lung and bone.

26.16 Surgical Treatment

The size separation of tumors is followed in the treatment recommendations. Patients with tumors <1 cm seldom have symptoms, have favorable outcome, and are generally cured by local excision. Thus, the smaller (<1 cm) and the larger (>2 cm) tumors have predictable outcome, whereas the intermediate tumors measuring 1–2 cm in diameter are unpredictable. These latter tumors need to be carefully followed and examined. Transrectal endosonography should be used for more precise assessment of tumor extension (possible infiltration into the muscularis propria layer) and to reveal regional lymph node metastases. CT or MRI can clarify local tumor growth in the pelvis, and also the presence of lymph node, and liver metastases. Owing to a general lack or presence of only few somatostatin receptors, somatostatin receptor analog-based PET is usually insensitive. However, since occasional cases (G1 > 1 cm and G2 regardless of size) may express high levels of somatostatin receptors leading to additional treatment options and imaging possibilities, it is recommended to perform a PET preoperatively for these tumors. Presence of local invasion or regional metastases favors aggressive approach with abdominoperineal or anterior resection with total mesorectal excision (TME). Incompletely removed polyps that are found to be NENs after removal may be re-excised using the same techniques.

However, results have documented more favorable survival rates than previously depicted, and local tumor removal may be advocated also in the presence of metastases. Five-year survival for rectal NENs with distant metastases is about 20–32%, which favors an aggressive approach for this group of patients, even in the presence of local pelvic invasion or distant lymph node, liver, lung, or skeletal metastases.

Our experience of individual patients with large tumors and distant metastases supports this view. Thus, we suggest surgery in these patients, often in combination with preoperative downstaging by chemotherapy, or in cases with PET-documented somatostatin receptor expression, **PRRT** with ^{177}Lutetium-labeled somatostatin analogues, which can be highly effective in some patients. However, patients with atypical histopathological features are less likely to benefit from the aggressive surgical treatment.

IFN-α and paclitaxel have in some patients resulted in reduced disease progression and also regression of metastases. Occasionally, patients with liver metastases may benefit from hepatic artery chemoembolization. In carefully selected cases, liver resection may be indicated, with the understanding, however, that these patients generally have poor outcome and short survival.

26.16.1 Recommendations

Patients with rectal NENs measuring >1 cm should be thoroughly investigated (MRT, CT, transrectal endosonography) for evidence of spread of disease, e.g., local or distant metastases. These patients should generally undergo surgery with the aim of achieving total tumor clearance, and the specimens should be thoroughly investigated for signs of atypical histopathology. Most rectal NENs <2 cm can be radically resected by endoscopic procedures. Tumors >1 cm should be investigated for invasion into the muscularis propriae since invasion is a contra-indication to endoscopic surgery. Tumors >2 cm may be resected by TEM or by a low anterior or abdomino-peritoneal resection depending on size, Ki67 index, muscular invasion, and presence of regional node metastases. The larger the tumor, the higher is the risk for metastatic disease. There are no studies demonstrating the benefit of preoperative medical or irradiation treatment. Patients with rectal NENs >1 cm, including those with infiltrative or disseminated disease, need follow-up, and if not removed may require palliation against pelvic pain. Selected individuals may be offered more aggressive medical (and surgical) treatment for distant metastases.

References

1. Janson ET, Knigge U, Dam G, Federspiel B, Gronbaek H, Stalberg P et al (2021) Nordic guidelines 2021 for diagnosis and treatment of gastroenteropancreatic neuroendocrine neoplasms. Acta Oncol 60(7):931–941
2. Elvin A (1993) Therapy evaluation and diagnostic accuracy in neuroendocrine tumours: assessment of radiological methods. Acta Radiol Suppl 390:1–25
3. Akerstrom G, Hellman P, Hessman O (2009) Gastrointestinal carcinoids. In: Lennard T (ed) Endocrine surgery, 4th edn. Elsevier Saunders, London, pp 147–176
4. Frilling A, Akerstrom G, Falconi M, Pavel M, Ramos J, Kidd M et al (2012) Neuroendocrine tumor disease: an evolving landscape. Endocr Relat Cancer 19(5):R163–R185
5. Lawrence B, Gustafsson BI, Chan A, Svejda B, Kidd M, Modlin IM (2011) The epidemiology of gastroenteropancreatic neuroendocrine tumors. Endocrinol Metab Clin N Am 40(1):1–18. vii
6. Granberg D, Wilander E, Stridsberg M, Granerus G, Skogseid B, Oberg K (1998) Clinical symptoms, hormone profiles, treatment, and prognosis in patients with gastric carcinoids. Gut 43(2):223–228
7. Dam G, Gronbaek H, Sorbye H, Thiis Evensen E, Paulsson B, Sundin A et al (2020) Prospective study of chromogranin a as a predictor of progression in patients with pancreatic, small-intestinal, and unknown primary neuroendocrine tumors. Neuroendocrinology 110(3–4):217–224
8. Adaway JE, Dobson R, Walsh J, Cuthbertson DJ, Monaghan PJ, Trainer PJ et al (2016) Serum and plasma 5-hydroxyindoleacetic acid as an alternative to 24-h urine 5-hydroxyindoleacetic acid measurement. Ann Clin Biochem 53(Pt 5):554–560
9. Johnbeck CB, Knigge U, Loft A, Berthelsen AK, Mortensen J, Oturai P et al (2017) Head-to-head comparison of (64)cu-DOTATATE and (68)Ga-DOTATOC PET/CT: a prospective study of 59 patients with neuroendocrine tumors. J Nuclear Med 58(3):451–457
10. Koopmans KP, Neels OC, Kema IP, Elsinga PH, Sluiter WJ, Vanghillewe K et al (2008) Improved staging of patients with carcinoid and islet cell tumors with 18F-dihydroxy-phenyl-alanine and 11C-5-hydroxy-tryptophan positron emission tomography. J Clin Oncol 26(9):1489–1495
11. Buchmann I, Henze M, Engelbrecht S, Eisenhut M, Runz A, Schafer M et al (2007) Comparison of 68Ga-DOTATOC PET and 111In-DTPAOC (Octreoscan) SPECT in patients with neuroendocrine tumours. Eur J Nucl Med Mol Imaging 34(10):1617–1626
12. Prasad V, Ambrosini V, Hommann M, Hoersch D, Fanti S, Baum RP (2010) Detection of unknown primary neuroendocrine tumours (CUP-NET) using (68)Ga-DOTA-NOC receptor PET/CT. Eur J Nucl Med Mol Imaging 37(1):67–77

13. Frilling A, Sotiropoulos GC, Radtke A, Malago M, Bockisch A, Kuehl H et al (2010) The impact of 68Ga-DOTATOC positron emission tomography/computed tomography on the multimodal management of patients with neuroendocrine tumors. Ann Surg 252(5):850–856
14. Binderup T, Knigge U, Loft A, Mortensen J, Pfeifer A, Federspiel B et al (2010) Functional imaging of neuroendocrine tumors: a head-to-head comparison of somatostatin receptor scintigraphy, 123I-MIBG scintigraphy, and 18F-FDG PET. J Nuclear Med 51(5):704–712
15. Modlin IM, Kidd M, Latich I, Zikusoka MN, Shapiro MD (2005) Current status of gastrointestinal carcinoids. Gastroenterology 128(6):1717–1751
16. Borch K, Ahren B, Ahlman H, Falkmer S, Granerus G, Grimelius L (2005) Gastric carcinoids: biologic behavior and prognosis after differentiated treatment in relation to type. Ann Surg 242(1):64–73
17. Ruszniewski P, Delle Fave G, Cadiot G, Komminoth P, Chung D, Kos-Kudla B et al (2006) Well-differentiated gastric tumors/carcinomas. Neuroendocrinology 84(3):158–164
18. Hopper AD, Bourke MJ, Hourigan LF, Tran K, Moss A, Swan MP (2009) En-bloc resection of multiple type 1 gastric carcinoid tumors by endoscopic multi-band mucosectomy. J Gastroenterol Hepatol 24(9):1516–1521
19. Burkitt MD, Pritchard DM (2006) Review article: pathogenesis and management of gastric carcinoid tumours. Aliment Pharmacol Ther 24(9):1305–1320
20. Campana D, Nori F, Pezzilli R, Piscitelli L, Santini D, Brocchi E et al (2008) Gastric endocrine tumors type I: treatment with long-acting somatostatin analogs. Endocr Relat Cancer 15(1):337–342
21. Fykse V, Sandvik AK, Qvigstad G, Falkmer SE, Syversen U, Waldum HL (2004) Treatment of ECL cell carcinoids with octreotide LAR. Scand J Gastroenterol 39(7):621–628
22. Jianu CS, Fossmark R, Syversen U, Hauso O, Fykse V, Waldum HL (2011) Five-year follow-up of patients treated for 1 year with octreotide long-acting release for enterochromaffin-like cell carcinoids. Scand J Gastroenterol 46(4):456–463
23. Lew EA, Pisegna JR, Starr JA, Soffer EF, Forsmark C, Modlin IM et al (2000) Intravenous pantoprazole rapidly controls gastric acid hypersecretion in patients with Zollinger-Ellison syndrome. Gastroenterology 118(4):696–704
24. Tomassetti P, Migliori M, Caletti GC, Fusaroli P, Corinaldesi R, Gullo L (2000) Treatment of type II gastric carcinoid tumors with somatostatin analogues. N Engl J Med 343(8):551–554
25. O'Toole D, Delle Fave G, Jensen RT (2012) Gastric and duodenal neuroendocrine tumours. Best Pract Res Clin Gastroenterol 26(6):719–735
26. Jensen RT, Rindi G, Arnold R, Lopes JM, Brandi ML, Bechstein WO et al (2006) Well-differentiated duodenal tumor/carcinoma (excluding gastrinomas). Neuroendocrinology 84(3):165–172
27. Wheeler MH, Curley IR, Williams ED (1986) The association of neurofibromatosis, pheochromocytoma, and somatostatin-rich duodenal carcinoid tumor. Surgery 100(6):1163–1169
28. Burke AP, Sobin LH, Federspiel BH, Shekitka KM, Helwig EB (1990) Carcinoid tumors of the duodenum. A clinicopathologic study of 99 cases. Arch Pathol Lab Med 114(7):700–704
29. Zyromski NJ, Kendrick ML, Nagorney DM, Grant CS, Donohue JH, Farnell MB et al (2001) Duodenal carcinoid tumors: how aggressive should we be? J Gastrointest Surg 5(6):588–593
30. Wilson RW, Gal AA, Cohen C, DeRose PB, Millikan WJ (1991) Serotonin immunoreactivity in pancreatic endocrine neoplasms (carcinoid tumors). Modern Pathol 4(6):727–732
31. Berge T, Linell F, Carcinoid tumours. (1976) Frequency in a defined population during a 12-year period. Acta Pathol Microbiol Scand Sect Pathol 84(4):322–330
32. Eriksson B, Kloppel G, Krenning E, Ahlman H, Plockinger U, Wiedenmann B et al (2008) Consensus guidelines for the management of patients with digestive neuroendocrine tumors—well-differentiated jejunal-ileal tumor/carcinoma. Neuroendocrinology 87(1):8–19
33. Norlen O, Stalberg P, Oberg K, Eriksson J, Hedberg J, Hessman O et al (2012) Long-term results of surgery for small intestinal neuroendocrine tumors at a tertiary referral center. World J Surg 36(6):1419–1431
34. Strosberg J (2012) Neuroendocrine tumours of the small intestine. Best Pract Res Clin Gastroenterol 26(6):755–773

35. Makridis C, Oberg K, Juhlin C, Rastad J, Johansson H, Lorelius LE et al (1990) Surgical treatment of mid-gut carcinoid tumors. World J Surg 14(3):377–383. discussion 84–5
36. Guo Z, Li Q, Wilander E, Ponten J (2000) Clonality analysis of multifocal carcinoid tumours of the small intestine by X-chromosome inactivation analysis. J Pathol 190(1):76–79
37. Åkerström G, Hellman P, Öhrvall U (2001) Midgut and hindgut carcinoid tumors. In: Doherty G, Skogseid B (eds) Surgical endocrinology. Lippincott Williams & Wilkins, Philadelphia, pp 447–459
38. Funa K, Papanicolaou V, Juhlin C, Rastad J, Akerstrom G, Heldin CH et al (1990) Expression of platelet-derived growth factor beta-receptors on stromal tissue cells in human carcinoid tumors. Cancer Res 50(3):748–753
39. Kidd M, Modlin IM (2011) Small intestinal neuroendocrine cell pathobiology: 'carcinoid' tumors. Curr Opin Oncol 23(1):45–52
40. Makridis C, Ekbom A, Bring J, Rastad J, Juhlin C, Oberg K et al (1997) Survival and daily physical activity in patients treated for advanced midgut carcinoid tumors. Surgery 122(6):1075–1082
41. Ohrvall U, Eriksson B, Juhlin C, Karacagil S, Rastad J, Hellman P et al (2000) Method for dissection of mesenteric metastases in mid-gut carcinoid tumors. World J Surg 24(11):1402–1408
42. Eckhauser FE, Argenta LC, Strodel WE, Wheeler RH, Bull FE, Appelman HD et al (1981) Mesenteric angiopathy, intestinal gangrene, and midgut carcinoids. Surgery 90(4):720–728
43. Sundin A, Arnold R, Baudin E, Cwikla JB, Eriksson B, Fanti S et al (2017) ENETS consensus guidelines for the standards of care in neuroendocrine tumors: radiological, nucsslear medicine & hybrid imaging. Neuroendocrinology 105(3):212–244
44. Strosberg J, Gardner N, Kvols L (2009) Survival and prognostic factor analysis of 146 metastatic neuroendocrine tumors of the mid-gut. Neuroendocrinology 89(4):471–476
45. Jacobs C (2009) Neuroendocrine tumors a rare finding: part I. Clin J Oncol Nurs 13(1):21–23
46. Mooney E (1985) The flushing patient. Int J Dermatol 24(9):549–554
47. Modlin IM, Lye KD, Kidd M (2003) A 5-decade analysis of 13,715 carcinoid tumors. Cancer 97(4):934–959
48. Matuchansky C, Launay JM (1995) Serotonin, catecholamines, and spontaneous midgut carcinoid flush: plasma studies from flushing and nonflushing sites. Gastroenterology 108(3):743–751
49. Kowlessar OD, Law DH, Sleisenger MH (1959) Malabsorption syndrome associated with metastatic carcinoid tumor. Am J Med 27:673–677
50. Vinik AI, McLeod MK, Fig LM, Shapiro B, Lloyd RV, Cho K (1989) Clinical features, diagnosis, and localization of carcinoid tumors and their management. Gastroenterol Clin N Am 18(4):865–896
51. Lundin L, Hansson HE, Landelius J, Oberg K (1990) Surgical treatment of carcinoid heart disease. J Thorac Cardiovasc Surg 100(4):552–561
52. Pellikka PA, Tajik AJ, Khandheria BK, Seward JB, Callahan JA, Pitot HC et al (1993) Carcinoid heart disease. Clinical and echocardiographic spectrum in 74 patients. Circulation 87(4):1188–1196
53. Westberg G, Wangberg B, Ahlman H, Bergh CH, Beckman-Suurkula M, Caidahl K (2001) Prediction of prognosis by echocardiography in patients with midgut carcinoid syndrome. Br J Surg 88(6):865–872
54. Orlefors H, Sundin A, Ahlstrom H, Bjurling P, Bergstrom M, Lilja A et al (1998) Positron emission tomography with 5-hydroxytryprophan in neuroendocrine tumors. J Clin Oncol 16(7):2534–2541
55. Hellman P, Lundstrom T, Ohrvall U, Eriksson B, Skogseid B, Oberg K et al (2002) Effect of surgery on the outcome of midgut carcinoid disease with lymph node and liver metastases. World J Surg 26(8):991–997
56. Makridis C, Rastad J, Oberg K, Akerstrom G (1996) Progression of metastases and symptom improvement from laparotomy in midgut carcinoid tumors. World J Surg 20(7):900–906. discussion 7

57. Daskalakis K, Karakatsanis A, Hessman O, Stuart HC, Welin S, Tiensuu Janson E et al (2018) Association of a Prophylactic Surgical Approach to stage IV small intestinal neuroendocrine tumors with survival. JAMA Oncol 4(2):183–189
58. Elias D, Sideris L, Liberale G, Ducreux M, Malka D, Lasser P et al (2005) Surgical treatment of peritoneal carcinomatosis from well-differentiated digestive endocrine carcinomas. Surgery 137(4):411–416
59. Kianmanesh R, Ruszniewski P, Rindi G, Kwekkeboom D, Pape UF, Kulke M et al (2010) ENETS consensus guidelines for the management of peritoneal carcinomatosis from neuroendocrine tumors. Neuroendocrinology 91(4):333–340
60. Dohan A, Hoeffel C, Soyer P, Jannot AS, Valette PJ, Thivolet A et al (2017) Evaluation of the peritoneal carcinomatosis index with CT and MRI. Br J Surg 104(9):1244–1249
61. Frilling A, Modlin IM, Kidd M, Russell C, Breitenstein S, Salem R et al (2014) Recommendations for management of patients with neuroendocrine liver metastases. Lancet Oncol 15(1):e8
62. Jann H, Roll S, Couvelard A, Hentic O, Pavel M, Muller-Nordhorn J et al (2011) Neuroendocrine tumors of midgut and hindgut origin: tumor-node-metastasis classification determines clinical outcome. Cancer 117(15):3332–3341
63. Landerholm K, Zar N, Andersson RE, Falkmer SE, Jarhult J (2011) Survival and prognostic factors in patients with small bowel carcinoid tumour. Br J Surg 98(11):1617–1624
64. Knigge U, Hansen CP (2012) Surgery for GEP-NETs. Best Pract Res Clin Gastroenterol 26(6):819–831
65. Frilling A, Li J, Malamutmann E, Schmid KW, Bockisch A, Broelsch CE (2009) Treatment of liver metastases from neuroendocrine tumours in relation to the extent of hepatic disease. Br J Surg 96(2):175–184
66. Kianmanesh R, Sauvanet A, Hentic O, Couvelard A, Levy P, Vilgrain V et al (2008) Two-step surgery for synchronous bilobar liver metastases from digestive endocrine tumors: a safe approach for radical resection. Ann Surg 247(4):659–665
67. Mazzaferro V, Pulvirenti A, Coppa J (2007) Neuroendocrine tumors metastatic to the liver: how to select patients for liver transplantation? J Hepatol 47(4):460–466
68. Scigliano S, Lebtahi R, Maire F, Stievenart JL, Kianmanesh R, Sauvanet A et al (2009) Clinical and imaging follow-up after exhaustive liver resection of endocrine metastases: a 15-year monocentric experience. Endocr Relat Cancer 16(3):977–990
69. Steinmuller T, Kianmanesh R, Falconi M, Scarpa A, Taal B, Kwekkeboom DJ et al (2008) Consensus guidelines for the management of patients with liver metastases from digestive (neuro)endocrine tumors: foregut, midgut, hindgut, and unknown primary. Neuroendocrinology 87(1):47–62
70. Elias D, Lefevre JH, Duvillard P, Goere D, Dromain C, Dumont F et al (2010) Hepatic metastases from neuroendocrine tumors with a "thin slice" pathological examination: they are many more than you think. Ann Surg 251(2):307–310
71. Norlen O, Stalberg P, Zedenius J, Hellman P (2013) Outcome after resection and radiofrequency ablation of liver metastases from small intestinal neuroendocrine tumours. Br J Surg 100(11):1505–1514
72. Kennedy A, Coldwell D, Sangro B, Wasan H, Salem R (2012) Integrating radioembolization into the treatment paradigm for metastatic neuroendocrine tumors in the liver. Am J Clin Oncol 35(4):393–398
73. Lewis MA, Jaramillo S, Roberts L, Fleming CJ, Rubin J, Grothey A (2012) Hepatic artery embolization for neuroendocrine tumors: postprocedural management and complications. Oncologist 17(5):725–731
74. Oberg KE (2012) The management of neuroendocrine tumours: current and future medical therapy options. Clin Oncol 24(4):282–293
75. van Essen M, Krenning EP, Bakker WH, de Herder WW, van Aken MO, Kwekkeboom DJ (2007) Peptide receptor radionuclide therapy with 177Lu-octreotate in patients with foregut carcinoid tumours of bronchial, gastric and thymic origin. Eur J Nucl Med Mol Imaging 34(8):1219–1227

76. Garske-Román U (2012) 177Lu-DOTA-octreotate radionuclide therapy of neuroendocrine tumours: dosimetry-based therapy planning and outcome. Uppsala University, Uppsala
77. Krausch M, Raffel A, Anlauf M, Schott M, Lehwald N, Krieg A et al (2014) "Cherry picking", a multiple non-anatomic liver resection technique, as a promising option for diffuse liver metastases in patients with neuroendocrine tumours. World J Surg 38(2):392–401
78. Ahlman H, Westberg G, Wangberg B, Nilsson O, Tylen U, Schersten T et al (1996) Treatment of liver metastases of carcinoid tumors. World J Surg 20(2):196–202
79. McEntee GP, Nagorney DM, Kvols LK, Moertel CG, Grant CS (1990) Cytoreductive hepatic surgery for neuroendocrine tumors. Surgery 108(6):1091–1096
80. Norton JA, Kivlen M, Li M, Schneider D, Chuter T, Jensen RT (2003) Morbidity and mortality of aggressive resection in patients with advanced neuroendocrine tumors. Arch Surg 138(8):859–866
81. Touzios JG, Kiely JM, Pitt SC, Rilling WS, Quebbeman EJ, Wilson SD et al (2005) Neuroendocrine hepatic metastases: does aggressive management improve survival? Ann Surg 241(5):776–783. discussion 83–5
82. Eriksson J, Stalberg P, Nilsson A, Krause J, Lundberg C, Skogseid B et al (2008) Surgery and radiofrequency ablation for treatment of liver metastases from midgut and foregut carcinoids and endocrine pancreatic tumors. World J Surg 32(5):930–938
83. Akyildiz HY, Mitchell J, Milas M, Siperstein A, Berber E (2010) Laparoscopic radiofrequency thermal ablation of neuroendocrine hepatic metastases: long-term follow-up. Surgery 148(6):1288–1293. discussion 93
84. Hellman P, Ladjevardi S, Skogseid B, Akerstrom G, Elvin A (2002) Radiofrequency tissue ablation using cooled tip for liver metastases of endocrine tumors. World J Surg 26(8):1052–1056
85. Groeschl RT, Pilgrim CH, Hanna EM, Simo KA, Swan RZ, Sindram D et al (2013) Microwave ablation for hepatic malignancies: a multiinstitutional analysis. Ann Surg 31:218
86. Granberg D, Eriksson LG, Welin S, Kindmark H, Janson ET, Skogseid B et al (2007) Liver embolization with trisacryl gelatin microspheres (embosphere) in patients with neuroendocrine tumors. Acta Radiol 48(2):180–185
87. Lewis MA, Hubbard J (2011) Multimodal liver-directed management of neuroendocrine hepatic metastases. Int J Hepatol 2011:452343
88. Schell SR, Camp ER, Caridi JG, Hawkins IF Jr (2002) Hepatic artery embolization for control of symptoms, octreotide requirements, and tumor progression in metastatic carcinoid tumors. J Gastrointest Surg 6(5):664–670
89. Strosberg JR, Choi J, Cantor AB, Kvols LK (2006) Selective hepatic artery embolization for treatment of patients with metastatic carcinoid and pancreatic endocrine tumors. Cancer Control 13(1):72–78
90. Norlen O, Daskalakis K, Oberg K, Akerstrom G, Stalberg P, Hellman P (2014) Indication for liver transplantation in young patients with small intestinal NETs is rare? World J Surg 38(3):742–747
91. Akerstrom G, Falconi M, Kianmanesh R, Ruszniewski P, Plockinger U, Mallorca Consensus Conference P et al (2009) ENETS consensus guidelines for the standards of care in neuroendocrine tumors: pre-and perioperative therapy in patients with neuroendocrine tumors. Neuroendocrinology 90(2):203–208
92. Strosberg JR, Weber JM, Feldman M, Coppola D, Meredith K, Kvols LK (2013) Prognostic validity of the American joint committee on cancer staging classification for midgut neuroendocrine tumors. J Clin Oncol 31(4):420–425
93. Miller HC, Drymousis P, Flora R, Goldin R, Spalding D, Frilling A (2014) Role of Ki-67 proliferation index in the assessment of patients with neuroendocrine Neoplasias regarding the stage of disease. World J Surg 38:1353
94. In't Hof KH, van der Wal HC, Kazemier G, Lange JF (2008) Carcinoid tumour of the appendix: an analysis of 1,485 consecutive emergency appendectomies. J Gastrointest Surg 12(8):1436–1438

95. Yao JC, Hassan M, Phan A, Dagohoy C, Leary C, Mares JE et al (2008) One hundred years after "carcinoid": epidemiology of and prognostic factors for neuroendocrine tumors in 35,825 cases in the United States. J Clin Oncol 26(18):3063–3072
96. Goede AC, Caplin ME, Winslet MC (2003) Carcinoid tumour of the appendix. Br J Surg 90(11):1317–1322
97. Plockinger U, Couvelard A, Falconi M, Sundin A, Salazar R, Christ E et al (2008) Consensus guidelines for the management of patients with digestive neuroendocrine tumours: well-differentiated tumour/carcinoma of the appendix and goblet cell carcinoma. Neuroendocrinology 87(1):20–30
98. Pape UF, Perren A, Niederle B, Gross D, Gress T, Costa F et al (2012) ENETS consensus guidelines for the management of patients with neuroendocrine neoplasms from the jejuno-ileum and the appendix including goblet cell carcinomas. Neuroendocrinology 95(2):135–156
99. Volante M, Grillo F, Massa F, Maletta F, Mastracci L, Campora M et al (2021) Neuroendocrine neoplasms of the appendix, colon and rectum. Pathologica 113(1):19–27
100. Vogelsang H, Siewert JR (2005) Endocrine tumours of the hindgut. Best Pract Res Clin Gastroenterol 19(5):739–751
101. Kang H, O'Connell JB, Leonardi MJ, Maggard MA, McGory ML, Ko CY (2007) Rare tumors of the colon and rectum: a national review. Int J Color Dis 22(2):183–189
102. Ramage JK, Goretzki PE, Manfredi R, Komminoth P, Ferone D, Hyrdel R et al (2008) Consensus guidelines for the management of patients with digestive neuroendocrine tumours: well-differentiated colon and rectum tumour/carcinoma. Neuroendocrinology 87(1):31–39
103. Kimura N, Sasano N (1986) Prostate-specific acid phosphatase in carcinoid tumors. Virchows Arch A Pathol Anat Histopathol 410(3):247–251

Liver-Directed Therapies in Neuroendocrine Tumors

27

Maxime Ronot, Marco Dioguardi Burgio, Lucas Raynaus, Luisa Paulatto, Lorenzo Garzelli, Jules Gregory, Jean-Charles Bijot, Magaly Zappa, Annie Sibert, Olivia Hentic, Louis de Mestier, Marie-Pierre Vullierme, Valérie Vilgrain, and Philippe Ruszniewski

27.1 Introduction

Neuroendocrine neoplasms are various tumors that develop at the expense of the diffuse neuroendocrine system. The World Health Organization (WHO) classifies these neoplasms according to their morphological characteristics (differentiation) and their degree of proliferation assessed by the mitotic index or Ki-67. Well-differentiated tumors are called "neuroendocrine tumors" (NETs), whereas tumors with little or no differentiation are called "neuroendocrine carcinomas" (NECs).

M. Ronot (✉) · L. Garzelli · J. Gregory · J.-C. Bijot · V. Vilgrain
Department of Radiology, Hôpital Beaujon, Assistance Publique-Hôpitaux de Paris, Clichy, France

Université de Paris, Paris, France
e-mail: maxime.ronot@aphp.fr; lorenzo.garzelli@aphp.fr; jules.gregory@aphp.fr; jeancharles.bijot@aphp.fr; valerie.vilgrain@aphp.fr

M. Dioguardi Burgio · L. Raynaus · L. Paulatto · A. Sibert · M.-P. Vullierme
Department of Radiology, Hôpital Beaujon, Assistance Publique-Hôpitaux de Paris, Clichy, France
e-mail: lucas.raynaud@aphp.fr; luisa.paulatto@aphp.fr; cayenne.fr.annie.sibert@aphp.fr

M. Zappa
Department of Radiology, Université de Paris, Paris, France

O. Hentic · L. de Mestier
Department of Gastroenterology, Hôpital Beaujon, Assistance Publique-Hôpitaux de Paris, Clichy, France
e-mail: olivia.hentic@aphp.fr; louis.demestier@aphp.fr

P. Ruszniewski
Université de Paris, Paris, France

Department of Gastroenterology, Hôpital Beaujon, Assistance Publique-Hôpitaux de Paris, Clichy, France
e-mail: philippe.ruszniewski@bjn.aphp.fr

S. Yalcin, K. Öberg (eds.), *Neuroendocrine Tumours*,
https://doi.org/10.1007/978-3-031-56968-5_27

Among NETs, grade (G) 1, 2, and 3 lesions are distinguished according to their degree of proliferation [1].

The liver is the predominant site for NET metastases, besides regional lymph nodes [2]. At diagnosis, about 65–95% of gastroenteropancretic (GEP) NET (excluding appendiceal, gastric and rectal NET) are associated with liver metastases [2]. NETs are metastatic at diagnosis in approximately 20%, 30%, and 50% of G1, G2, and G3 tumors, respectively, with metastatic status being the most important prognostic factor after tumor grade [3, 4]. Studies based on histological cohorts of untreated patients with NET have shown a dismal prognosis in patients with liver metastases compared to patients without. In fact, the 5-year survival is estimated at 13–54% in the event of metastases, against 75–99% in their absence [3–6]. Aside from the long-term prognosis, liver metastases also alter the quality of life of patients, regardless the primary site [2].

According to the recommendations of the European NeuroEndocrine Tumors Society (ENETS) [7], well-differentiated tumors, especially grade 1 or 2, are candidates for locoregional hepatic therapy, in particular when hepatic disease is isolated or dominant, while carcinomas are candidate for systemic treatment due to the rapid progression of the disease and usually widespread metastases. Locoregional treatments of liver metastases from GEP-NET include surgery-and image-guided therapies (ablative therapy and hepatic intra-arterial therapies that include chemoembolization, bland embolization, and radioembolization. Surgical resection of liver metastases is the standard of care and a curative-intent treatment. Surgery is recommended when complete resection or debulking more than 90% seems feasible [8]. This option justifies aggressive surgical approach that could require either 2-step surgery in synchronous bilobar tumors or patient preparation to surgery by portal vein ligation or embolization [9]. Complete R0 resection of liver metastases is the goal, with a 5-year survival of 80% when achieved [10]. Of note, the overall survival is still satisfactory in R1 resection with a 5-year survival of 70% [10]. However, surgery cannot be proposed to all patients, especially to those with diffuse liver metastases. In the study by Chamberlain et al., only 34 out of 85 patients could undergo surgical resection [11]. Hence, optimal selection of non-surgical treatments is crucial. In this setting, liver-directed treatments have two main objectives: oncologic (control of tumor growth) and symptomatic (control of secretory syndrome). For symptom control, liver-directed therapies are often second-line treatment considered after failure or insufficiency of somatostatin analogs. For control of tumor growth, treatments are often used when tumor progression is demonstrated or in case of large tumor burden.

This chapter addresses the various roles, technicalities, clinical efficacy, and safety of thermal ablation (radiofrequency, microwave, and cryotherapy) and transarterial procedures (bland embolization, chemoembolization, and radioembolization) as liver-directed therapies.

27.2 Thermal Ablative Techniques

Thermal ablation is based on the cytotoxic effects of local nonphysiologic temperature created by probes placed within the liver. Radiofrequency ablation (RFA) has been the most widely used and studied technique, but other techniques such as microwave ablation (MWA), laser, cryoablation or irreversible electroporation (IRE) have been developed. Radio-frequency ablation (RFA) is among the first techniques used for liver ablation and the one with the largest experience reported today in treatment of liver tumors; therefore, most of the studies reported in this publication refer to RFA.

Ablation can be performed percutaneously under computed tomography (CT), ultrasound (US), and rarely magnetic resonance imaging (MRI) guidance or intraoperatively mostly in combination with liver resection using either laparoscopic or open approach. In the latter setting, ablation is mostly used to destroy small metastases that either cannot be resected or would require extensive parenchymal resection, allowing for a most comprehensive surgery. In all cases, ablation can be considered curative intent when tumors are confined to the liver (Fig. 27.1).

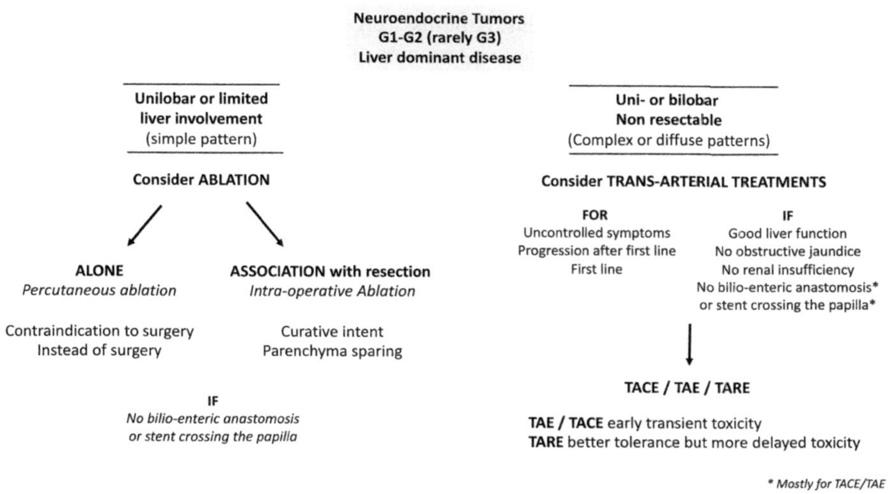

Fig. 27.1 Summary of the main indications and role of liver-directed treatments TACE/TAE/TARE: transarterial chemoembolization/embolization/radioembolization

27.2.1 Radiofrequency Ablation

With RFA, high-frequency current is transmitted to the liver through one or several electrode needles (uni- or multipolar technique). The ionic vibrations generated by the high frequency current induce heat that denatures intracellular proteins and leads to apoptosis and cell death. Pathologically, the destroyed tumor is replaced by coagulation necrosis. The thermal ablation area should include the tumor and sufficient safety margins to prevent from local progression (Fig. 27.2).

There are very few reports of ablation therapies in GEP-NET liver metastases, and most of them include a small number of patients. The size of the tumor is the factor that most influences the effectiveness of the treatment. In a study carried out in 34 patients with 234 metastases, the mean diameter of incompletely ablated tumors was 4.2 cm (vs 2.3 cm for the all studied groups) [12]. Therefore, the best candidates for ablation are patients with a low tumor volume (small numbers of tumors, usually ≤5, ideally with a diameter below 3–5 cm). This is due to the technical limitation of current RFA machines that allow a maximum volume of destruction around 5 cm that need to include, as mentioned above, the safety margins of 1–2 cm around the tumor.

The benefit of ablation or surgery alone for survival remains difficult to evaluate because patients eventually receive multiple subsequent lines of treatment. A retrospective study compared 103 patients who underwent RFA/resection and 273 patients with non-surgical treatment. Patients were matched on proliferation index, comorbidity, age, presence of symptoms, extent of metastases, and carcinoid heart disease. At 5 years, no difference in OS and disease-specific survival were observed [13].

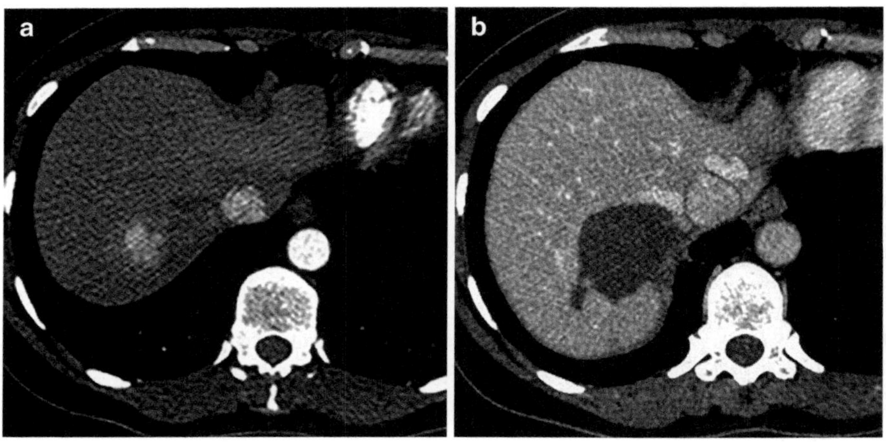

Fig. 27.2 Example of ablation in a 45-year-old man with small bowel neuroendocrine tumor liver metastases treated with prior left hepatectomy. (**a**) Axial CT scan (arterial phase) shows new metastases in the remnant right liver. (**b**) Axial CT scan (portal venous phase) obtained after radiofrequency ablation of the lesion shows the hypoattenuating ablation areas with no residual lesion

As discussed above, ablation is more frequently performed in association with resection. Ablation can also be discussed in tumor debulking and in controlling functional syndromes due to specific hormones excess. This explains why most series of patients with liver metastases from NET report more than five ablated tumors and use intraoperative RFA during one session [14, 15]. In the series by Elias et al., 16 patients had combined liver surgery and RFA [14]. A mean of 15 and 12 metastases per patient were surgically removed and RF ablated, respectively. Morbidity was observed in 69% of the cases. The 3-year overall survival and disease-free survival were similar to the previous experience of authors with of liver resection alone. In the study by Akyildiz et al., 119 laparoscopic RFA without liver resection were performed in 89 patients. The mean tumor size was 3.6 cm, and the mean number of tumors was six (range 1–16) [15]. Perioperative morbidity was 6% and 30-day morbidity was 1%. Forty-four patients had hormonal symptoms before the procedure. One week after RFA, 97% of these patients reported at least partial symptoms relief, and 73% had significant or complete relief. The symptomatic response lasted for a median of 14 ± 5 months [15]. Median disease-free survival was 1.3 year, and overall survival was 6 years after RFA.

Follow-up by imaging (CT and or MR imaging) is essential to assess complete tumor necrosis. One of the major issues is the recurrence of metastases within the liver as new tumors are reported up to 63% in the largest series of patients treated with RFA [15]. Conversely, local tumor progression is observed in 3.3–7.9% per lesion [15, 16]. Interestingly, in a meta-analysis including 5.224 ablated tumors of various origin, the rate of local progression was lower in neuroendocrine metastases than in other tumors [16]. This might be due to tumor characteristics such as well-circumscribed margins or a more indolent natural history of these tumors [16]. As with other liver malignancies, factors predictive of tumor recurrence are tumor size, presence of a safety margin, and blood vessel proximity [12]. In a multivariate analysis, statistically significant determinants of survival were only gender (with males having the worse prognosis) and size of the dominant liver metastasis (a tumor size exceeding 3 cm was associated with a higher mortality) [17].

Reported post-RFA death rates and major complication rates (pain, bile leakage, liver abscess, hemorrhage, bowel perforation pulmonary complications, portal vein thrombosis, and tumor seeding) are in the range of 0.5–1.5 and 3–5%, respectively [8, 12, 15, 17]. These complications are not specific to NET patients. Liver abscess is very rare in patients with no history of biliary-digestive anastomoses or a biliary stent crossing the ampulla (0.4% vs. 40% in patients with prior biliary intervention) [12]. Minor complications involve skin burns, segmental biliary dilatation, pleural effusions, and subcapsular hematoma of low abundance.

27.2.2 Microwave Ablation

MWA uses electromagnetic devices with frequencies ≥900 MHz. The principle of this technique is similar to RFA but has several theoretical advantages. First, the intratumoral temperatures are consistently higher than with RFA. Second, MWA is no sensitive to the "heat sink" effect observed in RFA that correspond to the cooling effect of blood flow in large vessels close to the tumor, both resulting in a theoretical better tumor control.

MWA has not been extensively evaluated in patient with liver metastases from NET [18]. As with RFA, most procedures are performed intraoperatively either with concomitant hepatic resection or not [19, 20]. For instance, in the study by Pickens et al., of the 50 patients (166 targeted lesions) who underwent MWA, 41 (82%) were treated with a minimally invasive approach, and 22 (44%) underwent MWA concomitant with hepatectomy and/or primary tumor resection. Recurrence-free survival at 1 and 5 years was 86% and 28%, respectively. Overall survival at 1 and 5 years was 94% and 70%, respectively (median follow-up 32 months, range 0–116 months) [19].

27.2.3 Cryotherapy

Cryotherapy is based on the decreased cell viability at low temperatures. The tissue temperature should reach at least −50 °C to achieve necrosis. Very few series have evaluated cryotherapy of liver metastases from NETs (the largest with 19 patients) [21–23]. As with other thermal ablative techniques, hormonal symptoms relief was observed in the vast majority of patients. Notably, postprocedural coagulopathy has been found in all patients of the two main series requiring transfusion of either platelets or fresh frozen plasma [22, 23]. In one of these series, two patients required intra-abdominal packing and transfusion of clotting factors [22]. The authors have not observed similar complications in any other liver malignancies and speculated that the necrosing tumors may release substances that disrupt the coagulation cascade [22]. Despite the efficacy on hormonal symptoms, cryotherapy has been gradually replaced by RFA, mainly for safety reasons.

27.2.4 Complications After Ablation Therapies

Death and major complications (bleeding, hollow organ perforation, portal vein thrombosis, and abscess) are rare after ablation, with reported rates around 0.5–1.5 and 3–5%, respectively. Liver abscess is very rare except in patients with a history of biliary-enteric anastomosis or of biliary intervention (e.g., biliary stent crossing the ampulla) for whom the risk is close to 50%. Consequently, a former biliary intervention constitutes a strong contraindication to ablation for most teams. Tumor seeding on the track of the needles is also very rare (<1%) and has been mostly reported with other tumors (e.g., hepatocellular carcinoma). Minor complications involve skin burns, pleural effusion, segmental biliary dilatation, and low-volume subcapsular hematoma.

27.3 Transarterial Treatments

27.3.1 Rationale

The rationale for transarterial hepatic treatments is based on the fact that liver metastases from NET derive their blood supply from the hepatic artery, while the normal liver has a dual vascular supply including 30% inflow from the hepatic artery and 70% inflow from the portal vein. Treatments lead to both the concentration of chemotherapy or radiation therapy (when used) in tumors and to ischemia thereby reducing hormone output and causing necrosis. Hepatic intra-arterial treatments include trans-arterial chemoembolization (TACE), trans-arterial embolization (TAE), and trans-arterial radioembolization (TARE).

27.3.2 Techniques

Intra-arterial hepatic treatments are most often performed during a short hospital stay, under light sedation or local anesthesia in patients who receive preventive pain relief and anxiolysis. The most frequent vascular access is the right femoral arterial, but the left radial artery is increasingly used.

The first step of all treatments is the production of a hepatic angiogram in two (digital subtracted angiography) and three dimensions (cone-beam CT or CT) to assess the arterial anatomy of patients. The obtained images are used for targeting (selection of the feeders that supply tumors) and for guidance (real-time control of the progression of endovascular devices). The treatments differ from each other by the nature of what is further injected.

TACE involves the injection of a chemotherapy drug followed by the embolization of the targeted arteries. It has been developed based on the principle that ischemia of tumor cells increases sensitivity to chemotherapeutic agents [24]. When the drug is injected as an emulsion in poppy seed oil (Lipiodol, Guerbet, Aulnay, France), it is called conventional chemoembolization. The attenuation of the oil allows fluoroscopic control of the injection and serves as drug carrier. This vectorization property makes it possible to reduce systemic exposure and to increase hepatic concentration, especially in tumors (up to 100 times that obtained by an intravenous injection). The drugs used in chemoembolization are numerous. The vast majority of teams use doxorubicin (around 1 mg/kg), but other teams use a combination of cisplatin, doxorubicin, and mitomycin C. Streptozotocin is also used. However, it should be noted that its injection requires general anesthesia due to severe pain during hepatic intra-arterial injection induced by acidic pH [25]. More recently, oxaliplatin has been reported as potentially interesting. Overall, based on current evidence, it is not possible to determine which drug is more efficient.

TAE is, as the name suggests, a targeted embolization of the blood vessels that supply tumors without injecting chemotherapy drugs.

Radioembolization is a vectorized internal selective radiation therapy. It consists of the injection of micron-sized calibrated biocompatible but nonbiodegradable resin or glass microbeads that contain a β-negative emitting radioisotope. The isotope is most often Yttrium-90 (90Y), a pure β emitter that decays to stable Zr-90 with a physical half-life of 64.1 h. New platforms using Holmium-166 (166Ho) are now available.

The treatment session is preceded by a first so-called "work-up" arteriography performed 7–14 days before the treatment. During the work-up, approximately 500 MBq are injected into the targeted area of the liver in the form of macro-aggregates of human albumin (MAA) labeled with metastable Technetium 99 (99mTc). A scintigraphy (or SPECT-CT) is further performed to estimate the fraction of pulmonary shunt (maximum tolerable dose to the lung of about 30 Gy), to check for the absence of extrahepatic perfusion and to calculate the estimated dose to the tumor and to the surrounding liver (personalized dosimetry). Tumor response is strongly associated with tumor absorbed dose, and hepatic toxicity with the dose received by the non-tumor liver and the non-target liver.

Treatment delivery is different from systemic therapy that is most often delivered at regular time interval until discontinued upon tumor progression or toxicity. As the hepatic metastases are most often diffuse or bilobar, intra-arterial treatment of the entire tumor burden generally requires two or three treatment sessions administered sequentially with 4-to-8-week intervals, to improve efficacy and limit toxicity. Of note, when tumors are small, selective catheterization of one or more arteries supplying the tumors is performed. Sequential procedures are performed depending on treatment tolerance, time required for liver function recovery, and signs of efficacy in the targeted areas. Intra-arterial treatments are usually discontinued when the entire tumor volume has been treated as planned, and when on objective tumor response has been obtained. Further intra-arterial treatments may be considered in case of disease progression (clinical and/or radiological) deemed technically accessible by an intra-arterial route. In the event of progression that cannot be treated by such an approach (extrahepatic progression, degraded arterial network, toxicity considered to be too great), another therapeutic option is preferred.

27.3.3 Patient Selection and Contraindications

The best candidates are patients with non-surgical liver predominant disease or those with major uncontrolled symptoms. The presence of small volume of lung, lymph node, or bone metastases is not considered an absolute contraindication (Fig. 27.1).

TACE and TAE lead to transient ischemia of the non-tumoral. Therefore, patients with impaired liver function should not be considered because treatment may lead to liver insufficiency. While TARE has no ischemic effect on the liver, transient radiation-induced decreased liver function is observed. Obstructive jaundice and history of biliary intervention (bilio-enteric anastomosis, biliary stent crossing the papilla) could expose to post-treatment infectious complications (cholangitis, bile duct necrosis, and liver abscess) [26]. This is especially true for TACE and TAE. TARE could be an interesting alternative with early results reporting low risk of post-treatment abscess [27]. TACE and TAE are contraindicated in patients with extensive portal vein thrombosis because the treatment can cause hepatic necrosis or infarction. However, segmental thrombosis is not a contraindication to TACE or TAE. TARE can be performed in patients with portal vein thrombosis. Other classical contra-indications are renal impairment, and altered (< 50%) left ventricular fraction ejection volume is doxorubicin is used. Patients with large tumor burden (e.g. >75% of liver involvement) must be treated with great caution, following a sequential approach that requires several treatment sessions.

27.3.4 Results of TACE and TAE

Intra-arterial treatments are among the most effective treatments for metastatic liver disease. Despite the large number of TACE or TAE studies performed in patients with liver metastases from NET, no randomized trials have been performed. Most studies have evaluated clinical, biological, and morphological responses. Partial or complete symptoms relief is observed in 42–100% and lasts between 9 and 24 months [28, 29]. Significant decrease in tumor markers occurs in 13–100% [28, 30]. The symptomatic response is higher when the treatment is used as first-line treatment with 70% complete symptomatic response and 20% partial response. Morphological response (either complete or partial) is depicted in 8–94% [30, 31] (Fig. 27.3) with, here again a greater benefit when the treatment is applied as first or

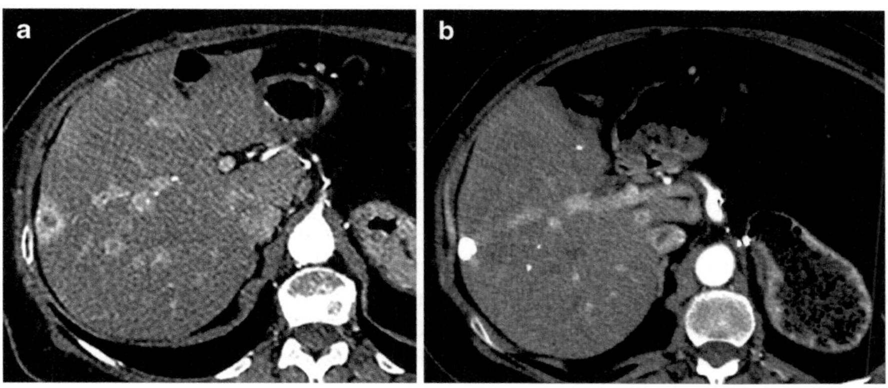

Fig. 27.3 Example of conventional chemoembolization in a 76-year-old man with pancreatic neuroendocrine tumor and multiple liver metastases. (**a**) Axial CT scan shows hyperenhancing lesions at the arterial phase. (**b**) Axial CT scan after conventional chemoembolization using streptozotocin shows marked lipiodol uptake with no residual enhancing tumor suggesting complete response

second line. Noticeably, imaging criteria for assessing tumor response have not been extensively evaluated. The overall survival is around 3 to 4 years [25, 32–35], up to 5 years in our experience. The improvement in survival reported by the most recent studies undoubtedly reflects a better selection of patients (treatment of G1 and G2 tumors only, treatment carried out at the onset of the disease) and a technical improvement (catheters, imaging 3D).

Predictive factors of tumor response after TAE or TACE have been identified. An hepatic tumor burden <30%, tumor enhancement on arterial phase CT images [36, 37], and primary tumor of the jejunum/ileum are associated with a better tumor response [25, 32, 36–38]. Other factors include tumor grade, the extent of extrahepatic disease, and the existence of previous treatment lines.

In the absence of randomized trials, individual predictors of survival are poorly understood. In retrospective series, a low tumor grade was associated with prolonged survival (54.5 months OS for patients with low-grade vs. 24 months for patients with high-grade tumors [35]. Midgut NETs have better outcomes than pancreatic NET higher response rate (66.7% vs 35.2%) and longer progression-free survival (PFS) (22.7 vs. 16.1 months), higher rate of symptoms control, and longer overall survival (median 80 vs 20 months) [32].

27.3.5 TACE and TAE: Technical Controversies

The superiority of TACE over TACE is not demonstrated. Historical data suggested that the use of intravenous chemotherapy in combination with arterial ligation or embolization improved objective responses rates of liver metastases from 56 to 75%, improved the duration of response from 6.6 to 19.8 months, and improved OS from 27 to 49 months [39].

In two retrospective studies, including one with close to 100 patients from three centers, no differences were observed in terms of patient survival and tumor response rate [40, 41]. In one study, chemoembolization demonstrated trends toward longer time-to-progression, symptom control and survival (although not significant) [42]. Of note, the toxicity profile of TACE and TAE was similar [42, 43]. In 2005, Gupta et al. performed a subgroup analysis comparing midgut and pancreatic tumors. Authors showed that the addition of intra-arterial chemotherapy to embolization did not improve overall survival or progression-free survival in patients with midgut tumors. Moreover, it had a deleterious effect on the morphologic response rate [25]. In contrast, a tendency toward prolonged survival and improved response rate was noted in patients with pancreatic tumors treated with TACE compared to TAE [25]. Only one prospective comparison of TAE and TACE in 26 patients with midgut metastases recruited over a 6-year period has been published [40]. The primary endpoint was progression-free survival. The expected number of enrolled patients was not achieved explaining that this study may suffer from a lack of power. Yet, no difference was observed between the two groups [40]. The 1-year progressive-free survival rates were 91.6% and 90% in the TAE and TACE groups, respectively. The median PFS was 24 months and 19 months in the TAE and TACE groups, respectively. There results suggest that the addition of intra-arterial chemotherapy to embolization may not prolong PFS in patients with midgut tumors. The question remains open in patients with pancreatic NET.

No comparison between absorbable and nonabsorbable particles has been conducted, and most studies have included patients treated with both particles [25, 41, 44, 45] (Fig. 27.4). Only one study has focused on TAE with triaxyl gelatin microspheres (embosphere®) (Fig. 27.5). Hepatic embolization was performed using either particles sized 300–500 μm, 500–700 μm, and/or 700–900 μm. Absence of disease progression was seen in 91% of the cases, and 35% of the patients had partial response on imaging using RECIST criteria despite the fact that some had

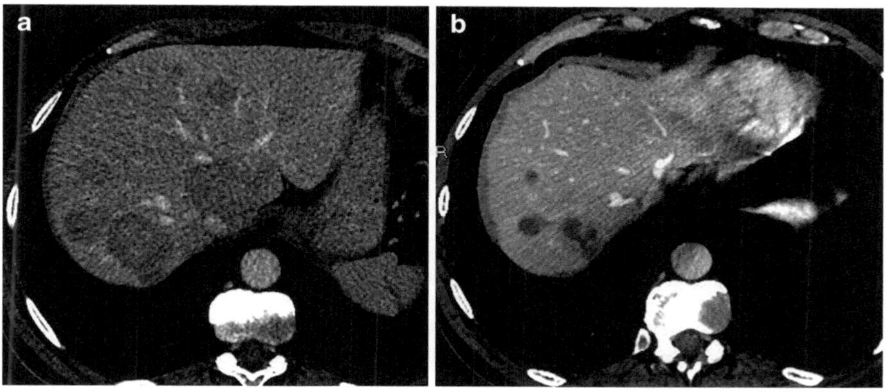

Fig. 27.4 Example of bland embolization with particles in a 56-year-old man with an history of resected small bowel neuroendocrine tumor. (**a**) Axial CT scan shows hypoattenuating liver metastases (portal venous phase). (**b**) Axial CT scan at the portal phase after bland embolization of the right liver with gel foam shows partial response with marked tumor necrosis and decrease in size of all lesions

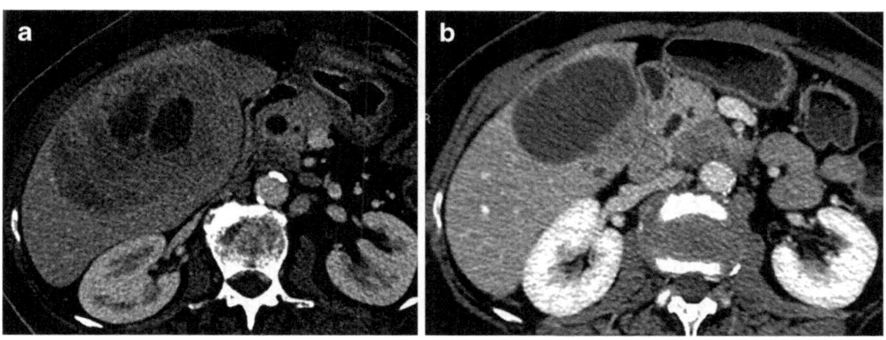

Fig. 27.5 67-year-old woman with a history of resected small bowel neuroendocrine tumor. (**a**) Axial CT scan shows a large hypoattenuating liver metastasis containing small area of necrosis (portal venous phase). (**b**) Axial CT scan at the portal venous phase after bland selective embolization shows complete response with marked necrosis and decrease in size of the lesion

extensive tumor necrosis [28]. No major complications occurred in this series. Notably, all patients with bilobar involvement were treated sequentially [28].

Drug-eluting beads (DEB) are particles that are preloaded with a chemotherapeutic agent. The principle is to deliver high dose and more sustained release of drug into the tumor compared to systemic chemotherapy. Drug-eluting bead (DEB)–TACE combines the theoretical advantages of embolization, high tumor exposure to a chemotherapy drug, and low systemic passage of the drug in animal tumor models [46, 47]. Initial reports of DEB–TACE with doxorubicin in patients with liver metastases reported stabilization or partial response on imaging in 95 and 100% of cases and a mean PFS of 14 and 15 months, respectively [48, 49]. No comparison has been made with conventional TACE in those patients. Later, biliary and liver injuries such as dilated bile ducts, portal vein narrowing, portal venous thrombosis, and bilioma/liver infarcts were reported in patients treated with DEB-TACE, with higher rates than in patients with hepatocellular developed on cirrhosis [50]. This first observation was largely confirmed by a study reported 7/13 (54%) patients with who developed bilomas [51]. This trial was therefore discontinued prematurely for seriousness of the adverse events. It is hypothesized that hypertrophied peribiliary plexus observed in cirrhosis could protect against the ischemic/chemical insult of bile ducts [50]. In the absence of randomized clinical trials, and no signal of better efficacy of DEB–TACE over conventional TACE, it is advisable to use Lipiodol–TACE especially when the total liver is treated.

27.3.6 Results of TARE

Few studies have analyzed the results of TARE in patients with hepatic NET metastases [52–59]. A multicenter retrospective review comprising 244 patients treated with 273 TARE sessions reported improvement of symptoms in 79% of patients (resolution 35%, improvement 44%), objective response and disease control rates of 62.9% and 91.4%, respectively (according to mRECIST criteria) [60]. Two recent meta-analyzes have confirmed these results, with objective response and tumor control rates of 50–51% and 86%, and a median overall survival of 28.5–32 months [61, 62] (Fig. 27.6). To date, no trial has compared TACE/TAE and TARE. Nevertheless, available evidence suggests that TACE have similar results to that reported with TACE or TAE [63–65].

27.3.7 Complications and Toxicity of Intra-Arterial Treatments

The most common and classical complication after TACE/TAE is the post-embolization syndrome that occurs in up to 80–90% of the patients [25] and includes fever, leukocytosis, abdominal pain, nausea, and a transient increase of liver enzymes. Post-embolization syndrome is best prevented by dexamethasone, and ondansetron is administered 6 h before and 30 min before treatment. Pain should be closely monitored, and pain control performed according to the severity of pain. Most of the time post-embolization syndrome is self-limited, improving within

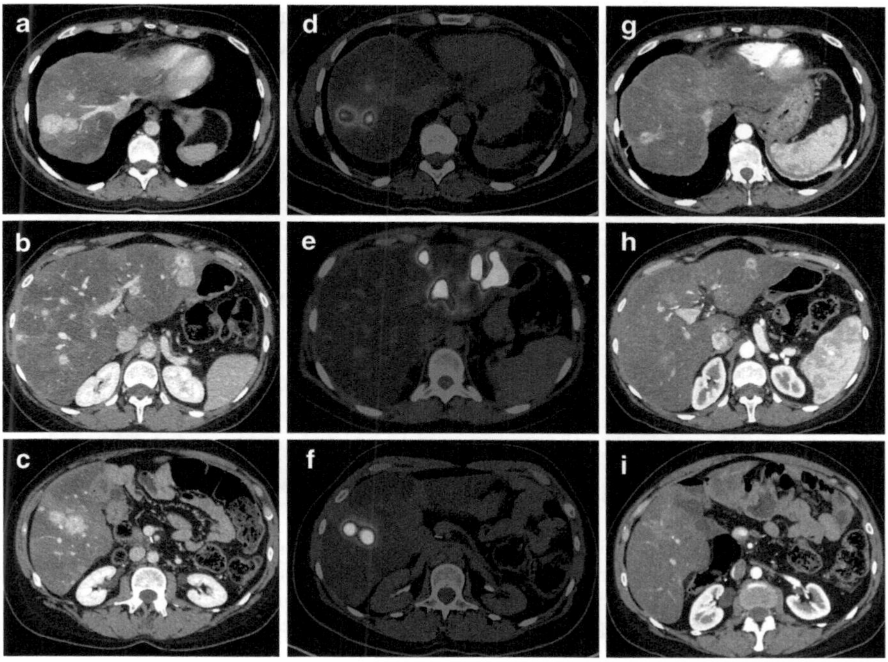

Fig. 27.6 Example of transarterial radioembolization in a 45-year-old woman with liver metastases from a pancreatic neuroendocrine tumor resected 17 years before. Liver metastases were bilobar and were treated with two sessions of TARE (resin microspheres, Yttrium 90). The left-hand side column (**a**–**c**) shows the baseline CT (portal venous phase), the central column (**d**–**f**) shows the SPECT CT performed after injection of 500 MBq activity in the form of macro-aggregates of human albumin (MAA) labeled with metastable Technetium 99 (99mTc), and the right-hand side column (**g**–**i**) shows sustained objective response at 2 years. The patient experienced no adverse event

3–5 days with conservative management. Locally, the toxicity of TACE/TAE is mainly hepato-biliary, with a risk of injury in up to 20–25% of patients. These lesions include biliary dilations, portal stenosis or thrombosis, the occurrence of bilioma, or even hepatic necrosis. In the vast majority of cases, these are moderate and subclinical damages. Severe complications include liver failure, liver abscess, cholecystitis, gastric ulcers and bleeding, and acute carcinoid crisis [8, 66–68] (Fig. 27.7). A prophylactic use of somatostatin analogs before TACE/TAE is therefore recommended in patients with functionally active tumors. Screening and treatment of carcinoid heart disease is also required in these patients.

The tolerance of radioembolization is significantly better than that of TACE/TAE. Moderate fatigue is common, post-embolization syndrome is virtually nonexistent. For the vast majority of patients, the quality of life is little or not altered and returns to its baseline level within 3–4 weeks [52, 56, 69]. Ulcer-type complications may occur when treatment is administered in extrahepatic arteries (gastroduodenal, right gastric, pancreatic-duodenal branches, etc.). Radiation lung disease has been

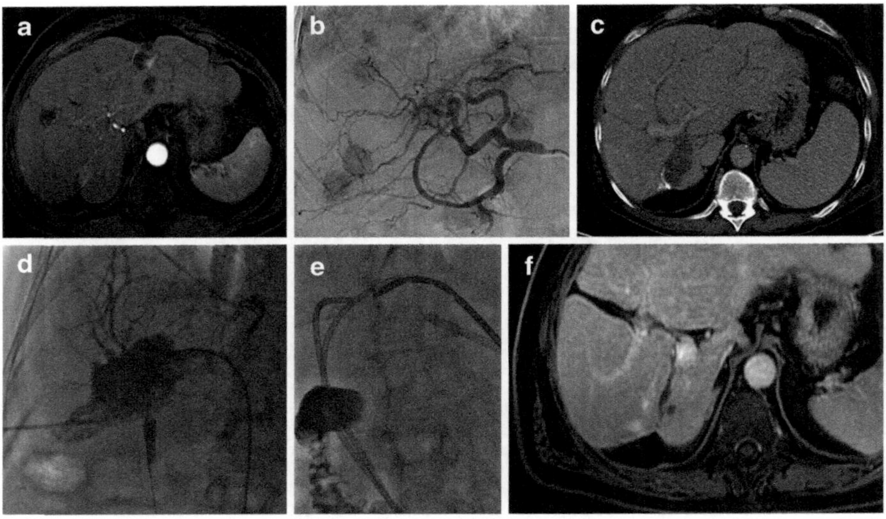

Fig. 27.7 Example of hepatobiliary toxicity in a 54-year-old patient with a grade 2 ileal neuroendocrine tumor and a history of right hepatectomy for liver metastasis and resection of the primary tumor. The MRI (**a**) shows recurrence of metastases in the remaining liver, appearing as tumor blushes on subtracted angiography images (**b**). The patient was treated with two sessions of conventional chemoembolization (doxorubicin and lipiodol) and one session of chemoembolization with beads loaded with doxorubicin. Subsequently, the patient developed mild bile ducts dilatation and bilioma in the right posterior sector (**c**), communicating with the bile ducts (**d**). The treatment consisted of the placement of percutaneous drains and drainage of the collection (**e**) which allowed the lesions to resolve (**f**)

reported in patients with major pulmonary shunting, as well as early hepatic decompensation when treatment targets a large liver volume in patients with preexisting impaired liver function. In the longer term, radioembolization exposes to a risk of post-radiation liver disease (cirrhotic-like dysmorphy, ascites, splenomegaly, and portosystemic shunts), especially when treatments are bilobar [70, 71], and eventually hepatic decompensation. Curie et al. recently reported similar long-term toxicity rates between TACE and TARE (22% and 29%, respectively), but a higher rate of treatment-related toxicity after TARE (14% versus 3%) [72]. The delayed toxicity associated with TACE appears less severe and manifests mainly as abnormal liver tests, whereas clinical hepatic decompensation dominates after TARE. A more selective approach, sparing hepatic segments and dosimetric analysis of both tumors and non-tumor parenchyma, can decrease hepatic exposure, and therefore the risk of radiation-induced liver disease.

27.4 In Conclusion

liver-directed therapies are widely performed in patients with liver metastases from neuroendocrine tumors. Due to its complexity, the metastatic liver disease requires medical expertise, and management in expert centers that provide high-quality care and the most recent type of imaging includes functional imaging with several tracers.

Within the current therapeutic armamentarium, interventional radiology offers a set of treatments (ablation, chemoembolization, bland embolization, and radioembolization) adapted to patients with liver dominant disease and oligometastatic lung and bone lesions. They are associated with very good clinical and symptomatic efficacy, high objective response rates with acceptable local toxicity. The choice of intra-arterial treatment is not standardized and should be part of a broader strategy in these patients who are often treated for long periods of time.

References

1. WHO (2019) Digestive system tumours, WHO classification of tumours, 5th edn. WHO, Geneva
2. Frilling A, Sotiropoulos GC, Li J, Kornasiewicz O, Plockinger U (2010) Multimodal management of neuroendocrine liver metastases. HPB (Oxford) 12(6):361–379
3. La Rosa S, Klersy C, Uccella S et al (2009) Improved histologic and clinicopathologic criteria for prognostic evaluation of pancreatic endocrine tumors. Hum Pathol 40:30–40
4. Yao JC, Hassan M, Phan A et al (2008) One hundred years after "carcinoid": epidemiology of and prognostic factors for neuroendocrine tumors in 35,825 cases in the United States. J Clin Oncol 26:3063–3072
5. McDermott EW, Guduric B, Brennan MF (1994) Prognostic variables in patients with gastrointestinal carcinoid tumours. Br J Surg 81(7):1007–1009
6. Zeitels J, Naunheim K, Kaplan EL, Straus F 2nd (1982) Carcinoid tumors: a 37-year experience. Arch Surg 117(5):732–737
7. Pavel M, Baudin E, Couvelard A et al (2012) ENETS consensus guidelines for the management of patients with liver and other distant metastases from neuroendocrine neoplasms of foregut, midgut, hindgut, and unknown primary. Neuroendocrinology 95:157–176
8. Auernhammer CJ, Goke B (2011) Therapeutic strategies for advanced neuroendocrine carcinomas of jejunum/ileum and pancreatic origin. Gut 60(7):1009–1021
9. Kianmanesh R, Sauvanet A, Hentic O, Couvelard A, Levy P, Vilgrain V, Ruszniewski P, Belghiti J (2008) Two-step surgery for synchronous bilobar liver metastases from digestive endocrine tumors: a safe approach for radical resection. Ann Surg 247(4):659–665
10. Elias D, Lasser P, Ducreux M, Duvillard P, Ouellet JF, Dromain C, Schlumberger M, Pocard M, Boige V, Miquel C, Baudin E (2003) Liver resection (and associated extrahepatic resections) for metastatic well-differentiated endocrine tumors: a 15-year single center prospective study. Surgery 133(4):375–382
11. Chamberlain RS, Canes D, Brown KT, Saltz L, Jarnagin W, Fong Y, Blumgart LH (2000) Hepatic neuroendocrine metastases: does intervention alter outcomes? J Am Coll Surg 190(4):432–445
12. Berber E, Siperstein AE (2007) Perioperative outcome after laparoscopic radiofrequency ablation of liver tumors: an analysis of 521 cases. Surg Endosc 21(4):613–618. https://doi.org/10.1007/s00464-006-9139-y13
13. Norlen O, Stalberg P, Zedenius J, Hellman P (2013) Outcome after resection and radiofrequency ablation of liver metastases from small intestinal neuroendocrine tumours. Br J Surg 100:1505–1514. https://doi.org/10.1002/bjs.9262
14. Elias D, Goere D, Leroux G, Dromain C, Leboulleux S, de Baere T, Ducreux M, Baudin E (2009) Combined liver surgery and RFA for patients with gastroenteropancreatic endocrine tumors presenting with more than 15 metastases to the liver. Eur J Surg Oncol 35(10):1092–1097. https://doi.org/10.1016/j.ejso.2009.02.017

15. Akyildiz HY, Mitchell J, Milas M, Siperstein A, Berber E (2010) Laparoscopic radiofrequency thermal ablation of neuroendocrine hepatic metastases: long-term follow-up. Surgery 148(6):1288–1293.; discussion 1293. https://doi.org/10.1016/j.surg.2010.09.014
16. Mulier S, Ni Y, Jamart J, Ruers T, Marchal G, Michel L (2005) Local recurrence after hepatic radiofrequency coagulation: multivariate meta-analysis and review of contributing factors. Ann Surg 242(2):158–171. https://doi.org/10.1097/01.sla.0000171032.99149.fe
17. Mazzaglia PJ, Berber E, Milas M, Siperstein AE (2007) Laparoscopic radiofrequency ablation of neuroendocrine liver metastases: a 10-year experience evaluating predictors of survival. Surgery 142(1):10–19. https://doi.org/10.1016/j.surg.2007.01.036
18. Martin RC, Scoggins CR, McMasters KM (2010) Safety and efficacy of microwave ablation of hepatic tumors: a prospective review of a 5-year experience. Ann Surg Oncol 17(1):171–178. https://doi.org/10.1245/s10434-009-0686-z
19. Pickens RC, Sulzer JK, Passeri MJ, Murphy K, Vrochides D, Martinie JB, Baker EH, Ocuin LM, McKillop IH, Iannitti DA (2020) Operative microwave ablation for the multimodal treatment of neuroendocrine liver metastases. J Laparoendosc Adv Surg Tech A 31:917. https://doi.org/10.1089/lap.2020.0558
20. Perrodin SF, Renzulli MM, Maurer MH, Kim-Fuchs C, Candinas D, Beldi G, Lachenmayer A (2020) Can microwave ablation be an alternative to resection for the treatment of neuroendocrine liver metastases? Endocr Pract 26(4):378–387
21. Bilchik AJ, Sarantou T, Foshag LJ, Giuliano AE, Ramming KP (1997) Cryosurgical palliation of metastatic neuroendocrine tumors resistant to conventional therapy. Surgery 122(6):1040–1047. discussion 1047-1048
22. Seifert JK, Cozzi PJ, Morris DL (1998) Cryotherapy for neuroendocrine liver metastases. Semin Surg Oncol 14(2):175–183. https://doi.org/10.1002/(SICI)1098-2388(199803)14:2<175::AID-SSU10>3.0.CO;2-2
23. Shapiro RS, Shafir M, Sung M, Warner R, Glajchen N (1998) Cryotherapy of metastatic carcinoid tumors. Abdom Imaging 23(3):314–317
24. Steward MJ, Warbey VS, Malhotra A, Caplin ME, Buscombe JR, Yu D (2008) Neuroendocrine tumors: role of interventional radiology in therapy. Radiographics 28(4):1131–1145. https://doi.org/10.1148/rg.284075170
25. Gupta S, Johnson MM, Murthy R, Ahrar K, Wallace MJ, Madoff DC, McRae SE, Hicks ME, Rao S, Vauthey JN, Ajani JA, Yao JC (2005) Hepatic arterial embolization and chemoembolization for the treatment of patients with metastatic neuroendocrine tumors: variables affecting response rates and survival. Cancer 104(8):1590–1602. https://doi.org/10.1002/cncr.21389
26. de Baere T, Roche A, Amenabar JM, Lagrange C, Ducreux M, Rougier P, Elias D, Lasser P, Patriarche C (1996) Liver abscess formation after local treatment of liver tumors. Hepatology 23(6):1436–1440
27. Devulapalli KK, Fidelman N, Soulen MC, Miller M, Johnson MS, Addo E, El-Haddad G, Nutting C, Morrison J, Farsad K, Lokken RP, Gaba RC, Fleming J, Brown DB, Kwan SW, Rose SC, Pennycooke KA, Liu DM, White SB, Gandhi R, Lazar AA, Kerlan RK Jr (2018) ⁹⁰Y Radioembolization for hepatic malignancy in patients with previous biliary intervention: multicenter analysis of hepatobiliary infections. Radiology 288(3):774–781
28. Granberg D, Eriksson LG, Welin S, Kindmark H, Janson ET, Skogseid B, Oberg K, Eriksson B, Nyman R (2007) Liver embolization with trisacryl gelatin microspheres (embosphere) in patients with neuroendocrine tumors. Acta Radiol 48(2):180–185. https://doi.org/10.1080/02841850601080440
29. Therasse E, Breittmayer F, Roche A, De Baere T, Indushekar S, Ducreux M, Lasser P, Elias D, Rougier P (1993) Transcatheter chemoembolization of progressive carcinoid liver metastasis. Radiology 189(2):541–547
30. Carrasco CH, Charnsangavej C, Ajani J, Samaan NA, Richli W, Wallace S (1986) The carcinoid syndrome: palliation by hepatic artery embolization. AJR Am J Roentgenol 147(1):149–154
31. Kress O, Wagner HJ, Wied M, Klose KJ, Arnold R, Alfke H (2003) Transarterial chemoembolization of advanced liver metastases of neuroendocrine tumors—a retrospective single-center analysis. Digestion 68(2–3):94–101. https://doi.org/10.1159/00007452274522

32. Eriksson BK, Larsson EG, Skogseid BM, Lofberg AM, Lorelius LE, Oberg KE (1998) Liver embolizations of patients with malignant neuroendocrine gastrointestinal tumors. Cancer 83(11):2293–2301. https://doi.org/10.1002/(SICI)1097-0142(19981201)83:11<2293::AID-CNCR8>3.0.CO;2-E
33. Kim YH, Ajani JA, Carrasco CH, Dumas P, Richli W, Lawrence D, Chuang V, Wallace S (1999) Selective hepatic arterial chemoembolization for liver metastases in patients with carcinoid tumor or islet cell carcinoma. Cancer Investig 17(7):474–478
34. Hur S, Chung JW, Kim HC et al (2013) Survival outcomes and prognostic factors of transcatheter arterial chemoembolization for hepatic neuroendocrine metastases. J Vasc Interv Radiol 24:947–956. (quiz 957
35. Sofocleous CT, Petre EN, Gonen M et al (2014) Factors affecting periprocedural morbidity and mortality and long-term patient survival after arterial embolization of hepatic neuroendocrine metastases. J Vasc Interv Radiol 25:22–30. (quiz 31)
36. Marrache F, Vullierme MP, Roy C, El Assoued Y, Couvelard A, O'Toole D, Mitry E, Hentic O, Hammel P, Levy P, Ravaud P, Rougier P, Ruszniewski P (2007) Arterial phase enhancement and body mass index are predictors of response to chemoembolization for liver metastases of endocrine tumours. Br J Cancer 96(1):49–55. https://doi.org/10.1038/sj.bjc.6603526
37. Roche A, Girish BV, de Baere T, Ducreux M, Elias D, Laplanche A, Boige V, Schlumberger M, Ruffle P, Baudin E (2004) Prognostic factors for chemoembolization in liver metastasis from endocrine tumors. Hepato-Gastroenterology 51(60):1751–1756
38. Ruszniewski P, Rougier P, Roche A, Legmann P, Sibert A, Hochlaf S, Ychou M, Mignon M (1993) Hepatic arterial chemoembolization in patients with liver metastases of endocrine tumors. A prospective phase II study in 24 patients. Cancer 71(8):2624–2630
39. Moertel CG, Johnson CM, McKusick MA, Martin J Jr, Nagorney DM, Kvols LK, Rubin J, Kunselman S (1994) The management of patients with advanced carcinoid tumors and islet cell carcinomas. Ann Intern Med 120:302–309. https://doi.org/10.7326/0003-4819-120-4-199402150-00008
40. Maire F, Lombard-Bohas C, O'Toole D, Vullierme MP, Rebours V, Couvelard A, Pelletier A-L, Zappa M, Pilleul F, Hentic O, Hammel P, Ruszniewski P (2012) Hepatic arterial embolization versus chemoembolization in the treatment of liver metastases of well-differentiated midgut endocrine tumors. A prospective randomized study. Neuroendocrinology 96(4):294–300. https://doi.org/10.1159/000336941
41. Pitt SC, Knuth J, Keily JM, McDermott JC, Weber SM, Chen H, Rilling WS, Quebbeman EJ, Agarwal DM, Pitt HA (2008) Hepatic neuroendocrine metastases: chemo—or bland embolization? J Gastrointest Surg 12(11):1951–1960. https://doi.org/10.1007/s11605-008-0640-6
42. Ruutiainen AT, Soulen MC, Tuite CM, Clark TW, Mondschein JI, Stavropoulos SW, Trerotola SO (2007) Chemoembolization and bland embolization of neuroendocrine tumor metastases to the liver. J Vasc Interv Radiol 18(7):847–855. https://doi.org/10.1016/j.jvir.2007.04.018
43. Fiore F, Del Prete M, Franco R, Marotta V, Ramundo V, Marciello F, Di Sarno A, Carratu AC, de Luca di Roseto C, Colao A, Faggiano A (2014) Transarterial embolization (TAE) is equally effective and slightly safer than transarterial chemoembolization (TACE) to manage liver metastases in neuroendocrine tumors. Endocrine 47:177. https://doi.org/10.1007/s12020-013-0130-9
44. Ho AS, Picus J, Darcy MD, Tan B, Gould JE, Pilgram TK, Brown DB (2007) Long-term outcome after chemoembolization and embolization of hepatic metastatic lesions from neuroendocrine tumors. AJR Am J Roentgenol 188(5):1201–1207. https://doi.org/10.2214/AJR.06.0933
45. Strosberg JR, Choi J, Cantor AB, Kvols LK (2006) Selective hepatic artery embolization for treatment of patients with metastatic carcinoid and pancreatic endocrine tumors. Cancer Control 13(1):72–78
46. Hong K, Khwaja A, Liapi E, Torbenson MS, Georgiades CS, Geschwind JF (2006) New intra-arterial drug delivery system for the treatment of liver cancer: preclinical assessment in a rabbit model of liver cancer. Clin Cancer Res 12:2563–2567. https://doi.org/10.1158/1078-0432.CCR-05-2225

47. Rao PP, Pascale F, Seck A, Auperin A, Drouard-Troalen L, Deschamps F, Teriitheau C, Paci A, Denys A, Bize P et al (2012) Irinotecan loaded in eluting beads: preclinical assessment in a rabbit VX2 liver tumor model. Cardiovasc Intervent Radiol 35:1448–1459. https://doi.org/10.1007/s00270-012-0343-y
48. de Baere T, Deschamps F, Teriitheau C, Rao P, Conengrapht K, Schlumberger M, Leboulleux S, Baudin E, Hechellhammer L (2008) Transarterial chemoembolization of liver metastases from well differentiated gastroenteropancreatic endocrine tumors with doxorubicin-eluting beads: preliminary results. J Vasc Interv Radiol 19(6):855–861. https://doi.org/10.1016/j.jvir.2008.01.030
49. Gaur SK, Friese JL, Sadow CA, Ayyagari R, Binkert CA, Schenker MP, Kulke M, Baum R (2011) Hepatic arterial chemoembolization using drug-eluting beads in gastrointestinal neuroendocrine tumor metastatic to the liver. Cardiovasc Intervent Radiol 34(3):566–572. https://doi.org/10.1007/s00270-011-0122-1
50. Guiu B, Deschamps F, Aho S, Munck F, Dromain C, Boige V, Malka D, Leboulleux S, Ducreux M, Schlumberger M, Baudin E, de Baere T (2012) Liver/biliary injuries following chemoembolization of endocrine tumours and hepatocellular carcinoma: Lipiodol vs. drug-eluting beads. J Hepatol 56(3):609–617. https://doi.org/10.1016/j.jhep.2011.09.012
51. Bhagat N, Reyes DK, Lin M, Kamel I, Pawlik TM, Frangakis C, Geschwind JF (2013) Phase II study of chemoembolization with drug-eluting beads in patients with hepatic neuroendocrine metastases: high incidence of biliary injury. Cardiovasc Intervent Radiol 36(2):449–459. https://doi.org/10.1007/s00270-012-0424-y
52. Kennedy AS, Dezarn WA, McNeillie P, Coldwell D, Nutting C, Carter D, Murthy R, Rose S, Warner RR, Liu D, Palmedo H, Overton C, Jones B, Salem R (2008) Radioembolization for unresectable neuroendocrine hepatic metastases using resin 90Y-microspheres: early results in 148 patients. Am J Clin Oncol 31(3):271–279. https://doi.org/10.1097/COC.0b013e31815e4557
53. Cao CQ, Yan TD, Bester L, Liauw W, Morris DL (2010) Radioembolization with yttrium microspheres for neuroendocrine tumour liver metastases. Br J Surg 97(4):537–543. https://doi.org/10.1002/bjs.6931
54. Kalinowski M, Dressler M, Konig A, El-Sheik M, Rinke A, Hoffken H, Gress TM, Arnold R, Klose KJ, Wagner HJ (2009) Selective internal radiotherapy with Yttrium-90 microspheres for hepatic metastatic neuroendocrine tumors: a prospective single center study. Digestion 79(3):137–142. https://doi.org/10.1159/000209849
55. King J, Quinn R, Glenn DM, Janssen J, Tong D, Liaw W, Morris DL (2008) Radioembolization with selective internal radiation microspheres for neuroendocrine liver metastases. Cancer 113(5):921–929. https://doi.org/10.1002/cncr.23685
56. Paprottka PM, Hoffmann RT, Haug A, Sommer WH, Raessler F, Trumm CG, Schmidt GP, Ashoori N, Reiser MF, Jakobs TF (2012) Radioembolization of symptomatic, unresectable neuroendocrine hepatic metastases using yttrium-90 microspheres. Cardiovasc Intervent Radiol 35(2):334–342. https://doi.org/10.1007/s00270-011-0248-1
57. Rhee TK, Lewandowski RJ, Liu DM, Mulcahy MF, Takahashi G, Hansen PD, Benson AB 3rd, Kennedy AS, Omary RA, Salem R (2008) 90Y Radioembolization for metastatic neuroendocrine liver tumors: preliminary results from a multi-institutional experience. Ann Surg 247(6):1029–1035. https://doi.org/10.1097/SLA.0b013e3181728a45
58. Saxena A, Chua TC, Bester L, Kokandi A, Morris DL (2010) Factors predicting response and survival after yttrium-90 radioembolization of unresectable neuroendocrine tumor liver metastases: a critical appraisal of 48 cases. Ann Surg 251(5):910–916. https://doi.org/10.1097/SLA.0b013e3181d3d24a
59. Benson AB 3rd, Geschwind JF, Mulcahy MF, Rilling W, Siskin G, Wiseman G, Cunningham J, Houghton B, Ross M, Memon K, Andrews J, Fleming CJ, Herman J, Nimeiri H, Lewandowski RJ, Salem R (2013) Radioembolization for liver metastases: results from a prospective 151 patient multi-institutional phase II study. Eur J Cancer 49(15):3122–3130. https://doi.org/10.1016/j.ejca.2013.05.012

60. Braat AJAT, Kappadath SC, Ahmadzadehfar H et al (2019) Radioembolization with ^{90}Y resin microspheres of neuroendocrine liver metastases: international multicenter study on efficacy and toxicity. Cardiovasc Intervent Radiol 42(3):413–425
61. Devcic Z, Rosenberg J, Braat AJAT et al (2014) J Nucl Med 55:1404–1410
62. Frilling A, Clift AK, Braat AJAT et al (2019) Radioembolization with 90Y microspheres for neuroendocrine liver metastases: an institutional case series, systematic review and meta-analysis. HPB (Oxford) 21(7):773–783
63. Engelman ES, Leon-Ferre R, Naraev BG, Sharma N, Sun S, O'Dorisio TM, Howe J, Button A, Zamba G, Halfdanarson TR (2014) Comparison of transarterial liver-directed therapies for low-grade metastatic neuroendocrine tumors in a single institution. Pancreas 43(2):219–225. https://doi.org/10.1097/MPA.0000000000000030
64. Whitney R, Valek V, Fages JF, Garcia A, Narayanan G, Tatum C, Hahl M, Martin RC 2nd (2011) Transarterial chemoembolization and selective internal radiation for the treatment of patients with metastatic neuroendocrine tumors: a comparison of efficacy and cost. Oncologist 16(5):594–601. https://doi.org/10.1634/theoncologist.2010-0292
65. Yang TX, Chua TC, Morris DL (2012) Radioembolization and chemoembolization for unresectable neuroendocrine liver metastases—a systematic review. Surg Oncol 21(4):299–308. https://doi.org/10.1016/j.suronc.2012.07.001
66. Kim W, Clark TW, Baum RA, Soulen MC (2001) Risk factors for liver abscess formation after hepatic chemoembolization. J Vasc Interv Radiol 12(8):965–968
67. de Baere T, Roche A, Amenabar JM, Lagrange C, Ducreux M, Rougier P, Elias D, Lasser P, Patriarche C (1996) Liver abscess formation after local treatment of liver tumors. Hepatology 23(6):1436–1440. https://doi.org/10.1002/hep.510230620
68. Woo S, Chung JW, Hur S, Joo SM, Kim HC, Jae HJ, Park JH (2013) Liver abscess after transarterial chemoembolization in patients with bilioenteric anastomosis: frequency and risk factors. AJR Am J Roentgenol 200(6):1370–1377. https://doi.org/10.2214/AJR.12.9630
69. Memon K, Lewandowski RJ, Mulcahy MF, Riaz A, Ryu RK, Sato KT, Gupta R, Nikolaidis P, Miller FH, Yaghmai V, Gates VL, Atassi B, Newman S, Omary RA, Benson AB 3rd, Salem R (2012) Radioembolization for neuroendocrine liver metastases: safety, imaging, and long-term outcomes. Int J Radiat Oncol Biol Phys 83(3):887–894. https://doi.org/10.1016/j.ijrobp.2011.07.041
70. Tomozawa Y, Jahangiri Y, Pathak P et al (2018) Long-term toxicity after Transarterial Radioembolization with Yttrium-90 using resin microspheres for neuroendocrine tumor liver metastases. J Vasc Interv Radiol 29(6):858–865
71. Su YK, Mackey RV, Riaz A et al (2017) Long-term hepatotoxicity of Yttrium-90 Radioembolization as treatment of metastatic neuroendocrine tumor to the liver. J Vasc Interv Radiol 28(11):1520–1526. https://doi.org/10.1016/j.jvir.2017.05.011
72. Currie BM, Nadolski G, Mondschein J et al (2020) Chronic hepatotoxicity in patients with metastatic neuroendocrine tumor: transarterial chemoembolization versus transarterial radioembolization. J Vasc Interv Radiol 31(10):1627–1635

Peptide Receptor Radionuclide Therapy (PRRT) 28

Murat Fani Bozkurt

28.1 Introduction

The theoretical basis of peptide receptor radionuclide therapy (PRRT) depends on delivering therapaeutic dose of radiation inside the tumor cells, owing to the internalization of the somatostatin receptor and radiolabeled somatostatin analog complex. Therefore, PRRT is actually an internal radiation therapy. Since Indium-111-labeled octreotide (^{111}In-Octreotide) was approved by the FDA as a diagnostic imaging agent for neuroendocrine tumors in 1994, studies have begun to assess whether it would be possible to apply radiolabeled somatostatin receptor analogs for therapy on the basis of the same molecular mechanism. The first trial to perform PRRT with radiolabeled octreotide dates back to early 1990s in a multicenter study in which high doses of diagnostic ^{111}In-Octreotide was administered to patients with neuroendocrine tumors, in whom somatostatin receptor overexpression was confirmed by a previous ^{111}In-Octreotide scintigraphy [1]. Although ^{111}In is only a gamma emitter radionuclide and does not emit any beta or alpha particles that are necessary for therapy, owing to its relatively high amount of Auger and conversion electrons which act like beta particles, it was expected to exert therapeutic effect if it is administered at high doses. This was the first approach to PRRT. However, ^{111}In-Octreotide therapy did not result with promising results and even partial remissions were exceptional. These disappointing results have given rise to use higher-energy and longer-tissue range radionuclides instead of ^{111}In, such as Yttrium-90 (^{90}Y). ^{90}Y is a pure beta emitter radionuclide with a high maximum energy (Emax:2,27 MeV), long tissue range (Rmax:11 mm), and a relatively long physical half-life (T1/2:64 h), which make this radionuclide a quite suitable agent to be used as a therapeutic radiopharmaceutical. Along with ^{90}Y, another radionuclide Lutetium-177 (^{177}Lu) has also been introduced as having suitable therapeutic characteristics (Emax:0,49 MeV, Rmax:2 mm, T1/2:6.7 days). The main difference of

M. F. Bozkurt (✉)
Department of Nuclear Medicine, Hacettepe University Faculty of Medicine, Ankara, Turkey

S. Yalcin, K. Öberg (eds.), *Neuroendocrine Tumours*,
https://doi.org/10.1007/978-3-031-56968-5_28

^{177}Lu from is that ^{90}Y is that ^{177}Lu is not a pure beta emitter, and it emits both beta radiation for therapy and gamma radiation for imaging. Both radionuclides are tagged to somatostatin analogs with bridging macrocyclic chelator 1,4,7,10-tetraaz acyclododecane-n, N′,N″,‴-tetraacetic acid (DOTA) to form different forms of therapeutic radiopharmaceuticals according to their N-terminal amino acids such as ^{90}Y/^{177}Lu-DOTATOC/DOTATATE/DOTANOC. These radiopharmaceuticals have been studied in different trials since early 2000s to recent years [2, 3]. More recently, alpha-emitting radiopharmaceuticals have been introduced for PRRT. Among these, Actinium-125 (^{125}Ac)-DOTATATE is getting wide acceptance especially for patients who do not show good therapy response following ^{177}Lu-DOTATATE or ^{90}Y-DOTANOC PRRT [4].

This chapter focuses on the use of therapeutic radiopharmaceuticals, indications, practical aspects, and monitorization of PRRT for neuroendocrine tumors along with some related future perspectives.

28.2 Rationale of PRRT for Neuroendocrine Tumors

Neuroendocrine tumor cells are characteristically regulated by particular hormones that exert their actions by binding some specific transmembrane-domain G-protein-coupled membrane surface receptors. The most abundant and most studied receptor-ligand system in neuroendocrine tumors is somatostatin receptor system. PRRT basically depends on the presence of overexpression of somatostatin receptors on cell membranes of neuroendocrine tumor cells and after radiolabeled somatostatin analog binds to specific receptor, the radiopharmaceutical-recceptor complex is internalized into the cell, where therapeutic irradiation from the radiopharmaceutical is emitted. There are a number of somatostatin receptor subtypes, out of which subtype 2 (sstr2) is most frequently expressed on many kinds of neuroendocrine tumor cells. Therefore, radiolabeled somatostatin analogues which have high affinity to sstr2 are preferred as therapeutic use, based on the same rationale for diagnostic imaging [2, 3].

28.3 Indications of PRRT

1. Gastroenteropancreatic and bronchial tract neuroendocrine tumors, which mainly overexpress sstr2. Such tumors should display high radiopharmaceutical uptake (preferably equal to or more than the liver uptake) on somatostatin receptor imaging studies.
2. Pheochromocytomas and paragangliomas, which show uptake on diagnostic somatostatin receptor imaging.
3. Medullary thyroid carcinomas, which are positive on diagnostic somatostatin receptor imaging.
4. Any tumor is to be potentially treated if sstr2 overexpression is confirmed and documented on diagnostic somatostatin receptor imaging and/or confirmed histopathologically. The benefit of PRRT should be justified for such patient on an individual basis with multidisciplinary evaluation.

28.4 Patient Selection and Eligibility for PRRT

Ideally, a tumor board with a minimum number of different specialists including surgeon, pathologist, oncologist, radiologist-interventional radiologist, nuclear medicine physician, radiation oncologist, endocrinologist, gastroenterologist, and others who are interested in neuroendocrine tumor management should be established on the first referral of neuroendocrine tumor patients. Decision for PRRT should be made by the tumor board after evaluation of all other therapeutic options starting from surgery, proceeding to systemic and local therapies. A complete clinical history and informed consent should be obtained from all patients referred to PRRT. For patient eligibility, these following information is mandatory:

1. Patient has to have histopathologically proven and documented neuroendocrine tumor.
2. High somatostatin receptor expression has to be documented by diagnostic somatostatin receptor imaging study and/or by immunohistochemistry.

The density of receptors on tumor tissue versus healthy organs should also be considered. In routine practice, the receptor density can easily be evaluated by diagnostic somatostatin receptor imaging, according to a kind of visual scale known as "Rotterdam scale"[4]. Rotterdam scale is graded as follows:

Grade 1: Tumors that have an uptake on planar images lower than that of normal liver uptake.
Grade 2: Tumors with uptake equal to the liver uptake.
Grade 3: Tumors that show higher uptake than that of normal liver.
Grade 4: Tumors that show very high uptake, higher than kidneys and spleen (the hottest organs in ^{111}In-octreotide scintigraphy).

Generally, tumors with a Rotterdam grade 2–4 are candidates for PRRT.
Along with Rotterdam scale, the following criteria should also be met [2–4].

1. Karnofsky performance status >60 or ECOG<2.
2. Tumor differentiation, preferably in G1-G2.
3. Tumor proliferation rate, preferably Ki-67 mitotic index≤20%. The rate of tumor growth that is detected by CT and/or MRI may also be helpful. Generally, less differentiated tumors with high proliferation are more eligible to chemotherapy compared to PRRT.

28.4.1 Pretherapy Renal Function Evaluation

For PRRT with ^{90}Y-labeled somatostatin analogs, a normal renal function is essential, since this radiopharmaeutical has a potential to deteriorate renal parameters. However, patients with compromised renal function may still be candidates for

PRRT with ^{177}Lu-labeled somatostatin analogs, since this radiopharmaceutical has much less toxicity on renal function. For ^{177}Lu-labeled PRRT, a mild to moderate grade of renal impairment (creatinine ≤1.7 mg/dL) can be tolerated [2, 3, 5, 6].

Patients' renal function should be assessed by blood biochemistry (creatinine and blood urea nitrogen) and GFR calculation. In addition to blood biochemistry, the renal function should be assessed by renal scintigraphy. Both glomerular and tubular radiopharmacueticals can be used for this purpose. Technetium 99 m-diethy lenetriaminepentaacetic acid (^{99}mTc-DTPA) and Technetium99m-mercaptotriacylglycine (^{99m}Tc-MAG3) are the most common radiopharmaecuticals, which show glomerular and tubular renal function, respectively. Glomerular filtration rate (GFR) or tubular extraction rate (TER) should preferably be 60% of the mean-age adjusted normal values at minimum [5, 6].

28.4.2 Haematological Evaluation

1. For PRRT with ^{177}Lu-labeled somatostatin analogs, white blood cell (WBC) should be >3000/μl, and platelet (Plt) count should be >75.000/ μl [2, 3, 5]. A more recent procedural guideline allows PRRT with ^{177}Lu-labeled somatostatin analogs for patients with at least WBC 2000/μl and Plt 70.000/μL for the first treatment [6].
2. ^{90}Y-labeled somatostatin analogs have WBC > 3000/μL, Plt > 90.000/μL, and red blood cell count >3.000.000/μL [2, 3, 5].

28.5 Precautions for PRRT

1. Before PRRT, obstructive renal disease should always be ruled out, and if there is, it should be corrected before PRRT. Dynamic renal scintigraphy with either ^{99m}Tc-DTPA or ^{99m}Tc-MAG3 is useful to rule out obstructive renal disease.
2. Previous myelotoxic chemotherapy and radiation therapy that were given recently (especially in a couple of weeks before PRRT) can constitute a risk for bone marrow failure and serious bone marrow supression, particularly in repeated therapies or subsequent cycles. Platelet counts after each cycle of PRRT can determine whether an interruption would be needed.
3. Before PRRT, hepatic failure should be regarded with caution. Preferably, serum total bilirubin level should be lower than 3 mg/mL and albumin level higher than 3 gr/dL for eligibility [5, 6].

28.6 Absolute Contraindications for PRRT

1. Pregnancy and breastfeeding (if not quitted).
2. Acute or severe concomitant diseases.
3. Severe psychiatric disorder.

28.7 Therapeutic Dose Assessment for PRRT

Ideally, PRRT should be given on dosimetry-based regimens. However, this approach is rarely preferred in routine practice since it is cumbersome and needs complex calculations. Therefore, fixed-activity treatment cycles or individualized dosing which is adjusted on the basis of some clinical parameters such as body surface area, clinical status, and haematological and renal function are the most preferred dose calculation methods.

For ^{90}Y-labeled somatostatin analogs, cumulative acitivities up to 19 GBq (~500 mCi) can be administered in 2–4 cycles, providing that renal absorbed dose threshold is not exceeded. Reported cumulative activities for ^{177}Lu-labeled peptides are between 22 and 30 GBq (~600–800 mCi), which can be administered in 4–6 cycles, according to different protocols [2–3, 5–6].

28.8 Patient Preparation for PRRT

28.8.1 Withdrawal of Somatostatin Analogs

Somatostatin analogs (cold somatostatin) should be discontinued for a certain period before PRRT. The duration of interruption depends on whether the drug is long or short acting. For long-acting drugs 3–4 weeks and for short-acting ones 1 day withdrawal are advised, although there is still debate on this subject [2–3, 5–6].

28.8.2 Premedication for PRRT

1. Just before dose administration, serotonin 5-HT3 receptor anatagonists such as ondansetron, granisetron, or tropisetron should be given and can be repeated when necassary.
2. Corticosteroids such as dexametasone 4 mg or more may be given short before PRRT and can be repeated if necessary [2–3, 5–6].

28.8.3 Pretherapy Renal Protection for PRRT

The renal absorbed dose is higher for ^{90}Y-labeled peptides compared with ^{177}Lu-labeled peptides because of different beta radiation features. Positively charged amino acids such as L-lysine and/or L-arginine are commonly used to competitively inhibit the proximal tubular reabsorbtion of radiopharmaceutical to reduce renal absorbed radiation dose. At least 25 g of positively charged amino acid solution should be infused before PRRT, in order to exert a protective effect on kidneys. Four amino acid protection methods have been introduced so far as follows [5–9]:

1. Single-day 50 g amino acid protection.
2. Three-day 25 g amino acid protection.

3. Three-day 50 g amino acid protection.
4. Single-day 50 g amino acid plus gelofusin protocol.

28.9 Treatment Regimens

Treatment regimens according to different radiopeptides for patients with normal bone marrow and renal function are given in Table 28.1.

Treatment doses should be reduced and individualized for compromised patients according to clinical and biochemical parameters.

28.9.1 PRRT for Pediatric Patients

In children, ^{90}Y-DOTATOC can be given in 1.5–1.85 GBq/m^2 activities per cycle in up to 3 cycles. There is no widespread use of ^{177}Lu-DOTATATE in pediatric patients, and activities should be adjusted per body surface area [10].

28.9.2 Retreatment with PRRT

Retreatment should be considered for patients with well-documented disease progression, who previously responded. The decision of retreatment should be taken within tumor board and the same eligibility criteria apply like the first treatment. Retreatment can be done with the same or a different radiopeptide.

Table 28.1 Different treatment regimens for PRRT

Radiopharmaceutical	Administered activity	Number of cycles	Time interval between cycles
^{90}Y-DOTATATE/ ^{90}Y-DOTATOC	3,7 GBq (100 mCi)/m2	2	10–12 weeks
^{90}Y-DOTATATE/ ^{90}Y-DOTATOC (another protocol)	2.78–4.44 GBq (75–120 mCi)	2–4	10–12 weeks
^{177}Lu -DOTATATE/ ^{177}Lu DOTATOC	5,55–7,4 GBq (150–200 mCi)	3–5	10–12 weeks
^{177}Lu + ^{90}Y Combination-Coctail protocol	5,55–7,4 GBq (150–200 mCi) (for ^{177}Lu) 2,5–5 GBq (68–135 mCi) (for ^{90}Y)	2–6	10–16 weeks

28.10 Imaging after PRRT

Since ^{177}Lu emits gamma radiation in addition to therapeutic beta particles, scintigraphic imaging using gamma rays should always be done following each treatment cycle to confirm targeting of radiopharmaceutical and to assess functional response. Planar and SPECT and/or SPECT/CT tomographic images are acquired usually on days 1, 4, and 7 after PRRT with ^{177}Lu-DOTATATE.

Since ^{90}Y is a pure beta emitter, it does not permit direct scintigraphic imaging but even if it is poor in quality, Brehmstrahlung (braking radiation) rays can be used to obtain a post-therapy imaging. It is usually done in 24 hours following PRRT with ^{90}Y-DOTATOC.

28.11 Outcomes of PRRT for Neuroendocrine Tumors

28.11.1 Response

Response evaluation for PRRT includes functional and anatomic imaging to assess functional and morphological response as well as biochemical and symptomatic response to assess patients' quality of life. Posttherapeutic ^{177}Lu-DOTATATE imaging can succesfully be used to assess functional response between therapy cycles and at the end of the therapy. The time period for response evaluation depends on different situations according to clinical needs, but generally the first follow-up is recommended after 3 months and to be continued after 3–6 months. Functional imaging with gallium-68 (^{68}Ga) DOTA peptides (DOTATE/DOTANOC/DOTATOC), PET/CT is of great importance in order to assess treatment response mostly following 4 cycles. Since ^{68}Ga-DOTApeptide imaging is a PET imaging, it can display more lesions and provide more clear images with higher sensitivity and contrast resolution compared to ^{177}Lu-DOTATATE imaging. Preferably, in-terim ^{68}Ga-DOTApeptide imaging can be performed for early assessment of therapy response such as following the 2 cycles of therapy. ^{68}Ga-DOTA peptide PET/CT images should be interpreted in comparison with the baseline PET/CT and should be correlated with anatomical imaging and biochemical evaluation along with clinical findings of the patient [11].

In most of the patients, anatomic imaging should be performed 1–3 months, 6 months, and 12 months after the completion of all PRRT cycles. According to NCCN guidelines, the patients should be monitored with contrast-enhanced abdominal and pelvic CT or MRI along with chest CT with or without contrast in 3–12 months. Liver magnetic resonance imaging (MRI) can be considered for the patients with liver-dominant disease [6]. It should be taken into account that the first imaging studies after the completion of PRRT cycles can be complicated by pseudoprogression. In about 10% of patients with stable disease, the lesion volumes can show a transient increase on anatomic imaging, most probably due to edema because of radiation from PRRT. Functional imaging with 68Ga-DOTApeptides can be useful in this setting [12].

PRRT for neuroendocrine tumors with ^{177} Lu and ^{90}Y labeled somatostatin analogs has been in clinical use for more than a decade. Most of the studies in the literature conclude that PRRT can give high absorbed doses to neuroendocrine tumors with overexpression of sstr2, which results with partial and complete objective responses in up to 30% of patients. Gastroenteropancreatic neuroendocrine tumors have showed the best objective response rates, with partial responses ranging from 9% to 29% and complete remission rates from 2% to 9%. Almost similar response rates have been reported for neuroendocrine tumors of the lungs and neuroectodermal tumors such as paragangliomas. Dedifferentiated thyroid carcinomas, medullary thyroid cancers, and neuroendocrine tumors of the thymus have displayed less satisfactory response rates. Besides these, promising results have been reported for other sstr-positive tumor types such as astrocytomas, medulloblastomas, and meningiomas [13–19].

The NETTER-1 Trial demonstrated the treatment efficacy of ^{177}Lu-DOTATATE PRRT in patients with midgut NETs. In this phase 3 trial, the researchers compared the treatment efficacy of ^{177}Lu-DOTATATE plus low-dose long-acting somatostatin analog (octreotide LAR) for best supportive care with that of high-dose octreotide LAR alone as control group in a randomized setting. The progression-free survival was 65.2% at month 20 for the ^{177}Lu-DOTATATE group versus 10.8% in the control group and the response rate was 18% in ^{177} Lu-DOTATATE versus 3% in the control group ($p < 0{,}001$). Clinically significant myelosupression was reported in less than 10% in the 177Lu-DOTATATE group [20].

28.11.2 Survival

According to some seminal studies in which survival analyses have been reported, patients who have high somatostatin receptor expression at the beginning of PRRT shows significantly higher objective responses in correlation with significantly longer survival when compared with similar patients with lower receptor expression [18, 19, 21].

The NETTER-1 phase-3 trial demonstrated markedly longer progression-free survival and a significantly higher response rate of ^{177}Lu-DOTATATE PRRT compared to high-dose octreotide LAR among patients with advanced midgut neuroendocrine tumors [20]. Such objective results from a large-scale randomised study have led PRRT to gain wider acceptance and approval worldwide.

Some studies have reported that biochemical response is also good predictor for the overall survival of patients with dedifferentiated thyroid cancer and medullary thyroid cancer following ^{90}Y-DOTATOC therapy [14, 16, 21]. Bushnell et al. concluded that significant symptomatic response after ^{90}Y-DOTATOC therapy has had an impact on progression-free survival of patients [22].

28.11.3 Side Effects and Toxicity

The kidney is the dose-limiting organ for PRRT. Pretherapy renal protection protocols are mandatory, and they reduce renal absorbed doses significantly and avoid serious renal dysfunction due to PRRT [5–9]. Renal toxicity is more frequently seen with ^{90}Y-DOTATOC, especially the patients with the diagnosis of long-standing and poorly controlled hypertension have high risk for renal toxicity [19]. Despite kidney protection, renal dysfunction can occur following PRRT with approximate creatinine clearance loss of 3.8% per year for ^{177} Lu-DOTATATE and 7.3% per year for ^{90}Y-DOTATOC [22]. Some variations most probably due to individual kidney sensitivity to radiation may have a role in the development of renal toxicity. Long-standing diabetes and hypertension may be considered as major risk factors for renal toxicity after ^{177}Lu-DOTATATE PRRT [8]. However, the risk of renal toxicity is rare (<5%), when the therapy is applied in accordance with the general guideline suggestions [20, 23, 24].

Acute bone marrow toxicity may be seen in about 10%–13% of patients following ^{90}Y-DOTATOC and in 2–3% following ^{177} Lu-DOTATATE PRRT. Most of the bone marrow toxicities are reversible. Grade 3 and 4 thrombocytopenia and neutropenia may ocur in less than 5% of patients, and they mostly resolve in 8 weeks. In fact, the most important long-term hematologic toxicity is the development of myelodysplastic syndrome or acute leukemia, which may occur in about 2–3% of patients in a median of 2 years following therapy. Prior chemotherapy is the most attributed risk factor in the development of such significant bone marrow effects following PRRT [20, 25–28].

PRRT may cause a transient impairment in male fertility, and recovery is commonly complete within 2 years following the last cycle of the therapy [27].

PRRT may cause hepatic failure not in patients with extensive metastatic involvement of the liver. In these patients, ^{177} Lu-DOTATATE should be preferred to ^{90}Y-DOTATOC and administered activity should be reduced [25, 27].

Although there are somatostatin receptors in healthy pituitary, thyroid, and adrenal glands, PRRT has never been reported to alter endocrine function [29].

28.11.4 PRRT with Alpha-Emitters

Although the invention of alpha emitters dates back to many many years, it has gained wide acceptance in clinical nuclear medicine just in the recent years with the introduction of Actinium-125 labeled prostate-specific membrane antigen (^{125}Ac-PSMA) therapy for castration-resistant metastatic prostate cancer patients, alternative to commonly used ^{177}Lu-PSMA therapy [30]. However, they are not currently used for PRRT as commonly as they are used for prostate cancer.

Alpha particles are positively charged and have a very high particle energy (5–9 MeV) along with a very short tissue range (40–100 μm). Therefore, the range of an alpha particle is almost equivalent to the thickness of 1–3 cell widths. Owing to such physical properties, intracellular accumulation of the alpha particles is expected to provide a higher chance of target damage to the cell's nucleus [31]. Therefore, the advantage of an alpha-emitter labeled radiopharmaceutical is that it can give much more radiation hazard to the targeted cell compared with beta-emitting radiopharmaceutical, and it may cause double-stranded breaks on DNA. Besides, due to its very short tissue range, it does not affect the surrounding healthy cells, when properly targeted to tumor cells.

Currently, the two major therapeutic radionuclides used in preclinical and clinical studies on PRRT are Bismuth-213 ^{213}Bi and ^{225}Ac. ^{213}Bi has a short physical half-life of 45 minutes, whereas ^{225}Ac has a much longer half-life of 10 days. Despite its short half-life, ^{213}Bi has been successfully labeled with DOTA peptides with over 99% purity in preclinical and clinical studies and has first been used in NET patients who were refractory to 177Lu-DOTATATE PRRT in the year 2014 [32, 33]. The radiochemical purity of ^{225}Ac labeled with DOTATOC in two preclinical studies has been slightly less (92 and > 95%) compared with ^{225}Ac-PSMA [34, 35]. Its higher energy and longer half-life make ^{225}Ac more promising alpha emitter than the others for therapy.

Although there are currently very few studies, PRRT with alpha emitters seems as a promising alternative especially for patients who are resistant to ^{177}Lu-DOTATATE or ^{90}Y-DOTATOC PRRT. Miederer et al. assessed the efficacy of ^{225}Ac-DOTATATE in comparison with ^{177}Lu-DOTATATE in an animal study, and they reported that ^{225}Ac-DOTATATE PRRT resulted with a more pronounced reduction in the tumor weight compared with^{177}Lu-DOTATATE PRRT at a preclinical setting [35].

At present, there is only one clinical study on the use of alpha-emitters for PRRT. In this study, a total of 8 patients who were refractory to previously given ^{177}Lu-DOTATATE and ^{90}Y-DOTATOC PRRT were treated with ^{213}Bi-DOTATOC. The therapeutic dose was administered via hepatic intraarterial route to increase targeting in 7 patients and intravenously in 1 patient. At follow-up, 1 patient developed complete metabolic response, 2 patients showed partial metabolic response, and 3 patients stayed stable. There were no reported life-threatening bone marrow or renal toxicities [33]. Currently, there are no other published data on clinical use of alpha emitters for PRRT.

PRRT with alpha emitters may be a good alternative for neuroendocrine tumor patients who are refractory or not appropriate for PRRT with ^{177}Lu-DOTATATE or ^{90}Y-DOTATOC PRRT. However, much more studies are certainly warranted .

28.11.5 The Current Strategies to Increase the Efficacy of PRRT and Future Perspectives

Although PRRT with ^{177}Lu-DOTATATE and ^{90}Y-DOTATOC is considered as an efficient and safe therapy option for patients with differentiated neuroendocrine tumors, most of the patients relapse on average of 2–3 years following a succesful treatment. Therefore, some strategies may be proposed in summary to increase the therapeutic efficacy as follows:

- Instead of routinely used intravenous administrations, intraarterial administrations should be preferred in order to increase targeting, especially for liver metastases [36].
- Pretherapy dosimetry instead of fixed-dose methodology can provide more sufficient tumor doses to reach higher tumoricidal effect. Dosimetry can also make

it possible to predict radiation doses of the target organs such as kidneys and bone marrow more precisely and therefore toxicities and serious side effects can be avoided [37].

- ^{177}Lu-DOTATATE and ^{90}Y-DOTATOC PRRT should be given in a combined fashion for tumors with heterogenous size ranges. Owing to their different particle range in tissues, ^{177} Lu is definitely more efficient in small tumors, whereas ^{90}Y is more succesful in larger tumors with respect to radiation exposure [4–6, 8].
- PRRT with antagonist radiopharmaceuticals and alpha emitters can be used alternatively for patients who are refractory to previous PRRT with ^{177}Lu-DOTATATE and ^{90}Y-DOTATOC. Antagonist radiopharmaceuticals that target somatostatin receptors can provide much more number of binding sites and are known to be more stable compared to agonist receptor tracers [38]. More studies are warranted on this issue.
- Chemotherapy can be used as a radiosensitizer to enhance the effect of radiation hazard of PRRT at suitable patients [39].

PRRT is expected to serve in a more efficient way for patients with NET if such perspectives are deeply considered and widely accepted in near future.

References

1. Valkema R, De Jong M, Bakker WH et al (2002) Phase I study of peptide receptor radionuclide therapy with [in-DTPA]octreotide: the Rotterdam experience. Semin Nucl Med 32(2):110–122
2. Bodei L, Ferone D, Grana CM et al (2009) Peptide receptor therapies in neuroendocrine tumors. J Endocrinol Investig 32(4):360–369
3. Kwekkeboom DJ, de Herder WW, van Eijck CH et al (2010) Peptide receptor radionuclide therapy in patients with gastroenteropancreatic neuroendocrine tumors. Semin Nucl Med 40(2):78–88
4. Navalkissoor S, Grossman A (2019) Targeted alpha particle therapy for neuroendocrine Tumours: the next generation of peptide receptor radionuclide therapy. Neuroendocrinology 108(3):256–264. https://doi.org/10.1159/000494760. Epub 2018 Oct 23
5. Zaknun JJ, Bodei L, Mueller-Brand J et al (2013) The joint IAEA, EANM, and SNMMI practical guidance on peptide receptor radionuclide therapy (PRRNT) in neuroendocrine tumours. Eur J Nucl Med Mol Imaging 40(5):800–816. https://doi.org/10.1007/s00259-012-2330-6
6. Hope TA, Abbott A, Colucci K et al (2019) NANETS/SNMMI procedure standard for somatostatin receptor-based peptide receptor radionuclide therapy with 177 Lu-DOTATATE. J Nucl Med 60(7):937–943. https://doi.org/10.2967/jnumed.118.230607
7. De Jong M, Valkema R, Jamar F et al (2002) Somatostatin receptor-targeted radionuclide therapy of tumors: preclinical and clinical findings. Semin Nucl Med 32(2):133–140
8. Bodei L, Cremonesi M, Ferrari M et al (2008) Long-term evaluation of renal toxicity after peptide receptor radionuclide therapy with 90Y-DOTATOC and 177Lu-DOTATATE: the role of associated risk factors. Eur J Nucl Med Mol Imaging 35(10):1847–1856
9. Rolleman EJ, Valkema R, de Jong M et al (2003) Safe and effective inhibition of renal uptake of radiolabelled octreotide by a combination of lysine and arginine. Eur J Nucl Med Mol Imaging 30(1):9–15
10. Schmidt M, Baum RP, Simon T et al (2010) Therapeutic nuclear medicine in pediatric malignancy. Q J Nucl Med Mol Imaging 54(4):411–428

11. Hope TA, Bergsland EK, Bozkurt MF et al (2018) Appropriate use criteria for somatostatin receptor PET imaging in neuroendocrine tumors. J Nucl Med 59(1):66–74
12. Brabander T, van der Zwan WA, Teunissen JJM et al (2017) Pitfalls in the response evaluation after peptide receptor radionuclide therapy with [177 Lu-DOTA 0,Tyr 3]octreotate. Endocr Relat Cancer 24(5):243–251
13. van Essen M, Krenning EP, Bakker WH et al (2007) Peptide receptor radionuclide therapy with 177Lu-octreotate in patients with foregut carcinoid tumours of bronchial, gastric and thymic origin. Eur J Nucl Med Mol Imaging 34(8):1219–1227
14. Iten F, Muller B, Schindler C et al (2009) [(90)yttrium-DOTA]-TOC response is associated with survival benefit in iodine-refractory thyroid cancer: long-term results of a phase 2 clinical trial. Cancer 115(10):2052–2062
15. Kwekkeboom DJ, Kam BL, van Essen M et al (2010) Somatostatin-receptor-based imaging and therapy of gastroenteropancreatic neuroendocrine tumors. Endocr Relat Cancer 17(1):R53–R73
16. Bodei L, Handkiewicz-Junak D, Grana C et al (2004) Receptor radionuclide therapy with 90Y-DOTATOC in patients with medullary thyroid carcinomas. Cancer Biother Radiopharm 19(1):65–71
17. Bartolomei M, Bodei L, De Cicco C et al (2009) Peptide receptor radionuclide therapy with (90)Y-DOTATOC in recurrent meningioma. Eur J Nucl Med Mol Imaging 36(9):1407–1416
18. Kwekkeboom DJ, de Herder WW, Kam BL et al (2008) Treatment with the radiolabeled somatostatin analog [177 Lu-DOTA 0,Tyr3]octreotate: toxicity, efficacy, and survival. J Clin Oncol 26(13):2124–2130
19. Imhof A, Brunner P, Marincek N et al (2011) Response, survival, and long-term toxicity after therapy with the radiolabeled somatostatin analogue [90Y-DOTA]-TOC in metastasized neuroendocrine cancers. J Clin Oncol 29(17):2416–2423
20. Strosberg J, El-Haddad G, Wolin E et al (2017) Phase 3 trial of 177 Lu-Dotatate for midgut neuroendocrine tumors. N Engl J Med 376(2):125–135
21. Iten F, Müller B, Schindler C et al (2007) Response to [90Yttrium-DOTA]-TOC treatment is associated with long-term survival benefit in metastasized medullary thyroid cancer: a phase II clinical trial. Clin Cancer Res 13(22):6696–6702
22. Bushnell DL Jr, O'Dorisio TM, O'Dorisio MS et al (2010) 90Y-edotreotide for metastatic carcinoid refractory to octreotide.J. Clin Oncol 28(10):1652–1659
23. Bodei L, Cremonesi M, Grana CM et al (2011) Peptide receptor radionuclide therapy with ^{177}Lu-DOTATATE: the IEO phase I-II study. Eur J Nucl Med Mol Imaging 38(12):2125–2135
24. Vegt E, de Jong M, Wetzels JF et al (2010) Renal toxicity of radiolabeled peptides and antibody fragments: mechanisms, impact on radionuclide therapy, and strategies for prevention. J Nucl Med 51(7):1049–1058
25. Valkema R, Pauwels SA, Kvols LK et al (2005) Long-term follow-up of renal function after peptide receptor radiation therapy with (90)Y-DOTA(0),Tyr(3)-octreotide and (177) Lu-DOTA(0), Tyr(3)-octreotate. J Nucl Med 46(1):83S–91S
26. Kwekkeboom DJ, Mueller-Brand J, Paganelli G et al (2005) Overview of results of peptide receptor radionuclide therapy with 3 radiolabeled somatostatin analogs. J Nucl Med 46(1):62S–66S
27. Kwekkeboom DJ, Teunissen JJ, Bakker WH et al (2005) Radiolabeled somatostatin analog [177Lu-DOTA0,Tyr3]octreotate in patients with endocrine gastroenteropancreatic tumors. J Clin Oncol 23(12):2754–2762
28. Brabander T, van der Zwan WA, Teunissen JJM et al (2017) Long-term efficacy, survival, and safety of [177 Lu-DOTA 0,Tyr 3]octreotate in patients with gastroenteropancreatic and bronchial neuroendocrine tumors. Clin Cancer Res 23(16):4617–4624
29. Teunissen JJ, Krenning EP, de Jong FH et al (2009) Effects of therapy with [177Lu-DOTA 0,Tyr 3]octreotate on endocrine function. Eur J Nucl Med Mol Imaging 36(11):1758–1766
30. Kratochwil C, Bruchertseifer F, Giesel FL et al (2016) 225Ac-PSMA-617 for PSMA-targeted α-radiation therapy of metastatic castration-resistant prostate cancer. J Nucl Med 57(12):1941–1944

31. Kassis AI (2008) Therapeutic radionuclides: biophysical and radiobiologic principles. Semin Nucl Med 38(5):358–366
32. Nayak TK, Norenberg JP, Anderson TL et al (2007) Somatostatin-receptor-targeted alpha-emitting 213Bi is therapeutically more effective than beta(−)-emitting 177Lu in human pancreatic adenocarcinoma cells. Nucl Med Biol 34(2):185–193
33. Kratochwil C, Giesel FL, Bruchertseifer F et al (2014) (213)bi DOTATOC receptor-targeted alpha-radionuclide therapy induces remission in neuroendocrine tumours refractory to beta radiation:a first-in-human experience. Eur J Nucl Med Mol Imaging 41(11):2106–2119
34. Graf F, Fahrer J, Maus S et al (2014) DNA double strand breaks as predictor of efficacy of the alpha-particle emitter ac-225 and the electron emitter Lu-177 for somatostatin receptor targeted radiotherapy. PLoS One 9(2):e88239
35. Miederer M, Henriksen G, Alke A et al (2008) Preclinical evaluation of the alpha-particle generator nuclide 225Ac for somatostatin receptor radiotherapy of neuroendocrine tumors. Clin Cancer Res 14(11):3555–3561
36. Kratochwil C, López-Benítez R, Mier W et al (2011) Hepatic arterial infusion enhances DOTATOC radiopeptide therapy in patients with neuroendocrine liver metastases. Endocr Relat Cancer 18(5):595–602
37. Bison SM, Konijnenberg MW, Melis M et al (2014) Peptide receptor radionuclide therapy using radiolabeled somatostatin analogs: focus on future developments. Clin Translat Imaging 2(1):55–66
38. Wild D, Fani M, Fischer R et al (2014) Comparison of somatostatin receptor agonist and antagonist for peptide receptor radionuclide therapy: a pilot study. J Nucl Med 55(8):1248–1252
39. Claringbold PG, Price RA, Turner JH (2012) Phase I–II study of radiopeptide 177Lu-octreotate in combination with capecitabine and temozolomide in advanced low-grade neuroendocrine tumors. Cancer Biother Radiopharm 27(9):561–569

Carcinoid Syndrome

29

Burak Yasin Aktas, Saadettin Kilickap, and Suayib Yalcin

29.1 Introduction

Neuroendocrine tumors (NETs) which originate from neuroendocrine cells can occur in any parts of the body but are most commonly found in the gastrointestinal tract (appendices, ileum, and rectum), pancreas, and lungs [1]. NETs can secrete specific hormones and/or biogenic amines according to the cell origin. Carcinoid syndrome is a result of hormone-producing NETs, and clinical findings are closely related to secreted peptides.

The incidence of NETs is between 2 and 5 per 100,000. Its incidence has increased in recent years. According to SEER database, almost 20% of patients with neuroendocrine neoplasm had carcinoid syndrome [2]. The incidence of carcinoid syndrome is also increasing, nearly doubling in the last decade. This may be related to an increase in the frequency of NETs, improvements in diagnostic methods, or increased awareness. Carcinoid syndrome is reported more frequently in women, and overall survival is shorter in NETs with carcinoid syndrome [2].

29.2 Pathophysiology

Amines, polypeptides, and prostaglandins secreted from neuroendocrine tumors, especially serotonin, cause carcinoid syndrome [3]. Small intestine NETs, which most frequently metastasize to the liver, constitute this clinical picture. More than 30 different vasoactive peptides have been identified in various

B. Y. Aktas
Department of Medical Oncology, Ankara City Hospital, Ankara, Turkey

S. Kilickap
Department of Medical Oncology, Istinye University, Ankara, Turkey

S. Yalcin (✉)
Department of Medical Oncology, Hacettepe University Cancer Institute, Ankara, Turkey

S. Yalcin, K. Öberg (eds.), *Neuroendocrine Tumours*,
https://doi.org/10.1007/978-3-031-56968-5_29

gastroenteropancreatic neuroendocrine tumors (GEP-NETs) [4]. Products of well-differentiated neuroendocrine tumors are summarized in Table 29.1.

One of the main changes detected in carcinoid syndrome is tryptophan metabolism. However, not all NETs develop carcinoid syndrome due to differences in end products formed [5]. Serotonin which stimulates intestinal secretion and motility and inhibits intestinal absorption, is the most likely cause of the diarrhea in carcinoid syndrome [6]. Also, the diversion of tryptophan to the synthesis of serotonin in patients with widely metastatic tumors may result in niacin deficiency and clinical manifestations of pellagra [7]. However, the development of flushing is not related to serotonin. Some foregut NETs (gastric and lung) produce 5-hydroxytryptophan (and histamine) instead of serotonin because they do not synthesize the aromatic amino acid decarboxylase that converts 5-hydroxytryptophan to serotonin. Also, hindgut NETs (distal colon and rectum) uncommonly secrete serotonin or any other bioactive hormones, and they are not associated with hormonal syndromes.

Histamine may be responsible for the atypical flushing and pruritus associated with these tumors and mainly produced by gastric NETs [8]. Bradykinin which occurs while some NETs produce kallikrein is a potent vasodilator and may be responsible for flushing in some patients [9]. Increased production of tachykinins (substance P, neurokinin A, and neuropeptide K) may contribute to flushing and diarrhea in some patients.

Table 29.1 Products of well-differentiated neuroendocrine tumors

Amines	Polypeptides	Prostaglandins
Serotonin	Kallikrein	
5-Hydroxytryptophan	Pancreatic polypeptide	
Norepinephrine	Bradykinin	
Dopamine	Motilin	
Histamine	Somatostatin	
Serotonin	Vasoactive intestinal peptide	
5-Hydroxytryptophan	Neuropeptide K	
Norepinephrine	Substance P	
Dopamine	Neurokinin A	
Histamine	Neurokinin B	
Serotonin	Corticotropin (ACTH)	
5-Hydroxytryptophan	Gastrin	
Norepinephrine	Growth hormone	
	Peptide YY	
	Glucagon	
	Beta-endorphin	
	Neurotensin	
	Chromogranin A	

29.3 Clinical Features

The carcinoid syndrome clinic is associated with peptides secreted by the NETs. Serotonin and its metabolites account for the majority symptoms of carcinoid syndrome. Although skin, GI tract, heart, and respiratory system are most commonly affected, other clinical features due to involvement of various organs and systems are reported. The main symptoms and the frequencies are summarized in Table 29.2.

29.3.1 Flushing and Other Skin Findings

Recurrent episodes of flushing, which occurs almost 90% of patients, is the clinical hallmark of carcinoid syndrome. The flushing starts suddenly without any prodromal symptom and can last for different durations from 30 s to 30 min. It primarily involves the face, neck, and upper chest instead of extremities and is associated with a mild burning sensation. Cardiovascular findings such as hypotension and tachycardia may also be seen in severe attacks [10]. Although most flushing episodes occur spontaneously, they also can be provoked by eating, alcohol consumption, exercise, various drugs, emotional changes, and anesthesia. Episodes induced by anesthesia may last hours and be accompanied by severe hypotension ("carcinoid crisis"). This problem can be minimized by pretreatment with octreotide.

Venous telangiectasia are late-period findings of the disease. They most often occur on the upper lip and malar areas. In some patients with severe flushing episodes, persistent brawny edema is added to the finding in the later stages.

Table 29.2 Main clinical features of carcinoid syndrome

Symptom	Frequency (%)
Flushing	85
Telangiectasia	25
Cyanosis	18
Pellagra	2–25
Diarrhea	75–80
Abdominal cramp	75
Bronchospasm	20
Valvular lesions	50
Right heart	40
Left heart	13
Asthenia	<5
Neuropsychiatric symptoms	<5
Musculoskeletal	<5

29.3.2 Diarrhea

Diarrhea occurs in 75–80% of cases with carcinoid syndrome and, it is the main symptom affecting quality of life. The diarrhea observed in patients with carcinoid syndrome is a secretory diarrhea, and the episodes are up to 20 stool per day. Thus, it may cause fluid and electrolyte depletion. The diarrhea is described as watery and non-bloody and mostly accompanied by abdominal cramping [6]. The diarrhea is unrelated to nutrition and may continue during fasting.

29.3.3 Bronchospasm

The most common respiratory symptoms in patients with carcinoid syndrome are wheezing and dyspnea. Pulmonary symptoms develop due to bronchospasm and occur about 20% of these patients.

29.3.4 Carcinoid Heart Disease

Vasoactive substances secreted in carcinoid syndrome mostly affect the valves and endocardium of the right side of the heart and cause fibrosis. Almost half of the patients have to face cardiac disease throughout the course of the carcinoid syndrome [11]. Since the involvement progresses slowly and the signs of right heart failure show late symptoms, it is usually not detected in the early period of the disease [12]. Fatigue and dyspnea on exertion might be the only symptoms of cardiac involvement at the early course of disease but after the right-sided heart failure worsens dyspnea, edema, and ascites occur.

29.4 Diagnosis

Patients are evaluated in terms of carcinoid syndrome as a result of hospital admission when the frequency or severity of symptoms such as diarrhea and flashing increase, which generally do not require a doctor's examination for a long time when they are mild and intermittent. Blood and/or urine tests of secreted amines and peptides are crucial for identifying and following patients with carcinoid syndrome. Nonhormonal peptide biomarkers (e.g., chromogranin A [CgA]) markers are less useful in the diagnosis of carcinoid syndrome.

29.4.1 Urinary 5-HIAA

Although there are many different blood serotonin tests, the measurement of serotonin level is not a preferred method in the diagnosis of carcinoid syndrome due to the varying sensitivity and specificity of the tests and the high false-positive rate

[13]. However, 24-h urine-level determination of the more stable serotonin metabolism product 5-HIAA is a more reliable diagnostic test. This test has a sensitivity and a specificity of over 90% for carcinoid syndrome [14]. A 3-day diet is needed in which the consumption of foods rich in tryptophan is stopped before urine collection. The importance of the test is reduced in foregut or hindgut tumors with little or no 5-HIAA synthesis [15].

29.4.2 Chromogranin A

Chromogranins are proteins that are stored and released concurrently with peptides and amines in neuroendocrine tissues. Well-differentiated NETs, including carcinoids, are associated with elevated blood concentrations of chromogranins. The daily change in serum level and the effect of consumed foods and drugs limit its clinical use [16]. However, chromogranin level monitoring is important, especially in high-volume and metastatic disease and in monitoring the treatment response.

29.4.3 Imaging

Since NETs that most frequently metastasize to the liver cause carcinoid syndrome, abdominal imaging is the first step in radiological evaluation [17].

Multiphasic contrast-enhanced CT is recommended for evaluation of all patients with NETs. Most NET liver metastases are highly vascular and enhance iodinated contrast during the early arterial phase. Multiphasic helical CT with multiplanar reformations can improve detection of small jejunum and ileum tumors [18].

MRI may represent the most sensitive method for the detection of liver metastases. In one study of 64 patients with metastatic gastrointestinal NETs, multiphasic MRI showed superiority of detecting liver metastases over either CT or 111-In pentetreotide [19].

Most well-differentiated NETs express high levels of somatostatin receptors (SSTRs) and can therefore be imaged with radiolabeled SSAs.

By exploiting SSTRs, NETs visualize with scintigraphy method using 111-In pentetreotide, the addition of single-photon emission computed tomography (SPECT) to planar imaging or more recently, positron emission tomography (PET) [20, 21]. These scans have two main advantages comparing other imaging techniques. First, these scans allow for whole body imaging. And second, they also provide information on SSTR expression, which has important therapeutic implications.

29.5 Treatment

There are two main approaches at the basis of the treatment of carcinoid syndrome. The first one is interventions to reduce the tumor burden that causes the symptoms, and the second is the treatments that suppress the hormone synthesis that causes the findings. Many of the current treatment options often meet both of these goals.

29.5.1 Somatostatin Analog Therapy

Somatostatin, a small peptide molecule, is known as a regulatory hormone that inhibits the secretion of a wide range of other hormones. Since approximately 80% of carcinoid tumors express somatostatin receptors, somatostatin analogs (octreotide and lanreotide) are highly useful for controlling the symptoms of carcinoid syndrome. A long-term symptom control is achieved more then 80% of patients [22]. Although both of these agents were developed for reducing symptoms of carcinoid syndrome by inhibiting secretion of vasoactive hormones initially, they have also been shown to control carcinoid tumor growth in phase III trials [23, 24].

Both the short-acting and depot form of octreotide and the long-acting form of lanreotide are used in the treatment of carcinoid syndrome. Subcutaneous administration of short-acting octreotide can be used in the initial treatment for symptomatic carcinoid syndrome. For the short-acting form, suggested daily dosage ranges from 100 μg/d to 600 μg/d in two to four divided doses. An octreotide pen (2500 μg/mL) also has been developed for the treatment of carcinoid syndrome, and it is designed for patient or caregiver administration. However, long-acting release (LAR) formula of the octreotide is more comfortable for majority of patients unless they are severely symptomatic. In general, the initial dose of octreotide LAR is 20–30 mg and is administered intramuscularly [25]. For the patients who cannot achieve adequate symptom control with initial treatment, escalation of the dose or frequency of octreotide LAR or adding a short-acting octreotide may be necessary. For example, patients who complain of exacerbation of symptoms at the end of the monthly treatment cycle, drug administration interval can be reduced to every 3 weeks.

Lanreotide is also available in a long-acting formulation for monthly injections at 60, 90, and 120 mg doses every 4 weeks. Lanreotide shows similar clinical efficacy and tolerability as octreotide for the treatment of the carcinoid syndrome. In a randomized placebo-controlled phase III trial of depot lanreotide in patients with carcinoid syndrome, lanreotide meets the primary endpoint and significantly reduced the need for rescue doses of short-acting somatostatin analogs [26].

Octreotide and lanreotide are both tolerated well. However, nausea, abdominal discomfort, bloating, and/or steatorrhea are adverse effects reported in various studies. Pancreatic malabsorption is sometimes a contributing element, which can be mitigated with pancreatic enzyme supplementation. One more impact of somatostatin analogs is restraint of gallbladder contractility, which can prompt gallstones. Consequently, a prophylactic cholecystectomy might be suggested for patients who are going through a surgical procedure for different indications.

29.5.2 Liver-Directed Therapies

Liver is the main site of GEP-NET metastases. Therefore, therapies targeting the liver have increasingly become an area of interest. Surgical removal of all resectable tumor tissues is the best treatment option to provide long-term remissions among metastatic patients [27, 28]. Hepatic resection should be considered in liver metastases without diffused bilobar involvement, compromised liver function, or widespread extrahepatic metastases. Hepatic resection or metastasectomy may also help relieve symptoms in patients affected by a large tumor or carcinoid syndrome.

For surgically unresectable and/or inoperable patients, hepatic trans-arterial embolization is another option for local treatment. Embolization of the entire liver can usually be performed in two to three separate sessions. Up to 75% of patients with liver metastases from neuroendocrine tumors have significant symptomatic improvement of flushing and diarrhea with embolization procedures. Embolizations can be performed with microparticles alone (Bland embolization), with admixed chemotherapy (chemoembolization), or more recently with yttrium-90 (90Y)-labeled resin or glass microspheres (radioembolization) [29, 30]. There are no randomized trials comparing efficacy of different embolization techniques for controlling symptoms yet. Short-term side effects of liver embolization include abdominal pain, fever, nausea/vomiting, and fatigue. Carcinoid crisis must be kept in mind in patients with carcinoid syndrome undergoing embolization procedures, and prophylactic octreotide must be prescribed before and after embolization.

29.5.3 Management of Refractory Symptoms

29.5.3.1 Telotristat

Serotonin is the main peptide implicated in the development of carcinoid syndrome. The enzyme tryptophan hydroxylase, catalyzing the conversion of tryptophan to serotonin, which is the rate-limiting step in serotonin biosynthesis, is inhibited by telotristat ethyl. Oral telotristat can be used for uncontrolled diarrhea due to carcinoid syndrome in combination with somatostatin analogs. The approval is based on a placebo-controlled three-arm randomized trial evaluated two different doses of telotristat (250 mg and 500 mg, each taken three times daily) compared to placebo. Treatment with telotristat at both doses significantly reduced daily stool frequency and urinary 5-hydroxyindoleacetic acid (5-HIAA; a metabolite of serotonin) level compared with placebo. Nausea and vomiting were more common with the 500 mg dose of telotristat than with the lower 250 mg dose or placebo [31]. Based on phase 3 trial data, telotristat has been approved in combination with somatostatin analogs for the treatment of diarrhea in patients with carcinoid syndrome, unresponsive to monotherapy with somatostatin analogs. The recommended dose is 250 mg three times daily.

29.5.3.2 Interferon

Interferon alfa (IFNα) is another option for the treatment of uncontrolled symptomatic carcinoid syndrome refractory to somatostatin analogs. IFNα also has antiproliferative and anti-angiogenic effects. IFNa at the dose of three to five million units three times weekly reduces flushing and diarrhea in up to half of the patients who are refractory to somatostatin analogs [32]. However, clinical benefits are generally not persistent and adverse effects are common.

29.5.4 Other Symptomatic Treatments

Antidiarrheal agents loperamide and diphenoxylate-atropine (Lomotil) also can be used for refractory diarrhea. For more severe diarrhea, the opiates paregoric and tincture are other options. Serotonin receptor antagonists, such as ondansetron, are reported to be effective to control diarrhea in patients refractory to somatostatin analogs [33].

Diarrhea may also occur due to fat malabsorption or bile acid malabsorption. Pancreatic enzyme supplementation and bile acid binders are prescribed when other underlying causes are identified.

29.5.5 Management of Carcinoid Crisis

Carcinoid crisis is one of the most feared complications of hormone-activated carcinoid tumors. It occurs when the symptoms seen in carcinoid syndrome are exacerbated and cardiovascular (such as arrhythmias and hypotension) and respiratory (such as shortness of breath) symptoms are added. It can be life-threatening if it cannot be brought under control with the appropriate approach. Various factors, especially surgical interventions, alcohol intake, emotional stress, and drugs, can trigger the development of carcinoid crisis. Many undesirable situations can be prevented by infusion of octreotide before planned interventions. Octreotide is administered as a bolus dose of 500–1000 μg or a continuous dose of intravenously 50–200 μg/h [34, 35]. Antihistamines to inhibit histamine discharge, loperamide, and other antidiarrheal agents for diarrhea treatment can be used as adjunctive therapy.

References

1. Yao JC, Hassan M, Phan A, Dagohoy C, Leary C, Mares JE et al (2008) One hundred years after "carcinoid": epidemiology of and prognostic factors for neuroendocrine tumors in 35,825 cases in the United States. J Clin Oncol 26(18):3063–3072. https://doi.org/10.1200/jco.2007.15.4377
2. Halperin DM, Shen C, Dasari A, Xu Y, Chu Y, Zhou S et al (2017) Frequency of carcinoid syndrome at neuroendocrine tumour diagnosis: a population-based study. Lancet Oncol 18(4):525–534. https://doi.org/10.1016/s1470-2045(17)30110-9
3. Feldman JM (1987) Carcinoid tumors and syndrome. Semin Oncol 14(3):237–246
4. Modlin IM, Kidd M, Latich I, Zikusoka MN, Shapiro MD (2005) Current status of gastrointestinal carcinoids. Gastroenterology 128(6):1717–1751. https://doi.org/10.1053/j.gastro.2005.03.038
5. Kvols LK (1994) Metastatic carcinoid tumors and the malignant carcinoid syndrome. Ann N Y Acad Sci 733:464–470. https://doi.org/10.1111/j.1749-6632.1994.tb17296.x
6. von der Ohe MR, Camilleri M, Kvols LK, Thomforde GM (1993) Motor dysfunction of the small bowel and colon in patients with the carcinoid syndrome and diarrhea. N Engl J Med 329(15):1073–1078. https://doi.org/10.1056/nejm199310073291503
7. Swain CP, Tavill AS, Neale G (1976) Studies of tryptophan and albumin metabolism in a patient with carcinoid syndrome, pellagra, and hypoproteinemia. Gastroenterology 71(3):484–489

8. Roberts LJ 2nd, Marney SR Jr, Oates JA (1979) Blockade of the flush associated with metastatic gastric carcinoid by combined histamine H1 and H2 receptor antagonists. Evidence for an important role of H2 receptors in human vasculature. N Engl J Med 300(5):236–238. https://doi.org/10.1056/nejm197902013000506
9. Condron ME, Jameson NE, Limbach KE, Bingham AE, Sera VA, Anderson RB et al (2019) A prospective study of the pathophysiology of carcinoid crisis. Surgery 165(1):158–165. https://doi.org/10.1016/j.surg.2018.04.093
10. Maton PN (1988) The carcinoid syndrome. JAMA 260(11):1602–1605
11. Hassan SA, Banchs J, Iliescu C, Dasari A, Lopez-Mattei J, Yusuf SW (2017) Carcinoid heart disease. Heart 103(19):1488–1495. https://doi.org/10.1136/heartjnl-2017-311261
12. Lundin L, Norheim I, Landelius J, Oberg K, Theodorsson-Norheim E (1988) Carcinoid heart disease: relationship of circulating vasoactive substances to ultrasound-detectable cardiac abnormalities. Circulation 77(2):264–269. https://doi.org/10.1161/01.cir.77.2.264
13. Richter G, Stöckmann F, Conlon JM, Creutzfeldt W (1986) Serotonin release into blood after food and pentagastrin. Studies in healthy subjects and in patients with metastatic carcinoid tumors. Gastroenterology 91(3):612–618. https://doi.org/10.1016/0016-5085(86)90630-x
14. O'Toole D, Grossman A, Gross D, Delle Fave G, Barkmanova J, O'Connor J et al (2009) ENETS consensus guidelines for the standards of care in neuroendocrine tumors: biochemical markers. Neuroendocrinology 90(2):194–202. https://doi.org/10.1159/000225948
15. Modlin IM, Gustafsson BI, Moss SF, Pavel M, Tsolakis AV, Kidd M (2010) Chromogranin A—biological function and clinical utility in neuro endocrine tumor disease. Ann Surg Oncol 17(9):2427–2443. https://doi.org/10.1245/s10434-010-1006-3
16. Pregun I, Herszényi L, Juhász M, Miheller P, Hritz I, Patócs A et al (2011) Effect of proton-pump inhibitor therapy on serum chromogranin a level. Digestion 84(1):22–28. https://doi.org/10.1159/000321535
17. Levy AD, Sobin LH (2007) Gastrointestinal carcinoids: imaging features with Clinicopathologic comparison. Radiographics 27(1):237–257. https://doi.org/10.1148/rg.271065169
18. Ganeshan D, Bhosale P, Yang T, Kundra V (2013) Imaging features of carcinoid tumors of the gastrointestinal tract. AJR Am J Roentgenol 201(4):773–786. https://doi.org/10.2214/ajr.12.9758
19. Dromain C, de Baere T, Lumbroso J, Caillet H, Laplanche A, Boige V et al (2005) Detection of liver metastases from endocrine tumors: a prospective comparison of somatostatin receptor scintigraphy, computed tomography, and magnetic resonance imaging. J Clin Oncol 23(1):70–78. https://doi.org/10.1200/jco.2005.01.013
20. Sadowski SM, Neychev V, Millo C, Shih J, Nilubol N, Herscovitch P et al (2016) Prospective study of 68Ga-DOTATATE positron emission tomography/computed tomography for detecting gastro-Entero-pancreatic neuroendocrine tumors and unknown primary sites. J Clin Oncol 34(6):588–596. https://doi.org/10.1200/jco.2015.64.0987
21. Schillaci O, Corleto VD, Annibale B, Scopinaro F, Delle FG (1999) Single photon emission computed tomography procedure improves accuracy of somatostatin receptor scintigraphy in gastro-entero pancreatic tumours. Ital J Gastroenterol Hepatol 31(Suppl 2):S186–S189
22. Kvols LK, Moertel CG, O'Connell MJ, Schutt AJ, Rubin J, Hahn RG (1986) Treatment of the malignant carcinoid syndrome. Evaluation of a long-acting somatostatin analogue. N Engl J Med 315(11):663–666. https://doi.org/10.1056/nejm198609113151102
23. Rinke A, Müller HH, Schade-Brittinger C, Klose KJ, Barth P, Wied M et al (2009) Placebo-controlled, double-blind, prospective, randomized study on the effect of octreotide LAR in the control of tumor growth in patients with metastatic neuroendocrine midgut tumors: a report from the PROMID study group. J Clin Oncol 27(28):4656–4663. https://doi.org/10.1200/jco.2009.22.8510
24. Caplin ME, Pavel M, Ćwikła JB, Phan AT, Raderer M, Sedláčková E et al (2014) Lanreotide in metastatic enteropancreatic neuroendocrine tumors. N Engl J Med 371(3):224–233. https://doi.org/10.1056/NEJMoa1316158
25. Rubin J, Ajani J, Schirmer W, Venook AP, Bukowski R, Pommier R et al (1999) Octreotide acetate long-acting formulation versus open-label subcutaneous octreotide acetate in malignant carcinoid syndrome. J Clin Oncol 17(2):600–606. https://doi.org/10.1200/jco.1999.17.2.600

26. Vinik AI, Wolin EM, Liyanage N, Gomez-Panzani E, Fisher GA (2016) Evaluation of LANREOTIDE depot/AUTOGEL efficacy and safety as a carcinoid syndrome treatment (elect): a randomized, double-blind, placebo-controlled trial. Endocr Pract 22(9):1068–1080. https://doi.org/10.4158/ep151172.Or
27. Chen H, Hardacre JM, Uzar A, Cameron JL, Choti MA (1998) Isolated liver metastases from neuroendocrine tumors: does resection prolong survival? J Am Coll Surg 187(1):88–92.; discussion 3. https://doi.org/10.1016/s1072-7515(98)00099-4
28. Chamberlain RS, Canes D, Brown KT, Saltz L, Jarnagin W, Fong Y et al (2000) Hepatic neuroendocrine metastases: does intervention alter outcomes? J Am Coll Surg 190(4):432–445. https://doi.org/10.1016/s1072-7515(00)00222-2
29. King J, Quinn R, Glenn DM, Janssen J, Tong D, Liaw W et al (2008) Radioembolization with selective internal radiation microspheres for neuroendocrine liver metastases. Cancer 113(5):921–929. https://doi.org/10.1002/cncr.23685
30. Ruszniewski P, Malka D (2000) Hepatic arterial chemoembolization in the management of advanced digestive endocrine tumors. Digestion 62(Suppl 1):79–83. https://doi.org/10.1159/000051860
31. Pavel M, Gross DJ, Benavent M, Perros P, Srirajaskanthan R, Warner RRP et al (2018) Telotristat ethyl in carcinoid syndrome: safety and efficacy in the TELECAST phase 3 trial. Endocr Relat Cancer 25(3):309–322. https://doi.org/10.1530/erc-17-0455
32. Oberg K, Funa K, Alm G (1983) Effects of leukocyte interferon on clinical symptoms and hormone levels in patients with mid-gut carcinoid tumors and carcinoid syndrome. N Engl J Med 309(3):129–133. https://doi.org/10.1056/nejm198307213090301
33. Kiesewetter B, Duan H, Lamm W, Haug A, Riss P, Selberherr A et al (2019) Oral ondansetron offers effective antidiarrheal activity for carcinoid syndrome refractory to somatostatin analogs. Oncologist 24(2):255–258. https://doi.org/10.1634/theoncologist.2018-0191
34. Kvols LK, Martin JK, Marsh HM, Moertel CG (1985) Rapid reversal of carcinoid crisis with a somatostatin analogue. N Engl J Med 313(19):1229–1230. https://doi.org/10.1056/nejm198511073131915
35. Ito T, Lee L, Jensen RT (2018) Carcinoid-syndrome: recent advances, current status and controversies. Curr Opin Endocrinol Diabetes Obes 25(1):22–35. https://doi.org/10.1097/MED.0000000000000376

30 Somatostatin Analogs and Interferon in the Treatment of Neuroendocrine Tumors

Taymeyah Al-Toubah and Jonathan Strosberg

30.1 Introduction

Biotherapy for neuroendocrine tumors (NETs) emerged in the 1980s when somatostatin analogs (SSAs) and interferons (IFNs) were investigated in small series of patients with malignant carcinoid syndrome. While early clinical trials focused on palliation of hormonal symptoms, subsequent studies have been designed to assess the inhibitory effects of SSAs and IFNs on tumor progression. The recognition that biological therapies may be synergistic has led to several randomized studies investigating IFNα in combination with SSAs. This chapter will review the mechanism of action and key clinical trials investigating SSAs and IFNs in advanced, well-differentiated NETs.

30.2 Somatostatin Analogs

Native human somatostatin is a cyclic peptide hormone that exists in two natural forms consisting of 14 and 28 amino acids [1, 2]. It is widely distributed in multiple tissues, including the central nervous system, pancreas, and gastrointestinal tract. It has been characterized as a universal endocrine "off switch" due to its inhibitory paracrine, exocrine, and endocrine effects. In the digestive tract, somatostatin inhibits multiple intestinal functions such as bowel motility and absorption [3]. Somatostatin also inhibits secretion of other pancreatic and intestinal hormones, including gastrin, glucagon, and serotonin. The physiological actions of somatostatin are mediated through five subtypes of somatostatin receptors (sst_1-sst_5) belonging to a family of G-protein-coupled receptors with seven transmembrane domains

T. Al-Toubah · J. Strosberg (✉)
Department of GI Oncology, H. Lee Moffitt Cancer Center and Research Institute, Tampa, FL, USA
e-mail: Taymeyah.al-toubah@moffitt.org; jonathan.strosberg@moffitt.org

S. Yalcin, K. Öberg (eds.), *Neuroendocrine Tumours*,
https://doi.org/10.1007/978-3-031-56968-5_30

[4]. Approximately 80% of well-differentiated NETs express high levels of somatostatin receptors, particularly receptor subtypes 2 and 5 [5].

Native somatostatin is rapidly cleared in the circulation due to enzymatic cleavage sites, limiting its clinical utility [5, 6]. In order to improve somatostatin's pharmacokinetics, synthetic SSAs have been developed by truncating the polypeptide chain while retaining somatostatin receptor binding sites [7, 8]. Two commercially available analogs, octreotide and lanreotide, are cyclic peptide SSAs which bind with high affinity to sst_2 and with moderate affinity to sst_3 and sst_5. SSAs have had a profound impact on neuroendocrine tumor treatment. They were initially developed as antisecretory agents designed to control symptoms such as flushing and diarrhea associated with the carcinoid syndrome. In recent years, high-level data has emerged demonstrating that SSAs can also control neuroendocrine tumor growth [9–11].

The initial formulation of octreotide was as a subcutaneously administered drug with an elimination half-life of approximately 2 h. A landmark phase II trial evaluated octreotide 150 μg tid in 25 patients with malignant carcinoid syndrome [12]. Rapid palliation of flushing and diarrhea was reported in 22 patients (88%), associated with major reductions of urine 5-HIAA in 18 patients (72%). Multiple subsequent studies have confirmed that both octreotide and lanreotide are effective for palliation of the carcinoid syndrome [13–15]. A crossover study of 33 patients comparing octreotide to lanreotide demonstrated equivalency in control of flushing and diarrhea as well as improvement in quality of life [13]. Both drugs are also effective at controlling hormonal symptoms associated with pancreatic neuroendocrine tumors such as VIPomas, glucagonomas, and gastrinomas [16–20]. Patients with advanced insulinomas may also respond to SSAs; [21] however, there is potential for exacerbation of hypoglycemia due to inhibition of the counter-regulatory hormone glucagon [22].

During the past two decades, a long-acting repeatable (LAR) depot formulation of octreotide (octreotide LAR) has been available, which releases drug slowly by cleavage of a polymer ester linkage and enables monthly intramuscular dosing. A randomized phase III study compared subcutaneous octreotide every 8 h to octreotide LAR 10 mg, 20 mg, or 30 mg every 4 weeks [23]. Control of diarrhea was comparable in each of the four study arms; however, control of flushing was least effective in the 10 mg LAR cohort. Based on this trial, the recommended starting dose of octreotide LAR was set at 20 mg every 4 weeks with subsequent dose titration suggested for symptom control [24]. A second somatostatin analog, lanreotide, was licensed in Europe in 1998 for the treatment of hormonal symptoms of advanced NETs [25]. A long-acting depot formulation of lanreotide was subsequently developed as a deep subcutaneous injection. It is supplied as a prefilled syringe consisting of a viscous aqueous solution available at doses of 60 mg, 90 mg, and 120 mg every 4 weeks.

The ELECT study was the first randomized trial phase III study to evaluate the palliative effect of an SSA for control of carcinoid syndrome. Patients with carcinoid syndrome who were SSA-naïve or who had control of symptoms on prior SSA were randomized to lanreotide 120 mg every 4 weeks versus placebo for 16 weeks, with access to short-acting octreotide as a rescue medicine [26]. The primary endpoint was percentage of days in which short-acting octreotide was used. The study demonstrated a statistically significant decrease in use of short-acting octreotide (34% of days with lanreotide versus 49% of days on placebo). No new safety concerns were identified.

Side effects of SSAs are generally mild and include nausea, bloating, and steatorrhea. Most side effects resolve over time. Malabsorptive symptoms caused by SSAs can often be controlled with pancreatic enzyme supplementation. Inhibitory effects of SSAs on gallbladder function increase the long-term risk of gallstones. Therefore, prophylactic cholecystectomy should be considered in patients undergoing abdominal surgery [27]. Other reported side effects include bradycardia, pancreatitis, and hyperglycemia. However, it is important to note that the only randomized trial of octreotide LAR versus placebo did not identify any increase in serious adverse events [28].

30.2.1 Treatment and Prophylaxis of the Carcinoid Crisis

Carcinoid crisis is defined as an episode of severe hypotension caused by an acute release of serotonin and other vasoactive substances into the circulation. It occurs most commonly in the operative setting since triggers include general anesthesia, epinephrine, and physical manipulation of tumors. Patients with carcinoid syndrome or elevated urine 5-HIAA who undergo an invasive procedure should receive a supplementary dose of octreotide 250–500 μg subcutaneously or intravenously 1 h prior to the procedure [29]. While it is common to administer octreotide during surgery (i.e., intravenous infusion of 50–100 μg/h), it has not been proven that patients benefit from octreotide prophylaxis [30]. Hypotension occurring in the setting of carcinoid crisis can be managed with bolus intravenous doses of octreotide 500–1000 μg until control of symptoms is achieved. Alternatively, continuous intravenous infusion of 50–100 μg/h may be given after a bolus dose [31].

30.2.2 Antiproliferative Effects of SSAs

In recent years, SSAs have been proven to inhibit the growth of neuroendocrine tumors. Antitumoral activity, also known as the "antiproliferative effect" of SSAs, can occur via direct and indirect mechanisms [6, 9, 32]. Direct mechanisms involve the binding of SSAs to somatostatin receptors on tumor cells leading to activation of intracellular signaling transduction pathways. Multiple in vitro studies using cell lines transfected with somatostatin receptors indicate that all receptor subtypes (sst1–5) can participate in inhibition of cellular proliferation, and that specific receptor subtypes (sst2,3) mediate apoptosis [33, 34]. Indirect antiproliferative mechanisms include inhibition of circulating growth factors such as vascular endothelial growth factor (VEGF) and insulin-like growth factor (IGF) [35], as well as inhibition of tumor angiogenesis through interaction with somatostatin receptors on endothelial cells [36].

30.2.2.1 Direct Antiproliferative Mechanisms

In vitro studies in various cell lines, including breast, pancreatic, and prostate carcinomas, demonstrate that SSA binding to somatostatin receptors activates a subset of phosphotyrosine phosphatases (PTPs), including SHP-1 and SHP-2, leading to cell cycle arrest [37, 38]. In a pituitary adenoma cell line, activation of sst_2 arrested cell proliferation via stimulation of SHP-1 [39]. SHP-1 has also been implicated in sst_3-dependent apoptosis in transfected Chinese Hamster Ovary (CHO) cells [40]. The precise effects of SSAs on mitogen-activated protein kinase (MAP-kinase) signaling are uncertain, since both inhibition and stimulation of this pathway have been linked to the antiproliferative effects of SSAs. In a glioma cell line, the receptor-like PTP, PTPeta, mediated the antiproliferative effects of somatostatin through inhibition of ERK1/2 [41]. In another study, somatostatin activated MAP-kinase in sst_1-expressing CHO cells, thereby stimulating the cyclin-dependent kinase inhibitor (CKI) p21 and inhibiting cell proliferation [42].

30.2.2.2 Indirect Antiproliferative Mechanisms

Suppression of tumor growth may occur through inhibition of various circulating growth factors, including growth hormone (GH) [43]. Inhibition of GH is thought to be mediated through sst_2 and sst_5, which are expressed in the anterior pituitary [44]. Octreotide has been shown to suppress circulating levels of IGF-1, both by suppressing pituitary GH and by inhibiting IGF-1 production in the liver [35, 45]. SSAs also appear to have an inhibitory effect on tumor angiogenesis [36, 46]. Octreotide has been shown to inhibit proliferating endothelial cells that express sst_2 and sst_5 [47]. The primary antiangiogenic mechanism may be suppression of endothelial nitric oxide release [48]. Inhibition of circulating vascular endothelial growth factor (VEGF) appears to also play a role in suppression of peritumoral vessel growth [49].

30.2.3 Clinical Evidence of the Antiproliferative Effect

Multiple phase II and retrospective studies have investigated the effects of SSAs on tumor progression in patients with gastroenteropancreatic neuroendocrine tumors (GEP-NETs). In general, these studies have documented low rates of objective radiographic response (<5%) but high rates of disease stabilization [11, 14, 25, 50–52].

Definitive evidence of the antiproliferative effect of SSAs emerged with the PROMID trial, the first randomized placebo-controlled study performed in the field of neuroendocrine tumors [28]. Eighty-five patients with metastatic well-differentiated NETs originating in midgut were randomized to receive either octreotide LAR 30 mg or placebo. Patients with severe uncontrolled carcinoid syndrome were excluded. The primary endpoint was time to tumor progression. Median time to tumor progression (TTP) was 14.3 months in the octreotide LAR 30 mg group versus 6.0 months in the placebo group (HR 0.34; $P = 0.000072$). Serious adverse events were nearly evenly balanced (11 patients in the octreotide LAR 30 mg arm and 10 patients in the placebo arm). On multivariate analysis, patients with resected primary tumor and low hepatic tumor burden (<10%) appeared to benefit most significantly from octreotide treatment versus placebo. The CLARINET study was a larger phase III study of lanreotide in hormonally nonfunctioning well-differentiated enteropancreatic NETs [53]. Two hundred and four patients with low- and intermediate-grade tumors (ki-67 index ≤10%) and evidence of somatostatin receptor expression on somatostatin receptor scintigraphy (SRS) were randomized to receive lanreotide 120 mg every 4 weeks versus placebo, with progression-free survival (PFS) as the primary endpoint. Interestingly, the study had a 3–6 month "run-in" phase of observation designed to document baseline progression status, during which time 96% of patients were found to be stable. The trial demonstrated a 53% improvement in PFS ($p = 0.0002$): median PFS was 18 months on placebo and not reached with lanreotide at time of primary endpoint analysis. On a subsequent analysis of an open-label extension phase of the study, median PFS among patients initially randomized to lanreotide was 32.8 months [54]. A plurality of patients on CLARINET had primary pancreatic tumors. The hazard ratio for PFS in this subgroup was 0.58 and was borderline statistically significant ($p = 0.06$). The hazard ratio for midgut NETs was 0.35 ($p = 0.009$), an outcome that was nearly identical to the hazard ratio in the PROMID study of midgut NETs. It is important to emphasize that the CLARINET study was not powered for subgroup analysis of efficacy. Based on results of the CLARINET study, lanreotide was approved for control of tumor growth in gastroenteropancreatic NETs.

The efficacy of SSAs in lung NETs remains poorly studied. Compared to gastrointestinal NETs, lung NETs express fewer somatostatin receptors, on average. A phase III study of lanreotide versus placebo in lung NETs (SPINET) was terminated for poor accrual (NCT02683941). Most guidelines, however, endorse use of SSAs in metastatic somatostatin receptor positive well-differentiated lung NETs [55, 56].

Randomized data are limited to tumors with ki-67 ≤ 10%. Most guidelines endorse use of SSAs for low-intermediate grade NETs (i.e., ki67 index <20%). There is very limited information on use of SSAs in higher-grade NETs, although many well-differentiated high-grade NETs (generally with ki-67 20%–50%) can express abundant somatostatin receptors.

30.2.4 Above-Label Doses of SSAs

While the highest dose of octreotide LAR tested prospectively in patients with metastatic NET has been 30 mg every 4 weeks, higher doses and/or frequencies are often prescribed for patients with suboptimal control of hormonal syndromes. Data supporting this practice derives primarily from retrospective studies. In a longitudinal database conducted by the National Comprehensive Cancer Network (NCCN) encompassing seven cancer centers, 40% of carcinoid tumor patients and 23% of pancreatic NET patients who received SSAs underwent dose escalations beyond 30 mg every 4 weeks [57]. The most common dose/frequency combinations were 40 mg every 4 weeks and 40 mg every 3 weeks. In one retrospective institutional study, 100 patients out of a total of 338 with metastatic midgut NETs (30%) received octreotide LAR at doses and/or frequency above the standard label dose of 30 mg every 4 weeks [58]. Indications for dose increase were worsening carcinoid syndrome (60 patients), radiographic progression of tumors (33 patients), and rising urine 5-HIAA (6 patients). Among patients whose doses were increased for refractory carcinoid syndrome, 34 patients (62%) experienced improvement in diarrhea and 28 patients (56%) experienced improvements in flushing. A single prospective trial investigated octreotide LAR 30 mg every 3 weeks among 28 patients with disease progression on 30 mg every 4 weeks [59]. Complete and partial control of clinical symptoms was observed in 40% and 60% of treated patients, respectively.

30.3 Interferon

Interferon-α (IFN-α) was first introduced for the treatment of midgut NETs in 1983 when a small study reported symptom palliation in six patients with carcinoid syndrome treated at doses of three–six million units daily [60]. Subsequent single-arm studies have reported objective response radiographic rates in the range of 5–10%, with higher rates of disease stabilization and palliation of hormonal symptoms [10, 61, 62]. More recently, randomized studies have offered evidence for the antiproliferative activity of interferon combined with somatostatin analogs.

30.3.1 Mechanisms of Action

Interferons are a complex array of cytokines with antiviral and antitumoral properties. They are divided into several classes. Type I interferons consist of IFNα (leukocyte interferon) and IFNβ (fibroblast interferon) which bind to a unique interferon receptor [63]. IFNs activate STAT (signal transducer and activator of transcription) complexes including the Janus-kinase-STAT (JAK-STAT) signaling pathway leading to signaling cascades involving the tumor cell and the host immune system [64]. Immune-related mechanisms of action include induction of major histocompatibility complex (MHC) type I expression in tumor cells which leads to enhanced immune surveillance. Other effects of IFNs include promotion of dendritic cell proliferation and differentiation and alterations of T-cell CD4:CD8 ratios [65]. Angiogenesis inhibition appears to be another indirect mechanism of action. In a study of neuroendocrine tumor xenografts in nude mice, IFNα treatment reduced microvessel density and suppressed vascular endothelial growth factor (VEGF) gene expression [66].

IFNs may also exert a direct antiproliferative effect on tumor growth through induction of cell cycle arrest; however, the precise mechanism remains elusive. In one in vitro study of lymphoid cell lines, G0/G1 cell cycle arrest was mediated through induction of the cyclin-dependent kinase inhibitors (CKIs) p21 and p15 and the expression of p27 [67]. However, another in vitro study of neuroendocrine tumor cells demonstrated that IFNα delayed progression from S-phase to G2 due to reduction of cyclin B levels and inhibition of Cdc2 kinase activity [68]. A third study demonstrated that IFNα induced apoptosis through activation of caspases-1, −2, −3, −8, and − 9 in a variety of malignant cell lines [69].

30.3.2 Studies of IFNα Monotherapy

An early study of IFNα three–six million units/day reported objective tumor responses in 4 of 36 patients (11%) with advanced carcinoid tumors and major reductions in urine 5-HIAA in 16 patients (53%) [70]. Another study of 22 patients with pancreatic NETs reported high rates of symptomatic and biochemical responses [71]. A more recent phase II study of 49 patients with advanced NETs evaluated IFNα-2a at a daily dose of six million units daily for 8 weeks followed by the same dose 3 times a weekly thereafter [72]. Among 34 patients with carcinoid tumors, partial radiographic responses were observed in four patients (12%) and major improvements in carcinoid syndrome were reported in 64% of cases. The most frequently observed side effects were fever, flu-like symptoms, and leukopenia. In the United States, Moertel et al. treated 27 patients with metastatic carcinoid tumors with IFNα at a high dose of 24 million units/m2 [73]. Despite an objective radiographic response rate of 20% and major urine 5-HIAA reductions in 39% of patients, the authors concluded that any therapeutic gains seemed to be outweighed by severity of side effects which included fevers/chills, anorexia, weight loss, leukopenia, and liver function abnormalities.

30.3.3 Studies of IFNα Combined with SSAs

Studies evaluating the combination of IFNα and SSAs emerged in the 1990s, based on in vitro data demonstrating that interferons can upregulate the expression of somatostatin receptors. One trial of patients with carcinoid syndrome who had become refractory to octreotide reported symptomatic improvement in 49% of patients after the addition of IFNα [74]. Another study reported disease stabilization in 14 of 21 patients in whom IFNα was added to preexisting octreotide therapy [75]. A more recent trial investigated pegylated IFN (PEGIFN), a long-acting formulation which enables weekly dosing. Of 17 patients who progressed on SSA therapy, inhibition of tumor growth was observed in 13 patients. The side effect profile of PEGIFN appeared to be superior to that of IFNα [76].

Several randomized clinical trials have investigated SSAs alone versus in combination with IFNα. One study of 68 patients with metastatic midgut carcinoid tumors who had undergone prior hepatic embolization evaluated octreotide alone versus octreotide combined with IFNα three million units administered five times per week

[77]. The 5-year survival in the combination arm was 57% versus 37% in the octreotide monotherapy arm. The overall survival results were not statistically significant ($p = 0.13$), possibly due to the small number of patients. However, the hazard ratio of 0.28 for tumor progression was highly significant ($p = 0.008$). Another randomized study of 109 gastroenteropancreatic NET patients compared octreotide alone versus octreotide combined with alpha-interferon 4.5 million units administered three times per week [78]. The median survival was prolonged in the combination arm (51 vs. 35 months), but results did not achieve statistical significance ($p = 0.38$). Objective response rates in both arms were less than 6%. A three-arm trial of 80 therapy-naïve patients with advanced carcinoid and pancreatic NETs compared subcutaneous lanreotide alone to IFNα five million units three times weekly, or the combination of the two drugs [79]. In this trial, time to tumor progression was similar in all three arms. Among 11 patients who were treated with lanreotide monotherapy and crossed over to combination therapy, one patient showed measurable inhibition of tumor growth.

Given the underpowered nature of these randomized trials, it is difficult to draw any definitive conclusions regarding the effects of alpha-interferon on overall survival or PFS. The most compelling data favoring IFNα is in midgut NETs where data support its use in combination with SSAs for palliation of the carcinoid syndrome and inhibition of tumor growth. Enthusiasm for IFNα is somewhat tempered by potential toxicities which include chronic fatigue, flu-like symptoms, and depression. Other abnormalities in laboratory values can include anemia, thrombocytopenia, leukopenia, and increases in liver enzymes. However, it is important to note most neuroendocrine trials have studied low doses of IFNα which are fairly tolerable. With the emergence of new systemic treatments including ^{177}Lutetium-dotatate and everolimus, the role of IFNα has become even more uncertain [80, 81].

30.4 Conclusion

Biotherapy plays a vital role in neuroendocrine tumor treatment, both for control of hormonal syndromes and inhibition of tumor growth. SSAs are exceptionally well tolerated and are appropriate as first-line systemic therapy for most patients advanced well-differentiated gastroenteropancreatic NETs that express somatostatin receptors. Their role in lung NETs is less established; however, it is highly likely that the impact of SSAs is more dependent on somatostatin receptor expression than on primary tumor site.

IFNα can also inhibit tumor growth and control hormonal symptoms, but its use is somewhat more limited due to toxicity. It appears to be most highly active in well-differentiated midgut NETs where trials have demonstrated a significant improvement in PFS in combination with SSA. Some guidelines suggest that IFNα be considered as a second-line agent in patients with refractory carcinoid syndrome or tumor progression on SSA; however, consensus has yet to be reached on optimal dose and formulation.

References

1. Reichlin S (1983) Somatostatin. N Engl J Med 309(24):1495–1501
2. Brazeau P et al (1973) Hypothalamic polypeptide that inhibits the secretion of immunoreactive pituitary growth hormone. Science 179(68):77–79
3. Evers BM et al (1991) Somatostatin and analogues in the treatment of cancer. A review. Ann Surg 213(3):190–198
4. Maurer R, Reubi JC (1985) Somatostatin receptors. JAMA 253(18):2741
5. Lamberts SW et al (1996) Octreotide. N Engl J Med 334(4):246–254
6. Weckbecker G et al (2003) Opportunities in somatostatin research: biological, chemical and therapeutic aspects. Nat Rev Drug Discov 2(12):999–1017
7. Bousquet C et al (2001) Antiproliferative effect of somatostatin and analogs. Chemotherapy 47(Suppl 2):30–39
8. Bauer W et al (1982) SMS 201-995: a very potent and selective octapeptide analogue of somatostatin with prolonged action. Life Sci 31(11):1133–1140
9. Strosberg J, Kvols L (2010) Antiproliferative effect of somatostatin analogs in gastroenteropancreatic neuroendocrine tumors. World J Gastroenterol 16(24):2963–2970
10. Shah T, Caplin M (2005) Endocrine tumours of the gastrointestinal tract. Biotherapy for metastatic endocrine tumours. Best Pract Res Clin Gastroenterol 19(4):617–636
11. Ducreux M et al (2000) The antitumoral effect of the long-acting somatostatin analog lanreotide in neuroendocrine tumors. Am J Gastroenterol 95(11):3276–3281
12. Kvols LK et al (1986) Treatment of the malignant carcinoid syndrome. Evaluation of a long-acting somatostatin analogue. N Engl J Med 315(11):663–666
13. O'Toole D et al (2000) Treatment of carcinoid syndrome: a prospective crossover evaluation of lanreotide versus octreotide in terms of efficacy, patient acceptability, and tolerance. Cancer 88(4):770–776
14. di Bartolomeo M et al (1996) Clinical efficacy of octreotide in the treatment of metastatic neuroendocrine tumors. A study by the Italian trials in medical oncology group. Cancer 77(2):402–408
15. Oberg K et al (2004) Consensus report on the use of somatostatin analogs for the management of neuroendocrine tumors of the gastroenteropancreatic system. Ann Oncol 15(6):966–973
16. Maton PN (1993) Use of octreotide acetate for control of symptoms in patients with islet cell tumors. World J Surg 17(4):504–510
17. Wymenga AN et al (1999) Efficacy and safety of prolonged-release lanreotide in patients with gastrointestinal neuroendocrine tumors and hormone-related symptoms. J Clin Oncol 17(4):1111
18. Kvols LK et al (1987) Treatment of metastatic islet cell carcinoma with a somatostatin analogue (SMS 201-995). Ann Intern Med 107(2):162–168
19. O'Dorisio TM et al (1988) Somatostatin and analogues in the treatment of VIPoma. Ann N Y Acad Sci 527:528–535
20. Boden G et al (1986) Treatment of inoperable glucagonoma with the long-acting somatostatin analogue SMS 201-995. N Engl J Med 314(26):1686–1689
21. Usukura M et al (2007) Medical treatment of benign insulinoma using octreotide LAR: a case report. Endocr J 54(1):95–101
22. Healy ML et al (2007) Severe hypoglycaemia after long-acting octreotide in a patient with an unrecognized malignant insulinoma. Intern Med J 37(6):406–409
23. Rubin J et al (1999) Octreotide acetate long-acting formulation versus open-label subcutaneous octreotide acetate in malignant carcinoid syndrome. J Clin Oncol 17(2):600–606
24. Sandostatin (octreotide acetate) Injections prescribing information (PI). Novartis Pharmaceuticals Corp
25. Eriksson B et al (1997) High-dose treatment with lanreotide of patients with advanced neuroendocrine gastrointestinal tumors: clinical and biological effects. Ann Oncol 8(10):1041–1044
26. Vinik AI et al (2016) Evaluation of Lanreotide depot/autogel efficacy and safety as a carcinoid syndrome treatment (Elect): a randomized, double-blind, placebo-controlled trial. Endocr Pract 22(9):1068–1080

27. Eriksson B et al (2008) Consensus guidelines for the management of patients with digestive neuroendocrine tumors—well-differentiated jejunal-ileal tumor/carcinoma. Neuroendocrinology 87(1):8–19
28. Rinke A et al (2009) Placebo-controlled, double-blind, prospective, randomized study on the effect of octreotide LAR in the control of tumor growth in patients with metastatic neuroendocrine midgut tumors: a report from the PROMID Study Group. J Clin Oncol 27(28):4656–4663
29. Kvols LK et al (1985) Rapid reversal of carcinoid crisis with a somatostatin analogue. N Engl J Med 313(19):1229–1230
30. Massimino K et al (2013) Octreotide LAR and bolus octreotide are insufficient for preventing intraoperative complications in carcinoid patients. J Surg Oncol 107(8):842–846
31. Caplin ME et al (1998) Carcinoid tumour. Lancet 352(9130):799–805
32. Grozinsky-Glasberg S et al (2008) Somatostatin analogues in the control of neuroendocrine tumours: efficacy and mechanisms. Endocr Relat Cancer 15(3):701–720
33. Sharma K, Srikant CB (1998) G protein coupled receptor signaled apoptosis is associated with activation of a cation insensitive acidic endonuclease and intracellular acidification. Biochem Biophys Res Commun 242(1):134–140
34. Lattuada D et al (2002) The apoptotic effect of somatostatin analogue SMS 201-995 on human lymphocytes. J Neuroimmunol 133(1–2):211–216
35. Serri O et al (1992) Octreotide inhibits insulin-like growth factor-I hepatic gene expression in the hypophysectomized rat: evidence for a direct and indirect mechanism of action. Endocrinology 130(4):1816–1821
36. Florio T et al (2003) Somatostatin inhibits tumor angiogenesis and growth via somatostatin receptor-3-mediated regulation of endothelial nitric oxide synthase and mitogen-activated protein kinase activities. Endocrinology 144(4):1574–1584
37. Zapata PD et al (2002) Autocrine regulation of human prostate carcinoma cell proliferation by somatostatin through the modulation of the SH2 domain containing protein tyrosine phosphatase (SHP)-1. J Clin Endocrinol Metab 87(2):915–926
38. Thangaraju M et al (1999) Interdependent regulation of intracellular acidification and SHP-1 in apoptosis. Cancer Res 59(7):1649–1654
39. Theodoropoulou M et al (2006) Octreotide, a somatostatin analogue, mediates its antiproliferative action in pituitary tumor cells by altering phosphatidylinositol 3-kinase signaling and inducing Zac1 expression. Cancer Res 66(3):1576–1582
40. Sharma K, Patel YC, Srikant CB (1996) Subtype-selective induction of wild-type p53 and apoptosis, but not cell cycle arrest, by human somatostatin receptor 3. Mol Endocrinol 10(12):1688–1696
41. Massa A et al (2004) The phosphotyrosine phosphatase eta mediates somatostatin inhibition of glioma proliferation via the dephosphorylation of ERK1/2. Ann N Y Acad Sci 1030:264–274
42. Florio T et al (1999) Somatostatin activation of mitogen-activated protein kinase via somatostatin receptor 1 (SSTR1). Mol Endocrinol 13(1):24–37
43. Koch BD, Schonbrunn A (1984) The somatostatin receptor is directly coupled to adenylate cyclase in GH4C1 pituitary cell membranes. Endocrinology 114(5):1784–1790
44. Schettini G et al (1988) Somatostatin inhibition of anterior pituitary adenylate cyclase activity: different sensitivity between male and female rats. Brain Res 439(1–2):322–329
45. Ambler GR et al (1996) The effects of octreotide on GH receptor and IGF-I expression in the GH-deficient rat. J Endocrinol 149(2):223–231
46. Woltering EA et al (1997) Somatostatin analogs: angiogenesis inhibitors with novel mechanisms of action. Investig New Drugs 15(1):77–86
47. Adams RL et al (2005) Somatostatin receptors 2 and 5 are preferentially expressed in proliferating endothelium. Br J Cancer 92(8):1493–1498
48. Arena S et al (2005) Somatostatin receptor subtype-dependent regulation of nitric oxide release: involvement of different intracellular pathways. Mol Endocrinol 19(1):255–267
49. Kumar M et al (2004) Antiangiogenic effect of somatostatin receptor subtype 2 on pancreatic cancer cell line: inhibition of vascular endothelial growth factor and matrix metalloproteinase-2 expression in vitro. World J Gastroenterol 10(3):393–399

50. Aparicio T et al (2001) Antitumour activity of somatostatin analogues in progressive metastatic neuroendocrine tumours. Eur J Cancer 37(8):1014–1019
51. Arnold R et al (1993) Somatostatin analog sandostatin and inhibition of tumor growth in patients with metastatic endocrine gastroenteropancreatic tumors. World J Surg 17(4):511–519
52. Saltz L et al (1993) Octreotide as an antineoplastic agent in the treatment of functional and nonfunctional neuroendocrine tumors. Cancer 72(1):244–248
53. Caplin ME et al (2014) Lanreotide in metastatic enteropancreatic neuroendocrine tumors. N Engl J Med 371(3):224–233
54. Caplin ME et al (2016) Anti-tumour effects of lanreotide for pancreatic and intestinal neuroendocrine tumours: the CLARINET open-label extension study. Endocr Relat Cancer 23(3):191–199
55. Shah MH et al (2018) NCCN guidelines insights: neuroendocrine and adrenal tumors, version 2.2018. J Natl Compr Cancer Netw 16(6):693–702
56. Pavel M, de Herder WW (2017) ENETS consensus guidelines for the standard of care in neuroendocrine tumors. Neuroendocrinology 105(3):193–195
57. Strosberg J et al (2013) Dosing patterns for octreotide LAR in neuroendocrine tumor patients. American Society of Clinical Oncology, Chicago
58. Weber J et al (2012) Above-label doses of octreotide LAR in patients with metastatic small-intestinal carcinoid tumors. J Clin Oncol 30:e14579. (Suppl; abstre14579)
59. Ferolla P et al (2012) Shortened interval of long-acting octreotide administration is effective in patients with well-differentiated neuroendocrine carcinomas in progression on standard doses. J Endocrinol Investig 35(3):326–331
60. Oberg K, Funa K, Alm G (1983) Effects of leukocyte interferon on clinical symptoms and hormone levels in patients with mid-gut carcinoid tumors and carcinoid syndrome. N Engl J Med 309(3):129–133
61. Biesma B et al (1992) Recombinant interferon alpha-2b in patients with metastatic apudomas: effect on tumours and tumour markers. Br J Cancer 66(5):850–855
62. Schober C et al (1992) Antitumour effect and symptomatic control with interferon alpha 2b in patients with endocrine active tumours. Eur J Cancer 28A(10):1664–1666
63. Pestka S et al (1987) Interferons and their actions. Annu Rev Biochem 56:727–777
64. Platanias LC (2005) Mechanisms of type-I-and type-II-interferon-mediated signalling. Nat Rev Immunol 5(5):375–386
65. Ferrantini M, Capone I, Belardelli F (2007) Interferon-alpha and cancer: mechanisms of action and new perspectives of clinical use. Biochimie 89(6–7):884–893
66. von Marschall Z et al (2003) Effects of interferon alpha on vascular endothelial growth factor gene transcription and tumor angiogenesis. J Natl Cancer Inst 95(6):437–448
67. Sangfelt O et al (1999) Molecular mechanisms underlying interferon-alpha-induced G0/G1 arrest: CKI-mediated regulation of G1 Cdk-complexes and activation of pocket proteins. Oncogene 18(18):2798–2810
68. Rosewicz S et al (2004) Interferon-alpha: regulatory effects on cell cycle and angiogenesis. Neuroendocrinology 80(Suppl 1):85–93
69. Thyrell L et al (2002) Mechanisms of interferon-alpha induced apoptosis in malignant cells. Oncogene 21(8):1251–1262
70. Oberg K et al (1986) Treatment of malignant carcinoid tumors with human leukocyte interferon: long-term results. Cancer Treat Rep 70(11):1297–1304
71. Eriksson B et al (1986) Treatment of malignant endocrine pancreatic tumours with human leucocyte interferon. Lancet 2(8519):1307–1309
72. Bajetta E et al (1993) Treatment of metastatic carcinoids and other neuroendocrine tumors with recombinant interferon-alpha-2a. A study by the Italian trials in medical oncology group. Cancer 72(10):3099–3105
73. Moertel CG, Rubin J, Kvols LK (1989) Therapy of metastatic carcinoid tumor and the malignant carcinoid syndrome with recombinant leukocyte A interferon. J Clin Oncol 7(7):865–868
74. Janson ET, Oberg K (1993) Long-term management of the carcinoid syndrome. Treatment with octreotide alone and in combination with alpha-interferon. Acta Oncol 32(2):225–229

75. Frank M et al (1999) Combination therapy with octreotide and alpha-interferon: effect on tumor growth in metastatic endocrine gastroenteropancreatic tumors. Am J Gastroenterol 94(5):1381–1387
76. Pavel ME et al (2006) Efficacy and tolerability of pegylated IFN-alpha in patients with neuroendocrine gastroenteropancreatic carcinomas. J Interf Cytokine Res 26(1):8–13
77. Kolby L et al (2003) Randomized clinical trial of the effect of interferon alpha on survival in patients with disseminated midgut carcinoid tumours. Br J Surg 90(6):687–693
78. Arnold R et al (2005) Octreotide versus octreotide plus interferon-alpha in endocrine gastroenteropancreatic tumors: a randomized trial. Clin Gastroenterol Hepatol 3(8):761–771
79. Faiss S et al (2003) Prospective, randomized, multicenter trial on the antiproliferative effect of lanreotide, interferon alfa, and their combination for therapy of metastatic neuroendocrine gastroenteropancreatic tumors—the International Lanreotide and Interferon Alfa Study Group. J Clin Oncol 21(14):2689–2696
80. Strosberg J et al (2017) Phase 3 trial of 177Lu-Dotatate for midgut neuroendocrine tumors. N Engl J Med 376(2):125–135
81. Yao JC et al (2016) Everolimus for the treatment of advanced, non-functional neuroendocrine tumours of the lung or gastrointestinal tract (RADIANT-4): a randomised, placebo-controlled, phase 3 study. Lancet 387(10022):968–977

The Role of Chemotherapy in Neuroendocrine Tumors

31

Ece Esin, Omer Dizdar, and Suayib Yalcin

31.1 Introduction

Since neuroendocrine tumors (NETs) are neoplasms originating from various neuroendocrine cells throughout the body, the cell of origin, the embryologic relation, and the morphological behavious and functional status are important in terms of clinical and pathological aspects and treatment strategy. According to North American Surveillance Epidemiology and End Results (SEER) database, NETs are detected most frequently in the gastrointestinal (GI) tract (60.9%) followed by bronchopulmonary tract (27.4%) and then by the hepato-biliary system, testes, pancreas, and ovaries quite rarely [1]. Due to increasing incidence rate and the survival time, NETs have become the second most prevalent GI cancer after colorectal cancer [2].

The prognosis of the patients is related to the extent of the disease and presence of metastases (tumor–node–metastasis (TNM) stage) [3, 4], Ki-67 index, the degree of differentiation (well or poorly differentiated), vascular invasion, tumor size, slope of tumor growth, and the primary origin site [5, 6].

Since NET classification is changing, the results of previous trials should be carefully extrapolated to the newly diagnosed patients. The World Health Organization (WHO) classification from 2010 categorizes neuroendocrine neoplasms (NENs) of the gastrointestinal tract according to Ki-67 index into well-differentiated neuroendocrine tumors (NET) G1 (Ki-67 $\leq$ 2%), G2 (Ki-67 3–20%), and neuroendocrine carcinomas (NEC) G3 (Ki-67 > 20%) [7].

Ki-67 is a proliferation antigen, present in G1, S, G2, and M phases of the cell cycle, which helps to detect the ratio of proliferative cells in a tumor. For pancreatic NETs, a Ki-67 cutoff level of 5% has been suggested as a better prognostic marker

E. Esin
Department of Medical Oncology, Bayindir Söğütözü Hospital, Ankara, Turkey

O. Dizdar · S. Yalcin (✉)
Department of Medical Oncology, Hacettepe University Cancer Institute, Ankara, Turkey
e-mail: syalcin@hacettepe.edu.tr

S. Yalcin, K. Öberg (eds.), *Neuroendocrine Tumours*,
https://doi.org/10.1007/978-3-031-56968-5_31

compared to 2% [8]. Bronchial NENs are classified according to WHO [9] into typical and atypical "carcinoids": typical should have <2 mitoses per 2 mm^2 (10 High Power Fields (HPF)) and no necroses, whereas atypical have 2–10 mitoses per 2 mm^2 (10 HPF) with necroses present. A comparison between mitotic count and Ki-67 index in bronchial NETs has not yet been performed.

The therapeutic landscape has been expanded in recent years with somatostatin analogs (SSA), interferon, and new molecular targeted therapies, mainly everolimus and sunitinib. When used with surgery, locoregional ablative therapies yield better results; however, there is still a significant number of patients who derive benefit from cytotoxic drugs even in well-differentiated neuroendocrine tumors.

The use of cytotoxics in well-differentiated NETs can be controversial. Their slow-growing nature and low rate of mitoses in NENs contrast the mechanism of efficacy of cytotoxic drugs. However, as seen in the efficacy of metronomic chemotherapy in malignancies, the slow growth of tumors can be used against the tumor itself by specifically combined therapeutic options. The new biological and molecular targeted therapies, which exert cytostatic rather than cytotoxic effects on tumors, lead to changes in the concept of treatment benefit. The "disease control" or progression-free survival (PFS) is more accepted, whereby stable disease or a delay in progression is considered as a positive response to treatment. Hence, the primary endpoints of benefit in trials should be interpreted carefully.

Defining the right drug or drugs for right patients while treating NENs is difficult. Bulky disease, symptomatic disease with urgent need for alleviation, and aggressively progressive tumors are potential candidates among well-to moderate-differentiated NENs. Additionally, for patients with locally advanced tumors, resectability may be possible with proper chemotherapy. Apart from clinical factors, primary tumor location and the degree of tumor proliferation have been used to guide therapeutic decisions and therefore histological characterization has been assessed using WHO criteria and Ki-67 index. Although Ki-67 has been shown to predict biological behavior and correlate with survival [10], it has not been established as a predictive factor for drug selection.

The rarity of NETs results in lack of large size clinical trials, so most of the data is achieved from retrospective case series. Despite the rarity of high-level evidence of activity, cytotoxic drugs remain as an important component of treatment of NETs.

Among the cytotoxic drug family, the two groups of drugs are the most active agents for NENs: alkylating agents including streptozocin (STZ), dacarbazine (DTIC), and temozolomide (TEM), and antimetabolites such as 5-fluorouracil (5-FU) and capecitabine (CAP). Topoisomerase inhibitors such as etoposide as well as platinum derivatives have been reported with high response rates (RRs) in both panNETs and poorly differentiated NECs, while modest activity has been observed in foregut and midgut carcinoids, respectively.

In the following sections, the strategies of chemotherapeutic use in NENs will be discussed:

31.2 Systemic Chemotherapy in Well-Differentiated NEN

A number of chemotherapeutic agents have been tested in metastatic well-differentiated G1 and G2 NETs, mainly pancreatic and other foregut tumors. Until now, results of systemic chemotherapy in well-differentiated small intestinal NETs have been poor with response rates of about 15% [11]. There is also limited data on systemic chemotherapy in "hindgut" NETs.

Alkylating agents include streptozocin (STZ), dacarbazine (DTIC), and temozolomide (TEM), and antimetabolites such as 5-fluorouracil (5-FU) and capecitabine (CAP). Topoisomerase inhibitors such as etoposide as well as platinum derivatives (oxaliplatin, OXA) are potentially effective for NENs.

The alkylating agent streptozotocin, later renamed as streptozocin (STZ), has been used since 1967. Murray-Lyon et al. showed that there are improvements in both hypoglycaemic symptoms and tumor load in a malignant pancreatic NET in 1968 [12]. STZ is a glucose analog and is selectively incorporated into the β cells of the pancreas via GLUT2 transporters. STZ binds to DNA and inhibits DNA repair [10]. GLUT2 receptors are also expressed in the liver and in the kidney. Hence, STZ toxicities may commonly involve these organs. The US Food and Drug Administration approved the use of STZ for "islet-cell" carcinoma in 1982.

STZ has been tested as single agent or in combination with other alkylator doxorubicin. However, due to irreversible cardiomyopathy, this combination is fallen from agenda. STZ alone or mostly in combination with 5-FU (5 fluorouracil) are currently in practice as the Moertel protocol (500 mg/m^2 of STZ plus 400 mg/m^2 of 5-FU on day 1–5 every 6 weeks) or the Uppsala protocol (500 mg/m^2 of STZ on days 1–5 and 400 mg/m^2 of 5-FU on days 1–3 followed by 1-day infusion of 1000 mg/m^2 of STZ and 400 mg/m^2 of 5-FU, repeated every 3 weeks).

DTIC is a synthetic alkylator agent that exerts cytotoxic activity via its active metabolite 5-(3-methyl-triazeno)imidazole-4-carboxamide (MTIC). MTIC acts as an alkylator and methylator of the DNA primarily at the N^7 or O^6 positions of guanine residues. This process leads to base pair mismatch, DNA single-and double-strand breaks, and consequently, apoptosis.

DTIC has been used either as monotherapy or in combination with 5-FU and epirubicin for the treatment of NETs. DTIC monotherapy was better tolerated than the combination regimen. The most common and the most severe toxicities included nausea, vomiting, and diarrhea, respectively. The Eastern Cooperative Oncology Group (ECOG) tested the efficacy of dacarbazine (DTIC) [13] in 50 patients with pancreatic NETs in a phase II trial. The partial response (PR) rate was 34%, but a total of 16 patients (30%) developed grade ¾ toxicities and 2 (4%) lethal toxicity.

TEM is an oral alkylating agent derivative of DTIC, and its active metabolite is similar to DTIC. It is a relatively new oral chemotherapeutic agent with activity in metastatic melanoma and glioma [14, 15].

CAP-TEM represented by the combination of capecitabine (CAP) 1–14.days in addition with TEM 10–15.days. The synergistic activity relies on depletion of intracellular thymidine pools, exerted by both drugs. The safety and efficacy of single agent TMZ was explored in a study of 21 patients with progressive (within the past

3 months) digestive NETs [16]. The patients were heavily treated with at least one prior regimen. TMZ was administered orally at 200 mg/m^2/day for 5 days every 28 days. The response was tested according to RECIST criteria. It was show that PR was obtained in one patient (5%) and SD in 17 patients (81%) and the median time to progression was 9 months. Grade 3 hematological toxicity occurred in five patients. The efficacy and safety of TMZ in 31 patients with progressive metastatic bronchial NETs (14 typical, 15 atypical, and 2 unclassified) were studied in a retrospective analysis [17]. Partial response was seen in three patients (14%) and SD in 11 (52%) with a median profession-free survival (PFS) of 5.3 months. Overall survival was 23.2 months. Notably, all patients with PR had atypical carcinoids with a high proliferative activity (10%, 18%, and 25%, respectively). There was no grade 4 toxicity, but adverse events (grade 3) were noted in four patients (14%). Most commonly observed grade 3 toxicities were thrombocytopenia ($n = 3$) and leukopenia ($n = 1$).

Oxaliplatin has a mechanism of action similar to alkylators as it binds to DNA via positively charged reactive intermediates and cross-linking DNA strands. Oxaliplatin is generally used in combination with capecitabine or with infusional 5-FU and folinic acid for the treatment of NETs.

The well-known chemotherapeutic agents like paclitaxel, capecitabine, gemcitabine, and topotecan have modest single-agent activity in the treatment of advanced NETs [18–21]. These single agents or combined drug treatments will be discussed further in accordance with the localization of the primary NEN.

31.2.1 The Role of Chemotherapy in PanNETs

Pancreatic NETs are considered more sensitive to cytotoxic drugs. The reason for the increased efficacy of the drugs may be due to different DNA repair enzyme expressions of pancreatic tumors, different genomic mutational backgrounds, and cell cycle kinetics. There have been no significant studies on the treatment of PanNETs since 1980s–1990s, leading to lack of recent improvements in therapeutic options. One should be cautious in discussing and taking into account of the results of these older and underpowered clinical trials. Cytotoxic drugs can be used in palliative settings in advanced PanNETs and preoperative settings (neoadjuvant) of locally advanced tumors.

STZ has a clinical activity which was shown in clinical trials of patients with metastatic PanNETs: the combination of STZ with 5-FU over STZ alone was first reported in a small randomized trial in 1980 by Moertel [22]. STZ was given intravenously (IV) at 500 mg/m^2 and 5-FU at 400 mg/m^2 IV for 5 days every 6 weeks. The overall response rates (RRs) were 63% and 36%, respectively. STZ was subsequently approved by the FDA as a treatment for pancreatic NETs.

Moertel et al. then compared the two regimens, STZ plus Dox (given IV at 50 mg/m^2 D1 and D22) and STZ plus 5-FU [22]. STZ/Dox was shown to be superior with a median time to progression (20 vs. 6.9 months) and overall survival (2.2 vs. 1.4 years), respectively [23]. The doxorubicin arm has had frequent side effects, including alopecia, myelosuppression, and cardiotoxicity. The same results, unfortunately, cannot be reproduced in another groups trials, most likely because of the use of hormonal responses and clinical assessment as response criteria in the Moertel study.

The recent reports of results with STZ/Dox describe RR of 6–36%, and most of these studies also had radiological responses according to WHO or RECIST [24–26]. The low response rates in some of the recent studies may reflect the fact that in the last 20 years, chemotherapy was used in later lines of treatment after biotherapy (SSA and interferon).

It was hypothesized that cisplatin addition to STZ/5-FU combination may yield better results. Turner et al. tested triple combination in a mixed group of 79 patients, mainly pancreatic NETs but also gastrointestinal, lung, and patients with unknown primary [27]. The regimen FCiSt (5-FU 500 mg/m^2, STZ 1 g/m^2, and cisplatin 70 mg/m^2) was given IV on D1 of a 21-day cycle. The RR was 38% for pancreatic NETs and 25% for non-pancreatic NETs. Stable disease was observed in 51% of patients, and overall time to progression was 9.1 months. They concluded that the three-drug regimen was not superior to two-drug regimen with STZ/5-FU or STZ/Dox.

Given the encouraging results obtained in the Moertels trial, a subsequent three-arm study investigated the efficacy of the triple combination of STZ/5-FU/Dox [28]. An overall RR in 84 pancreatic NETs of 39% and SD in 50% were observed, with a median duration of response of 9.3 months and a PFS of 18 months [28]. Toxicity grade 3–4 was noted in 23% of patients, mainly hematological. Post hoc analysis showed that more than 75% of the liver volume involvement and prior chemotherapy was independently associated with inferior PFS.

Due to the cumulative dose-related toxicity of the replacement is necessary with 5-FU. STZ can cause nausea and vomiting, but these side effects nowadays can be almost completely avoided by modern anti-emetics, e.g., 5-HT3-receptor blockers. Bone marrow toxicity is not an observed side effect with STZ/5-FU. Renal dysfunction, including proteinuria and decreased creatinine clearance, which occurs in 20% of patients, is the dose-limiting toxicity, but no grade 3–4 toxicity has been described in recent series [26, 28–30]. Creatinine clearance should be checked before each course, and dehydration during or after the course should be avoided. In some tumors, especially those with production of vasoactive intestinal polypeptide (VIP), chemotherapy may induce hormonal crises, causing severe dehydration. Thus, in these cases, "protective" SSA treatment should be given.

High-dose DTIC (850 mg/m^2 every 4 weeks) has been investigated in a phase II study sponsored by ECOG [13]. According to the results, median OS was 19 months with an ORR 33% among 42 patients with measurable disease. There are grade 2–3 toxicities event reported deaths due to high-dose DTIC. At present, DTIC high-dose combinations are not frequently advised.

The use of TEM alone or in combination has gained popularity in recent years. Data on TEM efficacy is mainly derived from older retrospective series. In one of the reports including 12 heavily pretreated metastatic PanNET patients, disease control was reported in 9 out of 12 patients, and thrombocytopenia was the most common grade 3 side effect, observed in 14% of cases.(14).

TEM has been tested in various combinations with either targeted drugs, cytotoxic agents, or peptide receptor radionuclide therapy (PRRT): in a phase II prospective study, TMZ was combined with thalidomide, an agent with hypothesized antiangiogenic effect in metastatic NETs [31]. A dose-intensive TMZ regimen of 150 mg/m^2/d for 7 days every other week was administered together with thalidomide at 50–400 mg daily, median 100 mg. This trial included 29 patients (11 pancreatic NETs, 14 carcinoids, and 4 pheochromocytomas). Of the study population, 16 (55%) had received no prior treatment. Radiologic response was seen in 25% of patients: five out of 11 (45%) of pancreatic NETs and one of 14 (7%) with carcinoids. Stable disease was observed in 68% of patients, and the duration of response was 13.5 months. Thalidomide toxicity (neuropathy) was the dose-limiting leaded to drug withdrawal. Grade 3–4 lymphopenia occurred in 69% of patients and 10% developed opportunistic infections.

The efficacy of TMZ in combination with bevacizumab was evaluated in 34 heavily pretreated patients with locally advanced or metastatic NETs (carcinoids 19 and pancreatic 15) in a phase II trial [32]. TMZ was given at 150 mg/m^2 D1–7, D15–21, and Bv 5 mg/kg IV every other week in a 28-day cycle. Overall radiologic response was 15%. There was significant difference in RR between patients with pancreatic NETs (5/15(33%)) and those with carcinoid tumors (0 of 19). The median PFS was 11.0 months (14.3 months for pancreatic NETs vs. 7.3 months for carcinoid tumors). The median overall survival was 33.3 months (41.7 months for pancreatic NETs and 18.8 months for carcinoids). Grade 3–4 adverse events included lymphopenia, thrombocytopenia, and vomiting.

A phase I/II study investigating TEM and the mTOR inhibitor everolimus in a population of 40 patients with advanced panNETs [33]. Everolimus is a mammalian target of rapamycin (mTOR) inhibitor with single-agent activity in pancreatic NETs. It was shown to result in improvement in PFS by 6.4 months compared with placebo as shown in the RADIANT-3 trial [34]. In this everolimus PanNET trial, patients with pancreatic NETs were treated with TMZ at a dose of 150 mg/m^2 per day D1–7 and D15–21 in combination with everolimus daily in each 28-day cycle. In cohort 1, TMZ was combined with everolimus at 5 mg daily. Safety was shown, and subsequent patients in cohort 2 were treated with TMZ and everolimus 10 mg daily. The majority of patients (77%) had received no prior systemic treatment with the exception of octreotide (40% continued during study). A total of 43 patients were enrolled, 7 in cohort 1 and 36 in cohort 2. Among 40 patients who were evaluated, 16 (40%) experienced PR according to RECIST and 21 (53%) had SD. The median PFS was 15.4 months, and median overall survival was not reached. Biochemical responses with >50% reduction of chromogranin. Treatment discontuniation was observed in nine patients due to adverse events, including pneumonitis ($n = 3$), edema ($n = 1$), rash ($n = 2$), elevated creatinine ($n = 2$), and elevated liver enzymes ($n = 1$). Grade 3 or 4 lymphopenia was observed nearly in 50% and 16% grade 3 or 4 thrombocytopenia. One patient had a reactivated hepatitis B infection. Other toxicities included mild mucositis, hyperglycemia, hypercholesterolemia, or hypertriglyceridemia. The authors' conclusion was that patients with advanced pancreatic NETs can be safely and effectively treated with the combination. The optimal dosing schedule of TMZ and everolimus is, however, remained unrevealed due to high toxicity rates.

In in vitro studies, TMZ and CAP worked synergically on tumor cell lines via combined effect on apoptosis. The CAP-TEM regimen recently drew more attention in advanced PanNET patients. In two retrospective series, the response rates have been relatively high. In one such study, 17 patients with mixed NETs, 11 (65%) having received prior chemotherapy, were treated with TMZ at 150–200 mg/m^2 D10–14 every 4 weeks and CAP 1000 mg twice daily D1–14. Complete response (CR) was noted in one patient (9%) and PR according to RECIST in nine patients (53%) with a median duration of 9 months [35]. Toxicities mainly included grade 3 thrombocytopenia ($n = 2$) and hand-foot syndrome ($n = 1$). In the other study, the combination was given as first-line in 30 patients with pancreatic NETs (16 well-differentiated, 9 moderately differentiated, and 5 not graded). TMZ was given at 200 mg/m^2 D10–14 and CAP 750 mg/m^2 twice daily D1–14 [36]. Partial response was noted in 21/30 patients (70%) and SD in 8/30 (27%) with a median PFS of 18 months, median duration of response of 20 months (responders). Overall survival at 2 years was 92%.

A phase II, prospective, randomized trial investigated TEM versus CAPTEM dual therapy in 144 patients with grade 1 or 2 PanNETs. ECOG researchers reported that combination arm had better median PFS (22.7 months vs. 14.4 months, respectively; hazard ratio 0.58, $p = 0.023$). Consistent with PFS data, the median OS was 38 months in patients receiving temozolomide alone, while it was not reached in patients treated with CAPTEM (hazard ratio 0.41, $p = 0.012$) [37].

TEM has been tested alone or in combination with CAP as a radiosensitizer in patients undergoing radionuclide therapy. The preliminary results showed that dual or triple combination of CAP-TEM and ^{177}Lu-Octreotate is compatible and harmonious with manageable toxicity profile [38, 39]. A median PFS of 48 months and 80% ORR have been demonstrated with CAPTEM and ^{177}Lu-Octreotate. As potential long-term survivors, even advanced NEN patients should be carefully followed by myelodysplastic syndrome after chemo-radionuclide therapy [40].

In several series and studies, the efficacy of oxaliplatin and its combinations were analyzed. In a phase II trial, OXA with CAP (XELOX regimen) were used in 27 well-differentiated NETs progressive to first-line somatostatin analogs. According to the results of 11 PanNET patients, PR was recorded as 27% and stable disease was achieved in 45% [41]. In a retrospective series of 104 NEN patients, oxaliplatin with gemcitabine was assessed. These patients were treated with GEMOX for at least six cycles. GEMOX showed an ORR of 38% and a median PFS of 7.3 months among patients with panNETs [42].

In conclusion, there is no definite evidence to guide chemotherapy choice for PanNETs. CAPTEM and STZ/5-FU represent the most used regimens in clinical practice, but it is currently unknown whether one should be preferred over the other. Additionally, no studies have compared cytotoxic drugs with targeted agents in panNET patients, and thus no sequencing strategies have been validated. The two-arm, randomized, phase III SEQTOR study is currently investigating whether the sequence of STZ/5-FU followed by everolimus at tumor progression has a better efficacy profile with respect to the sequential treatment with everolimus followed by STZ/5-FU (NCT02246127). The study has completed accrual.

31.2.2 The Role of Chemotherapy in Foregut NETs

So far there is no established systemic treatment for foregut NETs. STZ combinations have been given with varying results. One publication described PR in 6/17 patients (35%) and SD in 5/17 patients (29%) with STZ/5-FU in patients with atypical bronchial carcinoids [43].

31.2.3 The Role of Chemotherapy in Midgut NETs

The indolent course of midgut NETs even in the presence of advanced tumors creates a chemo-resistant environment. Hence, the role is not clear and probably minor. ECOG investigators studied 64 progressive metastatic NETs to receive STZ/5-FU or IFN-α. In this phase III trial, only one of 23 midgut NET patients had a partial response [44]. Similarly, in a randomized phase II/III trial, FU-DOX versus STZ-5FU was tested in 176 NET patients. Response rate was 16% in both treatment arms, with a median PFS of only 4.5 and 5.3 months, respectively [11]. While highly effective in panNETs, treatment with temozolomide-based regimens has been associated with poor responses in midgut NETs [31, 33, 45, 46]. To date, there is no scientific data that a cytotoxic agent has an efficacy in intestinal NET. Hence, ENETS guidelines do not recommend chemotherapeutics for well-differentiated midgut NETs [47].

31.2.4 The Role of Chemotherapy in Bronchopulmonary NETs

The therapeutic management of bronchopulmonary NETs is controversial. To date, there is no evidence of survival benefit deriving from chemotherapy in patients with bronchopulmonary NETs. The only data present come from retrospective series that included a small number of patients and produced low-quality evidence. In these setups, etoposide-, temozolomide-, and oxaliplatin-containing regimens have demonstrated some activity in patients with BP-NETs, but the recommended standard therapy has yet to be determined. Everolimus is the only approved agent for bronchopulmonary NETs. Systemic chemotherapy with any of these agent/agents can be offered to patients with clinically aggressive, rapidly progressing, and/or bulky disease or for large-sized tumors that are symptomatic.

31.2.5 Predictive Value of MGMT Expression

Methylguanine-DNA methyltransferase (MGMT) is a DNA repair enzyme involved in induce cancer cell resistance to *O*6-alkylating agents, e.g., TMZ. The cytotoxic effect of TMZ was shown to be related to its ability to induce methylation of guanine which results in DNA mismatch, which in turn leads to apoptosis and cell death [48]. The sensitivity of tumor cells to alkylating agents, including TMZ, has been associated with decreased levels of MGMT [49]. Among patients with advanced melanoma or glioblastoma treated with TMZ, low MGMT expression was associated with longer survival [50, 51]. The prevalence of MGMT deficiency in NENs was investigated and correlated with treatment response to TMZ-based regimens in a recent trial [52]. MGMT deficiency was found in 19/37 of pancreatic NETs (51%) and none of the carcinoid tumors. Among patients who received TMZ-based treatment, 18 of 53 patients (34%) with pancreatic NETs but only 1 (bronchial carcinoid) of 44 with carcinoid tumors (2%) experienced CR or PR ($P < 0.001$). Among 21 patients with evaluable tumor tissue who had received TMZ treatment, four of five with MGMT-deficient tumor (all pancreatic) and none of 16 patients with tumors showing intact MGMT expression responded to treatment ($P = 0.001$). There is, however, controversy regarding the optimal method of MGMT analysis. It was also shown that there are disconcordant results with IH and methylation-specific PCR in other tumors.

Standardization of techniques assessing MGMT status in tumor tissue and prospective trials is warranted. This would allow for confirming a correlation between MGMT status and response to treatment with TMZ. This analysis may also serve as a predictive test for sensitivity to other alkylating agents, e.g., streptozocin and dacarbazine, since they have a common cytotoxic mechanism, i.e., induction of methylation at the O^6 position of guanine, and may have a similar resistance mechanism [52]. All three drugs seem to be more effective in pancreatic NET than in small intestinal tumors.

31.3 New Molecular Targeted Agents in NETs

Recently, the mTOR inhibitor everolimus and the tyrosine-kinase inhibitor sunitinib have been approved for the treatment of well-differentiated pancreatic NETs based on two multicenter placebo-controlled randomized trials [34, 53]. In both trials, the primary endpoint was PFS and progression within the past 12 months was required for inclusion. The results were very similar with an improvement in PFS from 4.6 to 11.0 (hazard ratio for disease progression, 0.35; 95% CI 0.27 to 0.45; $p < 0.001$) for everolimus and from 5.5 to 11.4 months (hazard ratio for progression, 0.42; 95% CI, 0.26–0.66; $p < 0.001$) for sunitinib. Overall survival as a secondary endpoint could not be assessed since about 70% of patients crossed over from the placebo to the active arm in both studies. Tumor stabilization was achieved in both trials, but the objective response rates according to RECIST were low, 5% for everolimus and 9.3% for sunitinib. The proliferative rate or Ki-67 was not assessed except for a small number of patients in the sunitinib trial. Sunitinib was associated with diarrhea, nausea, asthenia, vomiting, and fatigue in more than 30% of patients, and grade 3 or 4 neutropenia and hypertension occurred in 12% and 10%, respectively. With everolimus treatment, stomatitis, rash, diarrhea, and fatigue occurred in at least 30% and the most common grade 3 or 4 adverse events were anemia (6%), hyperglycaemia (5%), stomatitis (7%), and pneumonitis in 2%. The hyperglycemic effect has turned out to be beneficial in patients with hypoglycemia due to malignant insulinoma.

Everolimus was also studied in nonpancreatic NETs with the carcinoid syndrome in combination with octreotide long-acting repeatable (LAR) in the RADIANT-2 trial [54]. Compared with octreotide-LAR alone, the PFS improved from 11.3 to 16.4 months (hazard ratio 0.77; 95%CI 0.50–1.00, one-sided log-rank test $p = 0.026$) with the combination, but this did not reach the prespecified p-value of $p \leq 0.0246$. The lack of significance may be due to imbalances between treatment arms.

31.4 Conclusions

The rarity of the heterogenous tumors complicates prospective studies. Hence, limited quality data from retrospective series in NETs help to guide the treatment and lead to ambiguity of drug choices.

Alkylating agents including streptozocin (STZ), dacarbazine (DTIC), and temozolomide (TEM), antimetabolites such as 5-fluorouracil (5-FU) and capecitabine (CAP), and topoisomerase inhibitors such as etoposide and platinum derivatives (Oxaliplatin-OXA) are potentially effective drug options for PanNET.

Cytotoxic agents have consistently shown substantial antitumor activity in panNETs, with modest and negligible efficacy in foregut and midgut carcinoids, respectively. So far, no prospective study compared STZ-containing regimens with TEM-or platinum-based combinations in patients with panNETs. Hence, it is impossible to conclude to an optimal standard protocol. Moreover, studies have not compared cytotoxic agents with targeted agents. In other foregut tumors and in midgut and bronchopulmonary NETs, the efficacy of cytotoxic drugs is still being debated.

The combination of new molecular targeted therapies with chemotherapy is an immersing option, which may improve the survival results. Although the new drugs have been demonstrated to prolong PFS, patients with a high tumor burden may benefit from chemotherapy due to much higher response rates with chemotherapy. In such combinations, assessment of side effects and quality of life is essential. Such combinations could also prevent the development of escape or resistance mechanisms [55].

Precise treatment options need to be tailored for heterogenous and rare tumors. In this context, clinical, pathological, and molecular predictors of response to chemotherapy have been studied recently. Pancreatic primary site, the biology of the disease, symptoms, the volume of disease, quality of life, mitotic rate, and Ki67 should orient the physician to choose the optimal strategy.

The age of immunotherapy may have an impact in the treatment protocols in the future, especially if used in combination with chemotherapy. With further understanding of importance of neoantigens and emergence of new mutations, the immunotherapy-cytotoxic therapy combination is sure to be popular in the near future.

References

1. Modlin IM, Lye KD, Kidd M (2003) A 5-decade analysis of 13,715 carcinoid tumors. Cancer 97:934–959
2. Schimmack S, Svedja B, Lawrence B et al (2011) The diversity and commonalities of gastroenteropancreatic neuroendocrine tumors. Langerbeck's. Arch Surg 396:273–298
3. Rindi G, Klöppel G, Ahlman H et al (2006) TNM staging fo foregut (neuor)endocrine tumors: a consensus proposal including a grading system. Virchows Arch 449:395–401
4. Rindi G, Klöppel G, Couvelard A et al (2007) TNM staging of midgut and hindgut (neuro)endocrine tumors: a consensus proposal including a grading system. Virchows Arch 451:757–762
5. Garcia-Carbonero R, Capdevila J, Crespo-Herrero G et al (2010) Incidence, patterns of care and prognostic factors for outcome of gastroenteropancreatic neuroendocrine tumors (GEP-NET): results from National Cancer Registry of Spain (RGETNE). Ann Oncol 21:1794–1803
6. Pape UF, Berndt U, Koch M et al (2008) Prognostic factors of long-term outcome in gastroenteropancreatic neuroendocrine tumors. Endocr Relat Cancer 15:1083–1097
7. Rindi G, Arnold R, Bosman FT et al (2010) Nomenclature and classification of neuroendocrine neoplasms of the digestive system. In: Bosman FT, Carneiro F, Hruban H, Theise ND (eds) WHO classification of the digestive system. IARC Press, Lyon, pp 13–14
8. Scarpa A, Mantovani W, Capelli P et al (2010) Pancreatic endocrine tumors: improved TNM staging and histopathology grading permit a clinically efficient prognostic stratification of patients. Modern Pathol 23:824–833
9. Travis WD, Muller-Hermelink HK, Harris C et al (2004) Tumors of the lung, pleura, thymus and heart. Pathology and genetics. WHO Classification of tumors. IARC Press, Lyon
10. Ekeblad S, Skogseid B, Öberg K et al (2008) Pancreatic endocrine tumors: survival and prognostic factors. Clin Cancer Res 14:7798–7803
11. Sun W, Lipsitz S, Catalano P et al (2005) Phase II/III study of doxorubicin with fluorouracil or dacarbazine in the treatment of advanced carcinoid tumors: eastern cooperative oncology group study E1281. J Clin Oncol 23:4897–4904
12. Murray-Lyon IM, Eddleston AL, Williams R et al (1968) Treatment of multiple-hormone-producing malignant islet-cell tumor with streptozotocin. Lancet 2:895–898
13. Ramanathan RK, Cnaan RG, Hahn G et al (2001) Phase II trial of dacarbazine (DTIC) in advanced pancreatic islet cell carcinoma. Study of eastern cooperative oncology group—E6282. Ann Oncol 12:1139–1143
14. Middleton MR, Grob JJ, Aaronsson N et al (2000) Randomized phase III study of temozolomide versus dacarbazine in the treatment of patients with advanced metastatic melanoma. J Clin Oncol 18:158–166
15. Stupp R, Mason WP, Van den Bent MJ et al (2005) Radiotherapy plus concomitant and adjuvant temozolomide for glioblastoma. N Engl J Med 352:987–996

16. Maire F, Hammel P, Faiver S et al (2009) Temozolomide: a safe and effective treatment for malignant digestive endocrine tumors. Neuroendocrinology 90:67–72
17. Crona J, Fanola J, Lindholm D et al (2013) Effect of temozolomide in metastatic bronchial carcinoids. Neuroendocrinology 98:151–155
18. Ansell SM, Pitot HC, Burch PA et al (2001) A phase II study of high-dose paclitaxel in patients with advanced neuroendocrine tumors. Cancer 91:1543–1548
19. Krzyzanowska MK, Tsao MS, Oza AM et al (2006) Capecitabine plus rofecoxib show no activity in patients with metastatic neuroendocrine tumors. Clin Oncol 18:88–89
20. Kulke MH, Kim H, Clark JW et al (2004) A phase II trial of gemcitabine for metastatic neuroendocrine tumors. Cancer 101:934–939
21. Ansell SM, Mahoney MR, Green EM et al (2004) Topotecan in patients with advanced neuroendocrine tumors; a phase II study with significant haematological toxicity. Am J Clin Oncol 27:232–235
22. Moertel CG, Hanley JA, Johnson LA et al (1980) Streptozotocin alone compared with streptozotocin plus fluroruracil in the treatment of advanced islet-cell carcinoma. N Engl J Med 303:1189–1195
23. Moertel CG, Lefkopoulu M, Lipiz S et al (1992) Streptozotocin-doxorubicin, streptozotocin-fluorouracil, or chlorozotocin in the treatment of advanced islet-cell carcinoma. N Engl J Med 326:519–523
24. Cheng PN, Saltz LB (1999) Failure to confirm major objective antitumor activity for streptozotocin and doxorubicin in the treatment of patients with advanced islet-cell carcinoma. Cancer 86:944–948
25. Mc Collum AD, Kulke MH, Ryan DP et al (2004) Lack of efficacy of streptozotocin and doxorubicin in patients with advanced pancreatic endocrine tumors. J Clin Oncol 27:485–488
26. Delaunoit T, Ducreux M, Boige V et al (2004) The doxorubicin-streptozotocin combination for the treatment of advanced well-differentiated pancreatic endocrine carcinoma: a judicious option. Eur J Cancer 40:515–520
27. Turner NC, Strauss SJ, Sarker D et al (2010) Chemotherapy with 5-fluorouracil, cisplatin and streptozocin for neuroendocrine tumors. Br J Cancer 102:1106–1112
28. Kouvaraki MA, Ajani JA, Hoff P et al (2004) Fluorouracil, doxorubicin, and streptozotocin in the treatment of patients with locally advanced and metastatic pancreatic endocrine carcinomas. J Clin Oncol 22:4762–4771
29. Eriksson B, Öberg K (1993) An update of the medical treatment of malignant endocrine pancreatic tumors. Acta Oncol 32:203–208
30. Eriksson B, Annibale B, Bajetta E et al (2009) ENETS consensus guidelines for the standards for care in neuroendocrine tumors: chemotherapy for neuroendocrine tumors. Neuroendocrinlogy 90:214–219
31. Kulke MH, Stuart K, Enzinger K et al (2006) Phase II study of temozolomide and thalidomide in patients with metastatic neuroendocrine tumors. J Clin Oncol 24:401–406
32. Chan JA, Stuart K, Earle CC et al (2012) Prospective study of bevacizumab plus temozolomide in patients with advanced neuroendocrine tumors. J Clin Oncol 30:2963–2968
33. Chan JA, Blaskowsky L, Stuart K et al (2013) A prospective, phase I/II study of everolimus and temozolomide in patients with advanced pancreatic neuroendocirne tumors. Cancer 119:3212–3219
34. Yao JC, Shah MH, Bohas CL et al (2011) Everolimus for advanced pancreatic neuroendocrine tumors. N Engl J Med 364:514–523
35. Isacoff WH, Moss RA, Pecora AL et al (2006) Temozolomide/capecitabine therapy for metastatic neuroendocrine tumors of the pancreas ASCO Meeting Proceedings. J Clin Oncol 24:I4023
36. Strosberg JR, Fine RL, Choi J et al (2011) First-line chemotherapy with capecitabine and temozolomide in patients with metastatic pancreatic endocrine carcinomas. Cancer 117:268–275
37. Kunz PL, Catalano PJ, Nimeiri HS, Fisher GA, Longacre TA, Suarez CJ et al (2018) A randomized study of temozolomide or temozolomide and capecitabine in patients with advanced pan-

creatic neuroendocrine tumors: a trial of the ECOG-ACRIN cancer research group. (E2211) [abstract]. J Clin Oncol 33(15S):4004
38. Thakral P, Sen I, Pant V, Gupta SK, Dureja S, Kumari J et al (2018) Dosimetric analysis of patients with gastro entero pancreatic neuroendocrine tumors (NETs) treated with PRCRT (peptide receptor chemo radionuclide therapy) using Lu-177 DOTATATE and capecitabine/temozolomide (CAP/TEM). Br J Radiol 91(1091):20170172
39. Kesavan M, Claringbold PG, Turner JH (2014) Hematological toxicity of combined 177Lu-octreotate radiopeptide chemotherapy of gastroenteropancreatic neuroendocrine tumors in long-term follow-up. Neuroendocrinology 99(2):108–117
40. Claringbold PG, Turner JH (2016) Pancreatic neuroendocrine tumor control: durable response to combination ^{177}Lu-octreotate-capecitabine-temozolomide radiopeptide chemotherapy. Neuroendocrinology 103(5):432–439
41. Bajetta E, Catena L, Procopiv G et al (2007) Are capecitabine and oxilaplatin (XELOX) suitable treatments for progressing and high-grade neuroendocrine tumors? Cancer Chemother Pharmacol 59:637–642
42. Dussol AS, Joly MO, Vercherat C, Forestier J, Hervieu V, Scoazec JY et al (2015) Gemcitabine and oxaliplatin or alkylating agents for neuroendo-$_{60.}$ Crine tumours: comparison of efficacy and search for predictive factors guiding treatment choice. Cancer 121:3428–3434
43. Guigay J, Ruffié P, Leboulleux S et al (2007) Response of atypical carcinoids to chemotherapy. J Thoracic Oncol 2(8):5599
44. Dahan L, Bonnetain F, Rougier P, Raoul JL, Gamelin E, Etienne PL et al (2009) Phase III trial of chemotherapy using 5-fluorouracil and streptozotocin compared with interferon alpha for advanced carcinoid tumors: FNCLCC-FFCD 9710. Endocr Relat Cancer 16(4):1351–1361
45. O'Toole D, Couvelard A, Rebours V et al (2010) Molecular markers associated with response to chemotherapy in gastro-entero-pancreatic neuroendocrine tumors. Endocr Relat Cancer 17:847–856
46. de Mestier L, Walter T, Brixi H, Evrard C, Legoux JL, de Boissieu P et al (2019) Comparison of temozolomide—capecitabine to 5-fluorouracile-dacarbazine in 247 patients with advanced digestive neuroendocrine tumors using propensity score analyses. Neuroendocrinology 108(4):343–353
47. Pavel M, Baudin E, Couvelard A et al (2012) ENETS consensus guidelines for the management of patients with liver metastases from neuroendocrine neoplasms of foregut, midgut, hindgut and unknown primary. Neuroendocrinology 95:157–176
48. Liu I, Gerson SL (2006) Targeted modulation of MGMT: clinical implications. Clin Cancer Res 12:328–331
49. Gerson SL (2002) Clinical relevance of MGMT in the treatment of cancer. J Clin Oncol 20:2388–2399
50. Hegi ME, Diserens AC, Godard S et al (2004) Clinical trials substantiates the predictive value of O-6-methylguanine-DNA methyltransferase promoter methylation in glioblastoma patients treated with temozolomide. Clin Cancer Res 10:1871–1874
51. Hegi ME, Diserens AC, Gorlia T et al (2005) MGMT gene silencing and benefit from temozolomide in glioblastoma. N Engl J Med 352:997–1003
52. Kulke MH, Hornick JL, Frauenhoffer C et al (2009) O^6-methylguanine DNA methyltransferase deficiency and response to temozolomide-based therapy in patients with neuroendocrine tumors. Clin Cancer Res 15:338–345
53. Raymond E, Dahan L, Raoul JL et al (2011) Sunitinib malate for the treatment of pancreatic neuroendocrine tumors. N Engl J Med 364:501–513
54. Pavel M, Hainsworth J, Baudin E et al (2011) Everolimus plus octreotide long-acting repeatable for the treatment of advanced neuroendocrine tumors associated with carcinoid syndrome (RADIANT-2): a randomized, placebo-controlled phase 3 study. Lancet 378:2005–2012
55. Frilling A, Åkerstrom FM et al (2012) Neuroendocrine tumor disease. An evolving landscape. Endocr Rel Cancer 19:R163–R185

Targeted Therapies

32

Marianne Pavel, Suayib Yalcin, and Şahin Laçin

32.1 Introduction

Neuroendocrine neoplasms (NENs) represent a heteregenous group of tumors that need individualized approach according to their clinicopathological and as well as molecular and genetic characteristics [1, 2]. Although the vast majority of NEN (~90%) are well to moderately diferentiated neuroendocrine tumors (NET G1/G2) and display slow tumor growth, NENs vary widely in terms of secretuary, functionality, proliferative activity, and growth behavior. Except NEN with pancreatic primary tumor site, grade 3 neuroendocrine tumors (NETs), and poorly differentiated neuroendocrine carcinoma (NEC), gastrointestinal and lung NETs are rather resistant to systemic chemotherapy. Their special features, such as a high degree of vascularity and expression of somatostatin receptors as well as involvement of different signaling pathways in neuroendocrine tumor cell proliferation and angiogenesis, make these tumors potentially sensitive to relevant targeted drugs. However, molecular studies in NET so far indicate that somatic mutations are rare, especially in small intestinal NET [3–5]. However, pancreatic NETs contain a larger-than-expected proportion of germline mutations, such as mutations in the DNA repair genes *MUTYH*, *CHEK2*, and *BRCA2*. Together with mutations in *MEN1* and *VHL*, the rate of mutations reaches up to 17% of patients with pancreatic NETS. Somatic mutations that including point mutations and gene fusions were commonly found in genes involved in four main pathways such as chromatin remodeling, DNA damage repair, activation of mammalian target of rapamycin (mTOR) signaling, and telomere

M. Pavel
Erlangen University Germany, Erlangen, Germany
e-mail: marianne.pavel@uk-erlangen.de

S. Yalcin (✉)
Department of Medical Oncology, Hacettepe University Cancer Institute, Ankara, Turkey

Ş. Laçin
Department of Medical Oncology, Faculty of Medicine, Koç University, Istanbul, Turkey

S. Yalcin, K. Öberg (eds.), *Neuroendocrine Tumours*,
https://doi.org/10.1007/978-3-031-56968-5_32

maintenance. Mutations in the mTOR pathway have been identified in 15% of patients with pancreatic NET and ~ 2% of intestinal NET. Although mutations in mTOR pathway genes such as *TSC2*, *PTEN*, *PIK3CA*, and *MEN1* and chromatin remodeling genes such as DAXX and ATRX genes are frequently found in pancreatic NET, the therapeutic significance of these alterations is unclear, genotype–phenotype correlations are still lacking, and currently they seem not to be druggable targets. Therefore, targeted therapies are mostly related to inhibiton of known signaling transduction pathways involved in proliferation of tumor cells, angiogenesis, cell survival, and immune checkpoints [6]. NET expresses a variety of peptide receptors including somatostatin receptors (sstr) and interferon (IFN) receptors. Inhibition of sstr's and IFN signaling by somatostatin analogs (SSAs) and interferon-alpha is an established approach to control secretion and growth of NET. Introduced in the mid 1980s, both drug classes can be considered as the oldest targeted drugs in the management of NET (see Chapter Kos-Kudla, Welin, and Strosberg).

Several growth-promoting targets are expressed in neuroendocrine tumor cells [7, 8]. These comprise not only growth factor receptors but also their ligands or other moleculesincluding vascular endothelial growth factor (VEGF), platelet-derived growth factor-α (PDGFR-α), platelet-derived growth factor-ß (PDGFR-ß), insulin-like growth factor 1 (IGF-1), transforming growth factor-α (TGF-α) and TGF-ß, and their cognate receptors [9]. VEGF-driven angiogenesis may play an important role in neuroendocrine tumorigenesis and tumor progession [10]. High vascularity is however rather a feature of well differentiated than poorly differentiated NET. The epidermal growth factor (EGF) receptor (EGFR) is frequently expressed in NET and binding of EGF or TGF-α induces RAF/MAP-ERK signaling in tumor cells; however, mutations of the EGFR tyrosine kinase which are predictive of a response to EGFR tyrosin kinase inhibitors in other types of cancers are rather uncommon in NET [11]. Activation of the IGF-1R by IGF-1 and -2 plays an important role in tumor cell proliferation, and in neuroendocrine tumor cell lines it has been demonstrated that IGF-1 stimulates tumor cell growth by an autocrine loop. IGF-1 also plays a role in the upstream activation of the mammalian target of rapamycin (mTOR) pathway [12, 13].

The protein kinase mTOR exerts a central control function integrating multiple signaling pathways in response to growth factors and intracellular signaling by nutrients. mTOR is involved in the regulation of growth-related cellular functions, and the best-known function is the regulation of translation initiation [14]. Inhibiting the mTOR pathway may reduce cell growth and proliferation and impair the metastatic potential of tumor cells. It also acts at the endothelial cells [15]. In NET, constitutively activated PI3K-Akt-mTOR signaling seems to be a crucial event with 75% of NET expressing activated Akt and 45% mTOR [16]. Loss or downregulation of the expression of PTEN or TSC2 has been reported recently in a high percentage of pancreatic NET and may lead to loss of inhibition of mTOR to overactivation of this pathway [17].

In neuroendocrine tumors, mTOR and angiogenesis inhibitors have been most extensively studied. Recently, immune checkpoint inhibitors (ICIs) are also being tested in patients with NEN. The following sections focus on the results from clinical trials with targeted agents.

32.2 Targeted Therapies in Pancreatic NET

32.2.1 Inhibitors of the Mammalian Target of Rapamycin (mTOR) Pathway

Temsirolimus and everolimus are inhibitors of mTOR structurally related to rapamycin. Temsirolimus was the first mTOR inhibitor used in NET patients in a phase II study in advanced progressive NET. The objective response rate was less than 6% and the median TTP 6 months [18]. However, a significant percentage of patients experienced disease stabilization (~60%) with temsirolimus and the 1-year progression-free rate of 40% suggests drug activity beyond the natural course of the disease.

In a phase II trial, everolimus in combination with the long-acting somatostatin analog (SSA) octreotide long-acting release (LAR) (30 mg q 28 days) led to a tumor response rate of 22% (with a more favorable response rate in pancreatic NET compared to NET of other origins, 27% vs. 17%, respectively). In the majority of the patients (70%), stable disease was the best response in pts. treated with everolimus [19]. The higher remission rate in pancreatic NET might be explained by the pathophysiological findings related to the mTOR pathway [17].

Antitumor activity has been confirmed with everolimus in patients with progressive metastatic pancreatic NET after the failure of cytotoxic chemotherapy in the phase II RADIANT-1 trial. One hundred and sixty patients were included in two strata. The partial remission rate was low with 9.6 and 4.4%, respectively. The rate of disease stabilizations was, however, high with 67.8% and 80%, respectively. The corresponding figures for progression-free survival (PFS) were 9.7 and 16.7 months [20]. Although data of this study are in favor of combination therapy of everolimus with octreotide, it remains an open issue if combination therapy of everolimus and somatostatin analogs is indeed superior to everolimus alone to inhibit tumor growth.

The benefit of everolimus in advanced pancreatic neuroendocrine tumors (pNET) was confirmed in a randomized placebo-controlled phase III trial (RADIANT-3) recruiting 410 patients. PFS was 11 months with everolimus, and 5.4 months with placebo [21]. Tumor remissions occurred in 5% of the patients. Based on these data, everolimus was approved for progressive pNET patients. A survival benefit could not be demonstrated with everolimus compared to placebo; however, there was a high crossover rate from placebo to open-label drug upon progression. Treatment is a continuous oral intake of everolimus 10 mg per day. Treatment is stopped if the progressive disease or intolerable toxicity occurs. Most frequently reported adverse events include stomatitis (62%) and rash (37%). Patients have to be followed carefully for infections (20%) and pulmonary events (12%), such as pneumonitis [21].

To improve objective response rates and overcome acquired resistance to the drug, multiple combination therapies of everolimus with somatostatin analogs or angiogenesis inhibitors and dual inhibitors targeting upstream and downstream signaling of the mTOR pathway are currently under investigation. Since other treatments are available (somatostatin analogs, chemotherapy with either temozolomide or streptozotocin plus 5-fluorouracil, and angiogenesis inhibitors), it has still to be defined which patients will benefit most from targeted therapy with everolimus and in which sequence everolimus should be used.

32.2.2 Inhibitors of VEGF Receptor Signaling

32.2.2.1 Monoclonal Antibodies

The antiangiogenic strategies currently used in clinical practice in NET are specific monoclonal antibodies against VEGF (anti-VEGF A), such as bevacizumab, ramucirumab, and tyrosine kinase inhibitors (TKIs) targeting receptors for VEGF or PDGF expressed by tumor vessels. Antiangiogenic drugs have also been and also being evaluated in combination with somatostatin analogs (SSAs), everolimus, systemic chemotherapy, and tyrosine kinase inhibitors. SSAs and everolimus also display antiangiogenic properties that include inhibition of endothelial cell proliferation and inhibition of secretion of angiogenic factors such as VEGF synthesized by tumor cells or microenvironment among other mechanisms [10, 22]. Bevacizumab is a humanized monoclonal antibody that binds to circulating VEGF-A and has been explored in the management of NETs.

Results of larger and comparative studies (e.g. bevacizumab plus everolimus vs. everolimus) are still lacking [23]. In small studies, promising results were achieved with the combination of bevacizumab with either temozolomide or metronomic capecitabine plus octreotide [24, 25]. However, some combination therapies such as sorafenib and bevacizumab seem too toxic [26]. In a multicenter, phase II clinical trial, patients with histologically confirmed measurable advanced NETs were treated with sorafenib 200 mg bid (days 1–5 of each week) and bevacizumab 5 mg/kg once every 2 weeks (day 1, week 1). A total of 44 patients were included(70.5% carcinoid tumors and 29.5% pancreatic tumor). Baseline target lesions mainly in the liver (86.4%). Global progression free survival rate (PFSR) was 90.9% (91.7% carcinoid tumors and 88.9% pancreatic tumors). Median PFS was 12.4 months, median TTP was 14.5 months, objective response rate (ORR) was 9.4%, and DCR was 95.1%. Most common grade 3–4 toxicities were asthenia (11.4%) and hand-foot skin reaction (15.9%). Sorafenib and bevacizumab combination showed some clinical benefit but unfavorable safety results compared with drugs in monotherapy. Since bevacizumab has relatively favorable tolerability and can be combined with other targeted agents and chemotherapy, it may be expected to be further tested as a part of combination therapies in the future in order to increase objective response rates, PFS, and overall survival in pNET or GI NET (Table 32.1).

32.2.2.2 Tyrosine Kinase Receptor Inhibitors

Currently, a plethora of small-molecule tyrosine kinase inhibitors (TKIs) has been evaluated in NET, including sunitinib, surufatinib, pazopanib, cabozantinib, lenvatinib, axitinib, and sorafenib, all of which have activity against diverse VEGF receptors and PDGF receptors. Some have additional activity against c-kit, rearranged during transfection (RET), or fibroblast growth factor receptor (FGFR) (Table 32.2), thus blocking multiple targets involved in growth, proliferation, and metastatic spread of tumor cells [27–30].

Table 32.1 Molecular targeted drugs in pancreatic NET

Author	Drugs	Targets	Study phase	Patients (*n*)	Objective response (%)	PFS/ TTP (months)
Duran et al. (2006) [18]	Temsirolimus	mTOR	II	15	10.6	6.7
Yao et al. 2008 [19]	Everolimus + octreotide	mTOR	II	30	27	12.5
Yao et al. 2010 [20]	Everolimus Everolimus+ octreotide (RADIANT-1)	mTOR SSTR-2/ SSTR-5	II	115 45	9.6 4.4	9.7 16.7
Yao et al. 2011 [21]	Everolimus vs. placebo (RADIANT-3)	mTOR/-	III	207 203	5.0 2.0	11.04 4.6
[a]	Everolimus Vs. Everolimus + bevacizumab	mTOR VEGF	II	138	Results pending	
[a]	Everolimus vs. Everolimus + Pasireotide (COOPERATE-2)	mTOR SSTR-1,2,3,5	II	160	Results pending	
Kulke et al. 2008 [29]	Sunitinib	VEGFR-1,-2; PDGF-R, kit	II	66	17	7.7
Raymond et al. 2011 [31]	Sunitinib vs. placebo	VEGFR-1,-2; PDGF-R, kit	III	86 85	9.3 0	11.4 5.5
Hobday et al. 2007 [28]	Sorafenib	C-RAF, B-RAF, VEGFR-2, VEGFR-3, PDGFR-β; kit	II	41	10	–
Ahn et al. 2013 [30]	Pazopanib	VEGFR-1, −2, 3, PDGF-α, PDGF-β, c-kit	II	12	18.9[b]	15.5
Chan et al. 2012 [25]	Bevacizumab + Temozolomide	VEGF MGMT	II	15	33	14.3
Castellano et al. 2013 [26]	Bevacizumab + Sorafenib	VEGF C-RAF, B-RAF, VEGFR-2, VEGFR-3, PDGFR-β; kit	II	13		
Berruti et al. 2014 [24]	Bevacizumab + octreotide + Metronomic Capecitabine	VEGF C-RAF, B-RAF, VEGFR-2, VEGFR-3, PDGFR-β; kit; antimetabolite	II	19	26.3	14.3

[a]www.clinicaltrials.gov
[b]Other types of NET

Table 32.2 Molecular targeted drugs in non-pancreatic NET ("Carcinoids")

Author	Drugs	Targets	Study phase	Patients (*n*)	Tumor site	Objective response (%)	Median PFS/TTP (months)
Duran et al. 2006 [18]	Temsirolimus	mTOR	II	21	Carcinoids	4.8	6.0
Yao et al. 2008 [19]	Everolimus + octreotide	mTOR SSTR-1,2	II	30	GI Carcinoids	17	15.8
Pavel et al. 2011 [9]	Everolimus + octreotide vs. placebo + octreotide	mTOR SSTR-1,-2	II	429	GI Lung Others	2.3 1.9	16.4 (12.0) 11.3 (8.6)
[a]	Everolimus vs. placebo (RADIANT-4)	mTOR	III	279	GI Lung CUP	Results pending	
[a]	Bevacizumab + octreotide vs. interferon-α + octreotide	VEGF SSTR-1,-2; IFN-R SSTR-1,-2	III	400	Advanced NET	Results pending	
Kulke et al. 2008 [29]	Sunitinib	VEGFR, PDGFR	II	41	Carcinoids	2.4	10.2
Yao et al. 2008 [59]	Bevacizumab+octreotide	VEGF SSTR-2,-5	II	22	Carcinoids	18	–
Berruti et al. 2014 [24]	Bevacizumab+octreotide + metronomic Capecitabine	VEGF SSTR-2,-5	II	26	Intestinal NET; CUP	11.5	14.3
Reidy et al. 2012 [35]	MK 0646	IGF-1R	II	15	Carcinoids	0	2.7

[a]www.clinicaltrials.gov; *CUP* carcinoma of unknown primary

Sunitinib is the first TKI that has been evaluated in a placebo-controlled phase III study based on promising results in a phase II trial including 66 patients with pNET. The objective response rate was 17% in the latter study, and 68% had stable disease [29]. In the phase III study, progressive disease was required before enrollment and the objective response rate was <10%. The primary endpoint, median PFS, was 11.4 months with sunitinib compared to 5.5 months with placebo. Most frequently reported adverse events include diarrhea (59%), nausea (45%), and asthenia (34%). Patients need to be followed carefully for hypertension (27%) and leukopenia (29%) [31]. Based on these results, sunitinib was approved for the treatment of pancreatic NET. In an updated survival analysis, no survival benefit could be demonstrated; however, most patients crossed over from placebo to open-label drug upon progression, a finding that may have biased these results.

Surufatinib (HMPL-012), which was previously named sulfatinib, is a small-molecule kinase inhibitor targeting VEGFRs, FGFR 1, and colony-stimulating factor 1 receptor (CSF-1), which demonstrated encouraging efficacy in previous phase Ib/II study in patients with advanced NETs regardless of tumor origin. Surufatinib has demonstrated superior efficacy in extra-pancreatic neuroendocrine tumors (NETs) in a prior phase III study [32, 33]. In a phase 3 trial, surufatinib was tested in the treatment of patients with pathological grade 1 or 2, locally advanced, or metastatic well-differentiated pancreatic NETs. Inclusion criteria also included documented radiological disease progression within the past 1 year and progression on two or fewer kinds of prior systemic therapies for advanced disease without progression on prior VEGF/VEGFR inhibitors. Functional NETs that required treatment with long-acting SSAs were excluded. The study evaluated the efficacy and safety of patients with well-differentiated pathological grade 1 or 2, progressive, unresectable, or metastatic pNETs. Patients were randomized in a 2:1 ratio to receive surufatinib or placebo, 300 mg, orally, once daily, until disease progression or intolerable adverse events. Crossover at disease progression was allowed. The primary endpoint was investigator-assessed progression-free survival (PFS). A total of 172 patients were randomized, 113 patients to surufatinib, and 59 to placebo. The study met the primary endpoint; investigator-assessed median PFS was 10.9 versus 3.7 months in surufatinib and placebo arms, respectively, with a hazard ratio (HR) = 0.491; 95% $p = 0.0011$. Analysis by a blinded independent radiology committee confirmed PFS improvement (13.9 vs. 4.6 months; HR = 0.339; 95% CI: 0.209–0.549; $p < 0.0001$). The investigator-assessed objective response rate was 19.2% with surufatinib and 1.9% with placebo ($p = 0.0021$). Most common (≥5% in either arm) grade ≥ 3 treatment-emergent adverse events (TEAEs) were hypertension (38.9% in S arm vs. 8.5% in P arm), proteinuria (9.7% vs. 1.7%), hypertriglyceridaemia (7.1% vs. 0), and alanine aminotransferase increased and gamma-glutamyltransferase increased (both 2.7% vs. 5.1%). TEAEs leading to drug discontinuation occurred in 10.6% pts. versus 6.8% pts. in S and P arms, respectively. In conclusion, surufatinib significantly improved the PFS in Pts with progressive, well-differentiated advanced pNETs. The safety profile was manageable and consistent with observations in prior studies. Surufatinib represents a promising treatment option in the armamentarium against pNETs.

32.3 Targeted Therapies in Non-pancreatic NET (Carcinoids)

32.3.1 Inhibitors of the Mammalian Target of Rapamycin (mTOR) Pathway

Following promising results from a phase II study, combined therapy of everolimus plus the somatostatin analog octreotide LAR was evaluated in a large placebo-controlled phase III trial (RADIANT-2) enrolling 429 patients with progressive NETs from various disease sites with a history of carcinoid syndrome [9, 19]. Due to heterogeneity of tumor types (most frequent tumor site was intestine, followed by lung) included in this trial, but also differences in local and central reading of radiographs, the results of the study are less clear. Median PFS by central reading (primary endpoint) was 16.4 months with everolimus plus octreotide, and 11.3 months with placebo plus octreotide, but did not reach prespecified statistical significance, probably due to imbalanced informative censoring that occurred following earlier assessment of tumor progression by local reading compared to central reading of radiographs and imbalances in baseline characteristics of the study population. However, despite discrepancies in local and central reading, the risk reduction (hazard ratio) was similar for both assessments [9]. The study provides evidence that subgroups of patients with functioning progressive non-pancreatic NET may have the benefit of everolimus. The activity of everolimus as monotherapy was further evaluated in intestinal and lung NET within a placebo-controlled phase III trial (RADIANT-4). In this randomized, double-blind, placebo-controlled, phase 3 RADIANT-4 trial, adult patients (aged ≥18 years) with advanced, progressive, well-differentiated, nonfunctional neuroendocrine tumors of the lung or gastrointestinal origin were enrolled from 97 centers in 25 countries worldwide. Eligible patients were randomly assigned in a 2:1 ratio by an interactive voice response system to receive everolimus 10 mg per day orally or identical placebo, both with supportive care. Patients were stratified by tumor origin, performance status, and previous somatostatin analog treatment. Patients, investigators, and the study sponsor were masked to treatment assignment. The primary endpoint was progression-free survival assessed by central radiology review, analyzed by intention to treat. Overall survival was a key secondary endpoint. A total of 302 patients were enrolled, of whom 205 were allocated to everolimus 10 mg per day and 97 to placebo. Median progression-free survival was 11.0 months (95% CI 9.2–13.3) in the everolimus group and 3.9 months (3.6–7.4) in the placebo group. Everolimus was associated with a 52% reduction in the estimated risk of progression or death (hazard ratio [HR] 0.48 [95% CI 0.35–0.67], $p < 0.00001$). Although not statistically significant, the results of the first preplanned interim overall survival analysis indicated that everolimus might be associated with a reduction in the risk of death (HR 0.64 [95% CI 0.40–1.05], one-sided $p = 0.037$, whereas the boundary for statistical significance was 0.0002). Grade 3 or 4 drug-related adverse events were infrequent and included stomatitis (in 18 [9%] of 202 patients in the everolimus group vs. 0 of 98 in the placebo group), diarrhea (15 [7%] vs. 2 [2%]), infections (14 [7%] vs. 0), anemia (8 [4%] vs. 1 [1%]), fatigue (7 [3%] vs. 1 [1%]), and hyperglycaemia (7 [3%]

Table 32.3 Comparison of frequent side effects (>20%) of sunitinib and everolimus

Sunitinib		Everolimus	
Adverse event	Frequency	Adverse event	Frequency
Diarrhea	59%	Stomatitis	64%
Nausea	45%	Exanthema	49%
Asthenia	34%	Diarrhea	34%
Emesis	34%	Fatigue	31%
Fatigue	33%	Infections	23%
Gray hair	29%	Nausea	20%
Leukopenia	29%	Edema	20%
Hypertension	27%	Pneumonitis and lung infiltrates	17%

Data from Ref. Yao et al. NEJM 2011 [21], Raymond et al. NEJM 2011 [31]

vs. 0). The safety findings were consistent with the known side-effect profile of everolimus. Everolimus is the first targeted agent to show robust antitumor activity with acceptable tolerability across a broad range of neuroendocrine tumors, including those arising from the pancreas, lung, and gastrointestinal tract (Table 32.3).

32.3.2 Inhibitors of VEGF Receptor Signaling

All studies evaluating anti-VEGF therapies for GI NET are small in size and most deal with mixed patient populations, including pancreatic NET and carcinoids. In a phase 2 study with the multiple tyrosine kinase inhibitor sunitinib, the objective response rate was low (2%) in the subgroup of carcinoids. Its activity against carcinoid tumors could not be definitively determined in this nonrandomized study [29]. Sunitinib is currently evaluated in combination with lanreotide versus single-agent lanreotide in progressive advanced or metastatic midgut carcinoid tumors in a randomized phase II Sunland trial (SUNLAND study; www.clinical trials.gov). The combination therapy of bevacizumab and octreotide was assessed over a limited study period of 18 weeks in carcinoids. The objective response rate was 18% with this combination and superior to a combination therapy of octreotide and pegylated interferon-alpha [19]. The results of a large US trial including 400 patients with carcinoids to further explore the combination of bevacizumab plus octreotide versus interferon-alpha plus octreotide are still pending. Until the results of comparative trials reported, add-on value of bevacizumab therapy in types of non-pancreatic NET remains unclear.

Simultaneous targeting of angiogenesis through VEGFRs/FGFR1 and modulating tumor immune microenvironment through CSF-1R may be a uniquely potent strategy to enhance antitumor activity in gastrointestinal NETS. Encouraging efficacy of surufatinib treating patients with advanced pancreatic NETs was reported (ORR 19%). Surufatinib demonstrated significant improvement in PFS in patients with NETs originating outside the pancreas in the pivotal phase III SANET-extrapancreatic (ep) study SANET-ep was a randomized, double-blind, placebo-controlled, phase 3 trial done in China. Adult patients with unresectable or metastatic, well-differentiated, extrapancreatic NETs, with an Eastern Cooperative Oncology Group performance status of 0 or 1, and progression on no more than two types of previous systemic regimens were enrolled. Patients were randomized as a 2:1 manner to receive oral surufatinib at 300 mg per day or matching placebo. Randomisation was stratified by tumor origin, pathological grade, and previous treatment. Crossover to the surufatinib group was allowed for patients in the placebo group at disease progression. The primary endpoint was investigator-assessed PFS, which was analyzed in the intention-to-treat population. Between December 9, 2015, and March 31, 2019, 198 patients were randomly assigned to surufatinib (n = 129) or placebo (n = 69). Median follow-up was 13.8 months (95% CI 11.1–16.7) in the surufatinib group and 16.6 months (9.2-not calculable) in the placebo group. Investigator-assessed median progression-free survival was 9.2 months (95% CI 7.4–11.1) in the surufatinib group versus 3.8 months (3.7–5.7) in the placebo group (hazard ratio 0.33; 95% CI 0.22–0.50; $p < 0.0001$). As the trial met the predefined criteria for early discontinuation of the study at the interim analysis, the study was terminated early, as recommended by the independent data monitoring committee. The most common treatment-related adverse events of grade 3 or worse were hypertension (47 [36%] of 129 patients in the surufatinib group vs. nine [13%] of 68 patients in the placebo group) and proteinuria (25 [19%] vs. zero). Treatment-related serious adverse events were reported in 32 (25%) of 129 patients in the surufatinib group and nine (13%) of 68 patients in the placebo group. Treatment-related deaths occurred in three patients in the surufatinib group (disseminated intravascular coagulation and hepatic encephalopathy, liver injury, and death with unknown reason) and one patient in the placebo group (cachexia and respiratory failure). Surufatinib has a favorable benefit-to-risk profile in patients with progressive, advanced, well-differentiated extrapancreatic NETs. These results suggest that surufatinib might be a new treatment option for this population [32, 33].

32.4 New Drugs in Horizon

Other drugs targeting growth factor receptors or ligands that bind to growth factor receptors have been performed in NET [34]. There is one published negative study on the use of the insulin-like growth factor-1 (IGF-1) receptor inhibitor, a human monoclonal antibody that binds to the IGF-1R (MK-0646) in patients with metastatic well-differentiated NET [35] who had very advanced disease. While the drug was inactive as a single agent in well-differentiated NETs, the outcome of combined use of other IGF 1-receptor inhibitors and octreotide, or IGF 1-receptor inhibitors with octreotide and everolimus, are not reported yet.

32.4.1 Lenvatinib

Lenvatinib is an oral TKI that is directed against VEGFR 1–3, FGFR 1–4, PDGFR α, and RET. It has been approved for the treatment of radioiodine-refractory differentiated thyroid cancer and hepatocellular cancer. The TALENT trial was a prospective multicohort phase II study of lenvatinib in patients with well-differentiated, advanced digestive NETs; it recruited 111 patients (55 with panNETs and 56 with gastroenteropancreatic neuroendocrine tumors (GEP-NET)). Thirty percent of patients had received sunitinib previously. The ORR was 29% (42.3% for panNETs and 16.3% for GEP-NETs). With a median follow-up duration of 19 months, the PFS and OS durations were 15.5 months (95% CI = 11.3 months-not reached) and 29.2 months (95% CI = 23.2 months-not reached) for panNETs and 15.4 months (95% CI = 11.5–19.4 months) and not reached for GEP-NETs, respectively. The most frequent grade 3 or higher adverse events were hypertension (22%), fatigue (11%), and diarrhea (11%). Dose reductions and interruptions were required in 91.8%, with a median dose of 20 mg daily [36].

32.4.2 Nintedanib

Nintedanib is an oral TKI that targets VEGFR, PDGFR, and FGFR [37]. It has been approved for the treatment of advanced nonsmall-cell lung cancer and idiopathic pulmonary fibrosis. In preclinical mouse models of NETs, prolonged exposure to nintedanib led to strong suppression of angiogenesis, accompanied by a reduced tumor burden, which translated to significant prolongation of survival [38]. A phase II study of nintedanib in advanced non-pancreatic and lung NETs enrolled 30 patients [39]. The median PFS and OS durations were 11 and 27.6 months, respectively, but the ORR was only 4% (1 of 30), with stable disease in 83% (20 of 30). The incidence of grade 3 toxicities was 27% (hypertension and decreased appetite). In addition, the results of recent studies suggest that high-grade diarrhea and dose-dependent elevated transaminases are possible side effects of therapy [40].

32.4.3 Axitinib

Axitinib is a selective inhibitor of VEGFR-1, −2, and − 3 that is currently indicated in the management of renal cell carcinoma [41]. Axitinib induces growth inhibition in pancreatic endocrine cell lines and causes a reduction in tumor vasculature, with widespread hypoxia and significant mTOR pathway activation, leading to resistance (reference). A phase II trial of 5 mg of axitinib twice daily in patients with progressive advanced low-to-intermediate grade carcinoid tumors enrolled 30 patients [42]. In this study, a median PFS duration of 26.7 months (95% CI = 11.4–35.1 months), with a 12-month PFS rate of 74.5% (± 10.2) were reported. The median OS duration was 45.3 months (95% CI = 24.4–45.3 months). The ORR was however low, with a partial response in 1 of 30 patients (3%) and stable disease in 21 (70%). Hypertension was the most common toxicity observed in 27 patients [90%]), with grade 3 or 4 hypertension reported in 19 patients (63%). Six (20%) patients discontinued treatment because of hypertension. The authors concluded that axitinib has an inhibitory effect on tumor growth in patients with advanced, progressive carcinoid tumors, but the high rate of grade 3 or 4 hypertension may represent an impediment to its use in unselected patients. The AXINET trial is a phase II/III study of Octreotide LAR with axitinib or placebo in patients with extrapanNETs (n = 255) without prior exposure to anti-VEGF therapies. The primary endpoint is PFS and the trial has completed accrual, and the results are awaited (NCT01744249).

32.4.4 Cabozantinib

Cabozantinib is a TKI that is known to influence tumor growth, metastasis, and angiogenesis through inhibition of multiple tyrosine kinases, including MET, VEGFR-2, AXL, and RET [43]. The clinical activity of cabozantinib in patients with NETs was evaluated in a phase II study that included patients with advanced panNETs and carcinoid tumors, many of whom had experienced tumor progression on prior therapy [44]. Radiographic responses were observed in 3 of 20 (15%) patients with panNETs and 6 of 41 (15%) patients with carcinoid tumors. The PFS was 21.8 months in patients with panNETs and 31.4 months in patients with carcinoid tumors. Treatment-related adverse events that were associated with cabozantinib in NET patients were similar to those that had been reported in other diseases. Grade 3 and 4 toxicities included hypertension (13%), hypophosphatemia (11%), diarrhea (10%), lymphopenia (7%), thrombocytopenia (5%), fatigue (5%), and increased lipase or amylase (8%). Unexpected toxicities included heart failure and autoimmune hemolytic anemia, each in one patient. Based on these encouraging results, the Alliance cooperative group (A021602) is evaluating the efficacy of cabozantinib compared with placebo in patients with advanced NETs in the ongoing randomized phase III CABINET trial (NCT03375320).

32.4.5 Pazopanib

Pazopanib exerts antitumor and antiangiogenic effects by targeting VEGFR-1, − 2, and − 3, PDGFR α and β, FGFGR-1, −2, and − 3, and c-Kit [45]. It was approved by the FDA as a treatment for metastatic renal cell carcinoma and advanced soft tissue sarcoma. Data from clinical trials suggest that pazopanib has antitumor activity in advanced NENs. A multicenter, single-arm, phase II study evaluated patients with advanced, well-differentiated pancreatic or extra-panNENs who received 800 mg of pazopanib orally once a day plus octreotide LAR [46]. Fifty-two patients were enrolled, with an ORR of 21.9% (7 of 32) in patients with panNETs. The median PFS durations were 14.4 and 12.2 months for panNET and extrapanNET patients, respectively. Treatment was generally well tolerated. The most frequently observed toxic effects were fatigue (75%), nausea (63%), diarrhea (63%), and hypertension (54%). Another phase II study of pazopanib from Spain enrolled 44 patients with advanced NETs (18 pancreatic, 15 gastrointestinal, five pulmonary, and six other or unknown) who had experienced disease progression on prior therapies [47]. The disease control rate at 6 months was 59.5% (four partial responses and 21 stable disease), with a median PFS duration of 9.5 months. Pazopanib had higher activity in patients with panNETs, and its benefit was similar in patients who had been previously treated with TKIs and those who had been treated with mTOR inhibitors (73% and 60%, respectively).

Alliance A021202 was a multicenter, randomized, double-blind, phase II study of pazopanib (800 mg/day) versus placebo in progressive non-pancreatic GEP-NETs [48]. Of 171 accrued patients, most (66%) had small bowel primary tumors, and the majority (87%) were on concurrent somatostatin analogs. The median PFS duration in patients receiving pazopanib ($n = 97$) was 11.6 months compared with 8.5 months in those receiving placebo ($n = 74$; HR = 0.53; $P = 0.0005$). There was no improvement in OS duration; however, crossover at disease progression ($n = 49$) most likely confounded the OS endpoint.

32.4.6 Immune Checkpoint Inhibitors

While recent progress in immunotherapy has revolutionized the treatment of some cancers such as melanoma and lung cancer, its application in the management of GEP-NETs is still evolving. Common avenues for immune-based treatments include tumor-targeted antibodies, oncolytic viruses, cellular-based, cytokines, and checkpoint inhibitors. Interferon (IFN)-α and checkpoint inhibitors are the primary immunotherapy modalities that have been investigated in GEP-NETs thus far. IFN-α2b has been used for many years now in the treatment of low-grade NETs, mostly as a combination therapy. One randomized controlled trial, for example, showed reduced tumor progression among patients with midgut NETs and liver metastases treated with octreotide plus IFN-α2b compared to octreotide alone after debulking and hepatic artery embolization [49]. More recently, a phase III trial by the Southwest Oncology Group (SWOG) found that IFN-α2b results in comparable outcomes to bevacizumab when combined with octreotide [50]. Checkpoint inhibitors utilize antibodies to target the programmed cell death receptor 1 (PD)-1/PD-L1 or cytotoxic T lymphocyte antigen (CTLA)-4 inhibitory axis found on immune cells to lower their threshold for activation and generate a more robust antitumor response. Several PD-1/PD-L1 antibodies are available for clinical use, including pembrolizumab, nivolumab, and avelumab as well as ipilimumab for CTLA4 targets [51]. PDL1 is expressed in some GEP-NETs and has been associated with more advanced tumors as well as intermediate- to high-grade (G2–G3) GEP-NETs [52]. One published phase Ib study to date, KEYNOTE-028, is a basket study that looked at 475 patients with multiple types of tumors treated with pembrolizumab of which 23 were neuroendocrine and found 12% response rate among this subset of patients [53]. Interestingly, their study showed higher response rates in tumors that had high mutational burdens as well as microenvironments that were T-cell-enriched, suggesting potential criteria that will be helpful in predicting eligibility for these treatments [53]. Several other studies are currently underway to investigate the utility of PD-L1 inhibitors in NETs [54]. Checkpoint inhibitors are an exciting avenue that deserve further investigation.

32.4.7 Bevacizumab

Bevacizumab is a monoclonal antibody with anti-VEGF properties, commonly used for the treatment of primary colon, lung, and other cancers. Bevacizumab has been studied in combination with several other regimens, including octreotide long-acting release (LAR) [50], capecitabine [24, 55], 5-FU/ streptozocin [56], 5-FU/ oxaliplatin [23], temozolomide [25], interferon [50], and mTOR inhibitors [57]. Nevertheless, its use has not been widely adopted due to mixed data regarding its benefit as well as serious adverse reactions that have been documented associated with its use [58]. Bevacizumab is not approved currently for the treatment of GEP-NETs as additional phase III efficacy trials are needed to clarify the optimal combination regimen and patient population that would benefit from its use.

32.5 Combination Strategies

Bevacizumab is a monoclonal antibody with anti-VEGF properties, commonly used for the treatment of primary colon, lung, and other cancers. Bevacizumab has been studied in combination with several other regimens, including octreotide long-acting release (LAR) [50], capecitabine [24, 55], 5-FU/ streptozocin [56], 5-FU/ oxaliplatin [23], temozolomide [25], interferon [50], and mTOR inhibitors [57]. Nevertheless, its use has not been widely adopted due to mixed data regarding its benefit as well as serious adverse reactions that have been documented associated with its use [58]. Bevacizumab is not approved currently for the treatment of GEP-NETs as additional phase III efficacy trials are needed to clarify the optimal combination regimen and patient population that would benefit from its use.

Its activity was studied in a randomized phase II trial in which 44 patients with advanced carcinoids were assigned to 18 weeks of bevacizumab or pegylated IFNα-2b [59], followed by combination therapy with bevacizumab plus interferon. The ORR was 18% in the bevacizumab arm, and no responses were noted in the interferon arm; the 18-week PFS rates were 95% versus 68% for the bevacizumab versus the interferon arms. These results led to a large randomized study of octreotide plus bevacizumab versus octreotide plus interferon in 427 patients with progressive, advanced carcinoids [50]. Although the bevacizumab arm had a higher ORR (12% vs. 4%), there was no improvement in the primary endpoint of median PFS (16.6 months in the bevacizumab arm vs. 15.4 months in the interferon arm [HR = 0.93; 95% CI = 0.73–1.18; $P = 0.55$]) [50].

Bevacizumab is a humanized monoclonal antibody that binds to circulating VEGF-A and has been explored in the management of NETs. Its activity was studied in a randomized phase II trial in which 44 patients with advanced carcinoids were assigned to 18 weeks of bevacizumab or pegylated IFNα-2b [59], followed by combination therapy with bevacizumab plus interferon. The ORR was 18% in the bevacizumab arm, and no responses were noted in the interferon arm; the 18-week PFS rates were 95% versus 68% for the bevacizumab versus the interferon arms. These results led to a large randomized study of octreotide plus bevacizumab versus octreotide plus interferon in 427 patients with progressive, advanced carcinoids. Although the bevacizumab arm had a higher ORR (12% vs. 4%), there was no improvement in the primary endpoint of median PFS (16.6 months in the bevacizumab arm vs. 15.4 months in the interferon arm [HR = 0.93; 95% CI = 0.73–1.18; *P* = 0.55]) [50]. These and other studies have shown that interferon is an active drug in patients with NETs. Immune stimulation, angiogenesis inhibition, and the induction of cell cycle arrest are postulated mechanisms for its antisecretory and antiproliferative effects in GEP-NETs. However, its use is limited by its adverse effects: influenza-like symptoms, depression, and myelosuppression [60, 61]. There was initial interest in combination therapies using mTOR inhibitors, somatostatin analogs, and various VEGF-targeted therapies in NETs. However, their limited benefits and/or cumulative side effect profiles as discussed below have halted their further development. The phase II COOPERATE-2 study in which 160 patients with advanced panNETs were randomly assigned to receive everolimus plus pasireotide (a somatostatin analog with greater affinity to the somatostatin receptors 1, 3, and 5) versus everolimus [62]. Despite an improvement in the ORR (20% vs.6%), the combination did not confer a PFS benefit compared to everolimus alone (HR = 0.991; 95% CI = 0.64–1.54), thus limiting its clinical utility. The glycemic complication rates were also significantly higher with the combination (grade 3 or 4 fasting hyperglycemia: 37% vs. 11%; diabetes mellitus: 26% vs. 7%). The LUNA trial was a prospective randomized phase II study with three arms (everolimus vs. pasireotide vs. everolimus plus pasireotide) in 124 patients with advanced, well-differentiated carcinoids of lung and thymus origin [63]. The adverse event profile was in line with the reported toxicities from the individual drugs. However, there was one death in the everolimus group and two deaths in the combination group; both suspected to be related to everolimus treatment. The primary endpoint (disease control rate at 9 weeks) was met in all three arms. No one approach was found to be significantly more Curr. Treat. Options in Oncol. (2020) 21:96 Page 7 of 15 96 effective (39.0% in the long-acting pasireotide arm, 33.3% in the everolimus arm, and 58.5% in the combination arm). CALGB 80701 was a randomized phase II study that compared the combination of everolimus and bevacizumab to everolimus alone in 150 patients with advanced, progressive panNETs [64]. The primary endpoint, PFS, was marginally improved in the combination arm, per the prespecified statistical cutoff of P G 0.15 (16.7 months vs. 14 months; HR = 0.80; *P* = 0.12). The ORR was also improved significantly with the addition of everolimus (31% vs. 12%; *P* = 0.005). However, the toxicities were notable, with 81% of patients on the combination arm reporting grade 3 and 4 adverse events (compared to 49% in the everolimus arm). Grade 3 and 4 hypertension (38% vs. 8%), proteinuria (16% vs. 1%), diarrhea (11% vs. 1%), and hypophosphatemia (10% vs. 1%) were more common in the combination arm. Even though the study met its primary endpoint, the higher type 1 error rate and the significantly higher toxicity rate made it a less promising approach. Along similar lines, the toxicity of combining mTOR inhibitors with VEGF TKIs has hampered their development in clinical trials. A phase I study of sorafenib with everolimus in patients with advanced NETs resulted in a significant toxicity burden (thrombocytopenia, hand-foot skin reaction, and rash or allergic reaction), which precluded its further development [65]. Similarly, the combination of sorafenib and bevacizumab was accompanied by an unfavorable safety profile, despite some activity in a phase II study [26].

32.6 Summary & Conclusions

The approval of sunitinib and everolimus for the management of advanced pancreatic NET has extended therapeutic options in this rare type of tumor. In contrast to everolimus, the role of sunitinib is less clear in NET of other sites. Besides pancreatic NETs with the results of RADIANT trials, everolimus is approved for the treatment of low and intermediate GEP-NET and thoracic NETs. Both are functioning and nonfunctioning. There are other drugs which are currently evaluated in ongoing clinical trials. Unfortunately, partial tumor remissions occur in less than 10% of the patients with molecularly targeted drugs without CR; however, stabilization of the disease including minor tumor shrinkages is more frequently observed and prolongation of PFS may be achieved and considered as a clinically important outcome parameter. Although prolongation of PFS is the major benefit of these targeted drugs, and an impact on overall survival could not be demonstrated in clinical trials in part due to a high crossover rate from placebo to open-label treatment, the use of these drugs in sequencing different kind of treatments may prolong individual patients' life. However, the clinical results achieved with targeted therapies are limited by de novo or acquired drug resistance. In consequence, treatment strategies utilizing combinations of agents targeting multiple pathways have been initiated in an attempt to increase response rates and improve clinical outcomes. One of the major challenges is to improve the molecular understanding of these diverse types of NET and to validate biomarkers for the selection and stratification of patients for distinctly targeted therapies.

References

1. Bosman FT, Carneiro F, Hruban RH et al (2010) WHO classification of tumours of the digestive system. World Health Organization, Geneva
2. Rindi G, Bordi C, Rappel S et al (1996) Gastric carcinoids and neuroendocrine carcinomas: pathogenesis, pathology, and behavior. World J Surg 20:168–172
3. Scarpa A, Chang DK, Nones K et al (2017) Whole-genome landscape of pancreatic neuroendocrine tumours. Nature 543:65–71
4. Banck MS, Kanwar R, Kulkarni AA et al (2013) The genomic landscape of small intestine neuroendocrine tumors. J Clin Invest 123:2502–2508
5. Jiao Y, Shi C, Edil BH et al (2011) DAXX/ATRX, MEN1, and mTOR pathway genes are frequently altered in pancreatic neuroendocrine tumors. Science 331:1199–1203
6. Vijayvergia N, Dasari A (2020) Targeted therapies in the management of well-differentiated digestive and lung neuroendocrine neoplasms. Curr Treat Options in Oncol 21:96
7. Welin S, Fjallskog ML, Saras J et al (2006) Expression of tyrosine kinase receptors in malignant midgut carcinoid tumors. Neuroendocrinology 84:42–48

8. Chaudhry A, Funa K, Öberg K (1993) Expression of growth factor peptides and their receptors in neuroendocrine tumors of the digestive system. Acta Oncol 32:107–114
9. Pavel M, Wiedenmann B (2011) Novel therapeutic agents for the treatment of gastroentero-pancreatic neuroendocrine tumors. Horm Metab Res 43:844–853
10. Scoazec JY (2013) Angiogenesis in neuroendocrine tumors: therapeutic applications. Neuroendocrinology 97:45–56
11. Kidd M, Schimmack S, Lawrence B et al (2013) EGFR/TGFalpha and TGFbeta/CTGF signaling in neuroendocrine neoplasia: theoretical therapeutic targets. Neuroendocrinology 97:35–44
12. Wulbrand U, Wied M, Zofel P et al (1998) Growth factor receptor expression in human gastroenteropancreatic neuroendocrine tumours. Eur J Clin Investig 28:1038–1049
13. von Wichert G, Jehle PM, Hoeflich A et al (2000) Insulin-like growth factor-I is an autocrine regulator of chromogranin a secretion and growth in human neuroendocrine tumor cells. Cancer Res 60:4573–4581
14. Shaw RJ, Cantley LC (2006) Ras, PI(3)K and mTOR signalling controls tumour cell growth. Nature 441:424–430
15. Villaume K, Blanc M, Gouysse G et al (2010) VEGF secretion by neuroendocrine tumor cells is inhibited by octreotide and by inhibitors of the PI3K/AKT/mTOR pathway. Neuroendocrinology 91:268–278
16. Shida T, Kishimoto T, Furuya M et al (2010) Expression of an activated mammalian target of rapamycin (mTOR) in gastroenteropancreatic neuroendocrine tumors. Cancer Chemother Pharmacol 65:889–893
17. Missiaglia E, Dalai I, Barbi S et al (2010) Pancreatic endocrine tumors: expression profiling evidences a role for AKT-mTOR pathway. J Clin Oncol 28:245–255
18. Duran I, Kortmansky J, Singh D et al (2006) A phase II clinical and pharmacodynamic study of temsirolimus in advanced neuroendocrine carcinomas. Br J Cancer 95:1148–1154
19. Yao JC, Phan AT, Chang DZ et al (2008) Efficacy of RAD001 (everolimus) and octreotide LAR in advanced low—to intermediate-grade neuroendocrine tumors: results of a phase II study. J Clin Oncol 26:4311–4318
20. Yao JC, Lombard-Bohas C, Baudin E et al (2010) Daily oral everolimus activity in patients with metastatic pancreatic neuroendocrine tumors after failure of cytotoxic chemotherapy: a phase II trial. J Clin Oncol 28:69–76
21. Yao JC, Shah MH, Ito T et al (2011) Everolimus for advanced pancreatic neuroendocrine tumors. N Engl J Med 364:514–523
22. Danesi R, Del Tacca M (1996) The effects of the somatostatin analog octreotide on angiogenesis in vitro. Metabolism 45:49–50
23. Abdel-Rahman O, Fouad M (2015) Bevacizumab-based combination therapy for advanced gastroenteropancreatic neuroendocrine neoplasms (GEP-NENs): a systematic review of the literature. J Cancer Res Clin Oncol 141:295–305
24. Berruti A, Fazio N, Ferrero A et al (2014) Bevacizumab plus octreotide and metronomic capecitabine in patients with metastatic well-to-moderately differentiated neuroendocrine tumors: the XELBEVOCT study. BMC Cancer 14:1–10
25. Chan JA, Stuart K, Earle CC et al (2012) Prospective study of bevacizumab plus temozolomide in patients with advanced neuroendocrine tumors. J Clin Oncol 30:2963
26. Castellano D, Capdevila J, Sastre J et al (2013) Sorafenib and bevacizumab combination targeted therapy in advanced neuroendocrine tumour: a phase II study of Spanish neuroendocrine tumour group (GETNE0801). Eur J Cancer 49:3780–3787
27. Grillo F, Florio T, Ferraù F et al (2018) Emerging multitarget tyrosine kinase inhibitors in the treatment of neuroendocrine neoplasms. Endocr Relat Cancer 25:R453–R466
28. Hobday T, Rubin J, Holen K et al (2007) MC044h, a phase II trial of sorafenib in patients (pts) with metastatic neuroendocrine tumors (NET): a phase II consortium (P2C) study. J Clin Oncol 25:4504–4504
29. Kulke MH, Lenz HJ, Meropol NJ et al (2008) Activity of sunitinib in patients with advanced neuroendocrine tumors. J Clin Oncol 26:3403–3410

30. Ahn HK, Choi JY, Kim KM et al (2013) Phase II study of pazopanib monotherapy in metastatic gastroenteropancreatic neuroendocrine tumours. Br J Cancer 109:1414–1419
31. Raymond E, Dahan L, Raoul JL et al (2011) Sunitinib malate for the treatment of pancreatic neuroendocrine tumors. N Engl J Med 364:501–513
32. Xu J, Li J, Bai C et al (2019) Surufatinib in advanced well-differentiated neuroendocrine tumors: a multicenter, single-arm, open-label, phase Ib/II trial. Clin Cancer Res 25:3486–3494
33. Xu J, Shen L, Zhou Z et al (2019) Efficacy and safety of surufatinib in patients with well-differentiated advanced extrapancreatic neuroendocrine tumors (NETs): results from the randomized phase III study (SANET-ep). Ann Oncol 30:v911
34. Scoville SD, Cloyd JM, Pawlik TM (2020) New and emerging systemic therapy options for well-differentiated gastroenteropancreatic neuroendocrine tumors. Expert Opin Pharmacother 21:183–191
35. Reidy-Lagunes DL, Vakiani E, Segal MF et al (2012) A phase 2 study of the insulin-like growth factor-1 receptor inhibitor MK-0646 in patients with metastatic, well-differentiated neuroendocrine tumors. Cancer 118:4795–4800
36. Capdevila J, Fazio N, Lopez Lopez C et al (2019) Final results of the TALENT trial (GETNE1509): a prospective multicohort phase II study of lenvatinib in patients (pts) with G1/G2 advanced pancreatic (panNETs) and gastrointestinal (giNETs) neuroendocrine tumors (NETs). Am Soc Clin Oncol 37:4106
37. Roth GJ, Binder R, Colbatzky F et al (2015) Nintedanib: from discovery to the clinic. J Med Chem 58:1053
38. Bill R, Fagiani E, Zumsteg A et al (2015) Nintedanib is a highly effective therapeutic for neuroendocrine carcinoma of the pancreas (PNET) in the Rip1Tag2 transgenic mouse model. Clin Cancer Res 21:4856–4867
39. Iyer RV, Konda B, Owen DH et al (2018) Multicenter phase 2 study of nintedanib in patients (pts) with advanced progressing carcinoid tumors. Am Soc Clin Oncol 36:4105
40. Abdel-Rahman O, Bahie Eldin N, ElHalawani H (2016) Risk of selected gastrointestinal and hepatic toxicities in cancer patients treated with nintedanib: a meta-analysis. Future Oncol 12:2163–2172
41. Hu-Lowe DD, Zou HY, Grazzini ML et al (2008) Nonclinical antiangiogenesis and antitumor activities of axitinib (AG-013736), an oral, potent, and selective inhibitor of vascular endothelial growth factor receptor tyrosine kinases 1, 2, 3. Clin Cancer Res 14:7272–7283
42. Strosberg J, Cives M, Hwang J et al (2016) A phase II study of axitinib in advanced neuroendocrine tumors. Endocr Relat Cancer 23:411–418
43. Yakes FM, Chen J, Tan J et al (2011) Cabozantinib (XL184), a novel MET and VEGFR2 inhibitor, simultaneously suppresses metastasis, angiogenesis, and tumor growth. Mol Cancer Ther 10:2298–2308
44. Chan JA, Faris JE, Murphy JE et al (2017) Phase II trial of cabozantinib in patients with carcinoid and pancreatic neuroendocrine tumors (pNET). Am Soc Clin Oncol 35:228
45. Verheijen RB, Beijnen JH, Schellens JH et al (2017) Clinical pharmacokinetics and pharmacodynamics of pazopanib: towards optimized dosing. Clin Pharmacokinet 56:987–997
46. Phan AT, Halperin DM, Chan JA et al (2015) Pazopanib and depot octreotide in advanced, well-differentiated neuroendocrine tumours: a multicentre, single-group, phase 2 study. Lancet Oncol 16:695–703
47. Grande E, Capdevila J, Castellano D et al (2015) Pazopanib in pretreated advanced neuroendocrine tumors: a phase II, open-label trial of the Spanish task force Group for Neuroendocrine Tumors (GETNE). Ann Oncol 26:1987–1993
48. Bergsland EK, Mahoney MR, Asmis TR et al (2019) Prospective randomized phase II trial of pazopanib versus placebo in patients with progressive carcinoid tumors (CARC)(Alliance A021202). Am Soc Clin Oncol 37:4005
49. Fjällskog M-L, Sundin A, Westlin J-E et al (2002) Treatment of malignant endocrine pancreatic tumors with a combination of α-interferon and somatostatin analogs. Med Oncol 19:35–42

50. Yao JC, Guthrie KA, Moran C et al (2017) Phase III prospective randomized comparison trial of depot octreotide plus interferon alfa-2b versus depot octreotide plus bevacizumab in patients with advanced carcinoid tumors: SWOG S0518. J Clin Oncol 35:1695
51. Cunha LL, Marcello MA, Rocha-Santos V et al (2017) Immunotherapy against endocrine malignancies: immune checkpoint inhibitors lead the way. Endocr Relat Cancer 24:T261–T281
52. Kim ST, Ha SY, Lee S et al (2016) The impact of PD-L1 expression in patients with metastatic GEP-NETs. J Cancer 7:484
53. Ott PA, Bang YJ, Piha-Paul SA et al (2019) T-cell–inflamed gene-expression profile, programmed death ligand 1 expression, and tumor mutational burden predict efficacy in patients treated with pembrolizumab across 20 cancers: KEYNOTE-028. J Clin Oncol 37:318–327
54. Weber MM, Fottner C (2018) Immune checkpoint inhibitors in the treatment of patients with neuroendocrine neoplasia. Oncol Res Treat 41:306–312
55. Mitry E, Walter T, Baudin E et al (2014) Bevacizumab plus capecitabine in patients with progressive advanced well-differentiated neuroendocrine tumors of the gastro-intestinal (GI-NETs) tract (BETTER trial)–a phase II non-randomised trial. Eur J Cancer 50:3107–3115
56. Ducreux M, Dahan L, Smith D et al (2014) Bevacizumab combined with 5-FU/streptozocin in patients with progressive metastatic well-differentiated pancreatic endocrine tumours (BETTER trial)–a phase II non-randomised trial. Eur J Cancer 50:3098–3106
57. Crabtree JS (2017) Clinical and preclinical advances in gastroenteropancreatic neuroendocrine tumor therapy. Front Endocrinol 8:341
58. Ranpura V, Hapani S, Wu S (2011) Treatment-related mortality with bevacizumab in cancer patients: a meta-analysis. JAMA 305:487–494
59. Yao JC, Phan A, Hoff PM et al (2008) Targeting vascular endothelial growth factor in advanced carcinoid tumor: a random assignment phase II study of depot octreotide with bevacizumab and pegylated interferon alfa-2b. J Clin Oncol 26:1316–1323
60. Kölby L, Persson G, Franzen S et al (2003) Interferon treatment of carcinoid tumours. Br J Surg 90:687–693
61. Arnold R, Rinke A, Klose K-J et al (2005) Octreotide versus octreotide plus interferon-alpha in endocrine gastroenteropancreatic tumors: a randomized trial. Clin Gastroenterol Hepatol 3:761–771
62. Kulke MH, Ruszniewski P, Van Cutsem E et al (2017) A randomized, open-label, phase 2 study of everolimus in combination with pasireotide LAR or everolimus alone in advanced, well-differentiated, progressive pancreatic neuroendocrine tumors: COOPERATE-2 trial. Ann Oncol 28:1309–1315
63. Ferolla P, Brizzi MP, Meyer T et al (2017) Efficacy and safety of long-acting pasireotide or everolimus alone or in combination in patients with advanced carcinoids of the lung and thymus (LUNA): an open-label, multicentre, randomised, phase 2 trial. Lancet Oncol 18:1652–1664
64. Kulke MH, Niedzwiecki D, Foster NR et al (2015) Randomized phase II study of everolimus (E) versus everolimus plus bevacizumab (E+ B) in patients (pts) with locally advanced or metastatic pancreatic neuroendocrine tumors (pNET), CALGB 80701 (Alliance). Am Soc Clin Oncol 33:4005
65. Chan JA, Mayer RJ, Jackson N et al (2013) Phase I study of sorafenib in combination with everolimus (RAD001) in patients with advanced neuroendocrine tumors. Cancer Chemother Pharmacol 71:1241–1246

Immunotherapy for Neuroendocrine Neoplasms

33

Magnus Essand and Mohanraj Ramachandran

33.1 Activation of the Adaptive Immune System

The primary role of our immune system is to protect us from disease caused by infectious agents such as viruses, bacteria, parasites and fungi. Innate immune cells throughout our body are the first line of defence. They recognise foreign invaders through pattern recognition receptors (PRRs) such as toll-like receptors (TLRs), which can sense bacterial DNA, viral RNA and other foreign signatures, together known as pathogen-associated molecular patterns (PAMPs). In some cases, innate immune cells eradicate pathogens by themselves; while in most cases it is the adaptive immune system, that is, T cells and/or B cells, that are called upon in order to clear an infection. The focus in this chapter will be on T cells, as they appear to play the central for immunological control of both viruses and tumours.

T cells need to be educated in order to become effector cells, and the main educator is an innate professional antigen-presenting cell called the dendritic cell (DC). Immature DCs reside as guardians in tissues waiting for a reason to activate adaptive immune cells. They are phagocytic cells that can ingest debris of dead cells. Ingestion of cellular debris from virus-infected cells leads to PRR triggering by viral PAMPs, which results in maturation of the DC and migration through the lymphatics to a draining lymph node for interaction with naive T cells. Proteins from the cell debris are processed into small peptide fragments by the DC and presented on the cell surface on so-called major histocompatibility complex class II (MHC-II) molecules to interact with antigen-specific CD4+ helper T cells. Antigenic peptides are also

M. Essand (✉) · M. Ramachandran
Department of Immunology, Genetics and Pathology, Uppsala University, Uppsala, Sweden
e-mail: magnus.essand@igp.uu.se; mohanraj.ramachandran@igp.uu.se

S. Yalcin, K. Öberg (eds.), *Neuroendocrine Tumours*,
https://doi.org/10.1007/978-3-031-56968-5_33

cross-presented by DC on major histocompatibility complex class I (MHC-I) molecules to interact with CD8+ cytolytic T cells. Naïve T cells with an adequate T cell receptor (TCR) recognising the MHC with a viral (foreign) peptide gets triggered. The mature DC also delivers co-stimulatory signals and appropriate cytokines to turn the T cells into fully activated T cell. Activated cytolytic T cells undergo clonal expansion to large numbers, enter the blood circulation and traffic back to the inflamed tissue of the virus infection by transmigrating through the inflamed and activated endothelia and enter the tissue. At the site, they kill virus-infected cells presenting viral peptide on their MHC-I. The killing occurs through the release of perforin, which makes pores in the infected cell, and granzymes, which enter through the pores and induce caspase activation and apoptosis (programmed cell death) in the infected cell. Expansion of specific T cells also gives rise to memory T cells, which leads to immunologic memory against the specific viral antigen.

33.2 Antitumour Immune Responses

It is today fully appreciated that the immune system, and in particular T cells, plays an important role in protecting us from cancer, a threat that comes from within and in most cases not caused by foreign pathogens. Tumour cells are genetically altered from their normal counterparts, containing DNA mutations induced by carcinogenic damage of DNA that can lead to alterations of amino acid sequences in cellular proteins. Such altered cellular proteins can be processed into peptides and are referred to as a neoantigens or neoepitopes. If neoepitopes are presented on MHC-I, then the MHC-I/peptide complex can be recognised and targeted by $CD8^+$ T cells. $CD8^+$ T cells do not recognise non-altered self-peptides presented by MHC-I, as T cells with a TCR recognising self-antigens have been eliminated during T cell education in the thymus.

The situation for T cell recognition of tumours parallels T cell recognition of a viral infection. For naïve T cells to become activated against tumour-specific neoantigens, DCs must take up neoantigens from dying tumour cells and neoepitopes must be cross-presented on MHC-I molecules on the surface of DCs. The DC must also obtain maturation stimuli in order to mature and migrate to draining lymph nodes where it can interact with and activate naïve $CD8^+$ T cells. There are however differences between the immune response towards virus infections and cancer. Infected cells contain plenty of virus proteins and multiple viral epitopes that can be presented by MHC-I, thereby generating a broad T cell repertoire, whereas tumours cells have a limited number of mutations and only a small fraction of these mutations will give rise to immunogenic neoepitopes. Infected cells contain viral PAMPs that can activate DCs, while PAMPs are missing for cancers that are not caused by viruses. The quality and quantity of the mounted T cell response therefore differ between virus infections and cancer.

The immunogenicity of cancers relies on individual neoepitopes. Since each cancer is genetically different (caused by random genetic mutations), there is a huge variety in neoepitopes and the immune response mounted against individual cancers. Some cancer forms are more immunogenic than others, and there appears to be a correlation between mutational load and immunogenicity, which is logical considering that more mutations can give rise to more potential neoepitopes. Neuroendocrine tumours/cancers generally speaking has a rather low mutational load, and as a consequence they are not very immunogenic.

33.3 Tumours Evade Immune Recognition

For tumours to grow, they need to evade immune recognition. There are different mechanisms through which this occur. Tumour cells, stromal cells and recruited immune cells heavily influence the tumour microenvironment through secretion of immunosuppressive factors such as interleukin-10 (IL-10), transforming growth factor beta (TGF-β) and indoleamine-pyrrole 2,3-dioxygenase (IDO). The tumour microenvironment also lacks chemokines for CD8+ T cell recruitment but comprises chemokines for recruitment of immunosuppressive cells, including regulatory T cells (Tregs), myeloid-derived suppressor cells (MDSCs) and M2-polarised tumour-associated macrophages. The immunosuppressive tumour microenvironment can thus efficiently block cytolytic CD8+ T cell activity. Tumour cells can up-regulate the expression of a molecule called Programmed Death-Ligand 1 (PD-L1) which can interact with Programmed cell Death protein 1 (PD-1) receptors on activated T cells. Ligation of PD-1 on T cells leads to inhibitory signalling and deactivation.

When characterising the immune landscape of clinical tumour samples, three scenarios can in principal be depicted based on the CD8+ T cell infiltration status: (1) ***inflamed tumours***; (2) ***immune-excluded tumours***; and (3) ***immune deserts***. For T cell-inflamed tumours (Fig. 33.1, left panel), which are also referred to as being immunologically "hot" tumours, tumour cells have not been able to completely avoid immune recognition and activated T cells have infiltrated the tumour bed. Patients with T cell-inflamed tumours tend to survive longer than those patients where T cells are not present. For T cell-excluded tumours (Fig. 33.1, middle panel), it appears as T cells have been activated but that the tumour microenvironment either lacks appropriate chemokines for T cell recruitment or that the tumour stroma and tumour vasculature block entry of these T cells into the tumour bed. Such tumours effectively avoid neoantigen-reactive T cells by excluding them. For immune desert tumours (Fig. 33.1, right panel) where T cells are neither inside nor in the surroundings of the tumour, it appears that immune recognition was poor in the first place and that there is a total lack of neoantigen-reactive T cells. T cell-excluding tumour and immune desert tumours are also referred to as being immunologically "cold," and patients with cold tumours tend to do worst.

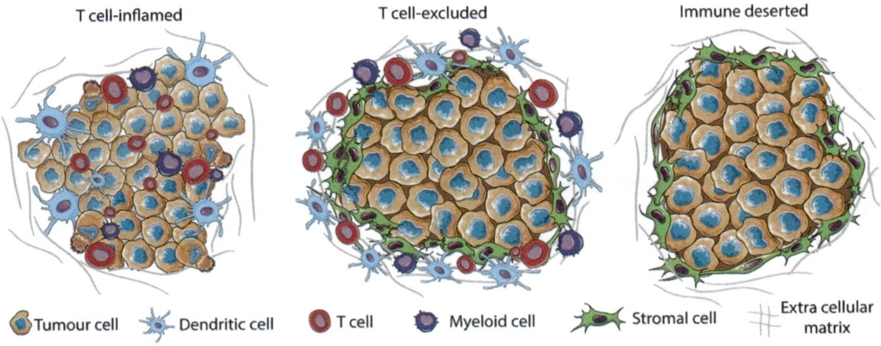

Fig. 33.1 The immune landscape of tumours correlates with prognosis and response to immune checkpoint inhibition therapy. *Left panel*) An illustration of a T cell-inflamed tumour, where T cells and other immune cells have infiltrated the tumour bed. Such tumours are also referred to as "immunologically hot" tumours. Patients with hot tumours generally has better prognosis than patients lacking T cell infiltration. Furthermore, patients with hot tumours generally respond better to immune checkpoint therapy than patients lacking infiltrating T cells. The response rate from immune checkpoint blockade may be further improved by combination treatments with drugs that can reduce immunosuppression in the tumour microenvironment. ***Middle panel***) An illustration of a T cell-excluded tumour, where T cells are residing at the edge of tumour but do not enter due to stromal and/or endothelial barriers. ***Right panel***) An illustration of an immune-deserted tumour with a complete absence of T cell activation and infiltration. Tumours illustrated in the middle and right panels are also referred to as "immunologically cold" tumours, and patients with such tumour immune landscape generally has poorer prognosis and do not respond to immune checkpoint blockade. Patients with a T cell-excluded tumour profile may improve from immune checkpoint blockade if it is combined with vascular targeting or targeting to reduce tumour stroma and extracellular matrix. Patients with tumours resembling an immune desert must first induce antitumour-directed T cells de novo before they can benefit from immune checkpoint blockade

33.4 Immunotherapy of Cancer

33.4.1 Checkpoint Inhibitors

Attempts to fight cancer with the cancer patient's own immune system has been tried for decades, but it is only in the last decade that cancer immunotherapy has been successfully implemented in the clinics and revolutionised the way we think about and treat cancer. The first success of cancer immunotherapy came from blocking inhibitory signalling in T cells and thus prolonging the active lifespan of tumour antigen-reactive T cells. James P. Allison was first to show that antibody blockade of a T cell inhibitory molecule known as CTLA-4 could lead to antitumour immune responses and rejection of tumours in mice [1]. Anti-CTLA4 antibodies later showed good clinical efficacy in refractory malignant melanoma, which represent the first real breakthrough of cancer immunotherapy. This concept of blocking T cell inhibitory pathways as a way of unleashing antitumour immune responses is termed "immune checkpoint blockade" and the antibodies used for immune checkpoint blockade are termed "checkpoint inhibitors." Tasuku Honjo later discovered PD-1 as another immune checkpoint molecule. Anti-PD1 and anti-PD-L1 antibodies have since been developed as checkpoint inhibitors. They have been approved for many forms of cancer and have completely revolutionised cancer treatment. Allison and Honjo were awarded the Nobel Prize in Medicine 2018, a sign that the field has matured. Antibodies blocking other inhibitory signalling pathways in T cells are currently being evaluated in clinical trials along with agonistic antibodies stimulating activating receptors in T cells.

As checkpoint inhibitors work by blocking inhibitory signalling in effector T cells, they require preexisting tumour antigen-reactive T cells to be effective. Although many cancer patients respond, the majority of patients unfortunately do not yet benefit from treatment with checkpoint inhibitors. It is becoming increasingly clear that patients with a T cell-inflamed tumour phenotype (Fig. 33.1, middle panel), characterised by the presence of T cell markers and chemokines related to T cell recruitment, are responding best to treatment with checkpoint inhibitors. Again, this is because checkpoint inhibitors act through reinforcement of preexisting tumour antigen-reactive T cells that have already infiltrated the tumour bed. Yet not all patients with inflamed tumours are responding to checkpoint inhibitors due to local immune suppression in the tumour microenvironment. Means to reduce immune suppression in the tumour microenvironment could make more patients susceptible and combination therapies with checkpoint inhibitors and for example IDO inhibitors are currently being evaluated in combination with checkpoint inhibitors. In cases where T cells can only be found in the periphery, i.e., excluded from the tumour bed (Fig. 33.1, middle panel) due to endothelial/stromal barriers and lack of chemokines for T cell recruitment, patients generally respond poorly to checkpoint inhibitors. In such cases, vascular normalising drugs could possibly help recruit T cells into the tumour bed and work synergistically with checkpoint inhibitors. Patients with tumour phenotypes without any signs of T cell infiltration (Fig. 33.1, right panel) do not respond at all to checkpoint inhibitors. In such cases, it is important to induce a strong T cell-mediated antitumour immune response de novo prior to treatment with checkpoint inhibitors.

As stated above, cell death in the presence of viral PAMPs can elicit potent immune responses. However, in the absence of PAMPs, damage-associated molecular patterns (DAMPs) emitted by tumour cells dying an immunogenic cell death can elicit antitumour immunity as well. DAMPs are molecules that have specific unrelated functions inside cells, but when released or exposed extracellularly they can trigger activation and maturation of DCs. Examples of such a DAMP is surface exposure of calreticulin, which acts as an eat-me signal to phagocytic cells, including DCs. Other examples are secretion of heat-shock proteins and extracellular ATP which together drives inflammation and activates DCs. Therefore, in order to induce T cell responses in immune desert tumours, one can aim to induce immunogenic cancer cell death. Ionising radiation is known to induce immunogenic cell death and so are certain cytostatic agents such as anthracyclines, oxaliplatin and bortezomib. Photodynamic therapy and oncolytic viruses are other therapies known to induce immunogenic cell death. Such therapies are currently being evaluated in combination with checkpoint inhibitors.

33.4.2 Oncolytic Viruses

Oncolytic viruses are engineered to selectively replicate in tumour cells and kill them through lysis, hence the name oncolytic viruses. When tumour cells are killed, progeny virus are released that can infect and kill neighbouring tumour cells. The tumour cell death caused by oncolytic viruses is in many instances highly immunogenic. It leads to release of both DAMPs, i.e., alarming molecules and PAMPs, i.e., viral signatures, from the dying tumour cells. The DAMPs and PAMPs activate tissue-resident DCs in the tumour microenvironment to take up material released from the dying tumour cells, including neoantigens (Fig. 33.2, left panel). The activation matures DCs and make them migrate to draining lymph nodes (Fig. 33.2, middle panel) where they can cross-present neoepitopes on their MHC-I for activation of naïve neoantigen-specific CD8+ T cells that can migrate to the tumour and specifically kill tumour cells (Fig. 33.2, right panel). This ability has led to the notion that oncolytic viruses can ignite immune activity in "immunologically cold tumours." An oncolytic virus infection is usually inflammatory. Therefore, it can also reduce immune suppression in otherwise "immunologically hot tumours" and make them even more responsive to immune checkpoint inhibitors. This notion has recently proven correct in a small-scale clinical trial for refractory malignant melanoma. Generally speaking, melanoma patients respond well to PD-1 inhibitors but when combined with T-VEC (Imlygic), an oncolytic herpes virus encoding granulocyte-macrophage colony-stimulating factor (GM-CSF) to induce a pro-inflammatory immune response, and the response rate was significantly higher [2]. This indicates a new direction of combination therapies with potentially much higher response rates to checkpoint inhibitors.

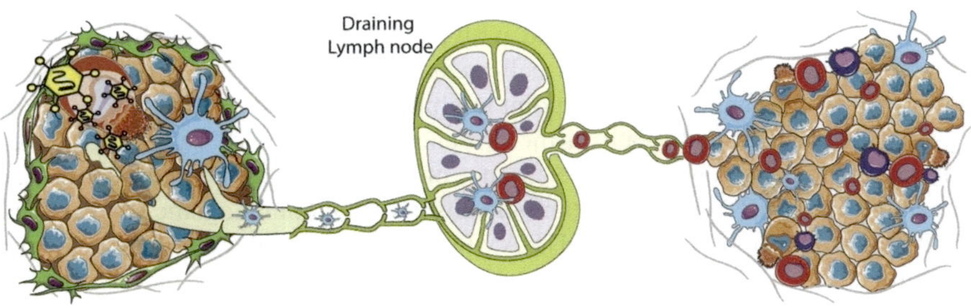

Fig. 33.2 Oncolytic viruses can induce antitumour-directed T cell responses and thereby increase response rates to immune checkpoint blockade. Patients with tumours lacking T cell infiltration generally have a poorer prognosis and respond to a lesser degree to checkpoint inhibitors. An oncolytic virus injected into a tumour can induce immunogenic cell death of tumours cells, with release of DAMPS and PAMPs, which leads to recruitment and activation of resident DCs to take up lysed tumour cell material. The activated DCs will migrate through the lymphatics to a draining lymph node and present tumour antigens to naïve tumour antigen-specific T cells. Stimulated cells become cytolytic T cells that exit the lymph node into the blood circulation, expand in numbers and infiltrate the tumour bed. The T cells can specifically kill tumours cells, and their efficacy may be enhanced by checkpoint inhibitors

33.4.3 Cancer Vaccines

Cancer vaccines based on non-mutated self-antigens, often oncofetal antigens and other antigens overexpressed by tumours are, generally speaking, safe but clinically inefficient. Cancer vaccines based on DCs loaded with such tumour-associated antigens or tumour cell lysates are safe but still not very efficient clinically. One reason may be that the tumour-associated antigens selected as vaccine are seldom essential for tumour progression and that tumour escape variants that lack the tumour-associated antigen can develop. Another explanation may be that the TCR affinities of a cancer patient's T cell repertoire may be too low against peptides from tumour-associated self-antigens.

DNA and RNA sequencing costs have decreased substantially in recent years, and it is today possible to sequence the DNA exons of healthy and malignant cells from a cancer patient to identify tumour-specific neoantigens caused by genetic mutations in tumour cells. RNA sequencing can be used to determine if the neoantigens are expressed. Computer algorithms can then be used to predict if a mutation has given rise to a neoepitope (peptide) that can in fact be processed and presented by the patient's MHC-I and then potentially being able to elicit a cytolytic T cell response. The affinities of TCRs for neoepitopes is usually significantly higher than the affinities of TCRs towards self-antigens, as T cells with TCRs able to recognise neoantigen are not depleted during thymic development. Patient-specific neoantigen vaccines based on the patient's cancer-specific "mutagenome" can then be developed in the form of synthetic peptides or synthetic mRNA. Such cancer vaccines can also be combined with autologous DCs, developed ex vivo from the cancer patient's blood cells.

If the neoepitope vaccine constitutes a so-called driver mutation, a mutation that confers a selective growth advantage (thus promoting or sustaining cancer development), there are good chances that the T cell response evoked in response to vaccination will be efficient and long-lasting. On the other hand, if the neoepitope is derived from a so-called passenger mutation, a mutation that does not cause growth advantage, there are high risks that escape variants of tumour cells lacking the mutation take over, leading to progression of cancer. Patient-specific neoantigen vaccinations are now being evaluated in early-phase clinical trials with promising efficacy data, especially for malignant melanoma [3, 4].

33.4.4 TIL and CAR T Cell Therapy

For most cancer forms, patients with T cell-inflamed tumours have better survival than patients lacking T cell infiltration [5]. Tumour infiltrating T lymphocytes (TILs) can be isolated from resected tumour samples or even biopsies and expanded before they are re-infused into the patient. Such personalised therapy leads to impressive response rates in refractory malignant melanoma, especially when the patients are pre-conditioned before the adoptive T cell transfer [6].

An alternative approach is to harvest T cells directly from the cancer patient's blood and genetically engineered them to express a new receptor that recognises a tumour-associated antigen. The transgene is typically delivered by a retroviral or lentiviral vector and can encode either a new TCR or a chimeric antigen receptor (CAR). TCRs are engineered to recognise an epitope of a tumour-associated antigen or neoepitope presented by MHC-I on the surface of tumour cells. CARs are chimeric molecules and consist of an extracellular antibody-based binding domain, a transmembrane domain and intracellular signalling domains from the TCR chain and co-stimulatory molecules, such as CD28 and 4-1BB. The antibody-based recognition features of the CAR make it recognise a tumour-associated antigen in an MHC-independent manner. For B cell malignancies (leukaemia and lymphoma), T cells isolated from cancer patients' blood can be engineered with a CAR recognising CD19, which is a pan B cell marker expressed on the cell membrane of malignant as well as normal B cells. The patient-derived CAR-engineered T cells are expanded ex vivo before being infused back into the patient. The complete response rates are very high for CD19 CAR T cell therapy, especially in acute lymphoblastic leukaemia. In 2017, CD19 CAR T cell therapies were approved by the Food and Drug Administration (FDA) in the United States for both B cell leukaemia and lymphoma. This was followed by approval by the European Medical Agency (EMA) in 2018.

CAR T cell therapy is not yet particularly effective against solid tumours. There are several reasons why. Solid tumours lack specific and homogenously expressed tumour-associated antigens, which can be targeted by antibody-based CAR molecules. Therefore, toxicity from targeting normal organs or cells may be dose-limiting. Heterogeneity within tumours also leads to that difficulties in targeting all tumours cells. Immunosuppression within solid tumours reduces both recruitment and activity of CAR T cells. The main challenge for CAR T cell therapy of solid tumours is to be able to engineer and produce CAR T cells that can migrate into solid tumours and withstand local immunosuppression. Ideally, they should also be able to induce bystander immunity, i.e., to recruit other immune cells that can target tumour cells that do not express the antigen targeted by the CAR. Combination therapies that can reduce immune suppression, break stromal barriers, and thereby pave the way for CAR T cell therapy are being investigated.

33.5 Neuroendocrine Neoplasms

33.5.1 The Immune Landscape of Neuroendocrine Tumours

Neuroendocrine neoplasms are rare tumours that develop in cells of the neuroendocrine system. There are a number of different types depending on the cell of origin and anatomic site where the tumour starts growing. Not too much is known about the immune landscape of neuroendocrine tumours with the exception of Merkel cell carcinoma where T cell infiltration can be found as the cancer is caused by the Merkel cell polyomavirus (MCPyV) (discussed below). Studies are currently looking at the immune profile of various neuroendocrine neoplasms, but as these studies are relatively small, the overall picture is not clear yet.

Tumours tend to upregulate PD-L1 in an attempt to send inhibitory signals to T cells and avoid being attacked. Expression of PD-L1 by tumour cells is often a sign that a T cell attack was launched against the tumour by the host immune system. In some situations, the degree of PD-L1 expression in tumour cells is an indication that checkpoint inhibitors may represent an effective treatment. It is therefore of interest to investigate PD-L1 expression levels in tumour samples as a biomarker to predict responses. These investigations have just begun when it comes to neuroendocrine tumours. For example, in gastric neuroendocrine tumours (foregut-derived and hindgut-derived), PD-L1 expression was observed in about 20% of the investigated cases. Two studies have reported that expression of PD-L1 is associated with high-grade classification and unfavourable prognosis [7, 8]. In pulmonary neuroendocrine tumours, PD-L1 expression is reported to be low (10% or lower) in large cell neuroendocrine carcinoma and small cell lung cancer and completely absent in lung carcinoids [9]. However, more and larger studies are needed to elucidate the potential clinical role of PD-1/PD-L1 blockage.

Another way by which tumours avoid T cell recognition is to down-regulate MHC-I, also known as human leukocyte antigen (HLA)-ABC in humans, expression in order not to present peptides from tumour-associated antigens. HLA expression has been investigated in neuroendocrine neoplasms, but also here larger studies are needed to draw any firm conclusions. One study found that HLA expression is lower in pancreatic neuroendocrine tumours (PNETs) than in the more common pancreatic adenocarcinoma [10]. The same study also analysed infiltration of immune cells in PNETs but did not find any correlation between the number of T cells at the primary disease site and disease-free survival or overall survival. Another study found strong HLA expression but modest T cell infiltration in liver metastases from gastrointestinal neuroendocrine tumours [11]. The same study sequenced the tumours and identified potential neoepitopes shared by multiple metastases that may constitute appropriate vaccine candidates for PNETs.

33.6 Immunotherapy of Neuroendocrine Cancer

33.6.1 Checkpoint Inhibitors

Merkel cell carcinoma is a rare but aggressive type of skin cancer of neuroendocrine origin. It is mainly seen in older individuals and occurs at increased frequency in persons with immunodeficiencies. Approximately 80% of all cases of Merkel cell carcinoma (MCC) in the United States and Europe is caused by a human polyomavirus that has been named Merkel cell polyomavirus (MCPyV). The remaining 20% of MCC tumours have large numbers of UV-associated mutations [12]. Importantly, both the UV-induced neoantigens in virus-negative tumours and the MCPyV T antigen oncogenes that are required for virus-positive tumour growth are immunogenic and can contain epitopes recognised by CD8+ T cells. Therefore, compared to most neuroendocrine cancers that are not caused by any known pathogen, MCPyV-induced Merkel cell carcinomas are highly immunogenic and tumour samples are often T cell-inflamed. There are reports stating that tumour-infiltrating MCPyV-specific T cells are associated with improved patient survival [13]. Perhaps not surprisingly, Merkel cell carcinoma patients are responding well to immune checkpoint inhibitors and hence the US FDA-approved checkpoint inhibitors as therapy for Merkel cell carcinoma in 2017.

Checkpoint inhibitors are currently being evaluated against other forms of neuroendocrine cancer, including gastroenteropancreatic NETs and pulmonary NETs. Ongoing studies with details can be found at a website by the United States National Institutes of Health (www.clinicaltrials.gov). One can expect many results to come out in the coming years. Case reports indicate that benefits may be achieved, especially when the mutational load is high [14, 15]. However, most neuroendocrine cancers contain only few genetic mutations and are seldom T cell-inflamed. In these cases, checkpoint inhibitors as a monotherapy may not be sufficient to generate durable clinical responses. Therefore, broader approaches will be needed to make immunotherapy effective in neuroendocrine neoplasms. Addition of agents that can induce immunogenic cell death and spark the immune system to induce T cells may help the situation.

33.6.2 Oncolytic Viruses

T-VEC (Imlygic), the gene-engineered herpes simplex virus approved for refractory malignant melanoma, is currently being evaluated for Merkel cell carcinoma. A report with two cases indicates that it may be effective [16]. Studies are ongoing wither with T-VEC used alone or in combination with hypofractionated radiotherapy. Another trial combines T-VEC with nivolumab (anti-PD-1 antibody) to augment the immune response in conjunction with T-VEC-mediated killing. So far, T-VEC has not yet been evaluated for other neuroendocrine tumours.

Seneca Valley Virus isolate 001 (SVV-001) is an oncolytic RNA virus of the *Picornaviridae* family with natural tropism for neuroendocrine cells. It has been evaluated in clinical trials both in adults [17] and children [18] with various forms of neuroendocrine tumours. The virus was administered once, intravenously in order to target also metastatic disease. The first phase I study on 30 adults [17] proved safety and feasibility of intravenous delivery to adult patients with heavily pretreated and metastatic neuroendocrine tumours. No objective responses were reported, but a feasible virus dose was established and a phase II study was opened. This study is however not recruiting any patients. The second study on 18 paediatric patients [18] of which 12 had neuroblastoma also showed good safety data but no clinical effects. All patients cleared the virus within the study period and mounted neutralising antibodies against the virus despite the addition of cyclophosphamide. The neutralising antibodies formed appeared to limit applicability. The recent discovery that SVV exploit tumour endothelial marker 8 (TEM8) for cellular entry [19] may open up for prescreening of patients in future clinical trials.

In order to induce a T cell-based antitumour immune response, it may be favourable to inject oncolytic virus into the tumours or if this is not possible deposit virus in close proximity to the tumours. This is the intention with the AdVince clinical trial. AdVince is an oncolytic adenovirus with has been modified in multiple ways to be adapted for treatment of liver metastasis from neuroendocrine tumours/cancers originating in the gastrointestinal tract, the pancreas or lungs. AdVince includes the gene promoter from human chromogranin A for selective replication in neuroendocrine cells, miR122 target sequences for reduced liver toxicity, and a cell-penetrating peptide in the capsid for increased infectivity of tumour cells and optimised spread within tumours [20]. I phase I trial, dose escalation trial has been initiated with primary endpoints to establish the maximum tolerable dose [20]. AdVince is administered through hepatic artery infusions to increase the amount of virus that is delivered to the liver metastases. It is given on four occasions over a period of 50 days, and patients are being evaluated 1 month later. There are indications that T cell immune responses can developed against the neuroendocrine tumours upon AdVince administration. Therefore, after finishing the phase I trial, it would be ideal to start a follow-up trial where AdVince is being combined with checkpoint inhibitors.

33.6.3 CAR T Cells

There are not yet any reports on CAR T cell therapy for neuroendocrine neoplasms, except for peripheral nervous system tumours such as childhood neuroblastoma, where the disialoganglioside GD2 is often targeted. GD2 CAR T cells have already shown promise in clinical trials for neuroblastoma with several objective responses seen in early phase studies. Whether GD2 CAR T cells can be used for other neuroendocrine cancers needs to be found out.

References

1. Leach DR, Krummel MF, Allison JP (1996) Science 271:1734–1736
2. Ribas A et al (2017) Cell 170:1109–1119 e1110
3. Ott PA et al (2017) Nature 547:217–221
4. Sahin U et al (2017) Nature 547:222–226
5. Fridman WH, Pages F, Sautes-Fridman C, Galon J (2012) Nat Rev Cancer 12:298–306
6. Rosenberg SA, Restifo NP (2015) Science 348:62–68
7. Kim ST et al (2016) J Cancer 7:484–489
8. Cavalcanti E, Armentano R, Valentini AM, Chieppa M, Caruso ML (2017) Cell Death Dis 8:e3004
9. Tsuruoka K et al (2017) Lung Cancer 108:115–120
10. Sato S et al (2014) Oncol Rep 32:2753–2759
11. Kosaloglu Z et al (2016) Onco Targets Ther 5:e1213931
12. Colunga A, Pulliam T, Nghiem P (2018) Clin Cancer Res 24:2035–2043
13. Miller NJ et al (2017) Cancer Immunol Res 5:137–147
14. Wang VE et al (2017) J Immunother Cancer 5:75

15. Ugwu JK, Nwanyanwu C, Shelke AR (2017) Case Rep Oncol 10:720–725
16. Blackmon JT, Dhawan R, Viator TM, Terry NL, Conry RM (2017) JAAD Case Rep 3:185–189
17. Rudin CM et al (2011) Clin Cancer Res 17:888–895
18. Burke MJ et al (2015) Pediatr Blood Cancer 62:743–750
19. Miles LA, Burga LN, Gardner EE, Bostina M, Poirier JT, Rudin CM (2017) J Clin Invest 127:2957–2967
20. Yu D et al (2017) Neuroendocrinology 105:54–66

Societies and Guidelines for Neuroendocrine Tumors

34

Kjell Öberg, Serkan Yaşar, and Suayib Yalcin

Neuroendocrine tumors (NETs) are increasing considerably in both incidence and prevalence over the last decades [1]. Beginning of the 1980s, there was very little interest in this field and only limited information and treatment options were available for a long time. There was also a lack of agreement on the definition of these tumors. There were discussions about whether these tumors should be called endocrine tumors or neuroendocrine tumors (NETs). The history of these tumors dates really back, and the term carcinoid was described first in an old publication from Obendorfer (1907). Later in the 1950s, description of Zollinger–Ellison syndrome and Verner Morrison Syndrome were described. Since then, there was very little added and written about this so-called rare disease till 1980s. In the late 1970s and early 1980s, the leading center in the United States taking care of patients with NETs was the Mayo Clinic with Professor Charles Moertel and Dr. Larry Kvols with a documented interest in managing these patients. There were a few therapeutic agents, such as streptozotocin plus 5-fluorouracil or doxorubicin, and healthcare professionals used these drugs for all different subtypes of metastatic NETS, especially for metastatic pancreatic NETS (pNETs). For symptom control and slow-growing neuroendocrine tumors, somatostatin analogs were developed. First, alpha-interferon has also the benefits for symptom and tumor growth control. Later on, in the 1990s, long active formulations of somatostatin analogs were developed. At the beginning of 2000, a new drug that temozolomide used for the treatment, following this agent, used targeted agents, everolimus, and sunitinib were integrated

K. Öberg
Department of Endocrine Oncology, Uppsala University Hospital, Uppsala, Sweden
e-mail: kjell.oberg@medsci.uu.se

S. Yaşar · S. Yalcin (✉)
Department of Medical Oncology, Hacettepe University Cancer Institute, Ankara, Turkey
e-mail: syalcin@hacettepe.edu.tr

S. Yalcin, K. Öberg (eds.), *Neuroendocrine Tumours*,
https://doi.org/10.1007/978-3-031-56968-5_34

into the therapeutic armamentarium as new treatment options. New imaging techniques' somatostatin receptor scintigraphy and positron emission tomography also achieved useful information for management diagnosis, treatment, and surveillance.

During this last decade, there were some developments, prospective randomized controlled trials (Promid Study with octreotide for carcinoids), the RADIANT 2 AND 3 trials with everolimus as well as the sunitinib trial for pancreatic NETs, and more recently CLARINET study for nonfunctioning enteropancreatic tumors, and radioactive treatment with peptide receptor radionuclide therapy (PRRT) also the most important general biomarker Chromogranin A was established worldwide. All these factors contributed to the accelerated increase in the incidence and prevalence of neuroendocrine tumors together with increased awareness. NETs have become an interesting and developing field thanks to the contribution of the training programs and the efforts of the organizations.

The first and oldest NET community, the European Neuroendocrine Tumor Society (ENETS), was founded in 2004 in Budapest, Hungary, and currently has more than 1500 members and Annual ENETS Conferences started. Now the center of the society is in Berlin. Founder members of the society are as follows: Hakan Ahlman Sweden; Bertram Wiedenmann, Germany; Ola Nilsson, Sweden; Barbro Eriksson, Sweden; Kjell Öberg, Sweden; Ursula Plöckinger, Germany; Philippe Ruszniewski, France; Guido Rindi, Italy; Martyn Caplin, United Kingdom; Rudolf Arnold, Germany; Wouter de Herder, The Netherlands; and Gianfranco Delle Fave, Italy. There is a diverse group of researchers from many medical disciplines, in this society, including oncology, gastroenterology, endocrinologist, pathology, radiology, nuclear medicine, surgery, and basic/translational science [2]. In 2005, the ENETS guideline makes recommendations for the diagnosis and treatment. That was published by expert members and has been updated according to the emergence of new scientific data [3, 4].

Various scientific activities are carried out within this society. ENETS has developed a set of standardized report templates to complement its guidelines and standards of care initiatives. The aim was to create a common perspective and some standards in the field of science and medicine. The members can access this publication from The Journal of Neuroendocrinology (vol. 34, issue 3) in March 2022 (free of charge in My ENETS). Furthermore, ENETS collaborates with the International Neuroendocrine Cancer Alliance (INCA) aim is to raise awareness, early diagnosis, optimal treatment, support, and care of net patients.

There are some ENETS-supported clinical trials that are ongoing. One of them is ASPEN study (prospective and observational), and its aim is Evaluation of the Management of Sporadic Asymptomatic Nonfunctioning Pancreatic Neuroendocrine Neoplasms ≤2 cm. The clinical trial started on 1 September 2017 and will end on 31 August 2023. SEQTOR, another interventional, randomized clinical trial, is currently investigating the antiproliferative efficacy and safety of everolimus, followed by STZ/5-FU in advanced pancreatic NET (pNET). Finally, ENETS-endorsed Trial SurvivApp (Observational) is investigating the frequency of distant metastases and clinically relevant relapse and mortality, respectively, of a NEN (Neuroendocrine Neoplasms of the Aprendix) measuring 1–2 cm.

An accreditation program for ENETS Centers of Excellence (CoE) was established in 2009 at six pilot centers for hospitals dealing with patients with neuroendocrine tumors and was officially launched in 2010. Sixty-five CoEs have been accredited since 2009. Three centers of excellence received their first accreditation in the winter of 2021–2022: Universitätsklinikum Erlangen, Erlangen, Germany—leading Prof Marianne Pavel, Hospital General Universitario Gregorio Marañón Servicio de Endocrinología y Nutrición & Hospital Universitario Infanta Sofia, Madrid, Spain—leading Dr. Juan Carlos Percovich Hualpa & Dr. Ana María Jiménez Gordo, and South Wales Neuroendocrine Cancer Service, University Hospital of Wales, Cardiff, United Kingdom—leading Mohid S. Khan.

There is a new database project for NENs, ENETS, since 2008 has a professional NEN registry for gastroenteropancreatic (GEP) NENs in Europe and non-European countries. It does this together with Centers of Excellence (CoE), such as the United States, Australia, and others. In 2020, the new database aims to collect epidemiological data on rare diseases. This project aims to create a platform for retrospective and prospective clinical information collection on patients with NEN.

ENETS decided to take the project to new academic levels with a new partner—the Coordinating Center for Clinical Trials at the Philipps-University of Marburg (KKS). KKS is an independent institution of the Faculty of Medicine of Philipps-Universität Marburg.

In order to induce international and global collaboration, ENETS works with sister communities around the world. A world-class scientific program was planned with the NET communities (including NANETS, APNETS, COMMNETS, CSNET, CNETS, JNETS, Argentum, NET Initiatives in South America, and INCA) in order to bring together scientists in the field of neuroendocrine neoplasms and more development planned the first World NET Forum and 19th Annual ENETS Conference in 2022, in Spain [2].

Another organization is North American Neuroendocrine Tumor Society (NANETS). In 2005, NET experts across America began discussing a new society for well understanding a more awareness of NEN. And on February 21, 2007, NANETS was established officially. Larry Kvols, MD, became the first chair of NANETS. first Annual Symposium met "New Horizons in NET Management" in Southampton, Bermuda, in 2008. NANETS changed its center from the state of Washington to New York state İn 2017. 2020–2021 president of the society is Emily K. Bergsland, Professor of Clinical Medicine, University of California, San Francisco School of Medicine, Helen Diller Family Comprehensive Cancer Center. Every year, new guides are published with the most updated information, and this information is available on the official website. NANET organizes annual symposiums and training programs with the participation of experts in this field, nonprofit making. NANETS provides grants to young investigators. NANETS supports research in four areas: Basic/Translational Science Investigator (BTSI), NANETS

Clinical Investigator Scholarship (NCIS), NANETS Theranostics Investigator Grant (NTIG), and NANETS Young Investigator (YI) Award [5].

The Asia-Pacific Association of Neuroendocrine Tumors (AP-NET) is an organization established to increase awareness and improve the care of patients with neuroendocrine tumors. A meeting to review the formation of APNETS was held by Dr. Organized Harjit Singh (Malaysia) and Dr. P. Jagannath (India) on the sidelines of the Asia Pacific Oncology Summit on July 7, 2012, at the Intercontinental Hotel in Kuala Lumpur. During this meeting, the formation framework and basic objectives of the society were determined. A committee has been temporarily appointed under the chairmanship of Dr. Harjit Singh, and the Asia Pacific Neuroendocrine Tumor Society (APNETS) was officially established on January 31, 2013, in Kuala Lumpur [6].

The Carcinoid-Neuroendocrine Tumor Society (CNETS) was founded in 2007 to assist the Canadian community with a particular focus on neuroendocrine tumors. In January 2020, the organization was renamed the Canadian Neuroendocrine Tumor Society (CNETS). CNETS has a Scientific and Medical Advisory Board (SMAB) functioning within this organization, and its purpose is to provide strategic advice to the Canadian Neuroendocrine Tumor Society (CNETS) Board of Directors on scientific and medical issues related to the CNETS mission. In addition, CNETS executes regular NET patient group meetings for patient education and information [7].

The British Society for Neuroendocrinology (BSN) was organized in 1984 by Gareth Leng, John Bicknell, Richard Dyer, and Bill Mason and began its work as the "British Neuroendocrine Group".The British Society for Neuroendocrinology (BSN) annually publishes the Journal of Neuroendocrinology, and current ideas are introduced by the two arms of the publication, Fundamental and Mechanistic Neuroendocrinology (FMN) and 'Translational and Clinical Neuroendocrinology' (TCN). The Editor-in-Chief of the FMN and TCN are Professor Julian Mercer and Professor Robert (Bob) Millar. Journal of Neuroendocrinology started to be published in 1989. It has since been the official journal of the organization. The journal also has a website where you can access publications from the newest to the oldest. *Journal of Neuroendocrinology* is also an official journal of the Pan American Neuroendocrine Society (PANS), Hypothalamic Neuroscience and Neuroendocrinology Australasia (HNNA), the International Regulatory Peptide Society (IRPS), and the International Neuroendocrine Federation (INF) [8].

Also, the society organizes the 'Masterclass in Neuroendocrinology' and Neuroendocrine Briefings that are important for both awareness and education. It has been published for more than 20 years. Annual meetings are held either separately or jointly with European or with other UK societies with similar interests [9].

The Carcinoid Cancer Foundation began as the Carcinoid Tumor and Serotonin Research Foundation in 1968 when the American National Institute of Health terminated the funds for rare cancers including neuroendocrine tumors. The name of the foundation was changed to the Carcinoid Cancer Foundation in 1995. This

New York-centered organization helps to promote education and research on carcinoid and related neuroendocrine cancers. The website https://www.carcinoid.org/ is constantly updated so that both patients and physicians can follow and benefit from current developments. Special events that benefit the neuroendocrine tumor community are published regularly. Current support groups, clinical research, current articles, and references for physicians can be found on the organization's website [10].

Founded in 1993, the National Comprehensive Cancer Network (NCCN) is an alliance of 31 cancer centers in the United States, most of which are designated by the National Cancer Institute as comprehensive cancer centers. It is a nonprofit organization with offices in Plymouth Meeting, Pennsylvania. Starting in 1996, NCCN publishes guidelines for the management of cancer. In addition to many other cancer types, the National Comprehensive Cancer Network, also has published guidelines for neuroendocrine tumors and regularly revises these guidelines for up-to-date treatment and follow-up of patients with all types of different cancers [11].

34.1 Conclusion

The development of professional and patient-oriented societies contributed to the development of the field and also improved the quality of life and survival of many patients. Many researchers had the opportunity to benefit from published guidelines. Patients with these diseases may get contact with professionals from different organizations to get the latest developments in the field of diagnosis and treatment of neuroendocrine tumors. Since the 1980s when there were only a few options for treatment, various treatments are now available, like radioactive treatment with peptide receptor radionuclide therapy (PRRT), targeted agents with everolimus, and sunitinib, and liver-directed therapies. These societies and guidelines will be beneficial for health professionals and patients in the future for NETs, which are constantly increasing incidence and prevalence [1, 11].

References

1. Yao JC, Hassan M, Phan A, Dagohoy C, Leary C, Mares JE et al (2008) One hundred years after "carcinoid": epidemiology of and prognostic factors for neuroendocrine tumors in 35,825 cases in the United States. J Clin Oncol 26(18):3063–3072
2. ENTS. (ENETS) European Neuroendocrine Tumor Society (ENETS) (2021) https://www.enets.org
3. Rindi G, de Herder WW, O'Toole D, Wiedenmann B (2006) Consensus guidelines for the management of patients with digestive neuroendocrine tumors: why such guidelines and how we went about it. Neuroendocrinology 84(3):155–157
4. Kulke MH, Anthony LB, Bushnell DL, de Herder WW, Goldsmith SJ, Klimstra DS et al (2010) NANETS treatment guidelines: well-differentiated neuroendocrine tumors of the stomach and pancreas. Pancreas 39(6):735–752

5. NANTS (NANETS). North American Neuroendocrine Tumor Society (NANETS) (2021). https://nanets.net
6. A-PNTS. (APNETS). Asia-Pacific Neuroendocrine Tumors Society (2021). https://apnets.org
7. CNTS (CNETS). Canadian Neuroendocrine Tumor Society (CNETS) (2021). https://cnets.ca/
8. Library WO (2021) J Neuroendocrinol. https://onlinelibrary.wiley.com
9. Neuroendocrinology BSf. British society for Neuroendocrinology (2021). https://www.neuroendo.org.uk
10. Foundation CC, Carcinoid Cancer Foundation (2021). https://www.carcinoid.org
11. NCCN (NCCN). National Comprehensive Cancer Network (NCCN) (2021) https://www.nccn.org

GPSR Compliance

The European Union's (EU) General Product Safety Regulation (GPSR) is a set of rules that requires consumer products to be safe and our obligations to ensure this.

If you have any concerns about our products, you can contact us on ProductSafety@springernature.com

In case Publisher is established outside the EU, the EU authorized representative is:

Springer Nature Customer Service Center GmbH
Europaplatz 3
69115 Heidelberg, Germany

Batch number: 10732023

Printed by Printforce, the Netherlands